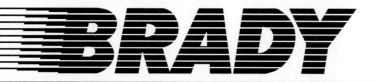

SEVENTH EDITION

Emergency Care

Harvey D. Grant
Robert H. Murray, Jr.
J. David Bergeron
Michael F. O'Keefe
Daniel Limmer

Contributors
Rick Buell
Edward T. Dickinson, M.D.
Bob Elling
Jonathan Politis
Andrew Stern
Owen Traynor, M.D.

Medical Editor
Edward T. Dickinson, M.D.

BRADY
Prentice Hall Education, Career & Technology
Englewood Cliffs, New Jersey 07632

Library of Congress Cataloging-in-Publication Data
Emergency care / Harvey D. Grant . . . [et al.].—7th ed.
     p.   cm.
     Revised based on US Department of Transportation EMT-B
National Standard Curriculum.
     Includes index.
     ISBN 0-89303-044-9.—ISBN 0-89303-009-0 (pbk.)
     1. Emergency medicine.   2. First aid in illness and injury.
3. Rescue work.   4. Emergency medical personnel.   I. Grant,
Harvey D.
RC86.7.G7   1995   94-37170
616.02′5—dc20   CIP

Publisher: *Susan Katz*
Managing Production Editor: *Patrick Walsh*
Editorial/Production Supervision: *Julie Boddorf*
Manufacturing Buyer: *Ed O'Dougherty*
Marketing Manager: *Judy Streger*
Managing Development Editor: *Lois Berlowitz*
Project Editor: *Sandy Breuer*
Development Editor: *Josephine Cepeda*
Proofreader: *Susan Shakhshir*
Managing Photography Editor: *Michal Heron*
Assistant Photography Editor: *Maura McGloin*
Photographers: *Steve Agricola, George Dodson,*
   Michael Gallitelli, Michal Heron
Cover Design: *Marianne Frasco*
Cover Photo: *Mitch Kezar/Phototake NYC*
Interior Design: *Lorraine Mullaney*
Composition and pre-press: *The Clarinda Company*
Printing and binding: *Von Hoffman*

© 1995 by Prentice-Hall, Inc.
A Division of Simon & Schuster
A Paramount Communications Company
Englewood Cliffs, New Jersey 07632

Printed in the United States of America
10 9 8 7 6 5 4 3 2 1

ISBN 0-89303-044-9
ISBN 0-89303-009-0 [pbk]

Prentice-Hall International (UK) Limited, *London*
Prentice-Hall of Australia Pty. Limited, *Sydney*
Prentice-Hall Canada Inc., *Toronto*
Prentice-Hall Hispanoamericana, S.A., *Mexico*
Prentice-Hall of India Private Limited, *New Delhi*
Prentice-Hall of Japan, Inc., *Tokyo*
Simon & Schuster Asia Pte. Ltd., *Singapore*
Editora Prentice-Hall do Brasil, Ltda., *Rio de Janeiro*

NOTICE ON CARE PROCEDURES

It is the intent of the authors and publisher that this textbook be used as part of a formal EMT-Basic education program taught by qualified instructors and supervised by a licensed physician. The procedures described in this textbook are based upon consultation with EMT and medical authorities. The authors and publisher have taken care to make certain that these procedures reflect currently accepted clinical practice; however, they cannot be considered absolute recommendations.

The material in this textbook contains the most current information available at the time of publication. However, federal, state, and local guidelines concerning clinical practices, including without limitation, those governing infection control and universal precautions, change rapidly. The reader should note, therefore, that the new regulations may require changes in some procedures.

It is the responsibility of the reader to familiarize himself or herself with the policies and procedures set by federal, state and local agencies as well as the institution or agency where the reader is employed. The authors and the publisher of this textbook and the supplements written to accompany it disclaim any liability, loss or risk resulting directly or indirectly from the suggested procedures and theory, from any undetected errors, or from the reader's misunderstanding of the text. It is the reader's responsibility to stay informed of any new changes or recommendations made by any federal, state, and local agency as well as by his or her employing institution or agency.

NOTICE ON GENDER USAGE

The English language has historically given preference to the male gender. Among many words, the pronouns "he" and "his" are commonly used to describe both genders. Society evolves faster than language, and the male pronouns still predominate in our speech. The authors have made great effort to treat the two genders equally, recognizing that a significant percentage of EMTs are female. However, in some instances, male pronouns may be used to describe both males and females solely for the purpose of brevity. This is not intended to offend any readers of the female gender.

NOTICE RE "ON THE SCENE"

The names used and situations depicted in "On the Scence" scenarios throughout this text are fictitious.

Brief Contents

Detailed Contents

Respiratory Emergencies 277

Cardiac Emergencies 293

Diabetes and Altered Mental Status 329

Allergies 343

Poisoning and Overdose Emergencies 357

Module 7

Operations 631

CHAPTER 30

Ambulance Operations 633

CHAPTER 31

Gaining Access 665

CHAPTER 32

Overviews 687

Elective:

Advanced Airway Management 705

CHAPTER 33

Advanced Airway Management 707

Appendices 739

APPENDIX A

ALS-Assist Skills 739

APPENDIX B

Infectious Diseases 747

APPENDIX C

Hazardous Materials 755

Basic Life Support: Airway, Rescue Breathing, and CPR 763

Reference Section 815

Patient Assessment Highlights

Photo Scans

Preface

You are about to begin your training to become an Emergency Medical Technician-Basic (EMT-B). EMT-B courses range from 110 to 150 hours in length. Regardless of the hours you spend in class, your course is most likely based on guidelines set by the U. S. Department of Transportation (DOT).

This is not to say that there is one universal EMT-B course. Using the DOT curriculum as a foundation, physicians and instructors in your local emergency medical services system have designed your course to meet specific training needs of your community. The basic training is the same, but there are differences in each state as to what materials are presented.

This textbook takes into account some of the variations in emergency care procedures used in different states. That is why you will find alternative methods cited throughout the text. There are some procedures that vary so much that only the most common methods in use are discussed. For such cases, you will be directed to follow local protocols.

Why is there no one method of providing care for certain illnesses and injuries? There are cases where more than one procedure works. Your EMS system may have tested only one procedure and decided that it was efficient, easy to learn, and simple to use. A different EMS system may have tested a second method and had the same results. This means that you will be trained to use the methods in which your own local EMS system has confidence based upon its own rigorous testing.

One thing is certain: Not all the methods you learn in your training will stay the same during your career as an EMT. You must keep up-to-date with local procedures. Your instructor will tell you how continuing education programs for EMT-Bs are presented in your locality, the prehospital emergency care journals and videos recommended by your EMS system, and any state- or locally-produced newsletters that are available to help the EMT-B stay current.

THE 1994 EMT-BASIC CURRICULUM

The Seventh Edition of *Emergency Care* is very different from previous editions. In 1994, the U.S. DOT released a revision of the EMT-B National Standard Curriculum. That newly revised curriculum has served as the foundation of this book. Some of the changes in the curriculum are summarized below.

The Job Title What was formerly the Emergency Medical Technician-Ambulance has become the Emergency Medical Technician-Basic. This reflects the fact that many EMT-Bs do not work on ambulances, but in other environments.

The Arrangement of Classroom Hours The total number of suggested minimum hours spent in the classroom remains unchanged at 110, but cardiopulmonary resuscitation (CPR) is now a prerequisite, and the 10 hours of clinical observation have been changed to supervised patient encounters without a requirement that a particular number of hours be spent doing so. Body substance isolation and other infection control procedures are, for the first time, incorporated into EMT-B training.

A few other worthwhile topics have also been included, but some were not. There is now an explicit acknowledgment in the curriculum that EMT-Bs cannot learn everything about assessing and treating patients in a classroom. The EMT-B course must provide them with the essential "need to know" information, skills, and judgments that they will need to start practicing as EMT-Bs. The course must also whet their appetites for more. Instructors must stress the importance of continuing education. Because there is so much to cover in this course, many EMT-B students without any previous EMS training or experience will need to spend more than the recommended minimum 110 hours learning this material.

The intent of the curriculum is for the student to follow a particular sequence in learning the knowledge and skills of an EMT-B. After completing CPR, the student begins the course with the preparatory module. This covers some of the foundation material the student will need to know in order to understand later topics. Airway management, because of its importance, comes next. Then the student learns how to assess patients. At this point, either trauma or medical emergencies could come next. The curriculum puts medical emergencies first, but instructors may alter this to meet local needs and suit local resources. The last two sections of the curriculum are on pediatrics and operations. The problems of infants and children are near the end, not because they are any less important than those of adults, but because at this point the students will have the background they need to understand the differences between adults and children.

The Educational Approach Previous EMT curricula used the diagnosis-based approach to teaching that is traditionally used in medicine. For a number of reasons, this approach is not needed and not very efficient in EMS. Instead, the approach that the 1994 curriculum uses is called assessment-based.

To see the differences between the two, consider the following example. An experienced EMT-A receives a call for an alert patient complaining of difficulty breathing not associated with an injury. After assessing the patient, he considers some causes of nontraumatic difficulty breathing: myocardial infarction, congestive heart failure, pulmonary edema, spontaneous pneumothorax, asthma, emphysema, chronic bronchitis, and hyperventilation. He may or may not come to a "diagnosis," but he probably gives the patient high concentration oxygen and transports him sitting up.

An EMT-B trained under the 1994 curriculum, on the other hand, assesses the patient and determines that he has an adult who is responsive, not injured, and complaining of difficulty breathing. Without hesitation, he gives the patient high concentration oxygen and transports him sitting up. A number of steps have been eliminated or streamlined to allow the EMT-B to come to the correct treatment decision. This is typically what good experienced EMT-As have actually been doing for years. Good EMT-As have never let their diagnosis-based EMT classroom training get in the way of patient care.

The Interventions The mainstays of EMT-A treatment have traditionally been oxygen, splinting, and spine immobilization. The 1994 curriculum includes some additional treatments. Medications the EMT-B will be able to assist patients in using are nitroglycerin, inhalers, and epinephrine auto-injectors. The EMT-B will be able to administer oral glucose and activated charcoal (activated charcoal has replaced syrup of ipecac). There is one new procedure, automated defibrillation.

Two pieces of equipment that receive special attention are the pneumatic anti-shock garment and the flow-restricted oxygen-powered ventilation device. Under the circumstances described in the curriculum and used appropriately, these devices should benefit patients. Two optional procedures are oral endotracheal intubation and pediatric gastric tubes. Like all of the medications in the curriculum, these require medical direction.

CONTENT OF *EMERGENCY CARE* SEVENTH EDITION

The authors have attempted to maintain a close alignment between the 1994 EMT-B curriculum and this text. A few additions have been made and some topics have been reorganized, but everything in the curriculum is included in the text. Each module in this textbook corresponds to a module in the 1994 curriculum. Each chapter corresponds to a lesson in the 1994 curriculum and addresses the objectives for that lesson. The content of *Emergency Care* Seventh Edition is summarized below.

Module 1, Preparatory: Chapters 1-6 This first module sets a framework for all the modules that follow by introducing some essential concepts, information, and skills. The Emergency Medical Services system and the role of the EMT-B within the system are introduced. Issues of EMT-B safety and well-being and legal and ethical issues are covered. Basic anatomy and physiology, vital signs, the skill of taking a patient history, and techniques of safe lifting and moving are also included in this first module.

Module 2, Airway Management: Chapter 7 There is only one chapter in Module 2, but it may be considered the most important module in the text, because no patient will survive without an open airway. Basic airway management techniques are covered in detail.

Module 3, Assessment: Chapters 8-15 Module 3 holds the key to the new 1994 assessment-based curriculum. The ability to perform a rapid but accurate assessment, treat for life-threatening conditions, and initiate transport to the hospital within optimum time limits are the essence of the EMT-B's job. In this module all of the steps of the assessment and their application to different types of trauma and medical patients, plus the skills of communication and documentation, are explained and illustrated.

Module 4, Medical Emergencies: Chapters 16-24 The Medical Emergencies module begins with a chapter on pharmacology in which the medications the EMT-B can administer or assist with under the 1994 curriculum are introduced. The module continues with chapters on respiratory, cardiac, diabetic, allergy, poisoning and overdose, environmental, behavioral, and obstetric/gynecological emergencies.

Module 5, Trauma: Chapters 25-28 The Trauma module begins with a chapter on bleeding and shock, then continues with chapters on soft tissue injuries, musculoskeletal injuries, and injuries to the head and spine.

Module 6, Infants and Children: Chapter 29 The difference between treating adult and pediatric patients often lies in understanding the differences in the anatomy, physiology, mental development, and psychology of infants and children. This module explores these special aspects of pediatric care, as well as medical conditions and injury patterns that are especially common to or critical for infants and children.

Module 7, Operations: Chapters 30-32 This module deals with nonmedical operations and special situations, including ambulance operations, motor vehicle collision rescues, and multiple-casualty and hazardous materials incidents.

Module 8, Advanced Airway Management (Elective): Chapter 33 In some states and regions, EMT-Bs will be trained to perform invasive airway management procedures, including orotracheal intubation and, in children, nasogastric intubation. Module 8 is included as an elective to cover these advanced airway management skills.

Appendices and BLS Review There are three appendices to this textbook, covering advanced life support assist skills, infectious diseases, and additional information on hazardous materials.

There is also a complete review of the basic life support course that is a prerequisite to the EMT-Basic course, entitled Basic Life Support: Airway, Rescue Breathing, and CPR.

FEATURES OF THE BOOK

The following features to make teaching, studying, and testing easier are part of the Seventh Edition of *Emergency Care*.

On the Scene Each chapter opens with a realistic "you-are-there" scenario in which EMT-Basics arrive on the scene to encounter a patient suffering from an injury or a medical or behavioral problem. The real-world setting is intended to catch your interest and to help you relate what you are reading to what you are likely to encounter in the field. Whenever possible, the chapter incorporates references to the On the Scene to help you see what you need to know and how it helps the patient.

Objectives The Objectives are presented as Knowledge and Attitude Objectives and also as Skills Objectives. Every objective from the 1994 EMT-Basic National Standard Curriculum is included. You should be able to master the Knowledge and Attitude Objectives by reading the chapter. Skills Objectives refer to key hands-on skills that are also covered in the chapter but that will require instructor-guided practice to master.

Scans Key information and step-by-step procedures are summarized and presented for easy reference in illustrated Scans. Patient Assessment and Care lists further describe the assessment and treatment you should provide for particular types of patients. Medication Scans give you all the information you need in order to administer or help administer medications. Procedure Scans list and describe the steps in performing particular procedures.

FYI Some chapters include an FYI—For Your Information—section. This includes material that goes beyond the chapter objectives. The information in an FYI section is intended to broaden your understanding of the chapter topic but is not essential to an understanding of your job as an EMT-B. Much of the diagnostic material that used to be included in the curriculum has been moved to this section.

Chapter Review Every chapter concludes with a Chapter Review, which consists of Key Terms, Summary, and Review Questions. Key Terms lists all terms that appear in bold type in the chapter with their definitions. The Summary is a concise review of important information. Review Questions ask you to give back certain information and to apply the principles you learned. Answers to the Review Questions appear in the Instructor Resource Manual. Together, Key Terms, Summary, and Review Questions provide a review of each chapter's objectives.

Special Notes Most chapters have an **Infants and Children Note** that describes what is different or special in children with regard to the chapter topic and how you should deal with these differences. Each chapter in the Medical Emergencies, Trauma, and Infants and Children modules also includes a **Documentation Tip** that explains or reminds you of important information to write on your prehospital care report. **Safety Notes** appear throughout the book as needed to point out situations where you need to take special care.

Skill Sheets The 1994 EMT-Basic curriculum includes a number of skill sheets designed to help students learn and instructors evaluate. At the time this book was going to press, the sheets were undergoing review and revision to improve them. When they become available, Brady Publishing will make them available to instructors.

THE EDUCATIONAL PACKAGE

The publisher of this text has provided several ancillary components as aids to instruction. There is a **Student Workbook**. The **Instructor's Resource Manual** contains detailed lesson plans that follow the 1994 curriculum and provides many ideas for making classroom time interesting and productive. It is keyed to this text. A set of **slides** and **videos** is also available.

IMPROVING FUTURE TRAINING AND EDUCATION

Some of the best ideas for better training and education methods come from students who can tell us what areas of study caused them the most trouble. Other sound ideas come from practicing EMT-Bs who let us know what problems they faced in the field and from instructors who have used our materials.

Emergency Care has undergone extensive revision in this Seventh Edition. The authors welcome any suggestions. Any student, practicing EMT-B, or EMS instructor who has an idea on how to improve this book or EMT-Basic training and education should write to the authors at

Brady Marketing Department
c/o Judy Streger
Prentice Hall
113 Sylvan Avenue
Englewood Cliffs, NJ 07632

If you have access to a computer with a modem, you can also reach the authors through America OnLine or Internet at either of the following addresses:

danlimmer@aol.com
mikeokvt@aol.com

Acknowledgments

The people who deserve our thanks are many, and we wish to thank them all.

Brady/Prentice Hall: Our publisher, Susan Katz, deserves credit for her belief in this project. Susan assembled the team that created this book and its supplements, a truly ambitious undertaking. She has made the process as smooth as possible and enjoyable as well.

Lois Berlowitz, managing development editor, provided energy, coordination, and dedication. The production team, including Pat Walsh and Julie Boddorf have done admirable work throughout all phases of production. Thanks also to Judy Streger, Judy Stamm, and Carol Sobel for their help and input throughout this project.

Sandy Breuer, our project editor, is amazing. While her EMS education comes primarily from working on *Emergency Care* Sixth Edition, she possesses a sense for EMS that many instructors wish their students had. Combining this with her talent for editing, she is an indispensable asset to this text. Her tireless work, dedication, and sense of humor are appreciated more than words can say.

Michal Heron, our managing photography editor, worked tirelessly to complete the extensive photo program on time. Her dedication, skill, creativity, and ability to handle the near-impossible task given to her are greatly appreciated. Mike Gallitelli, Steve Agricola, and George Dodson also provided photography for this text.

This edition of *Emergency Care* brings back last edition's Medical Advisor as Medical Editor. Edward T. Dickinson, M.D., REMT-P was involved each step of the way in developing this text. It was not unusual to call "Dr. Ed" during the writing process and photo shoots for his opinions and advice. His reviews were very detailed. We thank Ed and welcome him as Medical Editor to the Seventh Edition.

Our contributors: The following people contributed chapters and ideas to the Seventh Edition. They were an important part of the revision process. Our appreciation to Rick Buell, Edward T. Dickinson, M.D., Bob Elling, Jon Politis, Andy Stern, and Owen Traynor, M.D.

Our supplements team: In order to ensure a truly integrated supplements package, Allan Braslow, Ph.D., was brought aboard to coordinate the supplements to our textbook. Bob Elling authored the Student Workbook. John Bradley created an all-new Instructor's Resource Manual (IRM), which is especially important for the implementation of the new curriculum. Bob Brennan coordinated development of the Test Manager, written by Rick Buell, Elizabeth Delano, Bob Elling, and Dave Habben. Thanks also go to our slide and video production teams.

Reviewers

The following reviewers on the Seventh Edition provided invaluable feedback and suggestions.

Susan Barnes
Ohio Dept of Public Safety, EMS
Columbus, OH

Edgar Batsford
Training Coordinator
Division of EMS
Providence, RI

Chip Boehm
Training Coordinator
Maine Emergency Medical Sevices
Augusta, ME

Liza K. Burrill
Training Coordinator
Division of Public Health
Bureau of EMS
Berlin, NH

S. Gail Dubs
Pennsylvania Department of Health
Division of Emergency Medical Services
Harrisburg, PA

Cynthia S. Ehlers, Ralph Koretzky, Mary Ann Steckert, Nadja Vawryk Button, and Ralph Backenstoes; EHS Federation, New Cumberland, PA

John G. Grove
Assistant Principal
Selinsgrove Area High School
Selinsgrove, PA

JoAnne Palachick, Robert Doucette, Ralph Cope, and Barry Mutschler; Susquehanna EHS Council, Sunbury, PA

Jose V. Salazar
Jose Salazar & Associates
Reston, VA

Gail Stewart
EMS Program Director
Santa Fe Community College
Gainesville, FL

Donald White
Education & Training Coordinator
Board of EMS
Topeka, KS

Everitt F. Binns, Ph.D. and Stephen J. Martin, RN, BSN; Eastern Pennsylvania EMS Council, Allentown, PA

Cynthia S. Ehlers, Ralph Koretzky, Mary Ann Steckert, Nadja Vawryk Button, and Ralph Backenstoes; EHS Federation, New Cumberland, PA

JoAnne Palachick, Robert Doucette, Ralph Cope, and Barry Mutschler; Susquehanna EHS Council, Sunbury, PA

Photo Acknowledgments

Photo Sources The following photos are credited as follows: Scan 10-1a,h Michael Marks/ Timberwolf Studio; Figure 22-8 Breck P. Kent; Figure 22-9 Martha McGuffie, M.D.; Figure 24-4 Custom Medical Stock Photo; Figure 24-6 Phototake, © Doug Nobiletti; Figure 24-8 Custom Medical Stock Photo/SIU; Figure 24-12 Custom Medical Stock Photo; Scan 28-5 Robert Elling; Figures 32-10 a,b,c Jonathan Politis; Figure 33-13 Edward T. Dickinson, M.D.

We wish to thank the following companies for their cooperation in providing us with photos: Ferno, Inc., Wilmington, OH; Laerdal Medical Corporation, Armonk, NY; Marquette Electronics, Inc., Milwaukee, WI; Nonin Medical, Inc., Plymouth, MN; PhysioControl Corporation, Redmond, WA; Road Rescue, Inc., St. Paul, MN; SpaceLabs Medical, Inc., Redmond, WA; Wehr Engineering, Fairland, IN; and Westech Information Systems, Inc., Vancouver, BC

Organizations

We also wish to thank the following organizations for their assistance in creating the photo program for the Seventh Edition.

Colonie Department of EMS, Colonie, NY; Hudson Valley Community College, Troy, NY; Montgomery County Public Service Training Academy, Rockville, MD; North Bethlehem Fire Department, North Bethlehem, NY; Riverdale Fire Department, Riverdale, MD; Rockville Fire Station #3, Rockville, MD; Sandy Spring Volunteer Fire Department, Sandy Spring, MD.; Suburban Hospital, Bethesda, MD; Shady Grove Adventist Hospital, Shady Grove, MD; Town of Colonie Police Department, Colonie, NY; Town of Guilderland EMS, Guilderland, NY; Town of Guilderland Police, Guilderland, NY; Western Turnpike Rescue Squad, Albany, NY; and Wheaton Volunteer Rescue Squad, Wheaton, MD.

Technical Advisors

Thanks to the following people for providing technical support during the photo shoots.

Mark T. Beall, EMT-P Instructor, Career Firefighter, Paramedic
Maryland State EMS Instructor

Richard W. O. Beebe, BS, RN, EMT-Paramedic Instructor, EMS Program
Hudson Valley Community College

Gloria Bizjak, EMT-A, Curriculum Specialist
Maryland Fire and Rescue Institute

Steve Carter, Manager, Special Programs
Maryland Fire and Rescue Institute

Gail Collins, NR-EMT, EMT Instructor

Michael Collins, EMT-P

Ann Marie Davies, EMT-P

Bob Elling

Lt. Willa K. Little, EMS Training Officer
Montgomery County Public Service Training Academy

George Morgan, Industrial Training Specialist
Maryland Fire and Rescue Institute

Bruce Olsen, BS, RRT, EMT-P
Paramedic Program Coordinator
Hudson Valley Community College

Jonathan Politis, BA, EMT-P
Director, Emergency Medical Services
Town of Colonie

Jay Smith, EMT Class Coordinator
Montgomery County Public Service Training Academy

Christine Uhlhorn, EMT-A, EMT Instructor
Maryland Fire and Rescue Institute

Linda Zimmerman, EMT-A, EMT Instructor
Maryland Fire and Rescue Institute

Module 1

Preparatory

IN THIS MODULE

MODULE OVERVIEW

This book is divided into seven required modules and one elective module, each containing one or several chapters on a major aspect of emergency medical care. Upcoming modules will deal with airway management; the steps of patient assessment; medical emergencies (illnesses); trauma emergencies (injuries); infants and children; ambulance, rescue, and other operations; and (the elective) advanced airway management. This first module sets a framework for all the modules that follow and for your work as an Emergency Medical Technician-Basic by introducing some essential concepts, information, and skills.

Chapter 1 introduces you to the Emergency Medical Services system. As an EMT-Basic, you will be one of many persons and professions that come together to form an EMS system.

Your first concern as an EMT-B must be your own safety and well-being. Although you will face a number of potential hazards, including contact with infectious diseases, violence, and stress, you can have a long and safe career in EMS by learning and following the guidelines presented in Chapter 2.

Any medical career involves legal and ethical issues. "Can I get sued?" and "What's the right thing to do?" are questions you may often ask during your career as an EMT-B. Chapter 3 will help prepare you to deal successfully with these important issues.

Most people begin their EMT-B training with little or no medical knowledge. Chapter 4 provides basic information you will need about the structure and function of the human body. Chapter 5 will explain how to measure and assess vital signs, such as respirations, pulse, and blood pressure. This chapter will also cover the skill of interviewing your patient, family members, or bystanders to obtain information about the patient's current problem and past medical history.

As an EMT-B, you will often need to lift and move patients. Chapter 6 will provide information on body mechanics and techniques of lifting and moving without injuring (or further injuring) yourself or your patient.

You will use the information and skills you learn in this first module in every other module of this book, and you will find them to be vital to your safety and effectiveness as an EMT-B.

Introduction to Emergency Medical Care

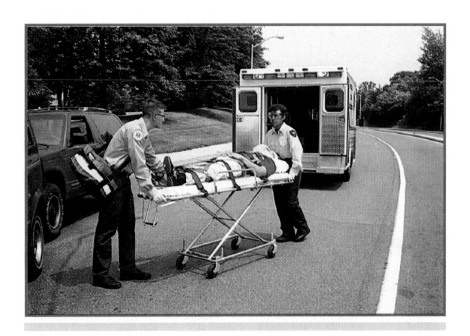

When a person is injured or becomes ill, it rarely happens in a hospital with doctors and nurses standing by. In fact, some time usually passes between the onset of the injury or illness and the patient's arrival at the hospital, time in which the patient's condition may deteriorate, time in which the patient may even die. The modern Emergency Medical Services (EMS) system has been developed to provide what is known as "pre-hospital" or "out-of-hospital" care. Its purpose is to get trained personnel to the patient as quickly as possible and to provide emergency care on the scene, en route to the hospital, and at the hospital. The Emergency Medical Technician-Basic (EMT-B) is a key member of the EMS team.

Objectives

Knowledge and Attitude *At the end of this chapter, you should be able to meet the following objectives.*

1. Define Emergency Medical Services (EMS) systems. (pp. 6–7)

2. Differentiate the roles and responsibilities of the EMT-Basic from other prehospital care providers. (p. 9)

3. Describe the roles and responsibilities related to personal safety. (p. 9)

4. Discuss the roles and responsibilities of the EMT-Basic towards the safety of the crew, the patient, and bystanders. (p. 9)

5. Define quality improvement and discuss the EMT-Basic's role in the process. (pp. 11–12)

6. Define medical direction and discuss the EMT-Basic's role in the process. (pp. 12–13)

7. State the specific statutes and regulations in your state regarding the EMS system. (p. 13)

8. Assess areas of personal attitude and conduct of the EMT-Basic. (pp. 10–11)

9. Characterize the various methods used to access the EMS system in your community. (p. 8)

On the Scene

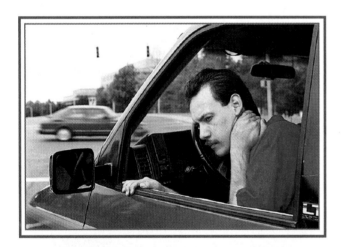

You are an EMT, and after working a long night of calls with the ambulance crew, you shower, change, and begin the drive home. Stopping at a red light not far from the station, you look forward to getting some sleep, but your thoughts are interrupted when another vehicle strikes yours from the rear.

A passing driver stops to see if she can help. You ask her to call 911. The dispatcher at the communication center alerts the fire department and the ambulance squad to respond.

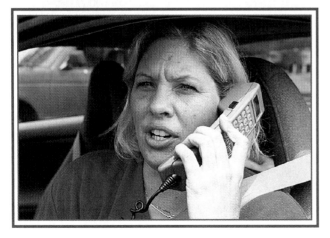

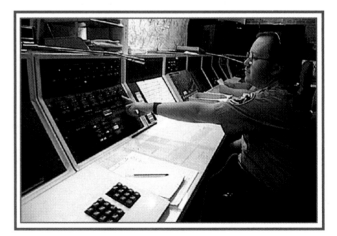

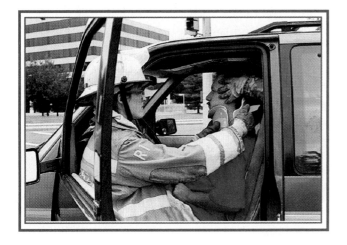

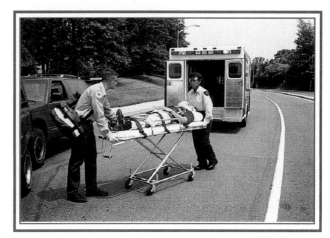

Along with surprise and shock at being struck, you have developed a pain in your neck. You know the fire-fighters who arrive first, because you often work with them. As trained and certified First Responders, they perform an assessment and immobilize your head and neck. When the EMT-Bs on the ambulance crew arrive, you know them too, of course. You left them at squad quarters only a few minutes ago. They immobilize your body on a spine board and bring you to the hospital.

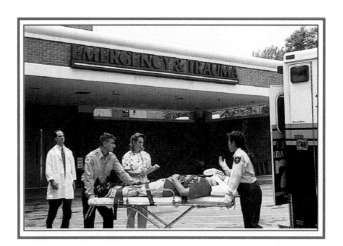

You know the people at the hospital as well, since you are often the person who brings them patients. This time, however, *you* are the patient. The EMT-Bs who bring you in give a report to the nurse who is waiting. The spinal immobilization equipment remains in place. The nurse begins to obtain a medical history and checks your vital signs. In comes the doctor, who examines you. "Better get some x-rays of your neck," he says.

You are taken to the radiology department for x-rays. After returning to the emergency department from radiology, your doctor tells you, "We've looked at the x-rays. We can't see any damage to the spinal column. You have a sprain. Stay out of work for awhile and we'll set you up with physical therapy." You are relieved when your doctor tells you that you can go home. But you are also feeling stiff and sore. You have been lying on a rigid backboard for over an hour, and you realize, "This is what a patient goes through!"

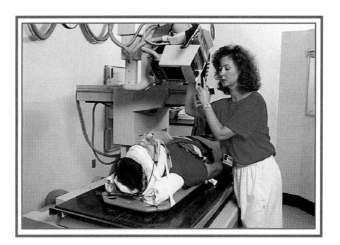

From the call to the dispatcher at the communication center, through your care by First Responders and fellow Emergency Medical Technicians, the ride to the hospital in the ambulance, and your treatment in the x-ray technician, all parts of the Emergency Medical Services system came together for you. You've been an EMT-B for quite awhile, but today you've seen the EMS system from a different aspect. You'll never look at a patient in quite the same way again.

As you begin to study for a career as an EMT-B, you will want to answer some basic questions. What is the EMS system? How did it develop? And what will be your role in the system? This chapter will help you begin to answer these questions.

THE EMERGENCY MEDICAL SERVICES SYSTEM

How It Began

In the 1790s, the French began to transport wounded soldiers so they could be cared for by physicians away from the scene of battle. This is the earliest documented emergency medical service. No medical care was provided for the wounded on the battlefield. The idea was simply to carry the victim from the scene to a place where medical care was available.

Other wars inspired similar emergency services. Clara Barton, a nurse, began such a service for the wounded during the American Civil War and later helped establish the American Red Cross. During World War I, many volunteers joined battlefield ambulance corps.

Nonmilitary ambulance services began in some major American cities in the early 1900s—again as transport services only, offering little or no emergency care. Smaller areas did not begin to develop ambulance services until the late 1940s, after World War II. Often the local undertaker provided a hearse for ambulance transport. Where services developed to offer emergency care along with transport to the hospital, the fire service was often the responsible agency.

During the Korean Conflict in the 1950s and the Vietnam War in the 1960s and '70s, medical teams produced advances in field care for trauma (injuries). Parallel advances in the civilian sector led to the first hospitals that were specialized emergency medical centers devoted to the treatment of trauma.

The importance of extending hospital-quality care to the sick and injured at the emergency scene—of beginning care at the scene and continuing it, uninterrupted, during transport to the hospital—became recognized. The need to organize systems for such emergency prehospital care and to train personnel to provide it was also recognized.

Keep in mind what emergency care must have been like in many areas of the country before medical direction, standards, and a national commitment were developed.

EMS Today

During the 1960s, the development of the modern Emergency Medical Services system began. In 1966 the National Highway Safety Act charged the United States Department of Transportation (DOT) with developing EMS standards and assisting the states to upgrade the quality of their prehospital emergency care. Most EMT-B courses today are based on models developed by the DOT.

In 1970, the National Registry of Emergency Medical Technicians was founded to establish professional standards and provide services to local EMS systems. In 1973, Congress passed the National Emergency Medical Services Systems Act as the cornerstone of a federal effort to implement and improve EMS systems across the United States.

Since then, the states have gained more control over their EMS systems, but the federal government continues to provide guidance and support. For example, the National Highway Traffic Safety Administration Technical Assistance Program has established an assessment program with a set of standards for EMS systems. The categories and standards set forth by NHTSA, summarized below, will be discussed in more detail throughout this chapter and the rest of this textbook.

- Regulation and Policy—Each state EMS system must have in place enabling legislation (laws that allow the system to exist), a lead EMS agency, a funding mechanism, regulations, policies, and procedures.
- Resource Management—There must be centralized coordination of resources so that all victims of trauma or medical emergencies have equal access to basic emergency care and transport by certified personnel, in a licensed and equipped ambulance, to an appropriate facility.
- Human Resources and Training—At a minimum, all transporting prehospital personnel (those who ride the ambulances) should be trained to the EMT-Basic level using a standardized curriculum taught by qualified instructors.
- Transportation—Safe, reliable ambulance transportation is a critical component. Most patients can be effectively transported by

ground ambulances. Other patients require rapid transportation, or transportation from remote areas, by helicopter or airplane.

- Facilities—The seriously ill or injured patient must be delivered in a timely manner to the closest appropriate facility.
- Communications—There must be an effective communications system, beginning with the universal system access number (911), dispatch-to-ambulance, ambulance-to-ambulance, ambulance-to-hospital, and hospital-to-hospital communications.
- Public Information and Education—EMS personnel may participate in efforts to educate the public about their role in the system, their ability to access the system, and prevention of injuries.
- Medical Direction—EMS physicians delegate medical practice to non-physician providers (such as EMT-Bs) and must be involved in all aspects of the patient care system.
- Trauma Systems—In each state, enabling legislation must exist to develop a trauma system including one or more trauma centers, triage and transfer guidelines for trauma patients, rehabilitation programs, data collection, mandatory autopsies (examination of bodies to determine cause of death), and means for managing and assuring the quality of the system.
- Evaluation—Each state must have a program for evaluating and improving the effectiveness of the EMS system, known as a quality improvement (QI) program, a quality assurance (QA) program, or total quality management (TQM).

With the development of the modern Emergency Medical Services (EMS) system, the concept of ambulance service as a means merely for transporting the sick and injured passed into oblivion. No longer could ambulance personnel be viewed as people with little more than the strength to lift a victim in and out of an ambulance. The hospital emergency department was extended, through the EMS system, to reach the sick and injured at the emergency scene. "Victims" became *patients*, receiving prehospital assessment and emergency care from highly trained professionals. The "ambulance attendant" was replaced by the *Emergency Medical Technician (EMT)*.

A current development in some areas is use of the term *out-of-hospital care*, rather than *pre-*

hospital care, in some areas, as EMS personnel begin to provide primary care for some conditions and in some circumstances without transport to a hospital. However, the term *prehospital care* will be used in the remainder of this text.

COMPONENTS OF THE EMS SYSTEM

To understand the EMS system (Figure 1-1), you must look at it from the view of the patient rather than from that of the EMT-B. For the patient, care begins with the initial phone call for help and continues far longer than emergency care performed at the scene and during transport to the hospital, as On the Scene, at the beginning of this chapter, illustrated.

From the ambulance, the patient is received by the Emergency Department. Here, the patient receives laboratory tests, diagnosis, and further treatment. The Emergency Department serves as the gateway for the rest of the services offered by the hospital. If a patient is brought to the Emergency Department with serious injuries, care is given to stabilize the patient, and the operating room is readied to provide further life-saving measures.

Some hospitals handle all routine and emergency cases but have a specialty that sets them apart from other hospitals. One specialty hospital is the *trauma center*. In some hospitals, a surgery team may not be available at all times. In a trauma center, surgery teams are available 24 hours a day.

In addition to trauma centers, there are also hospitals that specialize in the care of certain conditions and patients, such as burn centers, pediatric centers, and poison control centers.

As an EMT-B, you will become familiar with the hospital resources available in your area. Many EMS regions have specific criteria for transporting patients with special needs. It is important to consider the additional transport time that may be required to transport a patient to a specialized facility weighed against the condition of the patient. On-line medical direction (see below) may be available to help with this decision.

First Responders, EMT-Bs, and dispatchers are key members of the prehospital EMS team. Many others make up the hospital portion of the EMS system. These include physicians, nurses, physician's assistants, respiratory and physical therapists, technicians, aides, and more.

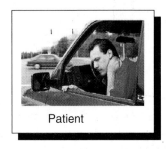
Patient

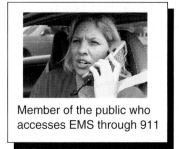
Member of the public who
accesses EMS through 911

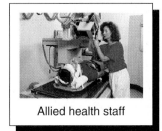
Allied health staff

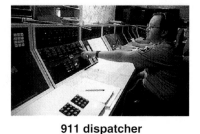
911 dispatcher

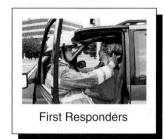
First Responders

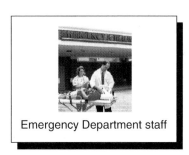
Emergency Department staff

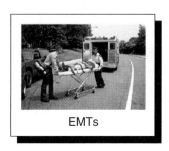
EMTs

FIGURE 1-1 The chain of human resources of the EMS system.

Accessing the System

Many localities have a **911** system for telephone access to report emergencies. A dispatcher answers the call, takes the information, and alerts EMS or the fire or police departments as needed. Still other localities are in the process of implementing the system. Since the number 911 is designed to be a national emergency number, there will be a time when 911 may be dialed from any phone in the country to be connected to the appropriate emergency center.

Some communications centers have **enhanced 911.** This system has the capability of automatically identifying the caller's phone number and location. If the phone is disconnected or the patient loses consciousness, the dispatcher will still be able to send emergency personnel to the scene.

Some communities do not have 911 systems. In these locations, a standard seven-digit telephone number must be dialed to reach the ambulance, fire, or police service. Dialing 911 where a 911 system is not in operation will usually connect the caller with an operator who will route the call to the appropriate dispatch center. This adds an extra step and extra time to the process, so it is important to make sure that the emergency numbers in use in the local area are prominently displayed on all telephones.

Another development in the communication and dispatch portion of the EMS system is the training and certification, in many localities, of Emergency Medical Dispatchers (EMDs). These specially trained dispatchers not only obtain the appropriate information from callers, they also provide medical instructions for emergency care. These include instructions for CPR, artificial ventilation, bleeding control, and more. Research has constantly pointed to the importance of early access and prompt initiation of emergency care and CPR. The Emergency Medical Dispatcher is one example of the EMS system providing emergency care at the earliest possible moment.

Levels of EMS Training

There are four general levels of EMS training and certification, as described below. These levels vary from place to place. Your instructor will explain any variations that may exist in your region or state.

- First Responder—This level of training is designed for the person who is often first at the scene. Many police officers, firefighters, and industrial health personnel are certified First Responders. The emphasis is on activating the EMS system and providing immediate care for life-threatening injuries, controlling the scene, and preparing for the arrival of the ambulance.
- EMT-Basic—The recently revised curriculum for the EMT-B deals with the assessment and care of the ill or injured patient. EMT-B in most areas is considered the minimum level of certification for ambulance personnel. Certification as an EMT-B requires successful completion of the DOT EMT-Basic National Standard Training Program or its equivalent and approval by a state emergency medical services program or other authorized agency. EMT-Basic is the level of certification for which this textbook and the course you are now taking are intended to help you prepare.
- EMT-Intermediate—An EMT-I is a basic-level EMT who has passed specific additional training programs in order to provide some level of advanced life support, for example the initiation of IV (intravenous) lines, advanced airway techniques, and administration of some medications beyond those the EMT-B is permitted to administer. In some states, this level includes those EMTs who are given the title of Shock-Trauma Technician or Critical Care Technician.
- EMT-Paramedic—Paramedic training includes or equals the DOT National Standard Paramedic Curriculum. Paramedics can generally perform relatively invasive field care, including insertion of endotracheal tubes, initiation of IV lines, administration of medications, interpretation of electrocardiograms, and cardiac defibrillation. Although some of these kinds of procedures are now performed by basic and intermediate level EMTs in many areas, the EMT-P may perform such procedures on a more advanced level.

Roles and Responsibilities of the EMT-B

As an EMT-B, you will be responsible for a wide range of activities. In addition to patient assessment and care, your responsibilities will include preparation for response, a safe response to the scene, safe transportation to the hospital, and transferring the patient to hospital personnel for continuity of care. The following are specific areas of responsibility for the EMT-B.

Personal Safety It is not possible to help a patient if you are injured before you reach the patient or while you are providing care, so *keeping yourself safe is your first responsibility.* Safety concerns include dangers from other human beings, animals, unstable buildings, fires, explosions, and more. Emergency scenes are usually safe, but they can also be unpredictable. You must take care at all times to stay safe.

Safety of the Crew, Bystanders, and Patient The same dangers that you face will also be faced by others at the scene. As a professional, you must also be concerned with the safety of others. This includes members of your crew, the patient, and bystanders.

Patient Assessment As an EMT-B, one of your most important functions will be assessment of your patient—that is, finding out enough about what is wrong with your patient to be able to undertake needed emergency care. To perform appropriate care, a proper assessment must come first.

Patient Care The actual care required for an individual patient may range from simple emotional support to life-saving CPR and defibrillation. Based on your assessment findings, patient care is an action or series of actions that your training will prepare you to take that will help the patient deal with and survive his illness or injury.

Lifting and Moving Since EMT-Bs are usually involved in transporting patients to the hospital, lifting and moving patients are important tasks. You must learn to do these procedures safely and efficiently to prevent injuring yourself. In addition, you must know how to lift and move without aggravating or adding to the patient's existing injuries.

Transport It is a serious responsibility to operate an ambulance at any time, but even more so when there is a patient on board. Securing and caring for the patient in the ambulance, as well as safe operation if you drive the ambulance, will be important parts of your job as an EMT-B.

Transfer of Care Upon arrival at the hospital, you will turn the patient over to hospital personnel. You will provide important information on the patient's condition, your observations of the scene, and other pertinent information to the hospital staff so that there will be continuity in the care of the patient. Although this part of patient care comes at the end of the call, it is very important. You must never abandon care of the patient at the hospital until transfer to hospital personnel has been properly completed.

Patient Advocacy As an EMT-B you are there for your patient. You are an *advocate*, the person who speaks up for your patient, who pleads your patient's cause. It is your responsibility to address the needs of the patient and to bring any concerns of the patient to the attention of the hospital staff. You will have developed a rapport with the patient during your brief but very important time together, a rapport that gives you an understanding of the patient's condition and needs. As an advocate, you will do your best to transmit this knowledge in order to help the patient continue through the EMS and hospital system. In your role as an advocate you may perform a task as important as reporting information that will enable the hospital staff to save the patient's life—or as seemingly simple as making sure a relative of the patient is notified. Acts that may seem minor to you may often provide major comfort to your patient.

Traits of a Good EMT-B

There are certain physical traits and aspects of personality that are desirable for an EMT-B.

Physical Traits Physically, you should be in good health and fit to carry out your duties. If you are unable to provide needed care because you cannot bend over or catch your breath, then all your training may be worthless to the patient who is in need of your help.

You should be able to lift and carry up to 125 pounds. Practice with other EMT-Bs is essential so that you can learn how to carry your share of the combined weight of patient, stretcher, linens, blankets, and portable oxygen equipment. For such moves, coordination and dexterity are needed, as well as strength. You will have to perform basic rescue procedures, lower stretcher patients from upper levels, and negotiate fire escapes and stairways while carrying patients.

Your eyesight is very important in performing your EMT-B duties. Make certain that you can clearly see distant objects as well as those close at hand. Both types of vision are needed for patient assessment, reading labels, controlling emergency scenes, and driving. Should you have any eyesight problems, they must be corrected with prescription eye glasses or contact lenses.

Be aware of any problems you may have with color vision. Not only is this important to driving, but it could also be critical for patient assessment. Colors seen on the patient's skin, lips, and nail beds often provide valuable clues to the patient's condition.

You should be able to give and receive oral and written instructions and communicate with the patient, bystanders, and other members of the EMS system. Eyesight, hearing, and speech are important to the EMT-B; thus any significant problems must be corrected if you are going to be an EMT-B.

Personal Traits Good personality traits are very important to the EMT-B. You should be

- Pleasant—to inspire confidence and help to calm the sick and injured
- Sincere—able to convey an understanding of the situation and the patient's feelings
- Cooperative—to allow for faster and better care, establish better coordination with other members of the EMS system, and bolster the confidence of patients and bystanders
- Resourceful—able to adapt a tool or technique to fit an unusual situation
- A self-starter—to show initiative and accomplish what must be done without having to depend on someone else to start procedures
- Emotionally stable—to help overcome the unpleasant aspects of an emergency so that needed care may be rendered and any uneasy feelings that exist afterwards may be resolved
- Able to lead—to take the steps necessary to control a scene, to organize bystanders, to deliver care, and, when necessary, to take complete charge of an emergency

- Neat and clean—to promote confidence in both patients and bystanders and to reduce the possibility of contamination (Figure 1-2)
- Of good moral character, having respect for others—to allow for trust in situations when the patient cannot protect his own body or valuables and so that all information relayed is truthful and reliable
- In control of personal habits—to reduce the possibility of rendering improper care and to prevent discomfort to the patient. This would include not smoking when providing care (Remember: smoking may contaminate wounds and is a danger around oxygen delivery systems) and never consuming alcohol within 8 hours of duty.
- Controlled in conversation—able to communicate properly, to inspire confidence, and to avoid inappropriate conversation that may upset or anger the patient or bystanders or violate patient confidentiality
- Able to listen to others—to be compassionate and empathetic, to be accurate with interviews, and to inspire confidence

Education An EMT-B must also maintain up-to-date knowledge and skills. Since ongoing research in emergency care causes occasional changes in procedure, some of the information you receive while you are studying to become an EMT-B will become out of date during your career. There are many ways to stay current. Some of these include

- Refresher training—Most areas require re-certification at regular intervals. Refresher courses present material to the EMT-B who has already been through a full course but now needs to receive updated information. Refresher courses are usually shorter than original courses. They are required at two- or three-year intervals.
- Continuing education—This type of training supplements the EMT-B's original course. It should not take the place of original training. For example, you may wish to learn more about pediatric or trauma skills or driving techniques. You can obtain this education in conferences and seminars, through lectures, classes, videos, or demonstrations.

It is important to realize that training is a constant process that extends long past your original EMT-B course.

Quality Improvement

Quality improvement is an important concept in EMS. It consists of continuous self-review with the purpose of identifying aspects of the system that require improvement. Once a problem is identified, a plan is developed and implemented to prevent further occurrences of the same problem. As implied in the name, quality improvement is designed and performed to assure that the public receives the highest quality prehospital care.

A sample quality improvement review might go as follows:

As part of a continuous review of the calls your ambulance squad makes, the Quality Improvement (QI) committee has reviewed all of the squad's run reports that involved trauma during one particular month. The committee has noted that the time spent at the scene of serious trauma calls was excessive. (You will later learn that time at the scene of serious trauma must be kept to a minimum, because the injured patient must be transported to the hospital for care that cannot be provided in the field.)

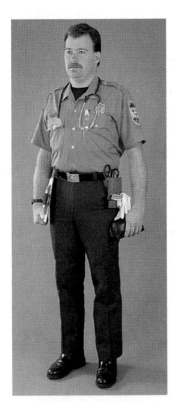

FIGURE 1-2 A professional appearance inspires confidence.

The QI committee has brought this fact to the attention of the leadership of the ambulance squad. As a result, monthly squad training has been developed that covers topics such as how to identify serious trauma patients and then requires skill practice to reinforce techniques of trauma care. (Later in the year, the QI committee will review the same criteria to assure that the extra training has been effective in improving the areas that were found to be deficient.)

During the review, the QI committee has also identified calls where the crews followed procedures and performed well. A letter was sent to these EMT-Bs commending them for their efforts.

As an EMT-B you will have a role in the quality improvement process. In fact, a dedication to quality can be one of the strongest assets of an EMT-B. There are several ways you can work toward quality care. These include

- Keeping careful written documentation—Call reviews are based on the prehospital care reports that you and other crew members write. If a report is incomplete, it is difficult for a QI team to assess the events of a call. If you are ever involved in a lawsuit, an inaccurate or incomplete report may also be a cause for liability. Be sure the reports you write are neat, complete, and accurate.
- Becoming involved in the quality process—As you gain experience, you may wish to volunteer for assignment to the QI committee. In addition, quality improvement has a place on every call. An individual ambulance crew can perform a critique after each call to determine things that went well and others that may need improvement. Have another EMT-B or advanced EMT look over your report before turning it in to assure that it is accurate and complete.
- Obtaining feedback from patients and the hospital staff—This may be done informally or, in some cases, formally. Your organization may send a letter to patients that asks for comments on the care they were given while under your care. Hospital staff may be able to provide information that will help strengthen your care-giving skills.
- Maintaining your equipment—It will be difficult to provide quality care with substandard, damaged, or missing equipment. While

the ingenuity of EMT-Bs should never be underestimated, it would be impossible to administer oxygen or provide cardiac defibrillation without the proper, functional equipment. Check and maintain equipment regularly.
- Continuing your education—An EMT-B who was certified several years ago and has never attended subsequent training will have a problem providing quality care. Seldom-used skills deteriorate without practice. Procedures change. Without some form of regular continuing education, it will be difficult to maintain standards of quality.

Quality improvement is another name for providing the care that you would want to have provided to yourself or a loved one in a time of emergency. That is the best care possible. Maintaining continuous high quality is not easy; it requires constant attention and a sense of pride and obligation. Striving for quality, both in the care you personally give to patients and as a collective part of an ambulance squad, is to uphold the highest standards of the EMS system.

Medical Direction

Each EMS system has a **Medical Director,** a physician who assumes the ultimate responsibility for **medical direction,** or oversight of the patient care aspects of the EMS system. The Medical Director also oversees training and develops **protocols** (lists of steps, such as assessment and steps and interventions to be performed in different situations). An EMT at a basic or advanced level is operating as a **designated agent** of the physician. This means that, as an EMT-B, your authority to give medications and provide emergency care is actually an extension of the Medical Director's license to practice medicine.

The physician obviously cannot physically be at every call. This is why EMS systems develop **standing orders.** The physician has issued a policy or protocol that authorizes EMT-Bs and others to perform particular skills in certain situations. An example may be the administration of glucose. Glucose is very beneficial to certain diabetic patients who are experiencing a medical emergency. The Medical Director issues an order that allows EMT-Bs to give glucose in certain circumstances without speaking to the Medical Director or another physician. This kind of "behind the scenes" medical direction is called **off-line medical direction.**

Certain other procedures that are not covered by standing orders or protocols require the EMT-B to contact the on-duty physician by radio or telephone prior to performing a skill or administering a medication. For example, EMT-Bs carry a medication called activated charcoal. This medication is beneficial to many, but not all, poisoning victims. Prior to administering activated charcoal, you may be required to consult with the on-duty physician. You would use a radio or cellular phone from the ambulance to provide patient information to the physician. After receiving the information, the physician would instruct you on how to proceed with care, including whether and how much activated charcoal to give. Orders from the on-duty physician given in this manner—by radio or phone—are called **on-line medical direction.**

On-line medical direction may be requested at any time you feel that medical advice will be beneficial to patient care.

Protocols and procedures for on-line and off-line medical direction vary from system to system. Your instructor will inform you what your local policies are. *Always follow your local protocols.*

Special Issues

In the coming weeks and through the chapters that follow in this textbook, you will be studying to become an EMT-Basic. As part of your course, your instructor will advise you on local issues and administrative matters, such as a course description, class meeting times, criteria including physical and mental requirements for certification as an EMT-B, as well as specific statutes and regulations regarding EMS in your state, region, or locality.

The Americans with Disabilities (ADA) act has set strict guidelines preserving the rights of Americans with disabilities. If you have a disability or have questions about the ADA, ask your instructor for more information.

CHAPTER REVIEW

KEY TERMS

You may find it helpful to review the following terms.

designated agent an EMT-B or other person authorized by a Medical Director to give medications and provide emergency care. The transfer of such authorization to a designated agent is an extension of the Medical Director's license to practice medicine.

medical direction oversight of the patient care aspects of an EMS system by the Medical Director. **Off-line medical direction** consists of standing orders issued by the Medical Director that allow EMTs to give certain medications or perform certain procedures without speaking to the Medical Director or another physician. **On-line medical direction** consists of orders from the on-duty physician given directly to an EMT-B in the field by radio or telephone.

Medical Director a physician who assumes the ultimate responsibility for the patient care aspects of the EMS system.

911 a system for telephone access to report emergencies. A dispatcher takes the information, and alerts EMS or the fire or police departments as needed. **Enhanced 911** has the additional capability of automatically identifying the caller's phone number and location.

protocols lists of steps, such as assessment and interventions, to be taken in different situations. Protocols are developed by the Medical Director of an EMS system.

quality improvement a process of continuous self-review with the purpose of identifying and correcting aspects of the system that require improvement.

standing orders A policy or protocol that is issued by a Medical Director that authorizes EMT-Bs and others to perform particular skills in certain situations.

SUMMARY

The EMS system has been developed to provide prehospital as well as hospital emergency care. The EMS system includes the 911 or other emergency access system, dispatchers, First Responders, EMTs, the hospital emergency department, physicians, nurses, physician's assistants, and other health professionals.

The EMT-B's responsibilities include safety; patient assessment and care; lifting, moving, and transporting patients; transfer of care; and patient advocacy. An EMT-B must have certain personal and physical traits to assure the ability to do the job.

Education (including refresher training and continuing education), quality improvement procedures, and medical direction are all essential to maintaining high standards of EMS care.

REVIEW QUESTIONS

1. Name the components of the Emergency Medical Services system.
2. List some of the special designations that hospitals may have. Name the special centers you have in your region.
3. List the four national levels of EMS training and certification.
4. List the roles and responsibilities of the EMT-B.
5. List several desirable personal and physical attributes of the EMT-B.
6. Define quality improvement (QI).
7. Describe the differences between on-line and off-line medical direction.

Application

- What qualities would you like to see in an EMT-B who is caring for you? How can you come closer to being this kind of EMT-B?
- You are devoting a considerable amount of time to becoming an EMT-B. How do you plan to refresh your knowledge and stay current once you are out of the classroom?

The Well-being of the EMT-Basic

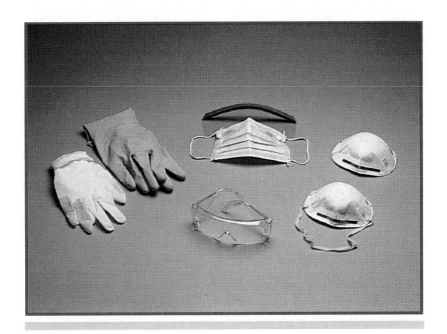

Learning how to safeguard your well-being as an EMT-Basic is critical. During your EMS service you will be exposed to all kinds of stress, including that which accompanies death and dying. You will also sometimes be exposed to dangerous situations. It is important to use equipment and learn strategies to help you stay physically safe and emotionally well.

Objectives

Knowledge and Attitude *At the end of this chapter, you should be able to meet the following objectives.*

1. List possible emotional reactions that the EMT-Basic may experience when faced with trauma, illness, death, and dying. (pp. 17–18)

2. Discuss the possible reactions that a family member may exhibit when confronted with death and dying. (p. 19)

3. State the steps in the EMT-Basic's approach to the family confronted with death and dying. (pp. 19–20)

4. State the possible reactions that the family of the EMT-Basic may exhibit due to their outside involvement in EMS. (p. 18)

5. Recognize the signs and symptoms of critical incident stress. (p. 18)

6. State possible steps the EMT-Basic may take to help reduce or alleviate stress. (pp. 18–19)

7. Explain the need to determine scene safety. (pp. 22–24)

8. Discuss the importance of body substance isolation (BSI). (p. 20)

9. Describe the steps the EMT-Basic should take for personal protection from airborne and bloodborne pathogens. (pp. 20–22)

10. List the personal protective equipment necessary for each of the following situations: (pp. 20–25)

- Hazardous materials
- Rescue operations.
- Violent scenes.
- Crime scenes.
- Exposure to bloodborne pathogens.
- Exposure to airborne pathogens.

11. Explain the rationale for serving as an advocate for the use of appropriate protective equipment. (p. 22)

Skills

1. Given a scenario with potential infectious exposure, the EMT-Basic will use appropriate personal protective equipment. At the completion of the scenario, the EMT-Basic will properly remove and discard the protective garments.

2. Given the above scenario, the EMT-Basic will complete disinfection/cleaning and all reporting documentation.

On the Scene

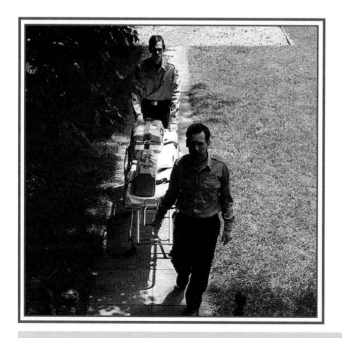

One Saturday afternoon, you are called to the scene of "a woman, injured." You and your partner reach the scene, a house in a residential neighborhood. There are no barking dogs or other pets that might pose a hazard. Everything appears to be quiet. You pull on gloves and grab your kit with supplies you may need, including additional personal protective equipment such as mask and protective eye wear.

As you approach the house, you realize that it is not as quiet as it had seemed at first. You can hear shouting from inside. Then you hear glass breaking and a scream. You know that you can't help anyone if you are injured yourself, and you know that the scene of domestic violence can be extremely dangerous to those who try to intervene.

You and your partner back off, retreating to the ambulance to call for police back-up. You will not approach the house again until the police have done their job and tell you that the scene is safe.

One of your most important jobs is to stay physically safe and emotionally well. Remember: If the EMT-B becomes a victim, he is of little or no use to a patient and may put other rescuers in jeopardy. Ways to safeguard your well-being include understanding and dealing with the stress that normally accompanies critical incidents, ensuring scene safety, and taking body substance isolation (BSI) precautions before treating a patient.

EMOTION AND STRESS

Causes of Stress

Emergencies are stressful. That is their nature (Figure 2-1). While most emergencies are considered "routine," some calls seem to have a higher potential for causing excess stress on EMS providers. They include the following.

- *Multiple-casualty incident (MCI).* A **multiple casualty incident** is a single incident in which there are multiple patients. Examples range from a motor vehicle accident in which two drivers and a passenger are injured to a hurricane that causes the injury of hundreds of people.
- *Calls involving infants and children.* Involving anything from a serious injury to sudden infant death syndrome (SIDS), these calls are known to be particularly stressful to all health-care providers.
- *Severe injuries.* Expect a stressful reaction when your call involves injuries that cause major trauma or distortion to the human body. Examples include amputations, deformed bones, deep wounds, and violent death.
- *Abuse and neglect.* Cases of abuse and neglect occur in all social and economic levels of society. You may be called to treat infant, child, adult, or elderly victims.
- *Death of a coworker.* A bond is formed among members of the public services. The death of another public safety worker—even if you do not know that person—can cause a stress response.

Stress may be caused by a single event or it may be the cumulative result of several incidents. Remember that any incident may affect

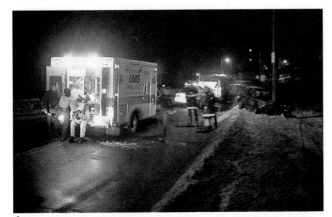

A.

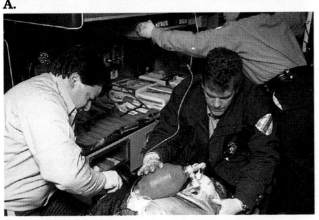

B.

FIGURE 2-1 Emergencies are often stressful for EMS providers.

you and coworkers differently. Two EMT-Bs on the same call may have opposite responses. Try never to make negative judgments about another person's reaction.

Stress may also stem from a combination of factors, including problems in your personal life. One common cause of stress is people who "just don't understand" the job. For example, your EMS organization may require you to work on weekends and holidays. Time spent on call may be frustrating to friends and family members. They may not understand why you can't participate in certain social activities or why you can't leave a certain area. You might get frustrated, too, because you can't plan around the unpredictable nature of emergencies. Then, after a very trying or exciting call, for instance, you may wish to share your feelings with a friend or someone you love. You find instead that the person does not understand your emotions. This can lead to feelings of separation and rejection, which are highly stressful.

Signs and Symptoms of Stress

There are two types of stress: *eustress* and *distress*. Eustress is a positive form of stress that helps people work under pressure and respond effectively. Distress is negative. It can happen when the stress of a scene becomes overwhelming. As a result, your response to the emergency will not be effective. Distress also can cause immediate and long-term problems with your health and well-being.

The signs and symptoms of stress include irritability with family, friends, and coworkers; inability to concentrate; changes in daily activities, such as difficulty sleeping or nightmares, loss of appetite, and loss of interest in sexual activity; anxiety; indecisiveness; guilt; isolation; and loss of interest in work.

Dealing with Stress

Life-Style Changes

There are several ways to deal with stress. They are called "life-style changes," and they include the following.

- *Develop more healthful and positive dietary habits.* Avoid fatty foods and increase your carbohydrate intake. Also reduce your consumption of alcohol and caffeine, which can have negative effects including an increase in stress and anxiety and disturbance of sleep patterns.
- *Exercise.* When performed safely and properly, this life-style change helps to "burn off" stress. It also helps you deal with the physical aspects of your responsibilities, such as carrying equipment and performing physically demanding emergency procedures.
- *Devote time to relaxing.* Try relaxation techniques, too. These techniques, which include deep-breathing exercises and meditation, are valuable stress reducers.

In addition to the changes you can make in your personal life to help reduce and prevent stress, there are also changes you can make in your professional life. If you are in an organization with varied shifts and locations, consider requesting a change to a different location that offers a lighter call volume or different types of calls. You may also want to change your shift to one that allows more time with family and friends.

There are many types of help available for EMT-Bs and others who are experiencing stress. Seek them out. It is not a sign of weakness. There are many professionals who can help you deal with the stress you feel, and much of the care may be covered by health insurance policies.

Critical Incident Stress Debriefing (CISD)

A **critical incident stress debriefing (CISD)** is a process in which a team of trained peer counselors and mental health professionals meet with rescuers and health care providers who have been involved in a major incident (Figure 2-2). The meetings are generally held within 24 to 72 hours after the incident. The goal is to assist emergency care workers in dealing with the stress related to that incident.

The CISD is an open discussion of the feelings experienced during and after the call. Participants are encouraged to talk about any fears or reactions they have had. It is critical that the CISD does not become a method of investigation of the events of the call. Everything discussed at the meetings is confidential and all participants are asked not to disclose information once the meeting is over. Any breech in the confidentiality of the discussion prevents others from sharing information that can help them. After the open discussion, the CISD team offers suggestions on how to deal with and overcome the stress. It is

- *The patient must sign a "release" form.* Such a form is designed to release the ambulance squad and individuals from liability arising from the patient's informed refusal.

Following the steps outlined above will not guarantee that you will be free from liability if the patient refuses care or transport. In addition to the liability factor, there is also an ethical issue. You would undoubtedly feel guilty if a patient was found unconscious or deceased after refusing care and you felt that transportation would have prevented the circumstance. If in doubt, do everything possible to persuade the patient to accept care and transport. Take all possible actions to persuade a patient who you feel should go to the hospital but refuses. These actions may include

- *Spending time speaking to the patient.* Use principles of effective communication. It may take reasoning, persistence, "dealing" (we'll call a neighbor to take care of your cat, but then you go to the hospital), or other strategies.
- *Informing the patient of the consequences of not going to the hospital, even if they are not pleasant.*
- *Consulting medical direction.* If you are in a residence, use the patient's phone to contact medical direction. If the on-line doctor is willing, let him speak to the patient when all else fails.
- *Contacting family members to help convince the patient.* Often family members can provide reasons for the patient to go to the hospital. Offers for a loved one to meet the patient at the hospital may be very helpful.
- *Calling law enforcement personnel if necessary.* Police may be able to order or "arrest" the patient who refuses care to force them to go to the hospital. This is done under the premise that the patient is temporarily mentally incompetent as demonstrated by refusing care that might save his life.
- *Trying to determine why the patient is refusing care.* Often the patient has a fear of the hospital, procedures, prolonged hospitalization, or even death. Refusal to go to the hospital may be a form of denial, or unwillingness to accept the idea of being ill. If you identify the cause of the refusal you may be able to develop a strategy to persuade the patient to accept your care and transportation to the hospital.

Bear in mind, however, that you do not have the right in most cases to force a competent patient to go to the hospital against his will. Doing so may result in assault and battery charges. Subjecting the patient to unwanted care and transport has actually been viewed as assault or battery in criminal and civil courts.

If all efforts fail and the patient does not accept your care or transportation, it becomes vital to document the attempts you made—to make your efforts a part of the official record—in order to prevent liability. Write into your records every step you took to persuade the patient to accept care or to go to the hospital. Include the names of any witnesses to your attempts and the patient's refusal. (A sample EMS patient refusal procedures checklist is shown in Figure 3-1.)

In all cases of refusal you should advise the patient that he should call back at any time if he has a problem or wishes to be cared for or transported. It is also advisable to call a relative or neighbor who can stay with the patient in case problems should develop. Leave phone stickers with emergency numbers so the patient will be able to call for help if necessary. You should also recommend that the patient or a relative call the family physician to report the incident and arrange for follow-up care. Document all actions you have taken for the patient.

While there may be patients who legitimately refuse care (for minor wounds, unfounded calls, and the like) a patient with any significant medical condition should be transported and seen at a hospital.

Do Not Resuscitate Orders

It will only be a matter of time before you come upon a patient who has a **do not resuscitate (DNR) order** (Figure 3-2). This is a legal document, usually signed by the patient and his physician, which states that the patient has a terminal illness and does not wish to prolong life through resuscitative efforts. A DNR order is called an "advance directive" because it is written and signed in advance of any event where resuscitation might be undertaken. It is more than the expressed wishes of the patient or family. It is an actual document.

There are varying degrees of DNR orders, expressed through a variety of detailed instructions that may be part of the order. Such an instruction might stipulate, for example, that resuscitation be attempted only if cardiac or respiratory arrest is observed, but not attempted if

EMS PATIENT REFUSAL CHECKLIST

PATIENT NAME:_____ AGE: _____

LOCATION OF CALL:_____ DATE: _____

AGENCY INCIDENT #:_____ AGENCY CODE: _____

NAME OF PERSON FILLING OUT FORM: _____

I. ASSESSMENT OF PATIENT (Circle appropriate response for each item)

   1. Oriented to:

Person?	Yes	No
Place?	Yes	No
Time?	Yes	No
Situation?	Yes	No

   2. Altered level of consciousness?   Yes   No

   3. Head injury?   Yes   No

   4. Alcohol or drug ingestion by exam or history?   Yes   No

II. PATIENT INFORMED (Circle appropriate response for each item)

Yes	No	Medical treatment/evaluation needed
Yes	No	Ambulance transport needed
Yes	No	Further harm could result without medical treatment/ evaluation
Yes	No	Transport by means other than ambulance could be hazardous in light of patient's illness/injury
Yes	No	Patient provided with Refusal Information Sheet
Yes	No	Patient accepted Refusal Information Sheet

III. DISPOSITION

_____ Refused all EMS services

_____ Refused field treatment, but accepted transport

_____ Refused transport, but accepted field treatment

_____ Refused transport to recommended facility

_____ Patient transported by private vehicle to _____

_____ Released in care or custody of self

_____ Released in care or custody of relative or friend

    Name: _____ Relationship: _____

_____ Released in custody of law enforcement agency

    Agency: _____ Officer:._____

_____ Released in custody of other agency

    Agency: _____ Officer: _____

IV. COMMENTS: _____

        _____

        _____

FIGURE 3-1 Certain procedures should be followed when a patient refuses care or transport. Above checklist from Spokane County Emergency Medical Services, Washington State.

Department of Health

Nonhospital Order Not to Resuscitate (DNR order)

Person's Name (Print) _____

Date of Birth ___/___/___

Do not resuscitate the person named above.

Person's Signature _____

Date ___/___/___

Physician's Signature _____

Print Name _____

License Number _____

Date ___/___/___

It is the responsibility of the physician to determine, at least every 90 days, whether this order continues to be appropriate, and to indicate this by a note in the person's medical chart. The issuance of a new form is **NOT** required, and under the law this order should be considered valid unless it is known that it has been revoked. This order remains valid and must be followed, even if it has not been reviewed within the 90 day period.

FIGURE 3-2 A do not resuscitate (DNR) order.

the patient is found already in arrest (to avoid the possibility of resuscitating a patient who may already have sustained brain damage). Many states also have laws governing living wills, statements signed by the patient, usually regarding use of long-term life-support and comfort measures such as respirators, intravenous feedings, and pain medications. Other states require naming a proxy—a person whom the signer of the document names to make health care decisions for him in case he is unable to make such decisions for himself. Living wills and health care proxies usually pertain to situations that will occur in the hospital rather than in the prehospital situation.

Become familiar with the legal DNR orders for your region or state and the laws and rules governing their implementation. It is important to know the forms and policies before you go to the call, since often the patient is in cardiac arrest (heart and breathing have stopped) or near death. These are stressful times for the family and for you, occasions when the window of time for making a resuscitation decision may be only a few moments.

If the patient himself refuses care, then becomes unconscious, implied consent usually takes over and care begins. It is a legal and ethical dilemma that is usually best resolved by providing care. It is better to be criticized or sued for saving a life than for letting a patient die. A legal DNR order prevents unwanted resuscitation and awkward situations. In most cases, the oral requests of a family member are not reason to withhold care.

Negligence

To the layperson, negligence means that something that should have been done was not done or was done incorrectly. The legal concept of negligence in emergency care is not that simple. A finding of **negligence,** or failure to act properly, requires that ALL of the following circumstances be proved.

- *The EMT had a duty to the patient (duty to act—see below).*
- *The EMT did not provide the standard of care (committed a breach of duty).* This may include the failure to act, that is, not providing needed care as would be expected of an EMT-B in your locality. Failure to act is a major cause of legal actions against EMS systems or EMTs.

- *The actions of the EMT in not providing the standard of care caused harm to the patient.* This harm can be physical or psychological.

Negligence is the basis for a large number of lawsuits involving prehospital emergency care. If the above circumstances are proved, the EMT may be required to pay damages if the harm to the patient is considered by the court to be a loss that requires reimbursement (compensable). The negligent EMT may be required to pay for medical expenses, lost wages (possibly including future earnings), pain and suffering, and various other factors as determined by the court.

Lawsuits against EMT-Bs are actually quite rare, especially when compared to the number of calls that are dispatched each day in this country. While liability and negligence should be important considerations, you should not live or work in fear of a lawsuit. When you perform proper care that is within your scope of practice and is properly documented, you will prevent most, if not all, legal problems.

Duty to Act

An EMT-B in certain situations has a **duty to act,** that is an obligation to provide emergency care to a patient. An EMT-B who is on an ambulance and is dispatched to a call clearly has a duty to act. If there is no threat to safety, the EMT-B must provide care. This duty to act continues throughout the call.

Once an EMT-B has initiated care, then leaves a patient without assuring that the patient has been turned over to someone with equal or greater medical training, **abandonment** exists.

The duty to act is not always clear. It depends on your state and local laws. In many states, an off duty EMT-B has no legal obligation to provide care. However, you may feel a moral or ethical obligation to act. An example of this would be if you observe a motor vehicle collision while off duty. You may feel morally bound to provide care, even if no legal obligation exists. If you are off duty and begin care and you leave before other trained personnel arrive, you may still be considered to have abandoned the patient.

Other situations are even more confusing. If you are an EMT-B in an ambulance, but you are out of your jurisdiction, the laws are again often unclear. In general, if you follow your conscience and provide care, you will incur less liability than if you do not act. Always follow your local protocols and laws. Your instructor will provide information about local issues.

Good Samaritan Laws

Good Samaritan laws have been developed in most states to provide immunity to individuals trying to help people in emergencies. Most of these laws will grant immunity from liability if the rescuer acts in good faith to provide care to the level of his training, to the best of his ability. These laws do not prevent someone from initiating a lawsuit, nor will they protect the rescuer from being found liable for acts of gross negligence and other violations of the law.

You must familiarize yourself with the laws that govern your state. Good Samaritan laws may not apply to EMT-Bs in your locality. In some states, the Good Samaritan laws only apply to volunteers. If you are a paid EMT-B, different laws and regulations may apply.

Some states have specific statutes that authorize, regulate, and protect EMS personnel. To be protected by such laws, you must be recognized as an EMT in the state where care was provided. Some states have specific licensing and certification requirements that must be met for recognition under Good Samaritan laws.

Confidentiality

When you act as an EMT-B you obtain a considerable amount of information about a patient. You also are allowed into homes and other personal areas that are private and contain much information about people.

Any information you obtain about a patient's history, condition, or treatment is considered confidential and must not be shared with anyone else. This principle is known as **confidentiality.**

The only time such information may be disclosed is when a written release is signed by the patient. Your organization will have a policy on this. Information should not be disclosed based on verbal permission, nor should information be disclosed over the telephone. You may be subpoenaed, or ordered into court by a legal authority, where you may also legally disclose information. You may be called to criminal trials or civil court to testify about an injury or incident. If you have a question about the validity of a legal document, contact a supervisor or your agency's attorney for advice.

Patient care information may be shared with other health care professionals who will have a role in care of the patient. It is appropriate to turn over information about the patient to the nurse and physician at the receiving hospital. This is necessary for continuity in patient care. It may also be necessary and permissible to supply patient care information for insurance billing forms.

Special Situations

You may respond to calls where a patient is critically injured, perhaps near death, and is an **organ donor.** An organ donor is a patient who has completed a legal document that allows for donation of organs and tissues in the event of his death. Many people have benefited from the donation of organs by persons who have completed this paperwork before death.

You may find that the patient is an organ donor when told by a family member. Often an organ donor card is kept on the patient's person (Figure 3-3). The back of the patient's driver's license may also contain an indication that the patient wishes to donate organs upon his death.

The emergency care for a patient who is an organ donor must not differ from that for a patient who is not. All emergency care measures must be taken. If a patient is recognized as an organ donor, contact medical direction. The on-line physician may order you to perform CPR on a patient where you might normally not resuscitate due to fatal injuries. The oxygen delivered to body cells by CPR will help preserve the organs until they can be harvested for implantation in another person.

A patient may also wear a medical identification device (Figure 3-4). This device is worn to alert EMT-Bs and other health care professionals that the patient has a particular medical condition. If the patient is found unconscious, the device provides important medical information. The device may be a necklace, bracelet, or card and may indicate a number of conditions including

- Heart conditions
- Allergies
- Diabetes
- Epilepsy

**Valley General Hospital
Permission For
Organ Donation/Anatomical Gift
By An Individual Prior To Death**

PATIENT IDENTIFICATION PLATE

I, _____, currently residing at _____

_____, being eighteen (18) years of age or older, do hereby make the following organ donation/anatomical gift to take effect upon my death:

1.   I give, if medically acceptable:

       ☐ My body;
       ☐ Any needed organs or parts;
       ☐ The following organs or parts:

       _____

       _____

2.   I make this gift to Valley General Hospital or to physicians or institutions designated by them for the following purposes:

       ☐ Any purpose authorized by law;
       ☐ Transplantation;
       ☐ Therapy;
       ☐ Medical Research and/or Education

3.   I acknowledge that I have read this document in its entirety and that I fully understand it and that all blank spaces have either been completed or crossed off prior to my signing.

4.   I understand that Valley General Hospital and its authorized designees will rely upon this consent.

_____   _____
WITNESS TO SIGNATURE   DATE   SIGNATURE   DATE
(PRINT NAME & ADDRESS BELOW)

_____   _____
                                              PRINT NAME

_____   _____
                                              ADDRESS

WITNESS TO SIGNATURE   DATE   _____
(PRINT NAME & ADDRESS BELOW)   TELEPHONE NUMBER

_____

_____

FIGURE 3-3 An organ donor form.

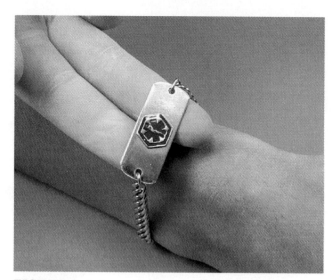

FIGURE 3-4 A medical identification device.

Crime Scenes

A crime scene is defined as the location where a crime has been committed or any place evidence relating to a crime may be found (Figure 3-5). Many crime scenes involve crimes against people. These crimes cause injuries that are often serious. *Once police have made the scene safe, the priority of the EMT-B at a crime scene is to provide patient care.*

While you are providing care at the crime scene there are actions that you can take to help preserve evidence. To preserve evidence, you must first know what evidence is, as described below.

The condition of the scene The way you find the scene is important evidence to the police. Should you arrive first, make a mental note of the exterior of the scene. Remember how you gained access. Doors that are found ajar, pry

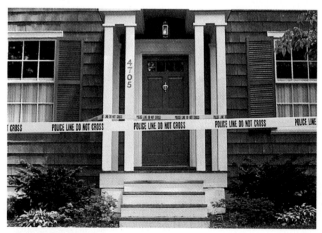

FIGURE 3-5 A crime scene.

marks, and broken windows are signs of danger for you and important evidence for the police. Make a note of whether the lights were on or off and the condition of the TV and radio.

The patient The patient himself provides valuable information. The position the patient is found in, condition of clothing, and injuries are all valuable pieces of evidence.

Fingerprints and footprints Fingerprints are perhaps the most familiar kind of evidence. They may be obtained from almost any surface. It is important for you to avoid unnecessarily touching anything at the scene in order to preserve prints. Since you will be wearing gloves at most scenes, you will not leave your fingerprints on objects. If you touch these objects, however, you may smudge fingerprints that were left by someone else.

Microscopic evidence Microscopic evidence is a wide range of evidence that is usually invisible to the naked eye. It consists of small pieces of evidence such as dirt and carpet fibers. To the eye, there may be no way to distinguish one from another. Under the microscope, scientists can develop valuable information. From just a few fibers, the materials and sometimes the brand name of carpets or clothes may be determined. Traces of blood may be enough to determine blood type or to be used for DNA comparison.

To preserve evidence at the crime scene, the following actions will be helpful to the police. *Remember that your first priority is always patient care.*

Remember what you touch It may be necessary to move the patient or furniture to begin CPR or other patient care. This cannot be avoided, but it is helpful to tell the police what you have touched or moved. Once you leave, if they find furniture moved or blood stains in two locations, they may think that a scuffle took place when in fact it did not. If you are forced to break a window to get to the patient and do not tell the police, they will think that a breaking-and-entering has occurred.

Minimize your impact on the scene If you are forced to move the patient or furniture to begin care, move as little as possible. Do not wander through the house or go to areas where it is not necessary to go. Avoid using the phone, which will prevent the police from using the "redial" button to determine who the victim called last. Do not use the bathroom since this may also destroy evidence.

Work with the police The police may require you to provide a statement about your actions or observations at the scene. While it may not be possible to make notes while patient care is going on, after you arrive at the hospital make notes about your observations and actions at the scene.

You may also wish to critique the scene—both with your crew and, if possible, with the police. Invite a member of your local or state police department to your agency for an in-service drill on crime scenes. Evidence recovery methods and procedures vary from area to area. The police officer who comes to your station will brief you on local procedures.

Interestingly enough, police are often as unfamiliar with EMS procedures as you are with evidence procedures. The police may ask you to delay your work at the scene so they can take photographs or interview the patient. They may do this because they don't understand—as you will learn in later chapters—that the time that elapses before on-scene care and transport to the hospital, in the case of serious injuries, must be kept to a minimum for the patient to have the best chance of survival. Education and critiques can be beneficial to both EMT-Bs and police officers.

Special Crimes and Reporting Many states require EMT-Bs and other health care professionals to report certain types of incidents. Many areas have hotlines for reporting crimes such as child, elderly, or domestic abuse. This may be mandatory in your area. Failure to report certain incidents may actually be a crime. There is also a strong moral obligation to report these crimes. Many states offer immunity from liability for people who report incidents such as these in good faith.

Other crimes may also require reports. Violence (e.g., gunshot wounds or stabbings) and sexual assaults often fall into this category. If you are required by law to report such incidents, you are usually exempt from confidentiality requirements in making these reports.

You may also be required to notify police of other situations, such as cases where restraint may be necessary, intoxicated persons found with injuries, or mentally incompetent people who have been injured.

CHAPTER REVIEW

KEY TERMS

You may find it helpful to review the following terms.

abandonment leaving a patient after care has been initiated and before the patient has been transferred to someone with equal or greater medical training.

confidentiality the obligation not to reveal information obtained about a patient except to other health care professionals involved in the patient's care, or under subpoena, or in a court of law, or when the patient has signed a release of confidentiality.

consent permission from the patient for care or other action by the EMT-B. *See also* expressed consent; implied consent.

do not resuscitate (DNR) order a legal document, usually signed by the patient and his physician, which states that the patient has a terminal illness and does not wish to prolong life through resuscitative efforts.

duty to act an obligation to provide care to a patient.

expressed consent consent given by adults who are of legal age and mentally competent to make a rational decision in regard to their medical well-being. *See also* consent.

Good Samaritan laws a series of laws, varying in each state, designed to provide limited legal protection for citizens and some health care personnel when they are administering emergency care.

implied consent the consent it is presumed a patient or patient's parent or guardian would give if they could, as for example an unconscious patient or a parent who cannot be contacted when care is needed. *See also* consent.

liability being held legally responsible.

negligence a finding of failure to act properly in a situation in which there was a duty to act, needed care as would reasonably be expected of the EMT-B was not provided, and harm was caused to the patient as a result.

organ donor a person who has completed a legal document that allows for donation of organs and tissues in the event of death.

scope of practice a set of regulations and ethical considerations that define the scope, or extent and limits, of the EMT-B's job.

SUMMARY

Medical, legal, and ethical issues are a part of every EMS call. A number of such issues involve consent, the permission a patient or patient's parent or guardian gives for care or transport. Consent may be expressed or implied. If a competent patient refuses care or transport, you should make every effort to persuade the patient, but you cannot force the patient to accept care or go to the hospital.

Negligence is failing to act properly when you have a duty to act. As an EMT-B, you have a duty to act whenever you are dispatched on a call. You may also have a legal or moral duty to act even when off duty or outside your jurisdiction. Abandonment is leaving a patient after you have initiated care and before you have transferred the patient to a person with equal or higher training. Confidentiality is the obligation not to reveal personal information you obtain about a patient except to other health care professionals involved in the patient's care or under legal subpoena or when the patient signs a release. As an EMT-B you may be sued or held legally liable on any of these issues. However, EMTs are rarely held liable when they have acted within their scope of practice and have carefully documented the details of the call.

Special situations include patients who are organ donors (care of the patient takes precedence; follow the advice of medical direction) and patients who wear medical identification devices. At a crime scene, care of the patient takes precedence over preservation of evidence, but you should make every effort not to disturb the scene unnecessarily and to report your actions and observations to the police.

REVIEW QUESTIONS

1. Define *scope of practice, negligence, duty to act, abandonment,* and *confidentiality.*
2. List several steps that must be taken when a patient refuses care or transportation.
3. List several types of evidence and ways you may act to preserve it at a crime scene.

Application

- You are called to the scene of a motor vehicle collision. An 8-year-old child has been struck by a vehicle and fortunately has sustained only slight injuries. Who can give consent for her care? How might you obtain consent?
- You respond to the scene of a terminally ill patient who appears to be near death. His family asks you to let the patient "go in peace" and not resuscitate the patient. Can you honor the family's request? What steps must you take in this situation, and why?

The Human Body

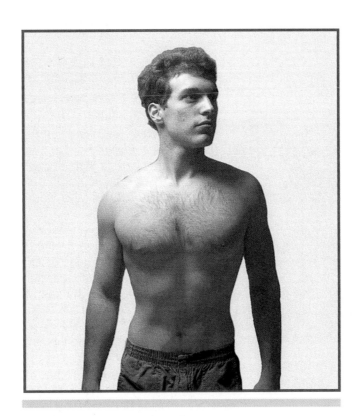

As an EMT-Basic, you will be called when a person has some problem with his body. The problem may be a traumatic injury, or it may be a medical problem such as chest pain. In any case, your assessment of the patient's condition will be based on your knowledge of the anatomy, or structure, of the body. You will also be required to know some of the body's functions, or physiology. Your knowledge will not only help you assess the patient but also will allow you to communicate your findings with other EMS personnel and hospital staff accurately and efficiently.

Objectives

Knowledge   *At the end of this chapter, you should be able to meet the following objectives.*

1. Identify the following topographic terms: medial, lateral, proximal, distal, superior, inferior, anterior, posterior, midline, right and left, mid-clavicular, bilateral, mid-axillary. (pp. 43–45)

2. Describe the anatomy and function of the following major body systems: respiratory (pp. 50–52), circulatory (pp. 52–56, 57), musculoskeletal (pp. 46–49), nervous (pp. 56, 58), and endocrine (pp. 59–60).

On the Scene

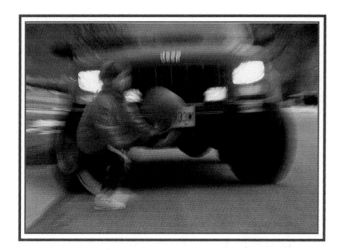

You are called to a street near a school playground. You arrive to find 10-year-old Janey lying in the street. She is crying and appears to be in pain. You notice that her left thigh appears oddly bent.

You: Hi, I'm Lisa from the ambulance. What's your name?
Janey: (through tears) Janey.
You: OK, Janey, we're going to take real good care of you. I want you to lie quietly while we see where you're hurt. My partner is going to hold onto your head to help you keep it still. We'll make sure someone calls your parents. Can you tell me what happened?
Janey: I ran into the street to get my ball and a car hit me.
You: Can you tell me where you hurt?
Janey: My leg hurts. And my belly hurts.
You: Can you point to where it hurts? (She does.)

At the hospital, you report to the triage nurse: "Janey was struck by a car. It doesn't appear as if she lost consciousness. She complains of pain in her left upper abdominal quadrant which radiates to her shoulder, and her left thigh is swollen and deformed but with no open wound. Her last vital signs were . . ."

Why did you use the term "left upper abdominal quadrant"? Couldn't you just have said "She has a pain in her stomach"? In this chapter you will learn about the importance of knowing the human body and being able to use correct terminology to describe it.

The human body has many different structures, forming a variety of systems with different functions. The term **anatomy** refers to body structures. The term **physiology** refers to body functions. It is important to be able to identify and correctly name the body's structures and functions in order to perform a proper assessment and report your findings to other medical professionals.

ANATOMICAL TERMS

The body is made up of a number of regions (Figure 4-1). Certain terms are used to describe directions and positions of the body.

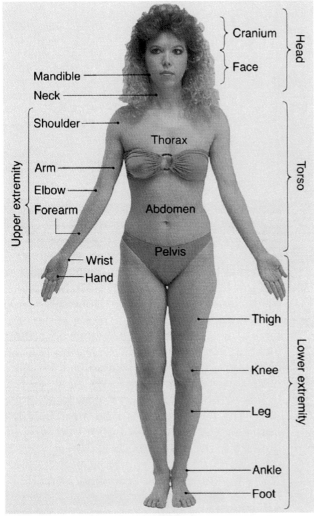

FIGURE 4-1 Body regions.

Directional Terms

There must be a standardized method of referring to places on the body when describing illness or injury. Standardized anatomical directional terms are used (Figure 4-2). For example, the directions left and right always refer to the *patient's* left and right.

- **Anatomical position**—All descriptions of the body start with the assumption that the body is in anatomical position, even if the patient is not in that position when found. Anatomical position is best described as a person standing, facing forward, with his palms facing forward (Figures 4-1 and 4-2). The importance of always referring to this standardized position is that all health care providers, anywhere, will use the same anatomical starting point when describing the body and will understand each other's references.
- **Planes**—The body may also be divided into planes. A plane is a flat surface, the kind of surface that would be formed if you sliced straight through a department store dummy or an imaginary human body. Cutting through from top to bottom, you could slice the body either into right and left halves or into front and back halves.

  The **midline** of the body is created by drawing an imaginary line down the center of the body passing between the eyes and extending down past the umbilicus (belly button, or navel). Slicing through the imaginary body at the midline devides the body into right and left halves. From this, the terms **medial** and **lateral** are developed. *Medial* refers to a position closer to the midline while *lateral* refers to a position farther away from the midline. An example of the use of these terms would be, "The bridge of the nose is medial to the eyes." As another example, an arm has a medial side (close to the body) and a lateral side (the outer arm, away from the body).

  You may also use the term **bilateral.** This refers to "both sides" of anything. Patients may have diminished lung sounds on both sides when you listen with a stethoscope. This would be reported as "The patient has diminished lung sounds bilaterally." Or, in a patient with chest pain, you might report that "the patient has pain in her chest that radiates bilaterally to the shoulders."

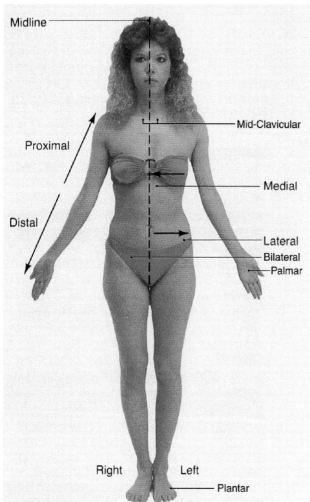
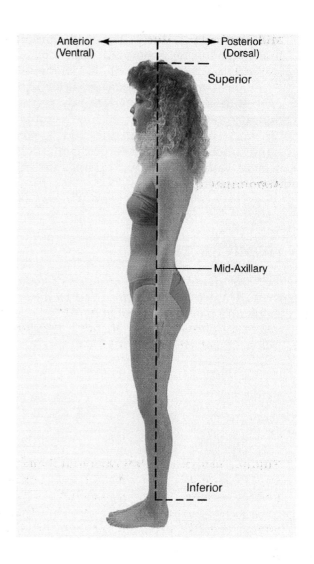

FIGURE 4-2 Directional terms.

The **mid-axillary line** is one that is drawn vertically from the middle of the armpit to the ankle. (The anatomical term for the armpit is the *axilla*, so *mid-axillary* means "middle of the armpit.") This divides the body into front and back halves. The term for the front is **anterior.** The term for the back is **posterior.** An example of these terms in use is "The patient has wounds to the posterior arm and the anterior thigh." A synonym for *anterior* is **ventral** (referring to the front of the body). A synonym for *posterior* is **dorsal** (referring to the back of the body).

- **Superior** and **inferior**—These terms refer to vertical, or up-and-down, directions. *Superior* means above, *inferior* means below. An example of this would be "The nose is superior to the mouth."
- **Proximal** and **distal**—These are relative terms. *Proximal* means closer to the **torso**

(the trunk of the body—the body without the head and the extremities), while *distal* means farther away from the torso. An example would be the elbow. The elbow is proximal to the hand because it is closer to the torso than the hand. The elbow is distal to the shoulder since the elbow is farther away from the torso than the shoulder. The terms are usually used when describing locations on extremities. For example, after splinting a leg or an arm, you will feel for a distal pulse—a pulse in the foot or the hand, points that are farther away from the torso than the splint—to be sure that the injury or the splint has not cut off circulation from the heart to the farthest part of the limb.

Two other terms you may sometimes hear are **palmar** (referring to the palm of the hand) and **plantar** (referring to the sole of the foot).

- **Mid-clavicular line**—The mid-clavicular line runs through the center of a clavicle (collar bone) and the nipple below it. Since there are two clavicles, there are two mid-clavicular lines. When you use a stethoscope to listen for breath sounds, you will place the stethoscope at the mid-clavicular lines to listen to each side of the chest and assess the function of both lungs.
- **Abdominal quadrants**—The abdomen is a large body region containing many vital organs. It is helpful, for example in describing the location of abdominal pain or an abdominal wound to divide the abdomen into four parts, or quadrants. This can be done by drawing horizontal and vertical lines through the navel. The quadrants would be the *right upper quadrant*, the *left upper quadrant*, the *right lower quadrant*, and the *left lower quadrant* (Figure 4-3).

Positional Terms

There are several positions for which you will also need to know the names.

- **Supine, prone,** and **lateral recumbent**—A supine patient is lying on his back. A prone patient is lying on his stomach. A person may also be lying on his right side (right lateral recumbent) or on his left side (left

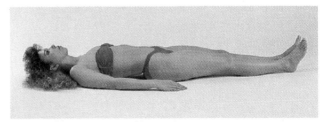

Supine

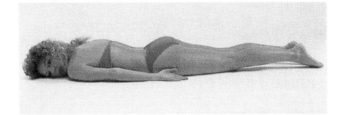

Prone

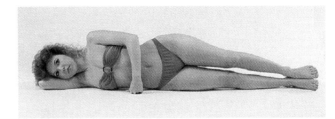

Right lateral recumbent

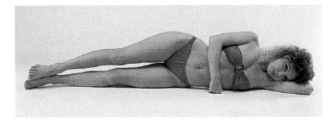

Left lateral recumbent

FIGURE 4-4 Anatomical postures.

lateral recumbent) or on his left side (left lateral recumbent) (Figure 4-4).

- **Fowler's position** and **Trendelenburg position**—When patients are transported on a stretcher there are several positions that they may be placed in. In the Fowler's position, the patient is seated (Figure 4-5). This is usually accomplished by raising the head end of the stretcher so the body is at a 45-to-60-degree angle. The patient may be sitting straight up or leaning slightly back. If leaning back in a semi-sitting position, this is sometimes called *semi-Fowler's*. In Fowler's position, the legs may be straight out or bent.

  In the Trendelenburg position, the patient is lying with the head slightly lower

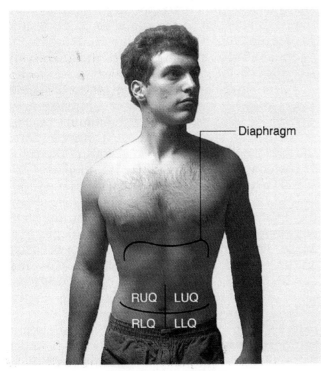

FIGURE 4-3 Abdominal quadrants.

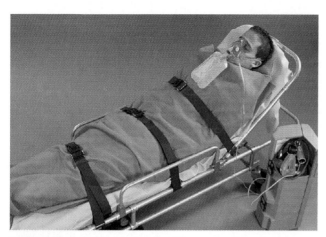

FIGURE 4-5 Fowler's position.

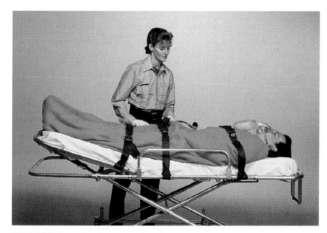

FIGURE 4-6 Trendelenburg position.

than the feet (Figure 4-6). This may be accomplished by having the patient lie flat and elevating the legs a few inches or, if the patient is on a spine board, by tilting the whole board so the legs are a few inches higher than the head. The Trendelenburg position is sometimes called the **shock position,** because it is used to treat patients in shock (those who have no possibility of head injury. Patients with head injuries must remain supine with the head and feet on the same level).

BODY SYSTEMS

The Musculoskeletal System

Unlike many other systems, the musculoskeletal system extends into all parts of the body. The skeleton consists of the skull and spine, the ribs and sternum, the shoulder and upper extremities, the pelvis and lower extremities (Figure 4-7).

Interacting with the skeletal system are muscles, ligaments (which connect bone to bone), and tendons (which connect muscle to bone).

The musculoskeletal system has three main functions:

To give the body shape
To protect vital internal organs
To provide for body movement

The Skull

To list the parts of the skeleton from top to bottom, you would begin with the skull (Figure 4-8). The skull is the bony structure of the head. A main function of the skull is to enclose and protect the brain.

The *cranium* consists of the top, back, and sides of the skull. The *face* is the front of the skull. The facial bones consist of the **orbits** which surround the eyes, the **nasal bone** which provides some of the structure of the nose, the **maxillae** or two fused bones of the upper jaw, and the **mandible** which is the lower jaw. The **zygomatic bones** are commonly referred to as the cheekbones.

The Spinal Column

The spinal column is an essential part of the anatomy. Not only does it provide structure and support for the body, it also houses and protects the spinal cord. You will see references throughout this text to "taking spinal precautions" for some patients. Since the spinal cord is essential for movement, sensation, and vital functions, injuries to the spine have the potential to be very serious, possibly resulting in paralysis or death.

The spinal column (also referred to simply as the spine), consists of 33 **vertebrae,** the separate bones of the spine. Like building blocks, vertebrae are stacked upon each other to form the spinal column. The five divisions of the spine are listed in Table 4-1 and shown in Figure 4-9.

The anatomy of the body allows some vertebrae to be injured more easily than others. Since the head is large and heavy, resting on the slender neck, incidents such as car accidents may cause the head to whip back and forth or strike an object such as the windshield. This frequently causes injuries to the cervical spine. Since the spine carries nerve impulses to the body, an injury to the spinal cord at this level may be fatal. The lumbar region is also subject to injury because it is not supported by other parts of the skeleton. The thoracic spine, to which the ribs are attached, and the sacral spine

The Skeleton

2ll bones   600 muscles

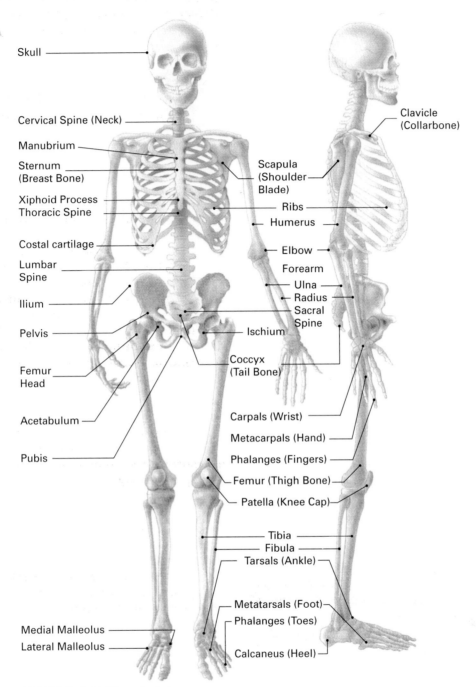

FIGURE 4-7 The skeleton.

and coccyx, which are supported by the pelvis, are less easily injured.

The Thorax

The **thorax** is the chest. It may also be called the *thoracic cavity*. This cavity contains the heart, lungs, and major blood vessels. An important function of the thorax is to protect these vital organs. This is accomplished by the twelve pairs of ribs that attach to the twelve thoracic vertebrae of the spine. In the front, ten of these pairs of ribs are attached to the **sternum** (breastbone) and two are called floating ribs since they have no anterior attachment. You will remember the sternum from your CPR training. This flat bone is divided into three sections: the **manubrium** (superior portion), the

The Skull: Cranium and Face

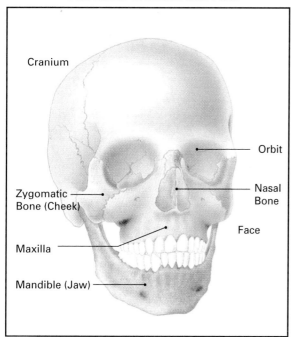

FIGURE 4-8 The skull: cranium and face.

TABLE 4-1 The Divisions of the Spine

Division	Corresponding Anatomy	Number of Vertebrae
Cervical	Neck	7
Thoracic	Thorax, ribs, upper back	12
Lumbar	Lower back	5
Sacral	Back wall of pelvis	5
Coccyx	Tailbone	4

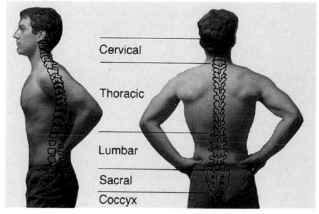

FIGURE 4-9 Divisions of the spine.

body (center portion), and the **xiphoid process** (inferior tip).

The Pelvis

The pelvis is commonly referred to as the hip, although the hip is actually the joint where the femur (thigh bone) and pelvis join. The pelvis contains bones that are fused together. The **ilium** is the superior bone that contains the *iliac crest*, the wide bony wing that can be felt near the waist. The **ischium** is the inferior, posterior portion of the pelvis. The **pubis** is formed by the joining of the bones of the anterior pubis. The pelvis is joined to the sacral spine.

The hip joint consists of the **acetabulum** (the socket of the hip joint) and the ball at the head of the femur.

The Lower Extremities

The pelvis and hip joint, described above, may be considered part of the lower extremities. Moving downward from the hip, the large thigh bone is the **femur.** Progressing down the leg, the **patella,** or kneecap, sits anterior to the knee joint. The knee connects with the femur superiorly and with the bones of the lower leg, the **tibia** and **fibula,** inferiorly. The tibia is the inner

and larger bone of the lower leg, also referred to as the "shin bone." The fibula is the outer and smaller bone of the lower leg.

The ankle connects the tibia and fibula with the foot. The ankle is a joint that consists of several small bones. Two distinct landmarks are the **lateral malleolus** and **medial malleolus.** These are the protrusions that you see on the lateral and medial aspects of your ankles. The ankle consists of bones called **tarsals.** The foot bones are called **metatarsals.** The heel bone is called the **calcaneus.** The toe bones are the **phalanges.**

The Upper Extremities

Each shoulder consists of several bones: the clavicle, the scapula, and the acromion. The **clavicle,** also known as the "collarbone," is located anteriorly. The **scapula** is the "shoulder blade," located posteriorly. The **acromion** is the highest portion of the shoulder. It forms the **acromioclavicular joint** with the clavicle and is a frequent area of shoulder injury.

The arm consists of three bones connected at the elbow. The bone between the shoulder and the elbow is the **humerus.** The **radius** and **ulna** are the two bones between the elbow and the hand. The radius is the lateral bone of the forearm. (The radial pulse is taken over the radius.) The ulna is the medial forearm bone.

The wrist consists of several bones called **carpals.** The bones of the hand are the **metacarpals.** The finger bones, like the toe bones, are called **phalanges.**

By this point in the chapter you are realizing the importance of anatomical terms such as *superior, inferior, medial, lateral, anterior,* and *posterior!* These terms will be used throughout the text, and you will need to use them correctly to properly document and report your patient's injuries and complaints.

Joints

Joints are where bones connect to other bones. There are several types of joints, including ball-and-socket joints and hinge joints. The hip is an example of a ball-and-socket joint, in which the ball of the femur rotates in a round socket in the pelvis. The elbow is an example of a hinge joint in which the angle between the two bones—which are connected by ligaments—bends and straightens, as the name suggests, like a hinge.

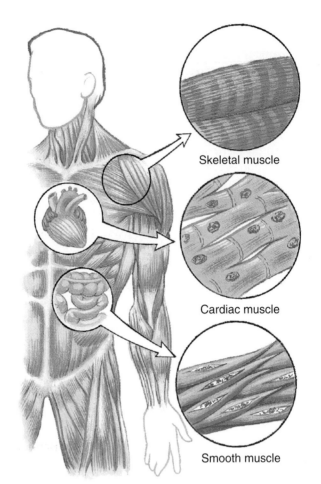

FIGURE 4-10 The three types of muscles.

The Muscles

Like the skeleton, the muscles protect the body, give it shape, and allow for movement. There are three types of muscle (Figure 4-10).

- **Voluntary** (skeletal) **muscle**—This type of muscle is under conscious control of the brain via the nervous system. Attached to the bones, the voluntary muscles form the major muscle mass of the body. They are responsible for movement. Voluntary muscle can contract and relax upon voluntary command of the individual. For example, if you want to, you can reach to pick up an item or walk about. These are examples of voluntary muscle use.
- **Involuntary** (smooth) **muscle**—Involuntary muscle is found in the gastrointestinal system, lungs, blood vessels, and urinary system and controls the flow of materials through these structures. Involuntary muscles respond automatically to orders from the brain. However, you do not have to consciously think about using these

muscles as you do with voluntary muscles. Fortunately, we do not have to tell our body to breathe, digest food, or perform other functions that occur under the control of the involuntary muscles. In fact, you have no direct control over the involuntary muscles. The involuntary muscles do respond to stimuli such as stretching, heat, and cold.
- **Cardiac muscle**—Cardiac muscle tissue is found only in the heart. It is a specialized form of involuntary muscle. Cardiac muscle is extremely sensitive to decreased oxygen supply and can tolerate interruption of blood supply only for very short periods. The heart muscle has its own blood supply through the coronary artery system.

The heart also has a property called **automaticity.** This means that the heart has the ability to generate and conduct electrical impulses on its own. The heartbeat (contraction) is controlled by these electrical impulses.

The Respiratory System

The purpose of the respiratory system is to move oxygen (O_2) into the blood stream through inhalation and pick up carbon dioxide (CO_2) to be excreted through exhalation. To review the anatomy (structure) of the respiratory system, we will follow the path of air through the system from the mouth and nose to its final destination in the blood stream.

Anatomy

There are a number of structures that make up the respiratory system (Figure 4-11). Air enters the body through the mouth and nose. It moves through the **oropharynx** (the area directly posterior to the mouth) and the **nasopharynx** (the area directly posterior to the nose). The **pharynx** is the area that includes both the oropharynx and the nasopharynx.

The air then proceeds on a path toward the lungs. A leaf-shaped structure called the **epiglottis** prevents foods and foreign objects from entering the trachea during swallowing. The **larynx,** also known as the voice box, contains the vocal cords. The **cricoid cartilage** is a ring-shaped structure that forms the lower portion of the larynx. The **trachea,** also known as the "windpipe," is the tube that carries inhaled air from the larynx down toward the **lungs.** At the level of the lungs, the trachea splits (bifurcates) into two branches called the **bronchi.** One bronchus goes to each lung. Inside each lung, the bronchi continue to branch and split and the air passages get smaller and smaller. Eventually, each branch ends at a group of **alveoli.** The alveoli are the small sacs within the lungs where gas exchange takes place with the blood stream.

The **diaphragm** is the muscular structure that divides the chest cavity from the abdominal cavity. During a normal respiratory cycle, the diaphragm and other parts of the body work together to allow the body to inhale and exhale. The role of the diaphragm and other muscles in the respiratory cycle is described below.

Physiology

Inhalation is an active process. The intercostal (rib) muscles and the diaphragm contract. The diaphragm lowers and the ribs move upward and outward. This expands the size of the chest cavity, causing air to flow into the lungs.

Exhalation is a passive process during which the intercostal muscles and the diaphragm relax. The ribs move downward and inward, while the diaphragm rises. This movement causes the chest cavity to decrease in size and causes air to flow out of the lungs.

Air moves into the lungs through the series of air passages that were described in the anatomy section (known as the *airway*). During inhalation, air is moved into the alveoli. These small sacs are where gas exchange with the blood takes place. From the air in the alveoli, oxygen is transferred to the blood while, at the same time, carbon dioxide enters the alveoli from the blood stream to remove this waste product from the body. The alveoli are very small. The blood vessels they interact with are also the smallest type of blood vessel, capillaries (described below under The Cardiovascular System).

When oxygenated blood leaves the lungs, it returns to the heart so it can be pumped into the circulatory system of the body. As the blood leaves the heart, it travels through a branching series of arteries that gradually become smaller and smaller until they are the smallest type of blood vessel, the capillary. Capillaries are found throughout the body. They exchange gasses with all the tissues of the body. Oxygen carried by the blood is given up to the cells and waste carbon dioxide is picked up from the cells and returned through veins to the heart and then to the lungs where it passes out of the body through exhalation.

This exchange of gases, both in the lungs and at the body's cells, is critical to support life.

Breathing (the process of inhaling and exhaling air) may be classified as adequate or inadequate. Simply stated, adequate breathing is sufficient to support life. Inadequate breathing is not. Adequate and inadequate breathing, and how you as an EMT-B should assess and care for breathing problems, will be discussed in detail in Chapter 17, Respiratory Emergencies.

Infants and Children

There are a number of special aspects of the respiratory anatomy of infants and children (Figure 4-12). In general, all structures in a child are smaller and more easily obstructed than in an adult. Infants' and children's tongues take up proportionally more space in the pharynx than do adults' tongues. The trachea is relatively narrower than in adults and, therefore, more easily obstructed by swelling or foreign matter. The trachea is also softer and more flexible in children and infants, so more care must be taken during any procedure when pressure

The Respiratory System

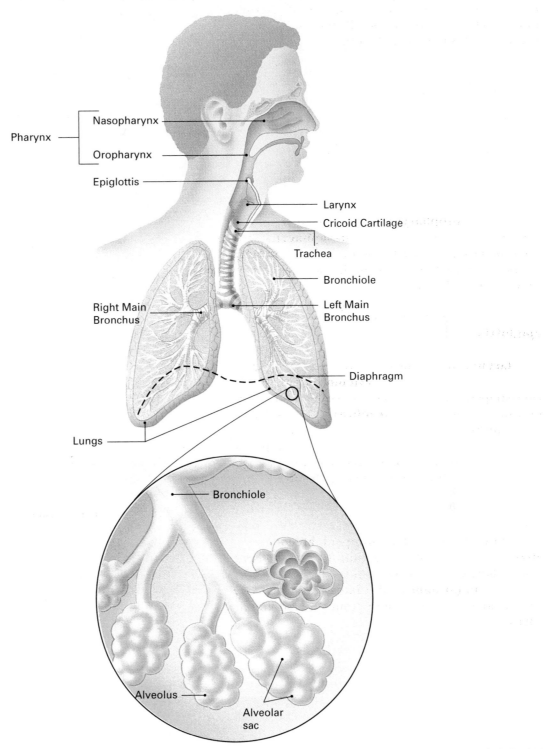

FIGURE 4-11 The respiratory system.

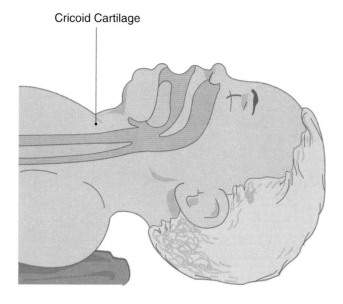

Cricoid Cartilage

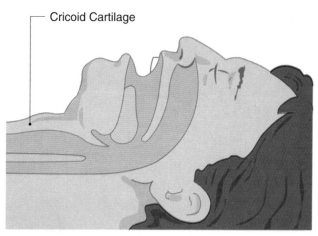

Cricoid Cartilage

FIGURE 4-12 Adult and child respiratory passages.

may be placed on the neck, such as in applying a cervical collar or during procedures to place a tube in the trachea. The cricoid cartilage is less developed and less rigid. Because the chest wall is softer, children and infants tend to rely more on the diaphragm for breathing, creating a visible "seesaw" breathing pattern when the infant or child is having difficulty breathing.

Special procedures that take into account the respiratory anatomy of infants and children will be discussed in later chapters on the airway and the respiratory system.

The Cardiovascular System

The Anatomy of the Heart

The human heart is a muscular organ about the size of your fist, located in the center of the thoracic cavity (Figure 4-13). The heart has four chambers: two upper chambers called **atria** (AY-tre-ah—the singular is *atrium*) and two lower chambers called **ventricles** (VEN-tri-kulz).

The atria both contract at the same time. When they contract, the blood is forced into the heart's lower chambers, the ventricles. Both ventricles receive blood from their respective atria and then contract simultaneously to pump blood out of the heart. The path the blood takes on its journey through the body is as follows: right atrium to right ventricle to lungs to left atrium to left ventricle to body—then back to the right atrium to start its journey all over again. Below, this path of the circulatory system is described in a little more detail.

- Right atrium—The **venae cavae** (the superior vena cava and the inferior vena cava) are the two large veins that return blood to the heart. The right atrium receives this blood and, upon contraction, sends it to the right ventricle.
- Right ventricle—The right ventricle receives blood from the chamber above it, the right atrium. When the right ventricle contracts, it pumps this blood out to the lungs via the pulmonary arteries. Remember, this blood is very low in oxygen and is carrying waste carbon dioxide that was picked up as the blood circulated through the body. While this blood is in the lungs, the carbon dioxide is excreted (taken out of the blood to be carried out of the body when the person exhales), and oxygen is obtained (taken into the blood from air the person has inhaled). The oxygen-rich blood is now returned to the left atrium via the pulmonary veins.
- Left atrium—The left atrium receives the oxygen-rich blood from the lungs. When it contracts, it sends this blood to the left ventricle.
- Left ventricle—The left ventricle receives oxygen-rich blood from the chamber above it, the left atrium. When it contracts, it pumps this blood into the **aorta,** the body's largest artery, for distribution to the entire body. Since the blood must reach all parts of the body, the left ventricle is the most muscular and strongest part of the heart.

The Heart

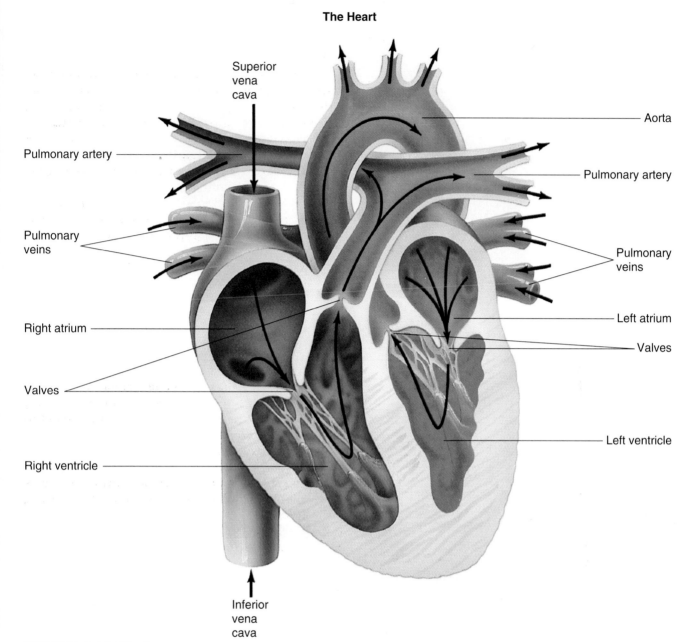

- Superior vena cava
- Aorta
- Pulmonary artery
- Pulmonary artery
- Pulmonary veins
- Pulmonary veins
- Right atrium
- Left atrium
- Valves
- Valves
- Left ventricle
- Right ventricle
- Inferior vena cava

FIGURE 4-13 The heart.

VAVA VAVA

Between each atrium and ventricle is a one-way valve to prevent blood in the ventricle from being forced back up into the atrium when the ventricle contracts. The pulmonary artery also has a one-way valve so that blood in the artery does not return to the right ventricle. The aorta also has a one-way valve to prevent backflow to the left ventricle. This system of one-way valves keeps the blood moving in the correct direction along the path of circulation.

The contraction, or beating, of the heart is an automatic, involuntary process. The heart has its own natural "pacemaker" and a system of specialized muscle tissues that conduct electrical impulses that stimulate the heart to beat. This network is called the **cardiac conduction system** (Figure 4-14). Regulation of rate, rhythm, and force of heartbeat comes, in part, from the cardiac control centers of the brain. Nerve impulses from these centers are sent to the pacemaker and conduction system of the heart. These nerve impulses and chemicals released into the blood (e.g., epinephrine) control the heart's rate and strength of contractions.

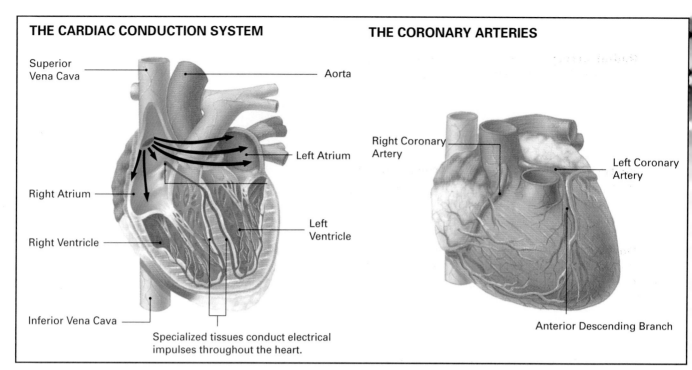

THE CARDIAC CONDUCTION SYSTEM

Superior Vena Cava
Aorta
Left Atrium
Right Atrium
Left Ventricle
Right Ventricle
Inferior Vena Cava
Specialized tissues conduct electrical impulses throughout the heart.

THE CORONARY ARTERIES

Right Coronary Artery
Left Coronary Artery
Anterior Descending Branch

FIGURE 4-14 The cardiac conduction system and coronary arteries.

Circulation of the Blood

When the blood leaves the heart, it travels throughout the body through several types of blood vessels. Blood vessels are described by their function, location, and whether they carry blood away from or to the heart. You will learn about arteries, veins, arterioles, venules, and capillaries.

Arteries The kind of vessel that carries blood away from the heart is called an **artery.** There are several arteries that you will find it important to know about.

- **Coronary arteries**—The coronary arteries (Figure 4-14) branch off from the aorta and supply the heart muscle with blood. Although the heart has blood constantly moving through it, it receives its own blood supply from the coronary arteries. Damage or blockage to these arteries usually results in chest pain.
- **Aorta**—The aorta is the largest artery in the body. It begins at its attachment to the left ventricle and continues inferiorly in front of the spine through the thoracic and abdominal cavities. At the level of the navel it splits into the iliac arteries.
- **Pulmonary artery**—This artery begins at the right ventricle. It carries oxygen-poor

blood to the lungs. You may note that this is an exception to the rule that arteries carry oxygen-rich blood while veins carry oxygen-poor blood. It does, however, follow the rule that arteries carry blood away from the heart while veins carry blood to the heart.

- **Carotid artery**—This is the major artery of the neck. You will be familiar with this vessel from your BLS CPR class. This is the artery that is palpated during CPR pulse checks for adults and children. It is the vessel that carries the main supply of blood for the head. There is a carotid artery on each side of the neck. Never palpate both at the same time because of the danger of interrupting the supply of blood to the head.
- **Femoral artery**—This is the major artery of the thigh. You can relate the name "femoral" to the bone in the thigh, the femur. Pulsations for this artery can be felt in the crease between the abdomen and the groin. This artery is the major source of blood supply to the leg.
- **Brachial artery**—This is an artery in the upper arm. This will also be familiar from BLS CPR because it is the pulse checked during infant CPR. The pulse can be felt anteriorly in the crease over the elbow and along the medial aspect of the upper arm. This is also the artery that is used when

determining blood pressure with a blood pressure cuff and a stethoscope.

- **Radial artery**—This artery travels through and supplies the lower arm. The radial artery is the artery felt when taking the radial pulse at the thumb side of the wrist. Again, you can relate the name "radial" to the radius, a bone in the forearm that the radial artery is near.
- **Posterior tibial artery**—This artery is often used when determining the circulatory status of the lower extremity. It may be palpated on the posterior aspect of the medial malleolus.
- **Dorsalis pedis artery**—This artery lies on the anterior portion of the foot, lateral to the large tendon of the big toe.

Arterioles, Capillaries, and Venules Arteries begin with large vessels, like the aorta. They gradually branch to smaller and smaller vessels. The smallest branch of an artery is called an **arteriole.** These small vessels lead to the capillaries. **Capillaries** are tiny blood vessels found throughout the body. As explained above, the capillaries are where gases, nutrients, and waste products are exchanged between the body's cells and the bloodstream. From the capillaries the blood begins its return journey to the heart by entering the smallest veins. One of these small veins is called a **venule** (Figure 4-15).

Veins The kind of vessel that carries the blood from the capillaries back to the heart is called a **vein.** Remember that the blood flow from the heart started in the largest arteries and moved into smaller and smaller arteries until it reached the capillaries. The blood takes an opposite course through the veins. The blood travels from the smaller to the larger vessels on its return trip to the heart.

- **Venae cavae**—Immediately after leaving the capillaries, the blood enters venules, the smallest veins. From the venules, the veins get gradually larger, eventually reaching the venae cavae. There are two venae cavae. The superior vena cava collects blood from the head and upper body. The inferior vena cava collects blood that is returned from the portions of the body below the heart. The superior and inferior venae cavae meet to return blood to the right atrium where the process of circulation begins again.
- **Pulmonary vein**—The pulmonary vein carries oxygenated blood from the lungs to the

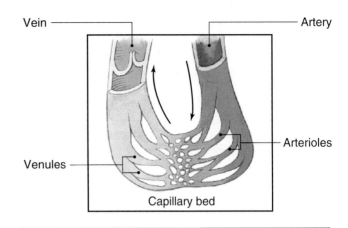

left atrium of the heart. This is an exception to the rule that veins carry oxygen-poor blood. It does follow the rule that arteries carry blood away from the heart while veins return blood to the heart.

FIGURE 4-15 The system of arteries, capillaries, and veins.

From the heart, oxygen-rich blood is carried out into the body by arteries. The arteries gradually branch into smaller arteries called arterioles. The arterioles gradually branch into tiny vessels called capillaries.

In the capillaries, the blood gives up oxygen and nutrients, which move through the thin walls of the capillaries into the body's cells. At the same time, carbon dioxide and other wastes move in the opposite direction, from the cells and through the capillary walls, to be picked up by the blood.

On its return journey to the heart, the oxygen-poor blood, now carrying carbon dioxide and other wastes, flows from the capillaries into small veins called venules which gradually merge into larger veins.

Composition of the Blood

The blood is made up of several components: plasma, red and white blood cells, and platelets.

- **Plasma**—Plasma is a watery, salty fluid that makes up over half the volume of the blood. The red and white blood cells and platelets are carried in the plasma.
- **Red blood cells**—also called RBCs, erythrocytes, or red corpuscles. Their primary function is to carry oxygen to the tissues and

CHAPTER 4 The Human Body **55**

carbon dioxide away from the tissues. These cells also provide the red color to the blood.

- **White blood cells**—also called WBCs, leukocytes, or white corpuscles. They are involved in destroying microorganisms (germs) and producing substances called antibodies that help the body resist infection.
- **Platelets** (PLATE-lets)—membrane-enclosed fragments of specialized cells. When these fragments are activated, they release chemical factors needed to form blood clots.

The Pulse

A **pulse** is formed when the left ventricle contracts, sending a wave of blood through the arteries. The pulse is felt by compressing an artery over a bone. This allows you to feel the wave of blood, or pulse, as it comes through the artery.

Earlier in this chapter, several arteries were named. Among them were the primary arteries where a pulse is taken for vital signs or CPR: the carotid, brachial, and radial arteries. You will also use the pulses at the ankles and feet (posterior tibial and dorsalis pedis) to check for adequate circulation to the lower extremities.

These points where a pulse can be felt may also be used for control of bleeding. Pressure applied to the brachial and femoral arteries can be used to control bleeding to the arm and leg respectively. You will learn about these techniques in Chapter 25, Bleeding and Shock.

The radial, brachial, posterior tibial, and dorsalis pedis pulses are called **peripheral pulses** because they can be felt on the periphery, or outer reaches, of the body. The carotid and femoral pulses are called **central pulses** because they can be felt in the central part of the body. Because they are at larger vessels closer to the heart, the carotid and femoral pulses can be felt even when peripheral pulses are too weak to be felt. Providing chest compressions during CPR is dangerous if the heart is beating, however weakly. This is why the carotid pulse, rather than a peripheral pulse, is used to determine pulselessness, the sign that CPR compressions can be begun. If a peripheral pulse site were felt when the heartbeat was weak but still present, the EMT-B might make an incorrect and potentially harmful decision to begin CPR.

The Blood Pressure

The pressure blood exerts against the walls of blood vessels is known as **blood pressure.** Usually, it is arterial blood pressure (pressure in an artery) that is measured.

Each time the left ventricle of the heart contracts it forces blood out into circulation. The pressure created in the arteries by this blood is called the **systolic** (sis-TOL-ik) **blood pressure.** When the left ventricle of the heart is relaxed and refilling, the pressure remaining in the arteries is called the **diastolic** (di-as-TOL-ik) **blood pressure.** The systolic pressure is reported first, the diastolic second, as in "120 over 80," written as "120/80."

Perfusion

The movement of blood through the heart and blood vessels is called circulation. In healthy individuals, circulation is adequate. That is, there is enough blood within the system and the means to pump and deliver it to all parts of the body efficiently (Figure 4-16). The adequate supply of oxygen and nutrients to the organs and tissues of the body, with the removal of waste products, is called **perfusion.**

Hypoperfusion (inadequate perfusion), also known as **shock,** is a serious condition. With hypoperfusion, there is inadequate circulation of blood through one or more organs or structures. Blood is not reaching and filling all the capillary networks of the body. Oxygen will not be delivered to, and waste products will not be removed from, all the tissues of the body. *Hypoperfusion may lead to death!* It is important to understand what hypoperfusion is, how it occurs, and how to recognize it. This will be discussed in depth in Chapter 25, Bleeding and Shock.

The Nervous System

The **nervous system** (Figure 4-17) is the system of brain, spinal cord, and nerves that transmits impulses and governs sensation, movement, and thought. The nervous system controls the voluntary and involuntary activity of the body.

The nervous system consists of the central and peripheral nervous systems.

- **Central nervous system**—The central nervous system is comprised of the brain and the spinal cord.

  The brain could be likened to a powerful computer that receives information from the body and, in turn, sends impulses to different areas of the body to respond to the changes in and outside the body.

  The spinal cord rests within the spinal column and stretches from the brain to the

The Circulatory System

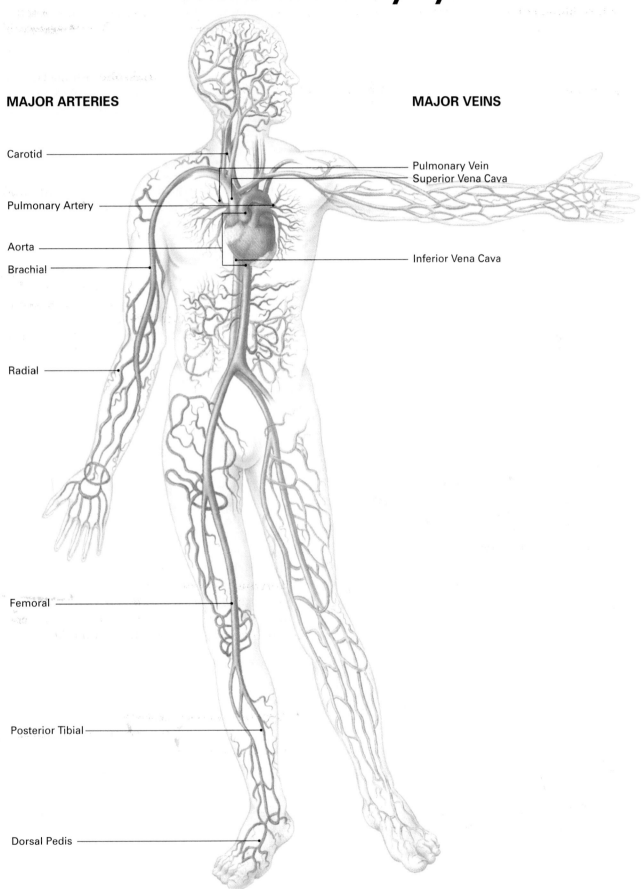

MAJOR ARTERIES

Carotid

Pulmonary Artery

Aorta

Brachial

Radial

Femoral

Posterior Tibial

Dorsal Pedis

MAJOR VEINS

Pulmonary Vein
Superior Vena Cava

Inferior Vena Cava

FIGURE 4-16 The circulatory system.

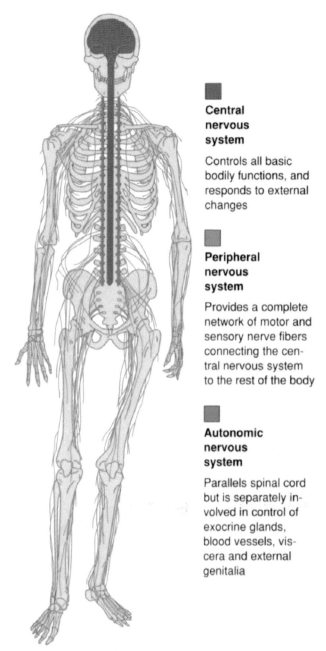

Central nervous system

Controls all basic bodily functions, and responds to external changes

Peripheral nervous system

Provides a complete network of motor and sensory nerve fibers connecting the central nervous system to the rest of the body

Autonomic nervous system

Parallels spinal cord but is separately involved in control of exocrine glands, blood vessels, viscera and external genitalia

FIGURE 4-17 The nervous system.

lumbar vertebrae. Nerves branch from each part of the cord and reach throughout the body.

- **Peripheral nervous system**—This system consists of two types of nerves:

  Sensory nerves—These nerves pick up information from throughout the body and transmit it to the spinal cord and brain. If you touch something hot, your sensory nerves transmit this to the brain so action may be taken.

Motor nerves—These nerves carry messages from the brain to the body. In the example given above, the brain would send a message to the part of the body that has just touched the hot item to pull away.

The **autonomic nervous system** is the division of the peripheral nervous system that controls involuntary motor functions and affects such things as digestion and heart rate.

The Skin

Functions

The skin performs a variety of functions, including protection, water balance, temperature regulation, excretion, and shock absorption.

- Protection—The skin serves as a barrier to keep out microorganisms (germs), debris, and unwanted chemicals. Underlying tissues and organs are protected from environmental contact. This helps preserve the chemical balance of body fluids and tissues.
- Water balance—The skin helps prevent water loss and stops environmental water from entering the body.
- Temperature regulation—Blood vessels in the skin can dilate (increase in diameter) to carry more blood to the skin, allowing heat to radiate from the body. When the body needs to conserve heat, these vessels constrict (decrease in diameter) to prevent heat loss. The sweat glands found in the skin produce perspiration, which will evaporate and help cool the body. The fat that is part of the skin serves as a thermal insulator.
- Excretion—Salts and excess water can be released through the skin.
- Shock (impact) Absorption—The skin and its layers of fat help protect the underlying organs from minor impacts and pressures.

Layers

The skin has three major layers: the epidermis, dermis, and subcutaneous layer (Figure 4-18).

- **Epidermis**—The outer layer of the skin is called the epidermis. It is composed of four layers (strata) except for the skin of the palms of the hands and soles of the feet. These two regions have five layers. The outermost layers are composed of dead cells,

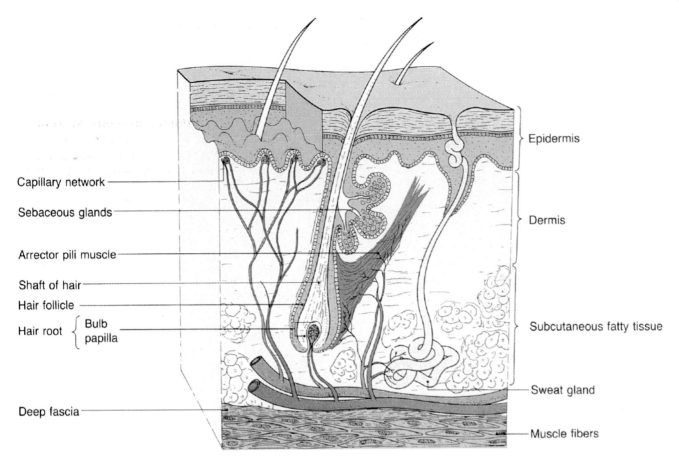

FIGURE 4-18 The layers of the skin.

Capillary network

Sebaceous glands

Arrector pili muscle

Shaft of hair

Hair follicle

Hair root { Bulb
papilla

Deep fascia

Epidermis

Dermis

Subcutaneous fatty tissue

Sweat gland

Muscle fibers

which are rubbed off or sloughed off and are replaced. The pigment granules of the skin and living cells are found in the deeper layers. The cells of the innermost layer are actively dividing, replacing the dead cells of the outer layers.

The epidermis contains no blood vessels or nerves. Except for certain types of burns and injuries due to cold, injuries of the epidermis present few problems in EMT-level care.

- **Dermis**—The layer of skin below the epidermis is the dermis. This layer is rich with blood vessels, nerves, and specialized structures such as sweat glands, sebaceous (oil) glands, and hair follicles. Specialized nerve endings are found in the dermis. They are involved with the senses of touch, cold, heat, and pain.

Once the dermis is opened to the outside world, contamination and infection become major problems. The wounds can be serious, accompanied by profuse bleeding and intense pain.

- **Subcutaneous layers**—The layers of fat and soft tissue below the dermis are called the subcutaneous layers. Shock absorption and insulation are major functions of this layer. Again, there are the problems of tissue and bloodstream contamination, bleeding, and pain when these layers are injured or exposed.

The Endocrine System

The endocrine system (Figure 4-19) produces chemicals called hormones which help to regulate many body activities and functions. You will later learn about a chemical called **insulin.** This substance is a hormone that is critical in the use of glucose, a sugar which fuels the body. **Epinephrine** is another example of a substance secreted by this system. Epinephrine (sometimes called adrenaline) allows us to respond to stressful situations.

The endocrine system is complex and interacts with many other body systems.

Endocrine System

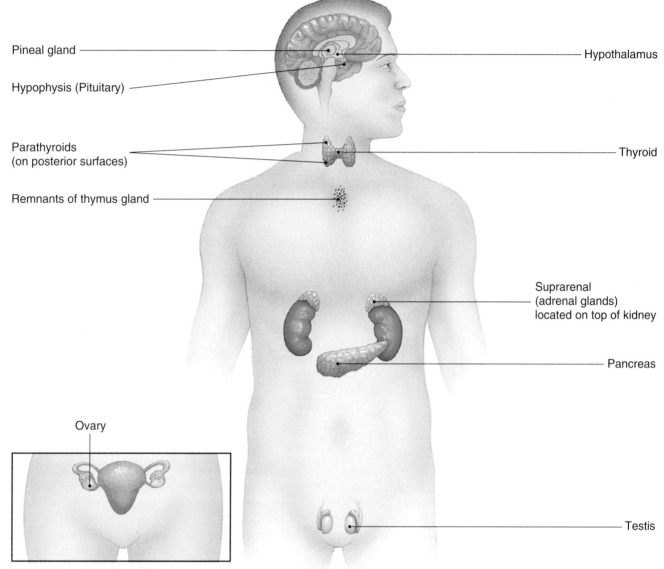

Pineal gland

Hypophysis (Pituitary)

Parathyroids
(on posterior surfaces)

Remnants of thymus gland

Hypothalamus

Thyroid

Suprarenal
(adrenal glands)
located on top of kidney

Pancreas

Testis

Ovary

FIGURE 4-19 The endocrine system.

LOCATING BODY ORGANS AND STRUCTURES

As an EMT-B, you will find it useful to understand the position of the body's major organs and structures. There are two ways to help locate organs and structures of the body.

- Visualizing—being able to picture organs and structures inside the body as you look at the external body.
- Topography—learning external landmarks: specific structures, notches, joints, and "bumps" on bones. Some are obvious

(navel, nipples), some you know by other names but will have to learn the medical terms (Adam's apple = thyroid cartilage), and some will probably be new to you (xiphoid process). It is important to learn where internal organs and structures are in relation to these landmarks, that you can easily see or feel from outside the body.

Figures 4-20 through 4-25 and Scan 4-1 show the positions of major organs and systems. Scan 4-2 shows the positions of major landmarks on the outer body (topography) and skeletal structures within the body.

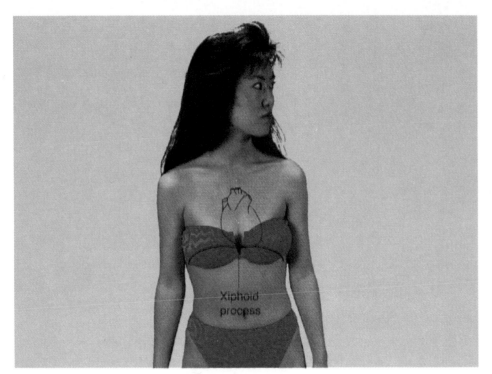

FIGURE 4-20 Position of the heart.

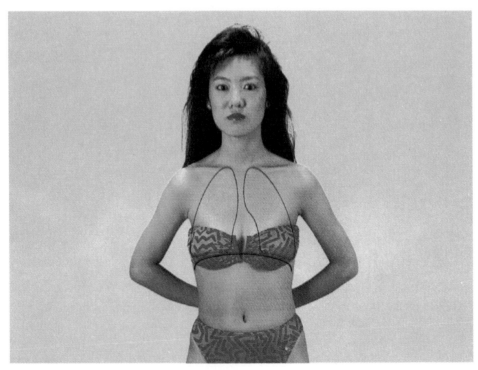

FIGURE 4-21 Position of the lungs.

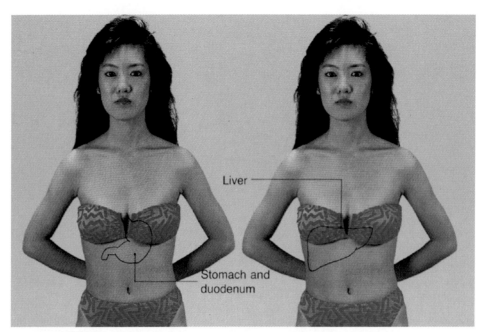

FIGURE 4-22 Position of the liver, stomach, and duodenum.

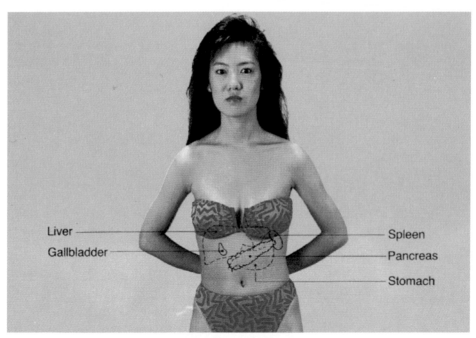

FIGURE 4-23 Position of the liver, gallbladder, spleen, pancreas, and stomach.

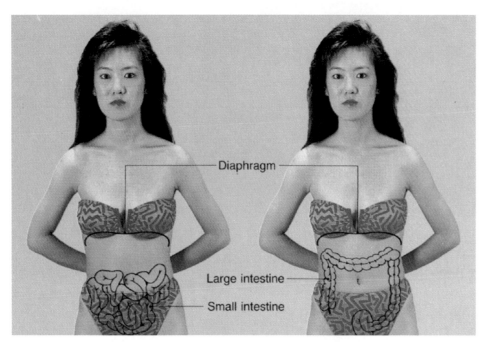

FIGURE 4-24 Position of the small and large intestine.

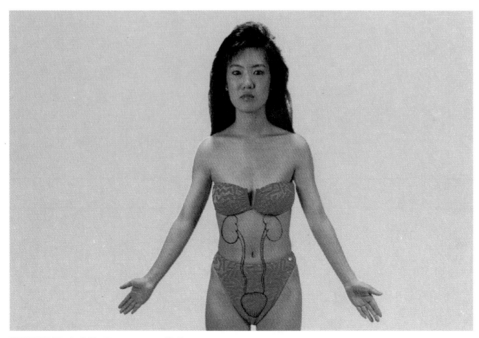

FIGURE 4-25 Position of the urinary system.

Scan 4-1
Major Body Organs

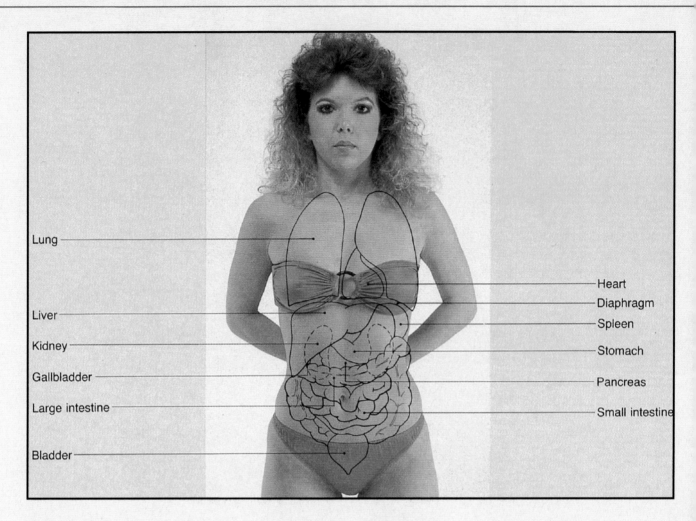

Lung

Liver

Kidney

Gallbladder

Large intestine

Bladder

Heart

Diaphragm

Spleen

Stomach

Pancreas

Small intestine

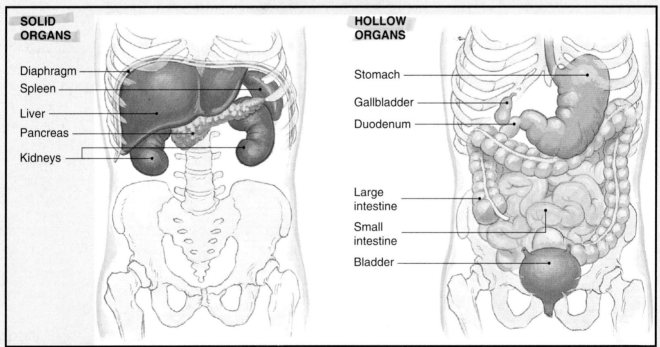

SOLID ORGANS

Diaphragm
Spleen
Liver
Pancreas
Kidneys

HOLLOW ORGANS

Stomach
Gallbladder
Duodenum

Large intestine
Small intestine
Bladder

Topography and Skeleton

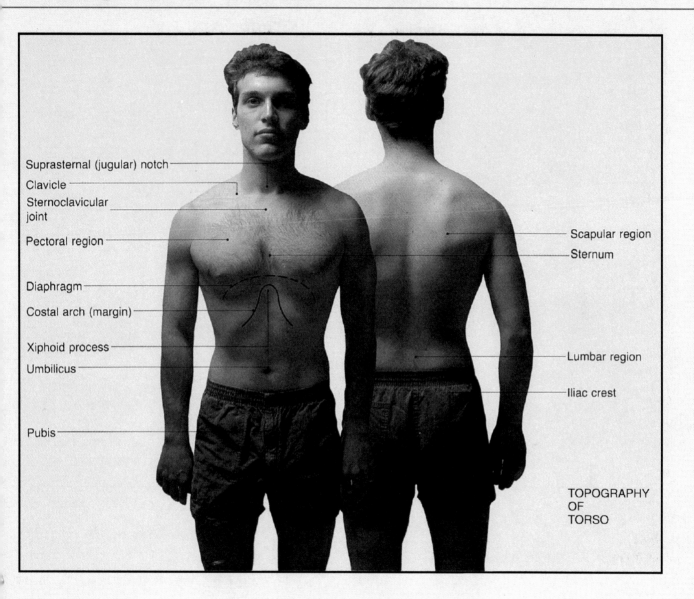

Suprasternal (jugular) notch

Clavicle

Sternoclavicular joint

Pectoral region

Diaphragm

Costal arch (margin)

Xiphoid process

Umbilicus

Pubis

Scapular region

Sternum

Lumbar region

Iliac crest

TOPOGRAPHY OF TORSO

HEAD AND NECK TOPOGRAPHY

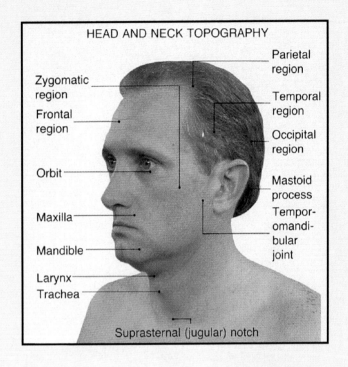

Zygomatic region

Frontal region

Orbit

Maxilla

Mandible

Larynx

Trachea

Parietal region

Temporal region

Occipital region

Mastoid process

Temporomandibular joint

Suprasternal (jugular) notch

LOWER BODY TOPOGRAPHY AND SKELETON

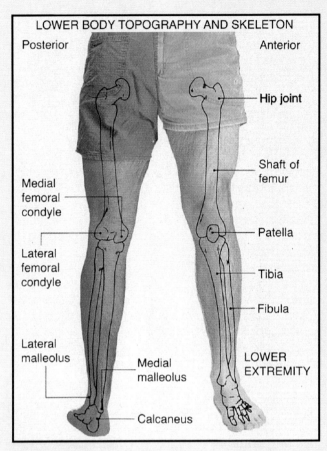

Posterior

Anterior

Hip joint

Shaft of femur

Medial femoral condyle

Lateral femoral condyle

Patella

Tibia

Fibula

Lateral malleolus

Medial malleolus

LOWER EXTREMITY

Calcaneus

UPPER BODY TOPOGRAPHY AND SKELETON

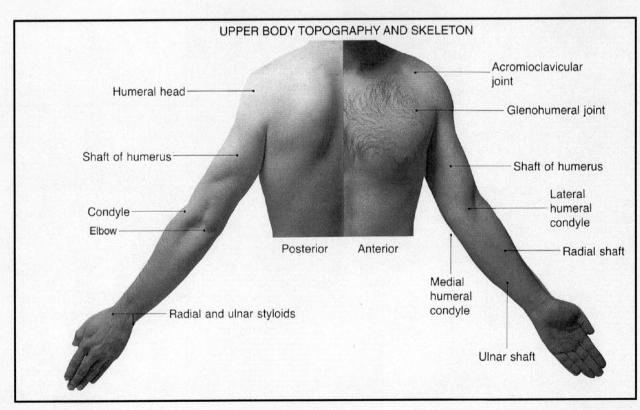

Humeral head

Shaft of humerus

Condyle

Elbow

Acromioclavicular joint

Glenohumeral joint

Shaft of humerus

Lateral humeral condyle

Radial shaft

Posterior   Anterior

Medial humeral condyle

Radial and ulnar styloids

Ulnar shaft

CHAPTER REVIEW

You may find it helpful to review the following terms.

abdominal quadrants four divisions of the abdomen used to pinpoint the location of a pain or injury: the right upper quadrant, the left upper quadrant, the right lower quadrant, and the left lower quadrant.

acetabulum (AS-uh-TAB-yuh-lum) the socket into which the head of the femur fits to form the hip joint.

acromioclavicular (ah-KRO-me-o-klav-IK-yuh-ler) **joint** the joint where the acromion and the clavicle meet.

acromion (ah-KRO-me-on) the highest portion of the shoulder.

alveoli (al-VE-o-li) the microscopic sacs of the lungs where gas exchange with the bloodstream takes place.

anatomical position the standard reference position for the body in the study of anatomy. The body is standing erect, facing the observer. The arms are down at the sides and the palms of the hands face forward.

anatomy the study of body structure.

anterior the front of the body or body part.

aorta (ay-OR-tah) the largest artery in the body. It transports blood from the left ventricle to begin systemic circulation.

arteriole (ar-TE-re-ol) the smallest kind of artery.

artery any blood vessel carrying blood away from the heart.

atria (AY-tree-ah) the two upper chambers of the heart. There is a right atrium (which receives unoxygenated blood returning from the body) and a left atrium (which receives oxygenated blood returning from the lungs).

automaticity (AW-to-mat-IS-it-e) the ability of the heart to generate and conduct electrical impulses on its own.

autonomic (AW-to-NOM-ik) **nervous system** the division of the peripheral nervous system that controls involuntary motor functions.

bilateral on both sides.

blood pressure the pressure caused by blood exerting force against the walls of blood vessels. Usually arterial blood pressure (the pressure in an artery) is measured.

brachial artery artery of the upper arm; the site of the pulse checked during infant CPR.

bronchi (BRONG-ki) the two large sets of branches that come off the trachea and enter the lungs. There are right and left bronchi. The singular is *bronchus.*

calcaneus (kal-KAY-ne-us) the heel bone.

capillary (KAP-i-lair-e) a thin-walled, microscopic blood vessel where oxygen/carbon dioxide and nutrient/waste exchange with the body's cells takes place.

cardiac conduction system a system of specialized muscle tissues that conduct electrical impulses that stimulate the heart to beat.

cardiac muscle specialized involuntary muscle found only in the heart.

cardiovascular (KAR-de-o-VAS-kyu-ler) **system** the system made up of the heart *(cardio)* and the blood vessels *(vascular);* the circulatory system.

carotid (kah-ROT-id) **arteries** the large neck arteries, one on each side of the neck, that carry blood from the heart to the head.

carpals (KAR-pulz) the wrist bones.

central nervous system (CNS) the brain and spinal cord.

central pulses the carotid and femoral pulses, which can be felt in the central part of the body.

circulatory system See *cardiovascular system.*

clavicles (KLAV-i-kulz) the collarbones.

coronary (KOR-o-nar-e) **arteries** blood vessels that supply the muscle of the heart (myocardium).

cricoid (KRIK-oid) **cartilage** the ring-shaped structure that forms the lower portion of the trachea.

dermis (DER-mis) the inner (second) layer of skin found beneath the epidermis. It is rich in blood vessels and nerves.

diaphragm (DI-uh-fram) the muscular structure that divides the chest cavity from the abdominal cavity.

diastolic (di-as-TOL-ik) **blood pressure** the pressure in the arteries when the left ventricle is refilling.

distal farther away from the torso. See also *proximal.*

dorsal referring to the back of the body. A synonym for *posterior.*

dorsalis pedis (dor-SAL-is PEED-is) **artery** artery supplying the foot, lateral to the large tendon of the big toe.

epidermis (ep-i-DER-mis) the outer layer of skin.

epiglottis (EP-i-GLOT-is) a leaf-shaped structure that prevents food and foreign matter from entering the trachea.

epinephrine (EP-uh-NEF-rin) a hormone produced by the body. As a medication it dilates respiratory passages and is used to relieve severe allergic reactions.

exhalation (EX-huh-LAY-shun) a passive process in which the intercostal (rib) muscles and the diaphragm relax, causing the chest cavity to decrease in size and causing air to flow out of the lungs.

femoral (FEM-o-ral) **artery** the major artery supplying the thigh.

femur (FEE-mer) the large bone of the thigh.

fibula (FIB-yuh-luh) the outer and smaller bone of the lower leg.

Fowler's position a sitting position.

humerus (HYU-mer-us) the bone of the upper arm, between the shoulder and the elbow.

hypoperfusion inadequate perfusion of the cells and tissues of the body caused by insufficient flow of blood through the capillaries. See also *perfusion*.

ilium (IL-e-um) the superior and widest portion of the pelvis.

inferior away from the head; usually compared with another structure that is closer to the head (e.g., the lips are inferior to the nose).

inhalation (IN-huh-LAY-shun) an active process in which the intercostal (rib) muscles and the diaphragm contract, expanding the size of the chest cavity and causing air to flow into the lungs.

insulin (IN-suh-lin) a hormone produced by the pancreas or taken as a medication by many diabetics.

ischium (ISH-e-um) the lower, posterior portions of the pelvis.

involuntary muscle muscle that responds automatically to brain signals but cannot be consciously controlled.

larynx (LAIR-inks) the voicebox.

lateral to the side, away from the midline of the body.

lateral recumbent (re-KUM-bunt) lying on one side.

lungs the organs where exchange of atmospheric oxygen and waste carbon dioxide take place.

malleolus (mal-E-o-lus) protrusion on the side of the ankle. The lateral malleolus is on the outer ankle, the medial malleolus is on the inner ankle.

mandible (MAN-di-bl) the lower jaw bone.

manubrium (man-OO-bre-um) the superior portion of the sternum.

maxillae (mak-SIL-e) the two fused bones forming the upper jaw.

medial toward the midline of the body.

metacarpals (MET-uh-KAR-pulz) the hand bones.

metatarsals (MET-uh-TAR-sulz) the foot bones.

mid-axillary (mid-AX-uh-lair-e) **line** a line drawn vertically from the middle of the armpit to the ankle.

mid-clavicular (mid-clah-VIK-yuh-ler) **line** the line through the center of each clavicle.

midline an imaginary line drawn down the center of the body, dividing it into right and left halves.

musculoskeletal (MUS-kyu-lo-SKEL-e-tal) **system** the system of bones and skeletal muscles that support and protect the body and permit movement.

nasal (NAY-zul) **bones** the nose bones.

nasopharynx (NAY-zo-FAIR-inks) the area directly posterior to the nose.

nervous system the system of brain, spinal cord, and nerves that govern sensation, movement, and thought.

orbits the bony structures around the eyes; the eye sockets.

oropharynx (OR-o-FAIR-inks) the area directly posterior to the mouth.

palmar referring to the palm of the hand.

patella (pah-TEL-uh) the kneecap.

perfusion the supply of oxygen to and removal of wastes from the cells and tissues of the body as a result of the flow of blood through the capillaries.

peripheral nervous system (PNS) the nerves that enter and leave the spinal cord and that travel between the brain and organs without passing through the spinal cord.

peripheral pulses the radial, brachial, posterior tibial, and dorsalis pedis pulses, which can be felt at peripheral (outlying) points of the body.

phalanges (fuh-LAN-jiz) the toe bones and finger bones.

pharynx (FAIR-inks) the area directly posterior to the mouth and nose. It is made up of the oropharynx and the nasopharynx.

physiology the study of body function.

plane a flat surface formed when slicing through a solid object.

plantar referring to the sole of the foot.

plasma (PLAZ-mah) the fluid portion of the blood.

platelets components of the blood; membrane-enclosed fragments of specialized cells.

posterior the back of the body or body part.

posterior tibial (TIB-ee-ul) **artery** artery supplying the foot, behind the medial ankle.

prone lying face down.

proximal closer to the torso. See also *distal*.

pubis (PYOO-bis) the medial anterior portion of the pelvis.

pulmonary (PUL-mo-nar-e) **arteries** the vessels that carry blood from the right ventricle of the heart to the lungs.

pulmonary veins the vessels that carry oxygenated blood from the lungs to the left atrium of the heart.

pulse the rhythmic beats caused as waves of blood move through and expand the arteries.

radial artery artery of the lower arm. It is felt when taking the pulse at the wrist.

radius (RAY-de-us) the lateral bone of the forearm.

red blood cells components of the blood. They carry oxygen to and carbon dioxide away from the cells.

respiratory (RES-pir-ah-tory-e) **system** the system of nose, mouth, throat, and lungs and muscles that brings oxygen into the body and expels carbon dioxide.

scapula (SKAP-yuh-luh) the shoulder blade.

shock See *hypoperfusion*.

shock position see *Trendelenburg position*.

sternum (STER-num) the breastbone.

subcutaneous (SUB-ku-TAY-ne-us) **layers** the layers of fat and soft tissues found below the dermis.

superior toward the head (e.g., the chest is superior to the abdomen).

supine lying on the back.

systolic (sis-TOL-ik) **blood pressure** the pressure created in the arteries when the left ventri-cle contracts and forces blood out into circulation.

tarsals (TAR-sulz) the ankle bones.

thorax (THOR-ax) the chest.

tibia (TIB-e-uh) the inner and larger bone of the lower leg.

torso the trunk of the body; the body without the head and the extremities.

trachea (TRAY-ke-uh) the "windpipe"; the structure that connects the pharynx to the lungs.

Trendelenburg (trend-EL-un-berg) **position** a position in which the patient's feet and legs are higher than the head. Also called *shock position*.

ulna (UL-nah) the medial bone of the forearm.

vein any blood vessel returning blood to the heart.

venae cavae (VE-ne KA-ve) the superior vena cava and the inferior vena cava. These two major veins return blood from the body to the right atrium. (*Venae cavae* is plural, *vena cava* singular.)

ventral referring to the front of the body. A synonym for *anterior*.

ventricles (VEN-tri-kulz) the two lower chambers of the heart. There is a right ventricle (which sends oxygen-poor blood to the lungs) and a left ventricle (which sends oxygen-rich blood to the body).

venule (VEN-yul) the smallest kind of vein.

vertebrae (VER-te-bray) the 33 bones of the spinal column.

voluntary muscle muscle that can be consciously controlled.

white blood cells components of the blood. They produce substances that help the body fight infection.

xiphoid (ZI-foid) **process** the inferior portion of the sternum.

zygomatic (ZI-go-MAT-ik) **bones** the cheekbones.

SUMMARY

As an EMT-Basic, your knowledge of the anatomy, or structure, of the body and the functions, or physiology, of the body will be important in allowing you to assess your patient and communicate your findings with other EMS personnel and hospital staff accurately and efficiently.

Major body systems with which you should be familiar include the musculoskeletal system, the respiratory system, the cardiovascular system, the nervous system, the skin, and the endocrine system.

REVIEW QUESTIONS

1. Define the following anatomical terms:

   medial   lateral

   anterior   posterior

   mid-clavicular   distal

2. List the three functions of the musculoskeletal system.

3. Name the five divisions of the spine and describe the location of each.

4. Describe the physical processes of inhalation and exhalation.

5. List four places a peripheral pulse may be felt.

6. Describe the central nervous system and peripheral nervous system.

7. List three functions of the skin.

Application

- As an EMT-B, you are called to respond to a teenage boy who has taken a hard fall from his dirt bike. He has a deep gash on the outside of his left arm about halfway between the shoulder and the elbow and another on the inside of his right arm just above the wrist. His left leg is bent at a funny angle about halfway between hip and knee, and when you cut away his pants leg, you see a bone sticking out of a wound on the front side. You take the necessary on-scene assessment and care steps and are on the way to the hospital in the ambulance. How do you describe your patient's injuries over the radio to the hospital staff?

Baseline Vital Signs and SAMPLE History

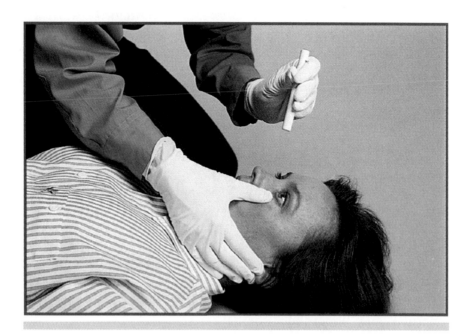

Two essential elements of patient assessment are vital signs and medical history. Vital signs are measurable things like pulse, blood pressure, and respirations. Because they reflect the patient's condition—and changes in the patient's condition—you will take them early and repeat them often. The medical history includes medical information about the present problem and facts about the patient that existed before the patient needed EMS. This information can affect the treatment you give a patient. It is called a SAMPLE history because the letters in the word SAMPLE stand for elements of the history.

Objectives

Knowledge and Attitude *At the end of this chapter, you should be able to meet the following objectives.*

1. Identify the components of vital signs. (p. 73)

2. Describe the methods used to obtain a breathing rate. (p. 77)

3. Identify the attributes that should be obtained when assessing breathing. (pp. 75–76)

4. Differentiate between shallow, labored, and noisy breathing. (p. 76)

5. Describe the methods to obtain a pulse rate. (p. 75)

6. Identify the information obtained when assessing a patient's pulse. (p. 74)

7. Differentiate between a strong, weak, regular, and irregular pulse. (p. 74)

8. Describe the methods used to assess the skin color, temperature, and condition (capillary refill in infants and children). (pp. 77–78)

9. Identify the normal and abnormal skin colors. (p. 77)

10. Differentiate between pale, blue, red, and yellow skin color. (p. 77)

11. Identify the normal and abnormal skin temperature. (pp. 77–78)

12. Differentiate between hot, cool, and cold skin temperature. (pp. 77–78)

13. Identify normal and abnormal skin conditions. (pp. 77–78)

14. Identify normal and abnormal capillary refill in infants and children. (p. 78)

15. Describe the methods used to assess the pupils. (p. 78)

16. Identify normal and abnormal pupil size. (p. 78)

17. Differentiate between dilated (big) and constricted (small) pupil size. (p. 78)

18. Differentiate between reactive and nonreactive pupils and equal and unequal pupils. (p. 78)

19. Describe the methods used to assess blood pressure. (pp. 78–81)

20. Define systolic pressure. (p. 78)

21. Define diastolic pressure. (p. 78)

22. Explain the difference between auscultation and palpation for obtaining a blood pressure. (pp. 80–81)

23. Identify the components of the SAMPLE history. (p. 82)

24. Differentiate between a sign and a symptom. (p. 82)

25. State the importance of accurately reporting and recording the baseline vital signs. (pp. 73–74)

26. Discuss the need to search for additional medical identification. (p. 82)

27. Explain the value of performing the baseline vital signs. (pp. 73–74)

28. Recognize and respond to the feelings patients experience during assessment. (p. 82)

29. Defend the need for obtaining and recording an accurate set of vital signs. (pp. 73–74)

30. Explain the rationale of recording additional sets of vital signs. (pp. 73–74)

31. Explain the importance of obtaining a SAMPLE history. (pp. 82–83)

Skills

1. Demonstrate the skills involved in assessment of breathing.

2. Demonstrate the skills associated with obtaining a pulse.

3. Demonstrate the skills associated with assessing the skin color, temperature, condition, and capillary refill in infants and children.

4. Demonstrate the skills associated with assessing the pupils.

5. Demonstrate the skills associated with obtaining blood pressure.

6. Demonstrate the skills that should be used to obtain information from the patient, family, or bystanders at the scene.

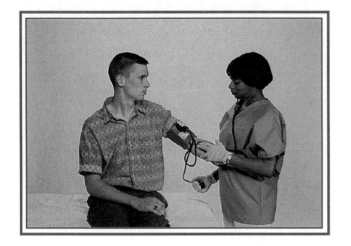

Just before you graduate from your EMT-Basic course, you find an EMS agency that has an opening and wishes to take you on. As part of pre-employment screening, you go to the agency's physician for a history and physical.

Vital Signs

Before the doctor sees you, a nurse comes into the examining room, places her fingers on your wrist, then puts a blood pressure cuff on your arm. She tells you that your pulse rate is 76, your respiratory rate is 20, and your blood pressure is 122 over 76.

History

Shortly after the nurse leaves, the doctor arrives, introduces himself, and chats with you for a minute or two about working in EMS. He then asks you what your health is generally like, whether you have any allergies to medications, what medications you take, and what medical conditions you have had in the past. He asks some additional questions and performs a physical examination. He also ensures that your vaccinations are up to date and orders some tests done on blood samples. Before he leaves, he tells you that he sees no medical reason to keep you from working in EMS and wishes you luck in your EMS career.

When you begin to assess a patient, some things are obvious or easy to discover. For example, the most important part of patient assessment is the chief complaint, the reason the patient called for EMS. Usually, the patient will tell you what his complaint is. Other parts of assessment that are usually apparent as soon as you see the patient are age and sex. Not all of your assessment is so obvious or so easy to find out, however. Two of the major components of assessment that will take a few minutes to complete are vital signs and medical history.

In the Assessment Module chapters, you will learn the other components of patient assessment and how they are integrated into the management of a patient. Vital signs and current and past medical history (SAMPLE history) are gathered on virtually every EMS patient. Occasionally a patient will be so seriously injured or ill that you are unable to get this information because you are too busy treating immediate threats to life. This is the exception, however. The vast majority of patients you will encounter as an EMT-B should have an assessment that includes, among other things, vital sign measurement and SAMPLE history gathering. If you do not get this information, you may remain unaware of important conditions, or trends in patient conditions, that require you to provide particular treatments in the field or prompt transport to a hospital.

VITAL SIGNS

Vital signs are outward signs of what is going on inside the body. They include respiration; pulse; skin color, temperature and condition (plus capillary refill in infants and children); pupils; and blood pressure. Evaluation of these indicators can give valuable information to the EMT-B. This is even more true when you repeat the vital signs. This allows you and other members of the patient's health care team to see trends in the patient's condition and to respond appropriately.

Another sign that gives important information about a patient's condition is mental status. It is not considered to be one of the vital signs; however, whenever you take the vital signs, you should also assess the patient's mental status. Chapter 9, The Initial Assessment, will describe how to evaluate mental status.

Note:

It is essential that you record the vital signs as you obtain them.

Pulse

The pumping action of the heart is normally rhythmic, causing blood to move through the arteries in waves—not smoothly and continuously at the same pressure like water flowing through a pipe. A fingertip held over an artery where it lies close to the body's surface and crosses over a bone can easily feel characteristic "beats" as the surging blood causes the artery to expand. What you feel is called the **pulse.** When taking a patient's pulse, you are concerned with two factors: rate and quality (Figure 5-1).

- The **pulse rate** is the number of beats per minute. The number you get will allow you to decide if the patient's pulse rate is normal, rapid, or slow (Table 5-1).

  Pulse rate varies among individuals. Factors such as age, physical condition, degree of exercise just completed, medications or substances being taken, blood loss, stress, and body temperature all have an influence on the rate. The normal rate for an adult at rest is between 60 and 100 beats per minute. Any pulse rate above 100 beats per minute is rapid, while a rate below 60 beats per minute is slow. A rapid pulse is called **tachycardia.** A slow pulse is called **bradycardia.** An athlete may have a normal at-rest pulse rate between 40 and 50 beats per minute. This is a slow pulse rate, but it is certainly not an indication of poor health. The same pulse rate in a non-athletic person or an elderly person may indicate a serious condition. As an EMT-B, you should be concerned about the typical adult whose pulse rate stays above 100 or below 60 beats per minute.

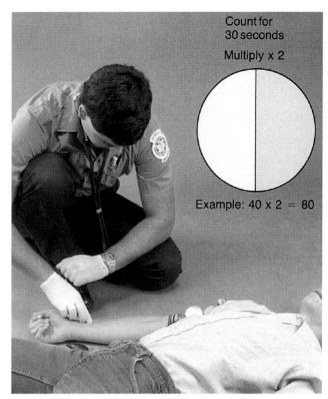

Count for 30 seconds

Multiply x 2

Example: 40 x 2 = 80

FIGURE 5-1 Pulse rate and quality are vital signs.

In an emergency it is not unusual for this rate *temporarily* to be between 100 and 140 beats per minute. If the pulse rate is higher than 150, or if you take a patient's pulse several times during care at the scene and find him *maintaining* a pulse rate above 120 beats or below 50 beats per minute, you must consider this to be a sign that something may be seriously wrong with the patient and that he should be transported as soon as possible.

- Two factors determine **pulse quality:** *rhythm* and *force. Pulse rhythm* reflects regularity. A pulse is said to be regular when intervals between beats are constant. When the intervals are not constant, the pulse is irregular. You should report and document irregular pulse rhythms.

  Pulse force refers to the pressure of the pulse wave as it expands the artery. Normally, the pulse should feel as if a strong wave has passed under your fingertips. This is a strong or *full pulse.* When the pulse feels weak and thin, the patient has a *thready pulse.*

  Many disorders can be related to variations in pulse rate, rhythm, and force (Table 5-1).

TABLE 5-1 Pulse

Normal Pulse Rates (beats per minute, at rest)	
Adults	60 to 100
Infants and Children	
Adolescent 11-14 years	60 to 105
School age 6-10 years	70 to 110
Preschooler 3-5 years	80 to 120
Toddler 1-3 years	80 to 130
Infant 6-12 months	80 to 140
Infant 0-5 months	90 to 140
Newborn	120 to 160

Pulse	Significance/ Possible Causes
Rapid, regular, and full	Exertion, fright, fever, high blood pressure, first stage of blood loss
Rapid, regular, and thready	Shock, later stages of blood loss
Slow	Head injury, drugs, some poisons, some heart problems
No pulse	Cardiac arrest (clinical death)

Infants and Children: A high pulse in an infant or child is not as great a concern as a low pulse. A low pulse (heart rate) may indicate imminent cardiac arrest (stoppage of heart function).

Pulse rate and quality can be determined at a number of points throughout the body. During the determination of vital signs, you should initially find a **radial pulse** in patients one year of age and older. This is the wrist pulse, named for the radial artery found on the lateral (thumb) side of the forearm. If you cannot measure the radial pulse on one arm, try the radial pulse of the other arm. When you cannot measure either radial pulse, use the **carotid pulse**, felt along the large carotid artery on either side of the neck, as you learned to do in cardiopulmonary resuscitation. Be careful when palpating a carotid pulse in a live patient. **Excess pressure can result in slowing of the heart,** especially in older patients. If you have difficulty finding the carotid pulse on one side, try the other side, but **do not assess the carotid pulses on both sides at the same time.**

In order to measure a radial pulse, find the pulse site by placing your first three fingers on the thumb side of the patient's wrist just above the crease (toward the shoulder). Do not use your thumb. It has its own pulse that may cause you to measure your own pulse rate. Slide your fingertips toward the thumb side of the patient's

radial pulse -80 / BIP
femoral pulse - 70 BIP
carotid pulse - 60 BIP

wrist, keeping one finger over the crease. Apply moderate pressure to feel the pulse beats. A weak pulse may require applying greater pressure. But take care—if you press too hard you may press the artery shut. Remember: If you experience difficulty, try the patient's other arm.

Count the pulsations for 30 seconds and multiply by 2 to determine the beats per minute. While you are counting, judge the rhythm and force. Record the information: for example, "Pulse 72, regular and full," and the time of determination.

If the pulse rate, rhythm, or character is not normal, continue with your count and observations for a full 60 seconds. The number counted is the rate in beats per minute.

Respiration

The act of breathing is called **respiration.** A single breath is considered to be the complete process of breathing in (inhalation or inspiration) followed by breathing out (exhalation or expiration). For the determination of vital signs, you are concerned with two factors: rate and quality (Figure 5-2).

15-30 child
25-50 Infant

- The **respiratory rate** is the number of breaths a patient takes in one minute (Table 5-2). The rate of respiration is classified as *normal, rapid,* or *slow.* The *normal* respiration rate for an adult at rest is between 12 and 20 breaths per minute. Keep in mind that age, sex, size, physical conditioning, and emotional state can influence breathing rates. Fear and other emotions experienced during an emergency can cause an increase in respiratory rate. However, if you have an adult patient maintaining a rate above 24 *(rapid)* or below 8 breaths per minute *(slow),* you must administer high concentration oxygen.

- **Respiratory quality,** the quality of a patient's breathing, falls into one of four categories: *normal, shallow, labored,* or *noisy. Normal* breathing means that the chest or abdomen moves an average depth with each breath and the patient is not using his accessory muscles (look for pronounced movement of the shoulder, neck, or abdominal muscles) to breathe. How can you tell if breathing is normal? Normal depth of respiration is something you can judge for yourself by watching people breathe when at rest.

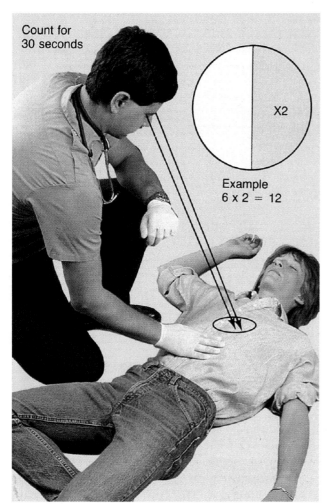

Count for
30 seconds

X2

Example
6 x 2 = 12

FIGURE 5-2 Respiration rate and quality are vital signs.

TABLE 5-2   Respirations

Normal Respiration Rates *(breaths per minute, at rest)*	
Adults	12 to 20 Above 24: Serious Below 8: Serious
Infants and Children	
Adolescent 11-14 years	12 to 20
School age 6-10 years	15 to 30
Preschooler 3-5 years	20 to 30
Toddler 1-3 years	20 to 30
Infant 6-12 months	20 to 30
Infant 0-5 months	25 to 40
Newborn	30 to 50

Respiratory Sounds	*Possible Causes/Interventions*
Snoring	Airway blocked/ Open patient's airway; Prompt transport
Wheezing	Medical problem such as asthma/Assist patient in taking presribed medications; Prompt transport
Gurgling	Fluids in airway/Suction airway; Prompt transport
Crowing (harsh sound when inhaling)	Medical problem that cannot be treated on the scene/Prompt transport

Shallow breathing occurs when there is only slight movement of the chest or abdomen. This is especially serious in the unconscious patient. It is important to look not only at the chest, but also at the abdomen when assessing respiration. Many resting people breathe more with their diaphragm (the muscle between the chest and the abdomen) than with their chest muscles.

Labored breathing can be recognized by signs such as an increase in the work of breathing (the patient has to work hard to move air in and out), the use of accessory muscles, nasal flaring (widening of the nostrils on inhalation), and retractions (pulling in) above the collarbones or between the ribs, especially in infants and children. You may also hear stridor (a harsh, high pitched sound heard on inspiration), grunting on expiration (especially in infants), or gasping.

Noisy breathing is obstructed breathing (when something is blocking the flow of air). Sounds to be concerned about (Table 5-2) include snoring, wheezing, gurgling and crowing. A patient with snoring respirations needs to have his airway opened. Wheezing may respond to medication the patient has and that you may be able to assist the patient in taking. Gurgling sounds usually mean that you need to suction the patient's airway. Crowing (a noisy, harsh sound when breathing in) may not respond to any treatment you give. The patient who is crowing needs prompt transport—as do all patients with difficulty breathing.

- **Respiratory rhythm** is not important in most of the conscious patients you will see. This is because the regularity of an awake patient's breathing is affected by their speech, mood, and activity, among other things. If you observe irregular respirations in an unconscious patient, however, you should report and document it.

Start counting respirations as soon as you have determined the pulse rate. Many individuals change their breathing rate if they know someone is watching them breathe. For this reason, do not move your hand from the patient's wrist or tell the patient you are counting the respiratory rate. After you have counted pulse beats, immediately begin to watch the patient's chest and abdomen for breathing movements. Count the number of breaths taken by the patient during 30 seconds and multiply by 2 to obtain the breaths per minute. While counting, note the rate, quality, and rhythm of respiration. Record your results. For example, "Respirations are 16, normal, and regular." Record the time of the assessment.

Skin

The color, temperature, and condition of the skin can provide valuable information about your patient's circulation. There are many blood vessels in the skin. Since the skin is not as important to survival as some of the other organs (like the heart and brain), the blood vessels of the skin will receive less blood when a patient has lost a significant amount of blood or the ability to adequately circulate blood. Constriction (growing smaller) of the blood vessels causes the skin to become pale. For this reason, the skin can provide clues to blood loss as well as a variety of other conditions.

The best places to assess skin color in adults are the nail beds, the inside of the cheek, and the inside of the lower eyelids. Tiny blood vessels called capillaries are very close to the surface of the skin in all of these places, so changes in the blood are quickly reflected at these sites. They are also more accurate indicators than other sites in adults with dark complexions. In infants and children, the best places to look are the palms of the hands and the soles of the feet. In patients with dark skin you can check the lips and nail beds.

Ordinarily, the color you see (Table 5-3) in any of these places is pink. Abnormal colors include pale, cyanotic (blue-gray), flushed (red) and jaundiced (yellow). Pale skin frequently indicates poor circulation of blood. A common cause of this in the field is loss of blood. Cyanotic skin is usually a result of not enough oxygen getting to the red blood cells. Flushed skin may be caused by exposure to heat. Jaundice is a yellowish tint to the skin from liver abnormalities. An uncommon skin color is mottling, a blotchy

TABLE 5-3   Skin Color

Skin Color	Significance/Possible Causes
Pink	Normal in light-skinned patients or at inner eyelids, lips, nail beds of dark-skinned patients
Pale	Constricted blood vessels possibly resulting from blood loss, shock, heart attack, emotional distress
Cyanotic (blue)	Lack of oxygen in blood cells and tissues resulting from inadequate breathing or heart function
Flushed (red)	Exposure to heat, high blood pressure, emotional excitement
Jaundiced (yellow)	Liver abnormalities
Mottling (blotchiness)	Occasionally in patients with shock

appearance that sometimes occurs in patients, especially children, in shock.

To determine skin temperature (Table 5-4), feel the patient's skin with the back of your hand. A good place to do this is the patient's forehead (Figure 5-3). Note if his skin feels normal (warm), hot, cool, or cold. At the same time, notice condition—if the skin is dry (normal), moist, or clammy (both cool and moist). Look for "goose pimples," which are often associated with chills. Many patient problems are exhibited by changes in skin temperature and condition. As you continue with the assessment and care of the patient, be alert for major temperature differences on various parts of the body. For example, you may note that the patient's trunk is

TABLE 5-4   Skin Temperature and Condition

Skin Temperature/ Condition	Significance/Possible Causes
Cool, clammy	Usual sign of shock, anxiety
Cold, moist	Body is losing heat
Cold, dry	Exposure to cold
Hot, dry	High fever, heat exposure
Hot, moist	High fever, heat exposure
"Goose pimples" accompanied by shivering, chattering teeth, blue lips, and pale skin	Chills, communicable disease, exposure to cold, pain, or fear

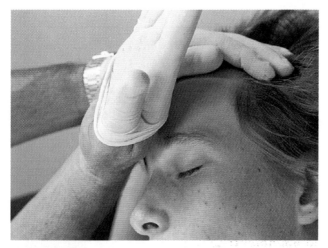

FIGURE 5-3 Determining skin temperature.

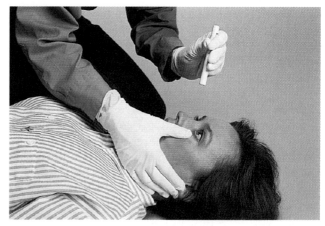

FIGURE 5-4 Examining the pupils.

warm but his left arm feels cold. Such a finding can lead you to a problem with circulation.

In infants and children, you should also evaluate capillary refill. Press on the nail bed—or the top of the hand or foot in a small child or infant—and watch how long it takes for the normal pink color to return after you release it. Normally, this takes no more than two seconds. If it takes longer than two seconds, the patient's blood is probably not circulating well. This sign is not reliable in children and infants who have been exposed to cold temperatures and in many adults, even under normal environmental conditions. Abnormal responses include prolonged and absent capillary refill.

Be sure to record your findings with regard to skin color, temperature, and condition.

Pupils

The **pupil** is the black center of the eye. One of the things that causes it to change size is the amount of light entering the eye. When the environment is dim, the pupil will **dilate** (get larger) to allow more light into the eye. When there is a lot of light, it will **constrict** (get smaller). So you will check a patient's pupils by shining a light into them (Figure 5-4). When you check pupils, you should look for three things: size, equality, and **reactivity** (reacting to light by changing size). Under ordinary conditions, pupils are neither large nor small, but midpoint. Dilated pupils are extremely large. In fact, it is usually difficult to tell what color eyes the patient has if his pupils are dilated. Both pupils are normally the same size, and when a light is shone into them, they react by constricting. The rate at which they constrict should be equal. Nonreac-

tive pupils do not constrict in response to a bright light.

When the patient is in bright light, using a penlight or flashlight will not work. Instead, cover the patient's eyes for a few seconds and then uncover them one at a time to observe for constriction of the pupil.

Pupils that are dilated, unequal in size or reactivity, or nonreactive may indicate a variety of conditions (Table 5-5) including drug influence, head injury, or eye injury. Any deviations from normal should be reported and documented.

Blood Pressure

Each time the ventricle (lower chamber) of the left side of the heart contracts, it forces blood out into the circulation. The force of blood against the walls of the blood vessels is called **blood pressure.** The pressure created when the heart contracts and forces blood into the arteries is called the **systolic** (sis-TOL-ik) blood pressure. When the left ventricle relaxes and refills, the pressure remaining in the arteries is called the **diastolic** (di-as-TOL-ik) blood pressure. These two pressures indicate the amount of pressure against the walls of the arteries and together are known as the blood pressure. When you take a patient's blood pressure, you report

TABLE 5-5 Pupils

Pupil Appearance	Significance/Possible Causes
Dilated (larger than normal)	Fright, blood loss, drugs, treatment with eye drops
Unequal	Stroke, head injury, eye injury, artificial eye
Lack of reactivity	Drugs, lack of oxygen to brain

the systolic pressure first, the diastolic second, as "120 over 80," or "120/80."

One blood pressure reading may not be very meaningful. You will need to take several readings over a period of time while care is provided at the scene and during transport. Changes in blood pressure can be very significant. The patient's blood pressure may be normal in the early stages of some very serious problems, only to change rapidly in a matter of minutes.

Just as pulse and respiratory rates vary among individuals, so does blood pressure (Table 5-6). There is a generally accepted rule for estimating blood pressure of adults up to the age of 40. For an adult male at rest, add his age to 100 to estimate his normal systolic pressure. For an adult female at rest, add her age to 90 to estimate her normal systolic pressure. Thus, using this formula, a 36-year-old man would have an estimated normal systolic blood pressure of 136 millimeters of mercury (mm Hg). (Millimeters of mercury refers to the units on the blood pressure gauge.) A 36-year-old woman would have an estimated normal systolic pressure of 126 mm Hg. Normal diastolic pressures usually range from 60 to 90 mm Hg. Serious low blood pressure is generally considered to exist when the systolic pressure falls below 90 mm Hg. High blood pressure exists once the systolic pressure rises above 150 or the diastolic above 90. Many individuals under stress (like that caused by having the ambulance come to your home) will exhibit a temporary rise in blood pressure. More than one reading will be necessary to decide if a high or low reading is only temporary. If the blood pressure drops, your patient may be developing shock (however, other signs are usually more important early indicators of shock). Report any major changes in blood pressure to emergency department personnel without delay.

To measure blood pressure with a **sphygmomanometer** (SFIG-mo-mah-NOM-e-ter—the cuff and gauge), first place the stethoscope around your neck. Position yourself at the patient's side and place the blood pressure cuff on his arm (Figure 5-5). The cuff should cover two-thirds of the upper arm, elbow to shoulder. Be certain that there are no suspected or obvious injuries to this arm. There should be no clothing under the cuff. If you can expose the arm sufficiently by rolling the sleeve up, do so, but make sure that this roll of clothing does not become a constricting band.

Wrap the cuff around the patient's upper arm so that the lower edge of the cuff is about one inch above the crease of the elbow. The

TABLE 5-6 Blood Pressure

Blood Pressure Normal Ranges		
	Systolic	Diastolic
Adults	90 to 150	60 to 90
Infants and Children	Approx. 80 plus 2 × age	Approx. 2/3 Systolic
Adolescent 11-14 years	average 115 (94 to 140)	average 59
School age 6-10 years	average 105 (80 to 122)	average 57
Preschooler 3-5 years	average 99 (78 to 116)	average 65
Blood Pressure	Significance/Possible Causes	
High blood pressure	Medical condition, exertion, fright, emotional distress or excitement	
Low blood pressure	Athlete or other person with normally low blood pressure; blood loss; late sign of shock	

Note: The systolic blood pressure usually parallels the pulse rate; that is, when the pulse (heart) rate increases, the systolic blood pressure increases, too.

Infants and children: Blood pressure is usually not taken on a child under 3 years. In cases of blood loss or shock, a child's blood pressure will remain within normal limits until near the end, then fall swiftly.

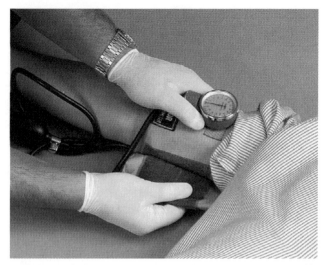

FIGURE 5-5 Positioning the blood pressure cuff.

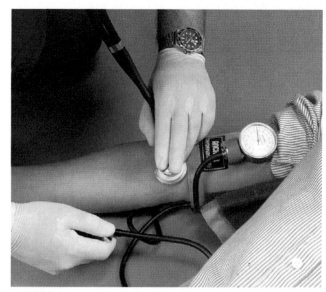

FIGURE 5-6 Measuring blood pressure by auscultation.

center of the bladder must be placed over the **brachial** (BRAY-key-al) **artery**, the major artery of the arm. The marker on the cuff (if provided) should indicate where you place the cuff in relation to the artery, but many cuffs do not have markers in the correct location. Tubes entering the bladder are not always in the right location, either. According to the American Heart Association, the only accurate method is to find the bladder center. Apply the cuff so it is secure but not overly tight. You are now ready to begin your determination of the patient's blood pressure.

There are two common techniques used to measure blood pressure with a sphygmomanometer: (1) **auscultation** (os-skul-TAY-shun), when a stethoscope is used to listen for characteristic sounds (Figure 5-6); and (2) **palpation,** when the radial pulse or brachial pulse is palpated (felt) with the finger tips (Figure 5-7).

• *Determining blood pressure by auscultation.* Begin by placing the ear pieces of the stethoscope in your ears (the ear pieces should be pointing forward in the direction of your ear canals). The patient should be seated or lying down. If the patient has not been injured, support his arm at the level of his heart. Place the cuff snugly around the upper arm so that the bottom of the cuff is just above the elbow. With your fingertips, palpate the brachial artery at the crease of the elbow. Position the diaphragm of the stethoscope directly over the brachial pulse or over the medial anterior elbow (middle of the front of the elbow) if no brachial pulse

can be found. Do not place the head of the stethoscope underneath the cuff, since this will give you false readings.

With the bulb valve (thumb valve) closed, inflate the cuff. As you do so, you soon will be able to hear pulse sounds. Inflate the cuff, watching the gauge. At a certain point, you will no longer hear the brachial pulse. Continue to inflate the cuff until the gauge reads 30 mm higher than the point where the pulse sound disappeared. Slowly release air from the cuff by opening the bulb valve, allowing the pressure to fall smoothly at the rate of approximately 5 to 10 mm per second. Listen for the start of clicking or tapping sounds.

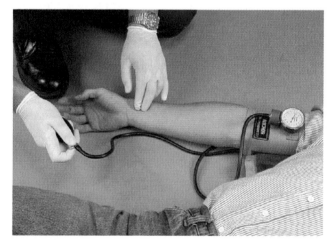

FIGURE 5-7 Measuring blood pressure by palpation.

When you hear the first of these sounds, note the reading on the gauge. This is the systolic pressure. Continue to deflate the cuff, listening for the point at which these distinctive sounds fade. When the sounds turn to dull, muffled thuds, the reading on the gauge is the diastolic pressure. Sometimes you will not be able to hear a change in these sounds. When this happens, the point at which the sounds disappear is the diastolic pressure. After obtaining the diastolic pressure, let the cuff deflate rapidly. If you are not certain of a reading, repeat the procedure. You should use the other arm or wait one minute before re-inflating the cuff. Otherwise, you will tend to obtain an erroneously high reading.

Record the measurements and the time of determination. For example, "B.P. is 140/90 at 1:10 p.m.." Blood pressure is reported in even numbers. If a reading falls between two lines on the gauge, use the higher number. If you are not sure of the reading you are getting, try again or get some help. Never make up vital signs!

Some patients who have high systolic blood pressures will have the pulse sounds disappear as you deflate the cuff, only to have these sounds reappear as you continue with deflation. When this happens, false systolic and diastolic readings may be obtained. If you determine a high diastolic reading, wait 1 to 2 minutes and take another reading. As you inflate the cuff, feel for the disappearance of the radial pulse to ensure that you are not measuring a false diastolic pressure. Listen as you deflate the cuff down into the normal range. The diastolic pressure is the reading at which the last clear sound takes place.

- *Determining blood pressure by palpation.* This method is not as accurate as the auscultation method, since only an approximate systolic pressure can be determined. The technique is used when there is too much noise around a patient to allow the use of the stethoscope.

Begin by finding the radial pulse on the limb to which the blood pressure cuff has been applied. Make certain that the adjustable valve is closed on the bulb and inflate the cuff to a point where you can no longer feel the radial pulse. Note this point on the gauge and continue to inflate the cuff 30 mm of mercury beyond this point.

Slowly deflate the cuff, noting the reading at which the radial pulse returns. This reading is the patient's systolic pressure. Record your findings as, for example, "blood pressure 140 by palpation" or "140/P" and the time of the determination. (You cannot determine a diastolic reading by palpation.)

As an EMT-B, you should obtain a blood pressure on every patient more than three years old. Blood pressures on infants and young children are difficult to obtain with any accuracy and have little bearing on field man-

Time	Pulse	Respirations	Blood Pressure
1410	88 str, reg	28	132 / 84

Pupils	Skin Color	Skin Temperature	Skin Condition
Equal ☑ Unequal ☐	Normal ☐	Cold ☐	Moist ☑
Reactive Ⓛ Ⓡ	Pale ☑	Cool ☑	Dry ☐
Nonreactive L R	Cyanotic ☐	Warm ☐	
Dilated ☐	Flushed ☐	Hot ☐	
Normal Size ☑	Jaundiced ☐		
Constricted ☐			

FIGURE 5-8 The prehospital care report (run sheet) provides spaces for recording vital signs.

agement of the patient. You can get more useful information about the condition of an infant or child by observing for conditions such as a sick appearance, respiratory distress, or unconsciousness.

Vital signs are usually taken more than once. How frequently they should be repeated depends on the condition of the patient and the patient care interventions you are performing. Stable patients need repeat vital signs at least every 15 minutes. Unstable patients need repeat vital signs at least every 5 minutes. You should also repeat vital signs after every medical intervention. Record every reading of the vital signs (Figure 5-8).

SAMPLE HISTORY

An EMT-B can gain two kinds of information about the patient's present problem: signs and symptoms. A **sign** is objective—something you see, hear, feel, and smell when examining the patient. The vital signs are, of course, signs, as are sweaty skin, staggering, and vomiting, for example. A **symptom** is subjective—an indication you cannot observe but that the patient feels and tells you about. Such things as chest pain, dizziness, and nausea are considered symptoms.

An important part of the information you should gain on all of your patients is information about the present problem (signs and symptoms) plus the past medical history—together called the **SAMPLE history.** To obtain it, ask these questions:

- **Signs/Symptoms.** What's wrong?
- **Allergies.** Are you allergic to medications, foods or environmentals? Is there a medical identification tag describing allergies?
- **Medications.** What medications are you currently taking (prescription, over the counter, or recreational)? (If the patient is a woman) Are you on birth control pills? Is there a medical identification tag with the names of medications on it?
- **Pertinent past history.** Have you been having any medical problems? Have you been feeling ill? Have you recently had any surgery or injuries? Have you been seeing a doctor? What is your doctor's name?
- **Last oral intake.** When did you eat last or drink? What did you eat or drink? (Food or liquids can cause symptoms or aggravate a

medical condition. Also, if a patient will need to go to surgery, the hospital staff must know when he has last had anything to eat or drink, since stomach contents can be vomited while a patient is under anesthesia, which is a very dangerous occurrence.)
- **Events leading to the injury or illness.** What sequence of events led up to today's problem (e.g., the patient passed out, then got into car crash versus got into car crash and then passed out)?

When conducting a patient interview

- *Position yourself close to the patient.* Depending on the patient's situation, kneel or stand close to him. If possible, position yourself so that the sun or bright lights are not at your back. That way the patient will not have to squint to see you. When practical, position yourself so the patient can see your face and your face is at a level close to the patient's face. This is especially important with children.
- *Identify yourself and reassure the patient.* It is important that the patient know he is in competent hands. Maintain eye contact with the patient and state your name, that you are an Emergency Medical Technician, and the organization you represent.
- *Speak in your normal voice.* When you ask a question, wait for a reply. Work to gain the patient's confidence through calm conversation. Avoid inappropriate remarks like "Don't worry," and "Everything is all right." The patient knows everything is not all right.
- *If you believe it to be appropriate, gently touch the patient's shoulder or rest your hand over his.* A simple touch is comforting to most people.
- *Learn your patient's name.* Once you know it, use it in the rest of your conversations. Children will expect you to use their first names. For adults, use the appropriate *Mr., Mrs., Miss,* or *Ms.* unless they introduce themselves by their first name. If you are unsure whether to addresss the patient as *Mr.,* ask the patient what he would like you to call him. You need the patient's name for completion of your forms and to give a personal touch that is often very reassuring to the patient. Having the patient's name could prove to be of great importance should he become unconscious and not be carrying any identification.

- *Learn your patient's age.* This will be needed for reports and communications with the medical facility.

The SAMPLE history gives valuable information about the patient's condition. This will sometimes influence the field management of the patient, but it will more often affect the patient's hospital treatment. If the patient should lose consciousness before arriving at the hospital, he will be unable to give his history. This is one of the most important reasons for the EMT to get this information.

Infants and Children

One of the most important factors that determines the normal range of vital signs is age. Infants and children have faster pulse and respiratory rates and lower blood pressures than adults. Compare the ranges for infants and children with those for adults in the tables in this chapter.

Another way in which infants and children differ from adults is that capillary refill can be a useful guide to the status of their circulation, which is not true of adults.

CHAPTER REVIEW

KEY TERMS

You may find it helpful to review the following terms.

auscultation (os-skul-TAY-shun) listening. A stethoscope is used to auscultate for characteristic sounds.

blood pressure the force of blood against the walls of the blood vessels.

brachial (BRAY-key-al) **artery** the major artery of the arm.

bradycardia (BRAY-duh-KAR-de-uh) a slow pulse; any pulse rate below 60 beats per minute.

carotid (kah-ROT-id) **pulse** the pulse felt along the large carotid artery on either side of the neck.

constrict (kon-STRIKT) get smaller.

diastolic (di-as-TOL-ik) **blood pressure** the pressure remaining in the arteries when the left ventricle of the heart is relaxed and refilling.

dilate (DI-late) get larger.

palpation touching or feeling. A pulse or blood pressure may be palpated with the fingertips.

pulse the rhythmic beats felt as the heart pumps blood through the arteries.

pulse quality the rhythm (regular or irregular) and force (strong or weak) of the pulse.

pulse rate the number of pulse beats per minute.

pupil the black center of the eye.

radial (RAY-de-ul) **pulse** the pulse felt at the wrist.

reactivity (re-ak-TIV-uh-te) in the pupils of the eyes, reacting to light by changing size.

respiration (res-puh-RAY-shun) the act of breathing in and breathing out.

respiratory (RES-puh-ruh-tor-e) **quality** the normal or abnormal (shallow, labored, or noisy) character of breathing.

respiratory rate the number of breaths taken in one minute.

respiratory rhythm the regular or irregular spacing of breaths.

SAMPLE history the present and past medical history of a patient, so called because the elements of the history begin with the letters of the word *sample*: signs/symptoms, allergies, medications, pertinent past history, last oral intake, events leading to the injury or illness.

sign an indication of a patient's condition that is objective, or can be observed by another person; an indication that can be seen, heard, smelled, or felt by the EMT-B or others.

sphygmomanometer (SFIG-mo-mah-NOM-uh-ter) the cuff and gauge used to measure blood pressure.

symptom an indication of a patient's condition that cannot be observed by another person but rather is subjective, or felt and reported by the patient.

systolic (sis-TOL-ik) **blood pressure** the pressure created when the heart contracts and forces blood out into the arteries.

tachycardia (TAK-uh-KAR-de-uh) a rapid pulse; any pulse rate above 100 beats per minute.

vital signs outward signs of what is going on inside the body, including respiration; pulse; skin color, temperature, and condition (plus capillary refill in infants and children); pupils; and blood pressure.

SUMMARY

As an EMT-B, you can gain a great deal of information about a patient's condition by taking a complete set of vital signs. These include pulse, respirations, skin, pupils and blood pressure. (See Tables 5-7, 5-8, and 5-9 for a summary of normal ranges for pulse, respirations, and blood pressure.) These must then be followed by repeat vital signs in order to recognize trends in the patient's condition. How often you repeat the vital signs will depend on the patient's condition. Another source of information is the SAMPLE history. By determining the Signs/symptoms, Allergies, Medications, Pertinent past history, Last oral intake, and Events leading to the injury or illness, you will gain information that may affect field treatment and will be important to the definitive treatment of the patient at the hospital.

REVIEW QUESTIONS

1. Name the vital signs.
2. Explain why vital signs should be taken more than once.
3. Explain the meaning of the letters S-A-M-P-L-E in patient assessment.

Application

- How might the EMT-B get a SAMPLE history when a patient is unconscious?

TABLE 5-7 Pulse, Normal Ranges

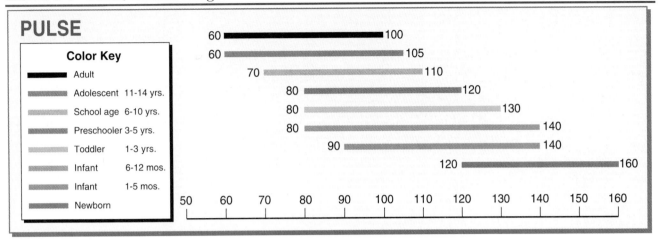

TABLE 5-8 Respirations, Normal Ranges

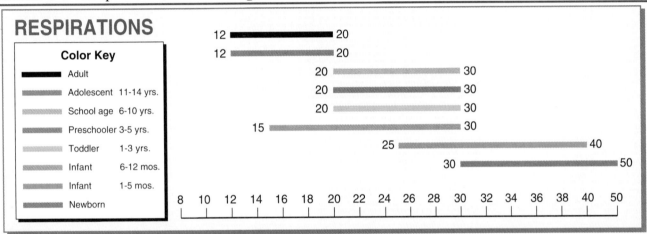

TABLE 5-9 Blood Pressure, Normal Ranges

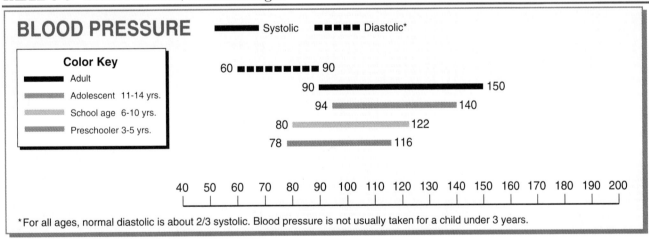

Concept for Tables 5-7, 5-8, and 5-9 by Christine M. Yuhas, practicing EMT, State of New Jersey.

Lifting and Moving Patients

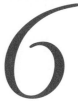

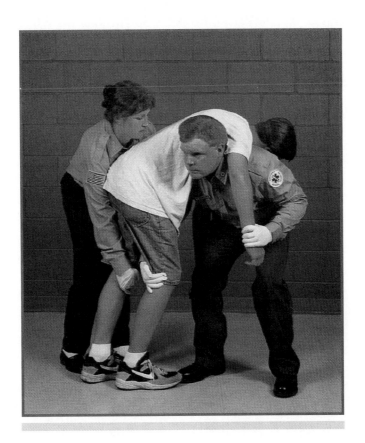

Lifting and moving patients is a part of almost every call. It will be an important part of your responsibilities to lift and move patients safely and effectively. You must perform these tasks without aggravating the patient's current condition or causing further injury. You must also be knowledgeable about methods of proper lifting and moving to prevent injury to yourself. Careful thought, planning, and knowledge of proper procedures must be used whenever a patient is lifted or moved.

Objectives

Knowledge and Attitude *At the end of this chapter, you should be able to meet the following objectives.*

1. Define body mechanics. (p. 89)

2. Discuss the guidelines and safety precautions that need to be followed when lifting a patient. (pp. 89–90)

3. Describe the safe lifting of cots and stretchers. (pp. 90–91)

4. Describe the guidelines and safety precautions for carrying patients and/or equipment. (pp. 89–91)

5. Discuss one-handed carrying techniques. (p. 90)

6. Describe correct and safe carrying procedures on stairs. (p. 90)

7. State the guidelines for reaching and their application. (pp. 90–91)

8. Describe correct reaching for log rolls. (p. 92)

9. State the guidelines for pushing and pulling. (p. 91)

10. Discuss the general considerations of moving patients. (p. 91)

11. State three situations that may require the use of an emergency move. (pp. 91–92)

12. Identify the following patient carrying devices: (pp. 96–98, 100–101)

On the Scene

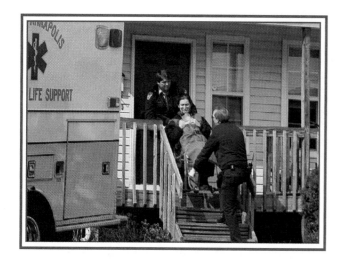

Your ambulance is one of two ambulances dispatched to the scene of a back injury. The location of the call sounds familiar to you—an ambulance was dispatched there about twenty minutes ago for chest pain.

The need for three ambulances at the scene confuses you, as does the nature of the call, but it all becomes clear when you arrive. An EMT-B from the first ambulance injured his back while lifting the stretcher into the ambulance. This meant that Mrs. Nagle, the patient with chest pain, could not be driven to the hospital and Lou Dolan, the injured EMT-B, now must also go to the hospital.

While Mrs. Nagle is being treated by EMT-Bs from the other ambulance, you move toward Lou Dolan. Lou explains that he has a terrible tearing pain in his lower back that developed when he tried to lift the stretcher. "I wasn't in a very good position," he said. "I tried to lift before I was square with the stretcher. I tried to turn a little while I lifted . . . and that was it."

Your colleague Lou is now your patient, and you carefully place him on a backboard. Seeing his pain, even with minor movements or bumps in the road, you tell yourself that you will always lift properly. "I'm going to start doing those back-strengthening exercises they showed us during in-service training," you promise yourself.

- wheeled ambulance stretcher
- portable ambulance stretcher
- stair chair
- scoop stretcher
- long spine board
- basket stretcher
- flexible stretcher.

13. Explain the rationale for properly lifting and moving patients. (p. 89)

Skills

1. Working with a partner, prepare each of the following devices for use, transfer a patient to the device, properly position the patient on the device, move the device to the ambulance, and load the patient into the ambulance:

- wheeled ambulance stretcher
- portable ambulance stretcher
- stair chair
- scoop stretcher
- long spine board
- basket stretcher
- flexible stretcher.

2. Working with a partner, the EMT-Basic will demonstrate techniques for the transfer of a patient from an ambulance stretcher to a hospital stretcher.

S peed is a major objective on many of the calls you will make as an EMT-Basic. At certain dangerous scenes, for example, you must rapidly move the patient to a safe place. When the patient has a life-threatening medical problem or a serious injury, getting the patient to the hospital quickly can mean the difference between life and death.

Doing things fast, however, can mean doing them wrong. You can be so focused on the need to hurry as you lift and carry the patient that you make careless moves. These can injure your patient. They can also injure you. Back injuries are serious and have the potential to end an EMS career as well as cause life-long problems. With the proper techniques, however, you can lift and move patients safely. Proper lifting and moving must be practiced on every call.

PROTECTING YOURSELF: BODY MECHANICS

Body mechanics is the proper use of your body to facilitate lifting and moving. There are several important things that you can do with your body to lift efficiently and prevent injury.

Planning is important before lifting a patient. Consider the following before lifting any patient or object.

- *What is the weight of the object?* Will we require additional help in lifting?
- *What are your physical characteristics?* Do I or my partner have any physical limitations that would make lifting difficult? While it may not always be possible to arrange, EMT-Bs of similar strength and height may lift and carry together more easily.
- *Communicate.* Communicate the plan for lifting and carrying to your partner. Continue to communicate throughout the process to make the move comfortable for the patient and safe for the EMT-Bs.

When it comes time to do the lifting, there are rules that must be followed to prevent injury. These include

- *Position your feet properly.* They should be on a firm, level surface and positioned shoulder-width apart.
- *When lifting, use your legs, not your back to do the lifting.*
- *When lifting, never twist or attempt to make any moves other than the lift.* Attempts to

turn or twist while you are lifting are a major cause of injury.

- *When lifting with one hand, do not compensate.* Avoid leaning to either side. Keep your back straight and locked.
- *Keep the weight as close to your body as possible.* This is part of good body mechanics and allows you to use your legs rather than your back while lifting. The farther the weight is from your body, the greater your chance of injury.
- *When carrying a patient on stairs, use a stair chair instead of a stretcher when possible.* Keep your back straight. Flex your knees and lean forward from the hips, not the waist. If you are walking backwards down stairs, ask a helper to steady your back (Figure 6-1).

There are many kinds of patient carrying devices, including stretchers, backboards, and stair chairs. (For more specifics, see Patient Carrying Devices later in this chapter). When possible, it is almost always safer as well as more efficient to move patients over distances on a wheeled device such as a wheeled stretcher or a stair chair. These devices allow the patient to be rolled along instead of carried.

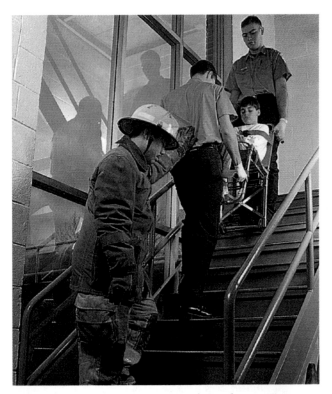

FIGURE 6-1 Moving a stair chair down steps.

When lifting a patient carrying device, it is best to use an even number of people. For a stretcher or backboard, one EMT-B lifts from the end near the patient's head, the other from the feet. If there are four rescuers available, one person can take each corner of a stretcher or board. If there are only three people available, never allow the third person to assist by lifting one side. This can cause the device to be thrown off balance, resulting in the stretcher tipping over and injuring the patient.

To prevent injury when lifting a patient carrying device, the general rules of body mechanics mentioned earlier apply. The following two methods can also help prevent injury.

- The **power-lift** is so named because it is used by power weight lifters. It is also known as the *squat-lift position* (Figure 6-2). In this position, you will squat rather than bending at the waist, and you will keep the weight close to your body, even straddling it if possible. When rising, your feet should be a comfortable distance apart, flat on the ground, with the weight primarily on the balls of the feet or just behind them. Your back should be locked in. You will raise your upper body before your hips.

  When you are lowering a patient, use the reverse order of this procedure.
- The **power grip** is a method of gripping with the hands. Remember that your hands are often the only portion of your body actually in contact with the object you are lifting, making your grip a very important element in the lifting process. As great an area of your fingers and palms as possible should be in contact with the object. All of your fingers should be bent at the same angle. Your hands, when possible, should be at least 10 inches apart.

There are situations where you will find yourself having to reach for patients or provide a considerable amount of effort pushing and pulling weight. These are moves that must be performed carefully to prevent injury. In general

When reaching

- Keep your back in a locked-in position.
- Avoid twisting while reaching.
- Avoid reaching more than 15 to 20 inches in front of your body.

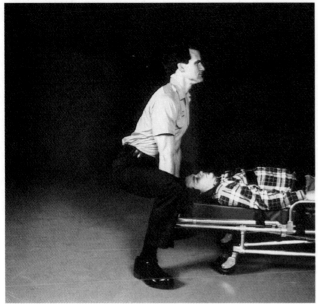

A.

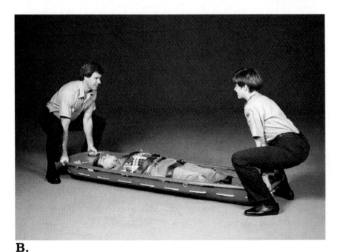

B.

FIGURE 6-2 The power lift, or squat lift.

- Avoid prolonged reaching when strenuous effort is required.

  When pushing or pulling

- Push, rather than pull, whenever possible.
- Keep your back locked-in.
- Keep the line of pull through the center of your body by bending your knees.
- Keep the weight close to your body.
- If the weight is below waist level, push or pull from a kneeling position.
- Avoid pushing or pulling overhead.
- Keep your elbows bent with arms close to your sides.

PROTECTING YOUR PATIENT: EMERGENCY, URGENT, AND NON-URGENT MOVES

How quickly should you move a patient? Must you complete your assessment before moving the patient? How much time should you spend on spinal protection and other patient safety measures? The answer is—it depends on the circumstances.

If the patient is in a building that is threatening to collapse or a car that is on fire, speed is the overriding concern. The patient must be moved to a safe place, probably before you have time to begin or complete an assessment, immobilize the patient's spine, or move a stretcher into position. In this situation, you would use what is known as an *emergency move.*

Sometimes the situation is such that you have time to carry out an abbreviated version of assessment and spinal immobilization although you must move the patient quickly, as when the patient's condition is so serious that he must be removed from wreckage and gotten to the hospital before there is time to do a full assessment. In this situation, you would use an *urgent move.*

Most of the time, you will be able to complete your on-scene assessment and care procedures and then move the patient onto a stretcher or other patient carrying device in the normal way, for example when you are called to the home of a patient with a non-life-threatening medical complaint. In this case, you would use a *non-urgent move.*

Emergency Moves

There are three situations that may require the use of an emergency move.

- *The scene is hazardous.* Hazards may make it necessary to move a patient quickly in order to protect you and the patient. This may occur when there is uncontrolled traffic, fire or threat of fire, possible explosions, electrical hazards, toxic gases, or radiation.
- *Care of life-threatening conditions requires repositioning.* You may have to move a patient to a hard, flat surface to provide CPR, or you may have to move a patient to reach life-threatening bleeding.
- *You must reach other patients.* When there are other patients at the scene requiring

care for life-threatening problems, you may have to move another patient to access the patient with life-threatening conditions.

The greatest danger to the patient in an emergency move is that a spinal injury may be aggravated. Since the move must be made *immediately* to protect the patient's life, full spinal treatment will not be possible. Whenever you suspect a possible spine injury, to minimize or prevent aggravation of the spine injury, *move the patient in the direction of the long axis of the body when possible.* The long axis of the body is the line that runs down the center of the body from the top of the head and along the spine.

There are several rapid moves called drags. In this type of move, the patient is dragged by the clothes, the feet, the shoulders, or a blanket. These moves are reserved only for emergencies because they do not provide protection for the neck and spine. Most commonly, a long-axis drag is made from the area of the shoulders. Dragging from the shoulder area causes the remainder of the body to fall into its natural anatomical position, with the spine and all limbs in normal alignment. Imagine dragging a patient from one side and the twisting and aggravation of injuries that could result.

Drags and other emergency moves known as carries and assists are illustrated in Scans 6-1, 6-2, and 6-3.

Urgent Moves

Urgent moves are required when the patient must be moved quickly to treat an immediate threat to life, but — unlike emergency moves — are performed with precautions for spinal injury. Examples of conditions where urgent moves may be required include the following.

- *Treatment of the patient's condition requires a move.* A patient must be moved in order to support inadequate breathing or to treat for shock or altered mental status.
- *Factors at the scene cause patient decline.* If a patient is *rapidly* declining because of heat or cold, for example, he may have to be moved.

Moving a patient onto a long spine board, also called a backboard, is an urgent move used when there is immediate threat to life and there is suspicion of injury to the spine. If the patient is supine on the ground, a log roll maneuver

must be performed to move him onto his side. The spine board is then placed next to the patient's body, and he is log-rolled back onto the spine board. After the patient is secured and immobilized on the spine board, spine board and patient are lifted together onto a stretcher and loaded into the ambulance. (When reaching across the patient to perform the log roll, remember the principles of body mechanics: Keep your back straight, lean from the hips, and use your shoulder muscles to help with the roll. See Figure 6-3.) Log rolls and immobilization on a long spine board will be discussed in Chapter 28, Injuries to the Head and Spine.

Another example of an urgent move is the rapid extrication procedure from a vehicle. If a patient has critical injuries, taking the time to apply an immobilizing short backboard or vest to the patient while he is still in the car may cause a deadly delay in removing the patient to the ambulance. During a rapid extrication, EMT-Bs use a quicker procedure, stabilizing the spine manually as they move the patient from the car onto a long spine board. The rapid extrication procedure will be discussed in Chapter 28, Injuries to the Head and Spine.

Non-Urgent Moves

When there is no immediate threat to life, the patient should be moved when ready for transportation, using a non-urgent move. On-scene assessment and any needed on-scene treatments, such as splinting, should be completed first. Non-urgent moves should be carried out in such a way as to prevent injury or additional

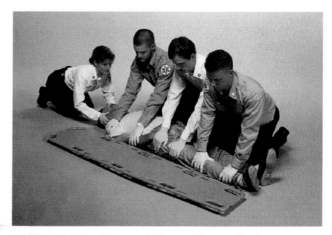

FIGURE 6-3 When doing a log roll, keep your back straight, lean from the hips, and use your shoulder muscles.

Emergency Moves—One Rescuer Drags

Caution: Always pull in the direction of long axis of patient's body. Do not pull patient sideways. Avoid bending or twisting the trunk.

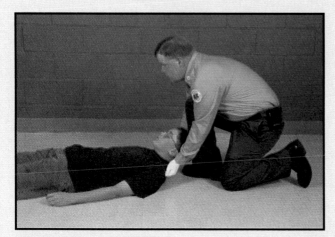

THE CLOTHES DRAG

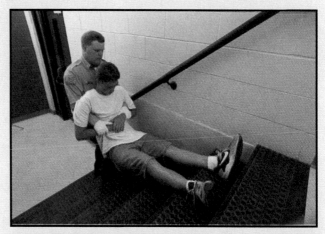

THE INCLINE DRAG Always head first.

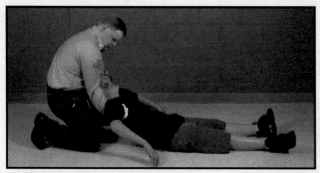

THE SHOULDER DRAG Be careful not to bump patient's head.

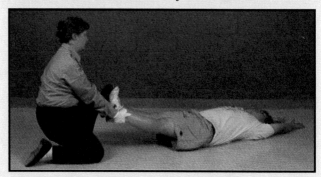

THE FOOT DRAG Be careful not to bump patient's head.

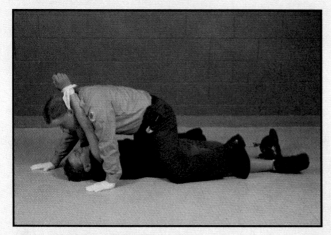

THE "FIREMAN'S DRAG" Place patient on his back and tie hands together. Straddle the patient, facing his head; crouch and pass your head through his trussed arms and raise your body. Crawl on your hands and knees. Keep the patient's head as low as possible.

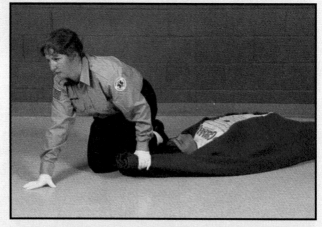

THE BLANKET DRAG Gather half of the blanket material up against the patient's side. Roll the patient toward your knees so that you can place the blanket under him. Gently roll the patient back onto the blanket. During the drag, keep the patient's head as low as possible.

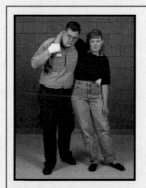

THE ONE-RESCUER ASSIST Place patient's arm around your neck, grasping her hand in yours. Place your other arm around patient's waist. Help patient walk to safety. Be prepared to change movement technique if level of danger increases. Be sure to communicate with patient about obstacles, uneven terrain, and so on.

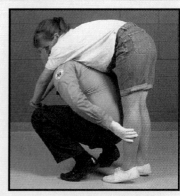

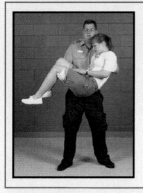

THE CRADLE CARRY Place one arm across patient's back with your hand under her arm. Place your other arm under her knees and lift. If patient is conscious, have her place her near arm over your shoulder. **Note:** This carry places a lot of weight on the carrier's back. It is usually appropriate only for very light patients.

THE PIGGY BACK CARRY Assist the patient to stand. Place her arms over your shoulder so they cross your chest. Bend over and lift patient. While she holds on with her arms, crouch and grasp each thigh. Use a lifting motion to move her onto your back. Pass your forearms under her knees and grasp her wrists.

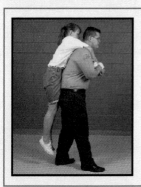

THE PACK STRAP CARRY Have patient stand. Turn your back to her, bringing her arms over your shoulders to cross your chest. Keep her arms as straight as possible, her armpits over your shoulders. Hold patient's wrists, bend, and pull her onto your back.

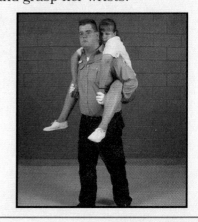

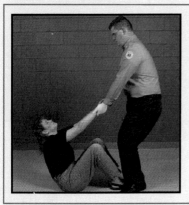

THE "FIREMAN'S CARRY" Place your feet against her feet and pull patient toward you. Bend at waist and flex knees. Duck and pull her across your shoulder, keeping hold of one of her wrists. Use your free arm to reach between her legs and grasp her thigh. Weight of patient falls onto your shoulders. Stand up. Transfer your grip on thigh to patient's wrist.

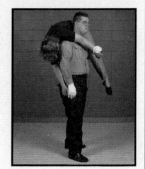

Emergency Moves—Two Rescuers

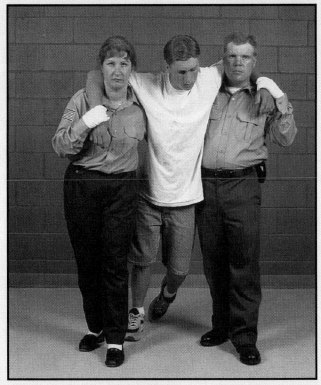

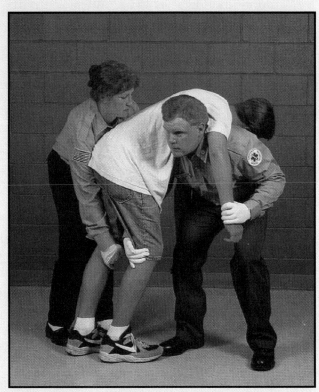

TWO-RESCUER ASSIST Patient's arms are placed around shoulders of both rescuers. They each grip a hand, place their free arms around patient's waist, then help him walk to safety.

"FIREMAN'S CARRY" WITH ASSIST Have someone help lift patient. The second rescuer helps to position patient.

injury to the patient and to avoid discomfort and pain.

In a non-urgent move, the patient is moved from the site of on-scene assessment and treatment (perhaps a bed or sofa, perhaps the floor or the ground outdoors) onto a patient carrying device.

Patient Carrying Devices

A patient carrying device is a stretcher or other device designed to carry the patient safely to the ambulance and/or to the hospital. The patient carrying devices described below are pictured in Scan 6-4.

Patient carrying devices are mechanical devices, and all EMT-Bs must be familiar with how to use them. Errors in use of these devices may result in injuries to yourself and the patient. For example, a stretcher that is not locked in position may collapse. Untended stretchers may simply roll away. Such an incident may be cause for a lawsuit if the patient is injured as a result of improper practices or faulty equipment. The devices must be regularly maintained and inspected. You should know the rating of each piece of equipment, that is, how much weight it will hold safely. Have alternatives available if the patient is too heavy or large for any device.

Wheeled Stretcher This device (Figure 6-4) is commonly referred to simply as "the stretcher" or "the cot." It is the device that is in the back of all ambulances. There are many brands and types of wheeled stretcher, but their purpose is the same: to safely transport a patient from one place to another, usually when the patient is in a reclining position. The head of the stretcher can be elevated, which will be beneficial for some patients, including cardiac patients, who have no suspected neck or spinal injuries.

Depending on the model, the stretcher will have variable levels. When moving the patient, the safest level is closest to the ground. Wheeling the stretcher in the elevated position raises the center of gravity, making it easier for the stretcher to tip over. The stretcher is ideal for level surfaces. Rough terrain and uneven surfaces may cause the stretcher to tip. Make sure to use proper body mechanics while placing the stretcher into or taking it out of the ambulance. Proper body mechanics are also important while wheeling the stretcher from place to place.

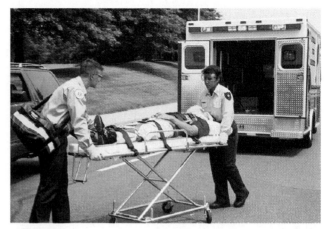

FIGURE 6-4 A wheeled stretcher is carried on every ambulance.

Remember, as discussed earlier in the chapter, odd numbers of EMT-Bs may cause the stretcher to become off-balance. When the stretcher is lifted, two EMT-Bs should lift at opposite ends of the stretcher—head and foot. The EMT-Bs should move to the sides of the stretcher to load it into the ambulance (Scan 6-5).

A stretcher can be carried by four EMT-Bs, one at each corner. This method can be useful on rough terrain because it helps keep the wheels from touching the ground and provides greater stability. It is also beneficial when carrying a patient a long distance because it divides the weight among four EMT-Bs instead of two.

The stretcher is the device that the patient will stay on during transport to the hospital. Make sure that it is always used in accordance with manufacturer's recommendations. Secure the patient to the stretcher before lifting or moving. After placing the patient into the ambulance, secure the stretcher to the ambulance. Ambulances have installed hardware for securing the stretcher while the ambulance is moving (Scan 6-5). Failure to secure the stretcher properly will cause it to shift during transit, causing an unsafe condition for the EMT-Bs as well as the patient.

Portable Stretcher Portable or folding stretchers may be beneficial in multiple-casualty incidents (incidents with many patients). The stretchers may be canvas, aluminum, or heavy plastic and usually fold or collapse.

Stair Chair The stair chair has many benefits for moving patients from the scene to the stretcher. The first benefit, as the name implies,

Patient Carrying Devices

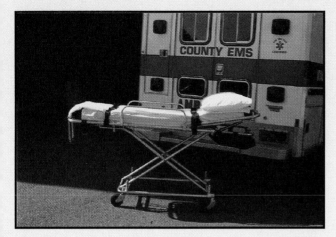

Wheeled Ambulance Stretcher

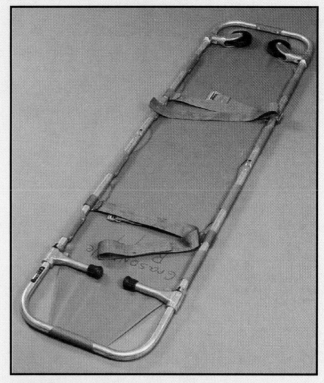

Portable Stretcher

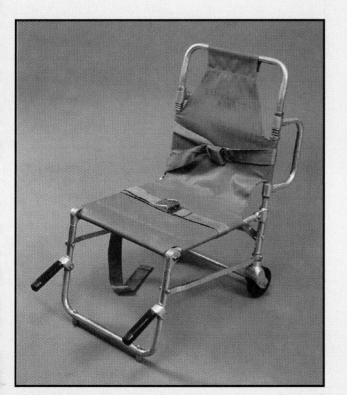

Stair Chair

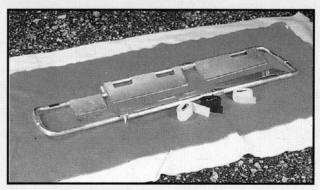

Scoop (Orthopedic) Stretcher

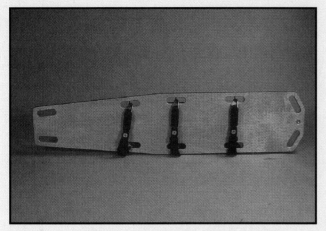

Long Spine Board

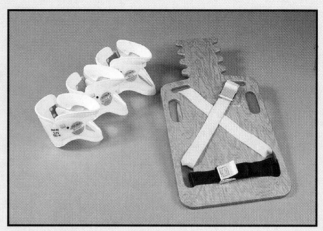

Short Spine Board

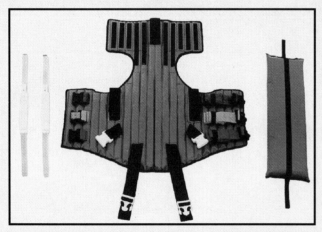

Vest-Type Extrication Device

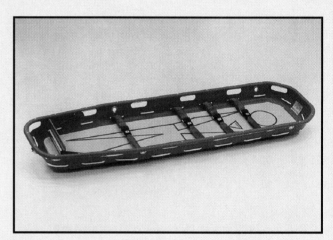

Basket Stretcher

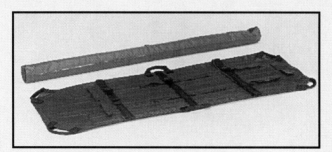

Flexible Stretcher

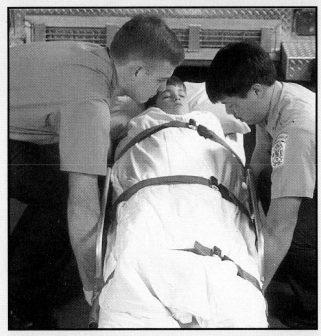

1. Clear interior of ambulance and lift rear step if necessary. Move stretcher as close to ambulance as possible. Lock stretcher in its lowest level before lifting. EMT-Bs position themselves on opposite sides of stretcher, bend at the knees, and grasp lower bar of stretcher frame.

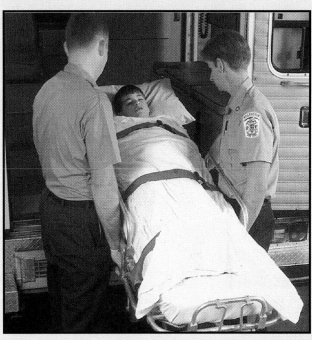

2. Both EMT-Bs come to a full standing position with their backs straight. Small sideways steps are used to move stretcher onto ambulance.

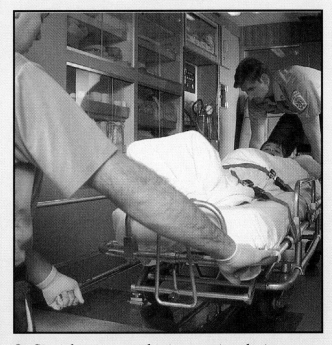

3. Stretcher is moved into securing device.

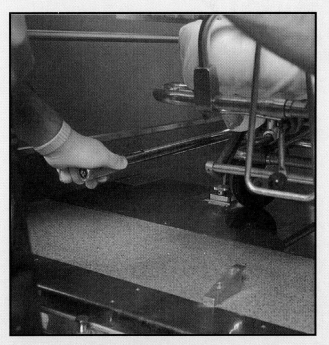

4. Both forward and rear catches are engaged.

is that it is excellent for use on stairs. Large stretchers often cannot be carried around tight corners and up or down narrow staircases. The stair chair transports the patient in a sitting position which greatly reduces the length of patient and device, allowing the EMT-B to maneuver around corners and through narrow spaces. It also has a set of wheels that allow the device to be rolled like a wheelchair over flat surfaces, preventing excess strain on the EMT-B and fatigue.

As with all devices in this chapter, there are times when the stair chair should be used and times when it shouldn't be used. The device is often ideal for patients with difficulty breathing. (You will learn about this in chapter 17, Respiratory Emergencies.) These patient usually find that they must sit up to breathe more easily, which the stair chair allows them to do. The stair chair must not be used for patients with neck or spinal injury because these patients must be placed supine on a backboard to prevent further injury.

Spine Boards There are two types of spine boards, or backboards: long and short. You will recall from On the Scene at the beginning of this chapter that the EMT-B who did not lift properly was placed on a long backboard. This device is used for patients who are found lying down or standing and must be immobilized. These devices are available in traditional wood as well as in plastics that resist splintering. (Splintered boards absorb body fluids, which may harbor infection.)

Short spine boards are used primarily for removing patients from vehicles when it is suspected that they have neck or spinal injuries. The short backboard can be slid between the patient's back and the seat back. Once secured to the short backboard, and wearing a rigid cervical collar, the patient can be moved from his sitting position in the vehicle to a supine position on a long spine board. Often, a vest-type extrication device is used in place of a short spine board. (You will learn more about extrication using short spine boards and vests in Chapter 28, Injuries to the Head and Spine.)

Scoop (Orthopedic) Stretcher This device is called the scoop stretcher because it splits into two pieces vertically. The scoop stretcher is favored by some since the patient can be "scooped" by the two halves of the stretcher (Figure 6-5). The scoop stretcher does not offer any support directly under the spine and is not rec-

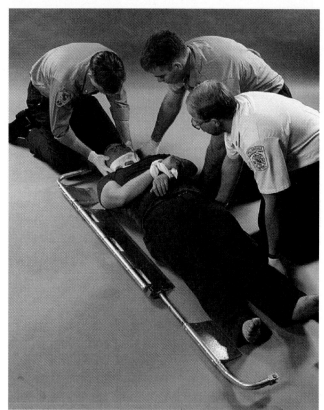

A.

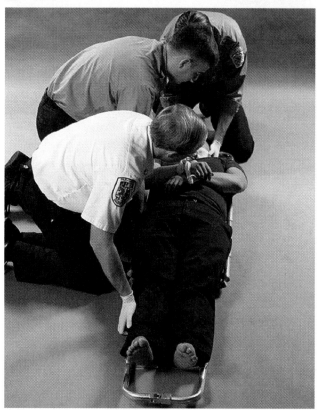

B.

FIGURE 6-5 Applying the scoop-style stretcher. **A.** One EMT carefully supports the patient's head while half of the stretcher is positioned. **B.** The stretcher halves are securely locked together and the head support is properly positioned.

ommended for patients with suspected spinal injury. Follow your local protocols on the use of this device.

Basket Stretcher A basket stretcher can be used to move a patient from one level to another or over rough terrain. The basket should be lined with a blanket before positioning the patient.

Flexible Stretcher A flexible stretcher is made of canvas or rubberized or other flexible material, often with wooden slats sewn into pockets and three carrying handles on each side. Because of its flexibility, it can be useful in restricted areas or narrow hallways.

Moving Patients onto Carrying Devices

There are several ways to move a patient onto a carrying device. You will choose a move based on the position the patient is in when it is time to move him to a carrying device and whether or not the patient is suspected of having a spine injury.

Patients with Suspected Spine Injury A patient who is suspected of having a spine injury must have his head, neck, and spine immobilized before being moved. After manual stabilization, you will place a rigid cervical collar on this patient. If he is seated in a vehicle, you will next immobilize him by a short spine board or vest and then on a long spine board (unless it is an urgent situation and you substitute the rapid extrication method with manual immobilization described under Urgent Moves, above). If the patient is lying down or standing, you will move him directly to a long spine board. The long spine board will then be placed on a wheeled ambulance stretcher for transport to the hospital. (You will learn more about cervical collars in Chapter 10, Focused History and Physical Exam—Trauma, and about immobilization for possible spine injury in Chapter 28, Injuries to the Head and Spine.)

Remember that immobilization is mandatory for any patient who has any possibility of a spine injury.

Patients with No Suspected Spine Injury The extremity lift, direct ground lift, bed-level lift, and draw-sheet method, listed below, are methods of moving a patient to a stretcher. *All are appropriate only for a patient with no suspected spine injury.* See Scan 6-6 for pictures and detailed descriptions of these methods.

- The **extremity lift** is used to carry a patient with no suspected spine or extremity injuries to a stretcher or a stair chair. It can be used to lift a patient from the ground or from a sitting position.
- The **direct ground lift** is performed when a patient with no suspected spine injury needs to be lifted from the ground to a stretcher.
- The **draw sheet method** is one of two methods (along with the direct carry method, below) that is performed during transfers between hospitals and nursing homes, or when a patient must be moved from a bed at home to a stretcher—for a patient with no suspected spine injury.
- The **direct carry method** is performed to move a patient with no suspected spine injury from a bed or from a bed-level position to a stretcher.

Patient Positioning

Positioning the patient during transfer to the ambulance and during transportation is a very important part of your care. Lifting, moving, and transportation must be performed as an integral part of your total patient care plan. The position in which the patient is transported depends on his medical condition and the device best designed to help this condition. Examples of patient conditions with the appropriate transportation position follow.

Unresponsive patients without suspected spinal injury should be placed in the recovery position (Figure 6-6). The patient should be on his side to aid drainage from his mouth and, if he vomits, to help prevent his breathing the vomitus into his lungs. This can be accomplished on a wheeled stretcher. You should avoid transporting the unresponsive patient in a chair-type device since the airway cannot be properly maintained.

Many patients who do not have suspected spinal injuries may be transported in a position of comfort. This includes many patients with medical complaints such as chest pain, nausea, or difficulty breathing. In this situation, allow the patient to choose a position he feels comfortable in. Breathing is often aided by raising the back of the stretcher so that the patient is in a semi-sitting position, also called Fowler's position (Figure 6-7). The position must be safe and not prohibit the proper use of any transportation device. The position of comfort must be used cautiously in case the patient vomits. Always

Non-Urgent Moves, No Suspected Spine Injury

Extremity Carry

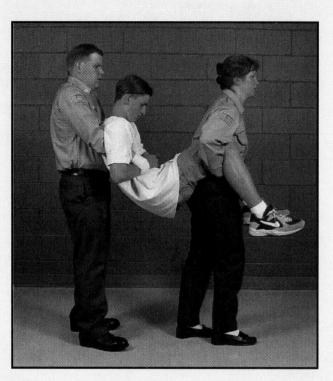

The extremity carry may be an emergency move or a non-urgent move for a patient with no suspected spine injury.

Place patient on back with knees flexed. Kneel at patient's head. Place your hands under his shoulders. Helper kneels at patient's feet and grasps patient's wrists. Helper lifts patient forward while you slip your arms under patient's armpits and grasp his wrists. Helper can grasp patient's knees while facing patient or turn and grasp patient's knees while facing away from patient. Direct helper so you both move to a crouch, then stand at the same time and move as a unit when carrying patient.

If patient is found sitting, crouch and slip your arms under patient's armpits and grasp his wrists. Helper crouches, then grasps patient's knees. Lift patient as a unit.

Draw Sheet Method

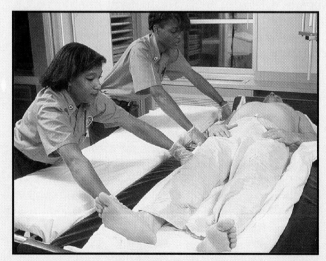

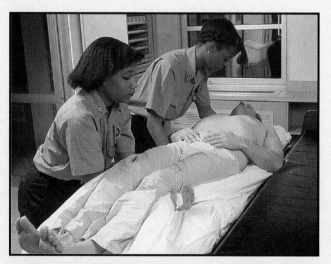

1. Loosen bottom sheet of bed and roll it from both sides toward patient. The stretcher, rails lowered, is placed parallel to bed, touching side of bed. EMT-Bs use their body and feet to lock the stretcher against the bed.

2. EMT-Bs pull on draw sheet to move patient to side of bed. They each use one hand to support patient while they reach under him to grasp draw sheet. EMT-Bs simultaneously draw patient onto stretcher.

Direct Ground Lift

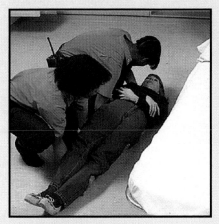

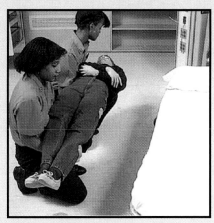

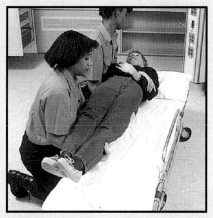

1. Stretcher is set in its lowest position and placed on opposite side of patient. EMT-Bs drop to one knee, facing patient. Patient's arms are placed on chest if possible. The head-end EMT-B cradles patient's head and neck by sliding one arm under patient's neck to grasp shoulder, the other arm under patient's lower back. The foot-end EMT-B slides one arm under the patient's knees and the other under the patient above the buttocks.

2. On a signal, they lift patient to their knees.

3. On a signal, they stand and carry patient to stretcher, drop to one knee, and roll forward to place patient onto mattress.

Note: If a third rescuer is available, he should place both arms under patient's waist while the other two slide their arms up to the mid back or down to the buttocks as appropriate.

Direct Carry

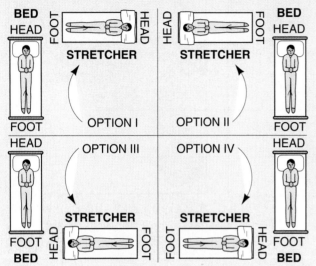

Stretcher is placed at 90° angle to bed, depending on room configuration. Prepare stretcher by lowering rails, unbuckling straps, and removing other items. Both EMT-Bs stand between stretcher and bed, facing patient.

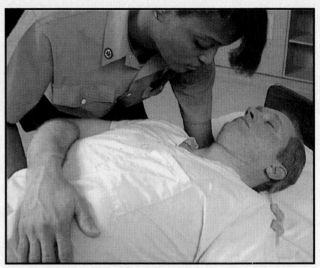

1. The head-end EMT-B cradles patient's head and neck by sliding one arm under patient's neck to grasp shoulder.

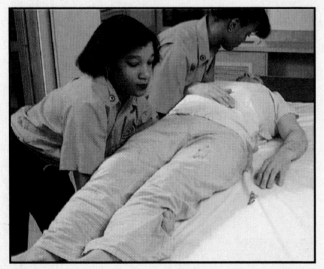

2. Foot end EMT-B slides hand under patient hip and lifts slightly. Head-end EMT-B slides other arm under patient's back. Foot-end EMT-B places arms under hips and calves.

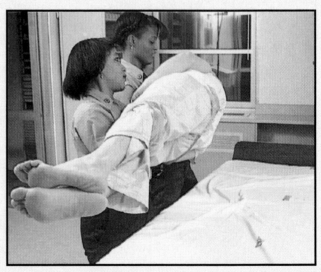

3. EMT-Bs slide patient to edge of bed and bend toward him with their knees slightly bent. They lift and curl patient to their chests and return to a standing position. They rotate and slide patient gently onto stretcher.

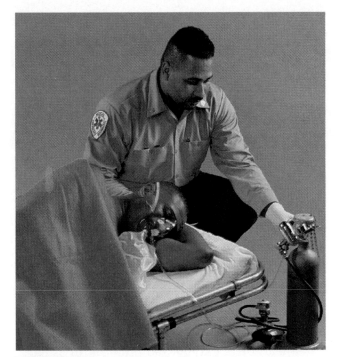

FIGURE 6-6 A patient in the recovery position.

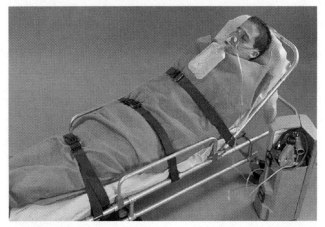

FIGURE 6-7 For many patients the position of comfort is a semi-sitting position.

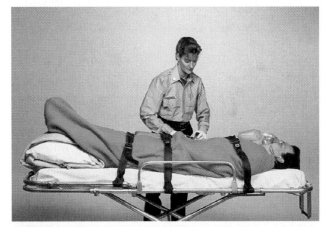

FIGURE 6-8 For a patient in shock, raise the legs 8 to 12 inches if there is no suspected spine injury.

monitor the patient's airway and level of consciousness. Place the patient into the recovery position at the first sign of a decreased level of consciousness.

If any patient has a suspected neck or spinal injury, he must be placed on a long backboard. Patients with spinal injuries who are found in a sitting position, such as in a vehicle, should also be affixed to a short backboard to prevent injuries while being moved.

Patients in shock for any reason require treatment for that condition (see Chapter 25, Bleeding and Shock). Elevate the patient's legs 8 to 12 inches. Do not risk harm to a spinal injury patient. For a patient with possible spinal injury, in general you should elevate the foot end of the backboard 8 to 12 inches so that the patient's entire body is inclined with the head 8 to 12 inches lower than the feet, often called the Trendelenburg position (Figure 6-8).

Transferring the Patient to a Hospital Stretcher

When you arrive at the hospital, you will move the patient from the ambulance stretcher to the hospital stretcher. You will probably use a modified draw sheet method to transfer the patient (Scan 6-7).

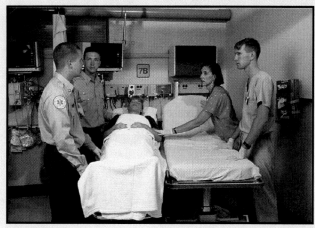

1. EMT-Bs position raised ambulance cot next to hospital stretcher. Hospital personnel adjust stretcher (raise or lower head) to receive patient from ambulance cot.

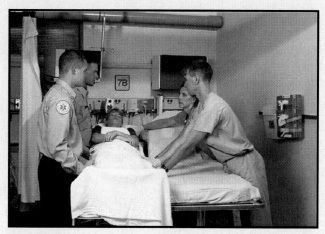

2. EMT-Bs and hospital personnel gather sheet on either side of patient and pull taut in order to transfer patient securely.

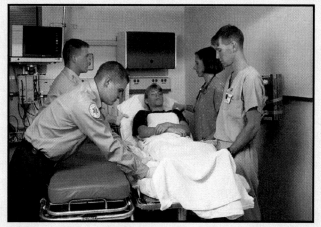

3. Holding gathered sheet at support points near shoulders, mid torso, hips, and knees, EMT-Bs and hospital personnel slide patient in one motion to hospital stretcher.

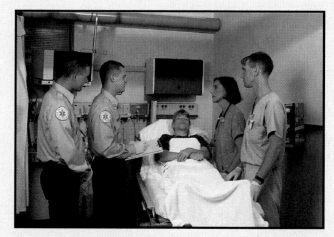

4. Assure patient is centered on stretcher. Make sure stretcher rails are raised before turning patient over to emergency department staff.

CHAPTER REVIEW

KEY TERMS

You may find it helpful to review the following terms.

body mechanics   the proper use of the body to facilitate lifting and moving and prevent injury.

direct carry method   a method of transferring a patient from bed to stretcher in which two or more rescuers curl the patient to their chests, then reverse the process to lower the patient to the stretcher.

direct ground lift   a method of lifting and carrying a patient from ground level to a stretcher in which two or more rescuers kneel, curl the patient to their chests, stand, then reverse the process to lower the patient to the stretcher.

draw sheet method   a method of transferring a patient from bed to stretcher by grasping and pulling the loosened bottom sheet of the bed.

extremity lift   a method of lifting and carrying a patient in which one rescuer slips hands under the patient's armpits and grasps the wrists, while another rescuer grasps the patient's knees.

power grip   gripping with as much hand surface as possible in contact with object being lifted, all fingers bent at the same angle, hands at least 10 inches apart.

power lift   also called the *squat lift position*. It is a lift from a squatting position with weight to be lifted close to the body, feet apart and flat on the ground, body weight on or just behind balls of feet, back locked in. The upper body is raised before the hips.

SUMMARY

Lifting and moving patients is a task that requires planning, proper equipment, and careful attention to body mechanics to prevent injury to yourself and your patient. While some may feel that this task is only secondary to patient care, *it is actually a critical part of your care.* Emergency moves are those that may aggravate spinal injuries and, therefore, are reserved for life-threatening situations. Urgent moves are used when the patient must be moved quickly but there is time to provide quick spinal stabi-

lization. Non-urgent moves are normal ways of moving a patient to a stretcher after complete on-scene assessment and any needed spinal stabilization have been completed.

Positioning the patient for transport should take into account the patient's comfort, medical needs, and safety. Remember the importance of correct lifting and moving techniques on every call. Protect your patient and protect yourself from injury to maintain a long and positive EMS experience.

REVIEW QUESTIONS

1. Define the term *body mechanics*. Describe several principles of body mechanics related to safe lifting and moving.
2. List several situations that may require an emergency move of a patient.
3. Describe several lifts and drags.
4. Define a long-axis drag and explain its importance.

Application

- For each of the following patients, use the knowledge gained in this chapter to identify the appropriate procedure or device for lifting and moving that patient.
  a. A patient who has fallen 18 feet and has suspected spinal injuries
  b. A patient with chest pain (without spinal injury) who lives on the fifth floor
  c. A patient who is found in an environment with a risk of immediate explosion

Module 2

Airway

MODULE OVERVIEW

There is only one chapter in this module, but it may be argued that it is the most important module in this textbook. *No patient will survive without an open airway.*

In your basic-life-support CPR course, you learned some fundamentals of airway care. This module reviews some of that material and includes new, important skills and information.

While your assessment of any patient begins with an examination of the airway, you should also understand that airway care must continue throughout the entire time you spend with a patient. This module will describe the use of devices and skills to improve the patient's airway and oxygen intake. These include oral and nasal airway adjuncts, suction, oxygen administration, and more. Devices to assist in ventilating a patient who is not breathing or is breathing inadequately are also covered.

Working hard to obtain the knowledge and skills presented in this chapter will surely mean the difference between life and death for many patients whom you treat in the field.

Airway Management

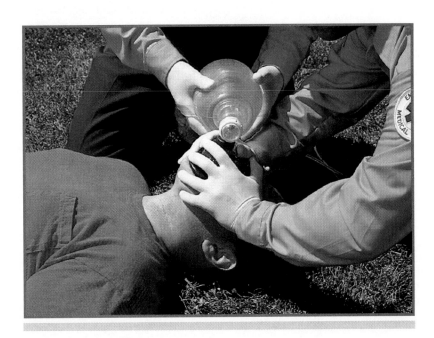

During your EMT-Basic course, you will learn the importance of the ABCs—airway, breathing, and circulation. It is no coincidence that the A for Airway in the ABCs is the first priority in treating every patient you will ever take care of as an EMT-B. Of all the skills you will learn in your EMT-B course, and subsequently use on real patients in the field, airway management is the most important. Simply stated, patients without an adequate airway die. No matter how good the care you may render to a critically ill or injured patient, if you cannot adequately clear and maintain the patient's airway, everything else you've done will be wasted because the patient will not be able to survive.

Knowledge and Attitude *At the end of this chapter, you should be able to meet the following objectives.*

1. Name and label the major structures of the respiratory system on a diagram. (pp. 114, 115)

2. List the signs of adequate breathing. (p. 115)

3. List the signs of inadequate breathing. (pp. 115–116)

4. Describe the steps in performing the head-tilt, chin-lift. (p. 119)

5. Relate mechanism of injury to opening the airway. (p. 119)

6. Describe the steps in performing the jaw thrust. (pp. 119–120)

7. State the importance of having a suction unit ready for immediate use when providing emergency care. (pp. 129–130)

8. Describe the techniques of suctioning. (pp. 131–133)

9. Describe how to artificially ventilate a patient with a pocket mask. (pp. 121–122)

10. Describe the steps in performing the skill of artificially ventilating a patient with a bag-valve mask while using the jaw thrust. (p. 123)

11. List the parts of a bag-valve-mask system. (p. 122)

12. Describe the steps in performing the skill of artificially ventilating a patient with a bag-valve mask for one and two rescuers. (pp. 123–124)

13. Describe the signs of adequate artificial ventilation using the bag-valve mask. (p. 120)

14. Describe the signs of inadequate artificial ventilation using the bag-valve mask. (p. 120)

15. Describe the steps in artificially ventilating a patient with a flow-restricted, oxygen-powered ventilation device. (pp. 124–125)

16. List the steps in performing the actions taken when providing mouth-to-mouth and mouth-to-stoma artificial ventilation. (pp. 120, 124)

17. Describe how to measure and insert an oropharyngeal (oral) airway. (pp. 126–128)

18. Describe how to measure and insert a nasopharyngeal (nasal) airway. (pp. 128–129)

19. Define the components of an oxygen delivery system. (pp. 134–138)

20. Identify a nonrebreather face mask and state the oxygen flow requirements needed for its use. (pp. 139, 143)

21. Describe the indications for using a nasal cannula versus a nonrebreather face mask. (pp. 139, 143)

22. Identify a nasal cannula and state the flow requirements needed for its use. (pp. 139, 143)

23. Explain the rationale for basic life support artificial ventilation and airway protective skills taking priority over most other basic life support skills. (pp. 111, 114)

24. Explain the rationale for providing adequate oxygenation through high inspired oxygen concentrations to patients who, in the past, may have received low concentrations. (p. 134)

Skills

1. Demonstrate the steps in performing the head-tilt, chin-lift.

2. Demonstrate the steps in performing the jaw thrust.

3. Demonstrate the techniques of suctioning.

4. Demonstrate the steps in providing mouth-to-mouth artificial ventilation with body substance isolation (barrier shields).

5. Demonstrate how to use a pocket mask to artificially ventilate a patient.

6. Demonstrate the assembly of a bag-valve-mask unit.

7. Demonstrate the steps in performing the skill of artificially ventilating a patient with a bag-valve mask for one and two rescuers.

8. Demonstrate the steps in performing the skill of artificially ventilating a patient with a bag-valve mask while using the jaw thrust.

9. Demonstrate artificial ventilation of a patient with a flow-restricted, oxygen-powered ventilation device.

10. Demonstrate how to artificially ventilate a patient with a stoma.

11. Demonstrate how to insert an oropharyngeal (oral) airway.

12. Demonstrate how to insert a nasopharyngeal (nasal) airway.

13. Demonstrate the correct operation of oxygen tanks and regulators.

14. Demonstrate the use of a nonrebreather face mask and state the oxygen flow requirements needed for its use.

15. Demonstrate the use of a nasal cannula and state the flow requirements for its use.

16. Demonstrate how to artificially ventilate the infant and child patient.

17. Demonstrate oxygen administration for the infant and child patient.

On the Scene

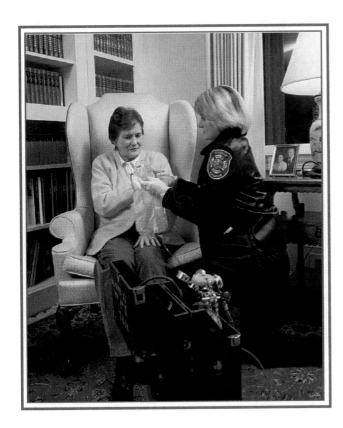

One evening, sixty-two-year-old Martha Quick is watching TV with her husband, Ralph, when she begins to feel chest pain. At first she tries to ignore it, but she finally tells Ralph, who immediately calls 911. On arrival, your *scene size-up* reveals no hazards. Mr. Quick leads you to his wife and introduces you to her. You ask Mrs. Quick if you may help her and she agrees. You quickly conduct your *initial assessment,* gaining a general impression of an alert older woman who is clutching at her chest and seems to be in pain. You discover no immediately life-threatening problems with her airway, breathing, or circulation. You begin the *focused history and physical exam.* As your partner takes her vital signs, you begin to take Mrs. Quick's history by asking about her chest pain.

You: Mrs. Quick, could you tell me about your pain?
Mrs. Quick: It's here. (She motions to the center of her chest.) It feels like something is squeezing my chest.
You: How bad is the pain?
Mrs. Quick: Oh! Well . . . it's bad. It's awful.
You: When you get chest pain, it may be your body's way of telling you that you need oxygen, so I'm going to put an oxygen mask on your face. This tube carries oxygen from the tank into the mask. It will provide a lot more oxygen than you get from breathing regular room air. The mask may feel a little uncomfortable, but it's important for you to get that extra oxygen, and it may help your pain.
Mrs. Quick: OK.

Mrs. Quick will continue to wear the oxygen mask throughout your exam and en route to the hospital.

You (as you prepare to transport her to the hospital): How is your pain now, Mrs. Quick?
Mrs. Quick (gratefully): It's a lot better.

En route to the hospital, you perform *ongoing assessment,* checking Mrs. Quick's vital signs, fit of the oxygen mask, and flow of the oxygen.

Oxygen is a drug. Since it is not in a pill or bad-tasting liquid, you may sometimes forget this fact. Oxygen is one of the best treatments you can provide as an EMT-B. In fact, you will probably administer oxygen on most emergency calls, since there are few patients who cannot benefit from oxygen—usually the sooner the better. Oxygen is used for many problems including injury, bleeding, shock, and—as the hospital confirmed in Mrs. Quick's case—heart problems.

Weeks later, you learn that Mrs. Quick is doing well under a doctor's guidance. The Quicks are both grateful for your prompt response and care.

T he cells of the human body must have oxygen. The reason the ABCs— airway, breathing, and circulation— are so important is that they are the means by which oxygen is brought into the body and carried to the cells. If the airway (the passageways that lead from the mouth and nose to the lungs) is not open, air cannot get into the body. If the patient is unable to breathe, air does not get into the body even if the airway is open. If the heart is not pumping blood through the lungs to pick up oxygen and circulate it around the body, an open airway and the ability to breathe are of no use. (In fact, breathing and heartbeat are so dependent on each other that if breathing stops first, heartbeat will stop very soon, or if heartbeat stops first, breathing will stop almost at once).

EMT-B training puts a great deal of emphasis on the airway—because it is so easy and so common for a patient's airway to become blocked and so easy to forget to monitor the patient's airway in the midst of an emergency when so many other details demand the EMT-B's attention.

The EMT-B's chief responsibilities (although not the only ones) are finding and correcting immediately life-threatening problems—airway, breathing, and circulation problems—and getting the patient to the hospital. As a prerequisite to your EMT-B course, you studied basic life support, including treating airway obstructions, performing rescue breathing, and performing cardiopulmonary resuscitation (CPR). You can review these topics by reading Basic Life Support: Airway, Rescue Breathing, and CPR in the back of this book.

In this chapter, you will learn additional EMT-B-level skills that relate to the airway, artificial ventilation, and oxygen therapy.

RESPIRATION

Another word for *breathing* is **respiration.** You learned about the respiratory system in Chapter 4. In preparation for this chapter, you should review the following structures of the respiratory system and be able to label them on a blank diagram of the respiratory system (Figure 7-1).

- Nose
- Mouth
- Oropharynx
- Nasopharynx
- Epiglottis
- Trachea
- Cricoid cartilage
- Larynx (voice box)
- Bronchi (right and left mainstem)
- Lungs
- Alveoli
- Diaphragm

Also review, in Chapter 4, how oxygen and carbon dioxide are exchanged through the alveoli of the lungs, and through the capillaries in the lungs and at the cells.

Adequate and Inadequate Breathing

The function of the respiratory system is to enable the body to inhale (breathe in) oxygen, which is then used by all the cells and organs in the body, and to exhale (breathe out) carbon dioxide, the major waste product of respiration. If either of these vital functions is disrupted, then the patient is likely to develop the sensation of shortness of breath and be at risk of respiratory failure.

Simply stated, **respiratory failure** is the reduction of breathing to the point where oxygen intake is not sufficient to support life. When breathing stops completely, the patient is in **respiratory arrest.** Respiratory arrest can develop during heart attack, stroke, airway obstruction, drowning, electrocution, drug overdose, poisoning, brain injury, severe chest injury, suffocation, and prolonged respiratory failure.

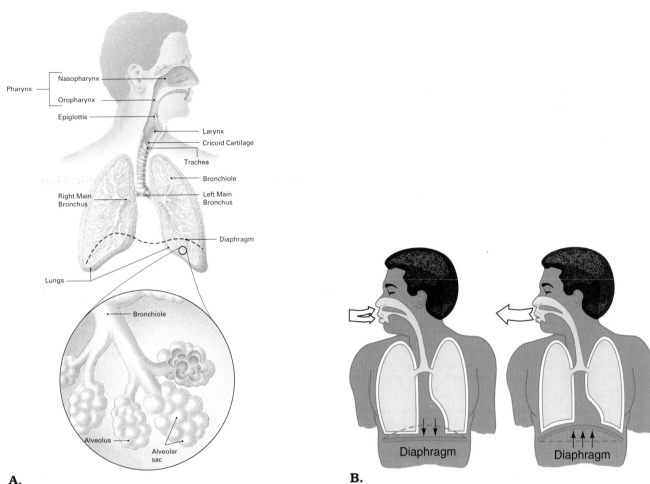

A.
B.

FIGURE 7-1 A. The respiratory system. B. The lungs and the diaphragm.

Patient Assessment—Respiratory Failure or Respiratory Arrest

As an EMT-B, you must be able to determine whether or not a patient is breathing adequately so that you can undertake appropriate airway management.

Signs

To determine the signs of ADEQUATE BREATHING, you should

☐ LOOK for adequate and equal expansion of both sides of the chest with inhalation.
☐ LISTEN for air entering and leaving the nose, mouth, and chest. The breath sounds should be present and equal on both sides of the chest. The sounds from the mouth and nose should be typically free of gurgling, gasping, crowing, and wheezing.

☐ FEEL for air moving out of the nose or mouth.
☐ Check for typical skin coloration. There should be no blue or gray colorations.
☐ Note a rate, rhythm, quality, and depth of breathing typical for a person at rest (Table 7-1).

The following are signs of INADEQUATE BREATHING.

☐ Chest movements are absent, minimal, or uneven.
☐ Movements associated with breathing are limited to the abdomen (abdominal breathing).
☐ No air can be felt or heard at the nose or mouth, or the amount of air exchanged is evaluated to be below normal.
☐ Breath sounds are diminished or absent.

TABLE 7-1 Adequate Breathing

Normal Rates
Adult—12-20 per minute
Child—15-30 per minute
Infant—25-50 per minute

Rhythm
Regular

Quality
Breath sounds—present and equal
Chest expansion—adequate and equal
Minimum effort

Depth
Adequate

☐ Noises such as wheezing, snoring, gurgling, or gasping are heard during breathing.

☐ The rate of breathing is too rapid or slow—above or below normal rates (see Table 7-1 and Chapter 5, Baseline Vital Signs).

☐ Breathing is very shallow, very deep, or appears labored.

☐ The patient's skin, lips, tongue, ear lobes, or nail beds are blue or gray. This is called **cyanosis** (SIGH-uh-NO-sis). The patient is said to be *cyanotic* (SIGH-uh-NOT-ik).

☐ Inspirations are prolonged (indicating a possible upper airway obstruction) or expirations are prolonged (indicating a possible lower airway obstruction).

☐ The patient is unable to speak, or the patient cannot speak full sentences because of shortness of breath.

☐ In children, there may be retractions (a pulling in of the muscles) above the clavicles and between and below the ribs.

☐ Nasal flaring (widening of the nostrils of the nose) may be present, especially in infants and children.

Patient Care—Respiratory Failure or Respiratory Arrest

When the patient's signs indicate inadequate or no breathing (respiratory failure or respiratory arrest), this is a life-threatening situation, and prompt action must be taken. The princi-

pal procedures by which life-threatening respiratory problems are treated are

☐ Opening and maintaining the airway
☐ Providing artificial ventilation to the non-breathing patient and the patient with inadequate breathing
☐ Providing supplemental oxygen to the breathing patient

These procedures will be discussed below.

OPENING THE AIRWAY

The **airway** is the passageway by which air enters or leaves the body. The structures of the airway are the nose, mouth, pharynx, larynx, trachea, bronchi, and lungs. The procedures for airway evaluation, opening the airway, and artificial ventilation are best carried out with the patient lying supine, or flat on his back. Often you will find a patient already supine in bed and can perform airway procedures with the patient in this position. Scan 7-1 illustrates the technique for positioning a patient found lying on the floor or ground. Patients who are found in positions other than supine or on the ground should be moved to a supine position on the floor or stretcher for evaluation and treatment (Figure 7-2).

Any movement of a trauma (injured) patient before immobilization of the head and spine can produce serious injury to the spinal cord. If injury is suspected, protect the head and neck as you position the patient. Airway and breathing, however, have priority over protection of the spine and must be assured as quickly as possible. If the trauma patient must be moved in order to open the airway or to provide ventilations, you will probably not have time to provide immobilization with a cervical collar or head immobilization device on a stretcher but, instead, will provide as much manual stabilization as possible, as shown in Scan 7-1.

Use the following as indications that head, neck, or spinal injury may have occurred—especially when the patient is unconscious and cannot tell you what happened.

- The mechanism of injury is one that can cause head, neck, or spinal injury. A patient who is found on the ground near a ladder or stairs, for example, may have such injuries. Motor vehicle collisions are

Positioning the Patient for Basic Life Support

This maneuver is used when the rescuer must act alone.

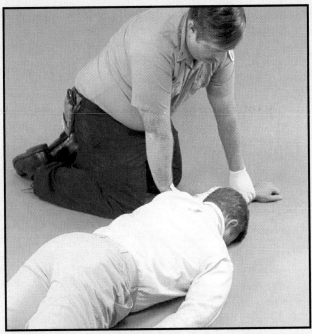

1. Straighten the legs and position the closest arm above the head.

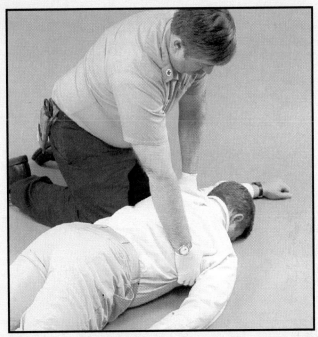

2. Cradle the head and neck. Grasp under the distant armpit.

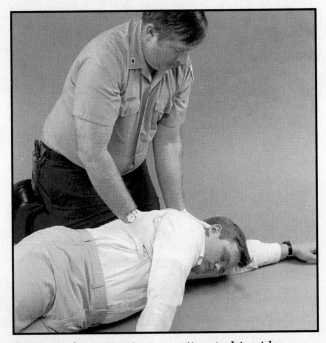

3. Move the patient as a unit onto his side.

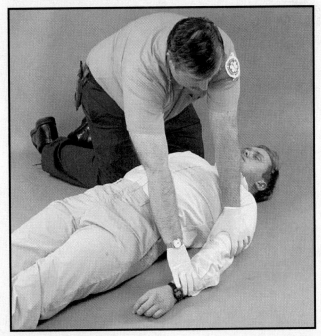

4. Move the patient onto his back and reposition the extended arm.

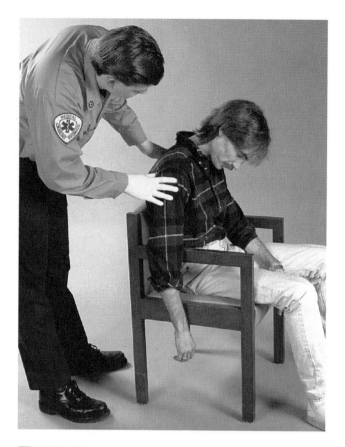

• Family or bystanders may tell you that an injury to the head, neck, or spine has occurred or may give you information that leads you to suspect it.

As an EMT-B you must open and maintain the airway in any patient who cannot do so for himself. This includes patients who have altered mental status, are unconscious, or are in respiratory or cardiac arrest.

Most airway problems are caused by the tongue. As the head flexes forward, the tongue may slide into the airway, causing an obstruction. If the patient is unconscious, the tongue loses muscle tone and muscles of the lower jaw relax. Since the tongue is attached to the lower jaw, the risk of airway obstruction by the tongue is even greater during unconsciousness. The basic procedures for opening the airway help to correct the position of the tongue (Figure 7-3).

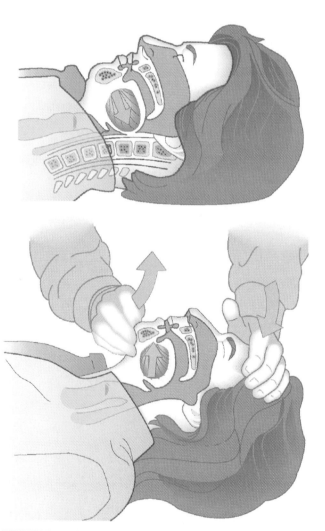

FIGURE 7-2 Positioning the patient for airway evaluation and care.

another common cause of head, neck, and spinal injuries.
• Any injury at or above the level of the shoulders indicates that head, neck, or spinal injuries may also be present.

FIGURE 7-3 Procedures for opening the airway to help reposition the tongue.

There are two procedures commonly recommended for opening the airway: the head-tilt, chin-lift maneuver and the jaw-thrust maneuver—the latter being recommended when head, neck, or spinal injury is suspected.

Head-Tilt, Chin-Lift Maneuver

The **head-tilt, chin-lift maneuver** (Figure 7-4) provides for the maximum opening of the airway. It is useful on all patients who are in need of assistance in maintaining an airway or breathing. It is one of the best methods for correcting obstructions caused by the tongue.

Warning: IF ANY INDICATION OF HEAD, NECK, OR SPINE INJURY IS PRESENT, DO NOT USE THE HEAD-TILT, CHIN-LIFT MANEUVER. Remember that any unconscious and many conscious trauma patients may be suspected of having an injury to the head, neck, or spine.

Follow these steps to perform the head-tilt, chin-lift maneuver.

1. Once the patient is supine, place one hand on the forehead and place the fingertips of the other hand under the bony area at the center of the patient's lower jaw.
2. Tilt the head by applying gentle pressure to the patient's forehead.

3. Use your fingertips to lift the chin and to support the lower jaw. Move the jaw forward to a point where the lower teeth are almost touching the upper teeth. *Do not* compress the soft tissues under the lower jaw, which can obstruct the airway.
4. *Do not* allow the patient's mouth to be closed. To provide an adequate opening at the mouth, you may need to use the thumb of the hand supporting the chin to pull back the patient's lower lip. *Do not* insert your thumb into the patient's mouth.

Jaw-Thrust Maneuver

The **jaw-thrust maneuver** (Figure 7-5) is most commonly used to open the airway of an unconscious patient or one with suspected head, neck, or spinal injuries.

Note: THE JAW-THRUST MANEUVER IS THE ONLY RECOMMENDED PROCEDURE FOR USE ON UNCONSCIOUS PATIENTS OR PATIENTS WITH POSSIBLE HEAD, NECK, OR SPINAL INJURIES.

Follow these steps to perform the jaw-thrust maneuver.

1. Carefully keep the patient's head, neck, and spine aligned, moving him as a unit as you place him in the supine position.

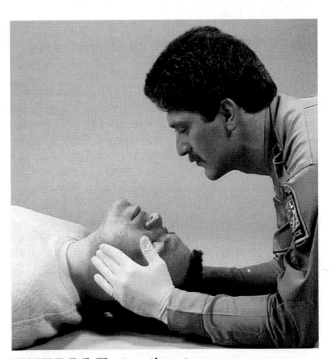

FIGURE 7-4 The head-tilt, chin-lift maneuver.

FIGURE 7-5 The jaw-thrust maneuver.

2. Kneel at the top of the patient's head, resting your elbows on the same surface on which the patient is lying.

3. Carefully reach forward and gently place one hand on each side of the patient's lower jaw, at the angles of the jaw below the ears.

4. Stabilize the patient's head with your forearms.

5. Using your index fingers, push the angles of the patient's lower jaw forward.

6. You may need to retract the patient's lower lip with your thumb to keep the mouth open.

7. *Do not* tilt or rotate the patient's head. REMEMBER, THE PURPOSE OF THE JAW-THRUST MANEUVER IS TO OPEN THE AIRWAY WITHOUT MOVING THE HEAD OR NECK.

In addition to physically opening the airway with the head-tilt chin-lift or the jaw-thrust maneuver, it is imperative that the airway also be cleared of any secretions, blood, or vomitus. The most effective way to clear the patient's airway is with a wide-bore, rigid-tipped suction device. For this reason it is crucial that a suction unit be ready for immediate use when opening and maintaining the airway. The specific equipment and techniques used for suctioning will be discussed later in this chapter.

TECHNIQUES OF ARTIFICIAL VENTILATION

If you determine that the patient is not breathing or that the respiratory efforts are so minimal that respiratory arrest is imminent, you will have to provide artificial ventilation. **Ventilation** is the breathing in of air or oxygen. **Artificial ventilation** is forcing air or oxygen into the lungs when a patient has stopped breathing or has inadequate breathing. There are various techniques available to you as an EMT-B with which you can provide artificial ventilations. In order of preference they are

1. Mouth-to-mask (preferably with high-flow supplemental oxygen at 15 liters per minute)

2. Two-person bag-valve mask (preferably with high-flow supplemental oxygen at 15 liters per minute)

3. Flow restricted, oxygen-powered ventilation device

4. One-person bag-valve mask

No matter what method is used to ventilate the patient, you should assure that the patient is being adequately ventilated. To determine the signs of ADEQUATE ARTIFICIAL VENTILATION, you should

- Watch the chest rise and fall with each ventilation.
- See the patient's heart rate return to normal with artificial ventilation.
- Assure that the rate of ventilation is sufficient—approximately 12 per minute in adults and 20 per minute in children.

INADEQUATE ARTIFICIAL VENTILATION occurs when

- The chest does not rise and fall with ventilations.
- The patient's heart rate does not return to normal with artificial ventilations.
- The rate of ventilation is too fast or too slow.

Techniques used for artificial ventilation should also assure adequate isolation of the rescuer from the patient's body fluids, including saliva, blood, and vomit. For this reason, mouth-to-mouth ventilation (described in Basic Life Support: Airway, Rescue Breathing, and CPR at the back of this book) is not recommended unless there is no alternative method of artificial ventilation available. There are a number of compact barrier devices available for personal use (Figure 7-6), which will be described below.

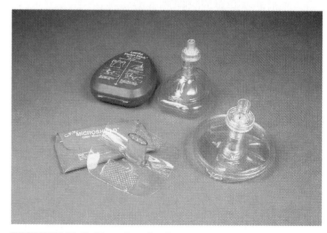

FIGURE 7-6 Barrier devices.

Mouth-to Mask Ventilation

Mouth-to-mask ventilation is performed using a **pocket face mask.** The pocket face mask is made of soft, collapsible material and can be carried in your pocket, jacket, or purse (Figure 7-7). Many EMT-Bs purchase their own pocket face masks for their workplace or automobile first aid kits.

Face masks have important infection control features. Your ventilations (breaths) are delivered through a valve in the mask so that you do not have direct contact with the patient's mouth. Most pocket masks have one-way valves that allow your ventilations to enter but prevent the patient's exhaled air from coming back through the valve and into contact with you.

Some pocket masks have oxygen inlets. When high concentration oxygen is attached to the inlet, an oxygen concentration of approximately 50% is delivered. This is significantly better than the 16% delivered by mouth-to-mask ventilations without oxygen.

Most pocket face masks are made of a clear plastic. This is important because you must be able to observe the patient's mouth and nose for vomiting or secretions that need to be suctioned. You also need to observe the color of the lips, an indicator of the respiratory status of the patient. Some pocket face masks may have a strap that goes around the patient's head. This is helpful during one-rescuer CPR, since it will hold the mask on the patient's face while you are performing chest compressions. However, it does not replace the need for proper hand placement described below.

To provide mouth-to-mask ventilation, you should

1. Position yourself at the patient's head and open the airway. It may be necessary to clear the airway of obstructions. If necessary, insert an oropharyngeal airway (see later in this chapter) to help keep the patient's airway open.
2. Connect oxygen to the inlet on the face mask. Oxygen should be run at 12 to 15 liters per minute. *If oxygen is not immediately available, do not delay mouth-to-mask ventilations.*
3. Position the mask on the patient's face so that the apex (top of the triangle) is over the bridge of the nose and the base is between the lower lip and prominence of the chin.
4. Hold the mask firmly in place while maintaining the proper head tilt (Figure 7-8) by placing

   - Both thumbs on the sides of the mask
   - Index, third and fourth fingers of each hand grasping the lower jaw on each side between the angle of the jaw and the ear lobe to lift the jaw forward

5. Take a deep breath and exhale into the mask port or one-way valve at the top of the mask port. Each ventilation should be delivered over 1½ to 2 seconds in adults, 1 to 1½ seconds in infants and children. Watch for the patient's chest to rise.
6. Remove your mouth from the port and allow for passive exhalation. Continue as you would for mouth-to-mouth ventilations or CPR (see Basic Life Support: Airway, Rescue Breathing, and CPR at the end of this book).

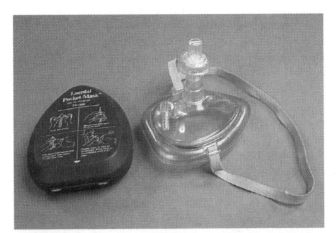

FIGURE 7-7 The pocket face mask has a chimney with a one-way valve for mouth-to-mask ventilations.

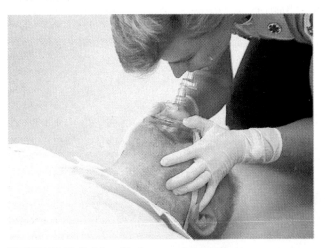

FIGURE 7-8 Mouth-to-mask ventilations.

When properly used, the pocket face mask will deliver higher volumes of air to the patient than the bag-valve-mask device.

The Bag-Valve Mask

The **bag-valve mask** is a hand-held ventilation device. It may also be referred to as a bag-valve-mask unit, system, device, resuscitator, or simply BVM. The bag-valve-mask unit can be used to ventilate a nonbreathing patient and is also helpful to assist ventilations in the patient whose own respiratory attempts are not enough to support life, such as a patient in respiratory failure or drug overdose. The BVM also provides an infection-control barrier between you and your patient. The use of the bag-valve mask in the field is often referred to as "bagging" the patient.

Bag-valve-mask units come in sizes for infants, children, and adults (Figure 7-9). Many different types of bag-valve-mask systems are available; however, all have the same basic parts as shown in Figure 7-10. The bag must be a self-refilling shell that is easily cleaned and sterilized. The system must have a non-jam valve that allows an oxygen inlet flow of 15 liters per minute. The valve should be nonrebreathing (preventing the patient from rebreathing his own exhalations) and not subject to freezing in cold temperatures. Most systems have a standard 15/22 mm respiratory fitting to ensure a proper fit with other respiratory equipment, face masks, and endotracheal tubes.

Warning: Many older bag-valve masks have "pop-off" valves. These valves were designed to

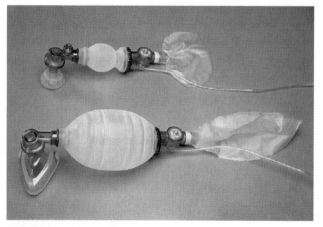

FIGURE 7-9 Pediatric and adult bag-valve-mask units.

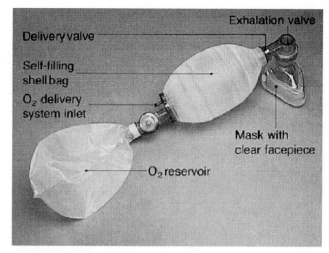

FIGURE 7-10 The typical bag-valve-mask system.

open after certain pressures were obtained. Studies have shown that pop-off valves may prevent adequate ventilations. BVM systems with pop-off valves should be replaced. BVM systems should also have a clear face mask so that you can observe the lips for cyanosis and monitor the airway in case suctioning is needed.

The mechanical workings of a bag-valve mask device are simple. Oxygen, flowing at 15 liters per minute, is attached to the BVM and enters the reservoir. When the bag is squeezed, the air inlet to the bag is closed, and the oxygen is delivered to the patient. BVM systems without a reservoir supply approximately 50% oxygen. Systems with an oxygen reservoir provide nearly 100% oxygen.

When the squeeze of the bag is released, a passive expiration by the patient will occur. While the patient exhales, oxygen enters the reservoir to be delivered to the patient the next time the bag is squeezed. The bag itself will hold anywhere from 1,000 to 1,600 milliliters of air, depending on the age of the BVM system. Newer models are designed to hold more air. According to American Heart Association guidelines, at least 800 milliliters of air must be delivered to the patient. This means that the bag-valve mask system must be used properly and efficiently.

The most difficult part of delivering BVM artificial ventilations is obtaining an adequate mask seal so that air does not leak in or out around the edges. It is difficult to maintain the seal with one hand while squeezing the bag with the other, and one-person bag-valve-mask operation is often unsuccessful or inadequate for this reason. Therefore it is recommended that BVM artificial ventilation be performed by two rescuers. In two-person BVM ventilation, one person is assigned to squeeze the bag while the other person uses two hands to maintain a mask seal.

The two-person technique can also be modified so that the jaw-thrust can be used during BVM ventilations. This technique is to be used when performing BVM ventilation on a patient with a suspected head, neck, or spinal injury.

To perform BVM ventilation when no trauma (injury) is suspected (Figure 7-11A)

1. Open the patient's airway USING THE HEAD-TILT, CHIN-LIFT TECHNIQUE. Suction and insert an airway adjunct (see later in this chapter) as necessary.
2. Select the correct bag-valve mask size (adult, child, or infant).
3. Kneel at the patient's head. Position thumbs over the top half of the mask, index and middle fingers over the bottom half.
4. Place the apex, or top, of the triangular mask over the bridge of the patient's nose, then lower the mask over the mouth and upper chin. If the mask has a large, round cuff surrounding a ventilation port, center the port over the patient's mouth.
5. Use ring and little fingers to bring the patient's jaw up to the mask and MAINTAIN THE HEAD-TILT, CHIN-LIFT.
6. The second rescuer should connect bag to mask, if not already done. While you maintain the mask seal, second rescuer should squeeze the bag with two hands until the patient's chest rises. Second rescuer should squeeze the bag ONCE EVERY 5 SECONDS FOR AN ADULT, ONCE EVERY 3 SECONDS FOR A CHILD OR INFANT.
7. The second rescuer should release pressure on the bag and let the patient exhale passively. While this occurs the bag is refilling from the oxygen source.

To perform BVM ventilation when trauma is suspected (Figure 7-11B)

1. Open the patient's airway USING THE JAW-THRUST TECHNIQUE. Suction and insert an airway adjunct (see later in this chapter) as necessary.
2. Select the correct bag-valve mask size (adult, child, or infant).

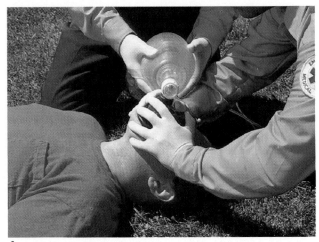

A.

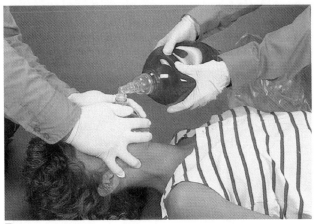

B.

FIGURE 7-11 A. Providing bag-valve-mask ventilations when there is no suspected trauma. B. Providing bag-valve-mask ventilations when trauma is suspected.

3. Kneel at the patient's head. Place thumbs over the nose portion of the mask and place your index and middle fingers over the portion of the mask that covers the mouth.
4. Use your ring and little fingers to bring the jaw upward, toward the mask, WITHOUT TILTING THE HEAD OR NECK.
5. The second rescuer should squeeze the bag to ventilate the patient as described above for the non-trauma patient.

As noted above, use of a bag-valve mask by a single rescuer is the last choice of artificial ventilation procedure behind use of a pocket mask with supplemental oxygen, a two-person bag-valve mask procedure, and use of a flow-restricted, oxygen-powered ventilation device (see below). You should provide ventilations with a one-person bag-valve-mask procedure only when no other options are available.

When using the bag-valve mask device alone you should

1. Position yourself at the patient's head and establish an open airway. Suction and insert an airway adjunct (see later in this chapter) as necessary.
2. Select the correct size mask for the patient. Position the mask on the patient's face as described above for the two-person BVM technique.
3. Form a "C" around the ventilation port with thumb and index finger. Use middle, ring, and little fingers under the patient's jaw to hold the jaw to the mask.
4. With your other hand, squeeze the bag *once every 5 seconds.* The squeeze should be a full one, causing the patient's chest to rise. For infants and children, squeeze the bag *once every 3 seconds.*
5. Release pressure on the bag and let the patient exhale passively. While this occurs the bag is refilling from the oxygen source.

If the chest does not rise and fall during BVM ventilation, you should

1. Reposition the head.
2. Check for escape of air around the mask and reposition fingers and mask.
3. Check for airway obstruction or obstruction in the BVM system. Resuction if necessary. Consider insertion of an airway adjunct if not already done.
4. If none of the above methods work, use an alternative method of artificial ventilation, such as a pocket mask or a flow-restricted, oxygen-powered ventilation device (see below).

The BVM may also be used during CPR (Figure 7-12). The bag is squeezed once each time a ventilation is to be delivered. In one-rescuer CPR, it is preferable to use a pocket mask with supplemental oxygen rather than a BVM system. A single rescuer would take too much time picking up the BVM and obtaining a face seal each time a ventilation is to be delivered, in addition to the normal difficulty in maintaining a seal with the one-person BVM technique.

Finally, the BVM can be used to artificially ventilate patients with a stoma or tracheostomy tube. Patients with stomas who are found to be in severe respiratory distress or respiratory arrest frequently have thick secretions blocking the stoma. It is recommended that you suction the stoma frequently in conjunction with BVM-

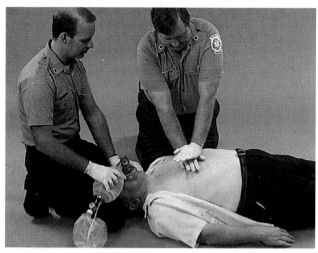

FIGURE 7-12 Two-rescuer CPR using a bag-valve-mask system.

to-stoma ventilations. As with other BVM uses, a two-person technique is preferred over a one-person technique. To provide artificial ventilation to a stoma breather with a BVM you should

1. Clear any mucus plugs or secretions from the stoma.
2. Leave the head and neck in a neutral position, as it is unnecessary to position the airway prior to ventilations in a stoma breather.
3. Use a pediatric-sized mask to establish a seal around the stoma.
4. Ventilate at the appropriate rate for the patient's age.
5. If unable to artificially ventilate through the stoma, consider sealing the stoma and attempting artificial ventilation through the mouth and nose. (This may work if the trachea is still connected to the passageways of mouth, nose, and pharynx. In some cases, the trachea has been permanently connected to the neck opening with no remaining connection to mouth, nose, or pharynx.)

Bag-valve mask devices should be completely disassembled and disinfected after each use. Because proper decontamination is often costly and time consuming, many hospitals and EMS agencies use single-use disposable BVMs.

The Flow Restricted, Oxygen-Powered Ventilation Device

A **flow-restricted, oxygen-powered ventilation device (FROPVD)** uses oxygen under pressure to deliver artificial ventilations through a mask placed over the patient's face. This device is similar to the traditional demand-valve resuscitator but includes newer features designed to optimize ventilations and safeguard the patient (Figure 7-13). Recommended features include

- A peak flow rate of 100% oxygen at up to 40 liters per minute
- An inspiratory pressure relief valve that opens at approximately 60 cm of water pressure
- An audible alarm when the relief valve is activated
- A rugged design and construction
- A trigger that enables the rescuer to use both hands to maintain a mask seal while triggering the device
- Satisfactory operation in both ordinary and extreme environmental conditions

Follow the same procedures for mask seal as recommended for the BVM. Trigger the device until the chest rises and REPEAT EVERY 5 SECONDS. If the chest does not rise, reposition the head, check the mask seal, check for obstructions, and consider the use of an alternative artificial ventilation procedure.

If neck injury is suspected, have an assistant hold the patient's head manually or use your knees to prevent movement. Bring the jaw up to the mask without tilting the head or neck.

The flow-restricted, oxygen-powered ventilation device should be used only on adults.

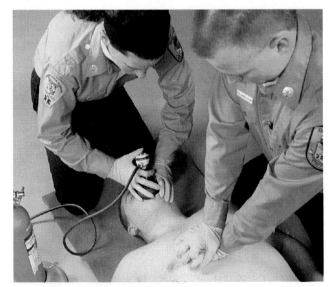

FIGURE 7-13 Providing ventilations with a flow-restricted, oxygen-powered ventilation device.

AIRWAY ADJUNCTS

Once you gain access to a patient and begin your initial assessment, your first course of action is to establish an open airway. This airway must be maintained throughout all care procedures.

The most common impediment to an open airway is the tongue. When a patient becomes unconscious, the muscles relax. The tongue will slide back into the pharynx and obstruct the airway. Even though a head-tilt, chin-lift or jaw-thrust maneuver will help open the airway of a patient, the tongue may return to its obstructive position once the maneuver is released. Sometimes even when the head-tilt, chin-lift or jaw-thrust is maintained, the tongue will "fall back" into the pharynx.

Airway adjuncts, devices that aid in maintaining an open airway, may be used early in the treatment of the unresponsive patient and continue throughout your care. There are several types of airway adjuncts. In this chapter, only the devices that are a part of the standard EMT-Basic course—those whose main function is to keep the tongue from blocking the airway—will be discussed.

The two most common airway adjuncts for the EMT-B to use are the **oropharyngeal airway** and the **nasopharyngeal airway.** The structure and use of these airways can be understood by analyzing their names. *Oro* refers to the mouth, *naso* the *nose,* and *pharyngeal* the throat. Oropharyngeal airways are inserted into the mouth and help keep the tongue from falling back into the throat. Nasopharyngeal airways are inserted through the nose and rest in the throat, also helping keep the tongue from becoming an airway obstruction.

Rules for Using Airway Adjuncts

Some general rules apply to the use of oropharyngeal and the nasopharyngeal airways.

- Use an airway on all unconscious patients who do not exhibit a **gag reflex.** The gag reflex causes vomiting or retching when something is placed in the throat. When a patient is deeply unconscious, the gag reflex usually disappears but may reappear as a patient begins to regain consciousness. A patient with a gag reflex who cannot tolerate an oropharyngeal airway may be able to tolerate a nasopharyngeal airway.

- Open the patient's airway manually before using an adjunct device.
- When inserting the airway, take care not to push the patient's tongue into the throat.
- Do not continue inserting the airway if the patient begins to gag. Continue to maintain the airway manually and *do not* use an adjunct device. If the patient remains unconscious for a prolonged time, you may later attempt to insert an airway to determine if the gag reflex is still present.
- When an airway adjunct is in place, YOU MUST MAINTAIN HEAD-TILT, CHIN-LIFT OR JAW THRUST AND MONITOR THE AIRWAY.
- When an airway adjunct is in place, YOU MUST STILL REMAIN READY TO SUCTION THE PATIENT'S AIRWAY to clear secretions as necessary.
- If the patient regains consciousness or develops a gag reflex, remove the airway immediately.
- Use infection control practices while maintaining the airway. Wear disposable gloves. In airway maintenance, there is a chance of a patient's body fluids coming in contact with your face and eyes. Wear mask and goggles or other protective eyewear to prevent this contact.

Oropharyngeal Airways

Once a patient's airway is opened, an oropharyngeal airway can be inserted to help keep it open. An oropharyngeal airway is a curved device, usually made of plastic, that can be inserted through the patient's mouth. The oropharyngeal airway has a flange that will rest against the patient's lips. The rest of the device holds the tongue as it curves back to the throat. The proper use of an oropharyngeal airway greatly reduces the chances of the patient's airway becoming obstructed.

There are standard sizes of oropharyngeal airways (Figure 7-14). Many manufacturers make a complete line, ranging from airways for infants to large adult sizes. An entire set should be carried to allow for quick, proper selection.

The airway adjunct *cannot* be used effectively unless you select the correct airway size for the patient. An airway of proper size will extend from the corner of the patient's mouth to the tip of the earlobe on the same side of the patient's face. An alternative method is to measure from the center of the patient's mouth to the angle of the lower jaw bone (mandible). *Do not* use an airway unless you have measured it

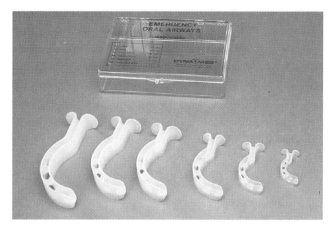

FIGURE 7-14 Various sizes of oropharyngeal airways.

against the patient and verified it as being the proper size. If the airway is not the correct size, do not use it on the patient (Figure 7-15).

To insert an oropharyngeal airway

1. Place the patient on his back. When caring for a medical patient with no indications of spinal injury, the neck may be hyperex-

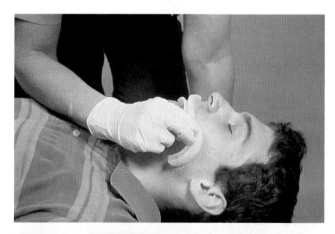

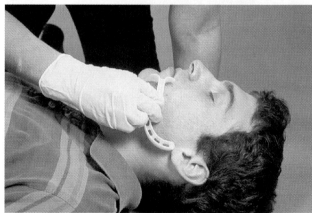

FIGURE 7-15 The oropharyngeal airway is chosen and checked for correct size.

tended. If there are possible spinal injuries, use the jaw-thrust maneuver, moving the patient no more than necessary to ensure an open airway (the airway takes priority over the spine). Extreme care must be taken.

2. Cross the thumb and forefinger of one hand and place them on the upper and lower teeth at the corner of the patient's mouth. Spread your fingers apart to open the patient's jaws (the crossed-fingers technique).

3. Position the correct size airway so that its tip is pointing toward the roof of the patient's mouth (Figure 7-16A).

4. Insert the airway and slide it along the roof of the patient's mouth, past the soft tissue hanging down from the back (the uvula), or until you meet resistance against the soft palate. Be certain not to push the patient's tongue back into the throat. Any airway insertion is made easier by using a tongue

blade (tongue depressor). In a few cases, you may *have* to use a tongue blade to hold the tongue in place. *Watch* what you are doing when inserting the airway. This procedure should not be performed by "feel" only.

5. GENTLY rotate the airway 180 degrees so that the tip is pointing down into the patient's throat (Figure 7-16B). This method prevents pushing the tongue back. Alternatively, insert the airway with tip already pointing "down" towards the patient's throat, using a tongue depressor to press the tongue down and forward to avoid obstructing the airway. *This is the preferred method for airway insertion in an infant or child.*

6. Place the nontrauma patient in a maximum head-tilt position. Minimize head movements if there are possible spinal injuries.

7. Check to see that the flange of the airway is against the patient's lips (Figure 7-17). If the airway is too long or too short, remove the airway and replace it with the correct size.

8. Place the mask you will use for ventilation over the in-place airway adjunct (Figure 7-18). If no barrier device is available, provide direct mouth-to-adjunct ventilation as you would provide mouth-to-mouth ventilation.

9. Monitor the patient closely. If there is a gag reflex, remove the airway adjunct at once. Remove the adjunct by following the

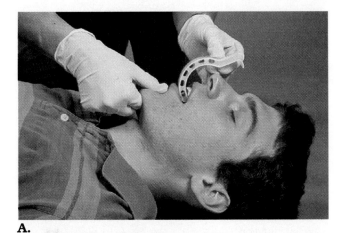

A.

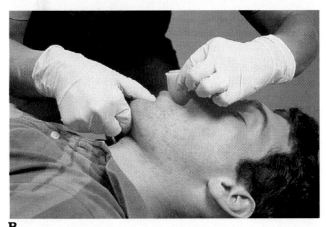

B.

FIGURE 7-16 A. The airway may be inserted with the tip pointing to the roof of the mouth and then . . . B. the airway is rotated into position.

Airway insertion

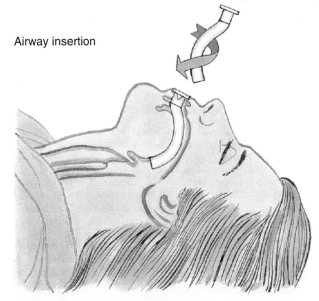

FIGURE 7-17 Note that when the airway is properly positioned, the flange rests against the patient's lips.

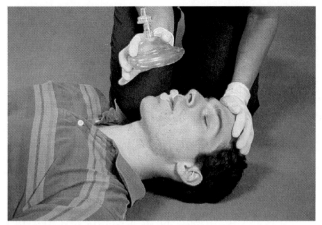

FIGURE 7-18 The patient is ready for ventilation.

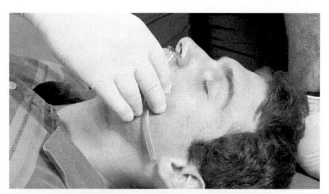

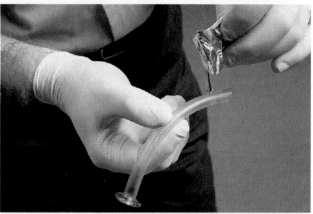

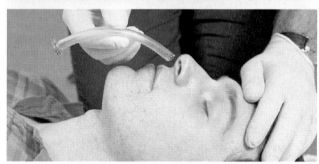

Airway insertion

anatomical curvature. You do not need to rotate the device when removing it.

Note: Some EMS systems allow an oropharyngeal airway to be inserted with the tip pointing to the side of the patient's mouth. The device is then rotated 90 degrees so that its tip is pointing down the patient's throat. Use this approach only if it is part of the protocol of your EMS system.

Nasopharyngeal Airways

The nasopharyngeal airway has gained popularity because it often does not stimulate the gag reflex. This allows the nasopharyngeal airway to be used in patients who have a reduced level of consciousness but still have an intact gag reflex. Other benefits include the fact that it can be used when the teeth are clenched and when there are oral injuries.

Use the soft flexible latex nasal airway and not the rigid clear plastic airway in the field. The soft ones are less likely to cause soft-tissue damage or bleeding. The typical sizes for adults are 34, 32, 30, and 28 French.

To insert a nasopharyngeal airway (Figure 7-19)

1. Select the largest nasopharyngeal airway that will fit into the patient's nostril without using any force. This is approximately the diameter of the patient's little finger.
2. Lubricate the outside of the tube with a water-based lubricant before insertion. *Do not* use a petroleum jelly or any other type of non-water-based lubricant. Such substances can damage the tissue lining the

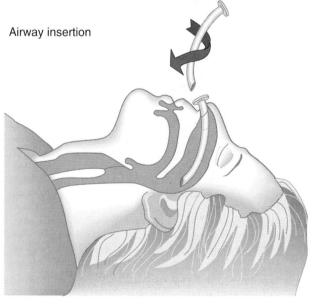

FIGURE 7-19 Measuring, lubricating, and inserting a nasopharyngeal airway.

nasal cavity and the pharynx and increase the risk of infection.

3. Gently push the tip of the nose upward. Keep the patient's head in a neutral position. Most nasopharyngeal airways are designed to be placed in the right nostril. The bevel (angled portion at the tip of the airway) should face toward the base of the nostril or toward the septum (wall that divides the two nostrils).

4. Insert the airway into the nostril. Advance the airway until the flange rests firmly against the patient's nostril. Never force a nasopharyngeal airway. If you experience difficulty advancing the airway, pull the tube out, rotate it 180 degrees, and try the other nostril.

Caution: Do not attempt the use of a nasopharyngeal airway if there is evidence of clear (cerebrospinal) fluid coming from the nose or ears. This may indicate a skull fracture in the area where the airway would pass.

Oropharyngeal and nasopharyngeal airways can be a tremendous asset to the EMT-B when used properly. However, no device can replace the EMT-B. The proper use of these airways or any other device depends on the appropriate use, good judgment, and adequate monitoring of the patient by the EMT-B. Oropharyngeal and nasopharyngeal airways prevent blockage of the upper airway by the tongue. To ensure an open airway to the level of the lungs, it is sometimes necessary to insert an endotracheal (through-the-trachea) tube. Endotracheal intubation is an advanced-life-support procedure that, in some jurisdictions, may be performed by EMT-Bs. The techniques for endotracheal intubation are discussed in Chapter 33, Advanced Airway Management (elective).

SUCTIONING AND SUCTION DEVICES

The patient's airway must be kept clear of foreign materials, blood, vomitus, and other secretions. Materials that are allowed to remain in the airway may be forced into the trachea and eventually into the lungs. This will cause complications ranging from severe pneumonia to complete airway obstruction. **Suctioning** is the method of using a vacuum device to remove such materials. A patient needs to be suctioned immediately whenever a gurgling sound is heard—whether before, during, or after artificial ventilation.

Before learning the techniques of suctioning we will discuss the types of suction equipment available and how each works.

Each suction unit consists of a suction source, a collection container for materials you suction, tubing, and suction tips or catheters. Systems are either mounted in the ambulance or are portable and may be brought to the scene.

Mounted Suction Systems

Many ambulances have a suction unit mounted in the patient compartment (Figure 7-20). These units are usually installed near the head of the stretcher so they are easily used. Mounted systems, often called "on-board" units, create a suctioning vacuum produced by the engine's mani-

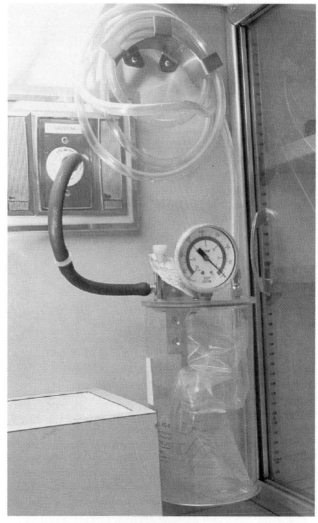

FIGURE 7-20 A mounted suction unit installed in the ambulance patient compartment.

fold or an electrical power source. To be effective, suction devices must furnish an air intake of at least 30 liters per minute at the open end of a collection tube. This will occur if the system can generate a vacuum of no less than 300 mm Hg (millimeters of mercury) when the collecting tube is clamped.

Portable Suction Units

There are many different types of portable suction units (Figure 7-21). They may be electrically powered (by batteries or household current), oxygen- or air-powered, or manually operated. The requirement for the amount of suction a portable unit must provide is identical to the fixed unit (30 liters per minute, 300 mm Hg). It is important to have the ability to suction anywhere. Portable suction provides that ability.

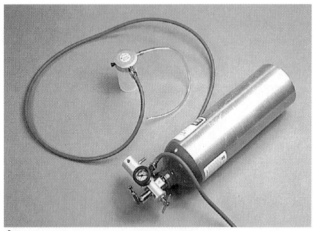

A.

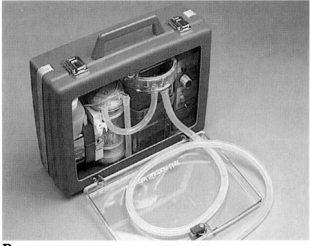

B.

FIGURE 7-21 A. An oxygen-powered portable suction unit. B. An electric-powered portable suction unit.

Tubing, Tips, and Catheters

For suctioning to be effective, the proper equipment must be used. While a suction unit might be the most powerful available, it will do no good unless used with the proper attachments.

- Tubing—The tubing attached to a suction unit must be thick-walled, non-kinking, wide-bore tubing. This is because the tubing must not collapse due to the suction, must allow "chunks" of suctioned material to pass, and must not kink, which would reduce the suction. The tubing must be long enough to comfortably reach from the suction unit to the patient.
- Suction Tips—Currently the most popular type of suction tip is the rigid pharyngeal tip, also called "Yankauer" or "tonsil sucker" or "tonsil-tip" suction. This rigid device allows you to suction the mouth and throat with excellent control over the distal end of the device. It also has a larger bore than flexible catheters. Most successfully used with an unresponsive patient, caution must be used with rigid tip suction, especially if the patient is not completely unresponsive or may be regaining consciousness. When the tip is placed into the pharynx, the gag reflex may be activated, producing additional vomiting. It is also possible to stimulate the vagus nerve in the back of the throat, which can slow the heart rate. So be careful not to suction more than a few seconds at a time with a rigid tip and never lose sight of the tip.
- Suction Catheters—Suction catheters are flexible plastic tubes. They come in various sizes identified by a number "French." The larger the number, the larger the catheter. A "14 French" catheter is larger than an "8 French" catheter. These catheters are usually not large enough to suction vomitus or thick secretions and may kink. Flexible catheters are designed to be used in situations when a rigid tip cannot be used. For example, a soft catheter can be passed through a tube such as a nasopharyngeal or endotracheal tube or used for suctioning the nasopharynx. (A bulb suction device may also be used to suction nasal passages.)

Another important part of a suction device is the collection container. All units should have a non-breakable container to collect the suctioned materials. These containers must be easily removed and decontaminated. Remember to wear gloves, protective eyewear, and mask not only while suctioning, but also while cleaning the equipment. Most newer suction devices have disposable containers to eliminate the time and risks involved in decontamination.

Suction units must also have a container of clean (preferably sterile) water nearby. This water is used to clear matter that is partially blocking the tubing. When this partial blockage of the tube occurs, place the suction tip or catheter in the container of water. This will cause a stream of water to flow through the tip and tubing, usually forcing the clog to dislodge. When the tip or tubing becomes clogged with an item that will not dislodge, replace it with a new tip or catheter.

In the event of copious, thick secretions or vomiting, consider removing the rigid tip or catheter and using the large bore, rigid suction tubing. After you are finished, place the standard tip back on for further suctioning.

Techniques of Suctioning

Although there may be some variations in suction technique (a suggested technique is shown in Scan 7-2), a few rules always apply.

- *Always use appropriate infection control practices while suctioning.* These practices include the use of protective eyewear, mask, and disposable gloves. Proper suctioning requires you to have your fingers around and sometimes inside the patient's mouth. Disposable gloves prevent contact between the EMT-B and the patient's bodily fluids. Protective eyewear and mask are also recommended since these fluids might splatter, or the patient may gag or cough, sending droplets to your face, eyes, and mouth.
- *Never suction for longer than 15 seconds at a time,* since supplemental oxygen or ventilations cease during suctioning, keeping oxygen from the patient. If the patient produces secretions as rapidly as suctioning can remove them, suction for 15 seconds, artificially ventilate for 2 minutes, then suction for 15 seconds, and continue the sequence. Consult medical direction in this situation.

Patients who need airway control and suctioning are often unconscious and may be in cardiac or respiratory arrest. Oxygen delivery to this patient is very important.

During suctioning, the ventilations or other method of oxygen delivery is discontinued to allow for the passage of the suction catheter. To prevent critical delays in oxygen delivery, limit suctioning to a few seconds, then resume ventilations or oxygen delivery.

You may **hyperventilate** a patient before and after suctioning. That is, you may ventilate a patient who is receiving artificial ventilations at a faster rate before and after suctioning to compensate for the oxygen not delivered during suctioning.

- *Place the tip or catheter where you want to begin the suctioning and suction on the way out.* Most suction tips and catheters do not produce suction at all times; you have to start the suctioning. The tip or catheter will have an open distal end where the suction is delivered. It will also have an opening, or port, in the proximal portion. When you put your finger over the proximal port, suctioning begins from the distal end.

It is not necessary to measure when using a rigid tip. Rather, you should be sure not to lose sight of the tip when inserting it. However, measure the suction catheter in a manner similar to an oropharyngeal airway. The length of catheter that should be inserted into the patient's mouth is equal to the distance between the corner of the patient's mouth and earlobe.

Carefully bring the tip of the catheter to the area where suctioning is needed. Never "jab" or force the suction tip into the mouth or throat. Then place your finger over the proximal opening to begin the suctioning, and suction as you slowly withdraw the tip from the patient's mouth, moving the tip from side to side.

Suctioning is usually delivered with the patient turned on his side. This allows free secretions to flow from the mouth while suctioning is being delivered. Caution must be used in patients with suspected neck or spinal injuries. If the patient is fully and securely immobilized, the entire backboard may be tilted to place the patient on his side. For the patient for whom such injuries are suspected but who is not immobilized, suction the best you can without turning the patient. If all other methods have failed, as a last resort you may turn the patient's body as a unit, attempting to keep the neck and spine in line. Suctioning should not be delayed to immobilize a patient.

Scan 7-2
Techniques of Suctioning

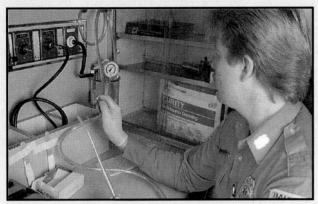

1. Turn unit on, attach a catheter, and test for suction at the beginning of your shift.

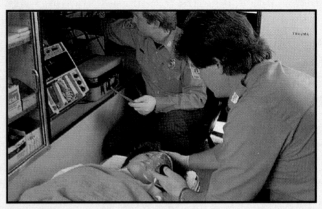

2. Position yourself at the patient's head and turn the patient to the side.

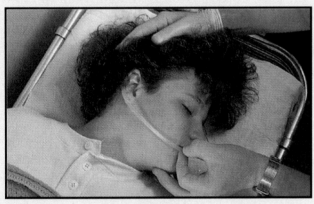

3. A rigid tip does not need to be measured; simply do not lose sight of the tip. Measure a flexible suction catheter: the distance between the patient's earlobe and the corner of the mouth, or center of the mouth to the angle of the jaw.

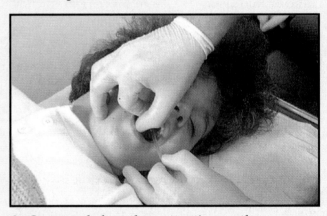

4. Open and clear the patient's mouth.

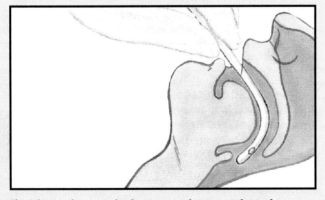

5. Place the rigid pharyngeal tip so that the convex (bulging-out) side is against the roof of the patient's mouth. Insert the tip just to the base of the tongue. Do not push the tip down into the throat or into the larynx.

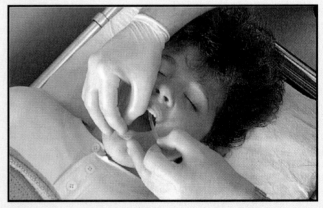

6. Apply suction *only* after the tip of the catheter or the rigid tip is in place. Suction on the way out, moving the tip side to side.

The rigid suction tip or flexible catheter should be moved into place carefully and not forced. Rigid suction devices may cause tissue damage and bleeding. Never probe into wounds or attempt to suction away attached tissue with a suction device. Certain skull fractures may actually cause brain tissue to be visible in the throat. If this occurs, do not suction near this tissue; limit suctioning to the mouth.

Suction devices may also cause activation of the gag reflex and stimulate vomiting. In a patient who already has secretions that need to be suctioned, vomiting only makes things worse. If you advance a suction catheter or rigid suction tip and the patient begins to gag, withdraw the tip to a position that does not cause gagging and begin suctioning.

The above techniques apply to suctioning of the upper airway. Techniques for orotracheal deep suctioning to the level of the lungs—an advanced life support procedure that may be performed by EMT-Bs in some jurisdictions—are discussed in Chapter 33, Advanced Airway Management (elective).

OXYGEN THERAPY

The Importance of Supplemental Oxygen

Administration of oxygen is often one of the most important and beneficial treatments an EMT-B can provide. The atmosphere provides approximately 21% oxygen. If a person is without illness or injury, that 21% is enough to support normal functioning. The fact is, however, people that EMT-Bs come in contact with *are* sick or injured and often require supplemental oxygen. Conditions that may require oxygen include

- Respiratory or Cardiac Arrest—CPR is only 25 to 33% as effective as normal circulation. High concentration oxygen administration provides a better chance of survival for the patient in respiratory or cardiac arrest.
- Heart Attacks and Strokes—These emergencies result from an interruption of blood to the heart or brain. When this occurs, tissues are deprived of oxygen. Providing extra oxygen is extremely important.
- Shock—Since shock is the failure of the cardiovascular system to provide sufficient blood to all the vital tissues, all cases of shock reduce the amount of oxygenated

blood reaching the tissues. Administration of oxygen helps the blood that does reach the tissues deliver the maximum amount of oxygen.
- Blood Loss—Whether bleeding is internal or external, there is a reduced amount of circulating blood and red blood cells, so the blood that is circulating needs to be saturated with oxygen.
- Lung Diseases—The lungs are responsible for turning oxygen over to the blood cells to be delivered to the tissues. When the lungs are not functioning properly, supplemental oxygen helps assure that the body's tissues receive adequate oxygen.
- Broken Bones, Head Injuries, and More—There are very few emergencies where oxygen administration would not be appropriate. All our body's systems work together. An injury in one part may cause shock that affects the rest of the body.

Hypoxia

Hypoxia is an insufficiency in the supply of oxygen to the body's tissues. There are several major causes of hypoxia. Consider the following scenarios where patients develop hypoxia.

- A victim is trapped in a fire. The air that the victim breathes contains smoke and reduced amounts of oxygen. Since the victim cannot breathe in enough oxygen, hypoxia develops.
- A patient has emphysema. This lung disease decreases the efficiency of the transfer of oxygen between the atmosphere and the body. Since the lungs cannot do their function properly, hypoxia develops.
- A patient overdoses on a drug that has a depressing effect on the respiratory system. The patient's respirations are only 5 per minute. In this case, the victim is not breathing frequently enough to support the body's oxygen needs. Hypoxia develops.
- A patient has a heart attack. The lungs function properly by taking atmospheric air and turning it over to the blood for distribution. The damaged heart, however, cannot pump the blood throughout the body, and hypoxia develops.

There are many causes of hypoxia, including the examples above, stroke, shock, and others. The most important thing to know is how to recognize signs of hypoxia so that it may be treated. Hypoxia may be indicated by cyanosis (blue or gray color to the skin). Additionally, when the brain suffers hypoxia, the patient's mental status may deteriorate. Restlessness or confusion may result.

As an EMT-B your concern will be to prevent hypoxia from developing or becoming worse and, when possible, to reduce the level of hypoxia. The way that this is done is with the administration of oxygen.

Hazards of Oxygen Therapy

Although the benefits of oxygen are great, oxygen must be used carefully. The hazards of oxygen therapy may be grouped into two categories: nonmedical and medical.

The nonmedical hazards of oxygen include

- The oxygen used in emergency care is stored under pressure, usually 2,000 to 2,200 pounds per square inch (psi) or greater in a full cylinder. If the tank is punctured, or a valve breaks off, the supply tank can become a missile (damaged tanks have been able to penetrate concrete walls). Imagine what would happen in the passenger compartment of an ambulance if such an accident occurred.
- Oxygen supports combustion, causing fire to burn more rapidly. It can saturate towels, sheets, and clothing, greatly increasing the risk of fire.
- Under pressure, oxygen and oil do not mix. When they come into contact, a severe reaction occurs which, for our purposes, can be termed an explosion. This is seldom a problem, but it can easily occur if you lubricate a delivery system or gauge with petroleum products, or allow contact with a petroleum-based adhesive (e.g., adhesive tape).

These nonmedical hazards are extremely rare and can be avoided totally if oxygen and oxygen equipment are treated properly.

The medical hazards of oxygen rarely affect the patients treated by the EMT-B. There are certain patients who, when exposed to high concentrations of oxygen for a prolonged time, may develop negative side effects. These situations are rare in the field.

- Oxygen Toxicity or Air Sac Collapse—These problems are caused in some patients whose lungs react unfavorably to the presence of oxygen and also may result from too high a concentration of oxygen for too long a period of time. The body reacts to a sensed "overload" of oxygen by reduced lung activity and air sac collapse. Like the other conditions listed here, these are extremely rare in the field.
- Infant Eye Damage—This condition may occur when premature infants are given too much oxygen. These infants may develop scar tissue on the retina of the eye. This does not occur from the infant's eyes being directly exposed to oxygen. Oxygen by itself does not cause this condition but it is the result of many factors. Oxygen should never be withheld from any infant with signs of inadequate breathing.
- Respiratory Depression or Respiratory Arrest—Patients with chronic obstructive pulmonary disease (COPD) may over time lose the normal ability to use the body's blood carbon dioxide levels as a stimulus to breathe. When this occurs, the COPD patient's body may use low blood oxygen as the factor that stimulates him to breathe. Because of this so-called *hypoxic drive,* EMTs have for years been trained to administer only low concentrations of oxygen to these patients for fear of increasing the patient's blood oxygen levels and wiping out their "drive to breathe." It is now widely believed that more harm is done by withholding high concentration oxygen than could be done by administering high concentration oxygen.

As an EMT-B you will probably never see oxygen toxicity or any other adverse conditions that can result from oxygen administration. The time required for such conditions to develop is too long to cause any problems during emergency care in the field. The bottom line is: ***Never withhold high concentration oxygen from a patient who needs it!***

Oxygen Therapy Equipment

In the hospital setting, oxygen is delivered to the patient from conveniently located oxygen tanks or regulators. In the field, oxygen equipment must be safe, lightweight, portable, and dependable.

Some field oxygen systems are very portable so they may be brought almost anywhere. Other systems are installed inside the ambulance so that oxygen can be delivered during transportation to the hospital. Most oxygen delivery systems contain several items (Figure 7-22): oxygen cylinders, pressure regulators, and a delivery device (face mask or cannula). When the patient is not breathing or is breathing inadequately, additional devices (such as a bag-valve mask) can be used to force oxygen into the patient's lungs.

Oxygen Cylinders

Outside a medical facility, the standard source of oxygen is the **oxygen cylinder,** a seamless steel or lightweight alloy cylinder filled with oxygen under pressure, equal to 2,000 to 2,200 psi when the cylinders are full. Cylinders come in various sizes, identified by letters (Figure 7-23). Those in common use in emergency care include

- D cylinder—contains about 350 liters of oxygen
- E cylinder—contains about 625 liters of oxygen
- M cylinder—contains about 3,000 liters of oxygen

Fixed systems on ambulances include the M cylinder and larger cylinders (Figure 7-24):

- G cylinder—contains about 5,300 liters of oxygen

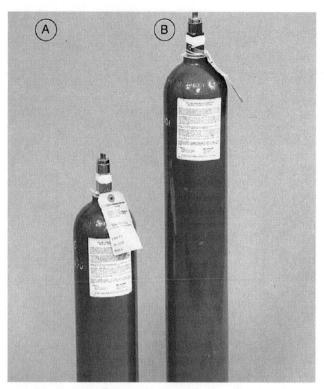

FIGURE 7-23 (A) A D cylinder and (B) an E cylinder. These cylinders still have the suppliers' plastic wrappers over the outlets. Do not use adhesive tape.

- H cylinder—contains about 6,900 liters of oxygen.

The United States Pharmacopoeia has assigned a color code to distinguish compressed gases. Green and white cylinders have been assigned to all grades of oxygen. Unpainted stainless steel and aluminum cylinders are also used for oxygen. Regardless of the color, always check the label to be certain you are using medical grade oxygen.

Part of your duty as an EMT-B is to make certain that the oxygen cylinders you will use are full and ready before they are needed to provide care. The length of time you can use an oxygen cylinder depends on the pressure in the cylinder and the flow rate. You cannot tell if an oxygen cylinder is full, partially full, or empty by lifting or moving the cylinder. The method of calculating cylinder duration is shown in Table 7-2. Oxygen cylinders should never be allowed to empty below the safe residual. The safe residual for an oxygen cylinder is when the pressure gauge reads 200 psi or above. Below this point there is not enough oxygen in the cylinder to allow for proper delivery to the patient. Before

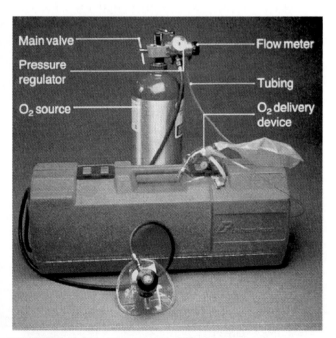

FIGURE 7-22 An oxygen delivery system.

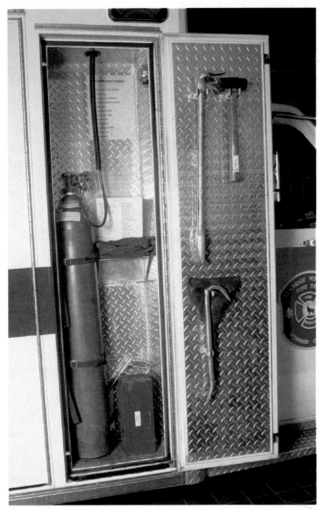

FIGURE 7-24 Larger cylinders are used for fixed systems on ambulances.

TABLE 7-2 Oxygen Cylinders: Duration of Flow

SIMPLE FORMULA:

Gauge pressure in psi (pounds per square inch) *minus* the safe residual pressure (always 200 psi) *times* the constant (see list below) *divided by* the flow rate in liters per minute = duration of flow in minutes.

CYLINDER CONSTANTS

D = 0.16	G = 2.41
E = 0.28	H = 3.14
M = 1.56	K = 3.14

EXAMPLE

Determine the life of an M cylinder that has a pressure of 2000 psi displayed on the pressure gauge and a flow rate of 10 liters per minute.

$$\frac{(2000 - 200) \times 1.56}{12} = \frac{2808}{12} = \text{234 minutes or 3 hours and 54 minutes}$$

the cylinder reaches the 200 psi reading, you must switch to a fresh cylinder.

SAFETY is of prime importance when working with oxygen cylinders. You should

- NEVER drop a cylinder or let it fall against any object. When transporting a patient with an oxygen cylinder, make sure the oxygen cylinder is strapped to the stretcher or otherwise secured.
- NEVER leave an oxygen cylinder standing in an upright position without being secured.
- NEVER allow smoking around oxygen equipment in use. Clearly mark the area of use with signs that read "OXYGEN—NO SMOKING."
- NEVER use oxygen equipment around an open flame.
- NEVER use grease, oil, or fat-based soaps on devices that will be attached to an oxygen supply cylinder. Take care not to handle these devices when your hands are greasy. Use greaseless tools when making connections.
- NEVER use adhesive tape to protect an oxygen tank outlet or to mark or label any oxygen cylinders or oxygen delivery apparatus. The oxygen can react with the adhesive and debris and cause a fire.
- NEVER try to move an oxygen cylinder by dragging it or rolling it on its side or bottom.
- ALWAYS use pressure gauges, regulators, and tubing that are intended for use with oxygen.
- ALWAYS use nonferrous metal oxygen wrenches for changing gauges and regulators or for adjusting flow rates. Other types of metal tools may produce a spark should they strike against metal objects.
- ALWAYS ensure that valve seat inserts and gaskets are in good condition. This prevents dangerous leaks. Gaskets on D and E oxygen cylinders should be replaced each time a cylinder change is made.
- ALWAYS use medical grade oxygen. Industrial oxygen contains impurities. The cylinder should be labeled "OXYGEN U.S.P." The oxygen must not be more than 5 years old.
- ALWAYS open the valve of an oxygen cylinder fully, then close it half a turn to prevent someone else from thinking the valve is closed and trying to force it open. The valve does not have to be turned fully to be open for delivery.

- ALWAYS store reserve oxygen cylinders in a cool, ventilated room, properly secured in place.
- ALWAYS have oxygen cylinders hydrostatically tested EVERY 5 YEARS. The date a cylinder was last tested is stamped on the cylinder. Some cylinders can be tested every 10 years. These will have a star after the date (e.g., 4M86*).

Pressure Regulators

The pressure in an oxygen cylinder (approximately 2000 psi in a full tank—varying with surrounding temperature) is too high to be delivered to a patient. A **pressure regulator** must be connected to the cylinder to provide a safe working pressure of 30 to 70 psi.

On cylinders of the E size or smaller, the pressure regulator is secured to the cylinder valve assembly by a yoke assembly. The yoke is provided with pins that must mate with corresponding holes in the valve assembly. This is called a pin-index safety system. Since the pin position varies for different gases, this system prevents an oxygen delivery system from being connected to a cylinder designed to contain another gas.

Cylinders larger than the E size have a valve assembly with a threaded outlet. The inside and outside diameters of the threaded outlets vary according to the gas in the cylinder. This prevents an oxygen regulator from being connected to a cylinder containing another gas. In other words, a nitrogen regulator cannot be connected to an oxygen cylinder, and vice versa.

Cylinder pressure can be reduced in one or two steps (Figure 7-25). For a one-step reduction, a single-stage pressure regulator is used. A two-step reduction requires a two-stage regulator. Most regulators used in emergency care are the single-stage variety.

Before connecting the pressure regulator to an oxygen supply cylinder, stand to the side of the main valve opening and open (crack) the cylinder valve slightly for just a second to clear dirt and dust out of the delivery port or threaded outlet.

Note: You must maintain the regulator inlet filter. It has to be free of damage and clean to prevent contamination of and damage to the regulator.

Flowmeters

A **flowmeter** allows control of the flow of oxygen in liters per minute. It is connected to the pres-

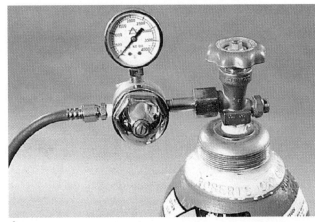

A.

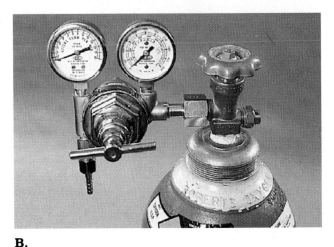

B.

FIGURE 7-25 A. A single-stage regulator. B. A two-stage regulator for D- and E-size cylinders.

sure regulator. Most jurisdictions keep the flowmeter permanently attached to the pressure regulator.

Three major types of flowmeters are available. For use in the field, the pressure-compensated flowmeter is considered to be superior to the Bourdon gauge flowmeter; however, it is more delicate than the Bourdon gauge and must be operated in an upright position. For these reasons, many EMS systems use the pressure-compensated flowmeter for fixed oxygen systems only.

- Bourdon Gauge Flowmeter (Figure 7-26A)— This unit is a pressure gauge calibrated to indicate flow in liters per minute. The meter is fairly inaccurate at low flow rates and has often been criticized as being unstable. However, it is rugged and will operate at any angle. It is a useful gauge for most portable units.

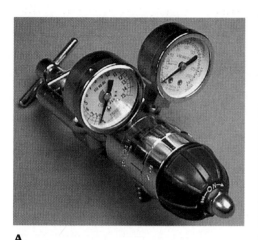
A.

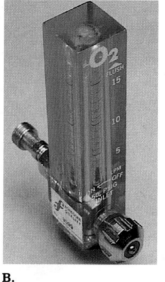
B.

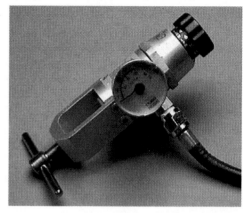
C.

FIGURE 7-26 A. Bourdon gauge flowmeter (pressure gauge). B. Pressure-compensated flowmeter. C. Constant flow selector valve.

The major fault with this type of flowmeter is its inability to compensate for back pressure. A partial obstruction (as from kinked tubing) will be reflected in a reading that is higher than the actual flow. The gauge may read 6 liters per minute and only be delivering 1 liter per minute. This type of gauge contains a filter that can become clogged, causing the gauge to read higher than the actual flow. Inspect and change the filter as recommended by the manufacturer.

• Pressure-Compensated Flowmeter (Thorpe tube-type flowmeter, Figure 7-26B)—This meter is gravity dependent and must be in an upright position to deliver an accurate reading. The unit has an upright, calibrated glass tube in which there is a ball float. The float rises and falls according to the amount of gas passing through the tube. This type of flowmeter indicates the actual flow at all times, even though there may be a partial obstruction to gas flow (as from a kinked delivery tube). If the tubing collapses, the ball will drop to show the lower delivery rate. This unit is not practical for many portable delivery systems.

• Constant Flow Selector Valve (Figure 7-26C)—This type of flowmeter is gaining in popularity. It has no gauge. It allows for the adjustment of flow in liters per minute in stepped increments (2, 4, 6, 8 . . .15 liters per minute). When using this type of flowmeter, make certain that it is properly

adjusted for the desired flow and monitor the meter to make certain that it stays properly adjusted. This type of meter should be tested for accuracy as recommended by the manufacturer.

Humidifiers

A **humidifier** can be connected to the flowmeter to provide moisture to the dry oxygen coming from the supply cylinder (Figure 7-27). Dry oxygen can dehydrate the mucous membranes of the patient's airway and lungs. In most short-term use, the dryness of the oxygen is not a problem; however, the patient is usually more comfortable when given humidified oxygen. This is particularly true if the patient has COPD.

A humidifier is usually no more than a non-breakable jar of water attached to the flowmeter. Oxygen passes (bubbles) through the water to become humidified. As with all oxygen delivery equipment, the humidifier must be kept clean. The water reservoir can become a breeding ground for algae, harmful bacteria, and dangerous fungal organisms. Always use fresh water in a clean reservoir for each shift. Sterile single-patient-use humidifiers are available and preferred.

In many EMS systems humidifiers are no longer used because they are not indicated for short transports and because of the infection risk. The devices may be beneficial on long transports and on certain pediatric patients with signs of inadequate breathing.

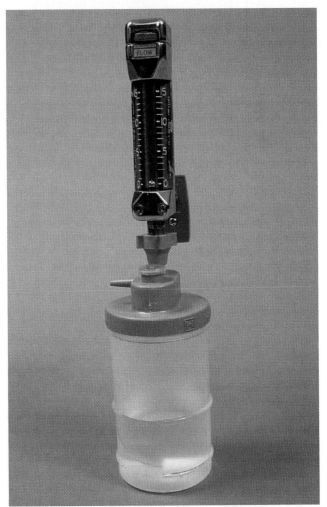

FIGURE 7-27 A simple oxygen humidifier.

Administering Oxygen

Scans 7-3 and 7-4 will take you step by step through the process of administering oxygen and discontinuing the administration of oxygen. Do not attempt to learn on your own how to use oxygen delivery systems. You should work with your instructor and follow your instructor's directions for the specific equipment you will be using.

Oxygen is administered to assist in the delivery of artificial ventilations to *nonbreathing patients*, as was discussed above under Techniques of Artificial Ventilation. Oxygen is also administered to *breathing patients* for a variety of conditions. A number of oxygen-delivery devices and systems are used. Each has benefits and drawbacks. A device that is good for one patient may not be ideal for another. The goal is to use the oxygen delivery device that is best for each patient.

Delivering Oxygen to the Breathing Patient

For the patient who is breathing and requires supplemental oxygen due to potential hypoxia, there are various oxygen delivery devices available. In general, however, the nasal cannula and the nonrebreather mask are the two devices most commonly used by the EMT-B to provide supplemental oxygen (Table 7-3).

- Nonrebreather Mask—Excluding the bag-valve mask used with oxygen and flow-restricted, oxygen-powered ventilation devices, the **nonrebreather mask** is the EMT-B's best way to deliver high concentrations of oxygen (Figure 7-28). This device must be placed properly on the patient's face to provide the necessary seal to ensure high concentration delivery. The reservoir bag must be inflated before the mask is placed on the patient's face. To inflate the reservoir bag, use your finger to cover the exhaust port or the connection between the mask and the reservoir. The reservoir must always contain enough oxygen so that it does not deflate by more than one third when the patient takes his deepest inspiration. This can be maintained by the proper flow of oxygen (15 liters per minute). Air exhaled by the patient does not return to the reservoir (is not

TABLE 7-3 Oxygen Delivery Devices

Oxygen Delivery Device	Flow Rate	% Oxygen Delivered	Special Use
Nonrebreather mask	12-15 liters per minute	80-90%	Delivery system of choice for patients with signs of inadequate breathing and patients who are cyanotic, cool, clammy, short of breath, or suffering chest pain, suffering severe injuries, or displaying an altered mental status.
Nasal cannula	1-6 liters per minute	24-44%	Patients who cannot tolerate a mask

Preparing the Oxygen Delivery System

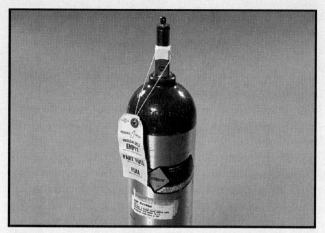

1. Select desired cylinder. Check label, "Oxygen U.S.P."

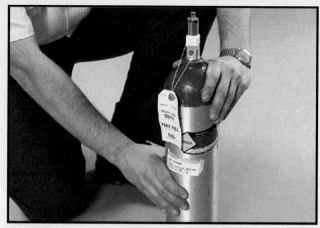

2. Place the cylinder in an upright position and stand to one side.

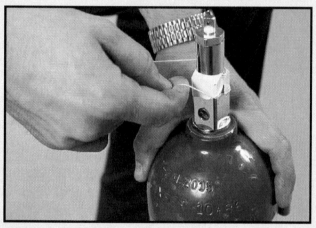

3. Remove the plastic wrapper or cap protecting the cylinder outlet.

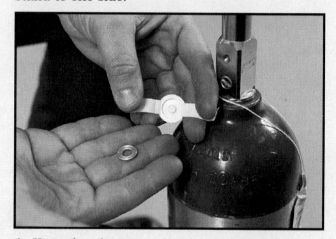

4. Keep the plastic washer (some set-ups).

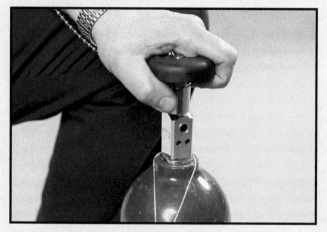

5. "Crack" the main valve for one second.

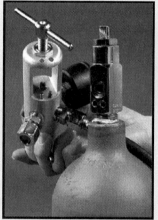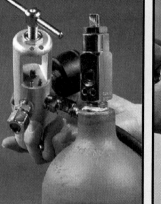

6. Select the correct pressure regulator and flowmeter. Pin yoke is shown on the left, threaded outlet on the right.

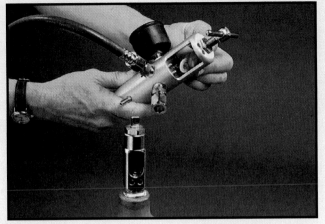

7. Place cylinder valve gasket on regulator oxygen port.

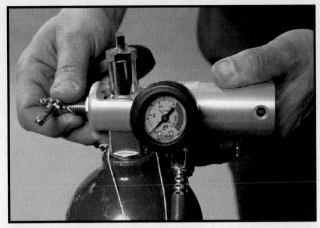

8. Make certain that the pressure regulator is closed.

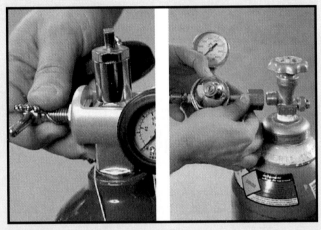

9. Align pins (left) or thread by hand (right).

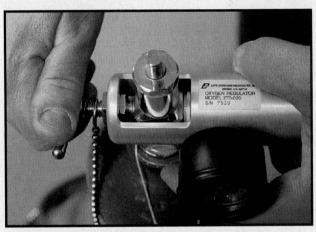

10. Tighten T-screw for pin yoke.

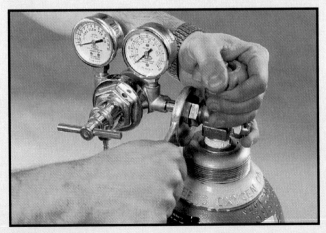

Tighten with a wrench for a threaded outlet.

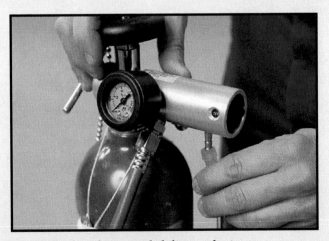

11. Attach tubing and delivery device.

Scan 7-4
Administering Oxygen

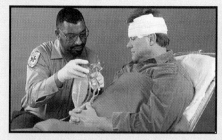

1. Explain to patient the need for oxygen.

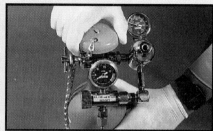

2. Open main valve and adjust flowmeter.

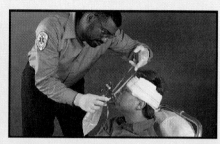

3. Place oxygen delivery device.

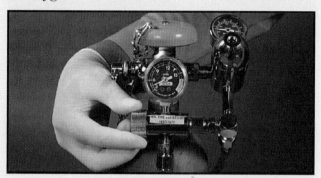

4. Adjust flowmeter.

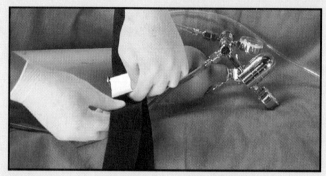

5. Secure during transfer.

Discontinuing Oxygen

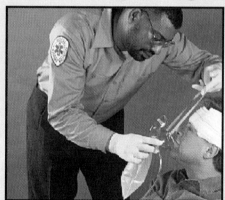

1. Remove delivery device.

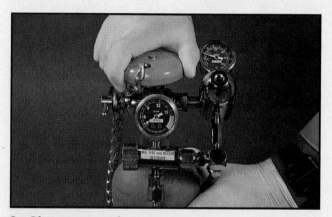

2. Close main valve.

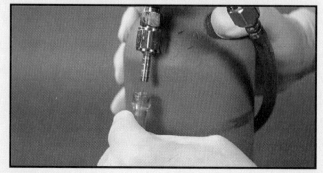

3. Remove delivery tubing.

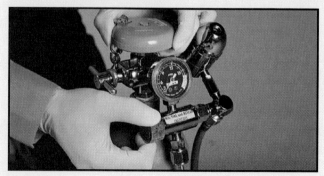

4. Bleed flowmeter.

142

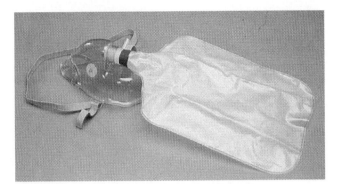

FIGURE 7-28 A nonrebreather mask.

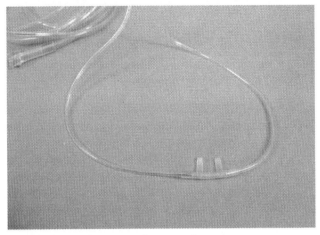

FIGURE 7-29 A nasal cannula.

rebreathed). Instead, it escapes through a flutter valve in the face piece.

This mask will provide concentrations of oxygen ranging from 80% to 90%. The minimum flow rate is 8 liters per minute. Depending on the manufacturer and the fit of the mask, the maximum flow can range from 12 to 15 liters per minute. New design features allow for one emergency port in the mask so that the patient can still receive atmospheric air should the oxygen supply fail. This feature keeps the mask from being able to deliver 100% oxygen but is a necessary safety feature. The mask is excellent for use in patients with inadequate breathing or who are cyanotic (blue or gray), cool, clammy, short of breath, or suffering chest pain, or displaying an altered mental status.

Nonrebreather masks come in different sizes for adults, children, and infants.

- Nasal Cannula—A **nasal cannula** provides low concentrations of oxygen (between 24% and 44%). Oxygen is delivered to the patient by two prongs that rest in the patient's nostrils. The device is usually held to the patient's face by placing the tubing over the patient's ears and securing the slip-loop under the patient's chin (Figure 7-29).

Patients who have chest pain, signs of shock, hypoxia, or other more serious problems need a higher concentration than can be provided by a cannula. However, some patients will not tolerate a mask-type delivery device because they feel "suffocated" by the mask. For the patient who refuses to wear an oxygen face mask, the cannula is better than no oxygen at all. The cannula should be used *only* when a patient will not tolerate a nonrebreather mask.

When a cannula is used, the liters per minute delivered should be no more than 4 to 6. At higher flow rates the cannula be-

gins to feel more uncomfortable and dries out the nasal mucous membranes.

SPECIAL CONSIDERATIONS

There are several special considerations in airway management.

- Facial Injuries—Take extra care with the airway when there have been facial injuries. Because the blood supply to the face is so rich, blunt injuries to the face frequently result in severe swelling or bleeding that may block or partially block the airway. Frequent suctioning may be required. Insertion of an airway adjunct or endotracheal tube (see Chapter 33, Advanced Airway Management) may be necessary.
- Obstructions—Many suction units are not adequate for removing solid objects like teeth and large particles of food or other foreign objects. These must be removed using manual techniques for clearing airway obstructions, such as abdominal thrusts, chest thrusts, or finger sweeps, which you learned in your basic life support course and which are reviewed in Basic Life Support: Airway, Rescue Breathing, and CPR at the end of this book. You may need to log roll the patient into a supine position to clear the oropharynx manually.
- Dental Appliances—Dentures should ordinarily be left in place during airway procedures. Partial dentures may become dislodged during an emergency. Leave a partial denture in place if possible, but be prepared to remove it if it endangers the airway.

Airway Considerations in Infants and Children

There are several special considerations that you must take into account when managing the airway of an infant or child.

Anatomic Considerations (Figure 7-30)

- The mouth and nose are smaller and more easily obstructed than in adults.
- In infants and children the tongue takes up more space proportionately in the mouth than in adults.
- The trachea (windpipe) is softer and more flexible in infants and children.
- The trachea is narrower and is easily obstructed by swelling.
- The chest wall is softer, and infants and children tend to depend more on their diaphragm for breathing.

Management Considerations

- Open the airway gently. Infants can be placed in a neutral neck position and children only require slight extension of the neck. Do not over extend the neck, because it may collapse the trachea.
- Avoid excessive bag pressure and volume. Use only enough to make the chest rise.
- Use properly sized face masks when providing BVM ventilations to assure a good mask seal.
- Flow-restricted, oxygen-powered ventilation devices are contraindicated (should not be used) in infants and children.
- Use pediatric-sized nonrebreather masks and nasal cannulas when administering supplemental oxygen.
- Infants and children are prone to gastric distention during ventilations or respiratory distress which may impair adequate ventilations. (See gastric tube insertion in Chapter 33, Advanced Airway Management.)
- An oral or nasal airway may be considered when other measures fail to keep the airway open.
- In suctioning infants and children, use a rigid tip but be careful not to touch the back of the airway.

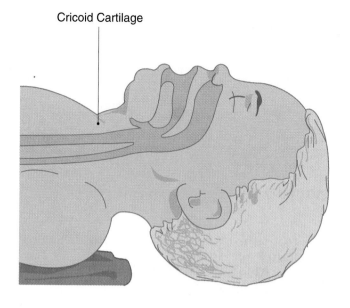

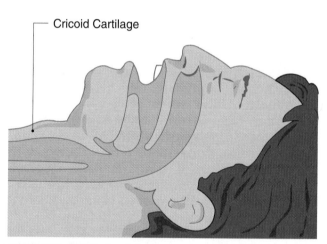

FIGURE 7-30 A child's airway structures differ from an adult's. A child's mouth and nose are smaller, the tongue takes up more space in the mouth, and the trachea is narrower than in an adult.

CHAPTER REVIEW

KEY TERMS

You may find it helpful to review the following terms.

airway the passageway by which air enters or leaves the body. The structures of the airway are the nose, mouth, pharynx, larynx, trachea, bronchi, and lungs.

artificial ventilation forcing air or oxygen into the lungs when a patient has stopped breathing or has inadequate breathing.

bag-valve mask a hand-held device with a face mask and self-refilling bag that can be squeezed to provide artificial ventilations to a patient. Can deliver air from the atmosphere or oxygen from a supplemental oxygen supply system.

cyanosis (SIGH-uh-NO-sis) a blue or gray color resulting from lack of oxygen in the body (*see* hypoxia).

flowmeter a valve that indicates the flow of oxygen in liters per minute.

flow-restricted, oxygen-powered ventilation device (FROPVD) a device that uses oxygen under pressure to deliver artificial ventilations. Its trigger is placed so that the rescuer can operate it while still using both hands to maintain a seal on the face mask. Has automatic flow restriction to prevent over-delivery of oxygen to the patient.

gag reflex vomiting or retching that results when something is placed in the throat.

head-tilt, chin-lift maneuver a means of correcting blockage of the airway by the tongue by tilting the head back and lifting the chin. Used when no trauma, or injury, is suspected. *See also* jaw-thrust maneuver.

humidifier a device connected to the flowmeter to add moisture to the dry oxygen coming from an oxygen cylinder.

hyperventilate (HI-per-VEN-ti-late) in suctioning, to provide ventilations at a higher rate to compensate for oxygen not delivered during suctioning.

hypoxia (hi-POK-se-uh) an insufficiency of oxygen in the body's tissues.

jaw-thrust maneuver a means of correcting blockage of the airway by moving the jaw forward without tilting the head or neck. Used when trauma, or injury, is suspected to open the airway without causing further injury to the spinal cord in the neck. *See also* head-tilt, chin-lift maneuver.

nasal cannula (NAY-zul KAN-yuh-luh) a device that delivers low concentrations of oxygen through two prongs that rest in the patient's nostrils.

nasopharyngeal (NAY-zo-fah-RIN-jul) **airway** a flexible breathing tube inserted through the patient's nose into the pharynx to help maintain an open airway.

nonrebreather mask a face mask and reservoir bag device that delivers high concentrations of oxygen. The patient's exhaled air escapes through a valve and is not rebreathed.

oropharyngeal (OR-o-fah-RIN-jul) **airway** a curved device inserted through the patient's mouth into the pharynx to help maintain an open airway.

oxygen cylinder a cylinder filled with oxygen under pressure.

pocket face mask a device, usually with a one-way valve, to aid in artificial ventilation. A rescuer breathes through the valve when the mask is placed over the patient's face. Also acts as a barrier to prevent contact with a patient's breath or body fluids. Can be used with supplemental oxygen when fitted with an oxygen inlet.

pressure regulator a device connected to an oxygen cylinder to reduce cylinder pressure to a safe pressure for delivery of oxygen to a patient.

respiration (RES-pir-AY-shun) breathing.

respiratory (RES-pir-uh-tor-e) **arrest** when breathing completely stops.

respiratory failure the reduction of breathing to the point where not enough oxygen is being taken in to sustain life.

suctioning (SUK-shun-ing) use of a vacuum device to remove blood, vomitus, and other secretions or foreign materials from the airway.

ventilation the breathing in of air or oxygen or providing breaths artificially. *See also* artificial ventilation.

The airway is the passageway by which air enters the body during respiration, or breathing. A patient cannot survive without an open airway. Maintaining an open airway is the first priority of emergency care.

Respiratory failure is inadequate breathing, breathing that is insufficient to support life. A patient in respiratory failure or respiratory arrest (complete stoppage of breathing) must receive artificial ventilations.

Airway adjuncts—the oropharyngeal and nasopharyngeal airway—can help keep the airway open during artificial ventilation. It may also be necessary to suction the airway or to use manual techniques to remove fluids and solids from the airway before, during, or after artificial ventilation.

Oxygen can be delivered to the nonbreathing patient as a supplement to artificial ventilation. Oxygen can also be administered as therapy to the breathing patient whose breathing is inadequate or who is cyanotic (blue), cool and clammy, short of breath, suffering chest pain, suffering severe injuries, or displaying an altered mental status.

REVIEW QUESTIONS

1. Name the main structures of the airway.
2. Explain why care for the airway is the first priority of emergency care.
3. Name the signs of adequate breathing and of inadequate breathing.
4. Explain when the head-tilt, chin-lift maneuver should be used and when the jaw-thrust maneuver should be used to open the airway—and why.
5. Name the techniques of artificial ventilation in the recommended order of preference.
6. Explain how airway adjuncts and suctioning help in airway management and artificial ventilation.
7. Name patient problems that would benefit from administration of oxygen and explain how to decide whether a nonrebreather mask or nasal cannula should be used to deliver oxygen to a patient.

Application

- On arrival at the emergency scene, you find an adult female patient with gurgling sounds in the throat and inadequate breathing slowing to almost nothing. How do you proceed to protect the airway and support the patient's breathing?

Patient Assessment

IN THIS MODULE

MODULE OVERVIEW

These chapters present the elements of assessment in almost the same order that you will do them. Before you reach the patient, you must perform a *scene size-up* (Chapter 8) to assess the scene, making sure there is no danger to you and your crew, the patient, or bystanders.

Once you have determined that the scene is safe (or made it safe), you need to determine whether the patient has any life-threatening problems and then correct them. This is called the *initial assessment* (Chapter 9) and will build on the ABCs you learned in your CPR course. Besides finding and correcting threats to life, the purpose of the initial assessment includes determining whether the patient has a trauma (injury) problem, a medical (non-injury) problem, or both. This will determine the next step in your assessment.

If the patient has a trauma problem (an injury), you will perform a *focused history and physical exam for a trauma patient* (Chapter 10). You will begin with the physical exam. This means one of two things. For the typical patient who does not have a mechanism of injury that leads you to suspect serious injury, you will focus the physical exam on the areas the patient tells you are injured. For the patient who has a serious mechanism of injury, you will do a rapid exam of the entire body to find potentially serious injuries. Then you will obtain vital signs and finally, if possible, obtain the patient's history.

If the patient has a medical problem, you will perform a *focused history and physical exam for a medical patient* (Chapter 11). For the medical patient—in contrast to the trauma patient for whom assessment began with a physical exam—you will first obtain a history. This means asking the patient questions and looking for certain signs and symptoms based on the chief complaint (the reason you were called). Then you will perform a physical exam focused on the problem area and obtain vital signs.

Later, if you have time, you will perform a *detailed physical exam* (Chapter 12) on the trauma patient. This means examining the patient from head to toe more slowly and thoroughly than in the rapid exam you did earlier.

Both medical and trauma patients will get *ongoing assessment* (Chapter 13) en route to a hospital. Here, you will repeat your initial assessment to find and correct any new life threatening problems, repeat vital signs, and make sure that your interventions (treatments) are working the way they should. You will *communicate* patient information to hospital personnel (Chapter 14), and you will carefully *document* details of the call in written reports (Chapter 15).

Patient assessment is the foundation of all that you will do for your patients. You need to be able to perform appropriate, timely assessments of your patients in order to treat them properly. Only with a systematic approach to this critical series of assessment steps will you be able to give quality care.

Scene Size-Up

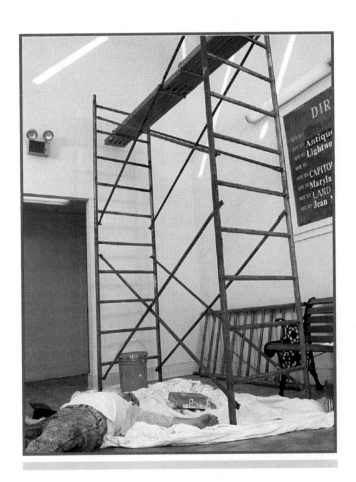

Scene size-up is the first part of the patient assessment process. It begins as you approach the scene, surveying it to determine if there are any threats to your own safety or the safety of your patients or bystanders, to determine the nature of the call, and to decide if you will need additional help.

Objectives

Knowledge and Attitude *At the end of this chapter, you should be able to meet the following objectives.*

1. Recognize hazards or potential hazards. (pp. 151, 152, 153–154, 156)

2. Describe common hazards found at the scene of a trauma and a medical patient. (pp. 153–154, 156)

3. Determine if the scene is safe to enter. (pp. 153–154, 156)

4. Discuss common mechanisms of injury or nature of illness. (pp. 156–159)

5. Discuss the reason for identifying the total number of patients at the scene. (pp. 151, 159–160)

6. Explain the reason for identifying the need for additional help or assistance. (pp. 151, 159–160)

7. Explain the rationale for crew members to evaluate scene safety prior to entering. (p. 151)

8. Serve as a model for others explaining how patient situations affect your evaluation of mechanism of injury or illness. (pp. 159–160)

Skills

1. Observe various scenarios and identify potential hazards.

On the Scene

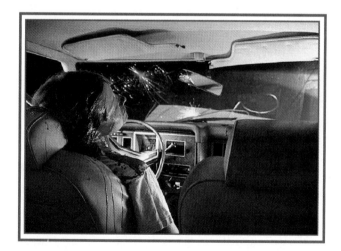

One afternoon, Rita Stocker veers to avoid hitting a squirrel and runs her car into a telephone pole. Moments later, while you are returning from the hospital after a call, you come upon the collision scene. You observe the car with its front end crumpled against the pole and a wire down across the hood. You can see Rita in the driver's seat with blood covering a considerable portion of her face. You notice that a portion of the driver's side windshield is damaged. Immediately, you put your scene size-up training into practice.

Body Substance Isolation

To protect yourself from Rita's blood and other body fluids, and those of any other patients you may encounter, you pull on disposable gloves as you exit the ambulance and grab your response kit containing protective eye wear and mask.

Scene Safety and Resources

You note that other motorists are slowing down to stare at the scene and that pedestrians are beginning to approach. The downed wires present a potential hazard to everyone, as does passing traffic. You will not approach the car until the wires are safely out of the way. You motion to the bystanders to stay clear of the car and off the road, and you signal Rita not to get out of the car. There is also the possibility that Rita's car will catch fire. Knowing that you will need assistance with the scene, you radio for the fire and police departments and the power company.

Mechanism of Injury and Number of Patients
The obvious impact of the car against the pole, the shattered windshield, and the blood on Rita's face alert you to the possibility of a variety of head, spine, and body injuries. For the moment, Rita is the only patient in sight, but you are watchful for passengers or pedestrians who may have been involved in the crash.

Scene size-up sets a foundation for the remainder of the patient assessment process, as well as the rest of the call. Do I have the personal protective equipment I may need? What potential hazards does this scene present? What is the likely mechanism of injury or the nature of the patient's illness? Will we need additional assistance? These are questions you will ask as you size up the scene and prepare for the safe and effective care of your patient.

THE SCENE SIZE-UP

Elements of the **scene size-up** (Scan 8-1) include

- *Body Substance Isolation (BSI) Precautions.* Your scene size-up will help determine exactly what BSI precautions are appropriate. A trauma patient with obvious bleeding will require different precautions than many medical patients.
- *Scene Safety.* This portion of the scene size-up is to determine whether there are dangers to yourself and all others at the scene. It includes

    Personal Safety—First determine if there are dangers to yourself or other EMS providers from sources such as unstable vehicles, machinery, toxic exposure, or violence.

    Patient Safety—Next determine if the patient is in danger or in an environment that may worsen his condition or impede recovery. Anything that may harm an EMT-B will certainly harm a patient.

    Bystander Safety—Are there bystanders who may be in danger? Are there bystanders or crowds that may endanger your safety or the safety of your patient?

- *Additional Resources.* Call for any needed additional resources, such as police department, fire department, or power company personnel.
- *Mechanism of Injury or Nature of Illness.* As you observe the scene, make note of the **mechanism of injury**—forces that may have caused injury to the patient—or evidence of a medical problem.
- *Determine the Number of Patients.* If there are more patients than you or your crew are able to handle, call for additional EMS resources.

Scene size-up is not confined to the first part of the assessment process. These considerations should continue throughout the call. Since emergencies are dynamic, always-changing events, you may find that patients, family members, or bystanders who were not a problem initially may become increasingly hostile later in the call. Vehicles or structures that seemed stable may suddenly shift and pose a danger.

After the initial scene size-up you will become more directly involved in patient assessment and care. However, it is a good idea to remember the parts of the size-up throughout the call to prevent dangerous surprises later.

At Rita Stocker's collision, described in On the Scene at the beginning of this chapter, important information was obtained in just a brief survey of the scene. The wires down across the car posed a potentially deadly situation for you as the EMT-B, your patient, and bystanders. Further observations of the scene revealed important information about the mechanism of injury. The damage to the windshield directly in front of the driver was a strong indicator of potential head and neck injury caused by the driver striking her head against the windshield.

Just as important as your observations were the actions you took to prevent further

Scene Size-up

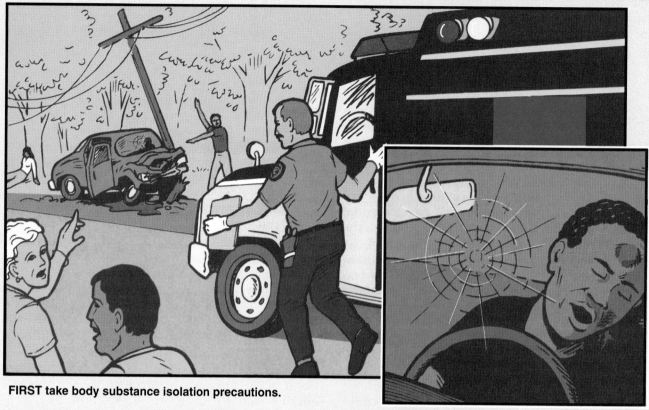

FIRST take body substance isolation precautions.

1. Determine scene safety. Look for possible threats to safety of EMTs, patient, and bystanders.

2. Determine the mechanism of injury or the nature of the patient's illness.

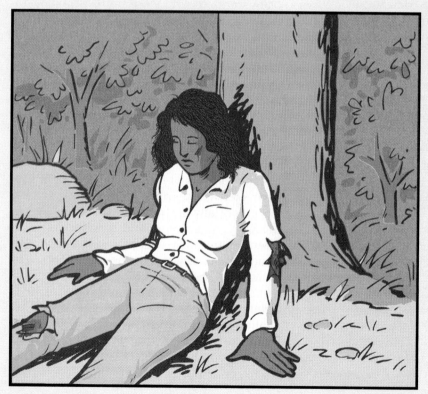

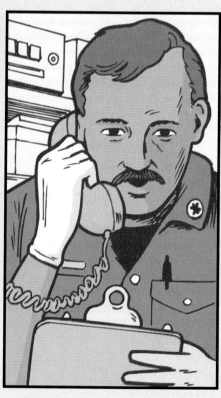

3. Determine the number of patients. Be alert for patients in addition to the first patient you see at the scene.

4. Request additional help if necessary.

Note: Consider whether spinal stabilization will be needed for the patient or patients.

injury to the patient by signaling her to stay in the vehicle (exiting the vehicle would have greatly increased the risk of electric shock) and to bystanders by motioning them to stay clear of the traffic and collision. Since the power lines were downed and there was some danger of fire, the power company and fire department, as well as the police department, were immediately notified.

Body Substance Isolation

As you perform your initial size-up of the scene, there are many important points to consider. One very important aspect of personal protection—and one that you will need long after you have addressed any physical dangers—is body substance isolation.

You learned about BSI precautions in Chapter 2, The Well-being of the EMT-Basic. To summarize: Body substances include blood, saliva, and any other body fluids or contents. All body substances can carry viruses and bacteria. Your patient's body substances can enter your body through cuts or other openings in your skin. They can also easily enter your body through your eyes, nose, and mouth. You are especially at risk of being infected by a patient's body substances when the patient is bleeding or coughing or sneezing or whenever you make direct contact with the patient as in mouth-to-mouth breathing. Infection is a two way street, of course. Your patient can also be infected by you. (For more information see Appendix B, Infectious Diseases.)

During the scene size-up in On the Scene, you observed that Rita Stocker had blood streaming down her face. This was a clear indication for all personnel to wear protective gloves. Since this potential hazard was spotted long before any contact with the patient, everyone should have been wearing gloves before beginning patient care. If Rita required suctioning or began spitting blood, protective eye wear, such as glasses with side protection, and a mask would also have been required. Whenever a patient is suspected of having tuberculosis, you will need to wear a high efficiency particulate air (HEPA) respirator that may filter out airborne particles the patient exhales or expels.

A key element of body substance isolation is always to have personal protective equipment readily available, either on your person or as the first items you encounter when opening a response kit. Remember that proper body substance isolation decisions early in the call will prevent needless exposure later on.

Scene Safety

The only predictable thing about emergencies is that they are often unpredictable. These situations may pose a great deal of danger to you if you are not careful. The scene of Rita Stocker's collision, for example, was very dangerous.

You will recall that you were returning from the hospital when you came upon the collision. The size-up you performed was especially important in that case since you were first on the scene. You observed a car into a utility pole, and this presented two very dangerous situations: the unstable pole and the wires that fell on the car. If you had ignored scene size-up procedures and rushed to the aid of the patient, the results could have been disastrous.

Often you will find scenes where there are police, fire, and even other ambulances present. In a situation like this, don't assume that the scene is safe because others have taken care of any hazards. Always perform your own size-up no matter who arrives first. Scan for dangers, infection control concerns, and hazardous materials. The scene size-up begins even before the ambulance comes to a stop. Observe the scene while you approach and again before you exit the vehicle.

The following are things to consider during the scene size-up portion of the assessment when approaching a crash or hazardous material emergency.

As you near the collision scene
- *Look and listen for other emergency service units approaching from side streets.*
- *Look for signs of a collision-related power outage*—e.g., darkened areas that will suggest that wires are down at the collision scene.
- *Observe traffic flow.* If there is no opposing traffic, suspect a blockade at the collision scene.
- *Look for smoke in the direction of the collision scene*—a sign that fire has resulted from the collision.

When you are within sight of the scene
- *Look for clues to escaped hazardous materials*—e.g., hazardous materials placards, a damaged truck, fumes, or vapor clouds. If you see anything suspicious, stop the

ambulance immediately and call your dispatcher to request advice, or consult your hazardous material reference book. (See more below under Establishing the Danger Zone.)

- *Look for collision victims on or near the road.* A person may have been thrown from a vehicle as it careened out of control, or an injured person may have walked away from the wreckage and collapsed on or near the roadway.
- *Look for smoke that you may not have seen at a distance.*
- *Look for broken utility poles and downed wires.* At night, direct the beam of a spotlight or handlight on poles and wire spans as you approach the scene. Keep in mind that wires may be down several hundred feet from the crash vehicles.
- *Be alert for persons walking along the side of the road toward the collision scene.* Curious onlookers (excited children in particular) are often oblivious to vehicles approaching from behind.
- *Watch for the signals of police officers and other emergency service personnel.* They may have information about hazards or the location of injured persons.

As you reach the scene
- *Sniff for odors* such as gasoline or diesel fuel or any unusual odor that may signal that a hazardous material has been released.

Establishing the Danger Zone

A **danger zone** exists around the wreckage of every vehicle collision, within which special safety precautions must be taken. The size of the zone depends on the nature and severity of collision-produced hazards (Scan 8-2). An ambulance should never be parked within the danger zone. Follow these guidelines in establishing the danger zone.

- *When there are no apparent hazards,* consider the danger zone to extend at least 50 feet in all directions from the wreckage. The ambulance will be away from broken glass and other debris, and it will not impede emergency service personnel who must work in or around the wreckage. When using highway flares to protect the scene, make sure that the person igniting

them has been trained in the proper technique.
- *When fuel has been spilled,* consider the danger zone to extend a minimum of 100 feet in all directions from the wreckage. In addition to parking outside the danger zone, park upwind, if possible. (Note the direction of the wind by observing flags, smoke, and so on.) Thus the ambulance will be out of the path of dense smoke if the fuel ignites. If fuel is flowing away from the wreckage, park uphill as well as upwind. If parking uphill is not possible, position the ambulance as far from the flowing fuel as possible. Avoid gutters, ditches, and gullies that can carry fuel to the ambulance. Do not use flares in areas where fuel has been spilled. Use orange traffic cones during daylight and reflective triangles at night.
- *When a collision vehicle is on fire,* consider the danger zone to extend at least 100 feet in all directions even if the fire appears small and limited to the engine compartment. If fire reaches the vehicle's fuel tank, an explosion could easily damage an ambulance parked closer than 100 feet.
- *When wires are down,* consider the danger zone as the area in which people or vehicles might be contacted by energized wires if the wires pivot around their points of attachment. Even though you may have to carry equipment and stretchers for a considerable distance, the ambulance should be parked at least one full span of wires from the poles to which broken wires are attached.
- *When a hazardous material is involved,* check the Department of Transportation *Emergency Response Guide* for suggestions as to where to park, or request advice from an agency such as CHEMTREC (Chemical Transportation Emergency Center, Washington, D.C., 24-hour hotline 800-424-9300 or 202-483-7616). In some cases you may be able to park 50 feet from the wreckage, as when no hazardous material has been spilled or released. In other cases you may be warned to park 2,000 feet or more from the wreckage, as when there is the possibility that certain high explosives may detonate. In all cases, park upwind from the wreckage when you discover that a hazardous material is present at a collision site. Park uphill if a liquid is flowing, but on the same level if there are gases or fumes

Establishing the Danger Zone

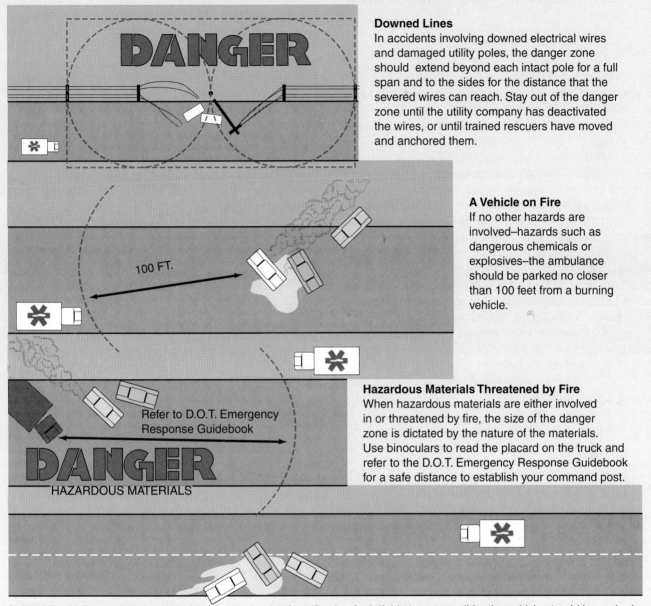

Downed Lines
In accidents involving downed electrical wires and damaged utility poles, the danger zone should extend beyond each intact pole for a full span and to the sides for the distance that the severed wires can reach. Stay out of the danger zone until the utility company has deactivated the wires, or until trained rescuers have moved and anchored them.

100 FT.

A Vehicle on Fire
If no other hazards are involved—hazards such as dangerous chemicals or explosives—the ambulance should be parked no closer than 100 feet from a burning vehicle.

Refer to D.O.T. Emergency Response Guidebook

DANGER
HAZARDOUS MATERIALS

Hazardous Materials Threatened by Fire
When hazardous materials are either involved in or threatened by fire, the size of the danger zone is dictated by the nature of the materials. Use binoculars to read the placard on the truck and refer to the D.O.T. Emergency Response Guidebook for a safe distance to establish your command post.

Spilled Fuel The ambulance should be parked uphill from flowing fuel. If this is not possible, the vehicle should be parked as far from the fuel flow as possible, avoiding gutters, ditches, and gullies that may carry the spill to the parking site. Remember, your ambulance's catalytic converter is an ignition source over 1000 degrees.

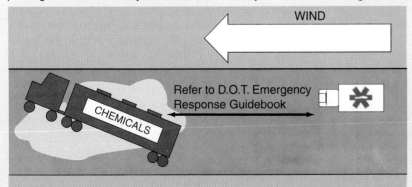

WIND

Refer to D.O.T. Emergency Response Guidebook

CHEMICALS

Hazardous Materials
Leaking containers of dangerous chemicals may produce a health as well as a fire hazard. When chemicals have been spilled, whether fumes are evident or not, the ambulance should be parked upwind. If the hazardous material is known, seek advice from experts through the dispatcher or CHEMTREC.

which may rise. Park behind some artificial or natural barrier if possible. (In Chapter 30, Ambulance Operations, you will learn more about parking the ambulance. In Chapter 32, Overviews, and in Appendix C you will learn more about hazardous materials.)

Crime Scenes and Acts of Violence

Another significant danger faced by the EMT-B is violence. Crime statistics vary, but it is certain that EMT-Bs working in the field are exposed to more dangerous situations than even a few years ago. While a majority of calls go by uneventfully, the EMT-B must be conscious of dangers from many sources, including other human beings. EMT-Bs often envision violence as occurring at bar fights or on the street, but *domestic violence,* violence in the home, is also a cause for concern.

Protection from violence is as important as protection from the dangers at a vehicle collision. As an EMT-B, you should never enter a violent situation to provide care. Safety at a violent scene requires a careful size-up as you approach. Just as the downed power lines signaled danger at the scene of Rita Stocker's collision, there are many signals of danger from violence that you may observe as you approach the scene. These signals include

- *Fighting or loud voices.* If you approach a scene and see or hear fighting, threatening words or actions, or the potential for fighting, there is a good chance that there will be a danger to you from this behavior.
- *Weapons visible or in use.* Any time you observe a weapon, you must use an extreme amount of caution. The weapon may actually be in the hands of an attacker (a grave danger), or simply in sight. Weapons include knives, guns, and martial arts weapons *as well as any other items that may be used as a weapon.* Table legs, kitchen utensils, pens, almost anything may be used as a weapon.
- *Signs of alcohol or other drug use.* When alcohol or other drugs are in use, a certain unpredictability exists at any scene. It will not take long for you to observe unusual behavior from a person under the influence of one of these substances. This behavior may result in violence toward emergency personnel at the scene. Additionally, there are hazards associated with the drug cul-

ture, such as street violence and the presence of contaminated needles.
- *Unusual silence.* Emergencies are usually active events. A call that is "too quiet" should also raise your suspicions. While there may be a good reason for the silence, extra care should be taken.
- *Knowledge of prior violence.* If you or a member of your crew has been to a particular location for calls involving violence in the past, extra caution must be used on subsequent calls to the same location.

Whether the call is residential or in the street, observe the scene for the signs of danger listed above and any others you may find. This brief danger assessment may be all that is required to prevent harm to you or your crew during the call.

If you observe signs of danger, there are actions that you must take to protect yourself. You learned about these actions in Chapter 2, The Well-being of the EMT-Basic. To summarize: The specific actions you should take depend on many factors including your local protocols, the type of danger, and the help available to you. In general you should *retreat to a position of safety, call for help, and return only after the scene has been secured by police.* Be sure to document the danger and your actions.

Mechanism of Injury

The mechanism of injury is what caused the injury (e.g., a rapid deceleration causing the knees to strike the dash of a car; a fall on ice causing a twisting force to the ankle) (Scan 8-3).

Certain injuries are considered "common" to particular accident situations. Injuries to bones and joints are usually associated with falls and vehicle collisions; burns are common to fires and explosions; penetrating soft tissue injuries can be associated with gunshot wounds, and so on.

Even if you cannot determine what injury the patient has sustained, knowing the mechanism of injury allows you to predict various injury patterns. For example, in many situations you will immobilize the patient's spine because the mechanism of injury, such as a forceful blow, is frequently associated with spinal injury. You do not need to know that the patient's spine is actually injured; you assume it is and treat accordingly. Knowing that the patient has fallen, you check for a painful, swollen, or deformed arm or leg.

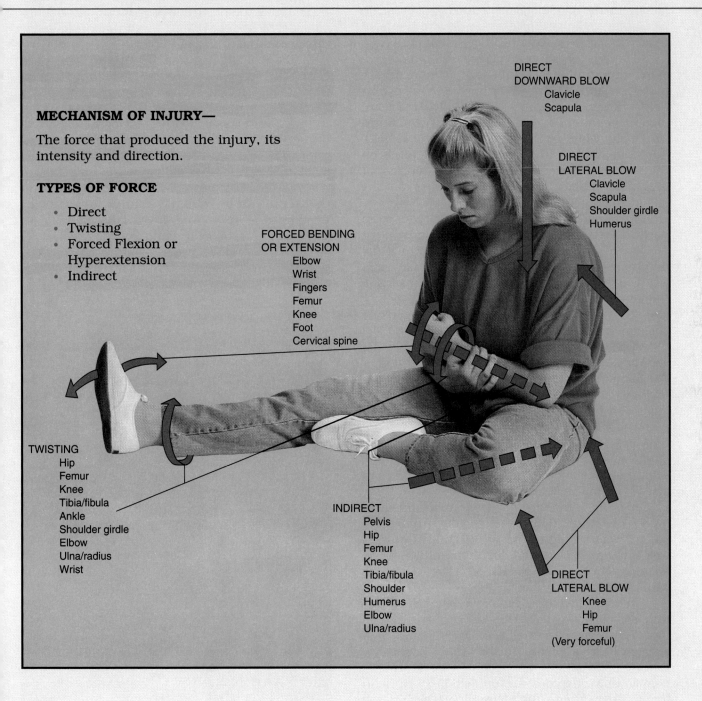

MECHANISM OF INJURY—

The force that produced the injury, its intensity and direction.

TYPES OF FORCE

- Direct
- Twisting
- Forced Flexion or Hyperextension
- Indirect

FORCED BENDING OR EXTENSION
Elbow
Wrist
Fingers
Femur
Knee
Foot
Cervical spine

DIRECT DOWNWARD BLOW
Clavicle
Scapula

DIRECT LATERAL BLOW
Clavicle
Scapula
Shoulder girdle
Humerus

TWISTING
Hip
Femur
Knee
Tibia/fibula
Ankle
Shoulder girdle
Elbow
Ulna/radius
Wrist

INDIRECT
Pelvis
Hip
Femur
Knee
Tibia/fibula
Shoulder
Humerus
Elbow
Ulna/radius

DIRECT LATERAL BLOW
Knee
Hip
Femur
(Very forceful)

Knowing the mechanism of injury is very important when dealing with motor vehicle collisions. A collapsed or bent steering column suggests that the driver has suffered a chest wall injury with possible rib or even lung or heart damage. A shattered, blood-spattered windshield points to the likelihood of a forehead or scalp laceration and possibly a severe blow to the head that may have caused a head or spinal injury.

The type of motor vehicle collision also provides important information on potential injury patterns. *Head-on collisions* have a great potential for injury to all parts of the body. It is common for a patient's head to strike the windshield (especially when he was not wearing a seat belt). Additionally, the patient may strike his chest on the steering wheel, causing chest injuries or breathing problems, and/or his knees on the dash, causing leg and knee injuries.

Rear end collisions are common causes of neck injury. *Side impact collisions* (broadside, or "T-Bone") have other injury patterns. Since the body is pushed laterally, the head often moves in a direction opposite the body, causing injuries to the head and neck. The chest, abdomen, pelvis, and thighs may be struck directly, causing skeletal and internal injuries.

Rollover collisions are potentially the most serious because of the forces involved and potential for multiple impacts. Rollover collisions frequently cause ejection of anyone who is not wearing a seat belt. Expect any type of serious injury pattern. *Rotational impact collisions* involve cars that are struck, then spin. The initial impact often causes subsequent impacts (the spinning vehicle strikes another vehicle or a tree). This can also cause multiple injury patterns.

It is an important aspect of mechanism of injury determination to find out where the patient was sitting in the vehicle and if he was wearing a seat belt. Note any deformities in the steering wheel, dash, pedals, or other structures within the vehicle.

Injuries involving motorcycles and all-terrain vehicles also have the potential to be serious. These vehicles offer the operator and passengers little protection in the event of collision. Determine whether the patient was wearing a helmet that offered some protection from head injury. Also attempt to determine whether the patient was ejected. In some cases, the operator will be thrown from the bike and strike and severely injure his hips, thighs, or legs.

Falls are another cause of injury where the extent and pattern of damage may be determined by the characteristics of the fall (Figure 8-1). Important factors to consider are the height from which the patient fell, the surface the patient fell onto, the part of the patient that hit the ground, and anything that interrupts the fall. Falls from heights of greater than 15 feet (or three times the height of the patient) are usually considered severe. Use this information to determine potential injury patterns.

Penetrating trauma, an injury caused by an object that passes through the skin or other body tissue, also has characteristics that may help in determining the extent of injury. These wounds are classified by the velocity, or speed, of the item that caused the injury. Low-velocity items are those that are propelled by hand, such as knives. Low-velocity injuries are usually limited to the area that was penetrated. Remember that there can be multiple wounds, or the blade may have been moved inside the patient, so there can be damage to multiple vital organs.

High-velocity wounds are caused by guns and can cause damage almost anywhere in the body. Bullets cause damage in two ways.

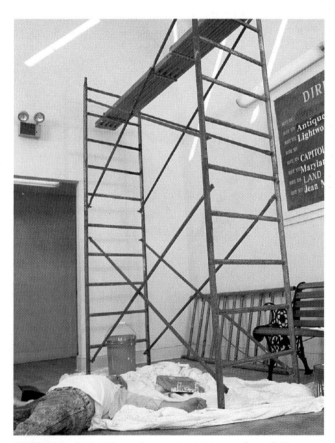

FIGURE 8-1 The characteristics of a fall may provide valuable clues to a patient's injuries.

- *Pressure related damage, or cavitation.* This means that the velocity of the bullet as it enters the body causes a cavity considerably greater than the size of the bullet. This cavity is temporary, but it may damage items in its path.
- *Damage directly from the projectile.* The bullet itself will damage anything in its path. The damage depends on the size of the bullet, its path, or whether it fragments (breaks up into smaller projectiles), the fragments taking different paths. The path of the bullet once it is inside the body is unpredictable since it may be deflected by bone or other tissue onto a totally different course.

Identifying the mechanism of injury should help you, as an EMT-B, to determine what injuries are possible and to treat these injuries accordingly, even if signs and symptoms are not present. *Never assume, based on the mechanism of injury, that there are no injuries.* Even very minor collisions may cause injuries.

Maintain a **high index of suspicion**—a keen awareness that there may be injuries—based on the mechanism of injury. Remember to maintain neck and spine stabilization as patient assessment progresses.

Nature of Illness

Identifying the nature of the illness for a medical patient serves the same purpose as identifying the mechanism of injury for a trauma patient: finding out what is or may be wrong with the patient. To begin identifying the nature of a patient's illness during the scene size-up, you must scan the entire scene. Information may be obtained from many sources.

- *The patient,* when conscious and oriented, is a prime source of information about his or her condition. Your dealings with the patient will continue throughout the assessment process.
- *Family members or bystanders* can also provide important information, especially for the unconscious patient. Even when the patient is conscious and able to tell you about his condition, however, always consider the information from others who are present. Patients who are disoriented or confused may provide information that is either partially true or even untrue. Use information from all sources to piece the patient assessment "puzzle" together.
- *The scene.* While you are sizing up the scene for safety, make note of other factors that may be clues to the patient's condition. You may observe medications, which you will make a mental note to examine later in your survey. You may be struck by dangerous or unsanitary living conditions for this particular patient. This is important to note and mention to the emergency department personnel later.

Number of Patients and Adequacy of Resources

The final part of the scene size-up is to determine if you have sufficient resources to handle the call. While you may not feel that a single-patient medical call could tax your resources, consider the following scenarios where you may find yourself needing extra help.

- Your ambulance is called to respond to an elderly woman with chest pain. You are greeted at the door by her husband, who doesn't look well. He denies any complaints but is sweaty and holding his chest. Your first patient tells you that her husband has a heart condition.
- A single patient experiences back pain. This is usually not a reason for additional assistance but this patient is immobilized on a backboard in a third floor apartment (no elevator) and weighs 425 pounds.
- Your ambulance is called for "general weakness." Upon the arrival of your two-person crew, two more persons in the same family develop the same flu-like symptoms. You appropriately suspect carbon monoxide poisoning, since they admit that they have been having furnace problems.

In each of these situations, what appeared to be a routine, one-patient call actually turned out to be more. An important part of the size-up is to immediately recognize these situations and *call for help immediately.* As the call progresses and you get more involved in patient care, it is less likely that you will remember to call for the additional help. It may also be too late when the help arrives if you do not call immediately.

Your response to these situations may range from simply calling for another ambulance to care for the ill husband in the first situation, or extra personnel to help move the 425-pound man in the second, to activating a Multiple Casualty Incident for the family with carbon monoxide poisoning. (You will learn about multiple casualty incidents in Chapter 32, Overviews.) Try to anticipate the maximum numbers of patients and radio for help accordingly. Follow local protocols.

CHAPTER REVIEW

KEY TERMS

You may find it helpful to review the following terms.

danger zone   the area around the wreckage of a vehicle collision or other accident within which special safety precautions should be taken.
high index of suspicion   keen awareness that there may be injuries.
mechanism of injury   a force or forces that may have caused injury.

penetrating trauma   an injury caused by an object that passes through the skin or other body tissues.
scene size-up   steps taken by an ambulance crew when approaching the scene of an emergency call: taking body substance isolation precautions, checking scene safety, noting the mechanism of injury or nature of the patient's illness, determining the number of patients, and deciding what, if any, additional resources to call for.

SUMMARY

Scene size-up is the first part of the patient assessment process. It is important during scene size-up to determine what, if any, threats there may be to your own safety and that of others at the scene and to institute appropriate body substance isolation procedures. Next it is important to determine the nature of the call by identifying the mechanism of injury or the nature of the patient's illness. Finally, you must take into account the number of patients and other factors at the scene to determine if you will need additional help.

REVIEW QUESTIONS

1. Describe several situations where it is appropriate to wear disposable gloves. Describe situations where you would additionally wear protective eye wear and mask. Describe situations where you would wear a HEPA respirator.
2. For each of the following dangers, describe actions that must be taken to remain safe at a collision scene.

   • Leaking gasoline
   • Toxic or hazardous material spill
   • Vehicle on fire
   • Downed power lines

3. List several indicators of violence or potential violence at an emergency scene.
4. Describe common mechanism-of-injury patterns.
5. List sources of information about the nature of a patient's illness.
6. List several medical and trauma situations where you may require additional assistance.

Application
   • You are called to the scene of a shooting at a fast food restaurant. En route, you plan your scene size-up strategy. What actions do you anticipate taking on arrival?

The Initial Assessment

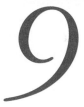

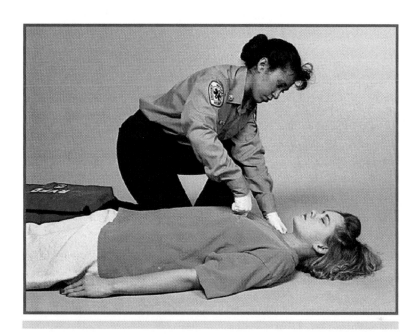

As an EMT-Basic, you will sometimes encounter a patient with a problem or problems that are immediately life-threatening, a patient who may die within minutes unless he or she receives immediate treatment and transport to a hospital. For such a patient, there is not enough time to go through all the steps of a thorough assessment. Therefore, every assessment begins with a process called the initial assessment, designed to identify and treat immediately life-threatening conditions and to set priorities for further assessment and treatment or immediate transport.

Objectives

Knowledge and Attitude *At the end of this chapter, you should be able to meet the following objectives.*

1. Summarize the reasons for forming a general impression of the patient. (pp. 164, 167)

2. Discuss methods of assessing altered mental status. (pp. 167–168, 169)

3. Differentiate between assessing the altered mental status in the adult, child, and infant patient. (p. 169)

4. Discuss methods of assessing the airway in the adult, child, and infant patient. (pp. 168, 169)

5. State reasons for management of the cervical spine once the patient has been determined to be a trauma patient. (pp. 174–175, 176)

6. Describe methods used for assessing if a patient is breathing. (pp. 168, 169)

7. State what care should be provided to the adult, child, and infant patient with adequate breathing. (pp. 168, 169)

8. State what care should be provided to the adult, child, and infant patient without adequate breathing. (pp. 168, 169)

9. Differentiate between a patient with adequate and inadequate breathing. (p. 168)

10. Distinguish between methods of assessing breathing in the adult, child, and infant patient. (p. 169)

11. Compare the methods of providing airway care to the adult, child, and infant patient. (pp. 168, 169)

12. Describe the methods used to obtain a pulse. (pp. 168, 169)

13. Differentiate between obtaining a pulse in an adult, child, and infant patient. (p. 169)

14. Discuss the need for assessing the patient for external bleeding. (pp. 168, 169)

15. Describe normal and abnormal findings when assessing skin color. (pp. 168–169))

16. Describe normal and abnormal findings when assessing skin temperature. (p. 168)

17. Describe normal and abnormal findings when assessing skin condition. (p. 168)

18. Describe normal and abnormal findings when assessing skin capillary refill in the infant and child patient. (p. 174)

19. Explain the reason for prioritizing a patient for care and transport. (pp. 169–170)

20. Explain the importance of forming a general impression of the patient. (pp. 164, 167)

21. Explain the value of performing an initial assessment. (p. 164)

Skills

1. Demonstrate the techniques for assessing mental status.

2. Demonstrate the techniques for assessing the airway.

3. Demonstrate the techniques for assessing if the patient is breathing.

4. Demonstrate the techniques for assessing if the patient has a pulse.

5. Demonstrate the techniques for assessing the patient for external bleeding.

6. Demonstrate the techniques for assessing the patient's skin color, temperature, condition, and capillary refill (infants and children only).

7. Demonstrate the ability to prioritize patients.

For futher information on these objectives . . .	See these chapters.
Objectives 4, 6, 7, 8, 9, 10, and 11 on assessment and management of the airway and breathing	See also Chapter 7, Airway Management
Objectives 12 and 13 on obtaining a pulse	See also Chapter 5, Baseline Vital Signs and SAMPLE History
Objective 14 on external bleeding	See also Chapter 25, Bleeding and Shock
Objectives 15, 16, 17, and 18 on assessing skin color, temperature, and condition and capillary refill in infants and children and on care for shock or possible shock	See also Chapter 5, Baseline Vital Signs and SAMPLE History; Chapter 25, Bleeding and Shock
Objectives 3, 4, 7, 8, 10, 11, 13, and 18 on special methods for infants and children	See also Chapter 29, Infants and Children

On the Scene

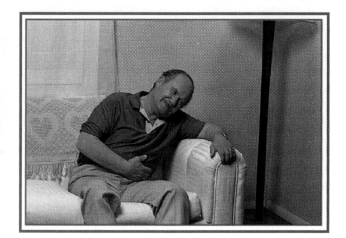

One spring afternoon, you are dispatched to "an elderly man whose stomach hurts."

Scene Size-up

You pull up to a quiet, well-kept house. The **scene appears safe.** You put on gloves for **body substance isolation** as you exit the ambulance. The door is opened by an older woman who appears a little anxious. The woman leads you to the patient as you find out that they are Mr. and Mrs. Schmidt. There is no apparent **mechanism of injury** and the dispatch message indicated a medical problem. The **number of patients** is just one: Mr. Schmidt. You immediately begin your initial assessment.

General Impression

As you approach the sofa where Mr. Schmidt is resting, you see that he is an older male who appears ill and in pain. You see nothing around him to suggest that he has been injured. All of this suggests a medical problem rather than an injury.

Mental Status, Airway, Breathing

You introduce yourself by saying, "Hello, Mr. Schmidt. I'm Gerry Jones. I'm an emergency medical technician from the Fairfield Ambulance Service. How can I help you?" "My stomach hurts," he replies. As you ask questions, you note that Mr. Schmidt is alert and answering clearly. The fact that he is speaking in a normal way indicates that his airway is open. You can hear that his breathing is not labored. You look at his chest and note that his breathing is normal in rate and depth.

Circulation

"I'm going to take your pulse," you explain as you reach for his wrist. You quickly assess Mr. Schmidt's circulation by palpating his radial pulse, observing his skin, and looking for bleeding. His pulse is normal in rate and strength and regular in rhythm. The skin at his wrist is pink, warm, and dry. No blood is evident anywhere around him.

Treatment and Transport Priority

With the information you have gathered in just a few seconds, you conclude that Mr. Schmidt has no problems that are likely to kill him in the next few minutes. No immediate life-saving measures are required, and neither is immediate transport to the hospital. You are able, instead, to move ahead with the next steps of your assessment as Mr. Schmidt continues to rest on the sofa.

The story of Mr. Schmidt's assessment will continue in Chapter 11.

Usually, you will take the time to do a thorough assessment (check of your patient), transporting your patient to the hospital only after the complete assessment is finished. But if the patient has an immediately life-threatening problem—such as a blocked airway, a stoppage of breathing or heartbeat, or severe bleeding—you must immediately perform **interventions**—actions to correct these problems—and consider whether you need to transport the patient without delay. The assessment steps you take for the purpose of discovering and dealing with any life-threatening problems are called the **initial assessment.** The initial assessment is always the first element in the total assessment of the patient.

In this chapter, you will learn the steps of the initial assessment. You will also read about several patients with different conditions in order to see how you would adjust the initial assessment to meet the requirements of a variety of situations. In later chapters we will return to some of these patients to see how the assessment process proceeds after the initial assessment and how the steps of patient assessment and patient management (care) are integrated.

THE INITIAL ASSESSMENT

The initial assessment has six parts (Scan 9-1).

- Forming a general impression
- Assessing mental status
- Assessing airway
- Assessing breathing
- Assessing circulation
- Determining the priority of the patient

Forming a General Impression

Forming a general impression is important because it helps you to determine how serious the patient's condition is and to set priorities for care and transport. It is based on your immediate assessment of the environment and the patient's chief complaint.

The environment can provide a great deal of information about the patient. It frequently gives clues—to the EMT-B who looks for them—about the patient's condition and history. One of the most important things it can sometimes tell you is what happened. Is there an overturned ladder, indicating that the patient may have fallen? Has the patient been exposed to a cold outdoor environment for a long time? Or is there no apparent mechanism of injury, leading you to presume that the patient has a medical problem rather than trauma (an injury)? Although the EMT-B cannot rely completely on the patient's environment to rule out trauma, when combined with the chief complaint (e.g., the patient complaining of symptoms that sound more like a medical problem than an injury), environmental clues become extremely useful.

The **chief complaint** is the reason EMS was called, usually in the patient's own words. It may be as obvious as abdominal pain or as vague as "not feeling good." In any case, it is the patient's description of why you were called.

FIRST take body substance isolation precautions.

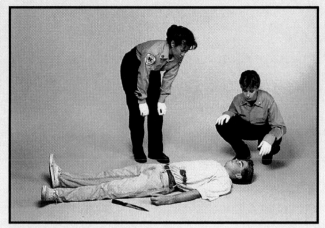

1. Form a general impression of patient and patient's environment.

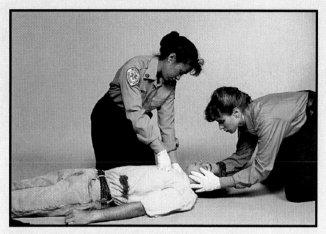

2. Assess patient's mental status.

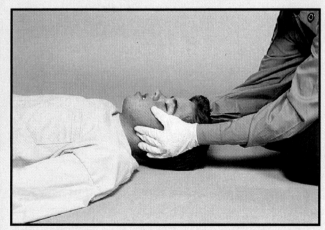

3. Assess airway. (Intervention: Perform appropriate maneuver to open and maintain airway. If necessary, insert oro- or nasopharyngeal airway.)

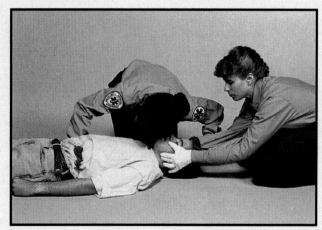

4. Assess breathing. (Interventions: If respiratory arrest or inadequate breathing, ventilate with 100% oxygen. If breathing above 24/min, give high concentration oxygen.)

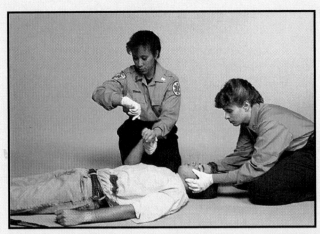

5. Evaluate circulation by taking the patient's pulse and evaluating skin temperature, color, and condition, and . . .

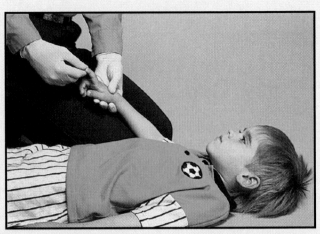

. . . in infants and children also assess circulation by testing capillary refill. (Interventions: For indications of poor circulation, treat for shock.)

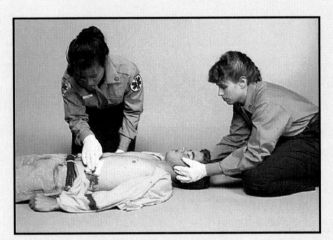

Assess and control severe bleeding.

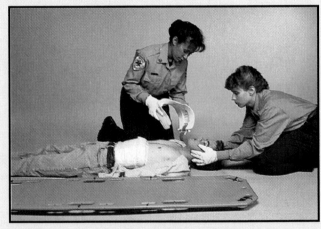

6. Make a decision about patient's priority for further assessment, interventions, or immediate transport.

You form a general impression by looking, listening, and smelling. You look for the patient's age and sex—easy to determine once the patient is in sight. You look at the patient's position to see if it indicates an injury, pain, or difficulty in breathing. You listen for sounds like moaning, snoring, or gurgling respirations. You sniff the air to detect any smells like hazardous fumes, urine, feces, vomitus, or decay.

Something that is more difficult to describe than your direct observations but just as important is the feeling or sense you get when you arrive at the scene or encounter the patient. You may become anxious when you see a patient who exhibits no outward signs of illness or injury, yet "just doesn't look right" to you. Or you may feel reassured when you are dispatched to a "sick baby," but see that the infant is alert and smiling. After you gain some practice assessing and managing patients, you may develop a "sixth sense" that clues you in to the severity of a patient's condition. This is part of what is called "clinical judgment"—judgment based on experience in observing and treating patients. Some people find it easier than others to cultivate this instinct, but even those who have excellent clinical judgment do not depend on it alone. A systematic approach to finding threats to life is the best way to make sure they are not missed.

Assessing Mental Status

After you form a general impression, the next step in the initial assessment is to determine the patient's **mental status,** or level of responsiveness. In most patients this will be quite easy, since most people are alert and responsive; that is, they are awake and will talk and

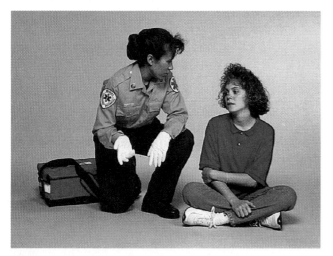
Alert

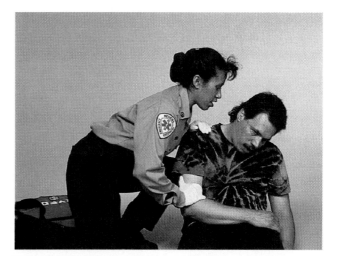
Verbal stimulus

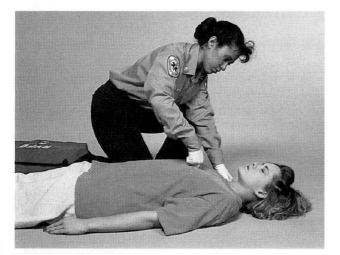
Painful stimulus

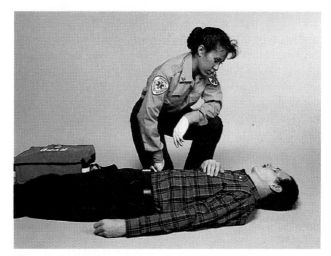
Unresponsive

FIGURE 9-1 The AVPU levels of responsiveness.

answer questions sensibly. Some patients, with a depressed level of responsiveness, are not awake but will respond to verbal stimuli, such as talking or shouting. A still more depressed level of responsiveness is indicated when the patient responds only to painful stimuli, such as pinching a toe or rubbing the sternum briskly. The lowest mental status, and the most serious, is unresponsiveness, when the patient will not respond even to a painful stimulus. An easy way to remember these levels of responsiveness is the letters **AVPU** (Figure 9-1), which stand for

Alert
Verbal
Painful
Unresponsive

A patient who is alert (awake) may still be confused. A good way to be more specific about an awake patient's level of responsiveness is to describe what the patient is "oriented to." Most EMS systems are concerned with orientation to three things: person, place, and time. A patient who can speak clearly can almost always tell you his name (orientation to person). A few patients are oriented to person, but can't tell you where they are (orientation to place). Some patients are oriented to person and place but can't tell you the day, date, or time (orientation to time). A few EMS systems include other questions in addition to those about person, place, and time to determine the patient's level of responsiveness or orientation.

A depressed level of responsiveness may indicate the possibility of a life-threatening problem such as severe bleeding or shock. If you find that the patient's level of responsiveness is below the Alert level, you will provide high concentration oxygen by nonrebreather mask. You will also take the patient's mental status into account when you make your priority decision. A depressed mental status will generally mean a higher priority for early transport.

Assessing the ABCs

When you learned cardiopulmonary resuscitation, you learned a new meaning for the ABCs: Airway, Breathing, and Circulation. Even when a patient is not in cardiac arrest, you will still check airway, breathing, and circulation as you look for life-threatening problems.

(See Table 9-1 for a summary of assessment steps for mental status and the ABCs for adults, children, and infants. You may also want to review Chapter 5, Baseline Vital Signs and SAMPLE History, and Chapter 7, Airway Management, in which you learned in detail about the airway, breathing, and circulation assessment management techniques that are mentioned below.)

In the alert patient, checking the airway is usually quick and easy. If the patient is talking clearly or crying loudly, you know that the airway is open. If the airway is not open, or if the patient is not alert, is supine, or is breathing noisily, indicating that his airway may be endangered, you will take measures to open the airway, such as the jaw-thrust maneuver, the head-tilt, chin-lift maneuver, suctioning, or insertion of an oro- or nasopharyngeal airway. If the airway is blocked, you will perform the Heimlich maneuver or back blows and chest thrusts.

If the airway is open, or as soon as you have corrected any airway problems, you will proceed to assessment of the patient's breathing. If the patient is in respiratory arrest, you will perform rescue breathing. If he is not alert (V, P, or U on the AVPU scale) and his breathing rate is slower than 8 breaths per minute, you will provide ventilations with a bag-valve mask and 100% oxygen. If the patient is alert and his breathing rate is faster than 24 breaths per minute, you will give high concentration oxygen by nonrebreather mask. If your patient is breathing without difficulty at a rate in the normal range, or after you have performed necessary interventions to correct any breathing problems, you will continue the initial assessment with an evaluation of circulation.

To begin your assessment of circulation, you will take the patient's pulse. If there is no pulse and the patient is in cardiac arrest, you will perform cardiopulmonary resuscitation.

Cardiac arrest, however, is not the only possible life-threatening circulation problem. Inadequate flow of blood throughout the body or severe loss of blood is also life threatening. Evaluating circulation involves assessment of three things: pulse, bleeding, and skin. If the patient is light-skinned, you can check pulse and skin at the same time: As you take the radial pulse, you can note whether the patient's skin at the wrist is warm, pink, and dry—indicating good circulation of blood—or whether the skin is, instead, pale and clammy (cool and moist)—

TABLE 9-1   Initial Assessment of Adults, Children, and Infants

	Adults	Children 1-6 yrs.	Infants to 1 yr.
Mental Status	AVPU: Is patient alert? responsive to verbal stimulus? responsive to painful stimulus? unresponsive? If alert, is patient oriented to person, place, and time?	As for adults	If not alert, shout as a verbal stimulus, flick feet as a painful stimulus. (Crying would be infant's response.)
Airway	Trauma: jaw thrust Medical: head-tilt, chin lift. Consider oro- or nasopharyngeal airway, suctioning.	As for adults, but see Chapter 7 and BLS Review for special child airway techniques. If performing head-tilt, chin-lift, do so without hyperextending (stretching) the neck.	As for children but see Chapter 7 and BLS Review for special infant airway techniques.
Breathing	If respiratory arrest, perform rescue breathing. If depressed mental status and inadequate breathing (slower than 8 per minute), ventilate with bag-valve mask and 100% oxygen. If alert and respirations are more than 24 per minute, give 100% oxygen by nonrebreather mask.	As for adults, but normal rates for children are faster than for adults. (See Chapter 5 for normal child respiration rates.) Parent may have to hold oxygen mask to reduce child's fear of mask.	As for children, but normal rates for infants are faster than for children and adults. (See Chapter 5 for normal infant respiration rates.)
Circulation	Assess skin, radial pulse, bleeding. If cardiac arrest, perform CPR. See Chapter 25 on how to treat for bleeding and shock.	Assess skin, radial pulse, bleeding, capillary refill. See Chapter 5 for normal child pulse rates (faster than for adults). If cardiac arrest, perform CPR. See BLS Review for special child techniques. See Chapter 25 on how to treat for bleeding and shock.	Assess skin, brachial pulse, bleeding, capillary refill. See Chapter 5 for normal infant pulse rates (faster than for children and adults). If cardiac arrest, perform CPR. See BLS Review for special infant techniques. See Chapter 25 on how to treat for bleeding and shock.

See Chapter 5, Baseline Vital Signs and SAMPLE History; Chapter 7, Airway Management; Chapter 25, Bleeding and Shock, Chapter 29, Infants and Children, and BLS Review for additional information.

indicating poor circulation. If your patient is dark-skinned, you can check the color of the skin at the lips or nail beds. You will also check for and control severe bleeding. If even one large blood vessel or several smaller ones are bleeding, a patient can lose enough blood in just a minute or two to die. Quick control of severe external bleeding can be life-saving.

You will take into account the potential for shock resulting from inadequate circulation and the amount of blood loss in making decisions about transport priority.

Determining Priority

When, during the initial assessment, you do encounter a life-threatening problem involving airway, breathing, or circulation, you will stop to treat the condition as soon as you discover it.

When the process of assessing and caring for life-threatening problems is complete, you will decide on the patient's priority for immediate transport to the hospital. Most patients don't need immediate transport, but a few do, and you must be able to distinguish between the two

TABLE 9-2 High Priority Conditions

Poor general impression
Unresponsive
Responsive, but not following commands
Difficulty breathing
Shock
Complicated childbirth
Chest pain with systolic blood pressure less than 100
Uncontrolled bleeding
Severe pain anywhere

TABLE 9-3 Patient Characteristics

A patient may have any of the following 12 combinations of characteristics.

	Responsive				Unresponsive		
	Adult	Child	Infant		Adult	Child	Infant
Medical				Medical			
Trauma				Trauma			

types of patients. If any life-threatening problem discovered and treated during the initial assessment continues or threatens to recur, or if the patient has a depressed level of responsiveness, you may decide that this patient has an immediate priority for transport, with assessment and care continuing en route.

Additional High Priority Conditions

In addition to the problems the initial assessment is designed to find and treat (depressed mental status or airway, breathing, or circulation problems), there are also a number of other conditions or findings that indicate patients should receive high priority for transport to the hospital (Table 9-2). These conditions are those for which, usually, there is little or no treatment that can be given in the field that will make a difference in how well the patient does. You will learn more about these conditions in later chapters.

PATIENT CHARACTERISTICS AND INITIAL ASSESSMENT

The initial assessment takes different forms, depending on the following characteristics of the patient.

- Whether the patient has a medical problem or a trauma problem (injury)
- Whether the patient is responsive or unresponsive
- Whether the patient is an adult, a child, or an infant

Over a series of calls, you will probably encounter patients with a variety of combina-

tions of these characteristics. In fact, twelve different combinations of these characteristics are possible, as shown in Table 9-3.

Even though the specific steps of the initial assessment will be different under different conditions, the goals and general approach of the initial assessment are always the same: find and correct immediately life-threatening problems and determine the patient's priority for treatment and transport.

Four patients with different combinations of characteristics are described on the following pages to give you an idea of how the six steps of the initial assessment might be carried out in a variety of situations.

A Responsive Adult Medical Patient

	Responsive				Unresponsive		
	Adult	Child	Infant		Adult	Child	Infant
Medical	▓			Medical			
Trauma				Trauma			

Mr. Schmidt, your patient from On the Scene at the beginning of this chapter, the older man who complained of abdominal pain, was a responsive adult with a medical problem. When you approached him, you followed all six steps of the initial assessment. You formed a *general impression* by looking at him. As you questioned him, you evaluated his *mental status, airway,* and *breathing.* You quickly assessed his *circulation* and determined that he had no immediately life-threatening problems.

The initial assessment of a responsive medical patient is summarized in Table 9-4, column one.

TABLE 9-4   Initial Assessment and Interventions

Responsive Medical Patient	Unresponsive Medical Patient	Responsive Trauma Patient	Unresponsive Trauma Patient
1. General impression	1. General impression	1. General impression Mechanism of injury Intervention: Manual head immobilization	1. General impression Mechanism of injury Intervention: Manual head immobilization
2. Mental Status—**A**VPU	2. Mental Status—**AVPU**	2. Mental Status—**A**VPU	2. Mental Status—**AVPU**
3. Airway is open.	3. Airway Interventions: Open airway with head-tilt, chin-lift; consider oro- or nasopharyngeal airway; suction as needed. For foreign body obstruction, use Heimlich maneuver or other blockage-clearing technique	3. Airway is open.	3. Airway Interventions: Open airway with jaw-thrust; consider oro- or nasopharyngeal airway; suction as needed. For foreign body obstruction, use Heimlich maneuver or other blockage-clearing technique
4. Breathing: Look for rise and fall of chest, listen and feel for rate and depth of breathing, look for work of breathing (use of accessory muscles, retractions) Interventions: If rate is greater than 24, high concentration oxygen by nonrebreather mask. If respiratory arrest, perform rescue breathing.	4. Breathing: Look for rise and fall of chest, listen and feel for rate and depth of breathing, look for work of breathing (use of accessory muscles, retractions) Interventions: If breathing is adequate, high concentration oxygen by nonrebreather mask. Position patient on side. If breathing is inadequate, ventilate with bag-valve mask and high concentration oxygen. If respiratory arrest, perform rescue breathing.	4. Breathing: Look for rise and fall of chest, listen and feel for rate and depth of breathing, look for work of breathing (use of accessory muscles, retractions) Interventions: If rate is greater than 24, high concentration oxygen by nonrebreather mask. If respiratory arrest, perform rescue breathing.	4. Breathing: Look for rise and fall of chest, listen and feel for rate and depth of breathing, look for work of breathing (use of accessory muscles, retractions) Interventions: If breathing is adequate, high concentration oxygen by nonrebreather mask. Position patient on side. If breathing is inadequate, ventilate with bag-valve mask and high concentration oxygen. If respiratory arrest, perform rescue breathing.
5. Circulation: Pulse; bleeding; skin color, temperature, condition (capillary refill in infants and children) Interventions: Control bleeding. Treat for shock. If cardiac arrest, perform CPR.	5. Circulation: Pulse; bleeding; skin color, temperature, condition (capillary refill in infants and children) Interventions: Control bleeding. Treat for shock. If cardiac arrest, perform CPR.	5. Circulation: Pulse; bleeding; skin color, temperature, condition (capillary refill in infants and children) Interventions: Control bleeding. Treat for shock. If cardiac arrest, perform CPR.	5. Circulation: Pulse; bleeding; skin color, temperature, condition (capillary refill in infants and children) Interventions: Control bleeding. Treat for shock. If cardiac arrest, perform CPR.
6. Priority	6. Priority	6. Priority	6. Priority

To review or preview specific assessments and interventions, see Chapter 7, Airway Management, Chapter 25, Bleeding and Shock, and BLS Review at the end of this book.

An Unresponsive Adult Medical Patient

	Responsive					Unresponsive		
	Adult	Child	Infant			Adult	Child	Infant
Medical					Medical	▨		
Trauma					Trauma			

On the Scene

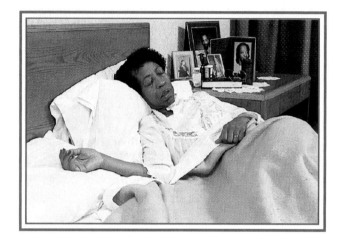

Your dispatcher sends you to an "unconscious" woman. As you approach the house and perform **scene size-up**, you draw on disposable gloves and make sure the scene is safe. Inside, the patient's daughter brings you to a bedroom. There is no evidence of any mechanism of injury.

Your **general impression** is formed as you go into the room and see an adult woman lying on her back in bed. She is not moving and her eyes are closed. You assess her **mental status** by saying, "Mrs. Malone, can you hear me?" In response to your question, she moans a little, so you know she responds to a verbal stimulus. In your report, you will describe both the stimulus (verbal) and the response (moaning). If Mrs. Malone had not responded to verbal stimulus, you would have inflicted a painful stimulus to try to get a response from her.

Because she is lying on her back, her **airway** is threatened by her tongue. Since patients with depressed responsiveness are always at risk for airway problems, you know that you need to be aggressive about opening and maintaining her airway. So even though you haven't heard any sounds indicating partial airway obstruction (like snoring or gurgling), you ask your partner to remove the pillow, tilt her head back, and lift her chin. Next, you evaluate

her **breathing** by bringing your ear next to her mouth and looking for movement of her chest and abdomen as you listen and feel for the movement of air with your ear. You determine the depth of Mrs. Malone's respirations and if her breathing rate is slow or fast. If you found that her breathing was inadequate you would ventilate Mrs. Malone with 100% oxygen.

Her respirations are in the normal range, but you will give Mrs. Malone high concentration oxygen by nonrebreather mask anyway because her level of responsiveness is depressed. You put in a nasopharyngeal airway and move Mrs. Malone onto her side in order to help protect her airway.

You next check **circulation.** Mrs. Malone's pulse is strong, regular, and in the normal range for rate. You look for blood, but find none. The skin at her wrist is cool and dry. Because Mrs. Malone is dark-skinned, you assess for skin color at her lips and nail beds, which are pale. Although the pulse and bleeding check are normal, the paleness and coolness of her skin are slightly abnormal.

The **priority** of this patient is high because her mental status is depressed, her airway is at risk, and her skin indicates a circulation problem. You arrange immediate transport to the hospital, planning to continue assessment and care en route.

In Chapter 11, we will continue the story of Mrs. Malone's assessment.

■

The initial assessment of Mrs. Malone, an unresponsive patient, looked very different from the initial assessment of Mr. Schmidt, a responsive patient, but in both cases the goal was the same: find and correct immediately life-threatening problems. Mrs. Malone had more problems to correct, so there were more actions to take, and the initial assessment took a little longer. Mrs. Malone's airway was at risk, and her level of responsiveness was depressed, although there was no suspicion of injury. So your partner used the head-tilt, chin-lift maneuver to keep Mrs. Malone's airway open until you were able to insert a nasopharyngeal airway, turn her on her side, and provide high concentration oxygen by nonrebreather mask.

In this text we will often group patients like Mrs. Malone whose mental status is less than "alert" on the AVPU scale—whether responsive to verbal or painful stimulus or completely unresponsive—in the general category of "unresponsive," because all will require oxygen and airway protection as were provided for Mrs. Malone.

What Mr. Schmidt and Mrs. Malone had in common was that both were suffering from medical conditions; in neither case was there any evidence of trauma, nor any need for the interventions trauma patients routinely require.

The initial assessment of an unresponsive medical patient is summarized in Table 9-4, column two.

A Responsive Child Trauma Patient

	Responsive				Unresponsive		
	Adult	Child	Infant		Adult	Child	Infant
Medical				Medical			
Trauma				Trauma			

On the Scene

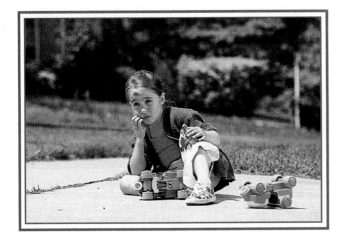

You respond to a scene where a child has fallen. Your **scene size-up** reveals nothing that looks threatening. Since the call came in as an injury, you assume that there will be blood at the scene and put gloves on as you arrive. As you approach the patient you begin to form your **general impression.** You see a girl who is about 5 years old sitting on the sidewalk. She is crying and holding a bloody cloth on her knee. A pair of skates gives you the idea that she has taken a tumble while skating.

When you reach the patient, you kneel next to her and introduce yourself. You ask what happened. She confirms your suspicion that she fell down while trying her new skates. When you ask her, she tells you her name is Clara Diller and that her head and knee hurt. Since she is crying and answers your question easily, you determine that her **mental status** is alert and her **airway** is clear.

Because there is a mechanism of injury indicating possible trauma, you explain to her that she should not move her head and that your partner is going to hold her head to help her keep it still. Her **breathing** is not labored and her respiratory rate and depth are in the normal range.

You start to evaluate her **circulation** by feeling her radial pulse. It is slightly rapid but strong and regular. You look around her and see no blood except on the cloth and on her knee. Since it is hard to tell how much bleeding may be under the cloth, you tell Clara you want to look at her knee. You see a 2-inch laceration which is oozing some blood, so you put the cloth back on and ask the neighbor who takes care of Clara to apply a little pressure to it. When you felt Clara's radial pulse, you noted that her skin is warm, pink, and dry. You also assess her capillary refill by pressing on the end of her fingernail. The color in the nail bed returns to pink in less than two seconds. So all indications are that Clara's circulation is good.

Based on the information you have gathered, you determine that Clara's **priority** for immediate transport is low. Clara has no significant mechanism of injury and no immediately life-threatening problems. There is no evidence that she was struck by a car or hit any object other than the sidewalk. However, since the sidewalk is a hard surface, you maintain a high index of suspicion for possible cervical spine injury. As soon as it is practical, you will apply a cervical collar and immobilize Clara on a backboard.

The story of Clara's assessment will continue in Chapter 10.

Trauma patients like Clara present a different kind of challenge during initial assessment. Here, there may be threats to your own safety and some new concerns for the condition of the patient.

Since this call came in as an injury, you anticipated the presence of blood and put on gloves as you arrived. You were also careful to look for potential dangers like oncoming traffic at the scene.

Cloth can absorb a lot of blood and cover a large bleeding wound, so it was necessary to look under the cloth for continuing bleeding. Fortunately, the wound was not bleeding heavily and direct pressure was enough to control it. The cloth was clean, so you did not need to replace it right away with a sterile dressing.

There was a mechanism of injury that made you suspect spinal injury, so you made sure that Clara's head was manually stabilized during your initial assessment. Clara did not have any immediately life-threatening problems, but you considered carefully how fast she was probably traveling and how hard she may have fallen. If serious injury had seemed possible, you would have treated her as a high priority. If, on the other hand, she was not traveling fast when she fell, there would probably have been more time to consider contacting her parents and getting consent for treatment and transport.

The initial assessment of a responsive trauma patient is summarized in Table 9-4, column three.

Infants and Children

Because Clara is a child, several other factors were different in her case than they were for your adult patients, Mr. Schmidt and Mrs. Malone.

Since children are often shy or distrustful of strangers or adults, you made a special effort to gain Clara's trust by kneeling to her level as you talked with her. Responsive children need to have some trust in the EMT-B. This may take a minute or two, but the general impression will guide you in determining how long to spend developing a rapport with the child.

Infants and children breathe faster than adults and their hearts beat faster, and you kept this in mind when you evaluated Clara's breathing and circulation.

A special part of the circulation check in infants and children is capillary refill. Nail beds are typically pink in healthy, normal people. When the end of the fingernail is gently pressed, it turns white. When the pressure is released, the nail bed turns pink again very quickly, usually in less than two seconds. In children, this is a good way to evaluate the circulation of blood. In an infant or small child with small nail beds, press the back of the hand or top of the foot instead. Count, "one-one thousand, two-one thousand" or say "capillary refill." If the nail or skin regains its pink color in the time it takes to say one of these, it is probably normal. Abnormal responses include prolonged and absent capillary refill (taking too long to turn pink again, or not turning pink again at all). These usually indicate problems with circulation.

Capillary refill is not a reliable sign for adults, so it is used only in infants and young children. In some adults, it is normal for capillary refill to take longer than two seconds, especially in the elderly. Even in infants and young children, it can be affected by factors such as the weather. Cold temperatures will prolong cap-illary refill. It should be used as one factor to consider in determining the priority of the young patient, but not the only one.

Like adult trauma patients, child and infant trauma patients need to have their heads immobilized in order to prevent injury to the cervical spinal cord.

An infant has an airway that is different from an adult's, so opening an infant's or child's airway means moving the head to a neutral position, not tilting it back the way an adult's airway is opened. The mental status of unresponsive infants is typically checked by talking to the infant and flicking the feet.

You will learn about other considerations in approaching and assessing pediatric patients in Chapter 29, Infants and Children.

Applying Manual Stabilization

Your partner held Clara's head still all during your initial assessment. You should apply manual stabilization to any patient who you suspect may have an injury to the spine based on mechanism of injury, or history, or signs and symptoms—that is, to virtually any trauma patient.

When you apply manual stabilization, your object is to hold the patient's head still in a neutral, in-line position. That is, the head should be facing forward and not turned to either side nor tilted forward or backward. You must be careful not to pull or twist the patient's head but rather to hold it perfectly still and to remind the patient not to try to move it.

When your patient is sitting up, position yourself just behind the patient and hold the head by spreading your fingers over the sides of the head and placing your thumbs on the back

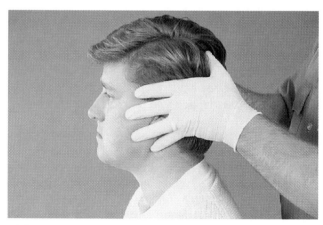

FIGURE 9-2 Stabilize a sitting patient's head from the rear.

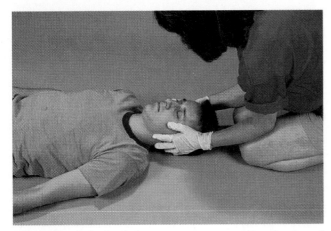

FIGURE 9-3 Stabilize a supine patient's head from the top.

of the head (Figure 9-2). When your patient is supine, kneel behind the patient and spread your fingers and thumbs around the sides of the head to hold it steady (Figure 9-3). If your patient is in another position, for example crumpled on his side, or is being moved by other EMS personnel, adapt the technique as practical to hold the head in a steady position in line with the spine.

An Unresponsive Adult Trauma Patient

	Responsive				Unresponsive		
	Adult	Child	Infant		Adult	Child	Infant
Medical				Medical			
Trauma				Trauma			

On the Scene

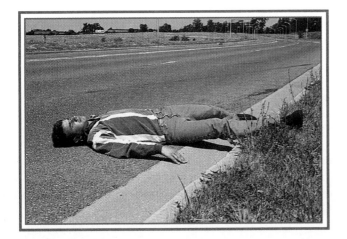

Driving too fast on a slick road, Brian Sawyer loses control of his car. You receive the call for "a motor vehicle collision."

As you approach and perform **scene size-up,** you see a police cruiser with its emergency lights on and firefighting apparatus just pulling up. You look for hazards and vehicles. You see no downed wires or other potential hazards, and there is only one vehicle at the scene other than the police and EMS vehicles, a compact car. It has sustained a lot of damage to the roof and sides, but is resting on its wheels, so you suspect it has rolled over. With your gloves on, you get out of your vehicle.

The police officer tells you that the only person who was in the car is lying beside the road approximately 20 feet from the vehicle. The officer recognizes him and tells you his name is Brian Sawyer. As you approach, you get a **general impression** of an approximately 25-year-old male who appears unresponsive and has snoring respirations. The mechanism of injury, the wrecked car, and the fact that Brian is quite a distance from his vehicle are obvious.

Your partner moves to stabilize Brian's head and to attend to the airway as you begin to check his **mental status.** He doesn't respond to your calling his name, and he is unresponsive to a brisk rub of your knuckles on his sternum. Your partner has started to treat the **airway** problem you both heard, snoring respirations that mean partial obstruction of the airway. Your partner manually stabilizes the head at the same time that he does a jaw thrust, which relieves the snoring sound. You listen closely and hear no other noises from his airway. If you heard gurgling or saw fluid in Brian's airway, you would suction him.

To evaluate **breathing,** you look, listen, and feel. Brian has respirations that appear normal in rate and depth. Because he is unresponsive but with adequate respirations, you give Brian high concentration oxygen by nonrebreather mask as soon as you finish checking circulation. You select an oropharyngeal airway and insert it, then apply a nonrebreather mask with 15 liters per minute of high concentration oxygen.

You start to assess **circulation** by feeling the radial pulse. It is rapid and weak. There is no blood on or near the patient that you can see. His skin is pale, cool, and sweaty.

The **priority** you assign Brian is high. He is unresponsive to pain and his rapid, weak pulse and pale, clammy skin are signs of diminished circulation. You will spend as little time on the scene as possible and plan to monitor his airway, place a cervical collar on him, immobilize him on a backboard, and to get him to an appropriate facility quickly. Since you and your partner will both be needed to care for this patient en route to the hospital, you radio for additional personnel to drive the ambulance.

In Chapter 10, we will continue the story of Brian Sawyer's assessment.

<hr>

With this unresponsive trauma patient, there were many things to pay attention to. There are many potential dangers at a scene like this, including gasoline spills, downed power lines, unstable vehicles, and traffic. In this case, fortunately, there is only one patient, but you need to think about and look for other patients when motor vehicles are involved.

Like Clara, the child who fell while skating, Brian has suffered trauma. Brian's mechanism of injury is more serious, but both patients need manual stabilization of the head and spine during the initial assessment. To further protect the spine, your partner used a jaw thrust to open the airway rather than a head-tilt, chin-lift. This allows the airway to be opened without the risk of worsening a trauma patient's injuries. Moving the head of a patient with a broken bone in the cervical spine may cause that bone to pinch or cut the spinal cord, paralyzing the patient, possibly for life, or even causing death. As soon as practical, you will apply a cervical collar and immobilize Brian on a spine board.

Unlike Clara, Brian had a depressed level of responsiveness, an airway problem, and indications of inadequate circulation. All of these signal possible life-threatening problems, so that

Brian's priority for immediate transport was high, while Clara's was low.

The initial assessment of an unresponsive trauma patient is summarized in Table 9-4, column four.

Other Types of Patients

Above, you have read about four types of patients you may encounter and how you would carry out an initial assessment on each of them. The chart below shows the eight types of patients you did not read about in this chapter.

	Responsive				Unresponsive		
	Adult	Child	Infant		Adult	Child	Infant
Medical				**Medical**			
Trauma				**Trauma**			

As you continue reading through the remainder of this text, you will encounter examples of all of these types of patients. In particular, you will read about adult, child, and infant patients with medical and trauma problems in the Medical module, Chapters 16-24, in the Trauma module, Chapters 25-28, and in the Infants and Children module, Chapter 29. As you read about these types of patients, consider how you would follow the six steps of the initial assessment to find and treat immediately life-threatening problems and to set priorities for treatment and transport.

<hr>

CHAPTER REVIEW

KEY TERMS

You may find it helpful to review the following terms.

AVPU a memory aid for *alert, verbal response, painful response, unresponsive* as a classification of a patient's level of responsiveness (see also mental status).

chief complaint in emergency medicine, the reason EMS was called, usually in the patient's own words.

initial assessment the first element in assessment of a patient; steps taken for the purpose of

discovering and dealing with any life-threatening problems. The six parts of initial assessment are forming a general impression, assessing mental status, assessing airway, assessing breathing, assessing circulation, and determining the priority of the patient for treatment and transport to the hospital.

interventions actions taken to correct a patient's problems.

mental status level of responsiveness (*see also* AVPU).

It is essential to assess patients in a systematic way that allows for quickly finding and treating immediate threats to life. This search is called the initial assessment. By forming a general impression, determining mental status, evaluating airway, breathing, and circulation, and determining the patient's priority, you can find and correct the problems that could otherwise end a patient's life in just a few minutes. You will also be able to determine how urgently the patient must be transported and how to conduct the rest of your assessment.

REVIEW QUESTIONS

1. List factors you will take into account in forming a general impression of a patient.
2. Explain how to assess a patient's mental status with regard to the AVPU levels of responsiveness.
3. Explain how to assess airway, breathing, and circulation during the initial assessment. Explain the interventions you will take for possible problems with airway, breathing, and circulation.
4. Explain what is meant by the term *priority decision.*
5. Explain what special interventions are required
   - if a patient has suffered trauma.
   - if a patient is unresponsive.

Application
   - You are called to respond to a "sick baby." When you arrive, you are led to a baby in its crib. Its eyes are closed. How do you conduct your initial assessment?

The Focused History and Physical Exam— Trauma Patient

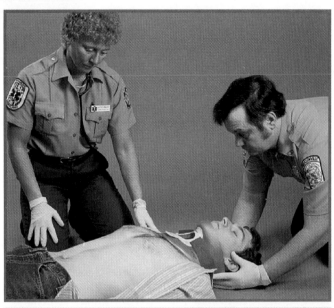

For the trauma patient—especially one whose injuries are serious—time must not be wasted at the scene. This patient needs to get to a hospital as quickly as possible. On the other hand, enough time must be spent at the scene to assess the patient adequately and give proper emergency care. How can you strike the right balance between care and speed? The key is focus. Instead of performing a time-consuming, comprehensive assessment on every patient, the EMT-B homes in on what is important for this particular patient. It is a process known as the focused history and physical exam.

Objectives

Knowledge and Attitude *At the end of this chapter, you should be able to meet the following objectives.*

1. Discuss the reasons for reconsideration concerning the mechanism of injury. (p. 182)

2. State the reasons for performing a rapid trauma assessment. (p. 190)

3. Recite examples and explain why patients should receive a rapid trauma assessment. (p. 190)

4. Describe the areas included in the rapid trauma assessment and discuss what should be evaluated. (p. 190)

5. Differentiate when the rapid assessment may be altered in order to provide patient care. (pp. 190, 201)

6. Discuss the reason for performing a focused history and physical exam. (p. 182)

7. Recognize and respect the feelings that patients might experience during assessment. (pp. 200–201)

Skills

1. Demonstrate the rapid trauma assessment that should be used to treat a patient based on mechanism of injury.

On the Scene

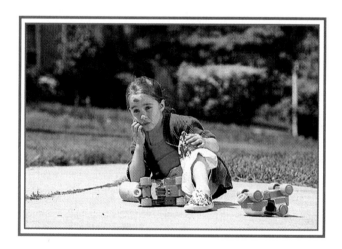

In Chapter 9, you began your assessment of Clara, the little girl who fell while roller skating. First you sized up the scene. Then you did the initial assessment.

Scene Size-Up (Review)

When you arrived on the scene, you put on gloves for **body substance isolation.** You evaluated **scene safety** and found nothing that could threaten your safety or that of anyone else at the scene. A **mechanism of injury,** Clara's fall to the sidewalk, was immediately obvious. The **number of patients,** as you could see, was just one: Clara.

Initial Assessment (Review)

Quickly, you did the initial assessment to look for and treat any immediate threats to Clara's life. First you got a **general impression** of an awake female child crying and holding a cloth on her knee. As your partner held her head still, you asked her what happened. She told you she fell while trying new skates. You could tell that her **mental status** was alert and her **airway** was clear. Her **breathing** was normal.

You evaluated her **circulation** by feeling her radial pulse, observing the blood on the cloth on her knee, and noting her skin condition. You also assessed her capillary refill by pressing on the end of her fingernail.

Based on the information you gathered, you determined Clara's *priority:* she had no significant mechanism of injury and no immediately life-threatening problems. So you will not transport Clara to the hospital immediately. There is time to do the next assessment step at the scene: the focused history and physical exam.

Focused History and Physical Exam—Trauma
No Significant Mechanism of Injury

Mechanism of Injury As you begin the focused history and physical exam, you consider Clara's mechanism of injury once again. Why? Because you will do a different version of the focused history and physical exam if the mechanism of injury is significant than if it is not. So you take a careful look around to make sure that Clara has only fallen to the sidewalk, not struck a pole or been hit by a car, for instance. A sidewalk is a hard surface to fall on. On the other hand a young child skating for the first time on level ground is unlikely to have built up enough speed to have sustained life-threatening injuries. Having confirmed your conclusion that there is *no significant mechanism of injury,* you proceed as follows.

Chief Complaint "Where do you hurt, Clara?" you ask her. You are not surprised when she says, "My knee hurts," because you can see that her knee is bleeding. Then she adds, "My head hurts, too." So you know that she may have struck her head. Based on the mechanism of injury, a fall to a hard surface, you suspect that she may have injured her spine as well. So you now *focus your assessment according to the chief complaint and mechanism of injury.* You focus not on Clara's whole body, but on her head, neck, spine, and knee.

Focused Physical Exam You look at Clara's head and the back of her neck, searching for injuries such as contusions (bruises), abrasions (scrapes), punctures or penetrations, burns, and lacerations (cuts). You find only some swelling on her forehead. Next, you gently press on her head and cervical spine, starting at the top, then moving to the back of her head and going down her neck to the big bump that indicates the lower end of the neck. You find no deformities, tenderness, or swelling. You now determine the proper size cervical spine immobilization collar for a child Clara's size. You put it around her neck without moving her head or neck while your partner continues to hold her head.

During the initial assessment, you controlled the bleeding from her knee. Now you tell her, "Clara, I need to lift up that cloth and look underneath. I'm going to feel around your knee, too. If it hurts, you can tell me, OK?" Clara agrees, and you look at her knee for contusions, abrasions, punctures or penetrations, burns, or lacerations. There is only the laceration you found earlier. It is bleeding very slowly and does not appear to be deep. You palpate (feel) the area around the knee. You find no deformities or swelling, but the lateral side (outside) of the knee is tender.

Vital Signs Next, you assess Clara's vital signs. Her *pulse* is 104 per minute, strong and regular. She has *respirations* of 24 per minute. They are normal in depth. You check her *skin* by looking at the palm of her hand and see that it is pink. You feel it and determine that it is warm and dry. You squeeze the end of her fingernail and find that her capillary refill is normal. After telling Clara what you are going to do, you shine a light into her eyes and find that her *pupils* are equal and reactive. Again, you tell Clara what to expect before you inflate a pediatric (for children) cuff on her arm and find her *blood pressure* is 90/60.

History While you are doing the focused exam, you ask Clara for more information. She is 5 years old, she tells you, and very scared because "my mommy told me not to try my new skates till later." The neighbor who takes care of Clara says, "I called Clara's mother at work when I saw her fall." You ask, "Did you see if Clara got knocked out? Even for a moment?" The neighbor tells you Clara did not lose consciousness.

Just now, Clara's mother arrives at the scene. You reassure her that Clara seems to have just an injury to her knee and a slight bump on her head. You also explain that you have put a special collar on her just in case she injured her neck and that she will be placed on a spine board for the ride to the hospital.

Clara's mother is a better source of medical information than a 5-year old, so you interview her for the *SAMPLE history.* You have already asked Clara what *symptoms* she has, so you ask her mother if Clara has any *allergies* or takes any *medicines.* You also ask about *pertinent past history.* She tells you that Clara has no allergies, takes no medicines and is healthy. The neighbor tells you Clara's *last food or drink* was lunch a couple of hours ago. When you ask her about *events leading to the injury,* she tells you Clara has been feeling fine and acting normal today.

You immobilize Clara on a backboard and transport her to the emergency department. Clara's visit to the hospital is brief. Any serious head or spine injury is ruled out. She gets some ointment and a cartoon bandage for her knee. She talks excitedly about her ambulance ride all the way home.

*I*n Chapter 9 you learned that you will encounter many kinds of patients in the field. There will be trauma and medical patients, alert and unresponsive patients, patients with serious problems and patients with less serious problems, situations in which the patient, family, and bystanders can all provide information, and situations in which there is no one who can provide information.

How can you tailor assessment procedures for such a bewildering variety of patients? The procedure known as the **focused history and physical exam** provides clear guideposts to help you achieve this goal. Once you have learned and thoroughly practiced the steps of the focused history and physical exam—the more thorough assessment that comes after the initial assessment for life-threatening problems—you will find that you can assess and treat any of these kinds of patients with optimum speed and effectiveness.

In this chapter, you will learn how to perform a focused history and physical exam for a trauma patient; in chapter 11 you will learn the procedure for a medical patient.

FOCUSED HISTORY AND PHYSICAL EXAM: THE TRAUMA PATIENT

Remember that *trauma* means "injury." Injuries can range from slight to severe, from a cut finger to a massive wound. Often you will not be able to see the injury—especially if it is internal—or know how serious it is. Usually, however, you will be able to see or find out the mechanism of injury—what caused the injury, such as a fall or a collision. If the mechanism of injury is significant (for example a gunshot or a motorcycle crash), you will do the focused history and physical exam differently than if the mechanism of injury is not significant (as when Clara, the child in On the Scene, fell down while skating).

No Significant Mechanism of Injury

The first step is to reconsider the mechanism of injury in order to determine how quickly you must transport the patient. If the patient has no significant mechanism of injury and no immediately life-threatening injuries, you will know that you have time to assess the patient more thoroughly at the scene. For a trauma

patient like Clara—one with no significant mechanism of injury—you will focus your assessment by evaluating just the areas that the patient tells you are painful or that you suspect may be injured because of the mechanism of injury. Then you will take a set of baseline vital signs and a SAMPLE history (Table 10-1).

Reconsidering the Mechanism of Injury

As part of scene size-up and the initial assessment, you will have already evaluated the mechanism of injury. Because mechanism of injury is so important in determining your next steps, you should now re-evaluate it. Why? When you first arrive on a scene and must take in a lot of information at once, it is easy to miss things. You are looking not only at how the patient was injured, but also for anything that might threaten you or your crew. You also have other concerns on your mind like whether you need to call for help. Combine that with the stress of knowing that you may have a patient with serious injuries and it is easy to see how an EMT-B can miss important information about the mechanism of injury. In Clara's case, you looked at the sidewalk where she fell and estimated her

TABLE 10-1 Focused History and Physical Exam—Trauma Patient

No Significant Mechanism of Injury	Significant Mechanism of Injury
After scene size-up and initial assessment:	After scene size-up and initial assessment:
1. Reconsider the mechanism of injury.	1. Reconsider the mechanism of injury.
	2. Continue spine stabilization. 3. Consider requesting advanced life support personnel. 4. Reconsider your transport decision. 5. Reassess mental status.
2. Perform focused physical exam based on chief complaint and mechanism of injury.	6. Perform rapid trauma assessment.
3. Assess baseline vital signs.	7. Assess baseline vital signs.
4. Obtain a SAMPLE history.	8. Obtain a SAMPLE history.

probable speed and force of impact. You determined that there was no vehicle involved in her accident and that she did not strike any other object.

Determining the Chief Complaint

The chief complaint is what the patient tells you is the matter. When you asked Clara where she hurt, she told you her knee and her head.

Performing a Focused Physical Exam

In deciding which areas of Clara's body to assess, you depended on what you could see (the knee injury) and what she told you (the chief complaint, the pain in her head and knee). But you did not rely just on these obvious signs and symptoms. You also paid attention to potential injuries the mechanism of injury caused you to suspect. In Clara's case, her fall on a hard surface caused you to suspect spinal injury. You looked at Clara's head and the back of her neck, making sure your partner was holding her head still. Then—because her complaint, mechanism of injury, and the bump you found on her forehead caused you to suspect possible neck or spine injury—you put a cervical collar on her. Finally you examined, then dressed and bandaged her knee.

When you assessed Clara's head, neck, and knee, you evaluated them in two ways: *inspecting* (looking) and *palpating* (feeling). You looked for contusions, abrasions, punctures, penetrations, burns, and lacerations. Then you palpated for deformities, tenderness (pain on pressure), and swelling. An easy way to remember what you are trying to find is the memory aid **DCAP-BTLS** (Scan 10-1). (You can pronounce it as "Dee-cap, B-T-L-S.")

- Deformities
- Contusions
- Abrasions
- Punctures/penetrations
- Burns
- Tenderness
- Lacerations
- Swelling

Deformities are just what they sound like, parts of the body that no longer have the normal shape. Common examples are broken or fractured bones that push up the skin where the bone ends are. Contusions are the medical term

for bruises. Abrasions, or scrapes, are some of the most common injuries you will see. Punctures and penetrations are holes in the body, frequently the result of gunshot wounds and stab wounds. When they are small, they are easy to overlook. Burns may be reddened, blistered, or charred-looking areas. Tenderness means that an area hurts when there is pressure on it, as when it is palpated. Pain (which is present even without any pressure) and tenderness frequently, but not always, go together. Lacerations are cuts, open wounds that sometimes cause significant blood loss. Swelling is a very common result of injured capillaries bleeding under the skin.

In order to find these signs, you will need to expose the patient. This means removing or cutting away clothing in order to see the area of the body you are assessing. Be sure to tell the patient what you are doing and to offer reassurance as necessary. Protect the patient's privacy and take steps to prevent unnecessarily long exposure to cold.

When you practice doing a physical exam, you can repeat *DCAP-BTLS* to yourself as you look at each body part, making sure to remember what each letter is prompting you to inspect or palpate for. You will also check each part for the special signs and symptoms listed in Table 10-3 and described under Performing the Rapid Trauma Assessment later in this chapter.

Obtaining Vital Signs and a SAMPLE History

For a trauma patient, you first conduct a physical exam to assess injuries. Next, you will assess baseline vital signs and get a SAMPLE history. (You learned these procedures in Chapter 5, Baseline Vital Signs and SAMPLE History.) In Clara's case, you were able to piece together her history by getting information from Clara herself, the neighbor who saw her fall, and Clara's mother.

Applying a Cervical Collar

You applied a cervical collar to Clara because she had an injury to her head and she had a mechanism of injury that suggested the possibility of a cervical spine injury. You should apply a cervical collar to any patient who you suspect may have an injury to the spine based on either mechanism of injury, or history, or signs and symptoms. (As you learned in Chapter 5, Baseline Vital Signs and SAMPLE History, signs are

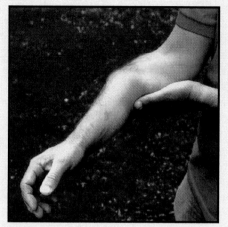

Deformities

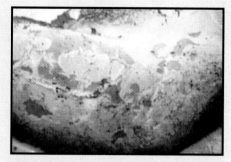

Burns

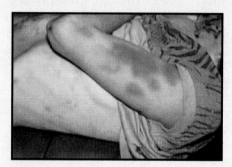

Contusions

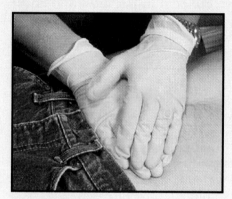

Tenderness

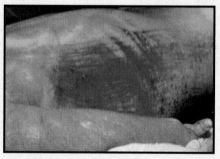

Abrasions

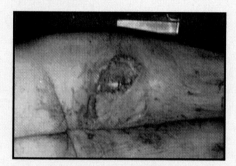

Lacerations

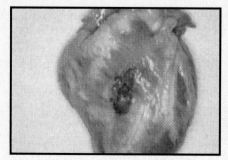

Punctures/Penetrations

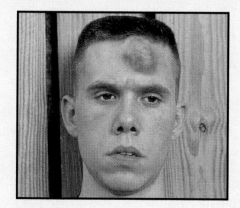

Swelling

184

what you observe, such as a bruise; symptoms are what the patient tells you he feels, such as pain.)

When is it appropriate to apply a cervical collar? There is a simple principle you can follow: If the mechanism of injury exerts great force on the upper body (Figure 10-1) or if there is any soft tissue damage to the head, face, or neck from trauma (e.g., a cut or bruise from being thrown against a dashboard), you may then assume that there is a possible cervical spine injury. Any blow above the clavicles (collarbones) may damage the cervical spine. If the patient has a depressed level of consciousness or if injury cannot be ruled out—even if the mechanism of injury is not known—suspect cervical spine injury. When any of these conditions exists, apply a cervical collar.

There are several types of cervical spine immobilization devices on the market. It is important when you select one that it be rigid (stiff, not easily movable) and that it be the right size. The traditional soft collar that you occasionally see someone wearing on the street has no role in immobilizing a prehospital patient's cervical spine. This type of collar provides so little restriction of neck motion that you may hear experienced EMTs refer to it as a "neck warmer."

The wrong size immobilization device may actually harm the patient by making breathing more difficult or obstructing the airway. Whatever device is used must not obstruct the airway. If the proper size collar is not available, it is better to place a rolled towel around the neck (to remind the patient not to move his head) and tape the patient's head to the backboard.

The techniques for selecting the right size cervical collar and for applying a cervical collar are presented in Scan 10-2. As you study the scan and practice applying a cervical collar, consider the following.

- *Make certain that you have completed the initial assessment and that you have cared for all life-threatening problems before you apply the collar.*
- *Use the mechanism of injury, level of consciousness, and location of injuries to determine the need for cervical immobilization.* Apply a rigid cervical collar whenever any of these factors lead you to believe that spine injury is a possibility.
- *Assess the patient's neck prior to placing the collar.* Once the collar is in place, you will not be able to inspect or palpate the back of the neck.
- *Reassure the patient.* Having a cervical collar applied around your neck can be a constricting and frightening experience. Explain the procedure to the patient.
- *Make sure the collar is the right size for the patient.* The proper size rigid collar depends more on the length of the patient's neck than on the width. A large patient may not be able to wear a large collar. A small patient with a long neck may need your largest collar. The front height of the collar should fit between the point of the chin and the chest at the suprasternal (jugular) notch—the U-shaped dip where the clavicles and sternum meet. Once in place, the collar should rest on the clavicles and support the lower jaw. It should be neither too high so that it stretches the neck, nor too short to support the chin, nor too tight so that it constricts the neck.
- *Remove necklaces and large earrings before applying the collar.*
- *Keep the patient's hair out of the way.*
- *Keep the head in the in-line anatomical position* (a neutral position with head facing front, not tilted forward or back or turned to either side) when applying manual stabilization and the collar.
- *Cervical immobilization collars alone do not provide adequate in-line immobilization.* Nor

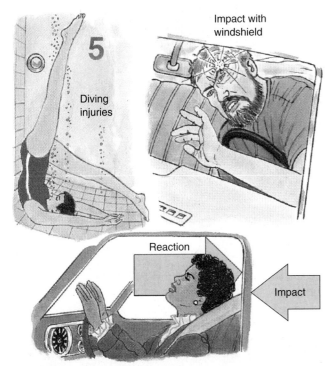

FIGURE 10-1 Mechanisms of cervical spine injury.

Scan 10-2
Cervical Collars

Rigid cervical collars are applied to protect the cervical spine. **Do not** apply a soft collar.

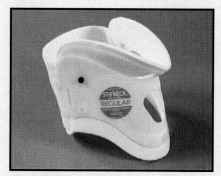

STIFNECK™—Rigid extrication

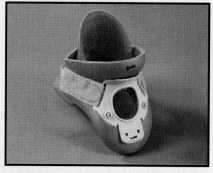

PHILADELPHIA CERVICAL COLLAR™

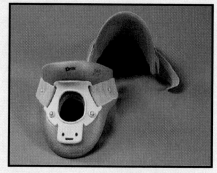

PHILADELPHIA CERVICAL COLLAR™—Opened

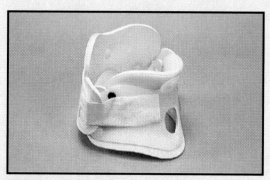

NEC-LOC™—Rigid extrication

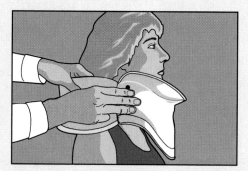

NEC-LOC™—Opened

Sizing a Cervical Collar

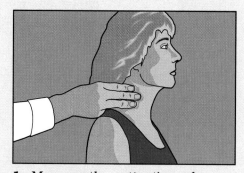

1. Measure the patient's neck.

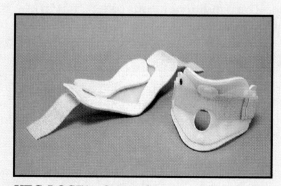

2. Measure the collar. Make sure that the chin piece of the collar will not lift the patient's chin and hyperextend the neck. Make sure the collar is not too small and tight, acting as a constricting band.

186

Stifneck™ Collar—Seated Patient

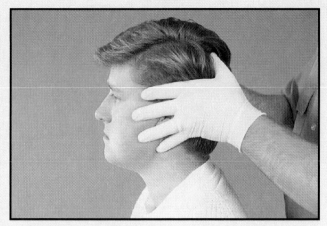

1. Stabilize the head and neck from the rear.

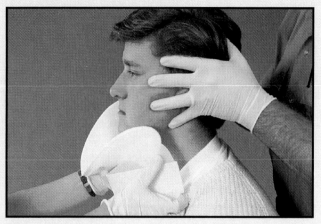

2. Properly angle the collar for placement.

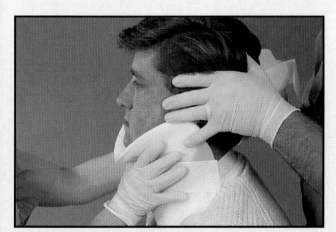

3. Position the collar bottom.

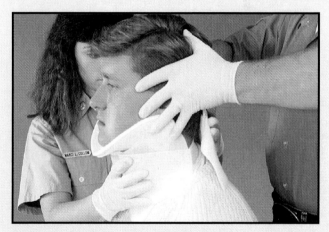

4. Set collar in place around neck.

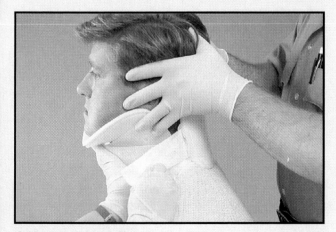

5. Secure the collar.

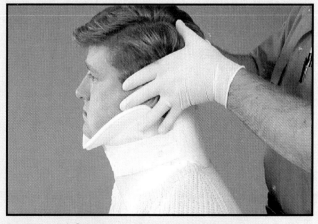

6. Spread fingers and maintain support.

187

Stifneck™ Collar—Supine Patient

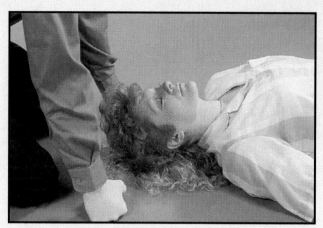

1. Kneel at patient's head.

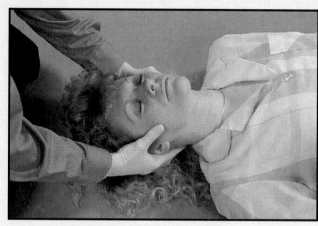

2. Stabilize the head and neck.

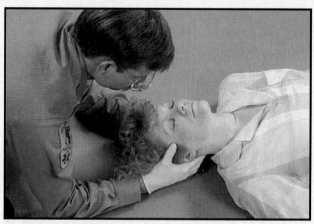

3. Maintain stabilization.

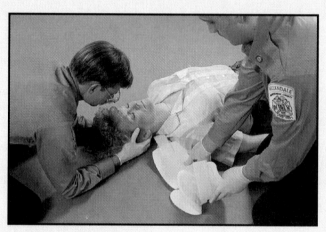

4. Set collar in place.

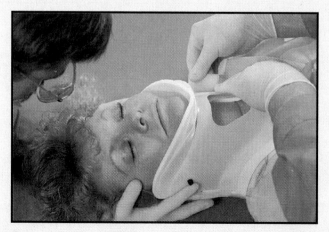

5. Secure the collar.

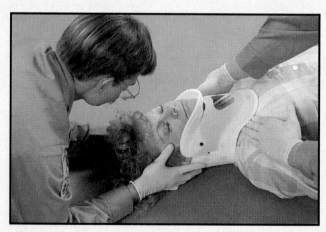

6. Continue to stabilize.

is applying the collar the first step in immobilization. You must manually stabilize the patient's head before the collar is applied, as you learned in Chapter 9, and continue to manually immobilize the head and neck until the patient is secured to a long backboard.

You will immobilize patients who have suspected head, neck, or spine injury not just with collars, but also with long backboards and sometimes short backboards. You learned about immobilization on a backboard in Chapter 6, Lifting and Moving, and will learn more in Chapter 28, Head and Spine, and in Chapter 31, Gaining Access.

Significant Mechanism of Injury

On the Scene

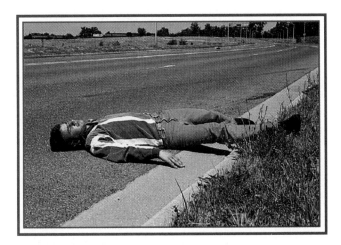

In Chapter 9, you began your assessment of Brian Sawyer, a man who apparently had been thrown from his car during a collision. First you sized up the scene. Then you did the initial assessment.

Scene Size-Up (Review)
As you responded to a motor vehicle accident, you put on gloves for **body substance isolation** and evaluated **scene safety.** The scene was safe. There was only one vehicle involved, a compact car which was resting on its wheels, but which had sustained a lot of damage to the roof and sides. The patient was a male who was found lying on his back approximately 20 feet from the vehicle. So the **mechanism of injury** was the impact of the collision and/or the impact of being thrown from the vehicle. The **number of patients** was just one: Brian.

Initial Assessment (Review)
You formed a **general impression** of an approximately 25-year-old male who appeared unresponsive and who had snoring respirations. You checked Brian's **mental status** at the same time that your partner started **airway** management. He immobilized Brian's head manually as he did a jaw thrust and relieved the snoring respirations. You evaluated Brian's **breathing** and **circulation.** You inserted an oropharyngeal airway and administered high concentration oxygen at 15 liters per minute by nonrebreather mask.

You assigned Brian a high **priority** because of the significant mechanism of injury and because he was unresponsive to pain and showed signs—rapid, weak pulse and pale, clammy skin—of diminished blood circulation. You decided to transport him quickly, taking just a few moments first to conduct a rapid version of the focused history and physical exam tailored for a patient, like Brian, with a significant mechanism of injury.

Focused History and Physical Exam—Trauma Significant Mechanism of Injury

Mechanism of Injury   You have no opportunity to take a closer look at the car Brian was in because it is 20 feet away from Brian, who needs your help. Instead, you ask a police officer on the scene to survey the car for any deformities that would indicate where Brian might have struck interior surfaces. The officer reports that there are no deformities in the interior of the car. However, the fact that Brian appears to have been thrown from the car is a *significant mechanism of injury.*

Spinal Stabilization   Your partner started manual immobilization of Brian's head during the initial assessment. He knows that his job now is to hold the head in a neutral in-line position and to keep the airway open.

Advanced Life Support Request   If you were in an area where paramedics are available to respond with EMT-Bs to certain types of patients, this would be a good time to call them. In your area, you do not have this option, so you continue your focused history and physical exam.

Transport Decision   The priority you assigned Brian at the end of your initial assessment was high. After you reconsider the mechanism of injury, you confirm your decision to transport him quickly—just as soon as you complete the focused history and physical exam.

Mental Status   Now you assess Brian's mental status. You determined during the initial assessment that he was unresponsive to a painful stimulus. You confirm that this is still the case by pinching his shoulder muscle. There is still no response.

Rapid Trauma Assessment   The physical exam you do on Brian is different from the one you did on Clara. Clara had no significant mechanism of injury. She was able to tell you what parts of her body hurt, and you were able to focus your physical exam on just the parts identified by her complaint and mechanism of injury. You examined only her head, neck, and knee. Then you put on a cervical collar and dressed and bandaged her knee.

Brian, on the other hand, is unresponsive and cannot tell you what hurts. Even if he could, you would want to give him a more thorough exam because he had a significant mechanism of injury. Being thrown from a car during a collision is likely to produce more than just a localized cut or scrape.

Yet, your examination of Brian must be speedy. You must do a more comprehensive exam than you did for Clara, but you must do it rapidly so that you can get Brian into the ambulance and en route to the hospital without delay.

So you now perform a rapid assessment of Brian. As you inspect and palpate each part of his body, you look and feel for the DCAP-BTLS signs and symptoms (deformities, contusions, abrasions, punctures/penetrations, burns, tenderness, lacerations, and swelling). In addition, with particular areas of Brian's body, you also look for certain additional signs. You expose each part of his body as necessary. So your rapid trauma assessment of Brian goes as follows.

1. *Head*—You assess Brian's head for DCAP-BTLS and the sound or feel of broken bones rubbing against each other. You find a laceration on the back of his head that is not bleeding.
2. *Neck*—You assess his neck for DCAP-BTLS, the sound or feel of broken bones rubbing against each other, and bulging or flat neck veins. There is no response from Brian when you palpate along his cervical spine. Brian's neck veins are flat, indicating possible blood loss, but no other abnormalities.
3. *Stabilization*—You now size and apply a cervical collar.
4. *Chest*—Next, you open Brian's shirt and assess his chest for DCAP-BTLS, the sound or feel of broken bones, breath sounds, and movements of part of the chest in a direction that is different from the rest of the chest. You find no abnormalities.

5. *Abdomen*—When you cut open Brian's trousers and assess his abdomen for DCAP-BTLS, you also check for firmness, softness, and distention. Brian's abdomen is very firm but does not look distended (larger than normal).
6. *Pelvis*—Next, you assess Brian's pelvis for DCAP-BTLS. You find no abnormalities. Since he is not able to complain of any pain in the pelvis, you compress it gently to determine tenderness or motion. You find nothing unusual, except for confirming that his level of responsiveness is still such that he does not respond to any pain from compression.
7. *Extremities*—Now you quickly assess all four extremities for DCAP-BTLS, distal pulse, sensation, and motor function. You find a deformity in Brian's right lower leg. You do not pause to splint the leg now but will tend to it en route to the hospital. He has weak pulses in all extremities and does not respond to a pinch there. Since he is not responsive, you cannot determine whether he has sensation or motor function.
8. *Posterior and immobilization*—A firefighter has gotten a backboard from your ambulance and places it next to Brian. You and your partner roll him onto his side as a unit and cut away his clothing to assess his posterior body, inspecting and palpating for DCAP-BTLS. You find nothing abnormal. The firefighter places the board next to Brian and you roll him back onto the board.

You have been able to conduct the entire assessment in just a few moments. If any life-threatening problem had been discovered before or during the rapid trauma assessment, you would have altered the procedure as needed to allow for treatment of the problem.

Vital Signs   You quickly assess Brian's baseline vital signs. He has a *pulse* of 120, regular and weak. His *respirations* are 20 per minute. His *skin* is pale, cool and sweaty. His left *pupil* is dilated and slow to react (the right pupil reacts normally to light). He has a *blood pressure* of 130/80.

History   No one is available to give you a SAMPLE history because Brian was apparently alone when this incident occurred. You did not come across any medical identification bracelet or necklace when you assessed the patient's extremities and neck.

In Chapter 12 we will continue the story of Brian Sawyer's assessment.

Focused History and Physical Exam–Trauma Patient

FIRST take body substance isolation precautions.

Mechanism of Injury

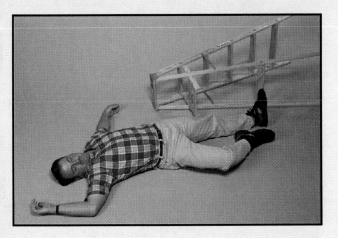

Reassess mechanism of injury.
If there is no significant mechanism of injury (e.g., patient has a cut finger), focus the physical exam (below) only on the injured part.

If mechanism of injury is significant:

- Continue spine stabilization
- Consider requesting ALS personnel
- Reconsider transport decision
- Reassess mental status and ABCs
- Perform rapid trauma assessment

Rapid Trauma Assessment

Rapidly assess each part of the body for the following problems (say "Dee-cap - B-T-L-S" as a memory prompt):

Deformities	Burns
Contusions	Tenderness
Abrasions	Lacerations
Punctures	Swelling

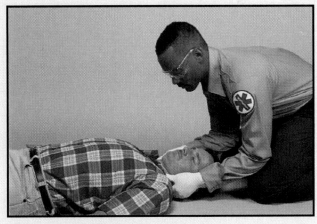

Head: DCAP-BTLS plus crepitation

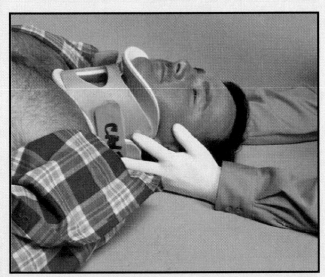

Neck: DCAP-BTLS plus jugular vein distention and crepitation (then place cervical collar)

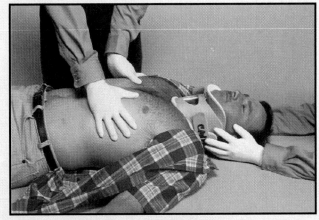

Chest: DCAP-BTLS plus crepitation and breath sounds (absent/present, equal)

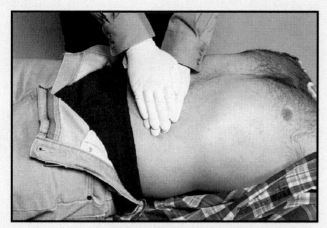

Abdomen: DCAP-BTLS plus firm, soft, distended

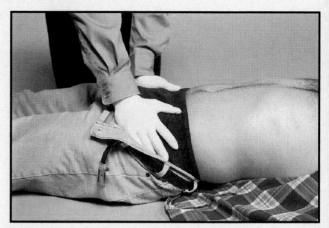

Pelvis: DCAP-BTLS. Gentle compression for tenderness

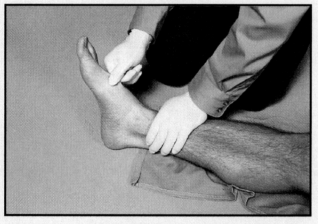

Extremities: DCAP-BTLS plus distal pulse, sensation, motor function

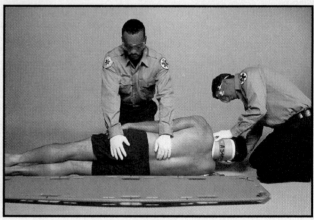

Posterior: DCAP-BTLS (To examine posterior, roll patient using spinal precautions.)

Vital Signs

Assess the patient's vital signs
  Respiration
  Pulse
  Skin color, temperature, condition (capillary refill in infants and children)
  Pupils
  Blood pressure

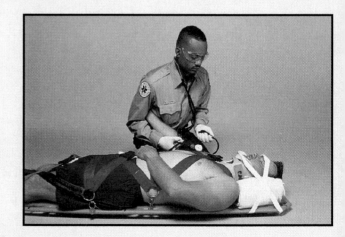

SAMPLE History

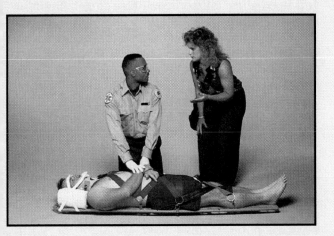

Interview patient or (if patient is unresponsive), interview family and bystanders to get as much information as possible about the patient's problem. Ask about:

S̲igns and symptoms
A̲llergies
M̲edicines
P̲ertinent past history
L̲ast oral intake
E̲vents leading to problem

Interventions and Transport

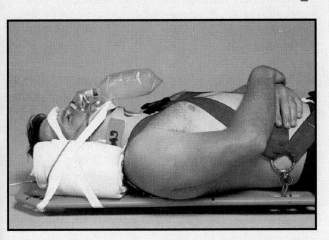

Contact on-line medical direction as needed, Perform interventions as needed.

Package and transport patient.

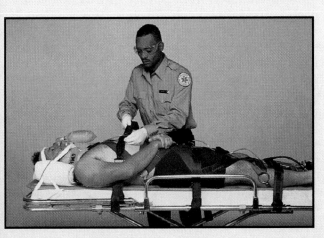

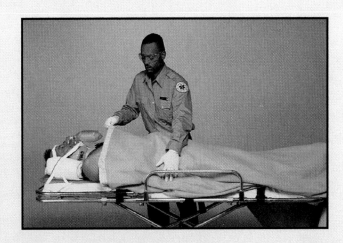

When you have a patient to whom you have assigned a high priority because of problems you found in the initial assessment or because of a *significant mechanism of injury,* you will do the following: continue spine stabilization, consider requesting advanced life support personnel, reconsider your transport decision, assess the patient's mental status, and perform a rapid trauma assessment (Table 10-1 and Scan 10-3).

Reconsidering the Mechanism of Injury

What is a significant mechanism of injury? Simply put, it is a way of getting hurt that carries a high risk of serious injury. A patient who has been ejected from a vehicle, for example, is several times more likely to have fatal injuries than a patient who is not thrown. A patient who is in a passenger compartment where another person died can be assumed to have sustained serious injury because of the amount of force that had to have been involved to kill the other person. A number of high risk situations are listed in Table 10-2. Brian Sawyer's injuries were caused by the first item on the list, ejection from a vehicle.

All of these mechanisms involve potentially large forces being exerted on a patient's body. In the case of a motor vehicle, you can gain a great deal of information by walking around the vehicle and looking at all of its outside surfaces. You should also look inside the vehicle, concentrating your attention on the steering wheel, pedals, dashboard, and rear-view mirror. Look for deformities that could have been caused by a person striking the surface (Figure 10-2). Also look for intrusion of the body of the car into the passenger compartment (i.e., Was the car crunched so that the inside is smaller than it used to be?). The preferred way to survey the mechanism of injury is, of course, to do it yourself. In Brian's case, because you couldn't walk away from him, you needed to ask someone else to get the information for you.

Some patients who undergo experiences like those in Table 10-2 will escape without serious injury, but many more will not be so lucky. For this reason, you should provide rapid assessment and treatment to any patient with a mechanism of injury listed in Table 10-2, which, in Brian's case, is what you did.

Although the mechanism of injury can provide a lot of information about the kinds of injuries a patient may have, there is still the possibility that patients will have "hidden injuries." These injuries are called hidden because patients may have no signs or symptoms initially but later develop serious conditions that may take time to become apparent.

Seat belt injuries are a good example. There is no doubt that properly used seat belts save lives by preventing drivers and passengers from hitting hard objects inside a vehicle and by preventing them from being thrown from vehicles. But seat belts can also cause injuries. When patients are in high velocity collisions, the force of being thrown forward against buckled seat belts will occasionally cause injury to the bowel and other abdominal organs. These injuries may not become apparent for several hours or even days. It is important to realize that even people who wear seat belts may have sustained serious injuries.

Airbags, too, save lives but do not provide total protection from injury. Airbags prevent occupants from going through the windshield and hitting hard objects inside the vehicle. They are most effective when used in combination with seat belts. However, the driver may hit the steering wheel after the bag deflates. When inspecting a vehicle in which an airbag has deployed, you should look at the steering wheel. Whenever you see a bent or broken steering wheel, you should treat the patient like every other patient who has a significant mechanism of injury. A good way to find this kind of damage is to remember to "lift and look" under the airbag after the patient has been removed from the vehicle.

TABLE 10-2   Significant Mechanisms of Injury

Significant Mechanisms of Injury
Ejection from vehicle
Death in same passenger compartment
Falls of more than 15 feet or 3 times patient's height
Roll-over of vehicle
High-speed vehicle collision
Vehicle-pedestrian collision
Motorcycle crash
Unresponsive or altered mental status
Penetrations of the head, chest, or abdomen, e.g., stab and gunshot wounds

Additional Significant Mechanisms of Injury for a Child
Falls from more than 10 feet
Bicycle collision
Vehicle in medium speed collision

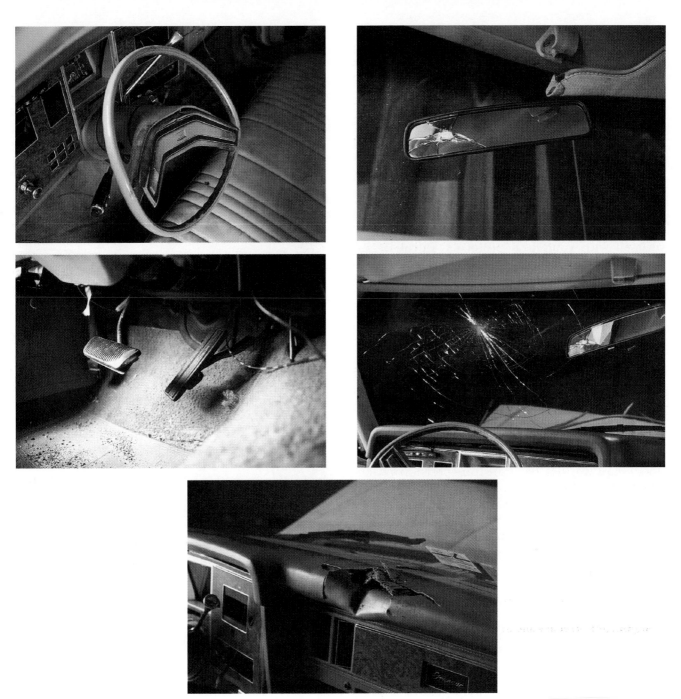

FIGURE 10-2 Deformities to the interior of a vehicle may show where a person has struck the surface, revealing a mechanism of injury.

Infants and Children

Infants and children are more fragile than adults. This means that a child may sustain the same injury as an adult, but from less force than was needed to cause the adult's injury. For this reason, there are additional mechanisms of injury that the EMT-B needs to consider significant when children and infants are concerned (Table 10-2).

Continuing Spine Stabilization

During the initial assessment you make sure that someone is manually stabilizing the patient's head to prevent any cervical spine injury from becoming a paralyzing cervical spinal cord injury. This manual immobilization must continue throughout the assessment until the patient is fully immobilized on a backboard. In Brian's case, your partner understood this

In Brian's case, your partner understood this and was committed to this important role.

Considering a Request for Advanced Life Support Personnel

Some areas of the country, particularly urban and suburban areas, have advanced life support personnel—paramedics who respond with EMTs when they are transporting patients who might benefit from the additional interventions paramedics can provide. If this is the case where you practice as an EMT-B, you should familiarize yourself with your local protocols. Rural EMTs do not usually have this option, but they may have other means by which to improve the patient's care before arrival at a hospital.

In some areas that are very distant from hospitals, local clinics have made arrangements to provide advanced care to certain kinds of patients. For example, if an ambulance is an hour away from the closest hospital, but a local clinic is only ten minutes away, the ambulance may be able to stop there with a patient in cardiac arrest. There are limits, though, on what can be done at health care centers like these. Many of them would not be able to provide additional care worth a delay in transport for awake trauma patients.

If arrangements like these exist where you work as an EMT-B, you must be familiar with the types of patients your clinic can help. The arrangements should be in writing in order to reduce confusion and prevent loss of precious time with critical patients.

In Brian's case, this was not an option.

Reconsidering Your Transport Decision

You assigned a high priority to Brian at the end of the initial assessment. This means you determined that he should be transported promptly. Assigning a high priority for transport is appropriate when the patient has a condition for which you cannot provide definitive treatment—treatment that can only be provided at the hospital. As you prepare to do the rapid trauma assessment (described below), it is a good time to reevaluate that decision. You will have had a chance to look at the mechanism of injury more closely and, if appropriate, to call for assistance from advanced life support personnel at the scene or by intercept en route to the hospital. At this point you should take just a moment to consider again how urgently you need to trans-

port the patient. After reconsideration, you confirmed your decision for Brian.

Reassessing Mental Status

You checked Brian's mental status again by pinching the muscle between his neck and shoulder. There was no response, so this confirmed that he was unresponsive to pain.

Performing the Rapid Trauma Assessment

A patient with a significant mechanism of injury needs a **rapid trauma assessment.** During the rapid trauma assessment, you will be able to detect injuries that may later threaten life or limb. You may also find life-threatening injuries, requiring immediate treatment, that you did not find during the initial assessment. When dealing with a responsive patient, you should ask the patient before and during the trauma assessment about any symptoms. You were unable to ask Brian about his symptoms because he was unresponsive.

During the rapid trauma assessment, you will use your sense of sight to inspect and your sense of touch to palpate different areas of the body. You may also use your sense of hearing to detect abnormal sounds, not just from the airway but also from other areas, such as the sound of broken bones rubbing against each other. You may use your sense of smell, as well, to detect odors like gasoline, urine, feces, or vomitus.

The rapid trauma assessment emphasizes evaluation of the areas of the body where the greatest threats to the patient are. You will evaluate the patient's head, neck, chest, abdomen, pelvis, extremities, and posterior. Remember that this is a quick evaluation, so you will not spend a lot of time on any one area.

The signs and symptoms you will assess each area for are summarized in Table 10-3.

Rapid Assessment of the Head You assessed Brian's head for DCAP-BTLS and also for the sound or feel of broken bones rubbing against each other, known as **crepitation.** When you ran your gloved fingers through his hair and palpated gently, you found only a laceration on the back of his head that was not bleeding. Since there was no bleeding, and so no life-threatening blood loss, you did not need to dress and bandage the wound right away. A good way to check the back of the head in a supine patient (a

TABLE 10-3 Rapid Trauma Assessment

Body Part	DCAP-BTLS	Plus
Head	DCAP-BTLS	crepitation
Neck	DCAP-BTLS	jugular vein distention crepitation
Chest	DCAP-BTLS	paradoxical motion crepitation breath sounds (present, absent, equal)
Abdomen	DCAP-BTLS	firmness softness distention
Pelvis	DCAP-BTLS	pain tenderness motion
Extremities	DCAP-BTLS	distal pulse sensation motor function
Posterior	DCAP-BTLS	——

patient on his back) is to start with your fingers at the top of the neck and carefully slide them upward toward the top of the patient's head. If there is blood on your gloves, there is an open wound. If you don't see any blood on the floor or ground, then you do not need to apply a dressing to the wound right away.

Rapid Assessment of the Neck You assessed Brian's neck for DCAP-BTLS, crepitation, and **jugular vein distention (JVD).** Jugular vein distention is present when you can see the patient's neck veins bulging. The neck veins are usually not visible when the patient is sitting up; however it is normal to see bulging of the neck veins when the patient is lying flat or with his head down. Although Brian was lying down, you found that his neck veins were flat. Flat neck veins in a patient who is lying down may be a sign of blood loss, showing that there is not enough blood to fill them. When you see FLAT neck veins in a FLAT patient, think "blood loss."

Other things you might find when assessing the patient's anterior neck are a **stoma** or a **tracheostomy.** A stoma is a permanent surgical opening in the neck through which the patient breathes. A tracheostomy is a surgical incision held open by a metal or plastic tube.

You may also find a medical identification medallion on a necklace when assessing the neck. Note the information on the necklace if you find one.

Cervical Collar Application After you assessed Brian's head and neck, you sized and applied a cervical spine immobilization collar. You used the same principles that you learned earlier in this chapter. Because Brian was supine, you used a special technique for applying the collar. (See Scan 10-2, Stifneck™ Collar—Supine Position].

Rapid Assessment of the Chest Next, you assessed Brian's chest for DCAP-BTLS, crepitation, breath sounds, and **paradoxical motion.** Paradoxical motion, movement of part of the chest in the opposite direction from the rest of the chest, is a sign of a serious injury. It usually occurs when a segment of ribs has broken at two ends and is "floating" free of the rest of the rib cage. (This condition is sometimes known as "flail chest.") The opposite motion of the broken section is obvious during respiration, moving inward when the lungs expand with air and outward when the lungs empty (Figure 10-3). Paradoxical motion also indicates that a great deal of force was applied to the patient's chest; in other words, there was a significant mechanism of injury.

You can check for crepitation (the sound or feel of broken bones) and paradoxical motion of the chest at the same time. Start by palpating the clavicles (collarbones). Next, gently feel the sternum (breast bone). Position your hands on the sides of the chest and feel for equal expansion of both sides of the chest. During this process you may feel broken bones or floating paradoxical segments.

Palpate the entire rib cage for deformities. Use your hands to apply gentle pressure to the sides of the rib cage. If there is an injured rib and the patient is able to respond, he will tell you that it hurts. Occasionally, you may detect a crackling or crunching sensation under the skin from air that has escaped from its normal passageways.

You listened for Brian's breath sounds (Scan 10-4) just under the clavicles in the mid-clavicular line and at the bases of the lungs in the mid-axillary line. You were listening to see if breath sounds were present and equal. A patient who has breath sounds that are absent or very hard to hear on one side may have a collapsed lung or other serious respiratory injury. There are many other characteristics of breath sounds, but in the trauma patient, presence and equality are the two things to look for at this time.

It is important to remember that when you reach the point of examining the patient's chest in the rapid trauma assessment, you need to

Assessing Breath Sounds

Listen to both sides of the chest. Is air entry present? absent? equal on both sides? Compare left side to right side.

Midclavicular

Midaxillary

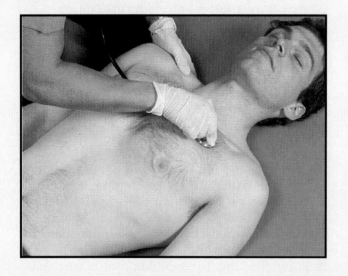

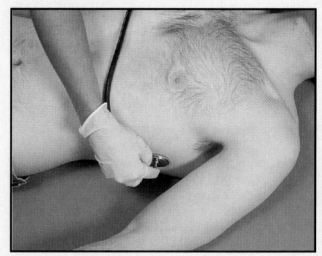

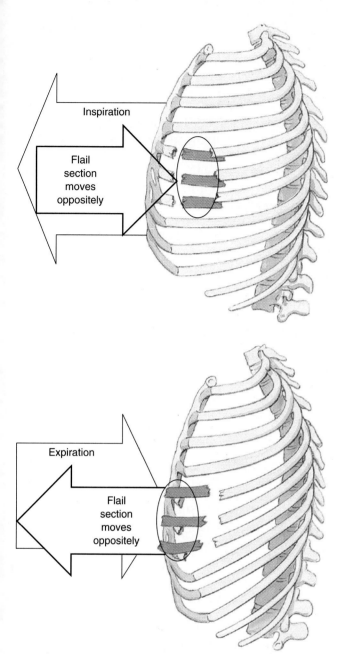

FIGURE 10-3 Paradoxical motion.

so do not spend a lot of time on it. You may also see a **colostomy** or **ileostomy** when you inspect the abdomen. This is a surgical opening in the wall of the abdomen with a bag in place to collect excretions from the digestive system. If you see such a bag, leave it in place and be careful not to cut it if you cut clothing away.

When you palpated, you found that Brian's abdomen was very firm (normally, the abdomen is soft). You did this by gently pressing down once on each quadrant of the abdomen. (You pictured the abdomen divided into four segments—upper left, upper right, lower left, lower right—and pressed on each quadrant in turn.) If the patient tells you he has pain in a specific area of the abdomen, palpate that site last. When practical, make sure your hands are warm. Press in on the abdomen with the palm side of your fingers, depressing the surface about one inch. Many EMTs prefer to use two hands, one on top of the other at the fingertips. Firmness of the abdomen can be a sign of injury to the organs in the abdomen. In Brian's case, this may be a sign that he is bleeding internally and may be the reason why he is showing signs of diminished circulation.

Another finding you may occasionally come across when palpating a patient's abdomen is a pulsating mass. This may be an enlarged aorta. If you do feel such pulsations, do not press any farther into the abdomen. Doing so could cause further injury to a weakened blood vessel.

Rapid Assessment of the Pelvis Next, you assessed Brian's pelvis for DCAP-BTLS. When you inspected the pelvis, you saw no bleeding or **priapism.** This is a persistent erection of the penis that can result from spinal cord injury or certain medical problems. For Brian, there were no abnormalities. Since he was unresponsive and not able to complain of any pain in the pelvis, you compressed it gently to determine tenderness or motion. You found nothing unusual.

If Brian had been awake, you would have asked him first if he had any pain in his pelvis. If he had been awake and complained of pain, you would NOT have compressed his pelvis. You would have considered his complaint of pain as reason enough to treat him for an injury to the pelvis. Compressing the painful pelvis of a conscious patient will not give you any more useful information, but it can produce excruciating pain and if done too strenuously may injure the patient. An unconscious patient cannot tell you if his pelvic area hurts. So you will gently com-

expose the chest if you have not already done so. However, keep the weather and the patient's privacy in mind when doing this.

Rapid Assessment of the Abdomen When you assessed Brian's abdomen for DCAP-BTLS, you also checked for firmness, softness, and distention. You looked and saw no distention or sign of external injury like bruises or protruding organs. The term **distention** is another way of saying the abdomen appears larger than normal. One of its causes can be internal bleeding. Whether the abdomen is abnormally distended or not may be a very difficult judgment to make,

press the pelvis of the unconscious patient to detect tenderness (if there is enough responsiveness to pain to cause him to flinch or groan) and motion of the bones (indicating instability or broken bones). These signs will help you determine whether you need to treat the unconscious patient for a pelvic injury.

Rapid Assessment of the Extremities You quickly assessed all four of Brian's extremities for DCAP-BTLS, distal pulse, sensation, and motor function—that is, whether there is a pulse, feeling, and the ability to move in the hands and feet. You found no deformities except in the middle of Brian's right lower leg. Because of his high priority for transport, you will not splint his leg at the scene but will treat it en route. He had weak pulses in all extremities, but did not respond to a pinch there. Since he was not responsive, you could not determine whether he had sensation or motor function. In a conscious patient, you would touch the patient's hand or foot and ask whether he could feel your touch. If you are not sure whether the patient is telling you the truth, you can ask where on the hand or foot you are touching him. You would also test movement in the extremities of a conscious patient by asking him to squeeze your fingers in his hands and to move his feet against your hands.

Rapid Assessment of the Posterior and Immobilization on Backboard While you were starting your assessment, a firefighter got a backboard from your ambulance and placed it next to Brian. This allowed you to roll him only once, instead of twice, in order to assess him and get him ready for transport. You rolled Brian onto his side as a unit (you will learn how to do a log roll maneuver in Chapter 28, Injuries to the Head and Spine) and assessed his posterior body, inspecting and palpating for DCAP-BTLS. Your inspection and palpation of his back (both the spine and the areas to the sides of the spine), buttocks, and lower extremities showed nothing abnormal. Meanwhile, the firefighter slid the backboard over so that, when you rolled Brian back into a supine position, he was on the backboard.

If Brian had shown signs or symptoms of an injury to the pelvis, you would have placed the pneumatic anti-shock garment on the board before you rolled the patient onto it. Your local protocol may direct you to place the anti-shock trousers on the backboard for other kinds of trauma patients, too. (You will learn about the

PASG in Chapter 27, Musculoskeletal Injuries.) Familiarize yourself with how local medical direction wishes you to manage these patients.

Obtaining Vital Signs

You quickly obtained a set of baseline vital signs for Brian. If you had had a third person available, this would have been an ideal thing for that person to do while your partner was stabilizing Brian's head and you were doing the rapid trauma assessment.

Taking a SAMPLE History

Brian was unresponsive, so you could not get a SAMPLE history from him. If there had been a friend or family member nearby, that person might have been able to give you information about Brian's medical history. In trauma situations, it is good to think of the S in SAMPLE as standing for not just "signs and symptoms" the patient is experiencing, but also for "story"—the history of the injury. This means information like the speed of the vehicle, whether seat belts were used, and whether the patient had a loss of consciousness. With patients who have been shot, information you should try to obtain includes the caliber of the gun, type of ammunition, and distance of the gun from the patient when the gun was discharged. When you are treating a patient who has been stabbed, try to find out the size and type of the knife.

Some General Principles

Several important principles to remember when examining a patient, mentioned throughout the chapter, are summarized here.

- *Tell the patient what you are going to do.* In particular, let the patient know when there may be pain or discomfort. Stress the importance of the examination and work to build the patient's confidence. Ask the patient if he understands what you are doing, and explain your actions again if needed. You were able to have this kind of conversation with Clara who fell while skating but not, of course, with Brian, who was unresponsive.
- *Expose any injured area before examining it so that you can see such things as bruises and puncture wounds.* Let the patient know when you must lift, rearrange, or remove

any article of clothing. Do all you can to ensure the patient's privacy. There was no clothing covering Clara's injuries. For Brian, you opened and cut away clothing to expose his body as you worked through the rapid trauma assessment.

- *Try to maintain eye contact.* Do not turn away while you are talking or while the patient is answering your questions. You were careful to maintain eye contact with Clara.
- *Assume spine injury.* Unless you are sure that you are dealing with a patient who does not have a spine injury (e.g., a medical patient with no mechanism of injury or reason to suspect trauma), assume the patient has such injuries. Always assume that the unconscious trauma patient has a spine injury. Both Clara and Brian were manually stabilized, fitted with properly-sized cervical collars, and will be immobilized on spine boards before transport to the hospital.
- *During the focused physical exam, or the rapid trauma assessment, you may stop or alter the assessment process to provide care that is necessary and appropriate for the priority of the patient.* In Clara's case, you took time to apply a cervical collar and to dress and bandage her bleeding knee before placing her on a backboard and transporting her to the hospital. In Brian's case, you

applied a cervical collar before immobilizing him on a backboard for transport. If you had found a wound that was bleeding, you would have controlled the bleeding. You did not, however, stop to bandage the non-bleeding laceration on his head or splint his deformed leg. These treatments, along with continued assessment, can take place en route.

Infants and Children

The focused history and physical exam of the pediatric (infant or child) trauma patient is very similar to the focused history and physical exam of the adult patient. One important difference is that you may need to spend more time reassuring children and explaining procedures to them. You will want to kneel or find another way to get on the same level with the child as you speak with him. Young children may be less frightened if you begin your assessment at the toes and work toward the head than proceeding in the usual head-to-toe direction.

A child's airway is narrower than an adult's and more susceptible to being closed. A cervical collar that is too tight can easily constrict a child's airway. A collar that is too high can close the airway by stretching the neck. So it is especially important to choose the correct size cervical collar for a child.

CHAPTER REVIEW

KEY TERMS

You may find it helpful to review the following terms.

colostomy [ko-LOS-to-me]   like an ileostomy, a surgical opening in the wall of the abdomen with a bag in place to collect excretions from the digestive system.

crepitation [krep-uh-TAY-shun]   the grating sound or feeling of broken bones rubbing together.

DCAP-BTLS   A memory aid to remember <u>d</u>eformities, <u>c</u>ontusions, <u>a</u>brasions, <u>p</u>unctures/penetrations, <u>b</u>urns, <u>t</u>enderness, <u>l</u>acerations, and <u>s</u>welling—signs and symptoms of injury found by inspection or palpation during patient assessment.

distention [dis-TEN-shun]   a condition of being stretched, inflated, or larger than normal.

focused history and physical exam   the step of patient assessment that follows the initial assessment.

ileostomy [il-e-OS-to-me]   See *colostomy*.

jugular [JUG-yuh-ler] **vein distention (JVD)** bulging of the neck veins.

paradoxical [pair-uh-DOCK-si-kal] **motion** movement of a part of the chest in the opposite direction to the rest of the chest during respiration.

priapism [PRY-ah-pizm]   persistent erection of the penis that may result from spinal injury and some medical problems.

rapid trauma assessment a rapid assessment of the head, neck, chest, abdomen, pelvis, extremities, and posterior of the body to detect signs and symptoms of injury.

stoma [STO-mah] a permanent surgical opening in the neck through which the patient breathes. See also *tracheostomy*.

tracheostomy [TRAY-ke-OS-to-me] a surgical incision held open by a metal or plastic tube. See also *stoma*.

SUMMARY

The focused history and physical exam of the trauma patient takes place immediately after the initial assessment. It starts with a reconsideration of the mechanism of injury. This allows you to determine which path you are going to take in assessing a patient.

The patient without a significant mechanism of injury receives a physical exam of areas that the patient complains about and areas that you think may be injured based on the mechanism of injury. It is important to have a high index of suspicion and evaluate any areas that you feel may have been injured. When in doubt, assess it. Next, you get a set of baseline vital signs and a SAMPLE history.

The patient who has a significant mechanism of injury receives a somewhat different assessment. You start by assuring continued immobilization of the spine, considering whether to call advanced life support personnel (if available), reconsidering how urgently to transport the patient, reassessing mental status, and then performing a rapid trauma assessment. The rapid trauma assessment looks for deformities, contusions, abrasions, punctures and penetrations, burns, tenderness, lacerations, and swelling plus certain additional signs appropriate to the part being assessed (as summarized in Table 10-3). You look for these in the areas where life-threatening injury is most likely to be found: the head, neck, chest, abdomen, pelvis, extremities, and posterior body. At the same time, you apply a cervical collar. Then you get a baseline set of vital signs and a SAMPLE history.

The findings of your focused history and physical exam will determine what you do next for the patient. You will treat the injuries you found on the patient without a significant mechanism of injury. You will immobilize the patient with a significant mechanism of injury on a backboard and stretcher so that you can begin transport and continue assessment and treatment en route to the hospital.

REVIEW QUESTIONS

1. Explain why it is important to reconsider the mechanism of injury at the beginning of the focused history and physical examination of a trauma patient.

2. Explain how the focused history and physical examination of a trauma patient with a significant mechanism of injury differs from that for a trauma patient with no significant mechanism of injury.

3. Name the signs and symptoms for which the letters DCAP-BTLS stand.

4. List the steps of the rapid trauma assessment and describe the kind of patient for whom the rapid trauma assessment is appropriate.

Application

- As an EMT-B, how would you balance the need for appropriate on-scene assessment and treatment with the need for speed in getting the patient to the hospital in each of the following situations?

  a. You arrive at a residence to find a patient who explains to you that he has accidentally cut his finger with a kitchen knife. The cut is bleeding profusely.

  b. You arrive at a schoolyard to find a girl who, bystanders tell you, was shot by a rival gang member. She is lying in a pool of blood but is able to speak to you.

The Focused History and Physical Exam—Medical Patient

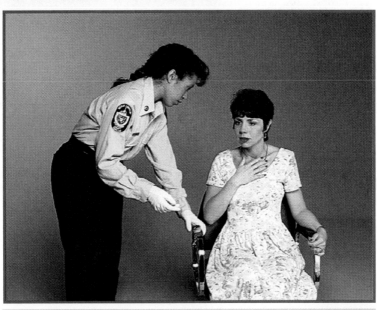

11

The responsive medical patient is the most common kind of patient you will encounter. With this patient, gathering information about the illness and the patient's history takes precedence over performing a physical exam. For the medical patient, like the trauma patient, the purpose of the focused history and physical exam is to provide adequate assessment and emergency care at the scene without unnecessarily delaying transportation to the hospital.

Objectives

Knowledge and Attitude *At the end of this chapter, you should be able to meet the following objectives.*

1. Describe the unique needs for assessing an individual with a specific chief complaint with no known prior history. (p. 203)

2. Differentiate between the history and physical exam that is performed for responsive patients with no known prior history and responsive patients with a known prior history. (pp. 207, 210)

3. Describe the needs for assessing an individual who is unresponsive. (pp. 207–216)

4. Differentiate between the assessment that is performed for a patient who is unresponsive or has an altered mental status and other medical patients requiring assessment. (pp. 206–212)

5. Attend to the feelings that these patients might be experiencing. (p. 210)

6. List the elements of the history of the present illness. [supplemental] (p. 207)

7. Given a chief complaint of a patient with a medical problem, list the elements of the physical exam for that patient. [supplemental] (pp. 206, 209, 210, 212, 214)

Skills

1. Demonstrate the patient assessment skills that should be used to assist a patient who is responsive with no known history.

2. Demonstrate the patient assessment skills that should be used to assist a patient who is unresponsive or has an altered mental status.

On the Scene

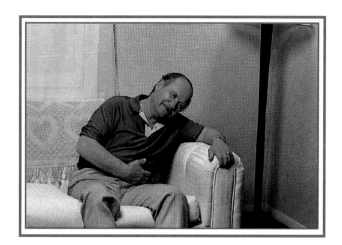

In Chapter 9, you began your assessment of Mr. Schmidt, the older man who complained that his stomach hurt. You were able to size up the scene and perform your initial assessment quickly.

Scene Size-up (review)

You put on gloves for **body substance isolation** as you exited the ambulance. **Scene safety** seemed assured as you approached the quiet home and were led to your patient. There was no **mechanism of injury,** and the **number of patients** was just one: Mr. Schmidt.

Initial Assessment (review)

Your **general impression** is of an awake older male. Your initial assessment told you that Mr. Schmidt's **mental status** was alert and that he had an open **airway,** was **breathing** adequately and without difficulty, and had good **circulation** without any visible bleeding. You assigned him a **priority** that indicated he is a medical (nontrauma) patient with no immediately life-threatening problems. With the initial assessment over, you have determined that Mr. Schmidt's complaint is medical in nature with no indication of any mechanism of injury, so you can now proceed to the focused history and physical exam for a medical patient.

Focused History and Physical Exam—Medical— Responsive Patient

History   You tell Mr. Schmidt that you need to get some information about his condition. You start by asking him questions that will give you the *history of the present illness.*

You: When did the pain start, Mr. Schmidt?
Mr. Schmidt: About two hours ago.
You: Can you describe it for me?
Mr. Schmidt: It's kind of a burning pain.
You: Has it changed at all since it started?
Mr. Schmidt: It's gotten worse, especially in the last hour.
You: Where exactly is the pain?
Mr. Schmidt: (points to his upper abdomen) Right here.
You: Does it seem to spread anywhere or does it stay right there?
Mr. Schmidt: It just stays right here.
You: What were you doing when it started?
Mr. Schmidt: I was talking with my wife.
You: Can you think of anything that might have triggered this pain?
Mr. Schmidt: No, not really.
You: You look uncomfortable. How bad is the pain?
Mr. Schmidt: Pretty bad. I've never had a pain this bad.

Now that you have the history of the present illness, you can find out the patient's age and proceed with the rest of the *SAMPLE history.*

You: How old are you, Mr. Schmidt?
Mr. Schmidt: I'm 68.
You: Have you had any other *symptoms?*
Mr. Schmidt: Well, I've been sick to my stomach.
You: Have you vomited?
Mr. Schmidt: No.
You: Have you had any diarrhea?
Mr. Schmidt: No.

You: Are you *allergic* to anything?
Mr. Schmidt: Just cats.
You: What *medicines* do you take?
Mr. Schmidt: Ibuprofen and Minipress.
You: What do you take those for?
Mr. Schmidt: I have arthritis and high blood pressure.
You: Do you have any other medical problems?
Mr. Schmidt: No.
You: Have you ever had this kind of problem before?
Mr. Schmidt: No.
You: Who is your doctor?
Mr. Schmidt: Dr. Anderson.
You: When was the last time you ate or drank anything?
Mr. Schmidt: I had dinner about three hours ago.
You: How have you felt today? Anything out of the ordinary?
Mr. Schmidt: No, it was a pretty normal day.

Focused Physical Exam   The next step in assessment is a focused physical exam. Since Mr. Schmidt is complaining of abdominal pain, you unbutton his shirt to expose his abdomen so you can inspect and palpate it. His abdomen does not appear distended, but there is some tenderness in the upper half.

Vital Signs   Next, you assess Mr. Schmidt's baseline vital signs. His *pulse* is 92, regular and full. *Respirations* are 20 and unlabored. *Skin* is normal (warm, pink and dry). *Blood pressure* is 140/86. Because his complaint is of abdominal pain, which has no relationship to the brain, you do not need to check his *pupils.*

You move Mr. Schmidt to your stretcher and put him in the position in which he is most comfortable: sitting. You and your partner move him to the ambulance and begin the trip to the hospital.

The story of Mr. Schmidt's assessment will continue in Chapter 13.

The key to moving from the initial assessment into the focused history and physical exam is reconsideration of the mechanism of injury, as well as of the patient's complaint. If there is a mechanism of injury, you will perform the focused history and physical exam for the trauma patient, which was described in Chapter 10. When the patient has a complaint that is medical in nature, and you have confirmed that there is no significant mechanism of injury, you will perform the focused history and physical exam for the medical patient—the subject of this chapter.

FOCUSED HISTORY AND PHYSICAL EXAM: THE MEDICAL PATIENT

As you learned in Chapter 9, Initial Assessment, it makes a great deal of difference in the assessment process whether the patient is responsive or unresponsive. This is especially true of the medical patient. In trauma patients, there are often many external signs of trauma, or injury, but this is not true of a medical condition. The most important source of information about a medical patient's condition is what the patient can tell you. This is why, when the patient is awake and responsive, obtaining the patient's history comes first.

The Responsive Patient

Mr. Schmidt is a good example of the kind of patient you will see often. He is awake, he has a medical problem, and he does not have any immediately life-threatening problems. You also confirmed that there was no mechanism of injury for Mr. Schmidt. In this kind of situation, after you finish the initial assessment, you proceed to gain more information by performing a focused history and physical exam for a medical patient. This will tell you what you need to know in order to administer the proper treatment.

The focused history and physical exam for a medical patient has four parts: history of the present illness, SAMPLE history, pertinent physical exam, and baseline vital signs (Table 11-1 and Scan 11-1).

Gathering a History

The interview you do with a patient is similar to the interview a physician conducts before a physical examination. It is a conversational information-gathering effort. Not only will you gain needed information from the interview, but you will also reduce the patient's fear and promote cooperation.

Relatives and bystanders may also serve as sources of information, but the most important source of information is the patient. Do not interview relatives and bystanders before the patient unless the patient is unconscious or unable to communicate (see later in this chapter). You may gain information from bystanders and medical identification devices later, while you are conducting the physical examination.

TABLE 11-1 Focused History and Physical Exam—Medical Patient

Responsive Patient	Unresponsive Patient
1. Gather the history of the present illness (OPQRST) from patient. Onset Provokes Quality Radiation Severity Time	1. Conduct a rapid physical exam. Assess head Assess neck Assess chest Assess abdomen Assess pelvis Assess extremities Assess posterior body
2. Gather a SAMPLE history from patient. Signs and symptoms Allergies Medications Pertinent past history Last oral intake Events leading to the illness	2. Obtain baseline vital signs. Respirations Pulse Skin Pupils Blood pressure
3. Conduct a focused physical exam (focusing on the area the patient complains of).	3. Gather the history of the present illness (OPQRST) from bystanders or family. Onset Provokes Quality Radiation Severity Time
4. Obtain baseline vital signs. Respirations Pulse Skin Pupils Blood pressure	4. Gather a SAMPLE history from bystanders or family. Signs and symptoms Allergies Medications Pertinent past history Last oral intake Events leading to the illness

Note: This table shows the general order of steps. You may alter this order in accordance with the situation and the number of EMTs available and when the patient's condition warrants immediate action due to immediate life threats.

One main purpose of talking to the patient is to find out his chief complaint, the one thing that seems most seriously wrong to him. When you ask the patient what is wrong, he may tell you that several things are bothering him. If this happens, ask what is bothering him the most. Find out if the patient is in pain and where he hurts. Unless the pain of one injury or medical problem masks that of another, most people will be able to tell you of painful areas.

Try to ask open-ended questions, that is, questions that the patient answers with responses other than "Yes" or "No." Instead of asking, "Is your chest pain dull and crushing?" ask "How would you describe your pain?" In this way, you will avoid giving the patient the impression that you want a particular answer. If the patient says that he cannot describe his pain, you can try giving him several choices: "Is your pain dull, or sharp, or burning?"

You asked Mr. Schmidt a number of questions to get the history of the present illness (a fuller description of the chief complaint and symptoms). An easy way to remember what questions to ask is to use the letters **OPQRST**

Onset	What were you doing when it started?
Provokes	Can you think of anything that might have triggered this pain?
Quality	Can you describe it for me?
Radiation	Where exactly is the pain?
	Does it seem to spread anywhere or does it stay right there?
Severity	You look uncomfortable. How bad is the pain?
Time	When did the pain start, Mr. Schmidt?
	Has it changed at all since it started?

After finding out Mr. Schmidt's age, you then got the rest of the SAMPLE history and the name of his personal physician.

Signs/ symptoms	Have you had any other symptoms? Have you vomited? Have you had any diarrhea?
Allergies	Are you allergic to anything?
Medications	What medicines do you take?
Pertinent past history	What do you take those for? Do you have any other medical problems? Have you ever had this kind of problem before? Who is your doctor?
Last oral intake	When was the last time you ate or drank anything?
Events leading to the illness	How have you felt today? Anything out of the ordinary?

A Patient with a Specific Chief Complaint and No Known Prior History Often the patient whose history you are gathering has no known prior history. Mr. Schmidt, your patient who complained of abdominal pain, answered "No" when you asked him if he had ever had this kind of problem before. This and other questions you ask as part of the SAMPLE history may tell you that the patient has not been under treatment for this problem and does not have any medicines on hand for the problem that you might want to assist him in taking. You will generally transport this patient to the hospital and provide the information to the emergency department staff.

A Patient with a Specific Chief Complaint and a Known Prior History Often, during the SAMPLE history interview, you will learn from your patient that he has a history relating to his chief complaint. Your patient has had this problem or something related to it before and may be under a physician's care for the problem. The patient can tell you what medical condition the current complaint probably relates to. For example, a woman with vaginal bleeding may be pregnant or have just undergone an abortion. A man who suffers a seizure may explain that he is an epileptic. Knowing this history may help you determine what interventions you can take at the scene or en route to the hospital, as well as providing information that you will give to the hospital staff. Chapters in the Medical Emergencies module later in this book will cover these and other situations in which there are prehospital interventions you can perform.

There are three situations involving a known prior history of the medical complaint that deserve special mention here. They are different from other medical emergencies because the patient may carry part of the treatment with him, and because the past medical history is essential in determining the prehospital treatment. The three situations are

- A patient with difficulty breathing who has an inhaler prescribed by his physician
- A patient with chest pain who has nitroglycerin prescribed by his physician
- A patient with an allergic reaction who has an epinephrine auto-injector prescribed by his physician.

In each of these cases, the patient has been evaluated by his physician, has been determined to have a condition that can be treated with

Focused History and Physical Exam—
Medical Patient—Responsive

First take body substance isolation precautions.

History of Present Illness

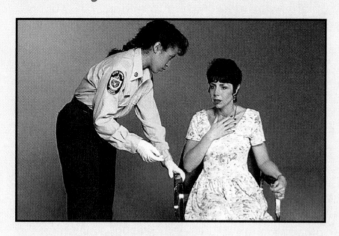

Ask the "OPQRST" questions:
Onset
Provokes
Quality
Radiation
Severity
Time

Sample History

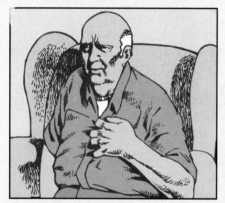

Signs and symptoms

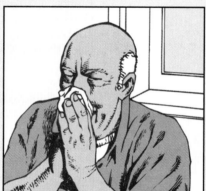

Allergies

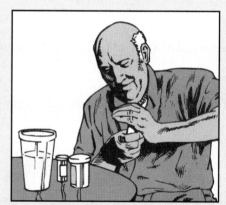

Medicines

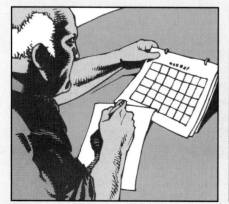

Pertinent past history

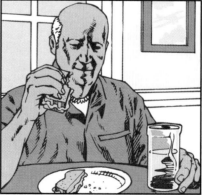

Last oral intake

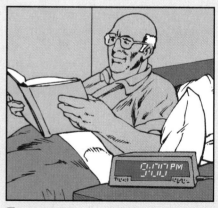

Events leading to illness

Focused Physical Exam

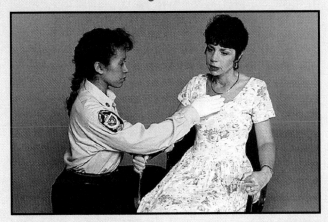

Quick exam of affected body part or system

Assess as needed:
Head
Neck
Chest
Abdomen
Pelvis
Extremities
Posterior

Vital Signs

Assess the patient's vital signs.

Respiration
Pulse
Skin color, temperature, condition
(capillary refill in infants and children)
Pupils
Blood pressure

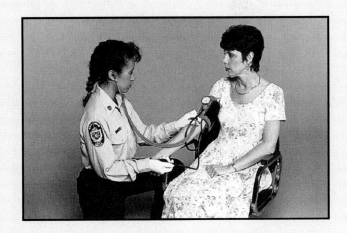

Interventions and Transport

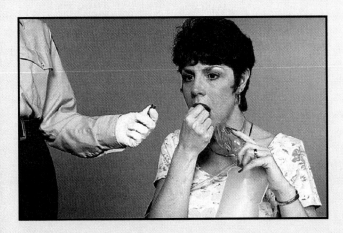

Contact on-line medical direction as needed. Perform interventions as needed.

Transport patient.

medication the patient can carry, and has filled a prescription for that medication. You will learn more about these conditions, also, in the Medical Emergencies module later in this book.

When a medical patient does not have a condition for which you have an intervention, you should generally transport the patient to the hospital. Similarly, when you have a patient with one of the conditions listed above, but the patient does not have his medication or has not received a prescription for a medication, you should generally transport the patient. *Note that you will generally transport the patient to the hospital even if he does have medication you can assist him in taking.* In fact, you may load the patient into the ambulance and assist him with his medication en route.

● Infants and Children

When gathering a history from a child, be sure to kneel or find another way to get on the same level with the child. Put the OPQRST and SAMPLE questions in simple language the child can understand.

Much of the history for a child and all of the information for an infant will need to be gathered from the parents, guardian, or other adult caretaker.

Performing a Focused Physical Exam

With responsive medical patients, the EMT-B's physical exam is usually brief. You will gather most of the important assessment information in this type of patient from the history and vital signs. The physical exam procedure will be the same as you learned for the trauma patient in Chapter 10. For each part of the body you examine, you will inspect and palpate for DCAP-BTLS (deformities, contusions, abrasions, punctures/penetrations, burns, tenderness, lacerations, swelling) plus the information that is specific to each body part. (Review Table 10-3 and Scan 10-1 in Chapter 10.) For the responsive medical patient, focus the exam on the body part that the patient has a complaint about. Mr. Schmidt complained of abdominal pain, so you inspected and palpated his abdomen. First, you looked at his abdomen. It did not appear distended. Next, you palpated each quadrant. It was soft (normal), but both upper quadrants were tender.

Obtaining Vital Signs

A complete set of vital signs is essential to the assessment of a medical patient. There was no reason to check Mr. Schmidt's pupils since he was alert and had a chief complaint (abdominal pain) not directly related to the brain. Examining the pupils is important when assessing a medical patient who has an altered mental status, headache, or complaint about his eye or vision.

Administering Interventions and Transporting the Patient

In later chapters, you will learn when to administer particular interventions, that is, treatments for the specific medical conditions that will be described in those chapters. The only treatment you have learned about so far that might be appropriate for a responsive patient is oxygen. Together, the initial assessment, history, physical exam, and vital signs did not give you any reason to believe that Mr. Schmidt needed oxygen. If your protocols tell you to, however, or if you wish, you may give Mr. Schmidt oxygen. It will not harm him. Throughout the exam you reassured Mr. Schmidt and tried to calm his fears. Now you will prepare to transport Mr. Schmidt to the hospital.

The Unresponsive Patient

On the Scene

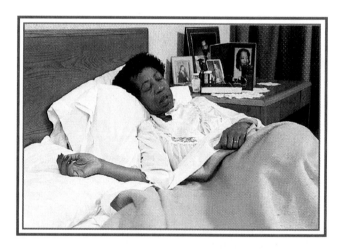

In Chapter 9, you began your assessment of Mrs. Malone, an adult woman reported to be unconscious. You sized up the scene and performed your initial assessment.

Scene Size-up (review)

You put on gloves for ***body substance isolation*** as you got out of the ambulance. You assessed ***scene safety*** as you approached a well-kept home and were led to your patient in her bedroom. There was no **mechanism of injury,** and the **number of patients** included only Mrs. Malone.

Initial Assessment (review)

Your **general impression** was of an adult woman lying on her back in bed. Mrs. Malone was not moving and her eyes were closed. Her **mental status** was responsive to verbal stimuli by moaning. Her **airway** was threatened by her tongue, so your partner tilted her head back and lifted her chin. Her **breathing** was in the normal range, with adequate movement of air in and out. You gave Mrs. Malone high concentration oxygen by nonrebreather mask and moved her onto her side in order to help protect her airway. **Circulation** check showed Mrs. Malone's pulse to be strong, regular, and in the normal range for rate. There was no visible blood. The skin at her wrist was cool and dry. The skin at her lips and nail beds was pale. The **priority** of this patient was high because of her depressed level of responsiveness and her threatened airway.

The next step in your assessment of Mrs. Malone is to perform a focused history and physical exam.

Focused History and Physical Exam—Medical—Unresponsive Patient

Rapid Physical Exam Because Mrs. Malone is unresponsive, you have no way of knowing what part of her body to focus on. So you do a rapid assessment of her head, neck, chest, abdomen, pelvis, extremities, and posterior in just the same way as you would for an unresponsive trauma patient. As you assess each area of her body, you remove enough clothing to be able to inspect and palpate it, then quickly replace the clothing. You find no abnormalities.

Vital Signs Your partner finds that Mrs. Malone has a **pulse** of 92, strong and regular. Her *respirations* are 20, full and non-labored. **Skin** is cool and dry. **Pupils** are equal and reactive. **Blood pressure** is 160/90. Everything is in the normal range except for her high blood pressure. You note this, but it does not require any action on your part.

You now check Mrs. Malone's airway again. Since you turned her on her side, you have not heard any abnormal sounds from her airway like snoring or gurgling. This, and the fact that she is breathing adequately, means that her airway is open. You check the oxygen and confirm that you are administering oxygen at 12 to 15 liters per minute by nonrebreather mask.

History Because Mrs. Malone has a decreased level of responsiveness and you could not get a history by interviewing her, you need to depend on others to provide as much of this information as possible. The family member who met you at the door is Mrs. Malone's daughter, Florence. You question her to find out what happened and what medical history her mother has.

You: What happened?
Florence: I think she had a convulsion.
You: What happened to make you say that?
Florence: Well, I heard some choking sounds from the room next door, and when I came in her arms and legs were moving around.
You: Was it both arms and both legs?
Florence: Yes, I think so.
You: Was anyone with her when this started?
Florence: No, no one else was home.
You: When did this happen?
Florence: About 10 minutes ago, just before I called 911.
You: How long did you see her arms and legs moving?
Florence: I think it was only about a minute, but it felt like a lot longer when it was happening.
You: Has she ever had anything like this happen before?
Florence: I don't think so, but my mother lives alone, so I'm not sure.
You: How old is your mother?
Florence: She's 60.
You: Is she allergic to anything?
Florence: Not that I know of.
You: Does she take any medicines?
Florence: No, I don't think so.
You: Is she generally healthy?
Florence: Yes, although sometimes she gets migraines.
You: Does she take any medicine for her migraines?
Florence: No, she used to, but she had to stop taking it because it made her feel so tired.
You: When did she stop taking the medicine?
Florence: Oh, that was months ago.
You: Do you know when she last ate?
Florence: We had lunch about four hours ago. I was starting to make dinner when this happened.
You: Can you think of anything unusual that happened today that might explain what happened to your mother?
Florence: No, it seemed like a normal day until just a little while ago.
You: I think you were right when you said she had a convulsion, or seizure. What you described sounds a lot like a seizure. We're going to take her to the hospital to be checked by a doctor in the emergency department.

Florence: Thank you. Should I come with you or drive to the hospital myself?

You: You're welcome to come with us, but it might be easier for you to get home if you drive.

Florence: OK. I'll meet you there.

You: Don't follow the ambulance too closely. Take your time and be careful.

You and your partner move Mrs. Malone to your stretcher and take her to the ambulance.

We will continue Mrs. Malone's story in Chapter 12.

For a responsive medical patient like Mr. Schmidt, the first step of your focused history and physical exam would be talking with the patient to obtain the history of his present illness and the SAMPLE history, followed by performing the physical exam and gathering the vital signs.

For an unresponsive patient, like Mrs. Malone, the process is turned on its head (Table 11-1 and Scan 11-2). Since you cannot obtain a history from the patient, you will begin with the physical exam and vital signs. After these procedures, you will gather as much of the patient's history as you can from any bystanders or family members who may be present, as you did by talking with Mrs. Malone's daughter, Florence.

Another difference between the focused history and physical exam for the responsive and for the unresponsive patient is the nature of the physical exam. For a responsive patient, you will be able to focus your exam on just the part of the body the patient complains of. For Mr. Schmidt, who complained of abdominal pain, you focused your physical exam on the abdomen. Since an unresponsive patient can't tell you where the problem is, you will need to do a rapid assessment of the entire body, as you did for Mrs. Malone.

Performing a Rapid Physical Exam

Your physical exam of Mrs. Malone was almost the same as the physical exam for a trauma patient like Brian Sawyer in Chapter 10, the young man who was thrown from a car. You rapidly assessed Mrs. Malone's head, neck, chest, abdomen, pelvis, extremities, and posterior. As you assessed each area, you looked for signs of injury like deformities, contusions, abrasions, penetrations, burns, tenderness, lacerations, and swelling (DCAP-BTLS). Other things to look for in the medical patient include

neck	jugular vein distention
	medical identification devices
chest	presence and equality of breath sounds
abdomen	distention
	firmness or rigidity
pelvis	incontinence of urine or feces
extremities	pulse
	sensation
	motor function
	medical identification devices

Medical ID Devices Medical identification devices can provide important information. One of the most commonly used medical-alerting devices is the Medic Alert emblem shown in Figure 11-1. Over one million people wear a medical identification device in the form of a necklace or a wrist or ankle bracelet. One side of the device has a Star of Life emblem. The patient's medical problem is engraved on the reverse side, along with a telephone number to call for additional information.

When doing the physical exam, look for necklaces and bracelets or wallet cards. Never assume you know the form of every medical identification device. Check any necklace or bracelet carefully, taking care when moving the patient or any of his extremities. You should alert the emergency department staff when you arrive that the patient is wearing or carrying medical identification and tell them what is on it, e.g., diabetes or heart condition.

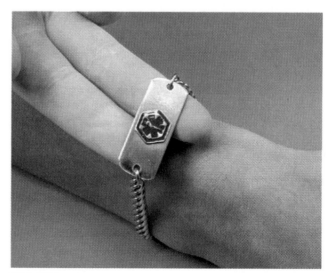

FIGURE 11-1 A medical identification device.

Obtaining Vital Signs

You assessed Mrs. Malone's pulse, respirations, skin, pupils, and blood pressure and noted any abnormalities. None required any action on your part at the scene.

Obtaining a History of the Present Illness and SAMPLE History

Since Mrs. Malone could not talk, you had to depend on her daughter, who was the only other source of information available. You asked her questions in order to get as much as possible of the information you would have gotten from the patient.

The history of the present illness that you obtain will not be as complete for an unresponsive patient as for a responsive patient. The only OPQRST questions (Onset, Provokes, Quality, Radiation, Severity, Time) that were pertinent in Mrs. Malone's case and could be answered by her daughter were onset (what happened) and time (when did it start and how long did it go on).

The SAMPLE history was a little easier to get. Mrs. Malone's daughter was able to supply information about her mother's signs and symptoms, allergies, medicines, pertinent past history, last oral intake, and events leading to the incident.

When interviewing bystanders, determine if any are relatives or friends of the patient. They usually have more information to provide about past problems than other bystanders would have. See which of the bystanders saw what happened. When questioning bystanders, you should ask

1. *What is the patient's name?* If the patient is obviously a minor, you should ask if the parent or guardian is present or if he or she has been contacted.
2. *What happened?* You may be told that the patient fell off a ladder, appeared to faint, fell to the ground and began seizing, was hit on the head by a falling object, or other possible clues.
3. *Did the bystander see anything else?* For example, was the patient clutching his chest or head before he fell?
4. *Did the patient complain of anything before this happened?* You may learn of chest pain, nausea, concern about odors where he was working, or other clues to the problem.

5. *Does the patient have any known illnesses or problems?* This may provide you with information about heart problems, alcohol abuse, allergies, or other problems that could cause a change in the patient's condition.
6. *Is the patient taking any medications?* Be sure to use the words "medications" or "medicines." If you say "drugs" or some other term, bystanders may not answer you, thinking that you are asking questions as part of a criminal investigation. In rare cases, you may feel that the bystanders are holding back information because the patient was abusing drugs. Remind them that you are an EMT-B and you need all the information they can give you so proper care can begin.

Vial of Life While gathering the patient's history, you should also see if there is a "Vial of Life" (Figure 11-2) or similar type of sticker on the main outside door, closest window to the main door, or the refrigerator door. If so, patient information and medications can usually be found in the refrigerator. (The Vial of Life is not used in all regions.)

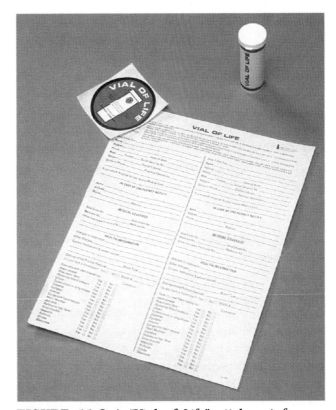

FIGURE 11-2 A "Vial of Life" sticker, information, and medication.

Focused History and Physical Exam—Medical Patient—Unresponsive

FIRST take body substance isolation precautions.

Rapid Physical Exam

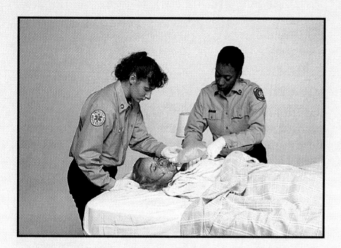

Rapid exam of entire body

Rapidly assess:
Head
Neck
Chest
Abdomen
Pelvis
Extremities
Posterior

Vital Signs

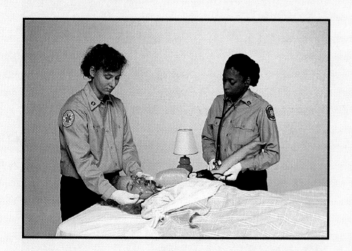

Assess the patient's vital signs.

Respiration
Pulse
Skin color, temperature, condition
   (capillary refill in infants and children)
Pupils
Blood pressure

SAMPLE History

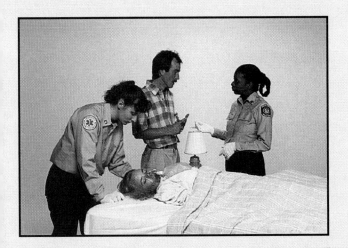

Interview family and bystanders to get as much information as possible about the patient's problem. Ask about:

Signs and symptoms (Ask the OPQRST questions regarding Onset, Provocation, Quality, Radiation, Severity, and Time)

Allergies
Medicines
Pertinent past history
Last oral intake
Events leading to problem

Interventions and Transport

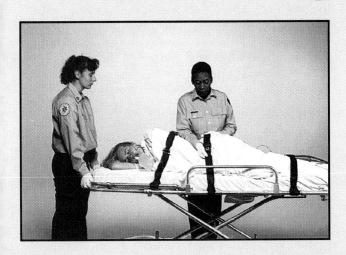

Contact on-line medical direction as needed.

Perform interventions as needed.

Transport patient.

Administering Interventions and Transporting the Patient

There is not usually much information gained from the focused history and physical examination of an unresponsive medical patient that will change treatment in the field. The most important thing to look for is mechanism of injury or signs of injury that would make you suspect a spine injury. Either of these would mean that you need to immobilize the patient's spine. Most of the time, the information you gather in your assessment of unresponsive medical patients will be particularly helpful to the staff in the emergency department. Emergency physicians and nurses depend on EMT-Bs to evaluate the scene carefully and to gather as much useful information as possible that they cannot get in the hospital.

Having completed the focused history and physical exam, you will prepare to transport Mrs. Malone to the hospital.

CHAPTER REVIEW

KEY TERMS

You may find it helpful to review the following term.

OPQRST questions a memory device for the questions asked to get a description of the present illness: Onset, Provokes, Quality, Radiation, Severity, Time.

SUMMARY

The focused history and physical exam of the medical patient takes two forms. You assess the responsive patient by getting a history of the present illness (a fuller description of the chief complaint), and a SAMPLE history, then performing a physical exam of affected parts of the body before getting baseline vital signs. The primary purpose of gathering this information is to determine the proper treatment of the patient.

In unresponsive medical patients, on the other hand, since the patient cannot communicate, history gathering will not provide as much useful information. In these patients, it is appropriate to start the assessment with a rapid physical exam. This exam looks almost the same as the trauma patient's rapid assessment. Baseline vital signs come next, and then you interview bystanders, family and friends to get any history that can be obtained. You may not change any field treatment as a result of the information gathered here, but the results of the assessment may be very important to the emergency department staff.

REVIEW QUESTIONS

1. Explain how and why the focused history and physical exam for a medical patient differs from the focused history and physical exam for a trauma patient.
2. Explain how and why the focused history and physical exam for a responsive medical patient differs from the focused history and physical exam for an unresponsive medical patient.

Application

- As an EMT-B, how would you deal with the following situations?
  a. What questions would you ask to get a history of the present illness from a patient with a chief complaint of chest pain?

b. You are trying to get information from the very upset son of an unresponsive man. He is the only available family member. He is so upset that he is having difficulty talking to you. How can you quickly get him to calm down and give you his father's medical history?

c. You are interviewing a very pleasant older woman. Unfortunately, your assessment is taking a long time because she doesn't answer your questions and instead starts talking about other things. She lives alone and appears to be lonely. How should you handle this?

The Detailed Physical Exam

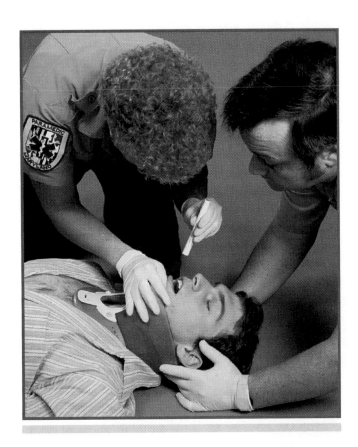

12

The initial assessment and the focused history and physical exam are done rapidly because of the necessity of getting the seriously injured or ill patient into the ambulance and to the hospital without delay. En route to the hospital, you may have time to do a more complete patient assessment, known as the detailed physical exam.

Objectives

Knowledge and Attitude *At the end of this chapter, you should be able to meet the following objectives.*

1. Discuss the components of the detailed physical exam. (pp. 222–227)

2. State the areas of the body that are evaluated during the detailed physical exam. (pp. 222–227)

3. Explain what additional care should be provided while performing the detailed physical exam. (pp. 222–227)

4. Distinguish between the detailed physical exam that is performed on a trauma patient and that of the medical patient. (pp. 226–227)

5. Given a part of the body, describe the procedure for assessing it. [supplemental] (pp. 222, 225–226)

6. Given a part of the body, describe the abnormalities that may be found when assessing it. [supplemental] (pp. 222, 225–226)

7. Explain the rationale for the feelings that these patients might be experiencing. (p. 226)

Skills

1. Demonstrate the skills involved in performing the detailed physical exam.

On the Scene

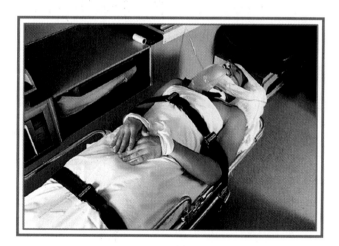

In Chapters 9 and 10, you began your assessment of Brian Sawyer, the man who had been thrown from his car during a collision. First you sized up the scene. Then you did the initial assessment. Then you performed a focused history and physical exam on Brian.

Scene size-up (review)

On arrival, you put on gloves for **body substance isolation** and evaluated **scene safety** and the **mechanism of injury,** which was the impact on Brian of the collision and/or the impact of being thrown from the vehicle. The **number of patients** was one: Brian.

Initial assessment (review)

You got a **general impression** of an unresponsive, approximately 25-year-old male with snoring respirations. His **mental status** was unresponsive to a painful stimulus. Your partner immobilized Brian's head manually as he opened the **airway** with a jaw thrust to relieve the snoring respirations. When you evaluated **breathing,** you found respirations that were normal in rate and depth. You assessed **circulation** and found a weak and rapid radial pulse with no blood on or near the patient. His skin was pale, cool, and sweaty. You assigned this patient a high **priority** because he was unresponsive to pain and showed signs of diminished circulation (rapid, weak pulse and pale, clammy skin).

Focused History and Physical Exam— Trauma Patient (review)

You reconsidered the **mechanism of injury** and made no changes in Brian's priority. Your partner **continued spine stabilization.** You did not call **advanced life support** personnel because your EMS system does not have such a team. You *reconsidered your transport decision* and confirmed that you should spend as little time as possible at the scene. You **reassessed mental status** and found Brian still unresponsive to pain (a pinch on his shoulder).

When you performed a **rapid trauma assessment,** you assessed Brian's head, neck, chest, abdomen, pelvis, extremities, and posterior. You found a laceration on the back of his head that was not bleeding. His neck veins were flat. You sized and applied a cervical collar. Breath sounds were present and equal. Brian's abdomen was firm but not distended. His pelvis was normal. You found a deformity in the middle of Brian's right leg. He had weak pulses in all extremities and did not respond to a pinch there. Since he was not responsive, you could not determine whether he had sensation. When you assessed his posterior body, you found nothing abnormal. You immobilized Brian on a backboard, which was also a quick, temporary way to immobilize his deformed leg. You hoped that you would be able to splint his leg en route, but realized that you might not get the chance because you might be too busy treating Brian's more severe problems.

In obtaining **vital signs,** you discovered that Brian had a pulse of 120, regular and weak, respirations of 20 per minute, skin that was pale, cool and sweaty, a left pupil that was dilated and slow to react, and a blood pressure of 130/80.

You could not obtain a **SAMPLE history** because Brian was apparently alone when the collision occurred, and he is unresponsive. You did not find any medical identification.

You and your partner immobilized Brian on a backboard before loading him onto the ambulance for transport.

Before the Detailed Physical Exam

Inside the ambulance, before conducting a detailed physical exam on Brian, you first ensure that any critical interventions are performed. You accomplish this by **repeating your initial assessment:** Your general impression is that Brian looks serious. His mental status is still unresponsive to pain. You are now managing his airway with an oropharyngeal airway and suction. His breathing is still adequate, so

you are giving him high concentration oxygen, but he is breathing adequately and you do not need to ventilate him. A check of his circulation shows that his radial pulse is still rapid and weak, there is no external bleeding you need to control, and his skin is pale, cool, and sweaty.

The Detailed Physical Exam

After you feel certain that Brian's ABCs are under control, you find that you have time before reaching the hospital to undertake a detailed physical exam. You accomplish this by **repeating the rapid trauma assessment in somewhat greater detail.**

You reassess Brian's head. The main difference from the rapid trauma assessment you did at the scene is that now you pay special attention to several areas you did not evaluate before: **the face, ears, eyes, nose, and mouth.**

You inspect and palpate Brian's face for DCAP-BTLS. You see no signs of injury, so you gently palpate his cheekbones, forehead, and lower jaw. You inspect and palpate his ears, searching for DCAP-BTLS and drainage. You see a little bit of blood in the left ear. You also gently bend each of his ears forward to look for bruising, but find none.

Next, you assess Brian's eyes, inspecting for the usual DCAP-BTLS and discoloration, unequal pupils, foreign bodies, and blood in the front of the eye. His left pupil is dilated and slow to react. You do not see any blood in the front of his eye or any other abnormalities.

Next, you assess Brian's nose, inspecting and palpating for injuries or signs of injury. In this case, you look not only for DCAP-BTLS, but also for drainage and bleeding. You do not find any.

When you assess his mouth, you open it and look for DCAP-BTLS, loose or broken teeth, other objects that could cause obstruction, swelling or laceration of the tongue, unusual breath odor, and discoloration. You do not find any of these.

You continue on to reassess Brian's neck, chest, abdomen, pelvis, extremities, and posterior body as you did during the rapid trauma assessment. You find no changes.

The last step in the detailed physical exam is to repeat Brian's **vital signs.** You obtain a pulse of 136, regular and weak, respirations of 14 per minute, skin that is still cool, pale and sweaty, a left pupil that is still dilated and slow to react, and a blood pressure of 100/70—indicating a more rapid pulse, slower respirations, and a lower blood pressure than during the rapid trauma assessment at the scene.

The story of Brian's assessment will continue in Chapter 13.

After you have performed the initial assessment and the focused history and physical exam, and after you have performed all necessary critical interventions, you may have the time to do a detailed physical exam. You will typically do the detailed physical exam en route to the hospital. If you are not on a transporting unit and the ambulance has not arrived, you may do the detailed physical exam at the scene.

THE DETAILED PHYSICAL EXAM

The purpose of the detailed physical exam is to gather additional information about the patient's injuries and conditions. Some of this information may help you to determine the proper treatment for the patient, and some of the information you gather in the detailed physical exam will assist the emergency department staff.

The detailed physical exam is performed most often on the trauma patient with a significant mechanism of injury, less often on a trauma patient with no significant mechanism of injury, and seldom on a medical patient.

The Trauma Patient with Significant Mechanism of Injury

For a trauma patient who is not responsive or has a significant or unknown mechanism of injury, you will have assessed almost the entire body during the rapid trauma assessment—but very quickly. For this patient, a detailed physical exam may reveal signs or symptoms of injury that you missed or that have changed since the rapid trauma assessment.

Before Beginning the Detailed Physical Exam

It is important to remember that you should perform the detailed physical exam *only after you have performed all critical interventions*. The best way to ensure this is to *repeat your initial assessment* before you begin the detailed physical exam. To do this, reassess your general impression of the patient, his mental status, plus airway, breathing, and circulation.

If you are treating a severely injured patient, you may be too busy to begin or com-

plete the detailed physical exam at all. This is not a failure on your part. Your responsibility is to give the patient the best care possible under the difficult conditions found in the field. If you do not do a complete assessment, but you keep a critical patient's airway, breathing, and circulation intact, you have helped the patient far more than if you had done the complete assessment. Performing a detailed physical exam is always a lower priority than addressing life-threatening problems. The place of the detailed physical exam among the priorities and sequence of assessment is shown in Table 12-1.

Performing the Detailed Physical Exam

If you haven't already exposed the patient, you need to do so now. Since you are now in the enclosed ambulance, it is much easier to protect the patient's privacy and protect him from exposure to the environment.

The **detailed physical exam** will look a lot like the rapid trauma assessment that you did during the focused history and physical exam. You will look for the familiar DCAP-BTLS signs (deformities, contusions, abrasions, punctures/penetrations, burns, tenderness, lacerations, and swelling—review Scan 10-1 in Chapter 10). You will also look for certain additional signs as you examine the head, neck, chest, abdomen, pelvis, extremities, and posterior body. The only areas you will assess in the detailed physical exam that you did not assess during the rapid trauma assessment portion of the focused history and physical exam will be the face, ears, eyes, nose, and mouth (Table 12-2 and Scan 12-1).

TABLE 12-1 The Detailed Physical Exam in the Sequence of Assessment Priorities

1. Scene size-up
2. Initial assessment for immediately life-threatening problems
   Critical interventions
3. Focused history and physical exam
   Interventions as necessary
4. Repeat initial assessment for immediately life-threatening problems
   Critical interventions
5. **Detailed physical exam (time and critical care needs permitting)**
6. Ongoing assessment for life-threatening problems, vital signs
   Critical interventions

TABLE 12-2 Detailed Physical Exam Compared with Focused History and Physical Exam

Focused History and Physical Exam: Rapid Trauma Assessment		Detailed Physical Exam	
Head	DCAP-BTLS* + crepitation	**Head**	
		Scalp and Cranium	DCAP-BTLS + crepitation
		Face	DCAP-BTLS
		Ears	DCAP-BTLS + drainage
		Eyes	DCAP-BTLS + discoloration, unequal pupils, foreign bodies, blood in anterior chamber
		Nose	DCAP-BTLS + drainage, bleeding
		Mouth	DCAP-BTLS + loose or broken teeth, objects that could cause obstruction, swelling or laceration of tongue, unusual breath odor, discoloration
Neck	DCAP-BTLS + jugular vein distention, crepitation	**Neck**	DCAP-BTLS + jugular vein distention, crepitation
Chest	DCAP-BTLS + paradoxical motion, crepitation, breath sounds	**Chest**	DCAP-BTLS + paradoxical motion, crepitation, breath sounds
Abdomen	DCAP-BTLS + firmness, softness, distention	**Abdomen**	DCAP-BTLS + firmness, softness, distention
Pelvis	DCAP-BTLS + pain, tenderness, motion	**Pelvis**	DCAP-BTLS + pain, tenderness, motion
Extremities	DCAP-BTLS + distal pulse, sensation, motor function	**Extremities**	DCAP-BTLS + distal pulse, sensation, motor function
Posterior	DCAP-BTLS	**Posterior**	DCAP-BTLS

*DCAP-BTLS = deformities, contusions, abrasions, punctures/penetrations, burns, tenderness, lacerations, swelling

In the case of Brian Sawyer, you inspected and palpated the face for DCAP-BTLS by looking and then gently palpating the cheekbones, forehead, and lower jaw. The bones in the face are fragile and may break when subjected to significant forces.

When you inspected and palpated the ears, searching for DCAP-BTLS and drainage, you found some blood in Brian's left ear. This is an important piece of information to pass on to the emergency department staff because it may be an indication of injury to the skull. You also gently bent each of Brian's ears forward to look for bruising, but found none. You were able to do this because you were careful when applying the cervical collar to make sure you did not enclose the ears in the collar. A bruise behind the ear of a patient is called Battle's sign (Figure 12-1) and indicates a serious injury to the head. This is another important sign of skull injury to tell hospital staff about.

Next, you assessed Brian's eyes, inspecting for the usual DCAP-BTLS and discoloration, unequal pupils, foreign bodies, and blood in the

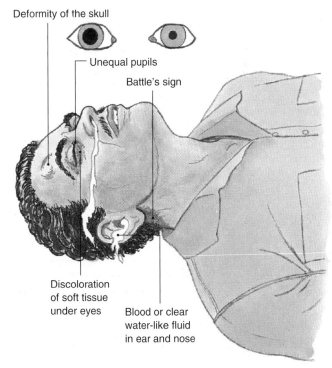

Deformity of the skull

Unequal pupils

Battle's sign

Discoloration of soft tissue under eyes

Blood or clear water-like fluid in ear and nose

FIGURE 12-1 Battle's sign and other signs of skull injury.

Basiler skull fracture most common skull fracture c̄ bruising behind ear.

Scan 12-1
Examining the Head During the Detailed Physical Exam

The detailed physical exam includes reexamination of the head, neck, chest, abdomen, pelvis, extremities, and posterior body, as was done during the rapid trauma assessment (review Scan 10-3 in Chapter 10). During the detailed physical examination of the head, however, the face, ears, eyes, nose, and mouth are given particular attention, as shown below.

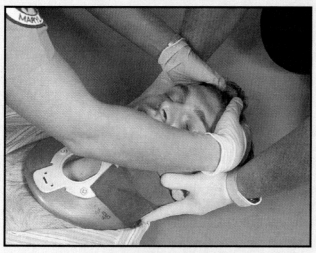

1. Examine the scalp, cranium, and face

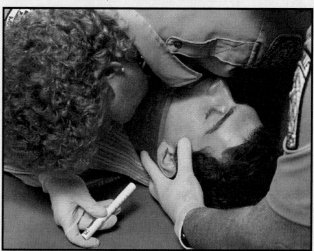

2. Examine the ears.

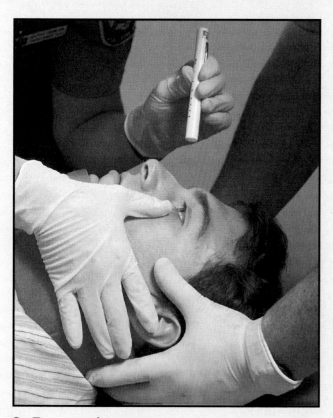

3. Examine the eyes.

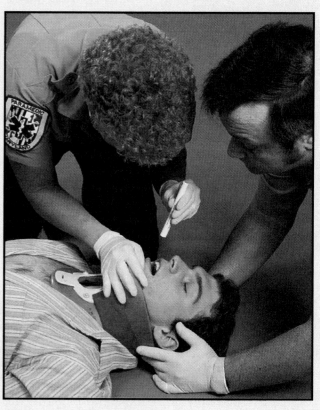

4. Examine the nose and mouth.

224

anterior chamber (front) of the eye. Blood in the anterior chamber is not common but, when present, is a sign that the eye sustained significant force and is bleeding inside (Figure 12-2). Brian's left pupil was dilated and slow to react. There was no blood in the anterior chamber of Brian's eye or any other abnormalities.

When you assessed Brian's nose, you inspected and palpated for injuries or signs of injury. You were looking not only for DCAP-BTLS, but also for drainage and bleeding. You did not find any.

When assessing the ears and nose, you may find blood or clear fluid draining from them. Blood may be from a laceration of that area or it may be coming from inside the skull. Clear fluid may be just from a runny nose or it may be cerebrospinal fluid (CSF). You should prevent an ear or nose that is draining blood or clear fluid from getting any dirtier than it already is. CSF surrounds the brain and spinal cord, and if it is leaking out then bacteria can get in to the brain. Similarly, a wound from inside the skull that is leaking blood can also provide a route for bacteria to get in.

You assessed Brian's mouth by opening it and looking for DCAP-BTLS, loose or broken teeth, other objects that could cause obstruction, swelling or laceration of the tongue, unusual breath odor, and discoloration. A foreign body like a broken tooth is a potential source of airway obstruction and must be removed as soon as possible from the patient's mouth. The most common unusual breath odor is from alcoholic beverages. Other conditions besides alcohol, though, can cause similar odors. You found none of these abnormalities in Brian's case.

There were only a few differences in the rest of the exam compared to what you did in the rapid trauma assessment. These differences result from either the different environment (the back of the ambulance) or from the treatment you have already given to the patient (e.g., cervical collar and immobilization on a backboard).

When you assessed the neck, you were limited by the cervical collar around Brian's neck. You couldn't inspect or palpate the back of the neck, but you were able to assess for DCAP-BTLS, jugular vein distention (JVD), and crepitation through the openings in the collar. You should make sure the collars you use have these openings.

Pupils constricted - Narcotics some drugs give pupil oval shape.

Racoon eyes - bruising around eyes. Indicates head injury. Epitaxes - bloody nose

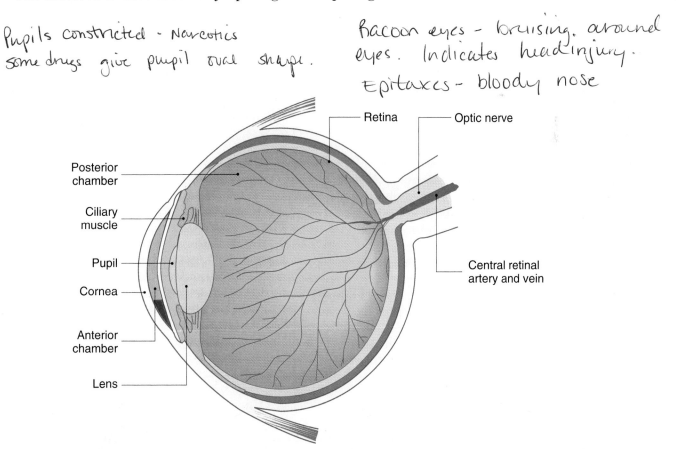

FIGURE 12-2 Blood in the anterior chamber of the eye is a sign that the eye has sustained considerable force.

Reassessing the chest can be challenge in a moving ambulance because road noise makes breath sounds difficult to hear. Just keep in mind that you are listening for the presence and equality of breath sounds in your trauma patient, not the different kinds of abnormal sounds that are more common in medical patients. If you are unable to hear breath sounds because of road noise, it is generally better to continue transporting the patient to the hospital. It makes little sense to stop the ambulance and delay transport unless you can do something to treat an abnormality you find.

When it came to reassessing the back, you did not roll Brian up off the backboard because that would have been inappropriate. By immobilizing a patient on a backboard, you are already treating for possible spine injury, so your primary concern at this point is to evaluate as much of the posterior body as you can reach for other injuries that may have been missed earlier. For Brian, you simply reassessed his flanks (sides) and as much of his spinal area as you could touch without moving him.

You found a deformity in Brian's right forearm during the rapid trauma assessment and strapped it next to him on the backboard. You would have liked to splint it (as you will learn how to do in Chapter 27, Musculoskeletal Injuries), but you realized that Brian had other more serious problems you needed to tend to. If Brian's other injuries were not keeping you so busy, a good time to apply a splint to that extremity would be after you perform the detailed physical exam. Keeping it strapped next to him is a good temporary means of preventing further injury to his forearm.

The rest of the detailed physical exam is essentially the same as the rapid trauma assessment, but you have more time, so you can be more thorough. This is especially true with long transports in rural or wilderness areas.

The final step of the detailed physical exam is to reassess the vital signs.

Your next priority is to make sure that the emergency department is ready for Brian. You do this by using the ambulance radio or cellular phone to notify the emergency department of Brian's condition. Depending on how far you are from the hospital and what your local protocols say, you may do this step before the detailed physical exam. If you have not yet notified the hospital, you should do it now. You will learn more about what to say and how to say it in Chapter 14, Communications.

The Trauma Patient with No Significant Mechanism of Injury

When caring for a trauma patient who is responsive and has no significant mechanism of injury, you will have focused your assessment on just the areas the patient tells you hurt plus those areas that you suspect may be injured based on the mechanism of injury.

This kind of patient received all the assessment he needed while still at the scene. He does not generally need a detailed physical exam. It is important to keep a high index of suspicion, though. When in doubt, do a detailed physical exam. Be aware of the responsive trauma patient's fear and need for emotional support.

The Medical Patient

On the Scene

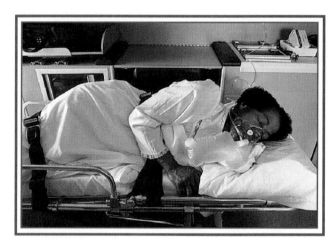

In Chapters 9 and 11, you did scene size-up, initial assessment, and focused history and physical exam for Mrs. Malone, an unresponsive patient with seizures resulting from an unknown problem but no mechanism of injury. You transport her to the hospital without doing a detailed physical exam en route because there is no reason to suspect injuries of the kind that a detailed physical exam would assess. Since Mrs. Malone is unresponsive, however, you maintain a high index of suspicion and remain ready to do a more detailed exam en route if anything about her condition should change in such a way as to cause you to suspect that she may have been injured.

Mrs. Malone's condition is potentially very serious. At the hospital, she is scheduled for a series of tests and referred to a specialist.

You should perform a detailed physical exam on a trauma patient who has a significant mechanism of injury. You should also do it on a patient who has an unclear or unknown mechanism of injury. But the detailed physical exam is not meant for medical patients. This is because there are usually few signs that you as an EMT-B can find in the physical exam of a medical patient that are significant or about which you can or should do anything. Most of the assessment information on medical patients comes from the history and the vital signs rather than from the physical exam.

Occasionally, you may come across a patient who could be either medical or trauma or both. For example, you respond to an elderly man who is found alone and unconscious slumped over the steering wheel of his car. The car is off the road and there is no damage to it. Did the patient lose consciousness first and then drive his car off the road, or did he drive off the road and then get knocked out from a blow to the head? The safest and best thing to do for a patient like this is generally to treat him as a trauma patient who gets a rapid trauma assessment and, if there is time, a detailed physical exam—but whenever possible, also get a history from any witnesses you can find.

CHAPTER REVIEW

KEY TERMS

You may find it helpful to review the following term.

detailed physical exam   an assessment of the head, neck, chest, abdomen, pelvis, extremities, and posterior of the body to detect signs and symptoms of injury. It differs from the rapid trauma assessment only in that it also includes examination of the face, ears, eyes, nose, and mouth during the examination of the head, that it may be done less rapidly than the rapid trauma assessment, and that it may be done en route to the hospital after earlier on-scene assessments and interventions are completed.

SUMMARY

Every assessment begins with a size-up of the scene. Every patient, as the first part of his assessment, receives an initial assessment. The medical patient gets a focused history and physical exam tailored to the medical patient. The trauma patient without a significant mechanism of injury gets an assessment of the areas the patient complains about and areas the EMT feels may have been injured based on the mechanism of injury. The trauma patient with a significant mechanism of injury receives a rapid trauma assessment. After the EMT has performed the appropriate critical interventions and transport has begun, the patient may receive a detailed physical exam en route to the hospital.

The detailed physical exam is very similar to the rapid trauma assessment, but it has several differences. A few more areas are assessed (face, ears, eyes, nose, and mouth). There is time to be more thorough in the assessment. And the detailed physical exam does not take place before transport unless transport is delayed.

The detailed physical exam is most appropriate for the trauma patient who is unresponsive or has a significant or unknown mechanism of injury. A responsive trauma patient with no significant mechanism of injury well seldom require a detailed physical exam. A detailed physical exam is not appropriate for most medical patients.

1. What are the additional areas that you assess in the detailed physical exam that you did not evaluate in the rapid trauma assessment?

2. List the areas covered in the detailed physical exam. What do you look and feel for as you assess each of these areas?

Application

- You are called to respond to a man who has been found unconscious on a sidewalk next to an apartment building in the middle of the night. There were no witnesses to explain what may have happened to him. Is it better to follow the assessment procedures for a trauma patient or for a medical patient? Why?

The Ongoing Assessment

13

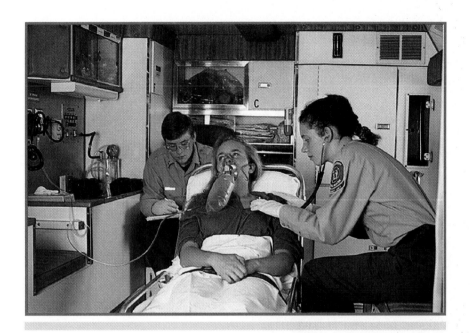

Your patient's condition can change. There may be a change for the better: An unresponsive patient regains consciousness, or a patient suffering from heat exposure improves once inside the air-conditioned ambulance. Or there may be a change for the worse: A patient who was alert and oriented becomes confused, or a child who seemed to be doing well suddenly goes into shock. So you must reevaluate your patient frequently, using the procedures of the ongoing assessment.

Objectives

Knowledge and Attitude *At the end of this chapter, you should be able to meet the following objectives.*

1. Discuss the reasons for repeating the initial assessment as part of the ongoing assessment. (pp. 232, 236)

2. Describe the components of the ongoing assessment. (p. 232)

3. Describe trending of assessment components. (pp. 232, 234, 236)

4. Explain the value of performing an ongoing assessment. (pp. 231–232, 234, 235)

5. Recognize and respect the feelings that patients might experience during assessment. (pp. 234, 237)

6. Explain the value of trending assessment components to other health professionals who assume care of the patient. (p. 232)

Skills

1. Demonstrate the skills involved in performing the ongoing assessment.

On the Scene

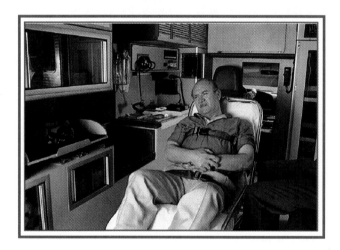

In Chapters 9 and 11, you began your assessment of Mr. Schmidt, a 68-year-old man complaining of abdominal pain. First you sized up the scene. Then you did the initial assessment, followed by a focused history and physical exam.

Scene size-up (review)

On arrival, you took **body substance isolation** precautions, assured **scene safety,** noted no **mechanism of injury** (confirming that this was probably a medical patient rather than a trauma patient), and saw that the **number of patients** included only Mr. Schmidt.

Initial assessment (review)

You formed a **general impression** of an elderly male with an alert **mental status** but who appeared to be uncomfortable. He had an open **airway,** was **breathing** adequately and without difficulty, and had good **circulation** without any visible bleeding. You assigned him a **priority** that indicated he was a medical patient with no immediately life-threatening problems.

Focused History and Physical
Exam—Medical (review)

You got a **history** of Mr. Schmidt's present illness by asking him the OPQRST questions. You found that the pain started about two hours before, was burning in nature, had gotten worse (especially in the last hour), was localized to his upper abdomen, did not spread anywhere, started when he was at rest, and was described by Mr. Schmidt as being "pretty bad." He could not think of anything that might have triggered this pain.

When you continued with the SAMPLE history, you learned that Mr. Schmidt felt sick to his stomach, had not had any episodes of vomiting or diarrhea, was allergic to cats (but no medications), was taking ibuprofen and Minipress for arthritis and high blood pressure, and had had no similar episodes in the past. His doctor was Dr. Anderson, the last time he ate was dinner about three hours ago, and he had been feeling fine that day.

When you performed the *physical exam,* you inspected and palpated his abdomen. It was not distended, but you found some tenderness in the upper quadrants.

Mr. Schmidt's baseline *vital signs* were pulse 92, regular and full, respirations 20 and unlabored, skin normal (warm, pink, and dry), and blood pressure 140/86. You did not examine his pupils because his complaint was one not related to the brain. You recorded your findings.

You moved Mr. Schmidt to the stretcher and put him in the position in which he was most comfortable, sitting. You and your partner moved him to the ambulance and began the trip to the hospital.

Ongoing Assessment—Stable Medical Patient

Once in the ambulance, you do not perform a detailed physical exam because Mr. Schmidt is an alert medical patient with a specific complaint, and further physical exam would be unlikely to reveal anything pertinent. So you move directly to the ongoing assessment—a repetition of key elements of the assessment procedures you have already done.

To begin the ongoing assessment, you *repeat the initial assessment* to check for any immediately life-threatening problems. You get a general impression of an older man who is in discomfort. By talking to him, you confirm that his mental status is alert and his airway and breathing are adequate. You check circulation by feeling his radial pulse and looking for external bleeding. His radial pulse is normal in rate and strength and regular in rhythm. The skin at his wrist is warm, pink, and dry. You do not see any blood around him. You conclude that Mr. Schmidt's condition has not changed and he is not a high priority patient.

Next, you *repeat and record the vital signs.* Mr. Schmidt has a pulse of 88, regular and full, respirations 20 and unlabored, skin normal (warm, pink, and dry), and blood pressure 134/88. His pulse and blood pressure are somewhat lower than when you assessed them during the focused history and physical exam, but well within normal ranges, probably indicating that he is somewhat calmer than before. You record your new findings.

Now you *repeat the focused history and physical exam.* When you ask Mr. Schmidt about his abdominal pain, he tells you there has been no change. He is still a little nauseated, but does not feel as though he will vomit. Nevertheless, you anticipate that he may vomit and keep a basin nearby. You very gently palpate his abdomen again. He reports no change in the amount of tenderness present, and you find no firmness or distention.

Next, you *check interventions* you have performed. In Mr. Schmidt's case, the only intervention that was appropriate was positioning. You ask Mr. Schmidt whether you can make him more comfortable, but he says he is fine sitting up.

The trip to the hospital takes about twenty minutes, so fifteen minutes after you leave the scene, you repeat the ongoing assessment and find no changes in Mr. Schmidt's condition.

At the hospital, Mr. Schmidt is diagnosed with an ulcer, given a prescription for medication, and advised to consult with Dr. Anderson, his regular physician.

An appropriate assessment at the scene and en route to the hospital allows you to detect and treat injuries and illnesses. Your job does not stop there, though. The patient's condition can change, either gradually or suddenly. You will be able to detect these changes by performing a series of steps called the ongoing assessment.

THE ONGOING ASSESSMENT

It is important to observe and reobserve your patient, not only to determine his condition when you first see him, but to detect any changes. The patient may exhibit an obvious change like loss of consciousness or more subtle differences such as restlessness, anxiety, or sweating. These may indicate a change in blood circulation. Most patients do not take a turn for the worse while in the field, so you may also see patient improvement.

During the **ongoing assessment,** you will perform the following four steps (see also Scan 13-1).

1. Repeat the initial assessment (to recheck for life-threatening problems)
   - Reassess mental status.
   - Maintain open airway.
   - Monitor breathing for rate and quality.
   - Reassess pulse for rate and quality.
   - Monitor skin color and temperature.
   - Reestablish patient priorities.
2. Reassess and record baseline vital signs.
3. Repeat the focused assessment regarding patient complaint or injuries.
4. Check the interventions you have performed for the patient.
   - Assure adequacy of oxygen delivery and artificial ventilation.
   - Assure management of bleeding.
   - Assure adequacy of other interventions.

You will perform the ongoing assessment on every patient after you have finished performing life-saving interventions and, often, after you have done the detailed physical exam. Sometimes you may skip doing a detailed physical exam because you are too busy taking care of life-threatening problems, or for a medical or non-critical trauma patient for whom the detailed physical exam would not yield useful information. The ongoing assessment, however, must never be skipped except when life-saving interventions prevent doing it. Even in the latter situation, one partner can often perform the ongoing assessment while the other continues performing life-saving interventions.

Because the ongoing assessment is a means of determining changes and trends, also known as **trending** in the patient's condition, you will need to do this reassessment frequently. The patient's condition and the length of time you spend with the patient will determine just how often and how you will conduct it. The more serious the patient's condition, the more often you will do it. The recommended intervals are *every fifteen minutes for a stable patient* (for example, a patient who is alert, has vital signs in the normal range, and has no serious injury) and *every five minutes for an unstable patient* (for example, a patient who has an altered men-

tal status, difficulty with airway, breathing, or circulation, including severe blood loss, or a significant mechanism of injury). Whenever you believe there may have been a change in the patient's condition, you should repeat the initial assessment. In this way, you will detect signs of life-threatening conditions as soon as possible. When in doubt, repeat the ongoing assessment every five minutes or as frequently as possible.

As you do each repetition of the ongoing assessment, be sure to record your findings. It is important to document and to remember any changes or trends in the patient's condition. Based on your findings, you may need to institute new treatments or adjust treatments you have already started. Your findings, especially any trends in the patient's condition, will also be important information for the hospital staff and will let them know if the patient's condition is improving or deteriorating.

Infants and Children

When reassessing the circulation of a young child or infant, don't forget to check capillary refill. Remember that when you press on a nail bed and then release the pressure, the pink color should return in less than two seconds. Counting "one-one thousand, two-one thousand" or saying "capillary refill" takes about two seconds, so the pink color should return before you finish saying either of these. In small children who have very small nail beds, press on the top of a hand or foot to check capillary refill. Mental status of an unresponsive child or infant can be checked by shouting (verbal stimulus) or flicking the feet (painful stimulus). An expected response would be crying.

Remember to keep eye contact with a conscious child, staying as much as possible on the child's level, and to explain what you are doing in a quiet and reassuring voice.

Ongoing Assessment—Medical Patient

You started the ongoing assessment of Mr. Schmidt, the medical patient in On the Scene, by repeating the initial assessment. You found that his mental status was still alert, his airway and breathing were fine, and his pulse and skin were still normal. He remained stable. Next, you took his vital signs again. All were in the normal range. You found that his pulse and blood pressure were somewhat lower than during the focused history and physical exam.

Ongoing Assessment

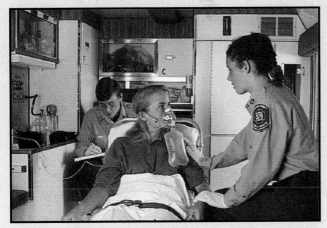

1. Repeat initial assessment.

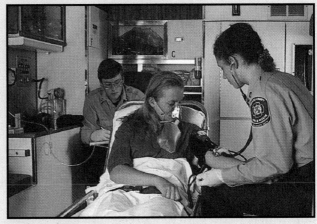

2. Reassess and record vital signs.

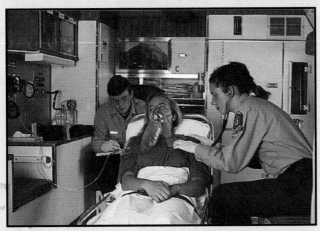

3. Repeat focused assessment.

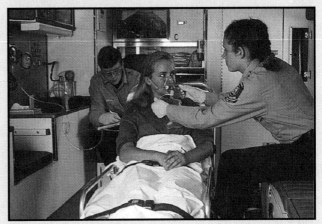

4. Check interventions.

An important part of the ongoing assessment is *recording,* or *documenting* your findings. In Chapter 5, you learned to record vital signs immediately after you take them. In this way, you will not need to worry about remembering the different numbers you get for pulse rate, blood pressure, and respiratory rate. When you have more than one set of vital signs, it becomes even easier to forget them if you have not written them down. Another reason to document your ongoing assessment is so that you can see trends. When you reach Chapter 25, Bleeding and Shock, you will learn more about the importance of seeing trends in the pulse rate and blood pressure. In Mr. Schmidt's case, the changes in his vital signs indicated an improvement in his condition, probably caused by a reduction of anxiety.

Since Mr. Schmidt's chief complaint was abdominal pain, you asked him about his pain and very gently palpated his abdomen again. It was the same as before, tender but not firm or distended. Repeatedly palpating a patient's painful abdomen can cause a significant amount of distress for the patient. For this reason, you should be very gentle when palpating the abdomen as part of your ongoing assessment.

The only intervention you performed for Mr. Schmidt was to place him in the position of comfort, sitting. He told you that he did not feel any other position would help him.

If you had given Mr. Schmidt oxygen, you would have checked. You would have made sure that the bag did not completely deflate and, if it did, checked that the oxygen tank had not run out or that the flow rate was high enough. If Mr. Schmidt had been bleeding, you would have checked to make sure that there was no bleeding from any wounds. Finally, you would have checked any other interventions to make sure they were still doing the job you wanted them to.

Whenever you check the interventions that you have performed for a patient, you should try to take a fresh look at the patient. Attempt to see the patient as though you had never seen him before. This may help you to more objectively evaluate the adequacy of your interventions and adjust them as necessary.

Throughout the assessment procedures that take place on the way to the hospital, remember to explain to a conscious patient what you are doing, to talk in a reassuring tone, and to consider the patient's feelings, such as anxiety or embarrassment.

Ongoing Assessment—Trauma Patient

On the Scene

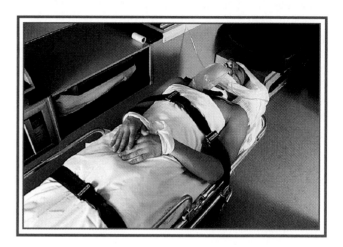

In Chapters 9, 10, and 12, you began your assessment of a critical trauma patient, Brian Sawyer, the young man who was thrown from a vehicle. First you sized up the scene. Then you did the initial assessment, followed by a focused history and physical exam, and—once in the ambulance and en route to the hospital—a detailed physical exam.

Scene Size-Up (Review)

You responded to a motor vehicle accident. You took appropriate **body substance isolation** precautions. The **scene was safe.** The **only patient** was Brian, a male you found lying on his back approximately 20 feet from the vehicle. The **mechanism of injury** was apparently ejection from his car.

Initial Assessment (Review)

You got a **general impression** of an approximately 25-year-old male who appeared unresponsive and who had snoring respirations. His **mental status** was unresponsive to a painful stimulus. Your partner immobilized the patient's head manually as he opened the patient's **airway** with a jaw thrust, which relieved his snoring respirations. When you evaluated **breathing,** you found respirations that were normal in rate and depth. You assessed **circulation** and found a weak and rapid radial pulse with no blood on or near the patient. His skin was pale, cool, and sweaty. You inserted an oral airway and applied oxygen through a nonrebreather mask at 15 liters per minute.

You assigned this patient a high **priority** because he was unresponsive to pain and showed signs of diminished circulation (rapid, weak pulse and pale, clammy skin).

Focused History and Physical Exam (Review)

Once you assessed and treated Brian for any life-threatening problems during the initial assessment, you began your focused history and physical exam. You **reconsidered the mechanism of injury** and made no changes in the priority you assigned to Brian. Your partner **continued spine stabilization.** You did not **call advanced life support** personnel because your EMS system does not have such a team to call. You **reconsidered your transport decision** and confirmed that you should spend as little time as possible at the scene with this patient. You **reassessed mental status** and found Brian unresponsive to pain (a pinch on his shoulder).

Next you performed a **rapid trauma assessment.** You assessed Brian's head, neck, chest, abdomen, pelvis, extremities, and posterior. You found a laceration on the back of his head that was not bleeding. His neck veins were flat. You sized and applied a cervical spine immobilization collar. Breath sounds were present and equal. Brian's abdomen was very firm, but did not look distended. His pelvis was normal. You found a deformity in the middle of Brian's right leg and stabilized it temporarily by placing him on the backboard. He had weak pulses in all extremities and did not respond to a pinch there. Since he was not responsive, you could not determine whether he had sensation. When you assessed his posterior body, you found nothing abnormal.

Finally, you took Brian's **vital signs.** He had a pulse of 120, regular and weak, respirations of 20 and unlabored, skin that was pale, cool and sweaty, a left pupil that was dilated and slow to react, and a blood pressure of 130/80. You recorded your findings.

You could not obtain a **SAMPLE history** because Brian was alone when the collision occurred. You did not find any medical identification bracelet or necklace when you assessed his extremities and neck.

Detailed Physical Exam (Review)

After moving Brian into the ambulance and leaving for the hospital, you **repeated the rapid trauma assessment.** This time, while examining his head, you also assessed his face, ears, eyes, nose, and mouth. You saw a little bit of blood in Brian's left ear. His left pupil was dilated and slow to react. The rest of your exam covered the neck, chest, abdomen, pelvis, extremities, and pelvis. You found no new injuries.

You then **repeated and recorded the vital signs.** You obtained respirations of 14 and normal in depth, a pulse of 136, regular and weak, skin that is still cool, pale and sweaty, a left pupil that is still dilated and slow to react, and a blood pressure of 100/70. As you record your findings, you note that his respirations are slowing, his pulse is more rapid, and his blood pressure is lower than when you assessed his vital signs during the focused history and physical exam before you loaded Brian into the ambulance.

Ongoing Assessment—Unstable Trauma Patient

You start the ongoing assessment by **repeating the initial assessment** to check for life-threatening problems. First you reassess Brian's mental status. When he does not respond to your shouting his name, you pinch his shoulder. There is no response. You reevaluate his airway by putting your ear next to his mouth and listening for abnormal sounds like snoring, gurgling, or stridor. There is a little bit of gurgling, so you suction his mouth. When you listen again, you hear no more abnormal sounds. You also look in Brian's mouth. You see nothing that could cause his airway to become obstructed. Next, you look at Brian's breathing. It is now slow (approximately 8 per minute) and shallow, so you get the flow-restricted oxygen-powered ventilation device for your partner, who starts to ventilate Brian at a rate of 12 per minute. Brian's pulse is rapid and weak. His skin is still pale, cool, and sweaty. You reconfirm that Brian is a high priority patient. In fact, his condition is even more serious than before, because you now need to assist his ventilations.

The next step in the ongoing assessment is to **repeat and record vital signs.** Brian has a pulse of 132, regular and weak, respirations of 8 and shallow, and a blood pressure of 100 by palpation. As you record these findings, you note that his pulse and blood pressure have not changed from your earlier readings, but—as you noted when repeating the initial assessment of respiration—his breathing has now slowed to a dangerous level that requires assisted ventilations.

Now you **repeat the rapid trauma assessment.** You find no additional injuries.

Finally, you **check the interventions** you performed for Brian. You confirm that oxygen is running into the flow-restricted oxygen-powered ventilation device and that Brian's chest is rising with each ventilation. When you checked the laceration on the back of Brian's head, you checked your gloves and found no fresh blood, so there is no need to control bleeding. Now you check the other interventions: the cervical collar, straps and long backboard. The collar is the right size and is in the right place (sometimes cervical collars can slip). The straps are snug, and Brian has not moved on the board. You find time now to splint Brian's leg.

During the ride to the hospital, you will repeat your ongoing assessment every five minutes (performing any needed interventions), recording your findings and noting any trends in his condition.

During the course of Brian's recovery, you check with hospital personnel from time to time to see how he's doing. You are told that the quick work you and your partner did in opening Brian's airway and assisting his ventilations have prevented any brain damage that might have occurred. Brian is transferred to the rehabilitation institute and, after several months, returns to work.

You and your partner both need to be with this critically injured patient on the way to the hospital. Fortunately, during your initial assessment, when you realized how seriously injured Brian might be, you asked dispatch to send another qualified driver so the two of you could continue to work on Brian en route to the hospital. In accordance with your local protocol, you told the driver to drive to the closest hospital able to provide quality trauma care.

The importance of the ongoing assessment became clear in Brian's case. Unlike Mr. Schmidt, the medical patient whose condition improved somewhat during the trip to the hospital, Brian took a turn for the worse. Because you closely reevaluated his airway, you discovered that he had some fluid in his pharynx (which caused the gurgling sound), and so you suctioned him. His respiratory rate had decreased to the point where his breathing was inadequate, and so your partner ventilated him with 100% oxygen.

The value of looking at trends also became apparent. If you look at Brian's vital signs in the form of a chart, you can see that his respiratory rate was decreasing, a bad sign in an unresponsive patient.

In later chapters, you will learn about other trends to look for in patients' vital signs.

After repeating the initial assessment (to recheck for life-threatening problems) and vital signs, you performed another rapid trauma assessment. Although you did not find any new injuries, you kept in mind the possibility that you might find something you missed before or might detect a sign of injury that was not present before.

You also checked the interventions you performed for Brian. Putting the patient on oxygen initially does not prevent the tank from running out later on, or the tubing from becoming disconnected. So you confirmed that oxygen was running into the flow-restricted oxygen-powered ventilation device and that Brian's chest was rising with each ventilation. Checking the oxygen flow into the oxygen-powered ventilation device was easy because the device will not run without oxygen. A nonrebreather mask, though, will require closer attention.

A good habit to develop is to check the entire path of the oxygen from the tank to the patient. This means you look at the regulator on the tank and confirm that it has sufficient oxygen and that the flowmeter is set to the proper flow. You make sure that the tube is firmly connected to the regulator. Follow the tubing and make sure there are no kinks that would prevent the flow of oxygen. Look at the mask. Make sure the tubing is connected to it, and that it is the proper mask, a nonrebreather (sometimes simple or rebreather masks are accidentally stocked in an ambulance). Confirm that the mask is snug on the patient's face and that the nonrebreather bag does not completely deflate when the patient inhales. Increase flow rate if it does. With practice, this sequence of steps will take just a few seconds.

Wounds that stopped bleeding can start bleeding again, so it is important to check them as part of the ongoing assessment. Check any bandage you have applied and make sure it is dry

Vital Signs Trends for Brian Sawyer			
Assessment Step	Pulse	Respirations	Blood Pressure
Focused History/ Physical Exam	120, reg. and weak	20 and normal	130/80
Detailed Physical Exam	136, reg. and weak	14 and normal	100/70
Ongoing Assessment	132, reg. and weak	8 and shallow	100/P (by palpation)

with no blood seeping through. When an unbandaged wound is in a location where you cannot see it, you should gently palpate it with gloved hands and check your gloves for blood. You also need to check other interventions, such as cervical collars, backboard straps, and splints. Each of these can slip and need adjustment.

There are many other changes you may find as you repeat the rapid trauma assessment. A chest injury may become apparent as muscles get tired and you see paradoxical motion that was not present when you first assessed the patient (paradoxical motion is present when a part of the chest goes in as the patient inhales and goes out as the patient exhales, opposite to the motion of the rest of the chest). The abdomen may become distended, a sign that you are especially likely to see if you have a long transport. As you learn about more injuries in other chapters, you will learn more signs to look for in your ongoing assessment.

Brian was not responsive, but if he had been awake, as with any responsive patient, you would have talked to him in a reassuring tone, explaining your actions, and taking into account his feelings, such as fear or embarrassment.

CHAPTER REVIEW

KEY TERMS

You may find it helpful to review the following terms.

ongoing assessment a procedure for detecting changes in a patient's condition. It involves four steps: repeating the initial assessment, repeating and recording vital signs, repeating the focused history and physical exam, and checking interventions.

trending evaluating and recording changes in a patient's condition, such as slowing respirations or rising pulse rate, that may show improvement or deterioration, and that can be shown by documenting repeated assessments.

SUMMARY

The ongoing assessment is the last step in your assessment of a patient. You will repeat it every fifteen minutes for stable patients and at least every five minutes for unstable patients. This means repeating the initial assessment, vital signs, focused assessment, and checking the interventions you performed for the patient. Interventions you need to check include oxygen, bleeding, spine immobilization, and splints.

To review all the assessment steps you have learned in Chapters 8 through 13, see Table 13-1.

REVIEW QUESTIONS

1. Name the four steps of the ongoing assessment and list what assessments you will make during each step.
2. Explain the value of recording, or documenting, your assessment findings, and explain the meaning of the term *trending*.

Application
- What do you need to do if your ongoing assessment turns up one of these findings?
  a. Gurgling respirations
  b. Bag on nonrebreather mask collapses completely when the patient inhales
  c. Snoring respirations

TABLE 13-2

Assessment Summary

In chapters 8 through 13 you have learned the assessment steps you will need to perform as an EMT-B and read about how these steps were applied to four patients: Clara Diller (responsive child trauma patient), Brian Sawyer (unresponsive adult trauma patient), Mr. Schmidt (responsive adult medical patient), and Mrs. Malone (unresponsive adult medical patient.) The assessments for these patients, and for patients like them, are summarized below.

Clara Diller

Clara was 5-year-old who fell on the sidewalk while skating. Her story was told in On the Scenes in Chapters 9 and 10. The following assessment steps were performed on Clara.

- Scene size-up. (BSI precautions. Scene was safe. Mechanism of injury [not significant]: fall to sidewalk.)
- Initial assessment. (Manual stabilization. Alert. Included capillary refill in circulation assessment. No life-threatening problems discovered. Low priority.)
- Focused history and physical exam. (Focused on head injury and knee injury. Cervical collar applied. Vital signs. History taken from Clara, bystanders, and mother.)
- (Immobilized on backboard. No detailed physical exam was necessary because her injuries were obvious and not severe.)
- Ongoing assessment. (Stable patient, so every 15 minutes en route to hospital.)

Brian Sawyer

Brian was the 25-year-old man who was thrown from his car during a collision. His story was told in On the Scenes in Chapters 9, 10, 12, and 13. The following assessment steps were performed on Brian.

- Scene size-up. (BSI precautions. Scene was safe. Mechanism of injury [significant]: apparently ejected from vehicle.)
- Initial assessment. (Manual stabilization. Unresponsive. Jaw thrust to open airway. Oxygen by nonrebreather mask. High priority.)
- Focused history and physical exam. (Rapid trauma assessment including DCAP-BTLS of head, neck, chest, abdomen, pelvis, extremities, posterior. Cervical collar applied. Vital signs. No witnesses so history could not be taken.)
- Detailed physical exam. (Immobilized on backboard. Repeat rapid trauma assessment with added attention to face, ears, eyes, nose, mouth. Repeat vital signs.)
- Ongoing assessment. (Unstable patient, so every 5 minutes en route to hospital.)

Mr. Schmidt

Mr. Schmidt was the 68-year-old man who complained of abdominal pain. His story was told in On the Scenes in Chapters 9, 11, and 13. The following assessment steps were performed on Mr. Schmidt.

- Scene size-up. (BSI precautions. Scene was safe. No mechanism of injury.)
- Initial assessment. (Alert. No life-threatening problems discovered. Low priority.)
- Focused history and physical exam. (SAMPLE history taken from patient. Physical exam focused on abdomen. Vital signs.)
- (No detailed physical exam was necessary because his complaint was medical, and information from a detailed physical exam would not be relevant.)
- Ongoing assessment. (Stable patient, so every 15 minutes en route to hospital.)

Mrs. Malone

Mrs. Malone was the 60-year-old woman whose daughter found her unconscious and having seizures. Her story was told in On the Scenes in Chapters 9, 11, and 12. The following assessment steps were performed on Mrs. Malone.

- Scene size-up. (BSI precautions. Scene was safe. No mechanism of injury)
- Initial assessment. (Responsive to verbal stimulus. Head-tilt, chin-lift to open airway. Oxygen by nonrebreather mask. High priority.)
- Focused history and physical exam. (Rapid assessment of head, neck, chest, abdomen, pelvis, extremities, posterior. Vital signs. Daughter provided partial SAMPLE history.)
- (No detailed physical exam was necessary because her complaint was medical, you had already done a thorough rapid physical exam, and information from a detailed physical exam would not be relevant.)
- Ongoing assessment. (Unstable patient, so every 5 minutes en route to hospital.)

Communications

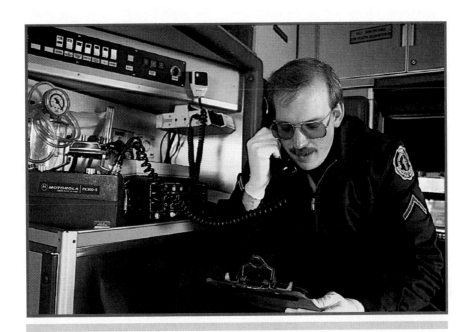

14

Communication is an important part of everyday life. For the EMT-Basic, effective communication may be critical in saving a life. Your communications will be person-to-person with patients and other members of the EMS system, as well as over the radio or telephone to dispatchers, medical direction, and receiving hospital staff. Your ability to communicate effectively will be crucial to the patient at the scene and en route to the hospital. Your ability to communicate effectively with hospital personnel about your patient may make an important difference in the care he receives.

Objectives

Knowledge and Attitude *At the end of this chapter, you should be able to meet the following objectives.*

1. List the proper methods of initiating and terminating a radio call. (pp. 243–244)

2. State the proper sequence for delivery of patient information. (p. 245)

3. Explain the importance of effective communication of patient information in the verbal report. (p. 246)

4. Identify the essential components of the verbal report. (p. 246)

5. Describe the attributes for increasing effectiveness and efficiency of verbal communications. (pp. 246–248)

6. State legal aspects to consider in verbal communication. (pp. 243, 244)

7. Discuss the communication skills that should be used to interact with the patient. (pp. 246–248)

8. Discuss the communication skills that should be used to interact with the family, bystanders, and individuals from other agencies while providing patient care, and the difference between skills used to interact with the patient and those used to interact with others. (pp. 246–248)

On the Scene

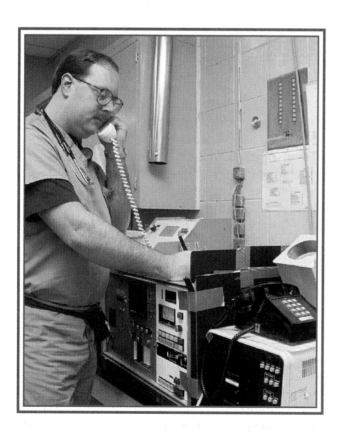

In Chapters 9 through 13, you followed several patients through an assessment sequence. Once more recall Mr. Schmidt, the older man who had abdominal pain. After completing your initial and focused assessment, you loaded him aboard the ambulance for the trip to the hospital. After transportation has begun and ongoing assessment and care undertaken, it is now time to radio the hospital to alert them to your arrival. Your radio transmission may go something like this:

You: Memorial Hospital, this is Community BLS Ambulance 6 en route to your location. How do you read this unit?

Hospital: Community Ambulance, you're loud and clear. Go ahead.

You: Memorial, we are en route to your location with a 15 minute ETA. We are transporting a 68-year-old male patient who complains of pain in his abdomen. Onset of pain was two hours ago and is accompanied by slight nausea. The patient has a history of high blood pressure and arthritis. He is alert and oriented, and never lost consciousness. His vital signs are pulse 88 regular and full, respirations 20 and unlabored, skin normal, and blood pressure 134 over 88.

9. List the correct radio procedures in the following phases of a typical call: (pp. 243–244)

- To the scene
- At the scene
- To the facility
- At the facility
- To the station
- At the station

10. Explain the rationale for providing efficient and effective radio communications and patient reports. (pp. 239, 242–243)

Skills

1. Perform a simulated, organized, concise radio transmission.

2. Perform an organized, concise patient report that would be given to the staff at a receiving facility.

3. Perform a brief, organized report that would be given to an ALS provider arriving at an incident scene at which the EMT-B was already providing care.

Our exam revealed tenderness in both upper abdominal quadrants. They did not appear rigid. For care we have placed him in a position of comfort. The level of pain has not changed during our care. Mental status has remained unchanged. Vital signs are basically unchanged. Does medical direction have any orders?

Hospital: No further orders. We'll expect your arrival in 15 minutes.

You have now provided a clear and concise report to the hospital. They have been able to "picture" the patient from your words. When you transfer Mr. Schmidt to the care of hospital personnel, you will provide them updated information about your patient in a verbal report.

You are also aware that your transmissions and verbal report to the hospital are only a part of your communications skills. During this call, you have used effective interpersonal communications to talk with Mr. and Mrs. Schmidt, to get Mr. Schmidt's history, to reassure the couple, and to persuade Mr. Schmidt to go to the hospital. In the ambulance you expressed your concern by asking him how you could make him more comfortable. You continue to maintain eye contact with Mr. Schmidt, inform him about what you are doing, and talk in a calm and reassuring tone as you conduct ongoing assessment and continue the trip to the hospital.

There are three types of communication that you will learn about in this chapter: radio communication, the verbal report at the hospital, and interpersonal communication. As the name implies, *radio communication* is conducted by radio. Technology has allowed the use of cellular phones and other equipment to be used where radio transmissions were previously the only choice. The *verbal report* is your chance to convey information about your patient directly to the hospital personnel who will be taking over his care. *Interpersonal communications* are important in dealing with other EMT-Bs, the patient, family and bystanders, medical direction, and other members of the EMS system.

COMMUNICATIONS SYSTEMS AND RADIO COMMUNICATION

Radio equipment is often taken for granted since it is now so common (Figure 14-1). However, the development of radio links between dispatchers, mobile units, and hospitals has been one of the key contributors to improvement in EMS over the years. Imagine if you had to call the dispatcher by phone every few minutes to see if there is a call! And without radio transmissions from ambulances, hospitals would be unable to prepare for the arrival of patients, as they do now.

Communications Systems

There are several components to any radio or communications system.

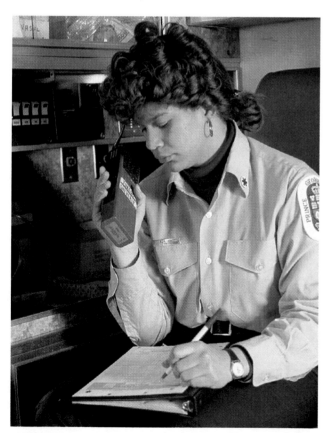

FIGURE 14-1 Communication from the ambulance can be by radio or cellular phone.

- **Base stations** are two-way radios that are at a fixed site such as a hospital or dispatch center.
- **Mobile radios** are two-way radios that are used or affixed in a vehicle. Most units are actually mounted inside the vehicle. These devices have lower transmitting power than base stations. The unit of measurement used in measuring output power of radios is the **watt.**
- **Portable radios** are hand-held two-way radios. This type of radio is important because it will allow you to be in touch with the dispatcher, medical direction, and other members of the EMS system while you are away from the ambulance.
- **Repeaters** are devices that are used when transmissions must be carried over a long distance. Repeaters may be in ambulances or placed in various areas around an EMS system. The repeater picks up signals from lower-power units, such as mobile and portable radios, and retransmits them at a higher power. The retransmission is done on another frequency.
- **Cellular phones** are phones that transmit through the air instead of over wires so that the phones can be transported and used over a wide area. These devices are becoming more widely available and popular around the country. In many areas where the distances or expense is too great to set up a conventional EMS radio system, cellular phones allow EMS communications through an already-established commercial system.
- **Other radio devices** New technology is developing almost constantly. Microwave radio transmissions are used in some areas. In other areas, radio communications are carried via phone lines for part of the signal's journey from one point to another. Digital radio equipment permits transmission of some standard messages, such as ambulance identification or arrival at the scene, by punching a key. The messages are transmitted in a condensed form that helps keep busy frequencies less crowded.

System maintenance

Radio systems require preventive maintenance and repair, just as the ambulance and your EMS equipment do. Radio equipment must be treated with care on a daily basis and not mishandled.

Since radios are so important to EMS today, many systems have *back-up radios.* This means that in the event of power failure or malfunction, another option is available. If the base station fails, there may be a back-up radio or alternative power supply available. If the mobile radio in your ambulance malfunctions, portable radios or phones may be used in its place.

Radio Communication

EMS is just one of many public services that use radio communication. To maintain order on the airwaves, the Federal Communications Commission (FCC) assigns and licenses radio frequencies. This is to prevent two or more agencies from trying to use the same frequency and interfering with each other's communications. There are also strict rules about interfering with emergency radio traffic and prohibiting profanities or offensive language.

General Rules

There are some general rules for radio transmissions that should always be followed. These rules prevent delays and allow all persons to use the frequencies. There may be some minor variations within your EMS system, but always keep in mind the principles shown in Table 14-1.

Radio Transmissions throughout the Call

The Emergency Medical Dispatcher (EMD) receives the initial call for help. The call most often comes via telephone but may also be radioed from another agency, such as the police. After proper information is obtained, the units are dispatched. The following is a sample flow of information between the dispatcher and units in the field. You are the EMT-B on ambulance number 6.

> **Dispatcher:** Ambulance 6 . . .
> **You:** Ambulance 6. Go ahead.

TABLE 14-1 Principles of Radio Communication

Follow these principles when using the EMS radio system.

- Make sure that your radio is on and the volume is adjusted properly.
- Reduce background noise by closing the vehicle window when possible.
- Listen to the frequency and ensure that it is clear before beginning a transmission.
- Press the "press to talk" (PTT) button on the radio, then wait one second before speaking. This prevents cutting off the first few words of your transmission.
- Speak with your lips about two to three inches from the microphone.
- When calling another unit or base station, use their unit number or name, followed by yours. "Dispatcher, this is Ambulance 2."
- The unit being called will signal that the transmission should start by saying "go ahead" or another regionally accepted term: "Ambulance 2, this is the dispatcher. Go ahead." If the unit you are calling tells you to "stand by," wait until they tell you they are ready to take your transmission.
- Speak slowly and clearly.
- Keep transmissions brief. If a transmission takes longer than 30 seconds, stop at that point and pause for a few seconds so that emergency traffic can use the frequency if necessary.
- Use plain English. Avoid codes.
- Do not use phrases like "be advised." These are implied and serve no purpose.
- Courtesy is assumed, so there is no need to say "please," "thank you," and "you're welcome."
- When transmitting a number that might be unclear (15 may sound like 16 or 50), give the number, then repeat the individual digits. Say "15, one-five."
- Anything said over the radio can be heard by the public on a scanner. Do not use the patient's name over the radio. For the same reason, do not use profanities or statements that tend to slander any person. Use objective, impartial statements.
- Use "we" instead of "I." As an EMT-B you will rarely be acting alone.
- "Affirmative" and "negative" are preferred over "yes" and "no" because the latter are difficult to hear.
- Give assessment information about your patient, but avoid offering a diagnosis of the patient's problem. For example, say "Patient complains of chest pain," but not "Probably having a heart attack."
- After transmitting, say "Over." Wait for acknowledgment that the person to whom you were speaking heard your message.
- Avoid codes, slang, or abbreviations that are not authorized.
- Use EMS frequencies only for authorized EMS communication.

Dispatcher: Ambulance 6, respond to 1243 Magnolia Boulevard—that's one-two-four-three Magnolia Boulevard—for an assault. The police are en route. Stand by at the corner of Magnolia and Third until the police report the scene secure.

You: Ambulance 6 received that. Will stand by at Magnolia and Third.

Without a prompt and efficient receipt and dispatch of information, the ambulance could easily be sent to the wrong location. In this situation, the dispatcher also relayed important safety information. Since the call was for an assault, the dispatcher "staged" the ambulance, or ordered it to stand by, until the scene is safe.

You respond to the assigned location, reporting your arrival to the dispatcher.

You: Dispatcher, Ambulance 6 is arriving at the staging area.

Dispatcher: Message received, Ambulance 6. I will advise you when the scene is secure.

Most scenes are safe. However, in this case the dispatcher has decided, from the nature of the call and other information she was able to obtain, that it wasn't. Police arrive at the scene and separate the parties involved in the assault. The police radio the dispatcher and advise that the scene is secure. The next transmission is to your ambulance.

Dispatcher: Ambulance 6, the police report that the scene is secure. Respond in.

You: Message received by Ambulance 6. (You drive two blocks to the scene and report to the dispatcher.) Dispatcher, Ambulance 6 is at the scene.

Dispatcher: Ambulance 6 at the scene (gives the time on the 24-hour clock) at 1310 hours.

The dispatcher records all the times from the time of the original call, the time dispatched, at the staging area, and finally at the scene. Should this case go to court, the records of the dispatch center, your care report, and the dispatch audio tape of the call may be subpoenaed. Unless there is a need for medical direction or assistance from the scene, the next call will be when you are en route to the hospital.

You: Dispatcher, Ambulance 6 is en route to Mercy Hospital with one patient.

Dispatcher: Ambulance 6 en route to Mercy Hospital at 1323 hours.

You will call the hospital via radio or phone to advise them of the status of your patient and the estimated time of arrival (ETA). When arriving at the hospital, you again advise the dispatcher.

You: Ambulance 6 is arriving at Mercy Hospital.

Dispatcher: Ambulance 6 at Mercy at 1334 hours.

You will note that the dispatcher gives the time after most transmissions. This will allow you to record times if they are required on your patient care record. The dispatcher also usually acknowledges by briefly repeating the message to assure that she has acknowledged the right unit. If two units happened to transmit at exactly the same time and the dispatcher simply acknowledged a transmission, both units would think that the dispatcher heard them when, actually, only one unit was able to get through.

After turning the patient over to the hospital staff and preparing the ambulance for the next run, you will advise the dispatcher that you are leaving the hospital. You may also find it part of your local procedure to advise the dispatcher when you are back in your district or area and when you are back in quarters (the station or ambulance garage).

A majority of these transmissions were made between the mobile radio within the ambulance and the dispatcher at a base station. Remember, when you have one available, bring your portable radio with you whenever you leave the ambulance. You may need to call for assistance during scene size-up if hazards or multiple patients are found, and the portable radio allows you to do it without running back to the ambulance to make the call on the fixed unit.

Medical Radio Reports

Reports must be made to medical personnel as part of almost every call. These reports may be by radio, verbal (in person), or in writing.

You will recall that in the On the Scene that started this chapter, you had presented a radio report to the receiving hospital about your patient, Mr. Schmidt. The report was specifically structured to present pertinent facts about the patient without telling more detail than necessary. Too much detail ties up the radio frequency and takes up the time of hospital personnel.

Experienced EMT-Bs often try to "paint a picture" of the patient in words. This requires knowledge of radio procedure and practice. If you have a critical patient, your radio report should make that clear. This can be done by describing the chief complaint, injuries, vital signs, treatments, and mechanism of injury. Even with critical patients you must keep a clear, steady tone to your voice. Resist the urge to talk fast or appear excited as it will prevent effective communication.

The medical radio report below is the report that you made from the ambulance to the hospital about Mr. Schmidt. Here, it is broken down into its twelve individual parts.

1. **Unit identification and level of provider**
   Memorial Hospital, this is Community BLS Ambulance 6 en route to your location . . .

2. **Estimated time of arrival**
   . . . with a 15-minute ETA.

3. **Patient's age and sex**
   We are transporting a 68-year-old male patient . . .

4. **Chief complaint**
   . . . who complains of pain in his abdomen.

5. **Brief, pertinent history of the present illness**
   Onset of pain was two hours ago and is accompanied by slight nausea.

6. **Major past illnesses**
   The patient has a history of high blood pressure and arthritis

7. **Mental status**
   He is alert and oriented, never lost consciousness.

8. **Baseline vital signs**
   His vital signs are pulse 88 regular and full, respirations 20 and unlabored, skin normal, and blood pressure 134 over 88.

9. **Pertinent findings of the physical exam**
   Our exam revealed tenderness in both upper abdominal quadrants. They did not appear rigid.

10. **Emergency medical care given**
    For care, we have placed him in a position of comfort.

11. **Response to emergency medical care**
    The level of pain has not changed during our care. Mental status has remained unchanged. Vital signs are basically unchanged.

12. **If your system requires contacting medical direction, or if you have questions**
    Does medical direction have any orders?

After giving this information, you will continue with ongoing assessment of the patient en route to the hospital. Additional vital signs will be taken, there may be changes in the patient's condition, or you may discover new information about the patient, particularly on long transports. In some systems, you should radio this additional information to the hospital in a follow-up radio call while en route (follow local protocols).

When medical direction is contacted, orders may be given to the EMT-B. The on-line physician may order you to assist in administering the patient's own medication, or order the administration of a medication you carry on the ambulance, or give other orders. In any case, the communication between you and medical direction must be clear and concise to avoid misinterpretations that can inadvertently harm the patient. For example, a patient may have a medication for chest pain called nitroglycerin. This medication, as you will learn in Chapter 16, General Pharmacology, is one that you may assist the patient in taking (according to local protocols). The medication should be given only if the patient's blood pressure is above a certain level. If there is a misunderstanding between you and the medical director and this medication is ordered improperly, harm may come to the patient.

To avoid misunderstanding and miscommunication, use the following guidelines when communicating with medical direction.

- *Give the information to medical direction clearly and accurately.* Speak slowly and clearly. The orders of the physician will be based on what you report.
- *After receiving an order for a medication or procedure, repeat the order word for word.* You may also ask to do a procedure or give a medication and be denied by medical direction. Repeat this also.
- *If an order is unclear, ask the physician to repeat it.* Once it is clearly received by you, repeat it back to the physician.
- *If an order appears to be inappropriate, question the physician.* There may have been a misunderstanding. Your questioning may prevent the inappropriate administration of a medication. If the physician verifies the order, he may explain to you why he has given you that particular order.

THE VERBAL REPORT

At the hospital, you will give a written report on your patient to hospital personnel. (See Chapter 16, Documentation.) However, it will take some time to complete your written report, so the first information you give to hospital personnel will be your verbal report.

As you transfer your patient to the care of the hospital staff, introduce the patient by name. Then summarize the same kind of information you gave over the radio, pointing out any information that is updated or different from your last radio report. Include the following in your verbal report.

- Chief complaint
- History that was not given previously
- Additional treatment given en route
- Additional vital signs taken en route

INTERPERSONAL COMMUNICATION

While communication between two or more human beings is a skill that you have learned over the years, many people still do not communicate as well as they could. Communicating with patients and others who are in crisis is even more difficult. While interpersonal communication could be presented as a course in itself, the following guidelines will help when dealing with patients, families, friends, and bystanders.

- *Use eye contact.* Make frequent eye contact with your patient. Eye contact shows that you are interested in your patient and that you are attentive. Failure to make eye contact signals that you feel uneasy around the patient. (If your patient is avoiding eye contact, consider that in some cultures eye contact is considered rude. You may want to match your behavior to the patient's in this situation.)
- *Be aware of your position and body language.* Your positioning in respect to the patient is important. If you are higher than the patient, you may appear intimidating. If possible, position yourself at or below the patient's eye level (Figure 14-2). This will be less threatening to the patient. Body language is also important. Standing with your

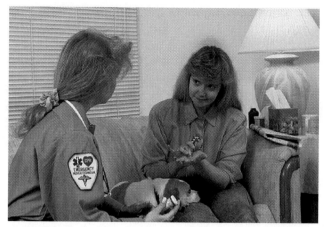

FIGURE 14-2 If possible, position yourself at or below the patient's eye level to be less intimidating and to aid communication.

arms crossed or not directly facing the patient (a closed stance) sends a signal to the patient that you are not interested. Use a more open stance (arms down, facing the patient), when it can be done safely, to communicate a warmer attitude.

A closed or more serious stance may sometimes be beneficial, however, when you need to calm or direct bystanders at the scene. Standing above a patient may indicate authority and can be done to gain control when necessary.

Watch the patient's body language to see how your communication with him is going. If the patient uses a closed stance, your communication efforts may not be working.

- *Use language the patient can understand.* Speak slowly and clearly. Do not use medical or other terms that the patient will not understand. Explain procedures before they are performed, to prevent anxiety.
- *Be honest.* Honesty is important. You will frequently be asked questions that you will not have the answer to: "Is my leg broken?" "Am I having a heart attack?" At other times you will know the answer to the question, but it is not pleasant: "Will it hurt when you put that splint on?" If the answer is yes, tell the truth. Explain that you will do it as gently as possible to reduce pain, but some pain may be experienced. It is much worse to lie to the patient and have them find out that you were not being truthful. This will erode confidence in you as well as other EMT-Bs and medical personnel the patient may meet later on.

- *Use the patient's proper name.* Especially with adults and senior citizens, do not assume familiarity. As a general rule, call patients as they introduce themselves to you. If a person many years older than you introduces himself as William Harris, it might be best to call him Mr. Harris as a sign of respect. Immediately calling him "Bill" when he clearly stated his name was "William" would be disrespectful. If, after you call him "Mr. Harris," he says "Please call me Bill," you have shown respect and can then use the less formal name. If in doubt, ask what the patient would like to be called.

- *Listen.* If you ask the patient a question, get an answer, then have to ask again, it will show the patient that you were not listening. If you are not listening, the patient will feel that you are not interested in what he has to say, or that you just don't care. If you ask a question, wait for the answer. Then write it down so you will not forget.

If a person has a mental disability or is hard of hearing, speak slowly and clearly. Do not talk down to the patient. If the patient has a hearing disability, he may read lips or, in any case, be much helped in understanding what you are saying if he can see your lips. So be sure that a deaf or hearing-impaired person can see your mouth when you talk.

Remember that a person who is blind or has a visual deficit can usually hear, so don't give in to the temptation to speak to him loudly or unnaturally. For the visually impaired person, you will want to take extra effort to explain anything that is happening that he can't see.

You may also find people who do not speak the same language as you. In this case use an interpreter (for example, a family member or friend who speaks both languages) or a manual that provides translations. You may also find that your communications center or medical direction may have someone available who speaks the patient's language.

The elderly are a rapidly growing segment of the population who often need EMS care. These older patients may have medical problems simply because of their age. They may also be more prone to falls and serious injury from trauma due to the condition of their bones and body systems.

Many elderly patients are well oriented and physically able. Others, however, may have

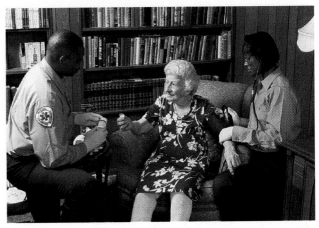

FIGURE 14-3 Be considerate of the elderly patient.

problems with hearing, sight, or orientation that have come on with age. These patients may seem confused or simply find it difficult to communicate. In spite of their sensory limitations, of course, these patients still have needs and feelings. They deserve patience, kindness, and understanding—along with proper emergency care (Figure 14-3).

Infants and Children

Children are sometimes difficult to assess and communicate with. It is often best to involve the parents of the child when communicating. Two rules of adult communication are critically important to children.

1. Always come down to the child's level (Figure 14-4). Never stand above a child. You literally tower over the child and appear very intimidating. Crouching down reduces

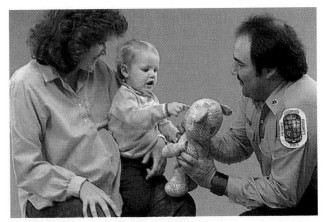

FIGURE 14-4 Always come down to the child's level or lower.

the size difference and greatly improves communication. If the child is not critically ill, you might even take the time to sit on the floor and get slightly below the child in the beginning.

2. Children often sense lies even faster than adults. It is important to tell the truth to children. Remember, you may be the first contact from the EMS system that the child has ever had. Work to make it positive.

CHAPTER REVIEW

KEY TERMS

You may find it helpful to review the following terms.

base station a two-way radio at a fixed site such as a hospital or dispatch center.
cellular phone a phone that transmits through the air instead of over wires so that the phone can be transported and used over a wide area.
mobile radio a two-way radio that is used or affixed in a vehicle.

portable radio a hand-held two-way radio.
repeater a device that picks up signals from lower-power radio units such as mobile and portable radios and retransmits them at a higher power. It allows low-power radio signals to be transmitted over longer distances.
watt the unit of measurement of the output power of a radio.

SUMMARY

Communication is not as tangible a skill as putting on a splint or taking a pulse, but it is a very important part of every call. Communication may be face-to-face with people—hospital personnel, other EMT-Bs, patients, family, bystanders, and others. Radio communication is important as your link to the dispatcher and medical direction. Use communication by any means or method carefully and accurately.

REVIEW QUESTIONS

1. List several guidelines for proper use of the EMS radio system.
2. List the steps of a medical radio report and describe the communication that may be necessary during each part.
3. List several guidelines for effective interpersonal communication with patients.

Application question

- The following information, describing a patient, is in random order. Organize the information and present a medical radio report as if you were radioing the hospital.

  Chest pain radiating to the shoulder
  56 years old
  Oxygen applied at 15 liters per minute via nonrebreather

  Alert and oriented
  Female
  Came on twenty minutes ago while mowing the lawn
  History of high blood pressure and diabetes
  20 minutes until arrival at hospital
  Pulse 86, respirations 22, skin cool and moist, blood pressure 110/66
  Oxygen relieved the pain slightly
  Denies difficulty breathing
  You are requesting orders from medical direction
  You are on Community BLS Ambulance 4
  Lungs sounds equal on both sides
  Placed in a position of comfort

Documentation

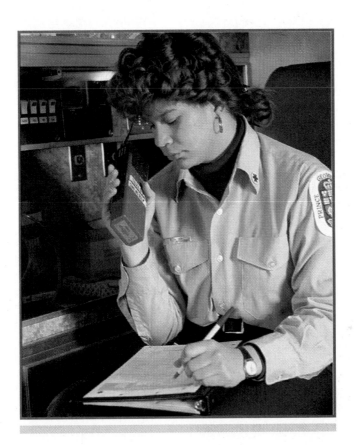

15

Documentation is an important part of the patient care process and lasts long after the call. The report you write will become a part of the patient's permanent hospital record. As records of your agency, your reports and those written by other EMT-Bs become a valuable source for research on trends in emergency medical care and a guide for continuing education and quality improvement. A report you have written may be used as evidence in a legal case. Documentation has short term benefits as well. Noting vital signs and patient history will help you remember important facts about the patient during the course of the call.

Objectives

On the Scene

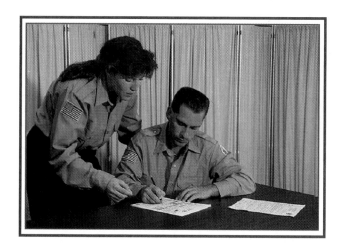

After completing a serious cardiac call, you complete the prehospital care report while your partner prepares the equipment and stretcher for the next call. You sit and begin writing. You record the patient's chief complaint, vital signs, and begin to do the handwritten portion, called the narrative. You stop for a minute. This pause is noticed by your partner, who comes over and asks how things are going.

You: The narrative is a tough part of the form to complete. How do you know what to write?
Your partner: Well, the report should paint a picture of the patient. It should tell the hospital and the quality improvement committee enough about the patient so they could picture the patient. That's a good report.
You: So how do I create a good report?
Your partner: A good report is complete and accurate. Those are probably the most important things. The way you present things is a matter of style and experience. I tell the story in the order that it happened. We got there and obtained the chief complaint. We performed an assessment, then we cared for the patient. If you can remember what happened and in what order, you can write a narrative. You don't have to duplicate things that are already in the fill-in boxes, like vital signs. Tell what happened. It'll work. Let's take a look at what you've got so far. . . .

As mentioned in the introduction to this chapter, documentation is an important part of patient care. Unfortunately, many experienced EMT-Bs do not document thoroughly or seriously. Documentation is more than a written conclusion to a call. The process called documentation actually begins early in the call, and the documents produced last for many years as the record of your call.

THE PREHOSPITAL CARE REPORT

The record that you produce during a call is called a prehospital care report or, informally, a "PCR." Your region or service may use a different name for the same kind of document, such as trip sheet, run report, or another name.

Prehospital care reports vary from system to system and state to state. While the information that is required to complete each is relatively similar, the method used to record the data may be somewhat different.

Written reports are those that have portions with narrative areas, areas to record vital signs in written number form, and check boxes (Figure 15-1).

Computerized reports are those that are completed by shading boxes to record data. These reports are scanned by computer for easy data storage and evaluation. In order to be scanned correctly, each box must be filled in completely with no stray marks (Figure 15-2)

A recent development in prehospital care reports is the "electronic clipboard." This device is a computer in a clipboard format. The computer is able to recognize handwriting and convert it to computer text. The data are stored and eventually downloaded to a larger computer. The computers, also called pen-based computers, may also be attached to printers at receiving hospitals to print out a hard copy of the report for the emergency department staff (Figure 15-3).

Functions of the Prehospital Care Report

The prehospital care report has many functions. It serves as the record of patient care, serves as a legal document, provides information for administrative functions, aids education and research, and contributes to quality improvement. These functions are discussed in the following paragraphs.

Patient Care Record

The prehospital care report conveys important information about the patient to members of the EMS system and beyond. Even though you provide a verbal report to the hospital staff before you leave the patient, the written record provides a means for the emergency department to look back at the status of the patient when you arrived on the scene, the care you gave, and how the patient's status may have changed during your care. An example of this would be the emergency department staff looking back at your original set of vital signs to compare the current condition of the patient with the condition of the patient when he was first found at the scene.

The prehospital care report becomes part of the patient's permanent hospital record.

Legal Document

The prehospital care report also serves as a legal document that may be called for at any legal proceeding resulting from the call. The person who wrote the report will ordinarily go to court with the form. If the patient was the victim or perpetrator of a criminal act, the report and the writer may be called into court to testify about the call during criminal proceedings. Civil law proceedings for negligence in injuries (e.g., a patient falls in a shopping mall and sues) are another reason that your report may be examined.

Unfortunately, there may be a time when the report is being examined because you are the subject of a law suit. Fortunately this is rare and usually preventable, but in this case too, the report in which you documented the circumstances and the care you gave will be very important.

Administrative

Depending on the service you belong to, you may have to obtain insurance and billing information from the patient or patient's family. This may be recorded on your prehospital care report, or on a separate form, or both.

Education and Research

Your report may be examined at a later date as part of a research project. Analysis of statistics compiled from prehospital care reports can reveal patterns and trends in EMS management and care. For example, analysts may see

MAINE EMS

PRESS DOWN, YOU ARE MAKING THREE COPIES

RUN REPORT #	Mo.	Day	Year	M T W Th	F S Sun	SERVICE NAME		SERVICE NO.	VEHICLE NO.	ALS ☐ Performed ☐ Back-up Called	SERVICE RUN NO.
746118											

NAME	BILLING INFORMATION
STREET OR R.F.D.	

CITY/TOWN	STATE	ZIP	

AGE / DATE OF BIRTH	☐ Male ☐ Female	PHONE	

INCIDENT LOCATION:	ADDRESS	CITY/TOWN

TRANSPORTED TO:	TREATING / FAMILY PHYSICIAN	CREW LICENSE NUMBERS

TRANSPORTATION / COMMUNICATIONS PROBLEMS

☐ Medical
  ☐ Cardiac
  ☐ Poisoning/OD
  ☐ Respiratory
  ☐ Behavioral
  ☐ Diabetic
  ☐ Seizure
  ☐ CVA
  ☐ OB/Gyn
  ☐ Other _____

☐ Trauma
  ☐ Multi-Systems Trauma
  ☐ Head
  ☐ Spinal
  ☐ Burn
  ☐ Soft Tissue Injury
  ☐ Fractures
  ☐ Other _____

☐ Code 99

R L LUNG SOUNDS
☐ ☐ CLEAR
☐ ☐ ABSENT
☐ ☐ DECREASED
☐ ☐ RALES
☐ ☐ WHEEZE
☐ ☐ STRIDOR

TYPE OF RUN
☐ Emergency Transport
☐ Routine Transfer
☐ Emergency Transfer
☐ No Transport
☐ Refused Transport

	TIME	CODE		ODOMETER
Call Received				
Enroute				
At Scene				
From Scene				
At Destination				
In Service				

☐ MEDICATIONS   ☐ ALLERGIES

CHIEF COMPLAINT:

TIME	PULSE	RESP	BP	PUPILLARY RESPONSE	SKIN	VERBAL RESPONSE	MOTOR RESPONSE	EYE OPENING RESPONSE	CAPILLARY REFILL
						5 4 3 2 1	6 5 4 3 2 1	4 3 2 1	☐ Normal ☐ Delayed ☐ None
						5 4 3 2 1	6 5 4 3 2 1	4 3 2 1	☐ Normal ☐ Delayed ☐ None
						5 4 3 2 1	6 5 4 3 2 1	4 3 2 1	☐ Normal ☐ Delayed ☐ None

☐ MVA   ☐ Concern AOB/ETOH   SEAT BELTS: ☐ Used   ☐ Not Used   ☐ N/A   ☐ Helmet Used

MUTUAL AID: Assisted/Assisted by Service # _____   Time Called: _____

PATIENT'S SUSPECTED PROBLEM:		**746118**	☐ Medication Administered	☐ Defib Lic #_____	**MEDICAL CONTROL** ☐ Written Order/Protocol ☐ Verbal Order/Protocol

		☐ Monitor	☐ Chest Decomp	IV ☐ SUC LIC.# _____ Total Attempts
Cleared Airway	Extrication	☐ Pacing	☐ Cricothyrotomy	☐ UNSUC LIC.# _____
Artificial Respiration/BVM	Cervical Immobilization	**EOA** Total Attempts		**ET** Total Attempts
Oropharyngeal Airway	KED/Short Board	☐ SUC LIC.# _____		☐ SUC LIC.# _____
Nasopharyngeal Airway	Long Board	☐ UNSUC LIC.# _____		☐ UNSUC LIC.# _____
CPR—Time:	Restraints	LIC #	EKG RHYTHM	TIME	MEDS / DEFIB / C-VERT	DOSE W/S	ROUTE
Bystander CPR	Traction Splinting						
AED	General Splinting						
Suction	Cold Application						
Oxygen—LPMin___ ☐ Nasal ☐ Mask	MAST Inflated						
Pulse Oximetry							
Autovent							

NAME OF E.D. TREATING PHYSICIAN   SIGNATURE OF CREW MEMBER IN CHARGE

COPY 1 HOSPITAL

FIGURE 15-1 The Maine prehospital care report has fill-in boxes and narrative space.

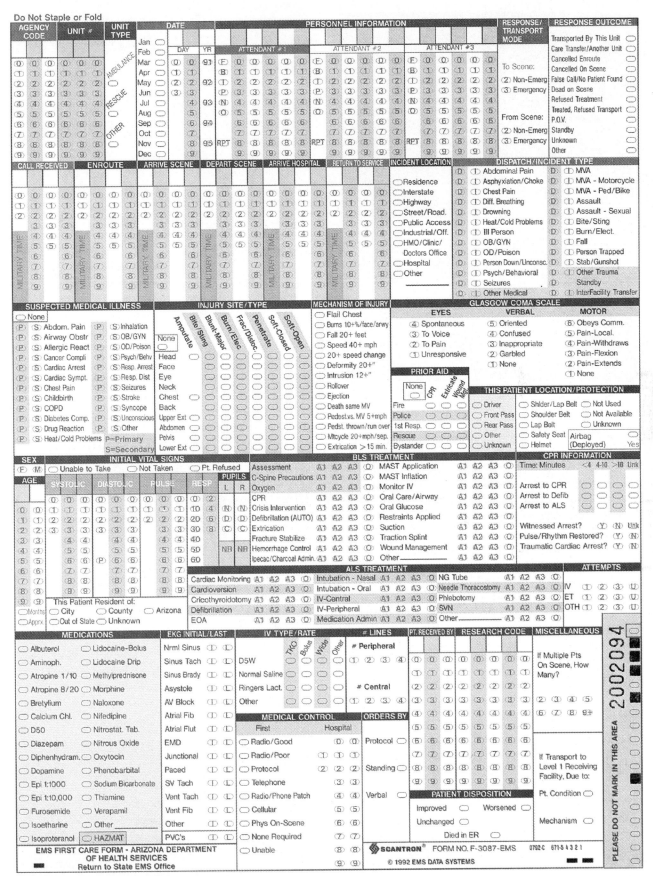

FIGURE 15-2 The Arizona prehospital care report has a scannible segment that can be read by a computer.

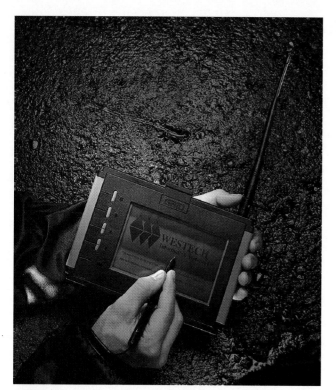

FIGURE 15-3 A pen-based computer can read handwriting and convert it to computer text.

instances in which response time could be improved or ways of scheduling and deploying units to prepare for busy areas and times. The statistics may justify a request for additional resources.

Prehospital care reports can also help management keep track of each EMT-B's experience and skills. Extra practice may be scheduled during continuing education sessions for skills that the reports reveal are underutilized, for instance. When an unusual or uncommon type of call has taken place, the prehospital care report may be used for demonstration of how to document such a case.

Quality Improvement

Most organizations have a Quality Improvement (QI)—or Quality Assurance (QA) or Total Quality Management (TQM)—system in place by which calls are routinely reviewed for conformity to current medical and organizational standards. Examination of prehospital care reports is one major way of conducting this review. At times, QI evaluations reveal excellent care by an EMT-B team that deserves special recognition and a "pat on the back."

Elements of the Prehospital Care Report

Data Elements

Each individual box in the prehospital care report is called a *data element*. While some elements may seem insignificant, each is actually an important part of the report and the description of the patient and response. These elements are necessary for research as well as for documenting the call.

To aid in research across many states and regions, the U. S. Department of Transportation has developed a *minimum data set*. These are the minimum elements that it is recommended be included in all prehospital care reports nationwide. There is also a standardized definition of what each element means. Over a period of time, it is hoped, the minimum data set will be widely adopted. The minimum data set is briefly summarized in Table 15-1.

The prehospital care report can be broken down into several sections, each containing different types of information. The sections include run data, patient data, check boxes, and the narrative section.

TABLE 15-1   The Minimum Data Set

Patient information *(Gathered at the time of the EMT-B's initial contact with patient on arrival at scene, following all interventions, and on arrival at facility)*
• Chief complaint • Level of consciousness (AVPU)—mental status • Systolic blood pressure for patients greater than 3 years old • Skin perfusion (capillary refill) for patients less than 6 years old • Skin color and temperature • Pulse rate • Respiratory rate and effort
Administrative information
• **Time of incident report** • **Time unit notified** • **Time of arrival at patient** • **Time unit left scene** • **Time of arrival at destination** • **Time of transfer of care**

Prehospital Care Report

		MILEAGE		USE MILITARY TIMES

Agency Name ARLINGTON RESCUE

Dispatch Information CARDIAC

Call Location 124 CYPRUS ST 2nd FLOOR

MILEAGE
END |2|4|4|9|6|
BEGIN |2|4|4|7|6|
TOTAL |0|0|0|2|0|

LOCATION CODE |0|1|2|4|

CHECK ONE
- ☒ Residence ☐ Health Facility ☐ Farm ☐ Indus. Facility
- ☐ Other Work Loc. ☐ Roadway ☐ Recreational ☐ Other

CALL TYPE AS REC'D
- ☒ Emergency
- ☐ Non-Emergency
- ☐ Stand-by

MECHANISM OF INJURY
- ☐ MVA (✓ seat belt used) N/A
- ☐ Fall of _____ feet N/A
- ☐ Unarmed assault
- ☐ GSW
- ☐ Knife
- ☐ Machinery
- ☐ _____

USE MILITARY TIMES
- CALL REC'D |0|7|0|5|
- ENROUTE |0|7|0|7|
- ARRIVED AT SCENE |0|7|1|9|
- FROM SCENE |0|7|3|8|
- AT DESTIN |0|7|5|4|
- IN SERVICE |0|8|1|0|
- IN QUARTERS |0|8|3|2|

FIGURE 15-4 One section of a prehospital care report contains run data.

Run Data

This section includes the agency name, unit number, date, times, run or call number, and crew members' names, certification levels, and numbers (Figure 15-4). Times recorded must be accurate and synchronous (by clocks or watches that show the same time). Be sure to use the time as given by the dispatcher when noting times on your report. Unless your watch or the ambulance clock displays exactly the same time as the dispatch center, the times on your report will not match. There may be a several-minute difference between the time displayed on your watch and the dispatch center's official time.

This time difference may seem insignificant but is actually very important in such areas as determining how long a patient has been in cardiac arrest, trends in patient condition, or measurement of system efficiency in response times.

Patient Data

This section contains information about the patient, the patient's condition throughout the call, and the care given to the patient (Figure 15-5). This is the major portion of your report. Specifically, it contains

- The patient's name, address, date of birth, age, sex
- Billing and insurance information (in many jurisdictions)
- Nature of the call
- Mechanism of injury
- Location where the patient was found
- Treatment administered before arrival of the EMT-B (by bystanders, first responders)
- Signs and symptoms, baseline and subsequent vital signs
- SAMPLE history

CHIEF COMPLAINT		TIME	RESP	PULSE	B.P.	LEVEL OF CONSCIOUSNESS	R PUPILS L	SKIN
"MY CHEST HURTS"	V I T A L	0724	Rate: 18 ☒Regular ☐Shallow ☐Labored	Rate: 88 ☐Regular ☒Irregular	148/88	☒Alert ☐Voice ☐Pain ☐Unresp.	☒Normal ☒ / ☐Dilated / ☐Constricted ☐ / ☐Sluggish / ☐No-Reaction ☐	☐Unremarkable ☒Cool ☒Pale ☐Warm ☐Cyanotic ☐Moist ☐Flushed ☐Dry ☐Jaundiced
PAST MEDICAL HISTORY ☐None ☒Allergy to ASPIRIN ☐Hypertension ☐Stroke ☐Seizures ☐Diabetes ☐COPD ☒Cardiac ☐Other (List) ☐Asthma	S I G	0730	Rate: 18 ☒Regular ☐Shallow ☐Labored	Rate: 84 ☐Regular ☒Irregular	144/86	☒Alert ☐Voice ☐Pain ☐Unresp.	☒Normal ☒ / ☐Dilated / ☐Constricted ☐ / ☐Sluggish / ☐No-Reaction ☐	☐Unremarkable ☒Cool ☒Pale ☐Warm ☐Cyanotic ☐Moist ☐Flushed ☐Dry ☐Jaundiced
Current Medications (List) CARDIZEM	N S	0745	Rate: 20 ☒Regular ☐Shallow ☐Labored	Rate: 88 ☐Regular ☒Irregular	144/86	☒Alert ☐Voice ☐Pain ☐Unresp.	☒Normal ☒ / ☐Dilated / ☐Constricted ☐ / ☐Sluggish / ☐No-Reaction ☐	☐Unremarkable ☒Cool ☒Pale ☐Warm ☐Cyanotic ☐Moist ☐Flushed ☐Dry ☐Jaundiced

FIGURE 15-5 One section of a prehospital care report is devoted to patient data.

☑ Moved to ambulance on stretcher/backboard
☐ Moved to ambulance on stair chair
☐ Walked to ambulance
☐ Airway Cleared
☐ Oral/Nasal Airway
☐ Esophageal Obturator Airway/Esophageal Gastric Tube Airway (EOA/EGTA)
☐ Endotracheal Tube (E/T)
☑ Oxygen Administered @ |1|5| L.P.M., Method NON-REBREATHER MASK
☐ Suction Used
☐ Artificial Ventilation Method _____
☐ C.P.R. in progress on arrival by: ☐ Citizen ☐ PD/FD/Other First Responder ☐ Other
☐ C.P.R. Started @ Time ▶ |__|__|__| Time from Arrest Until C.P.R. ▶ |__|__| Minutes

☐ Bleeding/Hemorrhage Controlled (Method Used: _____)
☐ Spinal Immobilization Neck and Back
☐ Limb Immobilized by ☐ Fixation ☐ Traction
☐ (Heat) or (Cold) Applied
☐ Restraints Applied, Type _____
☐ Baby Delivered @ Time _____ In County _____
  ☐ Alive ☐ Stillborn ☐ Male ☐ Female
☐ Transported in Trendelenburg position
☐ Transported in left lateral recumbent position
☑ Transported with head elevated
☐ Other _____

FIGURE 15-6 Most prehospital care reports have check boxes for some data elements.

- Care administered and the effect that the care had on the patient (e.g., improved, no change)
- Changes in condition throughout the call

Check Boxes

Many prehospital care reports have check boxes for many data elements. This can be an efficient way to document parts of the call. There will usually be several choices, and you will choose the appropriate box and check it. In some cases you will write a number or a few words into a short blank (Figure 15-6).

Narrative

The narrative section of a prehospital care report is less structured than the "fill-in-the-blank" and check box sections. It provides space to write information about the patient that cannot fit into fill-in blanks or check-off boxes (Figure 15-7).

Experienced EMT-Bs consider a good prehospital care report as one that "paints a picture" of their patient. The report, as mentioned previously, is read by many people and is a vital part of the patient's record. When hospital personnel or your quality improvement team reads your report, will it tell the patient's story fully and appropriately?

Remember, you were there throughout the call and are familiar with the patient, his chief complaint, and the care you gave. The people who read your report will have no prior knowledge of the call or the patient. It is imperative that you provide complete, accurate, and pertinent information about your patient and present the information in a logical order. The following guidelines will help you prepare narrative portions of your prehospital care reports.

- *Include both objective and pertinent subjective information.* Objective statements are those that are observable, measurable, or verifiable. An objective statement might be "The patient has a swollen, deformed extremity." This is backed up by your visual observation. Or it might be "The patient's blood pressure was 110/80," based on a measurement you took. Or it might be "Patient uses a prescribed inhaler," a verifiable fact provided by the patient.

  Subjective information is information from an individual point of view. It may be subjective information the patient provides, such as a symptom (e.g., "I feel dizzy"). It may also be subjective observations on the part of the EMT-B, such as your general impression of the patient (e.g., "Patient appears to have difficulty breathing") or

NARRATIVE THE PATIENT DEVELOPED A SUDDEN ONSET OF CHEST PAIN WHILE WATCHING TV. THE PAIN IS SUBSTERNAL, CRUSHING, AND RADIATES TO THE LEFT SHOULDER AND ARM. THE PATIENT STATES THAT THIS PAIN IS "EXACTLY THE SAME AS WHEN I HAD A HEART ATTACK 2 YEARS AGO." HE DENIES LOSS OF CONSCIOUSNESS OR DIFFICULTY BREATHING.

FIGURE 15-7 The narrative portion of a prehospital care report provides space to write information that will not fit into check-off boxes or fill-in blanks.

your evaluation of the patient's behavior or emotional state (e.g., "Patient appears agitated and hostile"). Avoid subjective statements that are merely opinions or are beyond your level of training or scope of practice (e.g., "I do not believe that the leg is broken," or "Patient is probably having a heart attack,") or are not relevant (e.g., "Patient's daughter was rude.").

Prehospital care reports are designed to be factual documents. Use objective statements whenever possible and only pertinent subjective statements. If you record something you did not observe yourself, put it in quotation marks (e.g., A bystander stated that "the patient passed out at the wheel before crashing."). Placing such a remark in quotation marks and identifying the source lets readers of the report know where the information came from.

The chief complaint is another piece of information that is usually given in quotes. If a patient is conscious and oriented, he will usually tell you why he or someone else called you (e.g., "My chest hurts."). If the patient is not conscious or oriented, the person who called EMS may provide the chief complaint (e.g., He said he "felt faint and then passed out."). Since the chief complaint is in someone else's words, it should be placed in quotes.

In documenting your assessment procedures, remember to document important observations about the scene, such as suicide notes, weapons, and any other facts that would be important for patient care but not available to the emergency department personnel.

- *Pertinent Negatives* are examination findings that are negative (things that are *not* true), but are important to note. For example, if a patient has chest pain, you will ask that patient if he has difficulty breathing. If the patient says he does *not* feel difficulty in breathing, that is an important piece of negative information. On your prehospital care report you would note "the patient denies difficulty breathing." Negative information often applies to trauma patients. For example, if the mechanism of injury indicates that there may be an injury to the arm but the patient says he feels no pain, you would note "the patient denies pain in right arm." Documenting pertinent negatives lets other medical professionals know that you thought to examine these areas and that the findings were negative. Not documenting them might leave the reader wondering if this area was explored at all.

Note: The simple fact that there is no pain or complaint of difficulty does not mean that the patient shouldn't be treated. If the patient's medical condition or if the mechanism of injury so indicates, treat the patient despite absence of pain or other symptoms.

- *Avoid radio codes and non-standard abbreviations.* Codes you may use on the radio may not be familiar to hospital personnel, so do not use them in written documentation. Abbreviations, when used properly, make writing efficient and accurate, but non-standard abbreviations will cause confusion and possibly lead to errors in patient care.
- *Write legibly and use correct spelling.* A prehospital care report will have absolutely no value if it cannot be read, so take the time to make your handwriting readable. Unclear writing, misread by others, may cause errors to be made that could harm the patient. Additionally, your QI team will be unable to read the report for review, and it will have no value for research or training. Spelling is also important. If you cannot properly spell a word, look it up (many ambulances and emergency departments have medical dictionaries) or use another word.
- *Use medical terminology correctly.* Be sure that any medical terms you use are used correctly. If you are not sure of the meaning of a term, look it up in a medical dictionary or use everyday language to describe the condition instead. Careless use of medical terms could make your report unclear or cause a misunderstanding that might result in harm to the patient.
- *If it's not written down, you didn't do it.* This is a statement that you will most likely hear from your instructor and experienced EMT-Bs in the field. It explains an important concept of EMS documentation. Make sure that you document all your interventions thoroughly. If you did not document them, it will appear as if they were never performed when the call is later reviewed.

The most important function of the prehospital care report is to present an accurate representation of the patient's condition throughout the call, the patient's history and vital signs, treatments performed, and changes or lack of changes in the patient's condition following treatments.

SPECIAL DOCUMENTATION ISSUES

Legal Issues

As mentioned earlier in this chapter, the prehospital care report serves as a legal document. There are several legal issues pertaining to prehospital care reports and other documents you may complete. These include issues of confidentiality, patient refusals, falsification, and error correction.

Confidentiality

The prehospital care report itself and the information it contains are strictly confidential. The information must not be discussed with or distributed to unauthorized persons. State or local regulations will indicate to whom the information may be distributed. Obviously, the receiving hospital must receive patient care information so they can treat the patient properly. Most reports have a copy that will be left at the hospital. Confidentiality has been discussed in Chapter 3, Medical/Legal and Ethical Issues.

Patient Refusals

In Chapter 3, the issue of liability when patients refuse treatment was discussed. It is one of the foremost causes of liability for EMT-Bs and their EMS systems. Several suggestions were presented in Chapter 3 on what to do when a patient refuses care or transportation.

All actions you have taken to persuade the patient to go to the hospital must be documented. Additionally, you will have to make notes on the patient's competency to make an informed, rational decision on his medical needs. If the patient was not capable of making this determination for any reason—including age, intoxication (alcohol and/or drugs), mental competency, or as a result of the patient's medical condition—actions you took to protect the patient must also be documented. The patient must be informed of the potential results of not going to the hospital or of refusing your care.

The fact that a patient does not wish to go to the hospital does not mean that you should not do an assessment. If the patient greets you with a statement such as "I don't know why my daughter called. I'm not going anywhere!" you may still be able to persuade the patient to get "checked out." Perform as much of a physical exam as possible, including vital signs. Document all of your findings and emergency care given on the prehospital care report. This information will be important to give to medical direction when you talk to them. Be sure to consult medical direction, according to your local protocols, whenever there is a patient refusal.

Most EMS agencies have a refusal-of-care form to use in the event that you have done your best to persuade the patient to accept care or transport and the patient still refuses. This form may be part of either the prehospital care report or a separate document. You should make sure the patient reads and signs this form (Figure 15-8). It is rare that a patient will refuse to sign the form, but if he does, be sure to document this, as well, and note the names of witnesses to the refusal. If possible, when a patient refuses to sign a refusal form, get the witnesses to sign a statement confirming that the patient has refused care or transport.

You should also include information about the patient refusal in the narrative section of the prehospital care report. A sample documentation of a patient refusal that might go into the narrative portion of the prehospital care report is shown in Figure 15-9.

You will note that the narrative shown in Figure 15-9 contains many points of information, including pertinent negatives. The report states that the patient "denies" chest pain or difficulty in breathing. Statements from the patient's daughter are noted as to the source: "according to her daughter. . ." "The daughter denies seeing any seizure activity."

Before you leave the patient who has refused care or transport, be sure to make alternative care suggestions, such as encouraging him to seek care from a doctor. Try to be sure that a responsible family member or friend remains with the patient. Make sure that person also understands that the patient should seek care. Never convey the impression that you are annoyed about being called to the scene "for nothing." Make certain the patient understands that if his condition worsens or if he changes his mind, he can call EMS and you or another EMT-B team will gladly come back.

REFUSAL INFORMATION SHEET

PLEASE READ AND KEEP THIS FORM!

This form has been given to you because you have refused treatment and/or transport by Emergency Medical Services (EMS). Your health and safety are our primary concern, so even though you have decided not to accept our advice, please remember the following:

1)   The evaluation and/or treatment provided to you by the EMS providers is not a substitute for medical evaluation and treatment by a doctor. We advise you to get medical evaluation and treatment.

2)   Your condition may not seem as bad to you as it actually is. Without treatment, your condition or problem could become worse. If you are planning to get medical treatment, a decision to refuse treatment or transport by EMS may result in a delay which could make your condition or problem worse.

3)   Medical evaluation and/or treatment may be obtained by calling your doctor, if you have one, or by going to any hospital Emergency Department in this area, all of which are staffed 24 hours a day by Emergency Physicians. You may be seen at these Emergency Departments without an appointment.

4)   If you change your mind or your condition becomes worse and you decide to accept treatment and transport by Emergency Medical Services, please do not hesitate to call us back. We will do our best to help you.

5)   DON'T WAIT! When medical treatment is needed, it is usually better to get it right away.

I have received a copy of this information sheet.

PATIENT SIGNATURE: _____ DATE: _____

WITNESS SIGNATURE: _____ DATE: _____

AGENCY INCIDENT #: _____ AGENCY CODE: _____

NAME OF PERSON FILLING OUT FORM: _____

G 11A

FIGURE 15-8 A refusal information sheet from Spokane County Emergency Medical Services, Washington State.

> The 49 year old female patient, according to her daughter, "passed out" suddenly. She was in that condition for about 3–5 minutes. The daughter stated that the patient "came to" gradually. Upon our arrival she was fully conscious and oriented. The daughter denies observing any seizure activity. She states that the patient passed out in a chair and did not fall or injure herself as a result of the incident. The patient denies any problems such as chest pain or difficulty breathing. She denies allergies. Her last oral intake was about 2 hours ago (sandwich and coffee). The patient denies any past medical history or current medications.
>
> Vital signs noted above show no abnormalities between two sets taken at a 15 minute interval. The patient refuses transportation to the hospital and has signed the refusal form attached to this report. Her daughter is present with her at her residence and witnessed the refusal. The patient appears competent and oriented. She was advised to call back at any time should she need our assistance or transportation to the hospital of her choice. She was also advised that her failure to go to the hospital may result in a return or worsening of the previous symptoms which, depending on the underlying cause, could result in a serious medical problem or even death.
>
> The patient's daughter will stay with her for several hours and then provide follow-up calls throughout the evening to make sure the patient is all right. The patient was encouraged to contact her family physician for follow-up care as soon as possible. Since the patient did not have one, a sticker listing our phone number was placed on her phone. We contacted medical direction about the situation and spoke to Dr. Baker at Mercy Hospital. She had no further suggestions.

FIGURE 15-9 Document a patient refusal of care thoroughly in the narrative portion of the prehospital care report.

Falsification

Prehospital care reports document the information obtained and the care rendered during the call. False entries or misrepresentations on a report are usually intended to cover up serious flaws in assessment or in care. However, falsification may actually make the problem look worse when it is uncovered.

There are two types of errors that may be committed during a call: omission and commission. Errors of omission are those in which an important part of the assessment or care was left out. An example is oxygen. If a patient is experiencing chest pain, oxygen is an appropriate treatment. If it is overlooked for any reason, never write that oxygen was administered when it wasn't.

Occasionally, because of events during the trip to the hospital, you may have only been able to get one set of vital signs. You realize that the change between two sets of vital signs is more important than an individual set, and you may be tempted to write down an extra set of vital signs when none were taken. Don't do it! Document only the vital signs that were take there is a reason why you have only tak set, document the reason (e.g., "The pa became combative and disoriented en route, p. venting a second set of vital signs.").

Errors of commission are actions performed on the patient that are wrong or improper. An example of this is incorrect administration of medication. There are certain medications that you will be able to administer or assist the patient in administering to himself. This is a great responsibility. If a medication was administered when it was not indicated, it is important to tell medical direction and document the incident on the prehospital care report. Failure to document exactly what happened may have a negative effect on the patient's care. The hospital may think that the patient's condition is due to some other cause. In other situations, the hospital may re-administer the medication, not realizing that it had already been given.

Document the situation surrounding any error of omission or commission and explain exactly what happened. Document what was done to correct the situation, including advising your medical direction and verbally notifying hospital personnel.

Falsification or misrepresentation on a prehospital care report leads to poor patient care because the facts were not documented, and hospital personnel may be misled about the patient's condition and the care he has received. *Falsification or misrepresentation may also lead to the suspension or revocation of your certification or license as an EMT-B.*

You will avoid falsifications if you follow this rule: *Write everything important that did happen and nothing that didn't.*

Correction of Errors

Prehospital care reports are not always written in ideal circumstances. You may even find yourself being dispatched to another call before you finish writing up your last one. In situations such as this you may inadvertently write incorrect information on the report.

Any time there is incorrect information on the report, it must be corrected. If the report is still intact (all copies attached and not yet distributed), draw a single horizontal line through the error, initial it, then write the correct information beside it (Figure 15-10). Do not completely cross out the error or obliterate it. This may be looked on by others as an attempt to cover a mistake in patient care.

If the error is discovered at a later date, after the report has been submitted, draw a single line through the error, mark the area with your initials and the date, and add the correct information to the end of the report or on a separate note. This should be done in a different color ink when possible so the change will be observed. Copies of the report may have already been distributed to other agencies, your quality improvement committee, insurance companies,

or attorneys, and a corrected copy may need to be sent. Make sure that you place the date on the changes so the most recent copy is identifiable. If information has been omitted and you wish to add it, be sure also to date this information and place your initials by the added information.

Special Situations

Multiple Casualty Incidents

An incident in which there are many patients or injuries—such as a multiple-vehicle collision, a major fire, or a plane crash—causes many logistical problems for an EMS system. Documentation of information for each individual patient may be difficult. A patient in a multiple casualty incident (MCI) will probably be moved from one treatment area to another at the scene and then receive transport to a hospital. Possibly patients will be transported to several different hospitals. It is very important to keep the information with the patient as he moves through the system. This is often done through the use of a triage tag (Figure 15-11). This tag is affixed to the patient and used to record chief complaint and injuries, vital signs, and treatments given. At a point later in the emergency, the tag will be used to complete a traditional patient care report.

When completing a prehospital care report for a patient involved in a multiple casualty incident, it will not be possible to provide the detail that you would normally provide for a single-patient call. This is an understandable consequence of the MCI. Your region or agency will have requirements for what information must be completed on the report during an MCI.

Special Situation Reports

Many states use a supplemental form for advanced-life-support calls or additional documentation for calls that were complex or involved (Figure 15-12).

Your activities as an EMT-B may also take you to some unusual situations that will require

COMMENTS PATIENT COMPLAINS OF PAIN IN HIS ~~RIGHT~~ DL LEFT SHOULDER THAT RADIATES TO THE LEFT ARM.

FIGURE 15-10 Cross out an error with a single line and initial the change.

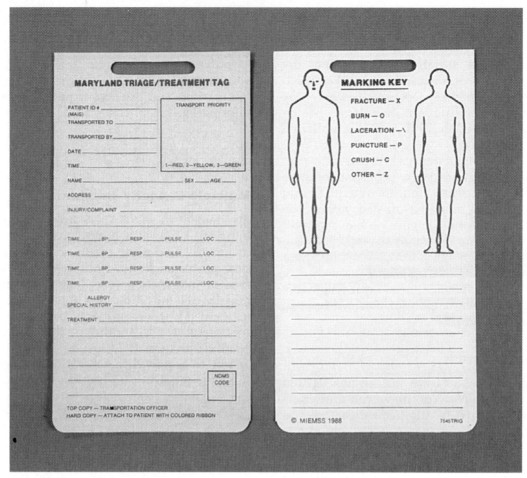

FIGURE 15-11 During a multiple casualty incident, triage tags are used to document information for each patient.

documentation on some form other than a prehospital care report. Such forms are usually specific to a local agency rather than mandated statewide (Figure 15-13). Some examples of situations that might require this kind of special report include

- Exposure to infectious disease
- Injury to yourself or another EMT-B
- Hazardous or unsafe scenes to which other crews should be alerted
- Referrals to social service agencies for elderly or other patients in need of home care.

- Mandatory reports for child or elderly abuse.

This list is not all-inclusive. If there is any situation that requires extra documentation, the special report form may be the place to note it. It is important to remain accurate and objective when filling out this type of report, especially in an unusual or emotional situation. Follow local guidelines for the documentation of confidential information in these reports and for distribution of copies to appropriate agencies or persons.

CONTINUATION FORM
for the
Prehospital Care Report

Press Down Firmly. You're Making 4 Copies.

| M | D | Y | | | | | | |

DATE RUN NO

AGENCY CODE VEH. ID

Name | Agency Name | Enter PCR ID# (Top Center of PCR)

ADDITIONAL HISTORY & PHYSICAL EXAM FINDINGS

Weight in Kilograms

R BREATH SOUNDS L	NECK VEINS	EDEMA	ABDOMEN
☐ Normal ☐	☐ Normal	☐ Pedal	☐ Normal
☐ Decreased ☐	☐ Distended	☐ Sacral	☐ Tender
☐ Absent ☐	**TRACHEAL SHIFT**	☐ Ascites	☐ Rigid
☐ Rales ☐	R L	☐ Other	☐ Distended
☐ Rhonchi ☐	☐ ☐		☐ Other
☐ Wheezes ☐			

SERIAL VITAL SIGNS, EKG, RHYTHMS, MEDICATIONS AND TREATMENT

TIME	RESP.	PULSE	B.P.	LEVEL OF CONSCIOUSNESS	EKG RHYTHMS	DEFIBRILLATION CARDIOVERSION	MEDICATIONS			DOSE	ROUTE
	Rate: ☐ Regular ☐ Shallow ☐ Labored	Rate: ☐ Regular ☐ Irregular		☐ Alert ☐ Voice ☐ Pain ☐ Unresp.	☐ NSR ☐ Brady. ☐ Asystole ☐ IVR ☐ V. Fib. ☐ V. Tach. ☐ PVC ☐ SVT ☐ Other		☐ Epinephrine ☐ Atropine ☐ Dextrose ☐ Lidocaine ☐ Lasix	☐ Dopamine ☐ Sodium Bicarb. ☐ Isoproterenol ☐ Other ___	☐ Naloxone ☐ Bretylium ☐ Nitroglyc.		☐ IV ☐ ET ☐ IM ☐ SL ☐ SQ ☐ PO ☐ Nebulizer
	Rate: ☐ Regular ☐ Shallow ☐ Labored	Rate: ☐ Regular ☐ Irregular		☐ Alert ☐ Voice ☐ Pain ☐ Unresp.	☐ NSR ☐ Brady. ☐ Asystole ☐ IVR ☐ V. Fib. ☐ V. Tach. ☐ PVC ☐ SVT ☐ Other		☐ Epinephrine ☐ Atropine ☐ Dextrose ☐ Lidocaine ☐ Lasix	☐ Dopamine ☐ Sodium Bicarb. ☐ Isoproterenol ☐ Other ___	☐ Naloxone ☐ Bretylium ☐ Nitroglyc.		☐ IV ☐ ET ☐ IM ☐ SL ☐ SQ ☐ PO ☐ Nebulizer
	Rate: ☐ Regular ☐ Shallow ☐ Labored	Rate: ☐ Regular ☐ Irregular		☐ Alert ☐ Voice ☐ Pain ☐ Unresp.	☐ NSR ☐ Brady. ☐ Asystole ☐ IVR ☐ V. Fib. ☐ V. Tach. ☐ PVC ☐ SVT ☐ Other		☐ Epinephrine ☐ Atropine ☐ Dextrose ☐ Lidocaine ☐ Lasix	☐ Dopamine ☐ Sodium Bicarb. ☐ Isoproterenol ☐ Other ___	☐ Naloxone ☐ Bretylium ☐ Nitroglyc.		☐ IV ☐ ET ☐ IM ☐ SL ☐ SQ ☐ PO ☐ Nebulizer
	Rate: ☐ Regular ☐ Shallow ☐ Labored	Rate: ☐ Regular ☐ Irregular		☐ Alert ☐ Voice ☐ Pain ☐ Unresp.	☐ NSR ☐ Brady. ☐ Asystole ☐ IVR ☐ V. Fib. ☐ V. Tach. ☐ PVC ☐ SVT ☐ Other		☐ Epinephrine ☐ Atropine ☐ Dextrose ☐ Lidocaine ☐ Lasix	☐ Dopamine ☐ Sodium Bicarb. ☐ Isoproterenol ☐ Other ___	☐ Naloxone ☐ Bretylium ☐ Nitroglyc.		☐ IV ☐ ET ☐ IM ☐ SL ☐ SQ ☐ PO ☐ Nebulizer
	Rate: ☐ Regular ☐ Shallow ☐ Labored	Rate: ☐ Regular ☐ Irregular		☐ Alert ☐ Voice ☐ Pain ☐ Unresp	☐ NSR ☐ Brady. ☐ Asystole ☐ IVR ☐ V. Fib. ☐ V. Tach. ☐ PVC ☐ SVT ☐ Other		☐ Epinephrine ☐ Atropine ☐ Dextrose ☐ Lidocaine ☐ Lasix	☐ Dopamine ☐ Sodium Bicarb. ☐ Isoproterenol ☐ Other ___	☐ Naloxone ☐ Bretylium ☐ Nitroglyc.		☐ IV ☐ ET ☐ IM ☐ SL ☐ SQ ☐ PO ☐ Nebulizer
	Rate: ☐ Regular ☐ Shallow ☐ Labored	Rate: ☐ Regular ☐ Irregular		☐ Alert ☐ Voice ☐ Pain ☐ Unresp	☐ NSR ☐ Brady. ☐ Asystole ☐ IVR ☐ V. Fib. ☐ V. Tach. ☐ PVC ☐ SVT ☐ Other		☐ Epinephrine ☐ Atropine ☐ Dextrose ☐ Lidocaine ☐ Lasix	☐ Dopamine ☐ Sodium Bicarb. ☐ Isoproterenol ☐ Other ___	☐ Naloxone ☐ Bretylium ☐ Nitroglyc.		☐ IV ☐ ET ☐ IM ☐ SL ☐ SQ ☐ PO ☐ Nebulizer
	Rate: ☐ Regular ☐ Shallow ☐ Labored	Rate: ☐ Regular ☐ Irregular		☐ Alert ☐ Voice ☐ Pain ☐ Unresp	☐ NSR ☐ Brady. ☐ Asystole ☐ IVR ☐ V. Fib. ☐ V. Tach. ☐ PVC ☐ SVT ☐ Other		☐ Epinephrine ☐ Atropine ☐ Dextrose ☐ Lidocaine ☐ Lasix	☐ Dopamine ☐ Sodium Bicarb. ☐ Isoproterenol ☐ Other ___	☐ Naloxone ☐ Bretylium ☐ Nitroglyc.		☐ IV ☐ ET ☐ IM ☐ SL ☐ SQ ☐ PO ☐ Nebulizer

COMMENTS:

MEDICAL FACILITY CONTACTED

CREW

ADDITIONAL NAME — CREW	ADDITIONAL NAME — CREW	ADDITIONAL NAME — CREW	ADDITIONAL NAME — CREW
☐ EMS-FR ☐ EMT ☐ AEMT #	☐ EMS-FR ☐ EMT ☐ AEMT #	☐ EMS-FR ☐ EMT ☐ AEMT #	☐ EMS-FR ☐ EMT ☐ AEMT #

EMS 100A (11/86) provided by NYS-EMS PROGRAM

AGENCY COPY/**WHITE**   HOSPITAL PATIENT RECORD COPY/**PINK**   RESEARCH COPY/**BLUE**   EXTRA SERVICE COPY/**GREEN**

PAGE _____ OF _____

FIGURE 15-12 A supplemental form from New York State.

Special Incident Report

Town of Colonie
Department of Emergency Medical Services

Date of Incident: _____ Time: _____ REMO #: _____

Town Run #: _____ Reported by: _____ Zone: _____

Type of Incident:
☐ MCI ☐ Rescue ☐ Personnel Matter ☐ Injury ☐ Accident with an EMS vehicle
☐ Infectious Disease Exposure ☐ Scene Conflict ☐ Other _____

Total # of Patients: ☐ #P-1: _____ ☐ #P-2: _____ ☐ #P-3: _____ ☐ #P-0: _____
Elapsed Scene Time: *(First unit arrival to last unit to hospital)* _____
Total Time of Incident: _____

Describe the Incident Below:
Attach any additional documentation such as news clippings and the pre-hospital care report.
Attach additional sheets if necessary.

_____
_____
_____
_____
_____
_____
_____
_____
_____
_____
_____
_____
_____
_____
_____
_____
_____
_____
_____

Signature: _____ Date: _____

Office Use Only
This incident relates to: ☐ Day Operation: TOT ☐ Night Operations: TOT: ☐ Administration: TOT:
_____ _____ _____

Disposition: _____
_____
_____ Date: _____

Notifications/Copies:
☐ Director ☐ Deputy Director ☐ Supervisors
☐ Deputy Supervisors ☐ Senior Medics ☐ Zone Coordinator (s)
☐ Other _____ Zone: ☐ 2 ☐ 3 ☐ 4

FIGURE 15-13 A special incident report from the Town of Colonie, New York.

CHAPTER REVIEW

SUMMARY

Documentation is an important skill. A properly completed prehospital care report provides important patient care and medical information about your patient. This form will become a permanent record in the patient's hospital chart as well as in the files of your agency. It may be used to help determine future treatments or as a legal document in a court proceeding. Your report will also be vital in charting trends, research, and quality improvement. Your report should "paint a picture" of your patient and his condition, accurately describing your contact with the patient throughout the call.

REVIEW QUESTIONS

1. Explain the term "minimum data set" and why it is important.
2. Explain what is meant by "objective" and "subjective" information in the narrative portion of the prehospital care report. Explain what is meant by "a pertinent negative."
3. Explain how spelling and the use of codes, abbreviations, and medical terms relate to writing a clear and accurate narrative report.
4. List some important steps to take and information to include when documenting a patient refusal.
5. Describe some possible consequences of falsifying information on a prehospital care report.
6. Describe how to properly correct an error in a prehospital care report.

Application

- Write a narrative report for a call you have been on. If you have not yet been on an ambulance, write one that describes an injury or illness that has happened to you or a family member. If a prehospital care report form is available, complete the whole form, including the check-off or fill-in boxes as well as the narrative portion.

Module 4

Medical Emergencies

IN THIS MODULE

MODULE OVERVIEW

Medical emergencies are often caused by a disease or malfunction within the body—in contrast to traumatic injuries, which are usually caused by an outside force.

This module contains information on a wide variety of medical emergencies that you will encounter as an EMT-Basic, beginning with a chapter on pharmacology, or the study of drugs and medicines. In the pharmacology chapter, you will learn something about the importance of medicines the patient may already be taking. During the pharmacology chapter as well as later chapters in this module, you will also learn how you may administer or assist a patient in taking certain medications—a great responsibility that is usually undertaken after consultation with medical direction.

The next two chapters of the module deal with respiratory and cardiac emergencies, which will account for a large number of the calls that you will respond to. As you might predict, emergencies concerning the ability to breathe and the actions of the heart can be not only life threatening but also extremely frightening to the patient. Even when they are not life threatening, respiratory and cardiac emergencies require careful observation, care, compassion, and concern for the patient's emotional as well as physical needs.

Diabetic emergencies, allergic reactions, and poisoning—also frequently life threatening—are the topics of the next three chapters in the module. The remaining chapters deal with behavioral emergencies (such as psychological emergencies and suicide attempts); with environmental emergencies, such as those caused by heat and cold, near-drowning, diving accidents, insect stings and snakebites; and with obstetrics (childbirth).

In this module, you will not only learn new information, you will also use the knowledge and skills from earlier modules—including knowledge of the human body, taking vital signs, obtaining a patient history, managing the airway, assessment, communication, and documentation—applying them to the care of patients who are experiencing specific kinds of medical emergencies.

General Pharmacology

16

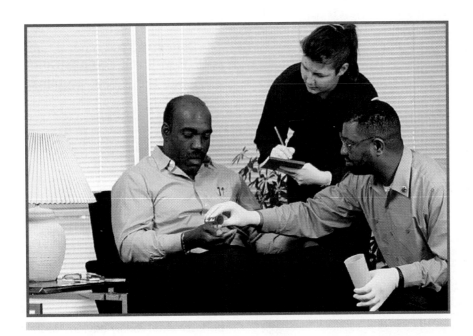

As an EMT-Basic, you will be carrying a few medications on your EMS unit that you will be able to give a patient under specific conditions. There will be another few medications that, when they have been prescribed for a patient, you will be permitted to assist the patient in taking himself. Being able to give the proper medication in an emergency situation can be critical to the well-being of your patient.

Objectives

Knowledge and Attitude *At the end of this chapter, you should be able to meet the following objectives.*

1. Identify which medications will be carried on the unit. (pp. 271–272)

2. State the medications carried on the unit by the generic name. (pp. 271–272)

3. Identify the medications which the EMT-Basic may assist the patient with administering. (pp. 272–274)

4. State the medications the EMT-Basic can assist the patient with by the generic name. (pp. 272–273)

5. Discuss the forms in which the medications may be found. (p. 274)

6. Explain the rationale for the administration of medications. (p. 274)

Skills

1. Demonstrate general steps for assisting patient with self-administration of medications.

2. Read the labels and inspect each type of medication.

On the Scene

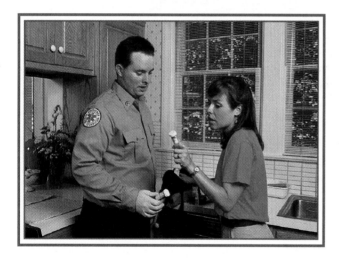

On a bright fall morning, Tracy Morris drops by her mother's apartment, finds her unconscious in bed, and dials 911. You pull on gloves as you arrive at the scene, ring the doorbell, and introduce yourself to Tracy when she answers the door. She leads you to a bedroom, nervously saying, "Mom's in here. I can't wake her up." Her mother's name, Tracy tells you, is Anita Foster.

Your *scene size-up* has revealed a safe scene and no apparent mechanism of injury. During your *initial assessment,* you find that Mrs. Foster is unresponsive but breathing and has a pulse. You work to protect her airway and give her oxygen by nonrebreather mask because of her depressed mental status. She is a high priority for quick transport to the hospital.

You begin your *focused history and physical exam* by gathering as much of a SAMPLE history as you can from Tracy Morris. She tells you that she found her mother unconscious in bed about 15 minutes ago but doesn't know how long she had been that way. Mrs. Foster has no allergies that her daughter knows of. So you have asked the S and A questions (about signs and symptoms and allergies) and have come to the *M* in *SAMPLE:* Medications.

"What medicines has your mother been taking?" you ask. "I don't know, but I'll get her purse," Tracy replies. She produces several containers of prescription medicines. You write down the information from the labels and say that you want to bring the medicines along to the hospital. You complete your on-scene assessment and load Mrs. Foster into the ambulance. En route, you include the information about the medicines in your *radio report* and *documentation* and perform *ongoing assessment* every five minutes until you arrive at the hospital. When you transfer Mrs. Foster to the emergency department staff, you also hand over the medicine containers.

In Mrs. Foster's case, the information provided by the medicine containers is critical. Tracy knew that her mother had been feeling "upset" lately, but she did not know that Mrs. Foster had been taking any medications. The medicines from her purse are tranquilizers on which, it turns out, she has accidentally overdosed. The M question in the SAMPLE history prompted Tracy to produce the tranquilizers, a clue that allows the hospital staff to treat Mrs. Foster quickly and effectively.

T he study of drugs—their sources, characteristics, and effects—is called **pharmacology.** You did not, however, ask Mrs. Foster's daughter, "Is your mother on drugs?" That is because the general public often associates the word *drugs* with illegal or abused substances. Among EMS personnel the terms *medications* and *drugs* are usually used interchangeably, but with the public the term *medications* or *medicines* is used.

In this chapter we will discuss the medications carried by EMT-Basics on the ambulance, as well as the medications the EMT-B may assist the patient in taking with approval from medical direction. You will learn the forms of medications as well as the names for common types of medications your patients may be taking and why they are used.

MEDICATIONS EMT-BASICS CAN ADMINISTER

There are six medications that you will be trained to administer in the field. They are *activated charcoal, oral glucose, oxygen, prescribed inhalers, nitroglycerin,* and *epinephrine.* The information below is a brief introduction to each of them.

Medications Carried on the Ambulance

As an EMT-B you will carry activated charcoal, oral glucose, and oxygen on the ambulance. Under specific circumstances that will be fully described in the chapters named below, you will be able to administer these medications to patients.

Activated Charcoal

Activated charcoal is a powder prepared from charred wood, usually pre-mixed with water for use in the field (Figure 16-1). It is used to treat a poisoning or overdose where a substance was swallowed and is in the patient's digestive tract. Activated charcoal will absorb some poisons and help prevent them from being absorbed by the body. The procedure for administering activated charcoal will be found in Chapter 21, Poisoning and Overdose Emergencies.

Oral Glucose

Glucose is a kind of sugar. **Oral glucose** is a form of glucose that can be taken by mouth as a

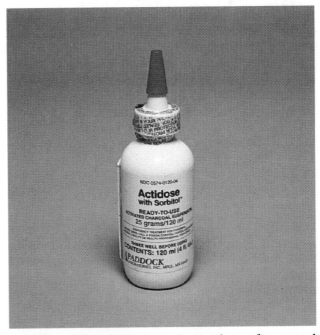

FIGURE 16-1 Activated charcoal is often used in poisoning cases.

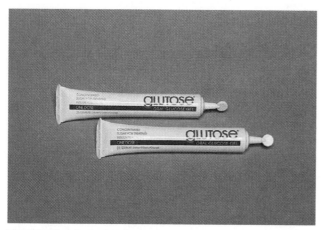

FIGURE 16-2 Oral glucose may help a diabetic.

treatment for an awake patient with an altered mental status and a history of diabetes. The brain is very sensitive to low levels of sugar, which may be caused by poorly managed diabetes, and this can be a cause of the altered mental status. Oral glucose usually comes as a tube of gel (Figure 16-2) that you can apply to a tongue depressor and place between the patient's cheek and gum. This area has many blood vessels, and the glucose is easily absorbed into the bloodstream, which carries it to the brain. This may begin to reverse the patient's potentially life-threatening condition. The procedure for administering oral glucose will be found in Chapter 19, Diabetic Emergencies and Altered Mental Status.

Oxygen

Oxygen is a gas commonly found in the atmosphere. Pure oxygen is used as a drug to treat any patient whose medical or traumatic condition causes him to be hypoxic, or low in oxygen (Figure 16-3). Throughout this text you have learned and will learn many situations in which a patient should be given oxygen. The specific methods of administering oxygen and various devices that can be used to do this are found in Chapter 7, Airway Management.

Prescribed Medications

The three medications described below—prescribed inhalers, nitroglycerin, and epinephrine—are drugs that, as an EMT-B, you may assist the patient in taking if they have been prescribed for the patient by a physician. The circumstances in which you might assist with each of these medications will be described in the chapters named.

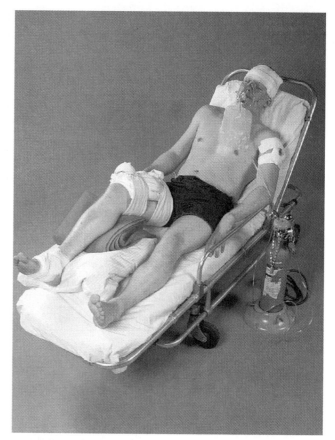

FIGURE 16-3 Oxygen is a powerful drug.

Prescribed Inhalers

There are various medications that patients may carry to help them through a period of difficulty breathing. Most often patients with diseases like asthma, emphysema, or chronic bronchitis carry a "bronchodilator," a medication designed to enlarge constricted bronchial tubes, making breathing easier. Many of these medications can be carried in an **inhaler,** which contains an aerosol form of a medication in a spray device with a mouth-piece so the patient can spray the medication directly into his airway (Figure 16-4).

You will need to have permission from medical direction to help a patient self-administer a prescribed inhaler. Be sure to determine that the inhaler is actually the patient's and not that of a family member or bystander. You may need to seek permission from your medical control physician by phone or radio, or there may be a standing medical order that permits you to assist a patient with this kind of medication. *Always comply with the protocols of your EMS system.* More detail on the use of a prescribed inhaler will be found in Chapter 17, Respiratory Emergencies.

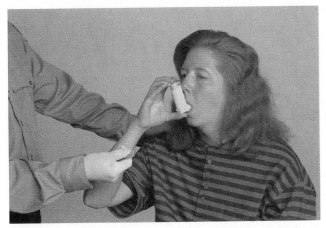

FIGURE 16-4 A prescribed inhaler may help a patient with respiratory problems.

Nitroglycerin

Many patients with problems such as recurrent chest pain, or who have had a heart attack, carry **nitroglycerin** pills or spray. Nitroglycerin (Figure 16-5) is a drug that helps to dilate the coronary vessels that supply the heart muscle with blood. It is often called just "nitro." This drug is taken by the patient when he begins to have chest pain he believes to be cardiac in origin. It is not uncommon for EMT-Bs to treat patients who have already taken a nitroglycerin pill or who are carrying a bottle of nitroglycerin and have not thought to try one of their pills. (Many patients are instructed by their physician to take up to three nitroglycerin pills for their chest pain and, if the chest pain persists, to call EMS.) You will need to have permission from medical direction to help the patient self-administer his nitroglycerin. Be sure to determine that the nitroglycerin is actually the patient's and not

that of a family member or bystander. You may need to seek permission from your medical control physician by phone or radio, or there may be a standing medical order that permits you to assist a patient with nitroglycerin administration. *Always comply with the protocols of your EMS system.* More detail on the administration of nitroglycerin will be found in Chapter 18, Cardiac Emergencies.

Epinephrine Auto-Injectors

When a patient is highly allergic to something like shell fish, penicillin, a bee sting, or a snake bite he may have a very severe reaction. This reaction may cause life-threatening changes in the airway and circulation. The reaction can be reversed by using a medication called **epinephrine.** Epinephrine is a medication that will help to constrict the blood vessels and relax passageways of the airway. Because severe allergic reactions may reach a life-threatening stage in a very short time, epinephrine must be administered quickly. Many patients who are prone to severe allergic reactions carry an epinephrine auto-injector (Figure 16-6). This is a syringe with a spring-loaded needle that will release and inject epinephrine into the muscle when the auto-injector is pushed against the thigh. If you need to assist a patient with the use of their epinephrine auto-injector, be sure to determine that the auto-injector is actually the patient's and not that of a family member or bystander. You may need to seek permission from your medical direction physician by phone or radio, or there may be a standing medical order that permits you to assist a patient with an epinephrine auto-injector. *Always comply with the protocols of your*

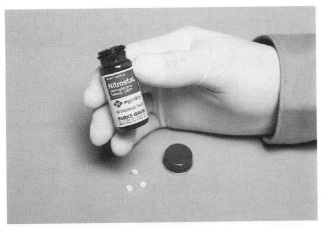

FIGURE 16-5 Nitroglycerin is often prescribed for chest pain.

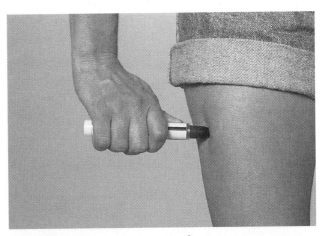

FIGURE 16-6 The Epi-Pen® is an epinephrine auto-injector.

EMS system. More detail on the use of the epinephrine auto-injector will be found in Chapter 20, Allergies.

GENERAL INFORMATION ABOUT MEDICATIONS

Drug Names

Every drug or medication is listed in the *U.S. Pharmacopoeia* (USP), which is a comprehensive government publication. Each drug is listed by its generic name (a general name that is not the brand name of any manufacturer), but, in fact, each drug actually has at least three names: the chemical name, the generic name, and one or more trade (brand) names given the drug by various manufacturers. For example, *epinephrine* is a generic drug name. Its chemical name is B-(e,4 dihydroxyphenyl)-a-methylaminoethanol. (Chemical names are technical formulas used only by scientists or manufacturers.) Epi-Pen® is the trade name of an epinephrine auto-injector.

What You Need To Know When Giving a Medication

Every drug has **indications,** or specific signs or circumstances under which it is appropriate to administer the drug to a patient. For example, nitroglycerin is indicated when a patient has crushing chest pain. Each drug also has **contraindications**, or specific signs or circumstances under which it is *not* appropriate, and may be harmful, to administer the drug to the patient. For example, nitroglycerin is contraindicated (should not be given) if the patient has low blood pressure, because nitroglycerin, in dilating the coronary arteries, causes a slight drop in the systolic blood pressure.

A **side effect** is any action of a drug other than the desired actions. Some side effects are predictable, like the drop in blood pressure from nitroglycerin. If you were not aware of the side effect of a drop in blood pressure and gave the drug to a patient who started out with low blood pressure, the results could be devastating. The patient's blood pressure might "bottom out"— definitely not a desirable effect for a cardiac patient.

Medications come in many different forms. A few examples are

- Compressed powders or tablets, such as nitroglycerin pills
- Liquids for injection, such as the epinephrine in an auto-injector
- Gels, such as the paste in a tube of oral glucose
- Suspensions, such as the thick slurry of activated charcoal in water
- Fine powder for inhalation, such as that in a prescribed inhaler
- Gases for inhalation, such as oxygen
- Sub-lingual (under-the-tongue) sprays such as a nitroglycerin spray.
- Liquid that is vaporized, such as a fixed-dose nebulizer.

Before administering a drug to any patient, you must confirm the order and write it down, then check the "four rights" by asking yourself the following questions as you select the medication and confirm that it is not expired.

- Do I have the **right patient?**
- Is this the **right medication?**
- Is this the **right dose?** Generally a dose is given in milligrams.
- And am I giving this medication by the **right route** of administration?

The route by which the drug is administered affects the rate that the medication enters the bloodstream and arrives at its target organ to achieve its desired effect. Methods of administration include

- Oral, or swallowed
- Intramuscular, or injected into a muscle
- Sublingual, or dissolved under the tongue
- Endotracheal, or sprayed directly into a tube inserted into the trachea, by which it reaches and is absorbed by the lungs
- Inhaled, or breathed into the lungs, usually in tiny aerosol particles as from an inhaler or as a gas such as oxygen

After any medication is given to a patient it is important that you reassess the patient to see how the drug has effected him. Obtain another set of vital signs and compare them to the baseline vital signs that you took before administering the medication. The ongoing assessment of the patient should include an evaluation of the changes in the patient's condition after administration of medicine. Be sure to document the response of the patient to each drug intervention. For example, "The patient's respiratory distress decreased after five minutes of high concentration oxygen by nonrebreather mask."

Topics included in the FYI—"For Your Information"—section are those that go beyond the chapter objectives. The information in this segment is intended to broaden your understanding of the chapter topic but is not essential to an understanding of your job as an EMT-B.

Medications Patients Often Take

It would be impossible to learn and carry around in your head all the types of medications you might discover your patients are taking. Mrs. Foster in On the Scene at the beginning of this chapter was taking tranquilizers. She might have been taking or misusing other medications that could have contributed to her altered mental status—perhaps insulin for diabetes, or Dilantin to control seizures, or morphine for pain, or Inderol for a heart rhythm disorder. The medications a patient is taking may be a clue to a preexisting medical condition or, if improperly used, a cause of their current problem.

It is a good idea to have a resource from which you can find out additional information about a patient's medications en route to the hospital. Many ambulances carry a *Physician's Desk Reference,* or *PDR,* for this purpose. Most EMT-Bs carry, or have available to them, a pocket guide that contains useful information such as commonly used abbreviations. These pocket guides usually list the most commonly prescribed medications along with the general category of that medication to help you understand what the medication may be used for. *However, remember that your main purpose in finding out what medications the patient is taking is not to make a diagnosis but to report this information to the medical director* and *hospital personnel.*

The following is a list of the six most common categories of medications you will find in the field that are relevant to patient care, with a few examples of medications in each category. There are many other drug categories in addition to those listed here.

- **Analgesics**—drugs prescribed for pain relief, fever control, and reducing inflammation. Examples: Darvon (propoxyphene), nalbuphine, morphine, Nubain (nalbuphine), Tylenol (acetaminophen), Advil (ibuprofen), aspirin, codeine, and methadone.
- **Antiarrhythmics**—drugs prescribed for heart rhythm disorders. Examples: Lanoxin (digoxin), Inderol (propranolol), Calan (verapamil), and Pronestyl (procainamide).
- **Anticonvulsants**—drugs prescribed for prevention and control of seizures. Examples: Dilantin (phenytoin), mephenytoin, Mysoline (primidone), primidone, Solfoton or Luminol (phenobarbital), and Tegretol (carbamazepine).
- **Antihypertensives**—drugs prescribed to reduce high blood pressure by controlling the sympathetic nervous system to relax the arterioles. They also work by increasing the elimination of salt and water throughout the body. Examples: Lasix (furosemide), Aprozide (hydrochlorothiazide), Bumex, Diuril (chlorothiazide), Aldomet (methyldopa), Capoten (captopril), and Procardia (nifediprine).
- **Bronchodilators**—drugs that relax the smooth muscles of the bronchial tubes. These medications provide relief of bronchial asthma and other allergies affecting the respiratory system. Examples: Alupent (metaproterenol), isoetharine, Proventil (albuterol), Slo-bid (theophylline), terbutaline, and Ventolin (albuterol).
- **Antidiabetic** agents—medications prescribed to help maintain the sugar level of the hypoglycemic (low blood surgar) patient and to provide insulin, which allows the body to transfer sugar into the cells. Examples: Novolin (insulin), Regular lletin I, glyburide, Orinase (tolbutamide), Tolinase (tolazamide), Ronase (tolazamide), Glucotrol (glipzide), Diabeta or Micronase (glyburide), Diabinese, and Insta-glucose.

CHAPTER REVIEW

KEY TERMS

You may find it helpful to review the following terms.

activated charcoal a powder, usually pre-mixed with water, that will absorb some poisons and help prevent them from being absorbed by the body.

contraindications (KON-truh-in-duh-KAY-shunz) specific signs or circumstances under which it is not appropriate and may be harmful to administer a drug to a patient.

epinephrine (ep-uh-NEF-rin) a drug that helps to constrict the blood vessels and relax passageways of the airway. It may be used to counter a severe allergic reaction.

indications specific signs or circumstances under which it is appropriate to administer a drug to a patient.

inhaler a spray device with a mouthpiece that contains an aerosol form of a medication that a patient can spray into his airway.

nitroglycerin (NEYE-tro-GLIS-uh-rin) a drug that helps to dilate the coronary vessels that supply the heart muscle with blood.

oral glucose (GLU-kos) a form of glucose (a kind of sugar) given by mouth to treat an awake patient with an altered mental status and a history of diabetes.

oxygen a gas commonly found in the atmosphere. Pure oxygen is used as a drug to treat any patient whose medical or traumatic condition may cause them to be hypoxic, or low in oxygen.

pharmacology (FARM-uh-KOL-uh-je) the study of drugs, their sources, characteristics, and effects.

side effect any action of a drug other than the desired action.

SUMMARY

The following are medications carried on the ambulance that the EMT-B may administer to a patient under specific conditions: activated charcoal, oral glucose, and oxygen. The following medications are those that, if prescribed for the patient, the EMT-B may assist the patient in taking: prescribed inhalers, nitroglycerin, epinephrine in auto-injectors. You may need to have permission from medical direction to administer or assist the patient with a medication. Follow local protocols.

There is a wide variety of medications that a patient may be taking. You will try to find out what medications a patient is taking when you take the SAMPLE history. These drugs may be identified by a variety of generic and trade names. Your main purpose in finding out what medications the patient is taking is to report this information to your medical director or hospital personnel.

REVIEW QUESTIONS

1. Name the drugs that are carried on the ambulance and may be administered by the EMT-B under certain circumstances.
2. Name the drugs that the EMT-B may assist the patient in taking if they have been prescribed for him and with approval by medical direction.
3. Medications may take the form of tablets. Name several other forms that medications may have.
4. Name the four "rights" you must check before administering a medication.
5. Name several routes by which medications may be administered.

Application

- A patient is complaining of chest pain. "Here's some nitroglycerin," says a family member. "Give him that." What do you do?

Respiratory Emergencies

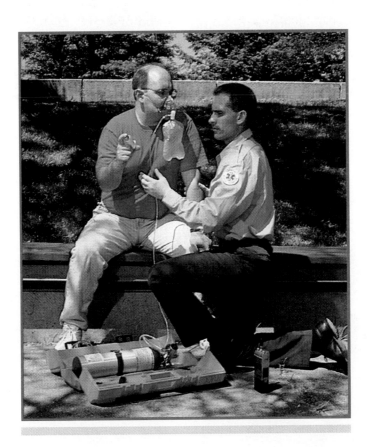

17

Respiratory complaints are one of the most common reasons that people call EMS. Complaints of respiratory problems are potentially serious calls for the EMT-B. In addition to the medical needs of the patient, you must remember that there are few feelings more frightening than not being able to breathe. Patients with respiratory complaints are often found to be anxious and require emotional as well as physical care. Children have a high incidence of respiratory problems. These problems, due to their smaller airway structures, can quickly become serious. A child with severe respiratory distress may rapidly deteriorate into respiratory failure. Your care for all patients in respiratory distress is critical for their physical and emotional well being.

Objectives

Knowledge and Attitude *At the end of this chapter, you should be able to meet the following objectives.*

1. List the structure and function of the respiratory system. (pp. 280–281)

2. State the signs and symptoms of a patient with breathing difficulty. (pp. 284–285)

3. Describe the emergency medical care of the patient with breathing difficulty. (pp. 285–289)

4. Recognize the need for medical direction to assist in the emergency medical care of the patient with breathing difficulty. (pp. 286–288)

5. Describe the emergency medical care of the patient with breathing distress. (pp. 281–284)

6. Establish the relationship between airway management and the patient with breathing difficulty. (pp. 283–284, 285–286)

7. List signs of adequate air exchange. (p. 281)

On the Scene

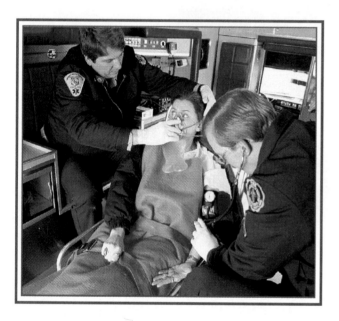

Your ambulance receives a call for a 58-year-old woman with breathing difficulty. As you arrive you perform a *scene size-up,* which includes evaluating the scene for safety, determining the need for BSI precautions, and noting the number of patients. You carefully approach the residence and do not observe any hazards to your safety. You observe a woman sitting upright in a chair just inside the front door. You bring your equipment inside and don protective gloves to begin your assessment.

As you begin your *initial assessment,* you introduce yourself and form a general impression of your patient, Olive McGillicutty, who is a conscious older female patient with apparent difficulty in breathing. She is aware of you and your purpose and responds appropriately to your introduction. As you begin to assess her airway you ask her the date and she replies correctly. Your patient has no unusual airway sounds. Her breathing is slightly labored. You observe adequate and equal chest expansion. She has a strong radial pulse and her skin at the wrist is warm, pink, and dry. You do not feel that this patient requires immediate transport and you begin the next assessment step, the *focused history and physical exam* for a medical patient.

While your partner applies a nonrebreather oxygen mask, you use the OPQRST format to find that Miss McGillicutty has had minor difficulty in breathing for several hours and decided to call EMS because the problem hasn't subsided. She was doing light housework when she first noticed that she was having some trouble breathing. The breathing problem does not change with inspiration or expiration. There

8. State the generic name, medication forms, dose, administration, action, indications, and contraindications for the prescribed inhaler. (p. 288)

9. Distinguish between the emergency medical care of the infant, child, and adult patient with breathing difficulty. (pp. 282, 283–284)

10. Differentiate between upper airway obstruction and lower airway disease in the infant and child patient. (pp. 283–284)

11. Defend EMT-Basic treatment regimens for various respiratory emergencies. (pp. 282–283, 285–286, 287, 288)

12. Explain the rationale for administering an inhaler. (pp. 282–283, 285–289)

Skills

1. Demonstrate the emergency medical care for breathing difficulty.

2. Perform the steps in facilitating the use of an inhaler.

---

is no pain associated with breathing. She tried resting but that did not change her level of distress.

The SAMPLE history reveals that she has had trouble catching her breath with no relief from rest (the symptoms that she explained in response to the OPQRST questions). She is allergic to penicillin and aspirin. She takes a medication for high blood pressure and also has an inhaler, which she shows you and says her doctor prescribed for her. She used her inhaler about one hour ago but her condition did not improve. Her past history includes high blood pressure and a recent diagnosis of emphysema, a long-term lung condition. Her last oral intake was about three hours ago when she had a glass of juice. The events leading to the problem were the light housework she described earlier.

You examine Miss McGillicutty and find that breath sounds are present and equal when you listen with a stethoscope. She denies pain when breathing and upon gentle palpation of her chest and back. You complete your physical exam. Your partner takes and records a set of vital signs, which are pulse 88 strong and regular, respirations 22 regular and slightly labored, blood pressure 140/88, and skin that is warm and dry. You use a stair chair to move her in a sitting position down the steps to the waiting stretcher, then to the ambulance. In the ambulance, you raise the head of the stretcher so that she can maintain a sitting position during the ride to the hospital.

You have brought Miss McGillicutty's inhaler along. She says that she has used her inhaler just once—an hour ago—since her breathing difficulty began. You examine the inhaler and assure that it is an inhaler that was prescribed for her. You radio medical direction en route for a consultation, informing the doctor of the time that the patient last used the inhaler. Medical direction advises you to help Miss McGillicutty use her inhaler, and you do.

You perform **ongoing assessment**—continuing to monitor Miss McGillicutty's breathing, checking her nonrebreather mask and oxygen flow, and recording vital signs every 15 minutes until arrival at the hospital.

Olive McGillicutty was a typical patient with a respiratory problem that was not immediately life threatening. Although she was experiencing some difficulty in breathing, her breathing was adequate; that is, it was enough to support life. You gave her oxygen by nonrebreather mask, you helped her to use her prescribed inhaler after consultation with medical direction, and you transported her to the hospital. Although she told you that her doctor had diagnosed her condition as a lung disease, emphysema, this information was not important to your determination of how to treat her. You would do the same for any patient with difficulty breathing but whose breathing was adequate:

provide oxygen, seek permission to help with a prescribed inhaler if the patient has one, and transport.

As an EMT-B, you will probably encounter some patients whose respiratory problems are more severe than Miss McGillicutty's. They may be having such extreme difficulty moving air in and out of their lungs that their breathing is no longer adequate to support life. These patients will require much more rapid care, probably including artificial respiration.

The difference between adequate and inadequate breathing is one of the most important concepts in this chapter.

RESPIRATORY ANATOMY AND PHYSIOLOGY

You learned about the respiratory system in Chapter 4, The Human Body, and in Chapter 7, Airway Management. In preparation for this chapter, you should review, in those chapters, the following structures of the respiratory system: nose, mouth, oropharynx, nasopharynx, epiglottis, trachea, cricoid cartilage, larynx, bronchi, lungs, alveoli, and diaphragm.

The diaphragm is a muscular structure that divides the chest cavity from the abdominal cavity. During a normal respiratory cycle, the diaphragm and other parts of the body work together to allow the body to inhale (breathe in) and exhale (breathe out) air. The respiratory cycle progresses as follows (Figure 17-1).

- Inspiration—**Inspiration** is an active process that uses the constriction of several muscles to increase the size of the chest cavity. The intercostal (rib) muscles and the diaphragm contract. The diaphragm lowers and the ribs move upward and outward. The expanding size of the chest cavity causes air to flow into the lungs. Another term for *inspiration* is **inhalation.**
- Expiration—**Expiration** is a passive process. It involves the relaxation of the rib muscles and diaphragm. The ribs move downward and inward, while the diaphragm rises. This movement causes the chest cavity to decrease in size and cause air to flow out of the lungs. Another term for *expiration* is **exhalation.**

Review in Chapter 4 how oxygen and carbon dioxide are exchanged through the alveoli of the lungs, and through the capillaries in the lungs and at the cells. The exchange of oxygen and carbon dioxide, both in the lungs and in the

INSPIRATIONS AND EXPIRATIONS

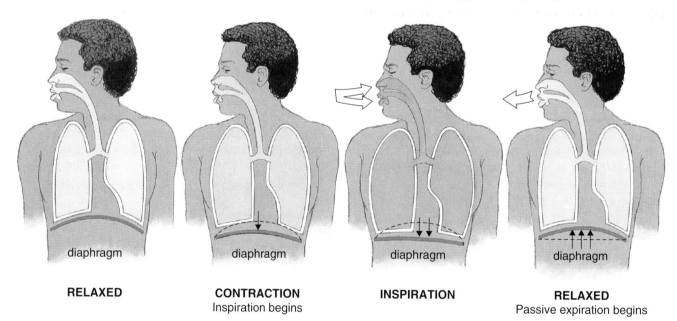

| RELAXED | CONTRACTION
Inspiration begins | INSPIRATION | RELAXED
Passive expiration begins |

FIGURE 17-1 The process of respiration. During inspiration, the diaphragm and rib muscles contract, causing air to flow into the lungs. During expiration, the muscles relax, causing air to flow out of the lungs.

body's cells, is critical to support life. There are many things that can go wrong within the body that will alter this vital exchange. Primarily, the problems are with the respiratory system or the circulatory system. This chapter will discuss the respiratory system, problems with breathing, and their effect on the body. Problems with the circulatory system will be discussed in Chapter 18, Cardiac Emergencies.

Breathing

It is easy to take breathing for granted. Fortunately, we do not consciously have to tell ourselves to inhale and exhale. The brain does that automatically.

As you learned in Chapter 7, Airway Management, breathing may be classified as adequate or inadequate. Simply stated, adequate breathing is breathing that is sufficient to support life. Inadequate breathing is not. Your assessment of the adequacy of a patient's breathing may be vital to his survival.

Adequate Breathing

Adequate breathing falls within certain ranges that are considered "normal." The patient will not appear to be in distress. He will be able to speak full sentences without having to catch his breath. His color, mental status, and orientation will be normal. Normal breathing may be determined by observing for *rate, rhythm,* and *quality.*

- *Rate*—Rates of breathing that are considered normal vary by age:
    - Adult: 12-20 breaths per minute
    - Child: 15-30 breaths per minute
    - Infant: 25-50 breaths per minute
- *Rhythm*—Normal breathing rhythm will usually be regular. The breaths will be taken at regular intervals, and will last for about the same length of time. Remember that talking and other factors may make normal breathing slightly irregular.
- *Quality*—Breath sounds, when auscultated with a stethoscope, will normally be present and equal when the lungs are compared to each other. When observing the chest cavity, both sides should move equally and adequately to indicate a proper air exchange. The depth of the respirations must be adequate.

INADEQUATE BREATHING

Inadequate breathing is breathing that is not sufficient to support life. If left untreated, this condition will surely lead to death. It is one of your most important tasks as an EMT-B to identify and treat patients with inadequate breathing. Assessment and treatment are begun early in the call and must be continued throughout your time with the patient. Patients who are breathing adequately at first may deteriorate into inadequate breathing later on (Table 17-1).

TABLE 17-1 Adequate and Inadequate Breathing

		Adequate Breathing	*Inadequate Breathing*
Rate		Adult: 12-20/min Child: 15-30/min Infant: 25-50/min	Above or below normal rates for the patient's age group
Rhythm		Regular	May be irregular
Quality			
	Breath sounds	Present and equal	Diminished, unequal, or absent
	Chest expansion	Adequate and equal	Inadequate or unequal
	Effort of breathing	Unlabored, normal respiratory effort	Labored; increased respiratory effort; use of accessory muscles (may be pronounced in infants and children and involve nasal flaring, seesaw breathing, grunting, and retractions between the ribs and above the clavicles)

Patient Assessment—Indaequate Breathing

If the patient is not breathing adequately to support life you may see any of the following conditions.

☐ *Rate*—The patient with inadequate breathing will have a breathing rate that is out of the normal ranges. Very slow breaths and very rapid breaths may not allow enough air to enter the lungs, resulting in not enough oxygen being distributed throughout the body.

Agonal respirations (also called dying respirations) are sporadic, irregular breaths that are usually seen just before respiratory arrest. They are shallow and gasping with only a few breaths per minute. This breathing pattern is clearly a sign of inadequate breathing.

☐ *Rhythm*—The rhythm of inadequate breathing may be irregular. However, rhythm is not an absolute indicator of adequate or inadequate breathing. Remember that someone who is talking or is aware that you are observing his respirations may have slight irregularities, even though his breathing is adequate. On the other hand, a patient may have a regular rate, even when his breathing is inadequate.

☐ *Quality*—When breathing is inadequate, breath sounds may be diminished or absent. The depth of respirations (tidal volume) will be inadequate or shallow. Chest expansion may be inadequate or unequal and respiratory effort increased. You may note the use of accessory muscles (muscles other than the diaphragm and the intercostal muscles, such as the muscles of the neck and abdomen) in breathing. Since oxygenation of the body's tissues is reduced, the skin may be pale or cyanotic (blue), and feel cool and clammy to the touch.

In patients who have a diminished level of consciousness or who are totally unresponsive, sounds such as snoring and gurgling also indicate a serious airway problem that requires immediate intervention.

Infants and Children

Respiratory problems can be very serious in infants and children. Since children rarely have heart attacks or other problems of adulthood, respiratory conditions, statistically, are a leading killer of infants and children. With this in mind, you must begin respiratory treatment of infants and children with a thorough and accurate assessment and prompt, proper care.

The structure of infants' and children's airways differs somewhat from that of adults.

- All airway structures are smaller in an infant or child than in an adult, and therefore are more easily obstructed.
- Infants' and children's tongues are proportionately larger and therefore take up more space in the mouth than an adult's tongue.
- The trachea is smaller, softer, and more flexible in infants and children, which may lead to obstruction from swelling or trauma more easily than in adults. The cricoid cartilage is less developed and less rigid.
- Infants and children depend more heavily on the diaphragm for respiration since the chest wall is softer. This is why infants and small children in respiratory distress exhibit "seesaw breathing" in which the movement of the diaphragm causes the chest and abdomen to move in opposite directions.

Signs of Inadequate Breathing in Infants and Children

- Nasal flaring (widening of the nostrils)
- Grunting
- Seesaw breathing
- Retractions (pulling in of the muscles) between the ribs (intercostal), above the clavicles (supraclavicular), and above the sternum (suprasternal).

Patient Care—Inadequate Breathing

There is a wide range of function between adequate respirations and complete stoppage of breathing (respiratory arrest). You must pay careful attention to the patient's breathing throughout the call. *It is not enough to simply make sure the patient is breathing. The patient must be breathing adequately!* If at any time you find that the patient is not breathing adequately, the treatment of this condition is your first patient care priority.

When you determine, by the signs discussed under Patient Assessment, above, that a patient's breathing is inadequate, you will

■ Provide artificial ventilation with supplemental oxygen.

In order of preference, the means of providing artificial ventilation are

1 Pocket face mask with supplemental oxygen
2 Two-person bag-valve mask with supplemental oxygen
3 Flow-restricted, oxygen-powered ventilator
4 One-person bag-valve mask with supplemental oxygen

The means of providing artificial ventilation were discussed in Chapter 7, Airway Management. Make sure that you are properly trained with the device that you are using for ventilation. If supplemental oxygen is not immediately available, begin artificial respirations without supplemental oxygen and attach the oxygen supply to the mask as soon as it is available.

If you are uncertain about whether a patient's breathing is inadequate and requires artificial ventilation, provide artificial ventilation. In the rare circumstance when a patient with inadequate breathing is conscious enough to fight artificial ventilation, transport immediately and consult medical direction.

Adequate and Inadequate Artificial Ventilation

Like breathing, artificial ventilation can be adequate or inadequate. When you are performing artificial ventilation adequately, the chest will rise and fall with each artificial ventilation. The adequate rate for artificial ventilation is 12 breaths per minute for adults, 20 per minute for infants and children.

When you are providing artificial ventilation without chest compression (patient has a pulse), monitor the pulse carefully. With adequate artificial ventilation, the pulse rate should return to normal. Since the pulse in adults will rise from a lack of oxygen, a pulse that remains the same or increases may indicate inadequate artificial ventilation. Naturally, if the pulse disappears this indicates that the patient is in cardiac arrest, and you will need to begin compressions (CPR).

● Infants and Children
Pediatric patients differ from adults in many ways. There are few differences that are more important in emergency care than those

within the respiratory system. When adult patients experience a decrease in oxygen in the bloodstream (hypoxia), their pulse increases.

In infants and children with respiratory difficulties you may observe a slight increase in pulse early, but soon the pulse will drop significantly. *A low (or bradycardic) pulse in infants and small children in the setting of a respiratory emergency usually means trouble!* This is a sharp contrast from adults where it is a good sign when their pulse lowers to a more normal level.

If you observe a pulse below the expected rates for infants and children, evaluate your ventilations or oxygen therapy thoroughly. In ventilations, make sure that you have an open airway and that the chest rises with each breath. In any situation make sure that the oxygen tank has not run out and that the tubing has not kinked or slipped off the delivery device or oxygen cylinder. *Nothing is more important for infants and children than adequate airway care!*

For any patient—adult, child, or infant—if the chest does not rise and fall with each artificial ventilation, or the pulse does not return to normal, increase the force of ventilations. If the chest still does not rise, check that you are maintaining an open airway by the head-tilt, chin-lift maneuver (if there is no suspected spine injury) or by the jaw-thrust maneuver (if spine injury is possible). Insert an oropharyngeal or nasopharyngeal airway as needed to prevent the tongue from blocking the airway. Suction fluids and foreign matter from the airway as necessary, or perform the Heimlich maneuver and finger sweeps as needed to clear large airway obstructions. (Deliver alternating series of back blows and chest thrusts to clear airway obstructions in infants. Do not perform blind finger sweeps—remove only visible objects—in infants and children.) If you are using supplemental oxygen, check that all connections are secure and that the tubing has not kinked.

Review the techniques of airway maintenance and artificial ventilation in Chapter 7, Airway Management, and in Basic Life Support: Airway, Rescue Breathing, and CPR in the back of this book.

● Infants and Children
In infants and children, it is especially important to try to distinguish between an upper airway obstruction and a lower airway disease if there appears to be a blockage of the airway. If the airway is blocked by the tongue,

blood, secretions or debris, you may consider suctioning the airway, performing finger sweeps, or inserting an oropharyngeal or nasopharyngeal adjunct to help maintain an open airway.

However, infants and children are also subject to lower respiratory diseases or infections that may result in swelling of the airway passages. With some of these diseases, it is dangerous to place anything in the patient's mouth or pharynx because this may set off spasms along the airway.

Refrain from placing anything in the patient's mouth and transport as quickly as possible if you see the following signs of a lower respiratory problem:

- Wheezing
- Breathing effort on exhalation
- Rapid breathing without stridor (a harsh, high-pitched sound)

For more about respiratory conditions in infants and children, see Chapter 29, Infants and Children.

BREATHING DIFFICULTY

Breathing difficulty is a frequent chief complaint, representing a patient's feeling of labored, or difficult, breathing. Although there are objective signs associated with breathing difficulty (listed below), the "difficulty" that is reported to you by the patient is a subjective perception of the patient. The amount of distress the patient feels may or may not reflect the actual severity of his condition. His breathing may be more adequate or less adequate than he feels it is. You should not rely entirely on the patient's report to decide how serious the condition really is. You will need to perform an assessment to help you make that determination

It is important to remember that a patient with breathing difficulty may have either adequate or inadequate breathing. You may encounter two patients, at different times, who tell you that they are having difficulty breathing ("I can't catch my breath" or a similar complaint). One patient may be having minor difficulty due to a preexisting respiratory condition but still have adequate breathing. His condition is not life threatening. The other patient, who has offered exactly the same complaint, may be having a problem such as an allergic reaction and severe difficulty breathing. Your examination of this patient may reveal inadequate breathing that requires immediate artificial ventilation.

Difficulty in breathing may have many causes ranging from ongoing medical conditions (for information on some of these respiratory diseases see the FYI section of this chapter), to illnesses such as pneumonia and other infections, to cardiac problems that cause disturbances in the respiratory system.

Patient Assessment—Breathing Difficulty

The following are signs and symptoms of breathing difficulty (Figure 17-2).

Signs

- [ ] Increased pulse rate
- [ ] Decreased pulse rate (especially in infants and children)
- [ ] Changes in the breathing rate (above or below normal levels)
- [ ] Changes in breathing rhythm
- [ ] Pale, cyanotic, or flushed skin
- [ ] Noisy breathing which may be described as
  - Audible wheezing (heard without stethoscope)
  - Gurgling
  - Snoring
  - Crowing
  - Stridor (harsh, high-pitched sound during breathing, usually due to upper airway obstruction)
- [ ] Inability to speak full sentences (or at all) due to breathing difficulty
- [ ] Use of accessory muscles to breathe (retractions)
- [ ] Altered mental status
- [ ] Coughing
- [ ] Flaring nostrils, pursed lips
- [ ] Patient positioning
  - Tripod position (patient leaning forward with hands resting on knees or another surface)
  - Sitting with feet dangling, leaning forward
- [ ] Unusual anatomy (barrel chest)

Symptoms

- [ ] Feeling of shortness of breath or difficult breathing or tightness in the chest
- [ ] Restlessness or anxiety

Patient History

The focused history and physical exam for patients with respiratory emergencies involves

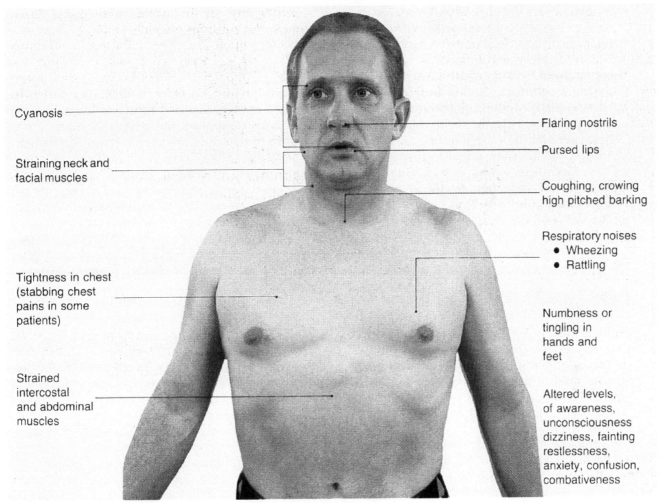

Cyanosis

Straining neck and
facial muscles

Tightness in chest
(stabbing chest
pains in some
patients)

Strained
intercostal
and abdominal
muscles

Flaring nostrils

Pursed lips

Coughing, crowing
high pitched barking

Respiratory noises
• Wheezing
• Rattling

Numbness or
tingling in
hands and
feet

Altered levels,
of awareness,
unconsciousness
dizziness, fainting
restlessness,
anxiety, confusion,
combativeness

FIGURE 17-2 Signs and symptoms of breathing difficulty

an appropriate interview and examination of the chest and respiratory structures.

Use the letters OPQRST to remember which questions to ask about the respiratory difficulty.

☐ Onset—When did it begin?
☐ Provocation—What were you doing when this came on?
☐ Quality—Can you describe the feeling you have?
☐ Radiation—Does the feeling seem to spread to any other part of your body? Do you have pain or discomfort anywhere else in your body?
☐ Severity—On a scale of 1 to 10, how bad is your breathing trouble? (10 is worst, 1 best)
☐ Time—How long have you had this feeling?

Ask if the patient has taken any prescribed medications or done anything else to help relieve his condition. This may affect the treatment provided by you and the treatment provided later at the hospital.

Patient Care—Breathing Difficulty

Emergency Care Steps

When a patient is suffering from breathing difficulty, provide the following care.

☐ *Assessment*—Assess the airway during the initial assessment and then frequently throughout the call. Assist respiration with artificial ventilations and supplemental oxygen whenever the patient has or develops *inadequate* breathing.
☐ *Oxygen*—Oxygen is the main treatment for any patient in respiratory difficulty. If the patient is breathing *adequately*, use a nonrebreather mask at 12 to 15 liters per minute to provide oxygen. Use a nasal cannula only

in cases where the patient will not tolerate a mask. If the patient has *inadequate* breathing, provide supplemental oxygen while performing artificial ventilations.

- *Positioning*—If the patient is experiencing breathing difficulty but is breathing *adequately*, place him in a position of comfort. Most patients with breathing difficulty feel they can breathe better sitting up. In the On the Scene that opened this chapter, Olive McGillicutty was carried out of the house to the stretcher on a stair chair for this reason. She was also placed in a sitting-up position during her ride in the ambulance. This would not be possible if the patient had *inadequate* breathing, since the patient would need to be supine to receive assisted ventilations.
- *Prescribed Inhaler*—If the patient has a prescribed inhaler, as Miss McGillicutty did, you may be able to assist the patient in taking this medication. This would be done after consultation with medical direction, often during transportation to the hospital.

You may hear from your instructor or other EMT-Bs that oxygen must be administered to some patients with caution—or not at all. This is because of a condition sometimes called *hypoxic drive.* (You read about hypoxic drive in Chapter 7 and will find more about this condition under FYI at the end of this chapter.) This occurs in some patients who have lung diseases such as emphysema or chronic bronchitis (which will also be discussed under FYI). For many years it was recommended that oxygen not be given, or be given cautiously, to such patients for fear that oxygen would destroy their "drive to breathe." It is now widely believed that more harm is done by withholding oxygen than could be done by administering oxygen. Even with patients who have these diseases, *never withhold oxygen from a patient in respiratory distress.*

Oxygen is a drug. Like all drugs, it must be administered responsibly and with careful monitoring of the patient. Occasionally, a patient may have an adverse reaction to oxygen. If the patient's respirations decrease or become shallow, or if the patient becomes increasingly sleepy, discontinue oxygen therapy and contact medical direction. If breathing becomes inadequate or stops, provide artificial ventilation. This kind of adverse response to oxygen, however, would rarely have time to develop during the short duration of prehospital care and is almost unheard-of during EMS calls.

The Prescribed Inhaler

You will recall that Olive McGillicutty in On the Scene had a prescribed inhaler. Because of her breathing difficulty, she was a possible candidate to receive this medication. You remembered to inform medical direction that she had used her inhaler one hour earlier. Patients may overuse the inhaler prior to your arrival, so it is important to determine exactly when and how many times the inhaler has been used.

The metered dose inhaler gets its name from the fact that each activation of the inhaler provides a metered, or exactly measured, dose of medication. Most patients simply refer to the device as their "inhaler" or "puffer." The inhaler is prescribed for patients with respiratory problems that cause **bronchoconstriction** (constriction, or blockage, of the bronchi that lead from the trachea to the lungs) or other types of lung obstructions. The inhalers contain a drug that dilates, or enlarges, the air passages, making breathing easier.

When patients use an inhaler, they often are excited or nervous because they are short of breath. Many do not use their inhaler properly. Some people have never had proper instruction in use of their inhaler. Make sure to calm the patient as best you can and coach him to use the inhaler properly, as follows.

- As with any medication, assure that you have the right patient, the right medication, the right dose, and the right route. Check the expiration date. Make sure the inhaler is at room temperature or warmer. Shake the inhaler vigorously several times.
- Make sure that the patient is alert enough to use the inhaler properly.
- Make sure the patient first exhales deeply.
- Have the patient put his lips around the opening and press the inhaler to activate the spray as he inhales deeply.
- After the patient inhales, make sure he holds his breath as long as possible so the medication can be absorbed. This may be difficult with a patient who is anxious, but unless the medication is held in the lungs, it will have minimal or no value.

Your role will involve more coaching than actually administering the medication. The proper sequence for administration of a prescribed

Scan 17-1
Prescribed Inhaler—
Patient Assessment and Management

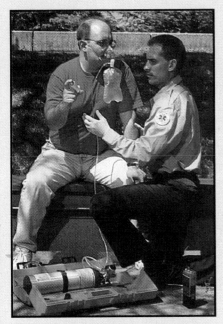

1. The patient has the indications for use of an inhaler: signs and symptoms of breathing difficulty and an inhaler prescribed by a physician.

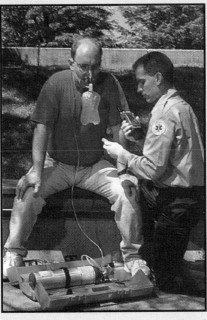

2. The EMT-B contacts medical direction and obtains an order to assist the patient with the prescribed inhaler.

3. The EMT-B assures the four "rights" for administration of a medication:

- Right patient
- Right medication
- Right dose
- Right route

EMT-B checks expiration date, shakes inhaler, makes sure inhaler is room temperature or warmer, makes sure patient is alert.

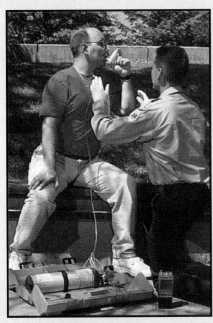

4. The EMT-B coaches the patient in use of the inhaler: Exhale deeply, press inhaler to activate spray, hold breath in so medication can be absorbed.

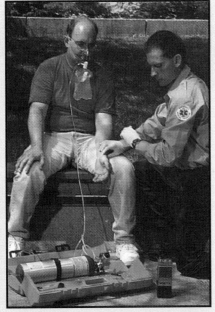

5. After use of inhaler, EMT-B reassesses the patient: takes vital signs, does a focused exam, determines if breathing is adequate.

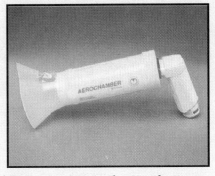

6. A "spacer" device between inhaler (shown inverted) and patient allows more effective use of medication. If the patient has a spacer, it should be attached to the inhaler before use.

Scan 17-2
Prescribed Inhaler

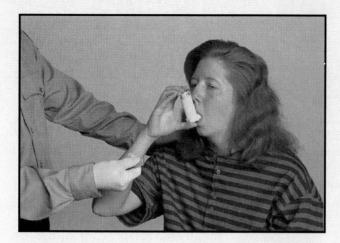

Medication Name
1. Generic: albuterol, isoetharine, metaprotaranol
2. Trade: Proventil, Ventolin, Bronkosol, Bronkometer, Alupent, Metaprel

Indications
Meets all of the following criteria:
1. Patient exhibits signs and symptoms of respiratory emergency.
2. Patient has physician-prescribed hand-held inhaler.
3. Medical direction gives specific authorization to use.

Contraindications
1. Patient is unable to use device (e.g., not alert).
2. Inhaler is not prescribed for patient.
3. No permission has been given by medical direction.
4. Patient has already taken maximum prescribed dose prior to EMT-B's arrival.

Medication Form
Hand-held metered dose inhaler

Dosage
Number of inhalations based on medical direction's order or physician's order

Administration
1. Obtain order from medical direction either on-line or off-line.
2. Assure right patient, right medication, right dose, right route, patient alert enough to use inhaler.
3. Check expiration date of inhaler.
4. Check if patient has already taken any doses.
5. Assure inhaler is at room temperature or warmer.
6. Shake inhaler vigorously several times.
7. Have patient exhale deeply.
8. Have patient put her lips around the opening of the inhaler.
9. Have patient depress the hand-held inhaler as she begins to inhale deeply.
10. Instruct patient to hold her breath for as long as she comfortably can so medication can be absorbed.
11. Put oxygen back on patient.
12. Allow patient to breathe a few times and repeat second dose if so ordered by medical direction.
13. If patient has a spacer device for use with her inhaler (device for attachment between inhaler and patient to allow for more effective use of medication), it should be used.

Actions
Beta agonist bronchodilator dilates bronchioles, reducing airway resistance.

Side Effects
1. Increased pulse rate
2. Tremors
3. Nervousness

Reassessment Strategies
1. Gather vital signs.
2. Perform focused reassessment of chest and respiratory function.
3. Observe for deterioration of patient; if breathing becomes inadequate, provide artificial respirations.

inhaler is shown in Scan 17-1. Inhalers are described in detail in Scan 17-2. Follow local protocols and consult medical direction, if required, before assisting a patient with an inhaler.

FYI

Topics included in the FYI—"For Your Information"—section are those that go beyond the chapter objectives. The information in this segment is intended to broaden your understanding of the chapter topic but is not essential to an understanding of your job as an EMT-B.

Chronic Obstructive Pulmonary Disease (COPD)

Emphysema—as well as chronic bronchitis, black lung, and many undetermined respiratory illnesses that cause the patient problems like those seen in emphysema—are all classified as chronic obstructive pulmonary disease (COPD). (*Chronic* refers to a disease that affects the patient continually and over a long period of time. *Obstructive* refers to the obstruction or blockage of airway passages. *Pulmonary* refers to the lungs.)

Chronic bronchitis can be seen in children and teenagers; however, COPD is mainly a problem of middle-aged or older patients. This may be because these are disorders that tend to develop over a long period of time as reactions of tissues in the respiratory tract to smoking, allergens, chemicals, air pollutants, or repeated infections.

Chronic bronchitis and emphysema are compared in Figure 17-3.

In chronic bronchitis, the bronchiole lining is inflamed. Excess mucus is formed. The cells in the bronchioles that normally clear away accumulations of mucus are not able to do so. The sweeping apparatus on these cells, the cilia, have been damaged or destroyed.

Usually the reason a COPD patient calls the ambulance is that a recent upper respiratory infection has caused an acute worsening of the disease.

In emphysema, the walls of the alveoli break down, greatly reducing the surface area for respiratory exchange. The lungs begin to lose elasticity, and the alveoli and bronchioles secrete excess mucus. These factors combine to

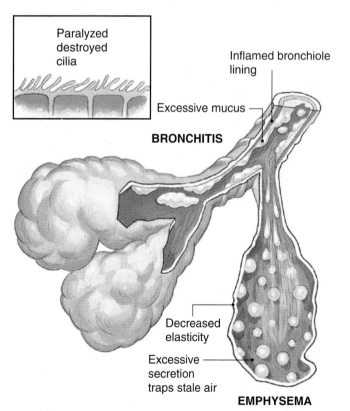

FIGURE 17-3 Chronic bronchitis and emphysema are chronic obstructive pulmonary diseases.

allow stale air to be trapped in the lungs, reducing the effectiveness of normal breathing efforts.

Many COPD patients will exhibit characteristics of both emphysema and chronic bronchitis.

COPD patients may be in hypoxic drive. This means they have developed a tolerance to high carbon dioxide levels and, instead, their bodies determine the need to breathe based on decreased blood levels of oxygen. The higher oxygen levels that result from oxygen administration may, in rare cases, signal the COPD patient to reduce breathing or even develop respiratory arrest.

In most cases, however, the hypoxic drive will not be a problem in the prehospital setting. The patient's need for oxygen will outweigh the risk involved with administration. If the patient has a possible heart attack or stroke, is developing shock, or has respiratory distress, a higher concentration of oxygen will be required in spite of the potential problems. *If oxygen is required by the COPD patient, do not withhold it.*

Constantly monitor the patient. If the patient's breathing becomes inadequate or stops, be prepared to assist respirations through artificial ventilation, and contact medical direction.

Asthma

Seen in young and old patients alike, asthma is an episodic disease (a disease that only affects the patient at irregular intervals). This is far different from chronic bronchitis and emphysema, both of which afflict the patient continually. Asthma also differs from chronic bronchitis and emphysema in that it does not produce a hypoxic drive. Between episodes, the asthmatic patient can lead a normal life.

An asthma attack may be triggered by an allergic reaction to something inhaled, swallowed, or injected into the body. Attacks can be precipitated by insect stings, air pollutants, infection, strenuous exercise, or emotional stress. When an asthma attack occurs, the small bronchioles that lead to the air sacs of the lungs become narrowed because of contractions of the muscles that make up the airway. To complicate matters, there is an overproduction of thick mucus. The combined effects of the contractions and the mucus cause the small passages to practically close down, severely restricting air flow.

The air flow is mainly restricted in one direction. When the patient inhales, the expanding lungs exert an outward pull, increasing the diameter of the airway and allowing air to flow into the lungs. During exhalation, however, the opposite occurs and the stale air becomes trapped in the lungs. This requires the patient to exhale the air forcefully, producing the characteristic wheezing sounds associated with asthma.

The discussion of these diseases and the concept of hypoxic drive is for your additional information only. There is no need to diagnose which respiratory disease or disorder the patient may have in order to provide the assessment and care described earlier in this chapter.

CHAPTER REVIEW

KEY TERMS

You may find it helpful to review the following terms:

bronchoconstriction constriction, or blockage, of the bronchi that lead from the trachea to the lungs.

exhalation (EX-huh-LAY-shun) another term for expiration.

expiration (EK-spuh-RAY-shun) a passive process in which the intercostal (rib) muscles and the diaphragm relax, causing the chest cavity to decrease in size and forcing air from the lungs.

inhalation (IN-huh-LAY-shun) another term for inspiration.

inspiration (IN-spuh-RAY-shun) an active process in which the intercostal (rib) muscles and the diaphragm contract, expanding the size of the chest cavity and causing air to flow into the lungs.

SUMMARY

Respiratory emergencies are common calls that require diligent assessment, care, and emotional support. It is very important to evaluate your patient for adequate breathing throughout the call. If at any time you find breathing inadequate, you must assist ventilations. Providing artificial ventilation to a patient promptly may prevent him from slipping into respiratory arrest—and death!

For a patient who is experiencing difficulty in breathing but whose breathing is adequate, administration of high concentration oxygen by nonrebreather mask, coaching the patient in the use of a prescribed inhaler if the patient has one, placing the patient in a position of comfort, and providing reassurance are the key treatments the EMT-B can provide.

REVIEW QUESTIONS

1. List the normal rates of breathing for adults, children, and infants. List the other signs of adequate breathing.
2. List the signs of inadequate breathing.
3. Explain the treatment you will give, as an EMT-B, when a patient's breathing is inadequate.
4. List the signs and symptoms of breathing difficulty.
5. Explain the treatments you may give, as an EMT-B, for breathing difficulty when breathing is adequate.
6. Explain the steps to follow before, during, and after helping a patient to use a prescribed inhaler.
7. List some differences between adult and infant/child respiratory systems.
8. List some special considerations in the assessment and treatment of infants and children with respiratory problems.

Application

• For each of the following patients, state whether the patient's breathing seems adequate or inadequate—and explain your reasoning.

a. A 45-year-old male patient experiencing severe difficulty in breathing. His respirations are 36/min. and very shallow. He has minimal chest expansion and can barely speak.

b. A 65-year-old female who tells you that she has trouble breathing. Her respirations are 20/minute and slightly labored. Her respirations are regular and there appears to be good chest expansion.

c. A 3-year-old patient who has had a respiratory infection recently. Her parents called because she is having difficulty breathing. You observe retractions of the muscles between the ribs and above the collarbones as well as nasal flaring. The child seems drowsy. Respirations are 40/minute.

Cardiac Emergencies

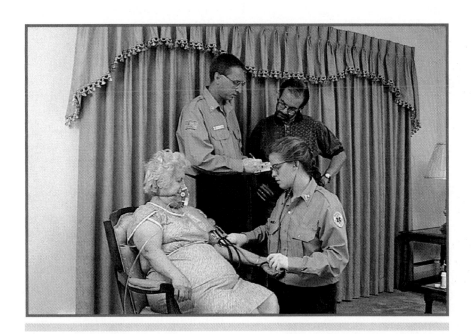

One of the most common types of call you will respond to in your EMS career is a patient with chest pain, the best known symptom of a heart problem. Over 600,000 Americans die each year from cardiovascular disease. Half of these deaths occur outside the hospital, with sudden collapse being the first sign of heart disease in half of those who die. As an EMT-B, you will, with medical direction, be able to assist patients who have chest pain in taking one of their medications and to defibrillate patients in cardiac arrest.

Objectives

Knowledge and Attitude *At the end of this chapter, you should be able to meet the following objectives.*

1. Describe the structure and function of the cardiovascular system. (p. 297)

Cardiac Compromise

2. Describe the emergency medical care of the patient experiencing chest pain or discomfort. (pp. 301–303)

3. Discuss the position of comfort for patients with various cardiac emergencies. (p. 301)

4. Recognize the need for medical direction of protocols to assist in the emergency medical care of the patient with chest pain. (pp. 301, 302)

5. List the indications for the use of nitroglycerin. (p. 304)

6. Explain the rationale for administering nitroglycerin to a patient with chest pain or discomfort. (p. 299)

7. State the contraindications and side effects for the use of nitroglycerin. (p. 304)

Defibrillation

8. List the indications for automated external defibrillation (AED). (pp. 310, 311)

9. List the contraindications for automated external defibrillation. (pp. 310, 311, 318–319)

10. Define the role of EMT-B in the emergency cardiac care system. (p. 308)

11. Explain the impact of age and weight on defibrillation. (p. 311)

12. Establish the relationship between airway management and the patient with cardiovascular compromise. (p. 318)

13. Predict the relationship between the patient experiencing cardiovascular compromise and basic life support. (p. 318)

14. Discuss the fundamentals of early defibrillation. (pp. 307–308)

15. Explain the rationale for early defibrillation. (pp. 307–308)

16. Explain that not all chest pain patients result in cardiac arrest and do not need to be attached to an automated external defibrillator. (pp. 297, 308)

17. Explain the importance of prehospital ACLS intervention if it is available. (pp. 308, 317)

18. Explain the importance of urgent transport to a facility with advanced cardiac life support if it is not available in the prehospital setting. (p. 308)

19. Discuss the various types of automated external defibrillators. (pp. 308–309)

20. Differentiate between the fully automated and the semiautomated defibrillator. (pp. 308, 319–320)

21. Discuss the procedures that must be taken into consideration for standard operations of the various types of automated external defibrillators. (pp. 311–317)

22. State the reasons for assuring that the patient is pulseless and apneic when using the automated external defibrillator. (pp. 310, 311)

23. Discuss the circumstances which may result in inappropriate shocks. (p. 310)

24. Explain the considerations for interruption of CPR when using the automated external defibrillator. (p. 311)

25. Discuss the advantages and disadvantages of automated external defibrillators. (pp. 320–321)

26. Summarize the speed of operation of automated external defibrillation. (pp. 321–322)

27. Discuss the use of remote defibrillation through adhesive pads. (pp. 320–321)

28. Discuss the special considerations for rhythm monitoring. (pp. 310–311, 321)

29. List the steps in the operation of the automated external defibrillator. (pp. 311–317)

30. Discuss the standard of care that should be used to provide care to a patient with persistent ventricular fibrillation and no available ACLS. (pp. 312, 316–317)

31. Discuss the standard of care that should be used to provide care to a patient with recurrent ventricular fibrillation and no available ACLS. (p. 318)

32. Differentiate between single rescuer and multi-rescuer care with an automated external defibrillator. (p. 318)

33. Explain the reason for pulses not being checked between shocks with an automated external defibrillator. (p. 317)

34. Discuss the importance of coordinating ACLS trained providers with personnel using automated external defibrillators. (p. 317)

35. Discuss the importance of post-resuscitation care. (pp. 317–318)

36. List the components of post-resuscitation care. (pp. 317–318)

37. Explain the importance of frequent practice with the automated external defibrillator. (pp. 322, 324)

38. Discuss the need to complete the Automated Defibrillator: Operator's Shift Checklist. (p. 322)

39. Discuss the role of the American Heart Association (AHA) in the use of automated external defibrillation. (pp. 306–308)

40. Explain the role medical direction plays in the use of automated external defibrillation. (p. 322)

41. State the reasons why a case review should be completed following the use of the automated external defibrillator. (pp. 322, 324)

42. Discuss the components that should be included in a case review. (pp. 322, 324)

43. Discuss the goal of quality improvement in automated external defibrillation. (pp. 322–324)

44. Define the function of all controls on an automated external defibrillator, and describe event documentation and battery defibrillator maintenance. (pp. 313–317, 322, 323)

45. Defend the reasons for obtaining initial training in automated external defibrillation and the importance of continuing education. (pp. 320, 324)

46. Defend the reason for maintenance of automated external defibrillators. (p. 322)

Skills

1. Demonstrate the assessment and emergency medical care of a patient experiencing chest pain or discomfort.

2. Perform the steps in facilitating the use of nitroglycerin for chest pain or discomfort.

3. Demonstrate the assessment and documentation of patient response to nitroglycerin.

4. Demonstrate the application and operation of the automated external defibrillator.

5. Demonstrate the maintenance of an automated external defibrillator.

6. Demonstrate the assessment and documentation of patient response to the automated external defibrillator.

7. Demonstrate the skills necessary to complete the Automated Defibrillator: Operator's Shift Checklist.

8. Practice completing a prehospital care report for patients with cardiac emergencies.

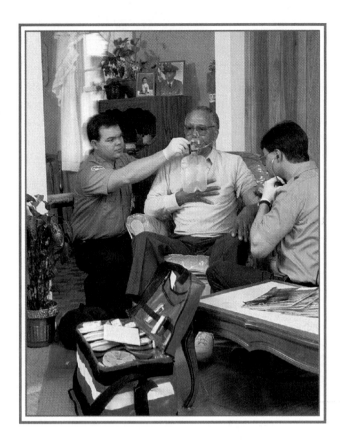

You begin your *focused history and physical exam* for a medical patient by questioning Mr. Sharpe. You discover that about half an hour ago, he started to feel some pressure in the middle of his chest when he was sweeping the floor. He denies having any pain but admits that the pressure radiates to his left arm. It feels like what he experienced two years ago when he had a heart attack. He took one of his nitroglycerin tablets a few minutes after the pressure started, but it didn't help. Your partner puts a nonrebreather mask with 12 liters per minute of oxygen on Mr. Sharpe as you continue your assessment.

Mr. Sharpe admits to a little difficulty breathing when you specifically ask him about it. His stomach is a little upset and he feels slightly nauseated, but he has not vomited. He has no allergies to medicines. His medications include digoxin, furosemide, and nitroglycerin. He has a history of a heart attack. The last thing he ate or drank was lunch about two and a half hours ago. He has been feeling fine and can't think of anything that might have caused this.

While you are getting Mr. Sharpe's history, your partner is taking baseline vital signs. Mr. Sharpe's pulse is 96, full and irregular. His blood pressure is 150/90. Respirations are 24 and unlabored. Skin is pale and sweaty.

Your partner has already started giving Mr. Sharpe oxygen. You consult medical direction and describe the patient, including his vital signs. The emergency department physician directs you to have the patient take another of his nitro tablets and check his blood pressure. He also tells you that if Mr. Sharpe continues to have chest pressure and his systolic blood pressure is still over 100 five minutes later, you should give one additional nitro after that. You help Mr. Sharpe take one of his nitroglycerin tablets and move him to the stretcher.

You transport the patient sitting up to the hospital and perform an *ongoing assessment* every five minutes. Five minutes after Mr. Sharpe's second nitro tablet, the pressure in his chest remains unchanged. His blood pressure is 140/90, so you help the patient take another nitro. His blood pressure and vital signs remain unchanged by the time you arrive at the hospital.

Mr. Sharpe is evaluated and treated in the emergency department for a possible heart attack. He is transferred to the coronary care unit where a heart attack is confirmed. He is discharged from the hospital a week later in good condition.

Jessie Sharpe is not having a good day. Things started out well enough, but a little while ago he started to feel a pressure in his chest. Fear goes through him, fear that he is having a heart attack like the one he had a few years ago. He sits down and takes one of his nitroglycerin tablets, but it doesn't help. His wife notices that he has stopped what he was doing and becomes concerned. Over his objections, she calls for EMS.

As you approach and *size up the scene,* you see nothing that appears hazardous. An older woman answers the door and shows you to her husband, Mr. Sharpe. She tells you he is 72 years old.

As you begin your *initial assessment,* you get a general impression of an older man who appears to be in some distress. Mr. Sharpe's mental status is alert. His airway is open and his breathing is adequate. You check his circulation by checking his pulse and skin and looking for bleeding. His radial pulse is slightly rapid and irregular, but strong. His skin is sweaty and his lips and nail beds are pale. You see no bleeding. You assign him a high priority.

ometimes a patient's chest discomfort will be the result of a cardiac (heart) problem—possibly a heart attack, possibly some other cardiac disorder. You will be able to provide these patients with oxygen, the most important drug in the treatment of heart problems. You may also be able to assist patients who have nitroglycerin in taking their medicine. Most patients having chest pain will not be having heart attacks—in fact may not have a heart problem at all. Oxygen will not harm patients who are not having heart problems and may be of great benefit to those who are.

Occasionally, you will encounter a patient who is in cardiac arrest—whose normal heartbeat and circulation of blood have completely stopped. Rapid defibrillation, which will be covered in the second part of this chapter, is the application of an electrical shock to the chest in order to restart the normal action of the heart. Cardiac arrest is one of the few situations in which you may actually be able to save someone's life by acting quickly and efficiently.

CARDIAC ANATOMY AND PHYSIOLOGY

You learned about the cardiovascular system and circulation of the blood in Chapter 4, The Human Body. Before continuing through this chapter on cardiac emergencies, you should review this material in Chapter 4. In particular, you should review

- The flow of blood through the chambers of the heart (the atria and ventricles), and the cardiac conductive system (the electrical impulses and specialized muscles that cause the heart to contract)
- The composition of the blood (red and white blood cells, platelets, and plasma)
- The flow of blood through the arteries, veins, arterioles, venules, and capillaries, and the names and positions of major blood vessels
- The circulation of blood between the heart and the lungs and between the heart and the rest of the body
- How heart function and the circulation of blood relate to pulse (review the peripheral and central pulses) and blood pressure (review systolic and diastolic pressure; also

review Chapter 5, Baseline Vital Signs and SAMPLE History)
- Shock (hypoperfusion)

You may also wish to review the diagrams of the heart, the cardiovascular system, the cardiac conductive system, and the circulatory system in Chapter 4 and the diagram of the cardiovascular system in the Anatomy and Physiology Plates at the end of this book.

CARDIAC COMPROMISE

Cardiac compromise is a blanket term that refers to any kind of problem with the heart. There are many different ways in which patients' hearts show that they are in trouble. One reason for this is that there are many different kinds of problems the heart can experience. A coronary artery may become narrowed or blocked, a one-way valve may stop working properly, or the specialized tissue that carries electrical impulses may function abnormally. Another reason is that there are no sensory nerves that go directly from the heart to the brain. If we had such nerves, patients' signs and symptoms would be much more similar and it would be a lot easier to determine that, for example, someone's heart wasn't getting enough oxygen.

Instead, there is a very wide variety of signs and symptoms that are associated with cardiac problems. Most of these signs and symptoms can also result from problems that have nothing to do with the heart. Many patients with heart trouble will complain of pain in the center of the chest. Others may have only mild chest discomfort or no pain at all. Some may experience difficulty breathing, while still others have only the sudden onset of sweating, nausea, and vomiting. Since the signs and symptoms of a heart problem can vary so greatly, it is much safer for the EMT-Basic to treat all patients with certain signs and symptoms as though they are having a heart problem—cardiac compromise—instead of trying to decide whether or not the patient has a heart problem or what kind of heart problem it might be.

The best known symptom of a heart problem is chest pain. Typically, a patient describes this pain as crushing, dull, heavy, or squeezing. Sometimes the patient will vehemently deny having pain, but may admit to some pressure, like Mr. Sharpe in On the Scene. Some patients will describe this sensation as just a discomfort. This is a good example of why you should have a patient describe in his own words how he is feeling. If you ask some of these patients whether they are having chest pain, they will tell you they are not because to them it is not pain. When a patient is having difficulty describing the sensation, try to give him several choices, as you learned in Chapter 11, Focused History and Physical Exam–Medical.

The pain, pressure, or discomfort commonly radiates along the arms, down to the upper abdomen, or up to the jaw. Patients complain of radiation to the left arm more than the right, but either (or both) is possible.

Another frequent complaint (and sometimes the only complaint in a patient with cardiac compromise) is difficulty breathing, called **dyspnea** (DISP-ne-ah). If the patient does not complain of difficulty breathing, you should specifically ask the patient about it. Sometimes the pain is so intense that patients focus their attention on that and don't mention other important symptoms.

When you see a patient with cardiac compromise, you will very often be able to tell that the patient is anxious. In some patients, this takes the form of a feeling of impending doom. Occasionally, you will see a patient whose anxiety displays itself through irritability and a short temper.

Other common symptoms in patients with cardiac compromise are nausea and pain or discomfort in the upper abdomen (epigastric pain). Some of these patients also vomit. A less common finding is loss of consciousness. This may result from the heart beating too fast or too slow for the brain to get enough perfusion. Usually, the patient regains consciousness quickly.

There are also several signs you will see in some of these patients. These include the sudden onset of sweating and an abnormal pulse or blood pressure. Many patients who have sudden onset of sweating think they are coming down with the flu, but denial is common in these patients. They refuse to acknowledge, at least consciously, that they may be having heart problems. You saw this with Mr. Sharpe. The pulse may be slower than 60 (bradycardia) or faster than 100 (tachycardia) and will frequently be irregular. Some patients complain of palpitations—irregular or rapid heartbeats that they can feel as a fluttering sensation in the chest. A few patients are hypotensive (systolic blood pressure less than 90), while others are hypertensive (systolic greater than 150 or diastolic greater than 90).

Patients with cardiac compromise can have many different presentations. Some, like Mr. Sharpe, complain of pressure or pain in the chest with difficulty breathing and a history of heart problems. Others may have just mild discomfort that they ignore for several hours or that goes away and returns. Between 10 and 20 percent of patients having heart attacks have no chest discomfort at all. Because of these many possibilities and because of the potentially severe complications of heart problems, it is important to have a high index of suspicion and treat patients with any of these signs and symptoms for cardiac compromise. The treatment will not hurt them and may help them.

Cardiovascular Disorders

Although you will treat all patients with signs and symptoms of cardiac compromise in the same manner (as will be detailed a bit later in this chapter)—without any need to diagnose what kind of heart problem the patient may be having—it is useful to have some background knowledge about the most common cardiovascular (heart and circulation) disorders: coronary artery disease, angina pectoris, acute myocardial infarction, and congestive heart failure.

Coronary Artery Disease

The heart is a muscle—a very active muscle. Like all other muscles, it needs oxygen to contract. When the coronary arteries are narrowed or blocked, blood flow is reduced, thereby reducing the amount of oxygen delivered to the heart. This might not be noticed when the body is at rest or at a low activity level. However, when the body is subject to stress or exertion, the heart rate (number of heartbeats per minute) increases. With the increased heart rate comes an increased need for oxygen. Arteries that are narrowed or blocked cannot supply enough blood to meet the demands of the heart.

Diseases that affect the arteries of the heart—often causing the narrowing or blockage through the deposit of cholesterol plaques on the interior wall of the arteries—are commonly called **coronary artery disease (CAD).** Coronary artery disease is a serious health problem that results in hundreds of thousands of deaths yearly in the United States.

There are factors that put a person at risk of developing CAD. Some of these risk factors, such as heredity (a close relative who has CAD) and age, cannot be changed. However, there are also many risk factors that can be modified to reduce the risk of coronary artery disease. These include hypertension (high blood pressure), obesity, lack of exercise, elevated blood levels of cholesterol and triglycerides, and cigarette smoking.

Many patients have more than one of these risk factors. Fortunately, the damage caused by the second group of risk factors may be reversed or slowed by changing behavior. Smokers can return to the risk level of a non-smoker soon after quitting. Medication and weight loss can lower high blood pressure. Improved diet and exercise can help the other controllable factors.

In the majority of cardiac-related medical emergencies, it is the reduced blood supply to the myocardium (heart muscle) that causes the emergency. The most common symptom of this reduced blood supply is chest pain. Patients may have symptoms that range anywhere from mild chest pain to sudden death (suddenly going into cardiac arrest). Angina pectoris (chest pain), acute myocardial infarction (heart attack), and congestive heart failure—all conditions that can be related to CAD—are discussed below.

Angina Pectoris

Angina pectoris means, literally, a pain in the chest. This condition is brought on by a reduced blood supply to the heart during times of exertion or stress (Figure 18-1). Coronary artery disease has caused a narrowing of the arteries that supply the heart. When the heart needs to beat faster because of some stress or exertion, more blood and oxygen are required. The narrowed coronary arteries cannot supply all the blood that is needed. As the heart works harder and doesn't get the oxygen it needs to do the work, the portion of the myocardium supplied by the narrowed artery becomes starved for oxygen. When the myocardium is deprived of the oxygen it needs, chest pain—angina pectoris—is the most frequent result. This pain is sometimes called an angina attack.

Since the pain of angina pectoris comes on after stress or exertion, frequently the pain diminishes when the patient stops the exertion. As the oxygen demand of the heart returns to normal, the pain subsides. Seldom does this painful attack last longer than 3 to 5 minutes.

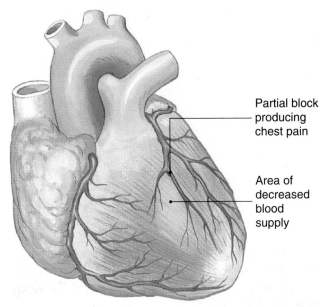

Partial block producing chest pain

Area of decreased blood supply

FIGURE 18-1 Angina pectoris produces pain in the chest that may be similar to that of a heart attack.

Another indication that the patient has a history of this condition is if the patient has the medication **nitroglycerin.** Nitroglycerin is a medication that dilates the blood vessels. This results in more blood staying in the veins of the body, so there is less blood coming back to the heart. With less blood to pump out, the heart does not have to work as hard. Nitroglycerin is available in tablets that are placed under the patient's tongue to dissolve, and also in sprays and patches (Figure 18-2). The patches have adhesive that keeps them on the skin. They gradually release nitroglycerin throughout the day.

Most angina patients are advised by their doctors to take nitroglycerin for their chest pain. Patients are usually told to rest and are allowed to take 3 nitroglycerin doses over a 10-minute period. If there is no relief of symptoms after that time they are instructed to call for help.

Acute Myocardial Infarction

The condition in which a portion of the myocardium dies as a result of oxygen starvation is known as **acute myocardial infarction (AMI)** (Figure 18-3). Often called a heart attack by lay persons, AMI is brought on by the narrowing or **occlusion** (blockage) of the coronary artery that supplies the region with blood. Rarely, the interruption of blood flow to the myocardium may be due to the rupturing of a coronary artery.

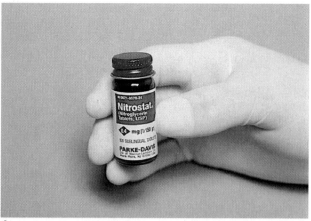

A.

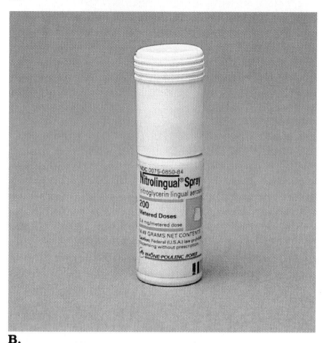

B.

FIGURE 18-2 A. Nitroglycerin tablets. B. Nitroglycerin spray.

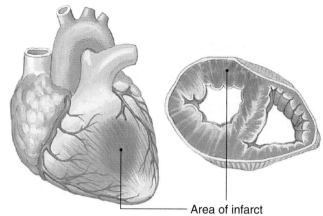

Area of infarct

FIGURE 18-3 Cross section of a myocardial infarction.

The American Heart Association reports over a million cases of AMI in the United States each year. Hundreds of thousands of deaths annually are the result of cardiovascular disease. A major portion of these are cases of **sudden death**, a cardiac arrest that occurs within two hours of the onset of symptoms. In most cases, sudden death occurs outside of hospitals. The patient may have no prior symptoms of coronary artery disease. Nearly 25% of these individuals have no previous history of cardiac problems.

A variety of factors can cause an AMI. Coronary artery disease is usually the underlying reason for the incident. However, for some patients, factors often regarded as harmless may trigger an AMI. These factors include chronic respiratory problems, unusual exertion, or severe emotional stress.

The treatment of AMI has changed radically over recent years. Previously, patients were admitted to coronary care units where they were observed and, when emergencies occurred, treated with varying degrees of success. Now, some patients receive treatment with medications called *thrombolytics* (throm-bo-LIT-iks) to dissolve the clot that is blocking the coronary artery. To be most effective, these medications must be administered early. With each hour that passes before they are administered, they become less and less likely to dissolve the clot. Many patients with myocardial infarctions are not candidates for this treatment, but those who are must reach the hospital quickly.

Another complication sometimes seen with AMI is mechanical pump failure. A lack of oxygen has caused the death of a portion of the myocardium. The dead area can no longer pump and contract. If a large enough area of the heart dies, the pumping action of the whole heart will be affected. This can lead to cardiac arrest, shock (see Chapter 25, Bleeding and Shock), pulmonary edema (fluids "backing up" in the lungs), congestive heart failure (edema of lungs and other body organs), and cell death in various regions of the body due to oxygen starvation. A few AMI patients suffer cardiac rupture as the dead tissue area of the myocardium bursts open. This occurs days after an AMI.

Congestive Heart Failure

Congestive heart failure (CHF) is a condition of excessive fluid buildup in the lungs and/or other organs and body parts. The fluid buildup causes edema, or swelling. The disorder is termed congestive because the fluids congest, or clog, the organs. It is termed heart failure because the congestion both results from and also aggravates failure of the heart to function properly. The congestion may also result from and aggravate failure of the lungs to function properly. More information on congestive heart failure is in the FYI section of this chapter.

Transportation of a patient with a heart condition must be carried out in a thoughtful, calm, and careful fashion. A rough ride with sudden starts, stops, and turns and siren wailing is likely to increase the patient's fear and apprehension, placing additional stress on the heart. Speed is important; the patient must reach the hospital quickly. However, the judicious use of siren or horn must be balanced against the possibility of worsening the patient's condition.

The management of a patient with cardiac compromise is detailed below and in Scan 18-1.

Patient Assessment—Cardiac Compromise

1. Perform the initial assessment.
2. Perform a focused history and physical exam. Inquire about onset, provocation, quality, radiation, severity, and time. Get a SAMPLE history.
3. Take baseline vital signs.

Signs and Symptoms

The following signs and symptoms are associated with cardiac compromise.

- [ ] pain, pressure, or discomfort in the chest or upper abdomen (epigastrium)
- [ ] difficulty breathing
- [ ] palpitations
- [ ] sudden onset of sweating with nausea or vomiting
- [ ] anxiety (feeling of impending doom, irritability)
- [ ] abnormal pulse
- [ ] abnormal blood pressure

Patient Care—Cardiac Compromise

Emergency Care Steps

1. *Place the patient in a position of comfort,* typically sitting up. This is especially true of patients with difficulty breathing. Patients who are hypotensive (systolic blood pressure less than 90) will usually feel better lying down. This position allows more blood to flow to the brain. Occasionally, you will see a patient who has both difficulty breathing and hypotension. It may be very difficult to find a good position in this case. The best way to determine the proper position is to ask the patient what position will relieve his difficulty breathing without making him weak or lightheaded.

2. *Apply high concentration oxygen through a nonrebreather mask* if not already done. If the patient has or develops an altered mental status, you will need to open and maintain the patient's airway. If the patient is not breathing adequately, you will also need to ventilate him. Always be prepared for the patient to go into cardiac arrest. (Procedures for cardiac arrest will be discussed later in this chapter.)

3. a. *Transport promptly* if the patient has <u>any one</u> of these things:

   - no history of cardiac problems, or . . .
   - a history of cardiac problems, but does not have nitroglycerin, or . . .
   - a systolic blood pressure of less than 100

   b. Give the patient (or help the patient take) nitroglycerin if <u>all of the following</u> conditions are met (Scan 18-2).

   - the patient complains of chest pain
   - the patient has a history of cardiac problems
   - the patient's physician has prescribed nitroglycerin (NTG)
   - the patient has the nitroglycerin with him
   - the systolic blood pressure is greater than 100 systolic and
   - medical direction authorizes administration of the medication

   c. *After giving one dose of the nitroglycerin, repeat another dose in 3-5 minutes* <u>if all of the following</u> conditions are met.

   - the patient experiences no relief, and . . .
   - the systolic blood pressure remains greater than 100 systolic, and . . .
   - medical direction authorizes another dose of the medication

Administer up to a maximum of three doses of nitroglycerin, reassessing vital signs and chest pain after each dose. If the blood pressure falls below 100 systolic, treat the patient for shock (hypoperfusion). Transport promptly.

Scan 18-1
Chest Pain Management

FIRST take body substance isolation precautions.

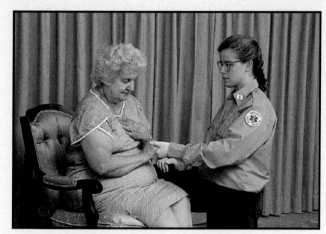

1. Perform the initial assessment.

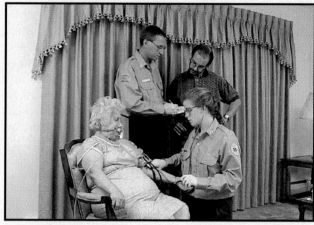

2. Provide high concentration oxygen by nonrebreather mask. Perform the focused history and physical exam for a medical patient. Document findings.

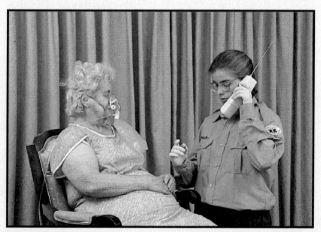

3. If patient meets nitroglycerin criteria and has prescribed nitroglycerin, ask the patient about the last dose taken. Consult medical direction with regard to assisting the patient in taking the medication.

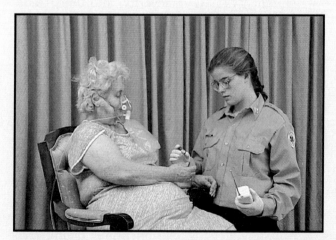

4. Check the four rights: right patient, right drug, right dose, right route. Check the expiration date.

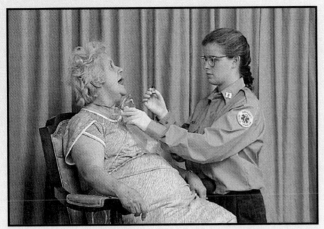

5. Remove oxygen mask. Ask patient to open mouth and lift tongue.

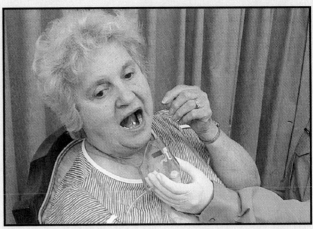

6. Place the nitroglycerin tablet under the tongue, or . . .

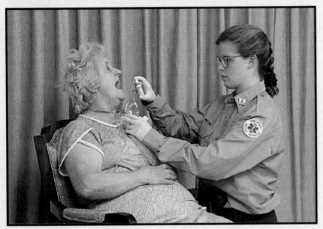

7. If the nitroglycerin is in spray form, spray the medication under the tongue according to label directions.

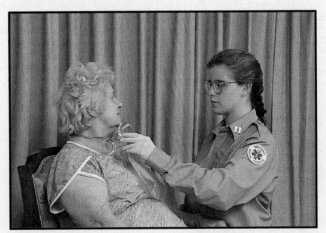

8. Have patient close mouth and hold the nitroglycerin under the tongue. This is an area where the medication will be quickly absorbed.

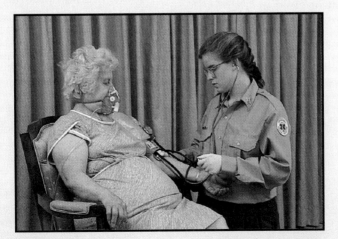

9. Replace oxygen mask. Reassess the patient. Document findings.

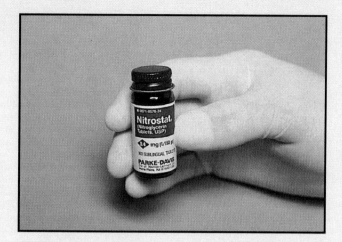

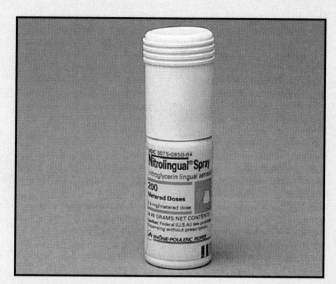

Medication Name
1. Generic: nitroglycerin
2. Trade: Nitrostat™

Indications
All of the following conditions must be met:
1. The patient complains of chest pain.
2. The patient has a history of cardiac problems.
3. The patient's physician has prescribed nitro-glycerin (NTG).
4. The systolic blood pressure is greater than 100 systolic.
5. Medical direction authorizes administration of the medication.

Contraindications
1. The patient has hypotension, or a systolic blood pressure below 100.
2. The patient has a head injury.
3. The patient is an infant or child.
4. The patient has already taken the maximum prescribed dose.

Medication Form
Tablet, sublingual (under-the-tongue) spray

Dosage
One dose, repeat in 3 to 5 minutes. If no relief, systolic blood pressure remains above 100, and if authorized by medical direction, up to a maximum of three doses.

Administration
1. Perform focused assessment for cardiac patient.
2. Take blood pressure. (Systolic pressure must be above 100.)
3. Contact medical direction if no standing orders.
4. Assure right medication, right patient, right dose, right route. Check expiration date.
5. Assure patient is alert.
6. Question patient on last dose taken and effects. Assure understanding of route of administration.
7. Ask patient to lift tongue and place tablet or spray dose under tongue (while wearing gloves) or have patient place tablet or spray under tongue.
8. Have patient keep mouth closed with tablet under tongue (without swallowing) until dissolved and absorbed.
9. Recheck blood pressure within 2 minutes.
10. Record administration, route, and time.
11. Perform reassessment.

Actions
1. Relaxes blood vessels
2. Decreases workload of heart

Side Effects
1. Hypotension (lowers blood pressure)
2. Headache
3. Pulse rate changes

Reassessment Strategies
1. Monitor blood pressure.
2. Ask patient about effect on pain relief.
3. Seek medical direction before readministering.
4. Record assessments.

Infants and Children

Children usually have very healthy hearts, so it is rare for an EMT-B to see a pediatric patient with a cardiac problem. Most such problems are congenital, i.e., the child is born with it, so they are discovered before the newborn leaves the nursery. You may see a child who has had cardiac surgery or has learned to live with his problem through changes in lifestyle or medication. In cases like these, parents are frequently very well informed and can be of great assistance.

Documentation Tip—
Nitroglycerin Administration

Be sure to document the patient's vital signs, especially blood pressure, before the first dose of nitroglycerin is administered and after each dose. Ask the patient about the effect of the medication on the chest pain or discomfort and record the patient's responses. It is vital information for hospital personnel to know if and how the patient has responded to nitroglycerin, since response or lack of response are important clues to the cause of the patient's difficulty.

CARDIAC ARREST

On the Scene

Fifty-six year old Krystal Courtney is mowing her front lawn on a Saturday afternoon as her husband Kevin does some gardening. Suddenly, Krystal feels lightheaded and collapses to the ground. Her husband rushes over and finds that he cannot wake her. Fearing the worst, he runs for the phone and calls 911. The dispatcher gets the necessary information and asks Kevin if he would like to do cardiopulmonary resuscitation. Kevin agrees, and takes the portable phone to his wife's side, where he follows the dispatcher's directions and starts CPR.

Four minutes after you received the call for a woman in cardiac arrest, you and your partner arrive and *size up the scene.* You see a middle-aged man doing CPR with a few neighbors standing nearby. You see nothing that appears to be potentially dangerous. You put on disposable gloves and other appropriate personal protective equipment. As you and your partner reach Mrs. Courtney with your oxygen, suction unit, airway kit, and automated external defibrillator, you ask Mr. Courtney to stop CPR.

As you begin your *initial assessment,* you get a general impression of an unresponsive middle-aged woman who actually appears to be dead. Her mental status is unresponsive to verbal stimuli. Your partner opens her airway with the head-tilt, chin-lift maneuver and finds that she is not breathing. You hand your partner an oral airway and the flow-restricted, oxygen-powered ventilation device and turn on the oxygen. Next, you check circulation by feeling at Mrs. Courtney's neck for a carotid pulse. There is none, so your partner quickly starts chest compressions. Both of you also note that Mrs. Courtney's skin is sweaty and blue (cyanotic). You see no bleeding. You assign the patient a high priority.

As your partner does one-rescuer CPR, you open the automated external defibrillator (AED). You turn it on and begin to describe for the voice recorder what the situation is and what you are doing as you do it.

You: (speaking into the AED recorder) This is Connie Reno at the scene of an approximately 60-year-old female in cardiac arrest. My partner has started CPR.

You remove a pair of monitoring-defibrillation pads from their package and attach them to the defib cables. Next, you peel the adhesive backing off the pads and place them on the patient's upper right chest and lower left ribs. At the same time that you are doing these things, you ask Mr. Courtney what happened.

You: (to the recorder) I'm putting the pads on the patient's chest. (As you attach the pads to cables and place them on Mrs. Courtney, you ask her husband a few questions.) Can you tell me what happened, sir?
Mr. Courtney: She was mowing the lawn when all of a sudden she collapsed.
You: Did she complain of anything? Pain?
Mr. Courtney: No, it happened too fast.
You: Has she ever had any heart problems?
Mr. Courtney: No, not that we knew of.
You: Does she take any medicines?
Mr. Courtney: No.
You: Her heart was stopped, so it's good that you were doing CPR. We're hooking her up to a heart monitor now to see if we can get her heart started again.

You ask your partner to stop CPR and cease contact with the patient, then press the button on your AED that allows it to analyze the rhythm. Almost immediately, you hear it start to charge up. Six or seven seconds later, the machine tells you to deliver a shock. After saying "Clear!" in a loud voice and making sure no one is touching the patient, you press the button that delivers the shock. You see Mrs. Courtney's muscles jerk. (There is a murmur of awe and appreciation from the neighbors. A patient's response to shock is quite dramatic.)

As soon as the AED tells you it has reset, you initiate another rhythm analysis and deliver another shock, again making sure everyone is clear of the patient. Once more, you initiate a rhythm analysis and deliver a third shock. Your partner checks for a carotid pulse and finds none, so she resumes CPR for one minute. You take this opportunity to check how effective the CPR is by feeling for a carotid pulse. There is a weak pulse beat with each compression and the chest rises with ventilations, so her CPR appears adequate.

After a minute of CPR, you again ask your partner to stop CPR and cease contact with the patient, then press the button on your AED that allows it to analyze the rhythm. It charges up and you deliver a fourth shock, making sure no one is touching the patient and saying "Clear!" in a loud voice. When you press the analyze button again, the AED gives you a message that no shock is indicated, so your partner checks for a carotid pulse. There is none, so she resumes CPR.

A back-up crew arrives to help you transport your patient, so you work with them to get Mrs. Courtney on a backboard and call for ALS intercept. A minute after your partner resumed CPR, she checks again for a pulse. This time, she finds a carotid pulse. Mrs. Courtney is only making occasional attempts to breathe, so she continues to ventilate her.

Mr. Courtney: Is she going to be OK?
You: Her heart was stopped, but we've started it beating again. She's doing better now, but she's still pretty serious. We're going to take her to the hospital now. Do you want to come with us?
Mr. Courtney: Yes, can I?
You: Sure. You can ride in the front seat.

You get Mrs. Courtney into the ambulance where you continue to ventilate her and perform ongoing assessment. En route to the hospital, she begins to wake up and breathe adequately, so you switch from the flow-restricted, oxygen-powered ventilation device to a nonrebreather mask. By the time you arrive at the emergency department, Mrs. Courtney has an irregular pulse of 120, a blood pressure of 130/80 and respirations of 20. After a week of tests and observation in the hospital, Krystal Courtney is discharged home, alert and in good condition.

In a typical ambulance service, only 1 to 2 percent of emergency calls are cardiac arrests, and most patients with heart problems do not go into cardiac arrest while they are under your care. Nonetheless, EMS systems exert a great deal of time and energy on attempts to resuscitate these patients. The odds of bringing a cardiac-arrest patient back to life have increased considerably over the last ten or fifteen years. As the problem of cardiac arrest has received more attention, EMS researchers, physicians, administrators, and providers have learned more about what is effective and what is not.

The Chain of Survival

The American Heart Association has summarized the most important factors that affect survival of cardiac arrest patients in its chain of survival concept. The chain (Figure 18-4) has four elements: (1) early access, (2) early CPR, (3) early defibrillation, and (4) early advanced care. An EMS system where each of these links is strong is much more likely to bring back a patient from cardiac arrest than a system that has weaknesses in the chain. This has been shown in systems that tried to strengthen just one link (early defibrillation) without strengthening the other links.

Early Access

Early access means that the person who sees someone collapse or finds someone unresponsive calls a dispatcher who quickly gets EMS responding to the emergency. Unfortunately, this is easier said than done. The lay public, unlike EMS providers, are not used to recognizing emergencies. It takes longer for them to realize that an emergency exists and that they need to call for help right away. Even when a layperson does decide to make the call for help, there may still be obstacles.

Many areas still do not have 911. This means that emergency services have seven digit telephone numbers that laypeople cannot be expected to remember. Even though many phone companies list emergency numbers on the inside cover of their directories, this adds an extra step to the process and delays even further the call for help. Many EMS agencies in this position have public information programs that include the distribution of telephone stickers with emergency numbers on them. Since Americans change residence frequently (and buy new tele-

Chain of Survival

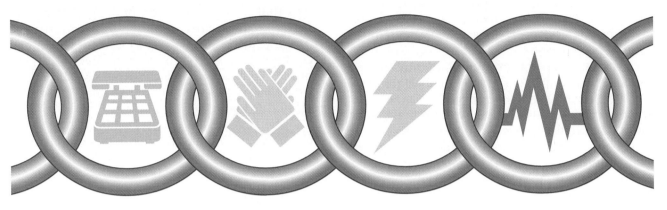

| EARLY | EARLY | EARLY | EARLY |
| ACCESS | CPR | DEFIBRILLATION | ADVANCED CARE |

FIGURE 18-4 The Chain of Survival (American Heart Association)

phones more often than that), emergency services must make these stickers available frequently and easily.

Early CPR

Early CPR can increase survival significantly. About the only time early CPR does not help is when defibrillation reaches the patient within approximately two minutes. Since this is rarely the case in real life, this means EMS agencies need to address this factor. There are at least three ways in which CPR can be delivered earlier: get CPR-trained professionals to the patient faster, train laypeople in CPR, and train dispatchers to instruct callers in how to do CPR.

An efficient way to get CPR to patients faster in many areas is to send CPR-trained professionals to the scene. This may mean police, firefighters, security officers, or lifeguards. Whoever it is needs to receive notification of the possible need for CPR as soon as possible. They also need to be in the right place and be able to respond quickly to where they are needed.

Some EMS agencies have CPR courses for the lay public as part of their public information and education programs, but too many do not. It is especially important to train the right laypeople. Teaching elementary and high school students CPR is good, especially in the long run, but they are not usually present when someone goes into cardiac arrest. The typical cardiac arrest patient is a male in his sixties, so it is not

surprising to learn that the typical witness of a cardiac arrest is a woman in her sixties. Middle aged and older people need CPR courses at least as much as children and adolescents.

A surprisingly effective way to get a layperson to perform CPR is for a dispatcher to instruct the caller over the phone. This has been done in a number of areas and has produced significant increases in the survival rate from cardiac arrest. The quality of CPR done by untrained laypeople instructed by dispatchers is comparable to CPR done by laypeople who were trained in CPR previously. Emergency Medical Dispatchers (EMDs) are trained to give such instructions. Pre-arrival dispatch instructions to guide other dispatchers in this step are available.

Early Defibrillation

Early defibrillation has received a great deal of attention the last few years. This is because it is the single most important factor in determining survival from cardiac arrest.

Although a lot of emphasis has been put on defibrillation, frequently there has not been enough attention paid to *early* defibrillation. With a few thousand dollars, an agency can purchase an automated defibrillator. The hard part is getting it to the patient in cardiac arrest early enough to be effective. If the response time of the defibrillator (time from call received to arrival of the defibrillator) is longer than eight minutes, virtually no one survives cardiac arrest. This is true even with early CPR. Although eight minutes is really the maximum response time where defibrillation is usually effective, the sooner the defibrillator arrives, the more likely it is that a patient will survive cardiac arrest. This is one time when it is literally true that every minute counts.

One way to get around long ambulance response times is to provide defibrillators to other emergency services providers. Some EMS systems have used innovative ways to make sure that a defibrillator arrives in time. In urban and suburban areas, police officers and firefighters have sometimes been equipped with the machines since they may arrive before the ambulance. In rural areas, some EMTs and first responders carry defibrillators in their personal vehicles so that the patient who needs a defibrillator gets it in time.

Early Advanced Care

Early advanced care is second only to defibrillation in the drama and excitement it stirs in laypeople. Putting a breathing tube into someone's throat (endotracheal intubation), putting a needle into someone's arm (starting an intravenous line), and administering medications into an IV line are all activities that laypeople may not understand, but they are actions that the public has come to expect. They are also apparently responsible for a higher survival rate.

The most common way for patients to get advanced cardiac life support (ACLS) is through paramedics who either respond to the scene or rendezvous with a basic life support unit en route to the hospital. In some areas, there are EMTs who have more training than EMT-Bs, but less than EMT-Paramedics. Their level of practice is frequently called EMT-Cardiac, EMT-Critical Care, or EMT-Intermediate. They may be able to perform interventions that can improve survival of these patients. Another method that is not quite as fast is for EMT-Bs to transport patients not to a hospital, but to a clinic or other medical facility that is closer. Any such arrangements need to be made before they are actually needed and should be in writing in the form of protocols. These protocols should be approved by your medical director.

Systems that have early access, early CPR, early defibrillation, and early advanced care have survival rates from cardiac arrest that are much higher than systems with one or more weak links in the chain of survival.

MANAGEMENT OF CARDIAC ARREST

As an EMT-B, the two links in the chain of survival that you can provide or help provide are early CPR and early defibrillation. You studied CPR in your basic life support course, which was required as a prerequisite to your EMT-Basic course. You can review CPR in Basic Life Support: Airway, Rescue Breathing, and CPR at the end of this book.

The rest of this chapter will emphasize the role of defibrillation in treating cardiac arrest patients. Managing a patient in cardiac arrest means you need to be able to

- Perform one- and two-rescuer CPR (Ordinarily, you will do two-rescuer CPR when you are on duty, but you must be able to do one-rescuer CPR while your partner is preparing equipment or while you are en route to a medical facility.)
- Use an automated external defibrillator
- Request advanced life support backup (when available) to continue the chain of survival
- Use a bag-valve-mask device with oxygen
- Use a flow restricted, oxygen-powered ventilation device
- Lift and move patients
- Suction a patient's airway
- Use airway adjuncts, i.e., oral and nasal airways
- Use body substance isolation equipment and techniques to protect yourself (and patients)
- Interview bystanders and family members to obtain facts related to the arrest

Most of the patients you see with chest pain or difficulty breathing will remain alert and in good condition while you are assessing or treating them, but a few will go into cardiac arrest before you arrive at the hospital. For this reason, you must be prepared for cardiac arrest whenever you have a patient with chest discomfort or difficulty breathing. This means bringing the defibrillator to the scene when you are dispatched to one of these calls and having the defibrillator nearby while you are transporting.

The Automated External Defibrillator (AED)

Types of AEDs

There are two ways someone can defibrillate. The traditional method (manual defibrillation) is for the operator to look at the patient's heart rhythm on a screen, decide the rhythm is shockable, lubricate and charge two paddles, and deliver a shock to the patient's chest. An automated defibrillator, on the other hand (Figure 18-5), contains a computer that analyzes the patient's heart rhythm after the operator applies two monitoring-defibrillation pads to the patient's chest.

There are two types of automated external defibrillators, semiautomatic and fully automatic. Semiautomatic defibrillators, the more common type, advise the EMT-B to press a button that will cause the machine to deliver a shock through the pads. Semiautomatic defibrillators are sometimes called shock advisory defibrillators. Fully automated defibrillators do not advise the EMT-B to take any action. They deliver the shock automatically once enough energy has been accumulated. All the EMT-B has to do to use a fully automatic defibrillator is assess the patient, turn on the power, and put the pads on the patient's chest. The information below about how to operate an AED applies principally to a semiautomatic AED.

How AEDs Work

Like all muscles, the heart produces electrical impulses. By putting two monitoring electrodes on the chest, it is possible to "see" the electrical activity of the heart. An AED can analyze this cardiac rhythm and determine whether it is a rhythm for which a shock is indicated. The microprocessors and the computer programs used to do this have been tested extensively and have been very accurate, both in the laboratory and in the field. Today's AEDs are very reliable

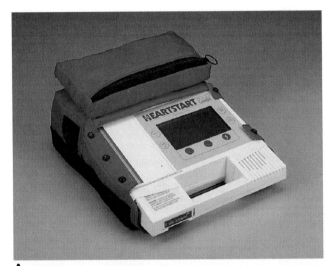

A.

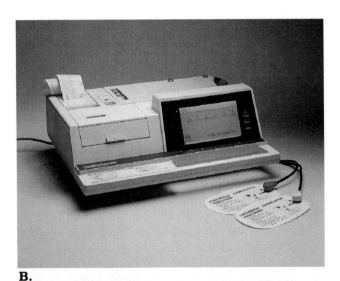

B.

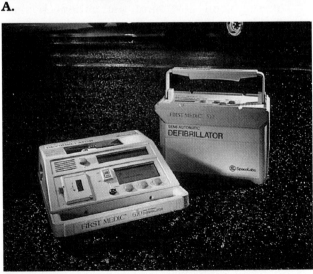

C.

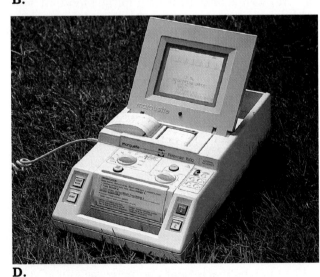

D.

FIGURE 18-5 AEDs from A. Laerdal, B. PhysioControl, C. SpaceLabs, and D. Marquette.

in distinguishing between rhythms that need shocks and rhythms that do not need shocks.

When AEDs deliver shocks inappropriately, it is almost always the result of human error. This occurs because the operator did not assess the patient properly (AEDs are designed only for use on patients in cardiac arrest), did not use the AED properly, or did not maintain the machine. The chance of mechanical error is always present, but it is small. Maintaining the AED in good operating order (see Defibrillator Maintenance later in this chapter), attaching an AED only to unresponsive, pulseless, nonbreathing patients, practicing frequently, and following your local protocols are the best ways to avoid making an error that could affect a patient.

Often, a cardiac event such as spasm or blockage of a coronary artery (myocardial infarction or heart attack) is associated with a disturbance of the heart's electrical, or conduction, system, which must function normally if the heart is to continue to beat with a regular rhythm. The most common conditions that result in cardiac arrest are

Shockable Rhythms
- Ventricular Fibrillation—The primary electrical disturbance resulting in cardiac arrest is called **ventricular fibrillation** (ven-TRIK-u-ler fib-ri-LAY-shun) **(VF)**. Between 50% and 60% of all cardiac arrest victims will be in VF if EMS personnel arrive in the first 8 minutes or so. The heart in VF may have plenty of electrical energy, but it is totally disorganized. Chaotic electrical activity originating from many sites in the heart prevents the heart muscle from contracting normally and thus pumping blood. If you could see a heart in VF, it would appear to be quivering like a bag of worms. VF is considered a shockable rhythm, one for which defibrillation is effective.
- Ventricular Tachycardia—Automated external defibrillators are also designed to shock a rhythm known as **ventricular tachycardia** (ven-TRIK-u-ler tak-i-KAR-de-uh) **(V-Tach)** if it is very fast. In ventricular tachycardia (a very unusual cardiac arrest rhythm observed in less than 10% of all out-of-hospital cases), the heart rhythm is organized, but it is usually quite rapid. The faster the heart rate, the more likely it is that ventricular tachycardia will not allow the heart's chambers to fill with enough blood between beats to produce blood flow sufficient to meet the body's needs, espe-

cially that of the brain. Pulseless V-Tach is considered a shockable rhythm.

Some patients with ventricular tachycardia are awake, even with very fast heart rates. If an AED was attached to one of these patients, it would charge up and advise a shock. Since the patient has a pulse and is awake, this would be inappropriate. This is one of the reasons the AED should be attached only to patients in cardiac arrest.

Nonshockable Rhythms
- **Pulseless Electrical Activity (PEA)**—In 15% to 20% of cardiac arrest victims, the heart muscle itself fails even though the electrical rhythm remains relatively normal. This condition of relatively normal electrical activity but no pumping action means that the heart muscle is severely and almost always terminally sick. Or it may mean that the patient has lost too much blood. The heart could pump if it had something to pump, but there is no fluid in the system. Defibrillation cannot help these people because their heart's electrical rhythm is already organized and slow (unlike ventricular tachycardia, where the rhythm is organized but very fast). PEA is not considered a shockable rhythm.
- **Asystole**—In the remaining 20% to 25% of cardiac arrest victims, the heart has ceased generating electrical impulses altogether. When this happens, a condition called **asystole** (ay-SIS-to-le), there is no electrical stimulus to cause the heart muscle to contract, and so it does not. As a result, there is no blood flow, and the patient has no pulse or respirations and is unconscious. (This condition is commonly called *flatline*, because the wavy line displayed on an ECG when there is electrical activity goes flat with asystole.) This condition can be the result of untreated ventricular fibrillation, a sick heart, a terminal illness, or severe blood loss. Asystole is not considered a shockable rhythm.

By adding up the numbers, you can see that automated defibrillators will shock at most only about six or seven of every ten cardiac arrest patients to whom they are attached: those suffering from the disturbed rhythms of ventricular fibrillation and ventricular tachycardia. For patients suffering from pulseless electrical activity (heart muscle failure) or asystole (complete lack of electrical activity), defibrillation will not be effective.

As an EMT-B you cannot diagnose heart ailments or causes of cardiac arrest. You must initiate CPR and defibrillation as rapidly as possible and, if defibrillation is not successful in restoring heart function, continue CPR to prevent biological death until the patient's care can be taken over at a medical facility or by those with advanced skills.

Coordinating CPR and AED for a Patient in Cardiac Arrest

During your course in cardiopulmonary resuscitation, you learned to interrupt CPR only when necessary and for as short a period as possible. Since you will be using a defibrillator on patients in cardiac arrest, you need to understand some additional circumstances when you should interrupt CPR.

If you are touching the patient when the AED is analyzing the rhythm, there can be interference from the electrical impulses of your heart and from movement of the patient's muscles. This can fool the computer in the AED into believing there is a shockable rhythm when there really isn't one or vice versa. It is also true that if a shock is delivered when you are touching the patient, the shock can be transmitted to you. Although it is not likely to cause you serious harm, you could be injured.

For these reasons, no one should ventilate, do chest compressions, or in any way touch the patient when the rhythm is being analyzed or a shock is being delivered.

Defibrillation is more effective than CPR in restoring a patient's pulse, so stopping CPR to allow for rhythm analysis and defibrillation is actually better for the patient. You may stop CPR for up to 90 seconds in order to give three shocks. You should resume CPR only after you deliver the first three shocks or you get a no-shock-indicated message (Figure 18-6 and Scan 18-3).

Patient Assessment—Cardiac Arrest

As with all calls, you should protect yourself from infectious diseases by using body substance isolation equipment and procedures. This is especially important in the case of a cardiac arrest where blood and other body fluids are commonly found.

1. Perform the initial assessment. If a bystander is doing CPR when you arrive,

have the bystander stop. Verify pulselessness (no carotid pulse) and **apnea** (AP-ne-ah—no breathing). Look for external blood loss.
2. After CPR has been resumed, you should perform a focused history and physical exam. Inquire about onset, trauma, and signs and symptoms that were present before the patient collapsed. Get a SAMPLE history if you can. Do not let history gathering interfere with or slow down defibrillation.

Emergency Care—Cardiac Arrest

Emergency Care Steps

1. Begin or resume CPR.
2. Determine whether the patient is a candidate for the AED.
   a. If the patient is an adult (at least 12 years old or 90 pounds for the purpose of defibrillation) who has not sustained trauma, proceed with the AED.
   b. If the patient is less than 12 years old and less than 90 pounds OR the patient has sustained trauma before collapse, do not attach the AED unless you are ordered to do so by medical direction. Continue CPR and transport.
3. Turn on the defibrillator power.
4. Begin the narrative if the AED has a voice recorder. You should describe who you are, what the situation is, and what you are doing as you do it. Do not delay your actions in order to describe them.
5. Attach the monitoring-defibrillation pads to the cables.
6. Bare the patient's chest (if not already done) and place the pads so that the one attached to the white cable is in the angle between the sternum and the right clavicle and the one attached to the red cable is over the lower left ribs ("white to right, red to ribs"). (This will be the patient's left and right, not your left and right.) Press the pads firmly on the chest to ensure good contact. Once in a while, you may have a male patient whose chest is so hairy that the pads do not make good contact. Use a hospital razor to quickly shave some of the hair away, and use a new pair of pads.
7. Stop CPR and clear the patient (make sure no one is touching the patient).

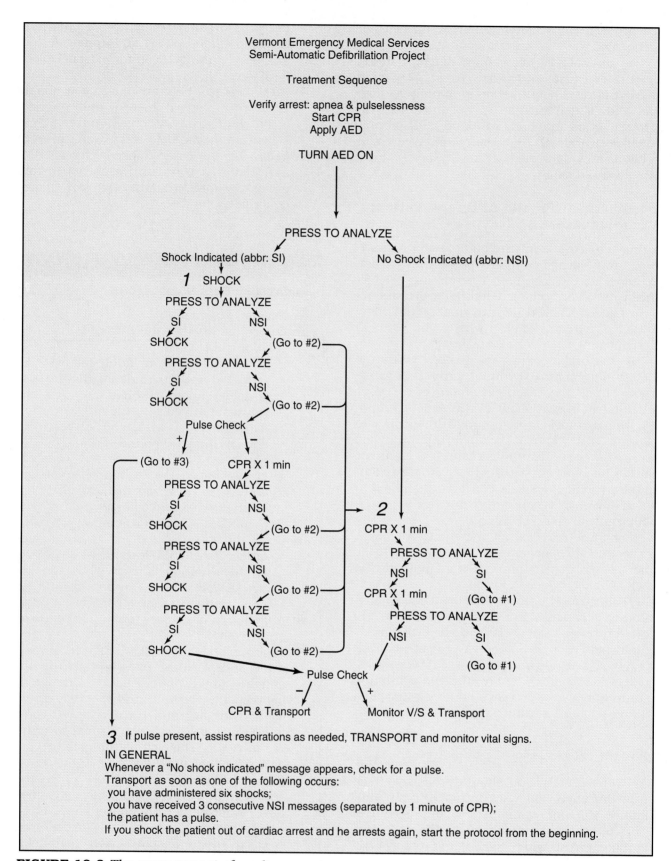

FIGURE 18-6 The management of cardiac arrest.

Note: No chart can show all possible sequences of events. The above is a general guide. Adapted from material originally provided by First Medic SpaceLabs.

Scan 18-3
Cardiac Arrest Assessment and Management

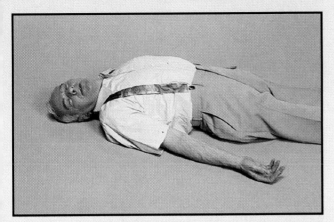

1. On arrival, briefly question those present about arrest events. (If a rescuer already on the scene is performing CPR, direct him to stop CPR.)

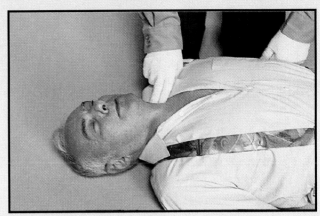

2. Verify absence of spontaneous pulse.

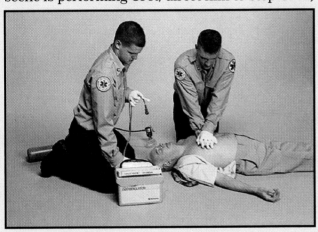

3. One EMT-B provides CPR while other sets up AED (automated external defibrillator).

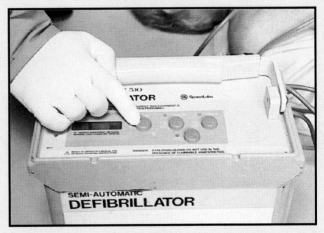

4. Turn on the AED power.

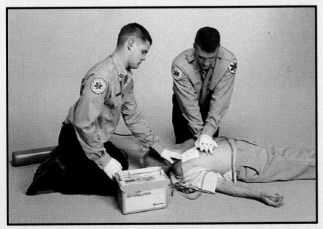

5. Connect two defibrillator pads to cables, following color code. Remove backing. Place one pad on upper right chest, one on lower left ribs.

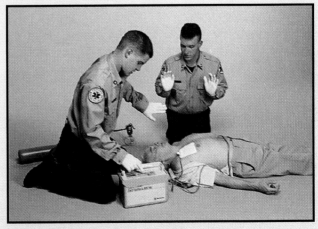

6. Say "Clear!" Ensure that all individuals are clear of patient.

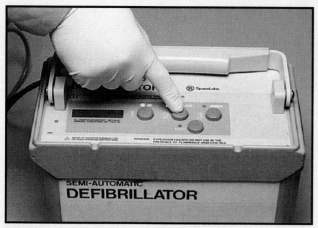

7. After everyone is clear, press the analysis button. Wait for the machine to analyze the rhythm.

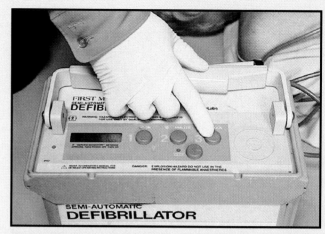

8. If advised by the defibrillator, press button to deliver shock. Repeat analysis and shock delivery until 3 shocks have been delivered.

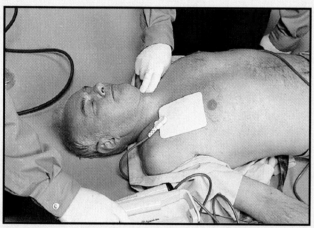

9. Check carotid pulse. Verify presence or absence of spontaneous pulse.

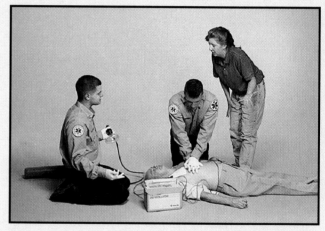

10. If pulse is absent, direct resumption of CPR. Gather additional information on arrest events.

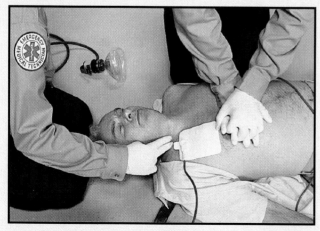

11. Check pulse during CPR to confirm effectiveness of CPR compressions.

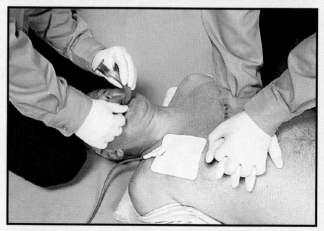

12. Direct insertion of airway adjunct.

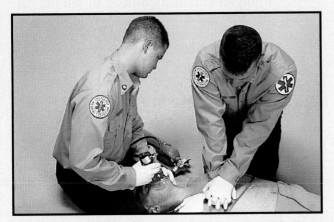

13. Direct ventilation of patient with high concentration oxygen.

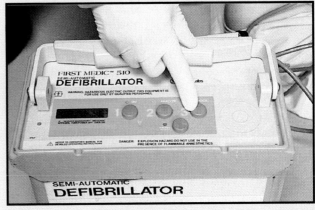

14. After 1 minute of CPR, have all individuals stand clear and repeat sequence of 3 analyses and shocks by AED.

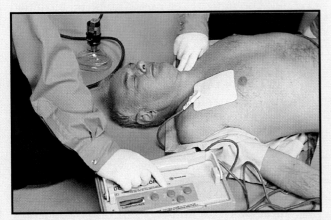

15. Check carotid pulse.

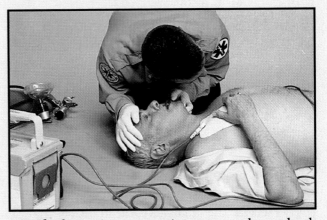

16. If there is a spontaneous pulse, check patient's breathing.

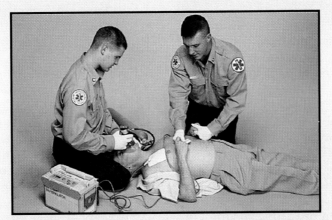

17. If breathing is adequate, provide high concentration oxygen by nonrebreather mask. If breathing is inadequate, ventilate patient with high concentration oxygen. Transport without delay.

Note: At earliest oportunity, call for ALS intercept.

Note: As noted earlier, about half of all patients in cardiac arrest have nonshockable heart rhythms. If this is the case, when you press the analysis button, the AED will give a "No shock" message. In other cases, the AED may give you a "Deliver shock" message and then, after one or more shocks are delivered, will give a "No shock" message on a subsequent try. (When the AED gives a "No shock" message, it may be very bad news—the patient has a nonshockable heart rhythm and cannot be helped by the defibrillator. Or it may be very good news—the electrical rhythm of the patient's heart has responded successfully to earlier shocks. In the latter case, even though the heart's electrical activity has recovered, another stint of CPR may be required to get enough oxygen into the muscle cells of the heart to start it beating again.)

Numbers 8 to 12 of the list you are now reading will explain how to proceed if you get a "Deliver shock" message every time you press the analysis button.

Number 13 will explain how to proceed if you get a "No shock" message when you press the analysis button.

If a "Deliver shock" message is received each time analysis button is pressed . . .

8 When you get a "Deliver shock" message

- Deliver the first shock.
- Press the analysis button to re-analyze the rhythm (get a "Deliver shock" message), deliver a second shock.
- Press the analysis button to re-analyze the rhythm (get a "Deliver shock" message), deliver a third shock.

The set of shocks you have just delivered is called a "set of three stacked shocks"—"stacked" because they are delivered with no pause for a pulse check or CPR between the three shocks.

9 After the first set of three stacked shocks, check the carotid pulse. If the patient has a pulse, check breathing.
   a. If the patient is breathing adequately, give high concentration oxygen by nonrebreather mask and transport.
   b. If the patient is not breathing adequately, provide artificial ventilations with high concentration oxygen and transport.

10 Repeat a cycle of three stacked shocks.

11 If the patient does not have a pulse, resume CPR for 1 minute. (Do not waste time checking the pulse again after the 1 minute of CPR. If there is a pulse, the AED will give you a "No shock" message.)

- Press the analysis button to analyze the rhythm (get a "Deliver shock" message), deliver the fourth shock.
- Press the analysis button to re-analyze the rhythm (get a "Deliver shock" message), deliver a fifth shock.
- Press the analysis button to re-analyze the rhythm (get a "Deliver shock" message), deliver a sixth shock.

You have now completed the second set of three stacked shocks.

12 Assuming there is no on-scene ACLS (such as paramedics), you should transport the patient when <u>any one</u> of the following occurs.
   a. The patient regains a pulse (determined during the pulse check before CPR or after the AED gives a "No shock" message), or . . .
   b. Six shocks have been delivered (two sets of three stacked shocks), or . . .
   c. The machine gives three consecutive messages (separated by one minute of CPR) that no shock is advised.

If a "No shock" message is received when analysis button is pressed . . .

13 After *any* rhythm analysis (whether the first time the analysis button is pushed or when the analysis button is pushed after one or more shocks have already been delivered), if the machine advises "No shock," check the pulse.
   a. If the patient has a pulse, check breathing.
      1. If the patient is breathing adequately, give high concentration oxygen by nonrebreather mask and transport.
      2. If the patient is not breathing adequately, artificially ventilate with high concentration oxygen and transport.
   b. If the patient has no pulse, resume CPR for one minute, then . . .
      1. Analyze the rhythm a second time. If the AED gives a "Deliver shock" message, deliver up to two sets of three stacked shocks (a total of six shocks), with one minute of CPR separating

the two sets. (Do not deliver more than a total of six shocks, including those you gave before receiving the "No shock" message. Consider that your first sequence was interrupted by the "No shock" message and now, having received a "Deliver shock message," you are going to continue the sequence. This will be your second try at completing the sequence of six shocks.)

2. If you get a "No shock" message at any point during the sequence and there is no pulse, resume CPR for one minute. Analyze the rhythm a third time. If the AED gives a "Deliver shock" message, deliver up to two sets of three stacked shocks separated by one minute of CPR. (Do not deliver more than a total of six shocks, including all those already delivered to this point. This will be your third try at completing the sequence of six shocks.) If you get a "No shock" message again, if there is no pulse, resume CPR and transport. Do not request any further analysis or deliver any further shocks with the AED machine.

Remember: If at any time you get a "No shock" message and determine that the patient has a pulse, check the patient's breathing. If breathing is adequate, provide high concentration oxygen by nonrebreather mask and transport. If breathing is inadequate, provide artificial ventilations with high concentration oxygen and transport.

General Principles of AED Use

- One EMT-B operates the defibrillator, one does CPR. This prevents the EMT-B who is operating the defibrillator from being distracted.
- Defibrillation comes first. Don't hook up oxygen or do anything that delays analysis of the rhythm or defibrillation.
- You must be familiar with the particular model of AED used in your area.
- All contact with the patient must be avoided during analysis of the rhythm.
- State "Clear!" and be sure everyone is clear of the patient before delivering every shock.
- No defibrillator is capable of working without properly functioning batteries. Check

the batteries at the beginning of your shift and carry an extra.
- If you have delivered six shocks (a rare occurrence) and you have no ALS back-up, you should prepare the patient for transport. You may deliver additional shocks at the scene or en route if local medical direction approves.
- An automated external defibrillator cannot analyze a rhythm in a moving emergency vehicle. You must completely stop the vehicle in order to analyze the rhythm if more shocks are ordered.
- It is not safe to defibrillate in a moving ambulance.
- Pulse checks should not occur during rhythm analysis. Typically there will be no pulse check after shocks 1 and 2 and shocks 4 and 5. Checking a pulse at these times would slow down defibrillation and is not necessary. If the AED makes a mistake, it is much more likely to fail to give a shock than it is to give an inappropriate shock.

Coordination with ALS Personnel

You do not need to have an advanced life support (ALS) team at the scene in order to use an AED, but the sooner the patient receives advanced cardiac life support (ACLS), the greater the patient's chance of survival. If you have an ALS team available, you should notify them of the arrest as soon as possible (preferably before you even arrive on the scene). Whether you postpone transport and wait for the ALS team at the scene or start transport and rendezvous with them should be in local protocols approved by your medical director. Your actions may depend on the location of the arrest and the estimated time of arrival of the ALS team.

If the ALS team arrives before you have finished the first cycle of stacked shocks, they should allow you to complete a cycle of three shocks. They should then institute the advanced care that they can give. They may allow you to defibrillate later, but that will be their decision. Since they are the most highly trained providers at the scene, they are responsible for the overall care of the patient.

Post Resuscitation Care

After you have run through the automated external defibrillation protocol, the patient will be in one of three conditions. (1) The patient may have a pulse. In this case, you will need to keep a close eye on his airway and be aggressive in keeping it open. You should keep the defibrillator on the patient during transportation in case the patient goes back into arrest. En route, you should perform a focused assessment based on what the patient tells you is bothering him and perform an ongoing assessment every five minutes. (2) If the patient has no pulse, the AED will have given you a "no shock indicated" message or (3) the AED may be prompting you to analyze the rhythm because it "thinks" there is a shockable rhythm. In either case, you will need to resume CPR. (You will not perform further defibrillation once you have completed the six shocks of the AED protocol unless the patient has recovered a pulse and then, later, goes back into cardiac arrest—see below).

For all of these patients, you will need to use the techniques of lifting and moving that you learned in Chapter 6. You will also need to consider how and where to meet ALS back-up (if available).

Patients Who Go Back into Cardiac Arrest

A patient who has been resuscitated from cardiac arrest is at high risk of going back into arrest. This change may be difficult to detect since most patients who have just been resuscitated are unconscious and many of them will need assisted ventilation. Since you are breathing for the patient, you may not notice that he no longer has a pulse. This is why, on unconscious patients who have recovered a pulse, you should check the pulse frequently (approximately every 30 seconds). A fully automated AED may alert you that it "thinks" the patient has a shockable rhythm. If you get such a prompt from the defibrillator, check for a pulse immediately. If you find that there is no pulse, then

1. If you are en route, stop the vehicle.
2. Have someone else start CPR if the AED is not immediately ready.
3. Analyze the rhythm.
4. Deliver a shock if indicated.
5. Continue with two sets of three stacked shocks separated by a minute of CPR or as your local protocol directs.

Witnessed Arrests in the Ambulance

Occasionally, you will be transporting a conscious patient with chest pain who becomes unconscious, pulseless, and apneic (not breathing). Although there are no guarantees, you have a very good chance of getting this patient back because you can defibrillate very shortly after the patient goes into a shockable rhythm. If this happens, you should stop the vehicle and treat him like any other patient in cardiac arrest.

Single Rescuer with an AED

Some EMT-Bs will be alone or have no one else nearby who can do CPR when they reach the patient. If this happens, the sequence of steps to take changes slightly. Since CPR is a way of supporting the body's organs until defibrillation is available, it makes little sense to start CPR instead of using the AED. In this situation, you should

1. Perform the initial assessment.
2. Assure pulselessness and apnea. Attempt ventilation, preferably with a pocket mask. Determine pulselessness but do not start chest compressions. In this way, you can be sure that the patient's arrest is not caused by a foreign body airway obstruction.
3. Turn on the AED and begin the narrative if the machine has a voice recorder.
4. Attach the device in the usual way.
5. Initiate analysis of the rhythm.
6. Deliver up to three shocks as advised by the AED.
7. Call for additional help, start CPR and follow your protocol. You should call for additional EMS help only after you get a "No shock" message, the patient regains a pulse, or you have delivered three shocks.

Contraindications

Unless your protocols state otherwise, you should apply an AED only to adult patients who are in cardiac arrest and have not suffered trauma prior to collapse. An adult, for the purpose of defibrillation, is someone who is over 12 years old or over 90 pounds. Neither children nor trauma patients will benefit from an AED.

The hearts of trauma patients in cardiac arrest are generally healthy. These patients are usually in arrest because they have lost too much blood. When this happens, the patient rarely goes into a shockable rhythm. Even in the hospital, more attention is paid to restoring the patient's blood volume than his heart rhythm.

Usually, you can tell very easily that a patient is in cardiac arrest because of trauma, but sometimes it is not so clear. For example, you find an elderly man in cardiac arrest in a car that went off the road. Did he go off the road and then go into cardiac arrest because of injuries, or did he go into arrest first and then go off the road? You may have protocols that address this issue. Even if you do, you will still have to exercise some judgment in determining how to treat the patient.

Children also have healthy hearts and rarely go into shockable rhythms. They do not need defibrillation—they need aggressive airway management and ventilation (with chest compressions) if they are to have any chance of survival.

Using an AED on either trauma patients or children will not help them. In fact, it will delay transport and the kind of treatment that may make a difference.

Safety

When you defibrillate a patient, you are delivering electrical current through a patient's chest. That current can be carried or conducted to you under certain conditions. Although it is unlikely to put you into cardiac arrest, this electricity can harm you. You can prevent this and other potentially harmful effects from occurring by following a few basic principles.

Do not defibrillate a soaking wet patient. Water is a very good conductor of electricity, so either dry the patient's chest or move him out of the wet environment (bring him inside, away from the rain).

Do not defibrillate the patient if he is touching anything metallic that other people are also touching. Metal is also a very good conductor of electricity. This means that you must be careful if the patient is on a metal floor or deck, and that you must make sure no one is touching the stretcher when you deliver a shock. It is also a good idea to make sure no one is touching anything, including a bag-valve-mask, that is in contact with the patient.

If you see a nitroglycerin patch on the patient's chest, remove it carefully before defibrillating. The plastic in the patch (not the nitroglycerin) may explode from the rapid melting that a defibrillatory shock can cause. This problem has been reported only when the patch is on the chest. Be sure to wear gloves when you remove the patch. It is designed to release nitroglycerin through the skin, and it will not discriminate between the patient's skin and yours.

The last thing you need at a cardiac arrest is a headache from nitroglycerin.

Be absolutely sure that before every shock you say "Clear!" and look from the patient's head to his toes to ensure no one is touching the patient or any conductive material that the patient is touching.

Cardiac Pacemakers When the heart's natural pacemaker does not function properly, an artificial pacemaker can be surgically implanted to perform the same function. This pacemaker helps the heart beat in a normal, coordinated function. A pacemaker is often placed below one of the clavicles, is visible as a small lump, and can be palpated. If you notice a lump under a clavicle, do not put a defibrillation pad over it. Try to put the pad at least several inches away while staying in the general area where you want the pad.

Implanted Defibrillators Cardiologists are sometimes able to identify patients who are at a high risk of going into ventricular fibrillation. These patients sometimes receive a miniature defibrillator surgically implanted in the chest. When the patient develops this lethal cardiac rhythm, the implanted defibrillator detects it and shocks the patient. These implanted devices are not as common as pacemakers but may be observed in the field. Since these defibrillators are directly attached to the heart, low energy levels are used for each shock. This should not pose a threat to the EMT-B. Emergency care and CPR for this patient are the same as for other cardiac patients.

Operating a Fully Automatic Defibrillator

A fully automatic defibrillator will assess the patient's rhythm and determine whether a shock is needed. If it senses that a shock is needed, a fully automatic defibrillator will automatically charge to a preset energy level and deliver the shock, all without any further action by the rescuer. Some models of fully automatic defibrillators have only two controls: an ON button and an OFF button. Fully automatic defibrillators also make use of voice synthesizers to verbally announce instructions and warnings such as "STOP CPR" and "STAND BACK" and "CHECK BREATHING AND PULSE."

Operating a fully automatic defibrillator is very similar to operating a semiautomatic defibrillator. You start with the initial assessment, begin CPR, turn on the machine, and attach it to the patient. The defibrillator will announce "STOP CPR" and begin analyzing the patient's rhythm. If a shock is indicated, the fully automatic defibrillator will repeatedly announce "STAND BACK," charge to 200 joules of energy, and deliver the shock. Do not touch or move the patient when you hear the warning "STAND BACK."

Remain clear of the patient. Immediately following delivery of the first shock, the fully automatic defibrillator will again analyze the rhythm. If the patient still has a rhythm for which a shock is indicated, the defibrillator will once again warn "STAND BACK" and charge to 200-300 joules of energy. The second shock will be delivered as soon as the charging process is complete.

Continue to remain clear of the patient. The process continues automatically until the third shock of 360 joules has been delivered or until the patient has a rhythm for which a shock is not indicated.

After three shocks have been delivered or if the patient has a rhythm that should not be shocked, the defibrillator will announce "CHECK BREATHING AND PULSE" and then enter an inactive monitoring mode. At this point, check for a spontaneous pulse and breathing.

If a pulse is present, immediately prepare the patient for transportation to a hospital. Leave the defibrillator connected to the patient. Continue life-support measures as necessary, including the administration of oxygen and assisting ventilations.

If there is no pulse, leave the defibrillator connected and resume CPR. After 60 seconds the fully automatic defibrillator will prompt you to "STOP CPR," following which it will again analyze the patient's rhythm. If a shock is indicated, the defibrillator will warn you to "STAND BACK" and then deliver up to three more shocks.

If a shock is not indicated or after the three additional shocks have been delivered, the fully automatic defibrillator will prompt you to "CHECK BREATHING AND PULSE," following which it will enter a perpetual monitoring mode. If there is no pulse, perform CPR. If the patient has a pulse, continue preparations for transportation.

During the perpetual monitoring mode, the fully automatic defibrillator will continually assess the patient's heart rhythm, although it will not be able to deliver additional shocks without further action on your part, even if a rhythm

develops for which a shock is indicated. If this should happen, you will hear a beep followed by the prompt "CHECK BREATHING AND PULSE." Stop immediately if you are performing CPR and carefully check for a spontaneous pulse and regular respirations. If there is no pulse, clear the area, press the ON button, and repeat the steps outlined above.

Remember: Not all models of fully automatic defibrillators function in exactly the same manner as described here. Consult the user's manual for the defibrillator you will be using for accurate and detailed instructions.

Advantages of Automated External Defibrillation

Only fifteen years ago, it was unthinkable for EMT-Bs to defibrillate patients in cardiac arrest. Now, EMT-Bs are expected to be trained and equipped to perform this potentially life-saving intervention. Probably the biggest reason this situation has changed is the improvement in technology that allows defibrillators to quickly and accurately determine whether a patient's rhythm is shockable.

This means that initial training and continuing education are much easier and simpler than that required for manual defibrillation in which the operator has to be able to read and analyze the heart rhythms that the AED does automatically. This is especially true in areas where EMT-Bs see few cardiac arrests, e.g., rural areas. Automated defibrillation is actually easier to learn and remember than CPR. This does not mean, though, that EMT-Bs are "well programmed robots." They still must carefully perform an initial assessment to assure that the patient is in cardiac arrest, they must memorize the treatment sequence, and they must always act with the safety of the patient and others in mind.

Another advantage of automated defibrillation is the speed of the procedure. An EMT-B can deliver the first shock within one minute of arrival at the patient's side. This is difficult to do with manual defibrillation.

Automation also requires that the operator defibrillate through adhesive pads instead of paddles. This is safer and allows for more accurate and consistent electrode placement. Since the operator does not have to hold paddles on the patient's chest, there is almost no chance of "arcing," the passage of electrical current outside the chest from too little paddle pressure. Certainly, the level of anxiety of the EMT-B is lower when he can push a button to deliver a shock instead of holding charged paddles on a patient's chest.

Some automated defibrillators may allow for monitoring of the rhythm of patients who are not in cardiac arrest. This can be confusing for the EMT-B since he is not trained in rhythm recognition and cannot treat any nonshockable rhythms anyway. A rhythm screen can be very distracting and take your attention away from the patient, where it belongs. If you monitor patients with chest pain or difficulty breathing, you should make sure that this is allowed by your medical director.

The Importance of Speed

Recall that a major factor in the survival of a person who is in cardiac arrest is the amount of time that elapses from the moment of collapse until the start of defibrillation. This time period has four phases.

1. EMS access time
2. Dispatch time
3. Ambulance response time
4. Assessment and shock time

For an EMS system to be effective, each of these time segments must be as short as possible (Table 18-1).

EMS Access Time   This is the time that passes from the time a person collapses in cardiac arrest until someone notifies the EMS system. A person who collapses in front of another person (witnessed arrest) should have a far greater chance of survival than a person who collapses in an isolated place away from other people; the person seeing the collapse can call for an ambulance. That someone sees a person collapse in cardiac arrest is no guarantee that an ambulance will be called immediately, however. In fact, most witnesses to a collapse delay calling for an ambulance for 2 minutes or more, and many delay calling for 4 to 6 minutes and longer.

Obviously, members of the public should be trained in CPR. But the public should also be trained to call for an ambulance immediately upon seeing someone collapse, even though they know CPR. Any delay in activating the community EMS system results in delayed defibrillation.

Dispatch Time   The second phase of a defibrillation effort begins with receipt of the call for help by a dispatcher and ends with the alerting of an ambulance crew. This time segment should be kept as short as possible. The dispatcher rapidly determines whether the call is for a cardiac problem (by asking the caller about difficult breathing, unconsciousness, unresponsiveness, and the like). Then the dispatcher immediately sends out an emergency medical service unit with a defibrillator. Once this is done, the dispatcher acquires additional information from the caller while the ambulance is on the way.

TABLE 18-1   Minimizing the Time from Collapse to Defibrillation

Time Component	Objective	Goal	Method
EMS access time	To minimize the time from collapse until someone places a call for help	1.0 min	An increased community awareness of the need for quickly calling for an ambulance; more public CPR programs
Dispatch time	To minimize the time it takes for an EMS dispatcher to elicit information from a caller and get a defibrillator-equipped unit on the road	.5 min	Better dispatcher training; improved call handling procedures
Response time	To minimize the time it takes to get a trained defibrillator team to the patient	3.0 min	Strategic placement of automated defibrillators with first-response personnel
Shock time	To minimize the time it takes to deliver the first shock	1.5 min	Use automated defibrillators; continually practice to maintain peak efficiency

Ambulance Response Time The third phase of the collapse-to-defibrillation period is the time from dispatch until the ambulance arrives at the location of the stricken person. Ambulance response time varies considerably from community to community, as well as from one area to another within large communities. Response times are often long in large cities where congested streets are a problem and in small communities where volunteers must respond to the ambulance garage from homes and places of business. The fastest ambulance response times are generally in towns and small cities that are large enough to have an ambulance service that is staffed around the clock by in-station crews, but small enough that traffic and response distances are not problems.

One way to shorten the time from dispatch to the arrival of a defibrillator in communities that do not have in-station crews is to station and equip a trained EMT in the community with an AED 24 hours a day. Thus, when a call for a potential cardiac problem is received, that trained individual can respond directly to the scene with the defibrillator while other EMTs respond to the station to get the ambulance. This approach works. In one group of small communities, the time it took to get a defibrillator on the road was reduced from 7.5 minutes to 2.5 minutes. Placing automated defibrillators with first responders in large cities has proved equally effective in reducing the response time of a trained individual with a defibrillator.

Assessment and Shock Time The final phase of a defibrillation period is the time that elapses from the time that a rescuer arrives at the side of the stricken person to the time the first shock is delivered. As with each of the other phases of the collapse to-defibrillation period, this time segment must be kept as short as possible if lifesaving efforts are to be effective—ideally 1 minute or less.

The shorter the collapse-to-defibrillation time, the greater the chance for survival. A person who can be shocked in 4 to 6 minutes or less after collapse has a good chance of surviving. A person who cannot be shocked within 8 minutes of the moment of collapse has only a slim chance of surviving.

Because the ambulance response time alone approaches 8 minutes in many communities, the importance of implementing creative approaches to shortening the various components of the time from collapse to shock cannot be overemphasized. The goals listed in Table 18-1, if achieved, should result in a witnessed VF survival rate of 25% or higher.

Defibrillator Maintenance

Because human error is so common, the U. S. Food and Drug Administration convened a panel of experts to review reports of defibrillator malfunctions. The experts drafted a checklist of actions that the defibrillator operator should complete on each shift (Figure 18-7). One of the most common problems with AEDs has been battery failure. It is especially important that you make sure the battery is charged and that you have a spare with the defibrillator. A defibrillator with a dead battery helps no one.

You should use the checklist at the beginning of every shift in order to be sure that you have all the supplies you will need and that the AED is functioning properly. The time to discover a problem is before you need the defibrillator, not when you are at the scene of a cardiac arrest.

Quality Improvement

There are many ways you can evaluate and improve your ability to resuscitate patients in cardiac arrest. These methods should be part of your service's quality improvement (QI) program. The defibrillation part of your QI program involves a number of things, including medical direction, initial training, maintenance of skills, case review, trend analysis, and strengthening the links in the chain of survival. Every participant in the EMS system has a role to play in QI, whether it is the patient who comes back to thank you, the physician who praises you for a job well done, the nurse who follows up on the patient's in-hospital course, or the EMT-B who uses the defibrillator and then documents the call.

Medical direction is an essential component of any defibrillation program. The medical director needs to be involved with all aspects of the program. This includes equipment selection (e.g., whether to get an AED with a voice recorder), initial training and evaluation, case review, continuing education, and skill maintenance. The EMT-B defibrillates under the medical director's license to practice medicine, so the medical director has a strong motivation to be involved.

An EMT-B who completes AED training in an EMT-Basic course is allowed to defibrillate

AUTOMATED DEFIBRILLATORS: OPERATOR'S SHIFT CHECKLIST

Date: _____ Shift: _____ Location: _____

Mfr/Model No.: _____ Serial No. or Facility ID No.: _____

At the beginning of each shift, inspect the unit. Indicate whether all requirements have been met. Note any corrective actions taken. Sign the form.

	Okay as found	Corrective Action/Remarks
1. Defibrillator Unit Clean, no spills, clear of objects on top, casing intact		
2. Cables/Connectors a. Inspect for cracks, broken wire, or damage b. Connectors engage securely		
3. Supplies a. Two sets of pads in sealed packages, within expiration date * g. Spare charged battery b. Hand towel * h. Adequate ECG paper c. Scissors * i. Manual override module, key, or card d. Razor * e. Alcohol wipes * j. Cassette tape, memory module, and/or event card plus spares * f. Monitoring electrodes		
4. Power Supply a. Battery-powered units (1) Verify fully charged battery in place (2) Spare charged battery available (3) Follow appropriate battery rotation schedule per manufacturer's recommendations b. AC/Battery backup units (1) Plugged into live outlet to maintain battery charge (2) Test on battery power and reconnect to line power		
5. Indicators/*ECG Display * a. Remove cassette tape, memory module, and/or event card * e. "Service" message display off b. Power-on display * f. Battery charging; low battery light off c. Self-test ok g. Correct time displayed—set with dispatch center * d. Monitor display functional		
6. ECG Recorder a. Adequate ECG paper b. Recorder prints		
7. Charge/Display Cycle * a. Disconnect AC plug—battery backup units * e. Manual override functional b. Attach to simulator f. Detach from simulator c. Detects, charges, and delivers shock for "VF" * g. Replace cassette tape, module, and/or memory card d. Responds correctly to non-shockable rhythms		
8. *Pacemaker a. Pacer output cable intact c. Inspect per manufacturer's operational guidelines b. Pacer pads present (set of two)		
☐ **Major problem(s) identified** **(OUT OF SERVICE)**		

* *Applicable only if the unit has this supply or capability*

P/N CL6721-00
rev 1.6 auto, 8/8/91

Signature: _____

FIGURE 18-7 An AED checklist from Laerdal.

only under certain conditions. He must meet the requirements of state laws and regulations and the medical director.

One of the best ways to improve your performance is by looking at how you performed when you actually managed an arrest. Every time an EMT-B uses an AED, the medical director or his designated representative must review the case. This can be done through several means, including the written report, voice ECG tape recorders in certain models of AED, and solid-state memory modules and magnetic tape recordings stored in the machine. The report should evaluate the timeliness of the EMT-B's actions, the accuracy of the machine, and any other factors that affect survival. The EMT-B should receive a copy of the medical director's report or other feedback each time he uses an AED.

Most EMT-Bs will not use an AED very often. It becomes very easy, then, for EMT-Bs to forget what they learned about defibrillation. This is one of the reasons continuing education and skill maintenance are so important. These sessions should occur at least every 90 days and should include review of past cases, descriptions of changes in the program, and demonstration of cardiac arrest management and defibrillation. The American Heart Association publishes a variety of guidelines and additional information on automated external defibrillation.

An important part of a QI program is looking at patient outcomes. Since cardiac arrests are uncommon events, few services will have enough arrest cases over a reasonable period of time to be able to conclude how well they are doing. Data collection over large regions, or even states, will give a better idea of how well things are going and where improvements need to occur. All of this depends on EMS agencies collecting and submitting the right data to the right place. This means that the information EMT-Bs collect and document has far-reaching consequences.

● Infants and Children

Since children usually have healthy hearts, cardiac arrest in children is rarely the result of heart problems. Instead, it usually is caused by respiratory problems like foreign body airway obstruction or drowning. For this reason, airway management and artificial ventilation are the best way to resuscitate these patients. Children rarely go into shockable rhythms, so automated external defibrillation is not appropriate for cardiac arrest in children

under 12 years of age and less than 90 pounds. It will almost always result in delays to definitive in-hospital care and rarely help the patient.

Documentation Tip—Cardiac Arrests

Cardiac arrests are stressful, strenuous calls, but after you have caught your breath and you are filling out your PCR, you should remember to document what you did and the patient's response to it. For example, it is a good idea to write that the patient's chest rose with ventilations and that a carotid pulse was palpable with chest compressions (assuming that that was the case).

FYI

Topics included in the FYI—"For Your Information"—section are those that go beyond the chapter objectives. The information in this segment is intended to broaden your understanding of the chapter topic but is not essential to an understanding of your job as an EMT-B.

The Nature of Cardiovascular Diseases

Most of the cardiovascular emergencies covered in this section are caused, directly or indirectly, by changes taking place in the inner walls of arteries. These arteries can be part of the systemic circulatory system, the pulmonary circulatory system, or the coronary system. Two conditions, atherosclerosis and arteriosclerosis, are involved in the changes found in these artery walls.

Atherosclerosis (ATH-er-o-skle-RO-sis) is a buildup of fatty deposits on the inner walls of arteries (Figure 18-8). This buildup causes a narrowing of the inner vessel diameter, restricting the flow of blood. Fats and other particles

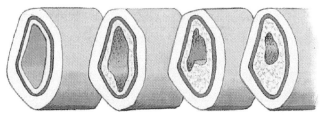

FIGURE 18-8 Atherosclerosis, the process of plaque formation.

combine to form this deposit, known as plaque. As time passes, calcium can be deposited at the site of the plaque, causing the area to harden. In **arteriosclerosis** (ar-TE-re-o-skle-RO-sis), the artery wall becomes hard and stiff due to calcium deposits. This hardening of the arteries causes the vessel to lose its elastic nature, changing blood flow and increasing blood pressure.

Throughout the entire process of both atherosclerosis and arteriosclerosis, the amount of blood passing through the artery is restricted. The rough surface formed inside the artery can lead to blood clots being formed, causing increased narrowing or occlusion (blockage) of the artery. The clot and debris from the plaque form a **thrombus** (THROM-bus). A thrombus can reach a size where it occludes (cuts off) blood flow completely, or it may break loose to become an **embolism** (EM-bo-lizm) and move to occlude the flow of blood somewhere downstream in a smaller artery. In cases of partial or complete blockage, the tissues beyond the point of blockage will be starved of oxygen and may die. If this blockage involves a large area of the heart or brain, the results may be quickly fatal (Figure 18-9).

Another cause of cardiovascular system disorder stems from weakened sections in the arterial walls. Each weak spot that begins to dilate (balloon) is known as an **aneurysm** (AN-u-rizm). This weakening can be related to other arterial diseases, or it can exist independently.

When a weakened section of an artery bursts, there can be rapid, life-threatening internal bleeding (Figure 18-10). Tissues beyond the rupture can be damaged because oxygenated blood they need is escaping and not reaching them. If a major artery ruptures, death from shock can occur very quickly. When an artery in the brain ruptures, a severe form of stroke occurs. The severity is dependent on the site of the stroke and the amount of blood loss.

Most AMI victims experience some sort of **arrhythmia** (ah-RITH-me-ah). Some of the arrhythmias associated with AMI include

- **Asystole** (ay-SIS-to-le) cardiac standstill, sometimes called flatline
- **Ventricular fibrillation** (ven-TRIK-u-lar fib-ri-LAY-shun) when the ventricles no longer beat with a full, steady, symmetrical pattern. Instead of producing a forceful contraction, the heart muscle quivers. This arrhythmia is common in adult AMI patients and may respond to defibrillation.
- **Bradycardia** (BRAY-di-KAR-de-ah) when the heart rate is slow, usually below 60 beats per minute.
- **Tachycardia** (tak-e-KAR-de-ah) when the heart rate is fast, above 100 beats per minute.

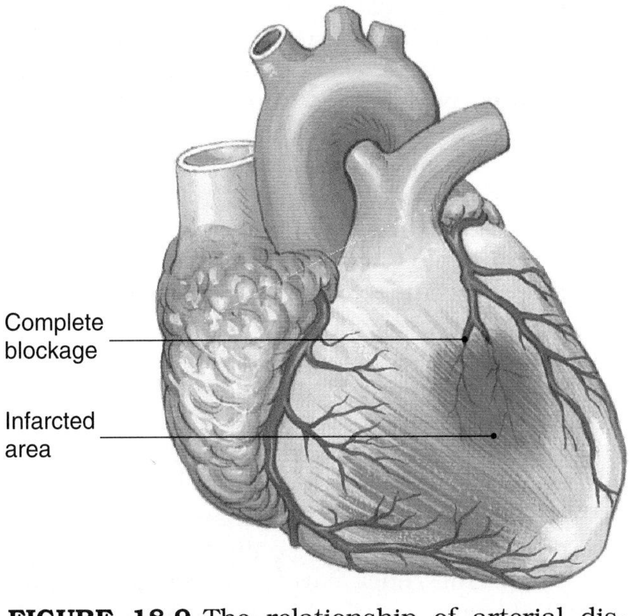

Complete blockage

Infarcted area

FIGURE 18-9 The relationship of arterial disease and heart disease.

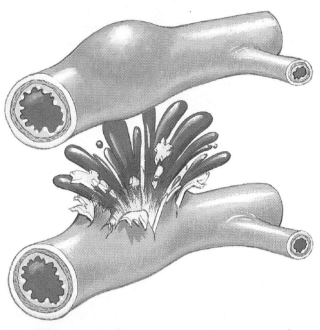

FIGURE 18-10 Formation and rupture of an aneurysm. A weakened area in the wall of an artery will tend to balloon out, forming a sac-like aneurysm, which may eventually burst.

Congestive Heart Failure

Congestive heart failure may be brought on by diseased heart valves, hypertension, or some form of obstructive pulmonary disease such as emphysema. CHF is often a complication of AMI. Congestive heart failure often progresses as follows.

1. A patient sustains an AMI. Myocardium in the area of the left ventricle dies. (Recall the function of the heart: The left is the side of the heart that receives oxygenated blood from the lungs and pulmonary circulation and pumps it to the rest of the body.)

2. Because of the damage to the left ventricle, blood backs up into the pulmonary circulation and then the lungs. Fluid accumulation in the lungs is called **pulmonary edema.** This edema causes a poor exchange of oxygen between the lungs and the bloodstream and the patient experiences shortness of breath or **dyspnea.** Listening to this patient's lungs with a stethoscope may reveal crackling or bubbly lung sounds called rales. Some patients cough up blood-tinged sputum from their lungs.

3. Left heart failure, if untreated, commonly causes right heart failure. The right side of the heart (which receives blood from the body and pumps it to the lungs) becomes congested because the clogged lungs cannot receive more blood. In turn, fluids may accumulate in the dependent (lower) extremities, the liver, and the abdomen. Accumulation of fluid at the feet or ankles is known as **pedal edema.** The abdomen may become noticeably distended, a condition known as **ascites** (as-SI-tez). In a bedridden patient, fluid collects in the sacral area of the spine.

Signs and Symptoms
- Tachycardia (rapid pulse, 100 beats per minute or more)
- Dyspnea (shortness of breath)
- Normal or elevated blood pressure
- Cyanosis
- Diaphoresis (profuse sweating), or cool and clammy skin
- Pulmonary edema, sometimes coughing up of frothy white or pink sputum
- Anxiety or confusion due to hypoxia (inadequate supply of oxygen to the brain and other tissues) caused by poor oxygen/carbon dioxide exchange
- Edema of the lower extremities
- Engorged, pulsating neck veins (late sign)
- Enlarged liver and spleen, with abdominal distention (late sign)

The CHF patient may be on medications for this condition. Often patients will tell you that they take a water pill for fluid buildup. This refers to a diuretic, a medication that helps remove fluid from the circulatory system. Other medications may increase the strength of the cardiac contraction to counteract the heart failure.

Electronic Implants and Bypass Surgery

With the rapidly expanding medical technology available, the EMT-B may be presented with patients who have undergone surgeries or had special electronic devices implanted in the body. The ABCs (including rescue breathing and CPR) and appropriate oxygen delivery will not change because of prior surgery or conditions. Some of the patients and devices you may observe in the field are

- Cardiac Pacemaker—Occasionally pacemakers malfunction. Although this situation is rare, it is possible. A malfunctioning pacemaker usually results in a slow or irregular pulse. The patient may have signs of shock due to the fact the heart isn't beating properly. Pacemaker failure can be life threatening. Care for patients with implanted pacemakers and signs of a cardiac emergency is the same as for those without a pacemaker. Arrange for ALS intercept and transport immediately.
- Cardiac Bypass Surgery—The coronary artery bypass has become a relatively common procedure in cardiac surgery. A blood vessel from another part of the body is surgically implanted to bypass an occluded coronary artery. This helps restore blood flow to a section of the myocardium. Should a patient with a suspected AMI tell you that he has had bypass surgery, or if you observe a midline surgical scar on the chest of an unconscious patient, provide the same emergency care and CPR as for any other patient.

CHAPTER REVIEW

KEY TERMS

You may find it helpful to review the following terms.

acute myocardial infarction (ah-KUTE MY-o-KARD-e-ul in-FARK-shun) **(AMI)** the condition in which a portion of the myocardium dies as a result of oxygen starvation; often called a heart attack by lay persons.

aneurysm (AN-u-rizm) the dilation, or ballooning, of a weakened section of the wall of an artery.

angina pectoris (AN-ji-nah [*or* an-JI-nah] PEK-to-ris) pain in the chest, occurring when blood supply to the heart is reduced and a portion of the heart muscle is not receiving enough oxygen.

apnea (AP-ne-ah) no breathing.

arrhythmia (ah-RITH-me-ah) a disturbance in heart rate and rhythm.

arteriosclerosis (ar-TE-re-o-skle-RO-sis) a condition in which artery walls become hard and stiff due to calcium deposits.

ascites (a-SI-tez) Notable distention of the abdomen.

asystole (ay-SIS-to-le) when the heart has ceased generating electrical impulses.

atherosclerosis (ATH-er-o-skle-RO-sis) a build-up of fatty deposits on the inner walls of arteries.

bradycardia (BRAY-di-KAR-de-ah) when the heart rate is slow, usually below 60 beats per minute.

cardiac compromise any heart problem.

congestive heart failure (CHF) the failure of the heart to pump efficiently, leading to excessive blood or fluids in the lungs, the body, or both.

coronary artery disease (CAD) diseases that affect the arteries of the heart.

dyspnea (DISP-ne-ah) shortness of breath; labored or difficult breathing.

embolism (EM-bo-lizm) a thrombus, or clot of blood and plaque, that has broken loose from the wall of an artery.

nitroglycerin a medication that dilates the blood vessels.

occlusion (uh-KLU-zhun) blockage, as of an artery by fatty deposits.

pedal edema accumulation of fluid at the feet or ankles.

pulmonary edema accumulation of fluid in the lungs.

pulseless electrical activity (PEA) a condition in which the heart's electrical rhythm remains relatively normal, yet the mechanical pumping activity fails to follow the electrical activity, causing cardiac arrest.

sudden death a cardiac arrest that occurs within two hours of the onset of symptoms. The patient may have no prior symptoms of coronary artery disease.

tachycardia (tak-e-KAR-de-ah) when the heart rate is fast, above 100 beats per minute.

thrombus (THROM-bus) a clot formed of blood and plaque attached to the inner wall of an artery.

ventricular fibrillation (ven-TRIK-u-ler fib-ri-LAY-shun) **(VF)** a condition in which the heart's electrical impulses are disorganized, preventing the heart muscle from contracting normally.

ventricular tachycardia (ven-TRIK-u-ler tak-i-KAR-de-uh) **(V-Tach)** a condition in which the heartbeat is quite rapid; if rapid enough, ventricular tachycardia will not allow the heart's chambers to fill with enough blood between beats to produce blood flow sufficient to meet the body's needs.

SUMMARY

Patients with cardiac compromise can have many different presentations. Some complain of pressure or pain in the chest with difficulty breathing and a history of heart problems. Others may have just mild discomfort that they ignore for several hours or that goes away and returns. Between 10 and 20 percent of patients having heart attacks have no chest discomfort at all. Because of these many possibilities and because of the potentially severe complications of heart problems, it is important to have a high index of suspicion and treat patients with these symptoms for cardiac compromise. The treatment will not hurt them and may help them.

These patients need high concentration oxygen and prompt, safe transportation to definitive care. You may be able to assist patients who have their own nitroglycerin in taking it, thereby relieving pain and anxiety.

Every EMS system should strive to strengthen the links in the chain of survival. It is not enough just to provide AEDs and train people how to use them. Only if there is *early* access, *early* CPR, *early* defibrillation, and *early* advanced care will EMS systems be able to save as many patients as possible from cardiac arrest. All of these things must be integrated with a quality improvement system that provides superb initial training, strong medical direction, individual case review, and encouragement to provide excellent care.

REVIEW QUESTIONS

1. What position is best for a patient with
   a. difficulty breathing and a blood pressure of 110/70?
   b. chest pain and a blood pressure of 180/90?
2. What is the best way to transfer down a flight of stairs a patient with difficulty breathing, chest pressure, and a blood pressure of 160/100?
3. Describe how to "clear" a patient before administering a shock.
4. List three safety measures to keep in mind when using an AED.
5. List the steps in the application of an AED.

Application Question

- Evaluate the system you work or live in with respect to the chain of survival. Which links are strong and which need work? How successful is your system in resuscitating patients from cardiac arrest?

Some of the material in this chapter on defibrillation and the AED has been adapted from material written by Kenneth R. Stults, M.S., Director of The University of Iowa Hospitals and Clinics, Emergency Medical Services Learning Resources Center.

Diabetic Emergencies and Altered Mental Status

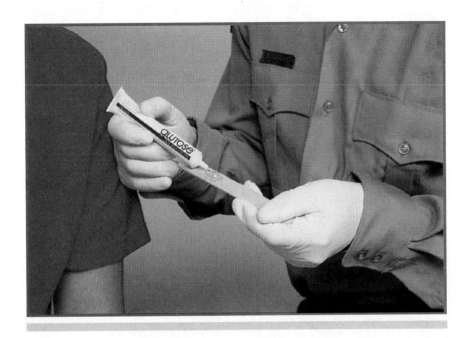

Diabetes is a prevalent disease in America. It has been estimated that between two and five percent of the population has either diagnosed or undiagnosed diabetes mellitus. When a diabetes patient has been diagnosed, is under a doctor's care, and is managing his condition, emergencies seldom arise. Diabetic emergencies most often result from a lapse in management of the disease. With prompt prehospital care, most diabetic emergencies can be successfully resolved.

Objectives

Knowledge and Attitude *At the end of this chapter, you should be able to meet the following objectives.*

1. Identify the patient taking diabetic medications with altered mental status and the implications of a diabetes history. (pp. 333–334)

2. State the steps in the emergency medical care of the patient taking diabetic medicine with an altered mental status and a history of diabetes. (pp. 333–337)

3. Establish the relationship between airway management and the patient with altered mental status. (pp. 332, 333, 334)

4. State the generic and trade names, medication forms, dose, administration, action, and contraindications for oral glucose. (p. 336)

5. Evaluate the need for medical direction in the emergency medical care of the diabetic patient. (p. 333)

6. Explain the rationale for administering oral glucose. (pp. 332, 336, 340)

On the Scene

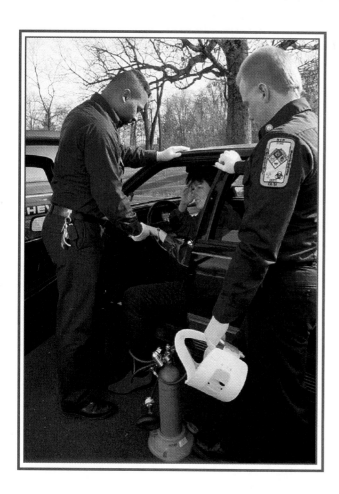

Twenty-five-year-old Rebecca Spicer begins to feel disoriented as she is driving. Before she knows it, she has run into the car in front of her. There isn't much damage, but as the driver of the other car comes back to see what happened, he notices that Rebecca appears intoxicated. "I knew it!" he mutters as he goes to call 911. The 911 dispatcher calls for both police and EMS response.

When you arrive, your ***scene size-up*** *tells* you that there is a mechanism of injury—the collision—but it doesn't seem to have been severe, and there is only one patient in view, a young woman at the wheel of one of the cars. You put on gloves and have your first-response kit with additional personal protective equipment handy in case there is severe trauma with blood and body fluids present. As you exit the ambulance, the other motorist hurries forward to tell you that the driver who caused the accident is drunk. The police officer on the scene tells you that, while Rebecca is acting "off the wall," he is not sure what the problem is. "Check her out and let me know if you smell alcohol," he says.

To begin your ***initial assessment,*** you approach Rebecca and introduce yourself. Rebecca slurs her words as she replies, "I'm almost there. Two more blocks, and it'll be on the right." You ask her name, and she replies, "Get out of the way! Can't you see I'm driving? How fast am I going?" Since the patient is talking and her breathing appears normal (without difficulty and between 8 and 24 times per minute), she has an open airway and is breathing adequately.

7. Identify causes and types of seizures. [supplemental] (pp. 337, 340–341)

8. Explain assessment and care procedures for seizures. [supplemental] (pp. 337–338)

Skills

1. Demonstrate the steps in the emergency medical care for the patient taking diabetic medicine with an altered mental status and a history of diabetes.

2. Demonstrate the steps in the administration of oral glucose.

3. Demonstrate the assessment and documentation of patient response to oral glucose.

4. Demonstrate how to complete a prehospital care report for patients with diabetic emergencies.

5. Demonstrate care of a seizure patient. [supplemental]

However, her mental status is altered. She is awake but confused, not oriented to person, place, or time. There is no sign of bleeding. You note that her pulse is rapid. Her skin is extremely sweaty.

Your partner begins manual stabilization of her head and neck as you begin your *focused history and physical exam.* As you begin the rapid trauma assessment, you find a necklace with a medical identification medallion. It confirms your suspicions that Rebecca is a diabetic. You advise the police officer of your findings.

You quickly take and record Rebecca's vital signs and prepare to give her oral glucose. You have confirmed the three criteria for giving this medication: Her medical identification necklace has revealed that she has a history of being diabetic, her mental status is altered, and she has an open airway and is able to swallow. You take a tube of oral glucose from your kit and persuade Rebecca to swallow the glucose.

The change in Rebecca's behavior is rapid. As she begins to return to her normal orientation, she explains that she had taken her insulin but had forgotten to eat. She thanks you profusely for pulling her out of hypoglycemia. It's a dangerous condition, but a satisfying one to treat. Few emergencies in the field have provided you the opportunity to care for a patient with such immediate and rewarding results.

Because she has been involved in a collision, your partner maintains manual stabilization of her head and neck as you complete your assessment, then put a cervical collar on her, immobilize her on a backboard, and transport her to the hospital with *ongoing assessment* en route. It turns out that she has not been seriously injured in the collision, and Rebecca vows, in the future, to remember to eat!

When you are called to the scene of a diabetic emergency, your task will not be to diagnose or treat diabetes but rather to recognize and treat a condition that diabetes, or the poor management of diabetes, can cause. The first indication that the patient is diabetic may be an altered mental status such as Rebecca's. There will often be other clues at the scene that the patient is a diabetic, such as Rebecca's medical identification necklace or the presence of insulin or other diabetic medication in the refrigerator or patient's purse, or information provided by family members, friends, or coworkers.

To do your job, you do not have to understand all the complications of diabetes but be ready to administer glucose if your assessment turns up a history of diabetes, an altered mental status, and assurance that the patient can swallow. However, having some information about diabetes and its possible effects can give you some perspective.

DIABETES

Glucose (GLU-kos), a form of sugar, is the body's basic source of energy. The sugars that a person eats are converted into glucose, which is then absorbed into the bloodstream. However, this blood sugar cannot simply pass from the bloodstream into the body's cells. To enter the cells, **insulin** (IN-suh-lin), a hormone produced by the pancreas, must be present. Without insulin the cells can be surrounded by glucose but still starve for this sugar. The insulin/glucose relationship has been described as a "lock and key" mechanism. Consider insulin the key. Without the insulin "key," glucose cannot enter the locked cells (Figure 19-1).

When sugar intake and insulin production are balanced, the body can effectively use sugar as an energy source. If, for some reason, insulin production decreases, the glucose cannot be used by the cells. This glucose remains in circulation, increasing in concentration as more sugars are digested by the person. The level of blood sugar climbs, eventually to be spilled over into the urine. High sugar leads to increased urine output, which in turn makes the patient abnormally thirsty.

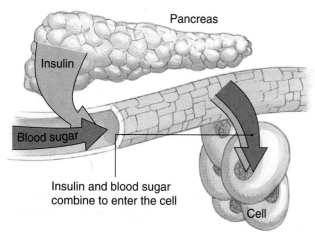

FIGURE 19-1 Insulin is needed to help the cells take in glucose.

The condition brought about by decreased insulin production is known as **diabetes mellitus** (di-ah-BEE-tez MEL-i-tus), or "sugar diabetes," often called just "diabetes." The person suffering from this condition is a diabetic.

Hypoglycemia

The most common medical emergency for the diabetic is a condition called **hypoglycemia,** or low blood sugar. (*Hypo* means "less than normal" or "deficient." *Glyc* means "sugar.") Hypoglycemia is caused when the diabetic

- takes too much insulin, (or, less commonly, oral medication used to treat diabetes), thereby putting too much sugar into the cells and leaving too little sugar in the blood, or . . .
- reduces sugar intake by not eating, or . . .
- over exercises or overexerts himself, thus using sugars faster than normal, or . . .
- vomits a meal, emptying the stomach of sugar as well as other food.

When sugar in the bloodstream is reduced by these causes, an altered mental status, possibly unconsciousness, can result. Permanent brain damage can occur quickly if the sugar is not replenished.

Rebecca, your patient in On the Scene, showed several typical signs of low blood sugar. Her condition came on in just a few minutes, so rapidly that she didn't even realize it was happening. Her skin was extremely sweaty. Her behavior was also abnormal. Like many diabetics whose blood sugar gets low, Rebecca became almost a completely different person. The hypoglycemic Rebecca was "off the wall" and could easily have been mistaken for someone who was drunk. The normal Rebecca, whom you saw after giving her glucose, is a pleasant, well-adjusted person who is rather embarrassed about what happened.

Rapid onset, abnormal behavior, and very sweaty skin are all typical of a sudden drop in blood sugar level and are indications of the need for prompt action by the EMT-B. Quick administration of glucose, when it can be done without threatening the airway (that is, if the patient is conscious and can swallow), is critical to this patient's outcome. Glucose must be given promptly, before the patient becomes unconscious.

Patient Assessment—Diabetic Emergencies

Prehospital treatment of the diabetic depends on rapid identification of the patient with an altered mental status and a history of diabetes. (See Scan 19-1.) To assess the patient

1. Perform the initial assessment. Identify altered mental status.
2. Perform a focused history and physical exam. In gathering the history of the present episode of altered mental status, attempt to discover from the patient or bystanders how the episode occurred, the time of onset, the duration, associated symptoms, any mechanism of injury or other evidence of trauma, whether there have been any interruptions to the episode, whether there have been seizures, whether the patient has a fever. In gathering the SAMPLE history attempt to determine
   - if the patient has a history of diabetes—by questioning the patient or bystanders, looking for medications, looking for a medical identification bracelet or other device
   - last meal
   - last medication dose
   - any related illness
   - whether the patient can swallow
3. Take baseline vital signs. (In some jurisdictions, oral glucose will be administered before the vital signs are taken.)

Signs and Symptoms

The following signs and symptoms are associated with a diabetic emergency.

- ☐ rapid onset of altered mental status
  - after missing a meal on a day the patient took prescribed insulin
  - after vomiting a meal on a day the patient took prescribed insulin
  - after an unusual amount of physical exercise or work
  - may occur with no identifiable predisposing factor
- ☐ Intoxicated appearance, staggering, slurred speech to complete unconsciousness
- ☐ Elevated heart rate
- ☐ Cold, clammy skin

- ☐ Hunger
- ☐ Seizures
- ☐ Insulin, or a trade name for insulin (Humulin, Lente) or an oral medication used to treat diabetes (Diabinese, Orinase, Micronase) found in refrigerator or at the scene
- ☐ Uncharacteristic behavior
- ☐ Anxiety
- ☐ Combativeness

Patient Care—Diabetic Emergencies

1. Give oral glucose in accordance with local protocol if *all three* of the following criteria are present (see Scans 19-1 and 19-2).
   - The patient has a history of diabetes, and . . .
   - The patient's mental status is altered, and . . .
   - The patient is awake enough to swallow.
   The glucose may be given by squeezing it from the tube onto a tongue depressor and placing it in the patient's mouth between the cheek and gum. Alternatively, if you think the patient is able to do so, let the patient squeeze the glucose from the tube directly into his mouth.
2. Reassess the patient.
   - If at any time the patient loses consciousness, remove the tongue depressor from his mouth and take steps to assure an open airway.
   - If the patient's condition does not improve, consult medical direction about whether to administer more glucose.
3. If the patient is not awake enough to swallow, treat him like any other patient with an altered mental status: Secure the airway, provide artificial ventilations if necessary, be prepared to perform CPR if needed. Position the patient appropriately. If the patient does not need to be ventilated, position him on his side so that he is less likely to choke on or to breathe fluids or vomitus into his lungs.

● Infants and Children

Children who have diabetes are more at risk for medical emergencies than adults. Children are more active than adults and may exhaust blood sugar levels—especially if they have taken their prescribed insulin—by playing

Scan 19-1
Diabetes Assessment and Management

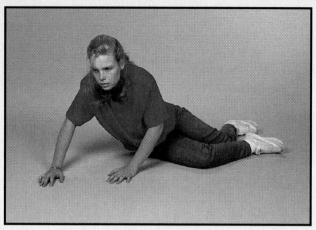

1. Perform an initial assessment. Determine if patient's mental status is altered.

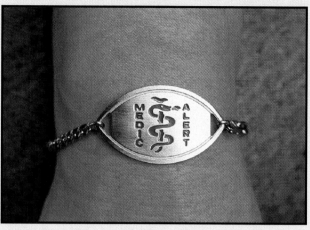

2. Obtain patient's history. Does patient have a history of diabetes?

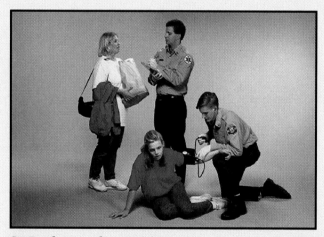

3. Perform a focused history and physical exam and take patient's vital signs.

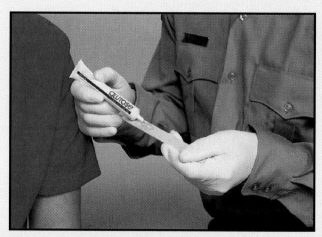

4. To administer oral glucose to a patient who is awake enough to swallow, squeeze glucose from tube onto tongue depressor.

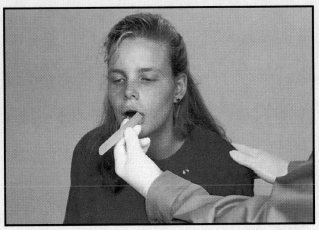

5. Insert the tongue depressor and oral glucose into patient's mouth between cheek and gum.

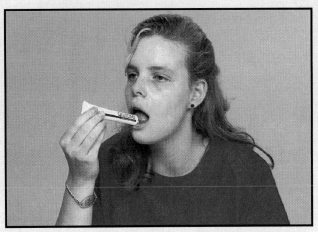

6. Alternatively, let patient squeeze the oral glucose into her own mouth.

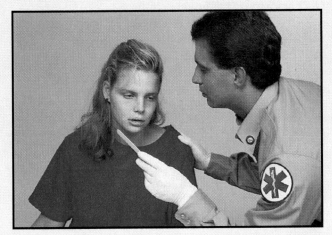

7. If patient is conscious, have her remove tongue depressor. Reassess patient.

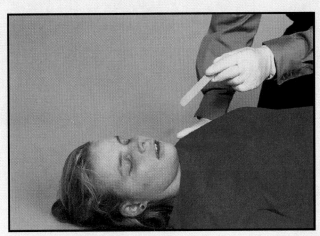

8. If patient loses consciousness, remove tongue depressor. Reassess patient.

Oral Glucose

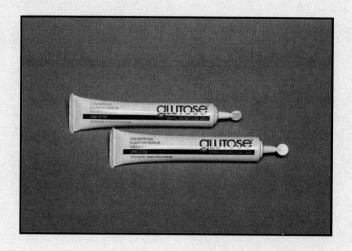

Medication Name
1. Generic: Glucose, oral
2. Trade: Glutose, Insta-glucose

Indications
1. Patients with altered mental status with a known history of diabetes mellitus

Contraindications
1. Unconsciousness
2. Known diabetic who has not taken insulin for days
3. Unable to swallow

Medication Form
Gel, in toothpaste-type tubes

Dosage
One tube

Administration
1. Assure signs and symptoms of altered mental status with a known history of diabetes
2. Assure patient is conscious
3. Administer glucose
   a. Place on tongue depressor between cheek and gum
   b. Self-administered between cheek and gum
4. Perform ongoing assessment

Actions
Increases blood sugar

Side Effects
None when given properly. May be aspirated by the patient without a gag reflex.

Reassessment Strategies
If patient loses consciousness or seizes, remove tongue depressor from mouth.

too hard. Children are also less likely to be disciplined about eating correctly and on time. As a consequence, children are more at risk of hypoglycemia than are adults.

Documentation Tips—Diabetic Emergencies

With diabetic emergencies, mental status is an important sign to watch. A change in mental status may indicate an alteration in the patient's blood sugar level. It is important to document mental status throughout the call, as well as to note the nature of the onset of altered mental status (rapid or gradual) according to the patient, friends, family, or bystanders.

To document mental status, use the AVPU scale (Alert, Verbal stimulus, Painful stimulus, Unresponsive). If alert, check for orientation to person, place, and time. The patient may be awake and responsive, but confused.

For some diabetic emergencies, you will administer oral glucose. This medication may have a dramatic effect in improving your patient's mental status. Make sure to document the patient's vital signs, as well as mental status, prior to and after administration of this or any medication.

SEIZURES

If the normal functions of the brain are upset by injury, infection, or disease, the electrical activity of the brain can become irregular. This irregularity can bring about a sudden change in sensation, behavior, or movement, called a **seizure** (also called a fit, spell, or attack by nonmedical people). Some seizures involve the uncontrolled muscular movements called *convulsions*.

A seizure is not a disease in itself, but rather a sign of some underlying defect, injury, or disease. The most common cause of seizures in adults is failure to take anti-seizure medication. The most common cause of seizures in infants and children 6 months to 3 years of age is high fever (febrile seizures). Other causes of seizures include

- Toxic—Drug or alcohol use or abuse or withdrawal can cause seizures (*toxic* means "poisonous"—the drug or alcohol has worked as a poison).
- Brain Tumor—A brain tumor may occasionally cause seizures.

- Congenital Brain Defects—Seizures due to congenital defects of the brain (defects one is born with) are most often seen in infants and young children.
- Idiopathic—Idiopathic seizures are those that occur spontaneously, with an unknown cause. This is often the case with seizures in children.
- Infection—Swelling or inflammation of the brain caused by an infection can cause seizures.
- Metabolic—Seizures can be caused by irregularities in the patient's body chemistry (metabolism).
- Trauma—Head injuries can cause seizures. So can scars formed at the site of previous brain injuries.

In addition, convulsive seizures may be seen with

- Epilepsy
- Stroke
- Measles, mumps, and other childhood diseases
- Hypoglycemia (One reason why diabetics sometimes have seizures.)
- Eclampsia (a severe complication of pregnancy)
- Hypoxia (lack of oxygen)

Epilepsy is perhaps the best-known of the conditions that result in seizures. Some people are born with epilepsy while others develop epilepsy after a head injury or surgery. Conscientious use of medications allows most epileptics to live normal lives without seizures of any type. Remember that, while a patient with seizures may be an epileptic, epilepsy is only one condition that causes seizures.

Not all seizures are alike. The type of seizure most people associate with epilepsy and other seizure disorders is the generalized tonic-clonic seizure—a seizure in which the person falls to the floor and has severe convulsions. This is the kind of seizure for which EMS will most likely be called. (For more information on types of seizures, see the FYI section later in this chapter.)

Patient Assessment—Seizure Disorders

As an EMT-B it is not your job to diagnose the cause of a seizure. However, it is very important to be able to describe the seizure to emergency department personnel. If you have not observed the seizure (usually you will be called to the scene after the seizure has taken place), always try to find out what the seizure was like by asking the following questions of bystanders. Be sure to record and report your findings.

☐ What was the person doing before the seizure started?
☐ Exactly what did the person do during the seizure—movement by movement—especially at the beginning? Was there loss of bladder or bowel control?
☐ How long did the seizure last?
☐ What did the person do after the seizure? Was he asleep (and for how long)? Was he awake? Was he able to answer questions? (If you are present during the seizure, use the AVPU scale to assess mental status.)

Patient Care—Siezure Disorders

Emergency Care Steps

If you are present when a convulsive seizure occurs

☐ Place the patient on the floor or ground. If there is no possibility that spine injury has occurred, position the patient on his side for drainage from the mouth.
☐ Loosen restrictive clothing.
☐ Remove objects that may harm the patient.
☐ Protect the patient from injury, but do not try to hold the patient still during convulsions (Figure 19-2).

After convulsions have ended

☐ Protect the airway. If there is no possibility of spine injury, position the patient on his side for drainage from the mouth. If necessary, suction the airway.
☐ If the patient is cyanotic (blue), assure an open airway and provide artificial ventilations with supplemental oxygen.
☐ Treat any injuries the patient may have sustained during the convulsions, or rule out trauma. Head injury can cause seizures, or the patient may have injured himself during the seizure. Immobilize the neck and spine if trauma is suspected.
☐ Transport to a medical facility, monitoring vital signs and respirations closely.

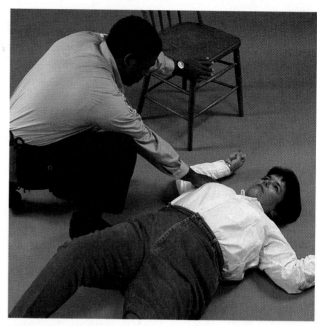

FIGURE 19-2 Protect the seizure patient from injury.

Note: Never place anything in the mouth of a seizing patient. Many objects can be broken and obstruct the patient's airway.

The epileptic is often very knowledgeable about his condition, medications, and history. Since seizures may be common for the patient, he may refuse transportation. The patient should be encouraged to accept transportation to a hospital for examination. Should the patient continue to refuse, he should not be left alone after the seizure, and he must not drive. A competent relative or other responsible person must remain with the patient.

Warning: Seizures usually last no more than 1 to 3 minutes. When the patient has two or more convulsive seizures without regaining full consciousness and lasting 5 to 10 minutes or more, it is known as **status epilepticus.** Some systems consider all patients who are still seizing when EMS arrives on the scene to be in status epilepticus. This is a high priority emergency requiring immediate transport to the hospital and possible ALS intercept (having an advanced life support team meet your ambulance en route). The airway must be opened and suctioned and a high concentration of oxygen should be administered at the scene and while en route.

Infants and Children

Seizures caused by high fevers are common in children. Children also often have idiopathic seizures, or seizures with no known cause. Seizures in children who frequently have them are rarely life-threatening. However, as an EMT-B, you should treat any seizure in an infant or child as if it is life-threatening.

FYI

Topics included in the FYI—"For Your Information"—section are those that go beyond the chapter objectives. The information in this segment is intended to broaden your understanding of the chapter topic but is not essential to an understanding of your job as an EMT-B.

Types of Diabetes

There are two major classifications of diabetes mellitus. Type I, or insulin-dependent, diabetes occurs in individuals with little or no ability to produce insulin. This type of diabetes has been called "juvenile diabetes" since it tends to begin in childhood. The Type I diabetic must inject daily doses of supplemental insulin.

Type II, or non-insulin-dependent, diabetes occurs in individuals who have the ability to produce insulin but are unable to develop enough of it or to use it effectively. This disorder usually develops in adults and has been called "maturity-onset diabetes." Diabetes in adulthood is usually associated with obesity and is seen more often in older than in younger people. Type II diabetes can often be controlled without supplemental insulin through supervised diets and oral medications.

The danger of undetected and untreated diabetes is severe. As the condition develops, the diabetic can become weak and lose weight even though he may increase his sugar and fat intake. Advanced diabetes is often associated with such complications as heart disease, kidney disease, and blindness.

Hyperglycemia

Although hypoglycemia, or low blood sugar (discussed earlier in this chapter), is the most common cause of diabetic emergency, another possible cause of emergency for the diabetic is too much sugar in the bloodstream, or **hyperglycemia.** Hyperglycemia is also known as high blood sugar. (*Hyper* means "more than normal" or "excessive." *Glyc* means "sugar.") Like hypoglycemia, hyperglycemia can prove to be life threatening.

Hyperglycemia occurs because the diabetic does not produce enough natural insulin to take sugar out of the blood and into the cells, and because . . .

- he has not taken enough insulin to make up for this deficiency, or . . .
- he has forgotten to take his insulin, or . . .
- he has overeaten, or . . .
- he has an infection that has upset his insulin/glucose balance.

With hyperglycemia, not only is there too much sugar in the blood, there is too little sugar in the cells. The body attempts to overcome the lack of sugar in the cells by using other foods for energy, particularly stored fats. However, fats are not an efficient alternative to glucose, and the waste products of fat utilization, ketones (compounds that are in the same class as those used to make fingernail polish remover), begin to concentrate in the blood, turning the blood acidic. The person will drink large quantities of water to offset the loss of fluids through excess urination, caused by the body's attempt to get rid of extra sugar. If allowed to go untreated, the acidity of the blood and the loss of fluids eventually lead to *diabetic ketoacidosis* (KEY-to-as-i-DO-sis), which can lead to death.

Differences Between Hypoglycemia and Hyperglycemia

Many students find that they confuse hypoglycemia and hyperglycemia. Fortunately, it is not necessary to distinguish between the two conditions in order to give the proper treatment.

There are three typical differences between hypoglycemia and hyperglycemia.

- Onset—Hyperglycemia usually has a slower onset, while hypoglycemia tends to come on suddenly. This is because some sugar still reaches the brain in hyperglycemic (high blood sugar) states. With hypoglycemia (low blood sugar), it is possible that no sugar is reaching the brain. Seizures may occur.

- Skin—Hyperglycemic patients often have warm, red, dry skin. Hypoglycemic patients have cold, pale, moist, or "clammy" skin.
- Breath—The hyperglycemic patient often has acetone breath (like nail polish remover), while the hypoglycemic patient does not.

Additionally, patients who are hyperglycemic frequently breathe very deeply and rapidly, as though they had just run a race. Dry mouth, intense thirst, abdominal pain, and vomiting are all common signs and symptoms of this condition. The proper treatment is given under close medical supervision in a hospital.

There appear to be clear-cut differences between the signs and symptoms of hyperglycemia and hypoglycemia, but distinguishing between them in the field can be difficult and is not necessary. Giving glucose will help the hypoglycemic patient by getting needed sugar into the bloodstream and to the brain. Although the hyperglycemic patient already has too much sugar in his blood, the extra dose of glucose will not have time to cause damage in the short time before he reaches the hospital and can be diagnosed and treated. This is why "sugar (glucose) for everyone" is the rule of thumb for diabetic emergencies, whether the patient is hypo- or hyperglycemic, and why you do not need to distinguish between the two conditions.

Note: Many hyperglycemic patients and some hypoglycemic patients will appear to be intoxicated. Always suspect a diabetic problem in cases that seem to involve no more than intoxication. Remember that the patient intoxicated on alcohol may also be a diabetic, with the alcohol breath covering over the acetone smell characteristic of diabetic ketoacidosis. The alcoholic diabetic is a good candidate for a diabetic emergency, because he tends to neglect eating and taking insulin during the course of prolonged drinking and usually has a low blood sugar level.

Types of Seizures

The generalized tonic-clonic seizure in which the person falls to the floor and has severe convulsions, described earlier in this chapter, is only one of four common types of seizures in two classifications: partial seizures and generalized seizures. The characteristics of these classifications and types of seizures are described below.

Partial Seizures
- Simple Partial Seizure (also called focal motor, focal sensory, or Jacksonian)—There is tingling, stiffening, or jerking in just one part of the body. There may also be an *aura* in which the person may experience sensations such as a smell, bright lights, a burst of colors, or a rising sensation in the stomach. There is no loss of consciousness. However in some cases the jerking may spread and develop into a generalized tonic-clonic seizure (see below).
- Complex Partial Seizure (also called psychomotor or temporal lobe)—Often preceded by an aura, this type of seizure is characterized by abnormal behavior that varies widely from person to person. It may involve confusion, a glassy stare, aimless moving about, lip smacking or chewing, or fidgeting with clothing. The person may appear to be drunk or on drugs, is not violent but may struggle or fight if restrained. Very rarely, a complex partial seizure may result in such extreme behavior as screaming, running, disrobing, or showing great fear. There is no loss of consciousness, but there may be confusion and no memory of the episode afterward. In some cases the seizure may develop into a tonic-clonic seizure.

Generalized Seizures
- Tonic-Clonic (also called grand mal)—There is often no aura or other warning. The person may cry out before falling to the floor. This type of seizure is characterized by unconsciousness and major motor activity. The patient will thrash about wildly, using his entire body. The convulsion usually lasts only a few minutes and has three distinct phases.
  1. Tonic phase—The body becomes rigid, stiffening for no more than 30 seconds. Breathing may stop, the patient may bite his tongue (rare), and bowel and bladder control could be lost.
  2. Clonic phase—The body jerks about violently, usually for no more than 1 or 2 minutes (some can last 5 minutes). The patient may foam at the mouth and drool. His face and lips often become cyanotic.
  3. Postictal phase—This begins when convulsions stop. The patient may regain consciousness immediately and enter a

state of drowsiness and confusion, or he may remain unconscious for several hours. Headache is common.

- Absence (also called petit mal)—The seizure is brief, usually only 1 to 10 seconds. There is no dramatic motor activity and the person usually does not slump or fall. Instead there is a temporary loss of concentration or awareness. An absence seizure may go unnoticed by everyone except the person and knowledgeable members of his family. A child may suffer several hundred absence seizures a day, severely interfering with his ability to pay attention and do well in school. Absence seizures often stop before adulthood but sometimes worsen and become tonic-clonic seizures.

Patient care for the generalized tonic-clonic seizure was described earlier in this chapter. For a simple or complex partial seizure, do not restrain the person; simply remove objects from his path and gently guide him away from danger. For an absence seizure, if you are aware that it has occurred, simply provide the patient with any information he may have missed.

Stroke

Another cause of altered mental status may be a *stroke*. Also called a *cerebral vascular accident*, or CVA, a stroke takes place when an artery in the brain becomes blocked, preventing oxygenated blood from reaching the areas supplied by the artery. The pathway of blood can also be disrupted when an artery ruptures, or bursts, often resulting in bleeding into the brain.

Age and physical condition influence the type of stroke suffered by a patient, as do the various sizes and locations of arteries involved. Sometimes the patient may have nothing more than a headache when first evaluated if the stroke is caused by bleeding from a ruptured vessel. However, most stroke patients do not experience headaches.

In many cases, you will find it difficult to communicate with the stroke patient. The damage to the brain sometimes causes a partial or complete loss of the ability to use words. The patient may be able to understand you but will not be able to talk, or will have great difficulty with speech. Sometimes, the patient will understand you and know what he wants to say, but he will say the wrong words. This difficulty with words is known as *aphasia* (ah-FAY-zhuh).

Signs and symptoms of stroke may include any of the following.

- Confusion
- Dizziness
- Impaired speech
- Numbness or paralysis (usually on one side of the body)
- Paralysis or weak, sagging muscles or loss of expression in the face (usually on one side)
- Headache (uncommon)
- Unequal pupils
- Impaired vision
- Rapid, full pulse
- Difficult respiration or snoring
- Nausea or vomiting
- Seizures
- Unconsciousness
- Loss of bowel or bladder control

It is not necessary to diagnose the patient's medical problem or to know that a stroke has taken place, although you may suspect it. You will treat the patient as you would any patient with similar symptoms.

- Conscious Patient—Do what you can to calm and reassure the patient. Ensure an open airway. Administer high concentration oxygen. Transport in semi-sitting position.
- Unconscious Patient—Maintain an open airway. Provide high concentration oxygen. Transport lying on side.

KEY TERMS

You may find it helpful to review the following terms.

diabetes mellitus (di-ah-BEE-tez MEL-i-tus) also called "sugar diabetes" or just "diabetes," the condition brought about by decreased insulin production. The person with this condition is a diabetic.

epilepsy (EP-uh-lep-see) a medical condition that sometimes causes seizures.

glucose (GLU-kos) a form of sugar, the body's basic source of energy.

hyperglycemia (HI-per-gleye-SEE-me-ah) high blood sugar.

hypoglycemia (HI-po-gleye-SEE-me-ah) low blood sugar.

insulin (IN-suh-lin) a hormone produced by the pancreas or taken as a medication by many diabetics.

seizure (SEE-zher) a sudden change in sensation, behavior, or movement. The most severe form of seizure produces violent muscle contractions called convulsions.

status epilepticus (STAY-tus or STAT-us ep-i-LEP-ti-kus) a prolonged seizure or when a person suffers two or more convulsive seizures without regaining full consciousness.

SUMMARY

Diabetic emergencies are usually caused by poor management of the patient's diabetes. Often this involves a condition brought about by hypoglycemia, or low blood sugar. The chief sign of this condition is altered mental status. Whenever a patient has an altered mental status and a history of diabetes and can swallow, the treatment to be administered by the EMT-B is oral glucose.

Seizures are sometimes experienced by diabetic patients but also have a number of other causes. When a patient experiences a seizure, assess and treat for possible spinal injury, protect the patient's airway, and provide oxygen as needed. Gather information about the seizure to give to hospital personnel.

REVIEW QUESTIONS

1. List the chief signs and symptoms of a patient who is having a diabetic emergency.
2. Explain how you can determine a medical history of diabetes.
3. Explain what treatment may be given by an EMT-B for a diabetic emergency and the criteria for giving it.
4. Tell whether treatment for a diabetic emergency should be given before or after baseline vital signs are taken. (Answer according to your local protocol.)
5. Explain the care an EMT-B will ordinarily give for a patient who has had a seizure.

Application

- You are dispatched to a "man behaving oddly" at a train station. When you arrive, you find that the man is unconscious. "He's drunk," a bystander tells you. "He was staggering and slurring his words." As you assess the patient, you find a medical identification bracelet that tells you he is a diabetic. Do you administer oral glucose? How do you proceed?

Allergies

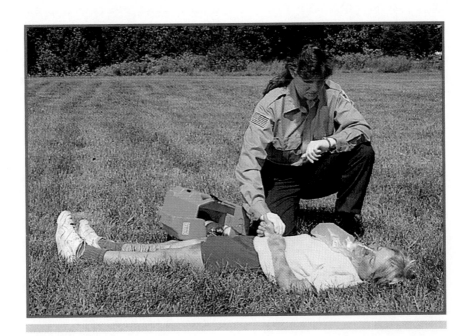

20

Almost everyone has an allergic reaction to something at some time, perhaps an itchy rash after contact with poison ivy or a sniffle during ragweed season. For most people, allergic reactions are an unpleasant nuisance. For some, however, allergic reactions can be far worse, developing into a life-threatening condition in just moments. As an EMT-B, your ability to recognize and manage a severe allergic reaction may make the difference between your patient's survival and death.

Objectives

Knowledge and Attitude *At the end of this chapter, you should be able to meet the following objectives.*

1. Recognize the patient experiencing an allergic reaction. (p. 348)

2. Describe the emergency medical care of the patient with an allergic reaction. (pp. 348–351)

3. Establish the relationship between the patient with an allergic reaction and airway management. (p. 349)

4. Describe the mechanisms of allergic response and the implications for airway management. (pp. 346–348)

5. State the generic and trade names, medication forms, dose, administration, action, and contraindications for the epinephrine auto-injector. (p. 353)

6. Evaluate the need for medical direction in the emergency medical care of the patient with an allergic reaction. (pp. 349, 350)

7. Differentiate between the general category of

On the Scene

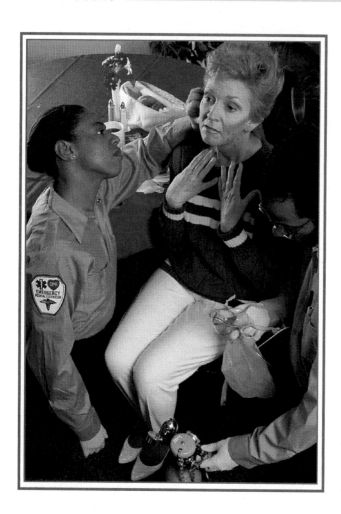

Allyson Wells has just had a promotion. To celebrate, she is having dinner with friends from work. Just into the main course, Allyson suddenly develops chest tightness and difficulty breathing. Initially, Allyson thinks it may be from the excitement of the promotion and the dinner. As the chest tightness worsens, she knows it is more serious.

A co-worker notices the look of concern on Allyson's face. Hives, too, are now visible on her face and neck. The co-worker asks Allyson if she wants an ambulance, and Allyson gasps "yes."

You are called to "a sick woman in a restaurant." As you arrive, you *size up the scene* and pull on disposable gloves. The restaurant manager points to Allyson's table and tells you her name. You begin your *initial assessment* even as you start toward Allyson. You form a general impression of an alert female patient who—you can see even from across the room—is having considerable difficulty breathing and is scratching her neck.

You: Ms. Wells, I'm Felicia Richardson, an emergency medical technician from the ambulance. Can you tell me what's wrong?
Allyson Wells: I can't catch my breath. My chest is tight and I'm itching all over, too.

Ms. Wells is alert and talking, so—at least right now—her airway is open. Although she is having difficulty breathing, she is breathing adequately. There is no indication of bleeding. Her pulse is rapid but

those patients having an allergic reaction and those patients having an allergic reaction and requiring immediate medical care, including immediate use of epinephrine auto-injector. (pp. 349, 352)

8. Explain the rationale for administering epinephrine using an auto-injector. (p. 352)

Skills

1. Demonstrate the emergency medical care of the patient experiencing an allergic reaction.

2. Demonstrate the use of epinephrine auto-injector.

3. Demonstrate the assessment and documentation of patient response to an epinephrine injection.

4. Demonstrate proper disposal of equipment.

5. Demonstrate completing a prehospital care report for patients with allergic emergencies.

---

strong. Because of her difficulty breathing, you assign her a high priority. As your partner prepares a nonrebreather mask and oxygen, you begin the *focused history and physical exam.* Since Ms. Wells is itching and has hives visible on her face and neck, you suspect an allergic reaction and ask her questions related to that kind of problem.

You: Do you have any allergies? Have you ever had an allergic reaction to any food?
Ms. Wells: Yes—to shellfish. But I didn't have any shellfish. I ordered chicken, but I only took a couple of bites before I started feeling sick.
You: (to the manager) Can you find out if there was any shellfish in Ms. Wells's meal? (to Allyson Wells) Have you had any other symptoms besides difficulty breathing, chest tightness, and itching from the hives on your neck and face?
Ms. Wells: I feel as though I have a lump in my throat.
You: When did the symptoms start?
Ms. Wells: About ten minutes ago.
You: How long after you started eating was that?
Ms. Wells: About five minutes.
You: Can you think of anything else you're allergic to or any other way you might have been exposed to shellfish?
Ms. Wells: No, I'm not allergic to anything else and I'm very careful about what I eat.
You: Have your symptoms changed since they started?

Ms. Wells: They seem to be getting worse. The itching started on my neck and seems to be spreading.
You: Have you taken any medicine to relieve your symptoms?
Ms. Wells: No.

Now that your partner has put oxygen on the patient, he starts to get a set of baseline vital signs. At the same time, you get a quick SAMPLE history. The patient has already told you her symptoms and allergies, and you can see the remains of her last oral intake on the table. She takes no medicines, has no pertinent past history, and can't tell you anything more about events leading up to this episode. You also find out that she is 48 years old.

Your partner tells you Ms. Wells has a pulse of 124, full and regular, a blood pressure of 110/80, and respirations of 26 and labored. You notice that she is wheezing with each breath and that she seems to have some flushing of the skin and swelling around her eyes and on her neck.

The manager hurries over to announce that the chef used shrimp in the sauce for the chicken. You put the pieces together: the patient is allergic to shellfish, she unknowingly ate some, she started having difficulty breathing with chest tightness, itching, and hives just a few minutes later, and she is feeling and looking worse by the minute. You recognize that this patient is having a serious allergic reaction, an anaphylactic reaction. You know that the best treatment for this condition is a medication that many patients subject to severe allergic reactions carry with them.

You: Has your doctor prescribed any medication to take for an allergic reaction?

Ms. Wells: I have an Epi-Pen in my purse, but I've never used it.

You: If you get it out, I'll call the doctor at the emergency department. I think he'll want us to use it.

You contact the emergency department and relay the information you have gathered to the physician there. He agrees that this is a serious allergic reaction and advises you to administer epinephrine with the patient's Epi-Pen.

The patient hands you the epinephrine syringe. You have already confirmed that it is hers, so you check the medication in the syringe. It is clear, the way it should be.

You: This should help you feel better, but you should know that sometimes people who get this kind of injection feel nauseated, get a headache, or experience trembling.

Ms. Wells: As long as I can breathe, I don't care.

You: This is also going to sting. After I give you the injection, I'm going to hold the Epi-Pen against your thigh so that all the medicine goes in.

You remove the safety cap and carefully but firmly press the end of the auto-injector against a spot midway between her waist and her knee on the lateral side (outside) of her left thigh. She winces a bit when the spring-loaded needle releases into her thigh.

You hold the injector against Ms. Wells's thigh. After you slowly count to 10, you remove it and put it into the sharps container your partner brought from the ambulance with the stretcher. You look at your watch and note the time on a patient information pad.

You and your partner get Ms. Wells onto the stretcher and transport her to the hospital. Epinephrine usually works very fast, so you re-assess Ms. Wells two minutes after the injection. She reports that she feels a little "jumpy" and that her breathing difficulty may be easing up a little bit. En route, you continue to perform an *ongoing assessment* at least every five minutes and note that her condition continues to improve. You ensure that she is still getting high concentration oxygen, re-assess vital signs and ABCs, and monitor her for signs and symptoms of both anaphylaxis and epinephrine administration.

When you arrive at the hospital, Ms. Wells is looking and feeling much better. You give a report to the nurse and physician who will be caring for her. After you write up your report, you step into the room

to see how the patient is doing. She looks fine. The doctor tells you your quick recognition that she was having an anaphylactic reaction—and your giving her epinephrine—probably saved Ms. Wells's life.

━━━━━━━━━━━━━━━━━━━━━━━━━━━ ■

When Allyson Wells had an allergic reaction to shellfish she unknowingly ate at the restaurant, she was lucky on several counts. First, she was lucky that her friend immediately recognized the seriousness of the problem and called 911. Second, she was lucky that the restaurant manager was able to find out right away that there had been shellfish in her meal. Finally, she was lucky that you, the EMT-Basic, recognized the signs of a serious allergic reaction and assisted her with her epinephrine auto-injector quickly enough to reverse what could have been a fatal episode.

ALLERGIC REACTIONS

A natural response of the human body is to react to any foreign substance—to defend the body by neutralizing or getting rid of the foreign material. An **allergic reaction** is an exaggerated response of the body's immune system. It is a natural, and usually harmless, function. Almost any of a wide variety of substances can be an **allergen,** something that causes an allergic reaction. For example, cat dander can be an allergen. A person who is allergic to cat dander will sneeze and itch whenever a cat is nearby. This is an unpleasant but minor allergic reaction.

In some people, however, contact with certain foreign substances triggers an immune response that gets out of hand. Consider bee stings. Most people have no reaction to a bee sting other than pain and some swelling at the sting site. A few people have very severe, life-threatening reactions to bee stings. This kind of severe allergic reaction is called **anaphylaxis,** or *anaphylactic shock.* In anaphylaxis, exposure to the allergen will cause blood vessels to dilate rapidly and cause a drop in blood pressure (hypotension). Many tissues may swell, including those that line the respiratory system. This swelling can obstruct the airway, leading to respiratory failure.

Something that all allergic reactions share is that people do not have them the first time they are exposed to an allergen. This is because the body's immune system hasn't "learned" to recognize the allergen yet. The first time someone is exposed to an allergen, the immune system forms antibodies in response. These antibodies are an attempt by the body to "attack" these foreign substances. A particular antibody will combine with only the allergen it was formed in response to (or another allergen very similar to the original one). The second time the person is exposed to the allergen, it combines with the antibody and results in dilation of the blood vessels, swelling, and difficulty breathing.

Causes of allergic reactions include (Figure 20-1)

- *Insects*—The stings of bees, yellow jackets, wasps, and hornets can cause rapid and severe reactions.
- *Foods*—Foods such as nuts, eggs, milk, and shellfish can cause reactions. In most cases, the effect is slower than that seen

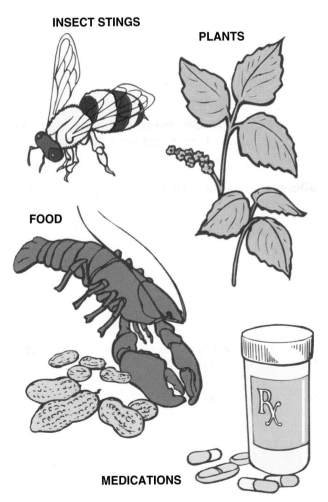

INSECT STINGS

PLANTS

FOOD

MEDICATIONS

FIGURE 20-1 Substances that may cause allergic reaction.

with insect stings. An exception to this is peanuts. Peanut allergies are frequently very severe and very rapid in onset. Many people with allergies to one food will have allergies to related foods, e.g., someone who is allergic to almonds is more likely to be allergic to walnuts. Again, peanuts are an exception. People who are allergic to peanuts do not necessarily have any other allergies, including nuts (in part because peanuts are legumes, not nuts).

- *Plants*—Contact with certain plants such as poison ivy can cause a rash that is sometimes severe. The rash associated with poison ivy is actually an allergic reaction. Approximately two thirds of the population is allergic to the oil on poison ivy leaves. Plant pollen also causes allergic reactions in many people, but rarely anaphylaxis.
- *Medications*—Antitoxins and drugs, especially antibiotics such as penicillin, may cause severe reactions. Just as with foods, people who are allergic to one kind of antibiotic can be allergic to related antibiotics. In the course of evaluating patients, you will hear many of them say they are allergic to penicillin or other antibiotics. Actually, many of these people are not allergic to these medications. They think that they are allergic because after they took the medication they had nausea, vomiting, abdominal cramps, or diarrhea. These are sometimes associated with allergic reactions, but they are not the same thing. These people were experiencing side effects of the medications but not necessarily an allergic reaction. A true allergic reaction involves hives, itching, difficulty breathing, or, in severe cases, shock.
- *Others*—Dust, chemicals, soaps, make-up, and a variety of other substances can cause allergic reactions, occasionally severe, in some people.

One particular product EMT-Bs should be aware of as a possible allergen is latex. Only in the last few years have health-care providers recognized allergic reactions to latex for what they are.

Two groups of people are especially likely to be allergic to latex. One of these groups is patients with conditions that require multiple surgeries. The repeated exposure to the latex in doctors' and nurses' gloves is probably the reason many such patients develop a severe allergy to latex. This is very important to understand, because if you wear latex gloves when treating a patient with a latex allergy you may actually cause an allergic or anaphylactic reaction in the patient.

The other group that is becoming more sensitive to latex is health care professionals—including EMT-Bs. Again, this is probably because of more frequent exposure to latex as a result of practicing body substance isolation. Fortunately, there are ways to avoid latex. Manufacturers of medical equipment are generally happy to provide information about which of their products contain latex and to suggest latex-free substitutes.

Safety Note

If you notice that your hands seem to be red and itchy after a call, you may be developing an allergy to latex. Whenever you see itching, the first thing you should think about is an allergy. You may also notice **hives** (red, itchy bumps) on the areas covered by your gloves. If you are allergic to latex, it is very important that you protect yourself from further exposure to this allergen. If you don't, these signs will get worse as you continue to wear latex gloves. Fortunately, gloves made of vinyl will also protect you from blood and other potentially infectious materials.

Some people become extremely sensitive to latex, so it is important that you tell this to any health care provider who is caring for you as a patient. You should also discuss this with your own physician so that you can become as informed as possible about this topic and learn how to protect yourself.

There is no way to predict the exact course of anaphylactic shock. Severe reactions most often take place immediately, but they are occasionally delayed 30 minutes or more. A mild allergic reaction may turn into more serious anaphylactic shock in a matter of minutes. When you have a patient with an exposure to a known allergen but who is displaying only minor signs and symptoms, you must closely monitor the patient for signs of the condition becoming more serious. This patient's airway may swell and close off in just a few minutes. Be prepared to manage the airway with the techniques you learned in Chapter 7, Airway Management, as well as to treat the patient with epinephrine.

The signs and symptoms of anaphylactic shock can include

Skin

- Itching
- Hives, especially around an insect sting
- Flushing (red skin)
- Swelling of face (especially the eyes and lips), neck, hands, feet, or tongue
- Warm, tingling feeling in the face, mouth, chest, feet, and hands.

Respiratory

- Patient may report a feeling of tightness in his throat or chest
- Cough
- Rapid breathing
- Labored, noisy breathing
- Hoarseness, muffled voice, or loss of voice entirely
- Stridor (harsh, high-pitched sound during inspiration)
- Wheezing (audible without a stethoscope)

Cardiac

- Increased heart rate
- Decreased blood pressure

Generalized findings

- Itchy, watery eyes
- Headache
- Runny nose
- Patient expresses a sense of impending doom

Decreasing mental status

Signs and symptoms of shock (hypoperfusion) or respiratory distress

Patient Assessment—Allergic Reaction

Conduct the usual assessment sequence, as follows.

1. Perform the initial assessment and care for any immediately life-threatening problems with the airway, breathing, or circulation.
2. Perform a focused history and physical exam. Inquire about
   - History of allergies
   - What patient was exposed to

- How patient was exposed (contact, ingestion, etc.)
- What signs and symptoms the patient is having
- Progression (what happened first, next? how rapidly?)
- Interventions (has any care been provided? has the patient taken any medication?)

3 Assess baseline vital signs and get the remainder of the SAMPLE history.

Important: *Suspect an allergic reaction whenever . . .*

☐ The patient has come in contact with a substance that has caused an allergic reaction in the past, and . . .
☐ The patient complains of itching, hives, or difficulty breathing, or shows signs or symptoms of shock (hypoperfusion)

Patient Care—Allergic Reaction

Emergency Care Steps

Manage the patient's airway and breathing.

■ Apply high concentration oxygen through a nonrebreather mask if you have not already done so during the initial assessment. If the patient has or develops an altered mental status, you will need to open and maintain the patient's airway. If the patient is not breathing adequately, you will also need to provide artificial ventilations.

If (1) the patient has come in contact with a substance that caused an allergic reaction in the past, and (2) the patient complains of respiratory distress or exhibits signs and symptoms of shock, and (3) **the patient has a prescribed epinephrine auto-injector . . .**

■ Contact medical direction and, if so ordered, assist the patient with the auto-injector (Scan 20-1).
■ Record the administration of the epinephrine auto-injector. Transport. Reassess two minutes after epinephrine administration and record reassessment findings.

If (1) the patient has come in contact with a substance that caused an allergic reaction in the past, and (2) the patient complains of respiratory distress or exhibits signs and symptoms of shock, and (3) **the patient has been prescribed an epinephrine auto-injector but does not have it available or has never had an epinephrine auto-injector prescribed . . .**

■ Care for shock and transport immediately.

If patient has come in contact with a substance that caused an allergic reaction in the past, **but the patient is not wheezing or showing signs of respiratory distress or shock (hypoperfusion)**

■ Continue with the focused assessment.
■ Consult medical direction. Administer epinephrine only if ordered.

You will probably not see many patients with allergic reactions, but most of them will be able to give you a history of allergies. Once in a while, you will see a patient who has no history and is having his first allergic reaction. In this case, the patient will not be carrying an epinephrine auto-injector because his physician has not prescribed one. Treat the patient for shock and transport immediately.

Remember: A patient with an allergic reaction may have a compromised airway or respiratory function, or these conditions may develop as the allergic reaction progresses. Carefully monitor the patient's airway and breathing throughout care and transport. Manage the airway and respiration as presented in Chapter 7, Airway Management.

In your ongoing assessment, you will frequently find that the patient's condition improves, but sometimes it will deteriorate. You may need to give additional doses of epinephrine in this case. You will be able to do this only if the patient has one or more extra auto-injectors AND you have remembered to ask the patient to bring them in the ambulance. Auto-injectors on the market today can give only one dose of epinephrine. WHENEVER A PATIENT HAS AN EPINEPHRINE AUTO-INJECTOR, BEFORE YOU LEAVE THE SCENE, ASK IF HE HAS ANY SPARES AND ATTEMPT TO GET THEM FOR THE TRIP TO THE HOSPITAL.

Scan 20-1
Epinephrine Auto-Injector

FIRST take body substance isolation precautions.

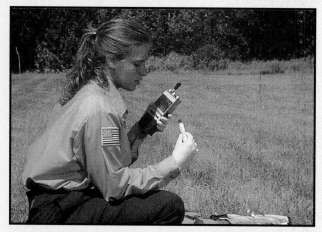

1. Patient suffers severe allergic reaction.

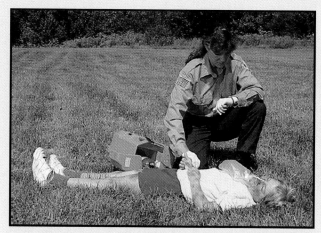

2. Perform an initial assessment. Provide high concentration oxygen by nonrebreather mask.

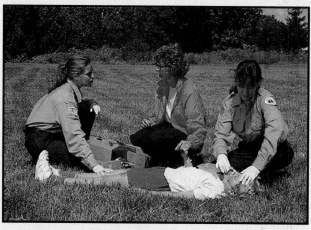

3. Obtain a SAMPLE history.

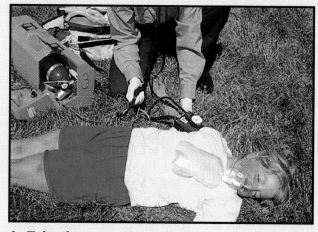

4. Take the patient's vital signs.

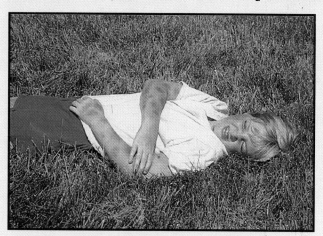

5. Ascertain if the patient has a prescribed epinephrine auto-injector. Check to be sure injector is prescribed for this patient. Check expiration date. Check for cloudiness or discoloration if liquid is visible. Contact medical direction.

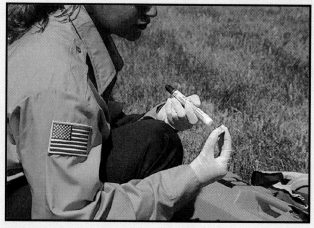

6. If medical direction orders use of the epinephrine auto-injector, prepare it for use. Remove the safety cap.

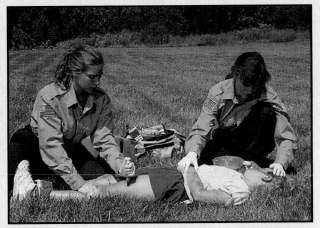

7. Press the injector against the patient's thigh to trigger release of the spring-loaded needle and inject the dose of epinephrine into the patient.

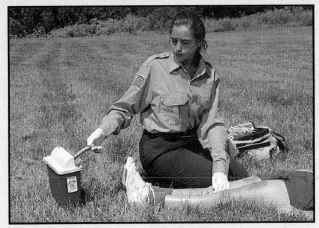

8. Dispose of the used injector in a portable biohazard container.

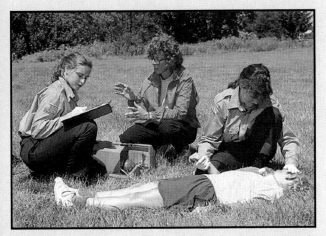

9. Document the patient's response to the medication.

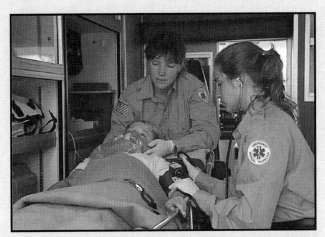

10. Perform ongoing assessment, paying special attention to the patient's ABCs and vital signs, en route to the hospital.

SELF-ADMINISTERED EPINEPHRINE

For years, physicians have prescribed **epinephrine** (EP-uh-NEF-rin) in the form of bee sting kits, AnaKits®, or EpiPens® for patients who are susceptible to severe allergic reactions. Epinephrine is a hormone produced by the body. When administered as a medication, it will constrict blood vessels (helping to raise the blood pressure and improve perfusion) and will dilate the bronchioles (helping to open the airway and improve respiration).

Many people who are subject to severe allergic reactions are prescribed an epinephrine auto-injector by their physician to carry with them and use when such a reaction occurs. The reason it is important for such a patient to carry an epinephrine auto-injector is that an allergic reaction can become life threatening so quickly that there is not enough time to transport the patient to a hospital to receive the medication. An **auto-injector** is a spring-loaded needle and syringe with a single dose of epinephrine that will automatically release and inject the medication.

When authorized by medical direction, you may administer or help the patient administer a dose of epinephrine from an auto-injector that has been prescribed for the patient by a physician. After you make sure that the auto-injector is prescribed for the patient and that the liquid is clear (if you can see it), you will remove the cap and press the injector firmly against the patient's thigh and hold it there until the entire dose is injected. (Injection on the outside of the thigh midway between waist and knee is recommended.) On reassessment two minutes after the epinephrine is administered, in addition to some relief of symptoms, expect the patient's pulse to have increased.

The procedure for administering an epinephrine auto-injector is shown in Scan 20-1. Information about epinephrine auto-injectors is summarized in Scan 20-2.

Epinephrine is a very powerful medication. It can not only save lives, it can also occasionally take lives. One of the good things epinephrine does for patients is make the heart beat more strongly. This is beneficial when the patient is hypoperfusing (i.e., the patient is in shock), because one reason for the hypoperfusion is that the patient's blood vessels are dilated and blood is not returning to the heart as quickly. Unfortunately, once you give a drug, you can't take it back. This means that if the dose of epinephrine in the auto-injector is more than the patient needs, the patient's heart will be working harder than it needs to. This can be dangerous in the patient with a heart condition or who is hypertensive (has high blood pressure).

This is one of the reasons why EMT-Basics are taught to *give epinephrine only to patients who have been prescribed auto-injectors by their physicians.* These patients have been evaluated by physicians who have considered the patient's history and physical condition. Once the physician was satisfied that the patient was a good candidate for epinephrine, he wrote a prescription. Some patients receive instruction from their physicians in how to use the auto-injector, but others will be uncomfortable or afraid to use one because of unfamiliarity with the device and will prefer to have you help them with it.

Ordinarily when a health care provider gives an injection, the clothing over the injection site is rolled up or down and the area is cleansed with an alcohol pad. These steps are nice but not necessary with an epinephrine auto-injector. The risk of giving the patient an infection because you did not do either of these things is extremely small. The risk is so small, in fact, that the manufacturer's instructions for auto-injectors do not advise patients to do these things. Your protocols may direct you to act differently. Follow your local protocols.

One of the most difficult things you may have to do is distinguish between the patient with a (localized) *allergic reaction,* when the patient *should not* receive epinephrine, and the patient with a (generalized) *anaphylactic reaction,* when epinephrine *should* be given. Patients can and do present in many different ways. One patient in anaphylaxis may have severe difficulty breathing without hives or hypotension, while another may be tachycardiac (with rapid heartbeat) and hypotensive without any difficulty breathing. *The important thing to recognize in any presentation is the presence of either respiratory distress or signs and symptoms of shock (hypoperfusion). One of these needs to be present for the patient to be in anaphylaxis.*

Infants and Children

Epinephrine auto-injectors come in two different sizes. The adult size contains an adult dose of 0.3 mg. The child size (for a child weighing less than 66 pounds) has 0.15 mg.

Infants rarely experience anaphylactic reactions because their immune systems have not

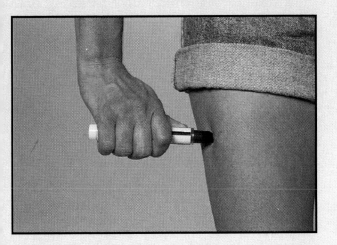

Medication Name
1. Generic: epinephrine
2. Trade: Adrenalin™, Epi-Pen®

Indications
Must meet the following three criteria:
1. Patient exhibits signs of a severe allergic reaction, including either respiratory distress or shock (hypoperfusion)
2. Medication is prescribed for this patient by a physician
3. Medical direction authorizes use for this patient

Contraindications
No contraindications when used in a life-threatening situation

Medication Form
Liquid administered by an auto-injector—an automatically injectable needle-and-syringe system

Dosage
Adult—One adult auto-injector (0.3 mg)
Infant and child—One infant/child auto-injector (0.15 mg)

Administration
1. Obtain patient's prescribed auto-injector. Ensure:
   a. Prescription is written for the patient who is experiencing the severe allergic reaction
   b. Medication is not discolored (if visible)

2. Obtain order from medical direction, either on-line or off-line
3. Remove cap from auto-injector.
4. Place tip of auto-injector against patient's thigh.
   a. Lateral portion of the thigh
   b. Midway between waist and knee
5. Push the injector firmly against the thigh until the injector activates.
6. Hold the injector in place until the medication is injected (at least 10 seconds).
7. Record activity and time.
8. Dispose of injector in biohazard container.

Actions
1. Dilates the bronchioles
2. Constricts blood vessels

Side Effects
1. Increased heart rate
2. Pallor
3. Dizziness
4. Chest pain
5. Headache
6. Nausea
7. Vomiting
8. Excitability, anxiety

Reassessment Strategies
1. Transport
2. Continue focused assessment of airway, breathing, and circulatory status.

If patient's condition continues to worsen (decreasing mental status, increasing breathing difficulty, decreasing blood pressure):

   a. Obtain medical direction for an additional dose of epinephrine
   b. Treat for shock (hypoperfusion)
   c. Prepare to initiate basic life-support procedures (CPR, AED)

If patient's condition improves, provide supportive care:

   a. Continue oxygen
   b. Treat for shock (hypoperfusion)

matured enough to develop the kinds of antibodies that cause anaphylactic reactions. Allergic reactions are common in older children, though. Fortunately, many children "grow out" of their allergies as they mature. Parents frequently will have a great deal of useful information about the child's medical history.

Documentation Tip—Allergic Reactions

The administration of epinephrine, like all medications, needs to be documented carefully. This is especially true with a medication this strong. Epinephrine can be lifesaving, but it can also occasionally be fatal. Epinephrine has powerful effects on the heart and will increase the workload of the heart significantly. It is very important that anyone caring for the patient, after you hand the patient over to more advanced providers, know how much epinephrine the patient has received, when and what effects the medication had on the patient, both good and bad. This will allow for better care of the patient after you are gone.

CHAPTER REVIEW

KEY TERMS

You may find it helpful to review the following terms.

allergen something that causes an allergic reaction.
allergic reaction an exaggerated immune response.
anaphylaxis (an-ah-fi-LAK-sis) a severe or life-threatening allergic reaction in which the blood vessels dilate, causing a drop in blood pressure, and the tissues lining the respiratory system swell, interfering with the airway. Also called *anaphylactic shock.*

auto-injector a syringe pre-loaded with medication that has a spring-loaded device that pushes the needle through the skin when the tip of the device is pressed firmly against the body.
epinephrine (EP-uh-NEF-rin) a hormone produced by the body. As a medication it constricts blood vessels and dilates respiratory passages and is used to relieve severe allergic reactions.
hives red, itchy bumps on the skin that often result from allergic reactions.

SUMMARY

Allergic reactions are common. Anaphylaxis, a true life-threatening allergic reaction, is rare. The most common symptom in all of these cases is itching. Patients with anaphylaxis, though, will also display life-threatening difficulty breathing or signs and symptoms of shock (hypoperfusion). These patients will also be extremely anxious. Their bodies are in trouble and are letting them know it.

Fortunately, most of these patients know about their condition and manage to avoid exposure to the allergens they are sensitive to. Their physicians have usually prescribed epinephrine auto-injectors for them for the times when they are exposed.

By quickly recognizing the condition, consulting medical direction, and administering the appropriate treatment, you can literally make the difference between life and death for these patients.

REVIEW QUESTIONS

1. What are the indications for administration of an epinephrine auto-injector?
2. List some of the more common causes of allergic reactions.
3. List signs or symptoms of an anaphylactic reaction associated with each of the following:

   - skin
   - respiratory system
   - cardiovascular system

Application

- You are treating an alert 5-year-old boy who has many environmental allergies and who now has hives on his neck, chest, and arms after playing inside the home of neighbors who own a cat. One of his many allergies is to cats. He has a pulse of 100, BP of 90/60, and respirations of 20 and unlabored. Capillary refill is normal. He has no other signs or symptoms. Do you think the physician in the emergency department will order the use of an Epi-Pen Jr.? If yes, why? If no, why not?

Poisoning and Overdose Emergencies

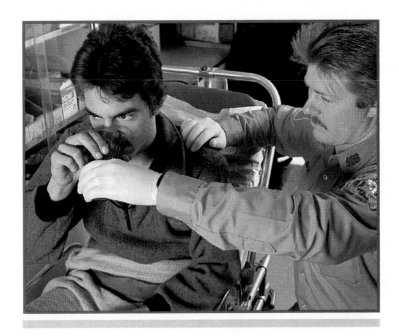

21

Poisoning is a frequent cause of medical emergencies. The largest number of poisoning victims are children who swallow or are exposed to poisons as they explore their environments. Many adults are poisoned by overdosing on medication, either accidentally or deliberately. Poisonous substances are common throughout the everyday environment and can be swallowed, breathed in, injected, or absorbed through the skin. With early prehospital management, the vast majority of poisoning patients have an excellent chance of recovery.

Objectives

On the Scene

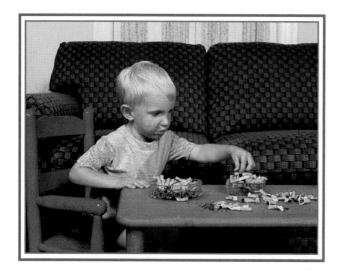

Early on a Saturday morning, you receive a call to respond to a two-year-old boy who has eaten an unknown number of cigarette butts. Your dispatcher tells you that the poison control center has requested administration of activated charcoal and EMS transport to an emergency department.

On arrival, your *scene size-up* reveals a quiet home with no dogs or other potential hazards. You pull on gloves, grab your kit, and approach the anxious-looking woman who has opened the door. Your *initial assessment* begins immediately. You get a general impression of an alert but scared-looking toddler in her arms. You introduce yourself to Mrs. Olson and the little boy tells you his name is Billy.

You follow Mrs. Olson as she carries Billy into the living room. There you see evidence of the present problem: an overturned ashtray with cigarette butts and ashes spilled around it. Mrs. Olson has refrained from cleaning it up, assuming that you would want to see it.

Mrs. Olson has seated herself on a chair with Billy in her lap. You talk to Billy quietly and reassuringly as you assess airway, breathing, and circulation. It's obvious that his airway is open, and you determine that his breathing is adequate and radial pulse is strong and slightly rapid. There is no visible external bleeding. His skin is warm, pink, and dry. Capillary refill is less than two seconds.

direction early in the prehospital management of the poisoning or overdose patient. (p. 367)

10. Describe assessment and care steps for alcohol abuse and withdrawal. (supplemental) (pp. 373–374)

11. Describe assessment and care steps for substance abuse and withdrawal. (supplemental) (p. 374)

Skills

1. Demonstrate the steps in the emergency medical care for the patient with possible overdose.

2. Demonstrate the steps in the emergency medical care for the patient with suspected poisoning.

3. Perform the necessary steps required to provide a patient with activated charcoal.

4. Demonstrate the assessment and documentation of patient response.

5. Demonstrate proper disposal of equipment for the administration of activated charcoal.

6. Demonstrate completing a prehospital care report for patients with a poisoning or overdose emergency.

Beginning the *focused history and physical exam* for a medical patient, you question Billy's mother and learn that, about 15 minutes ago, Billy came to her crying and vomiting cigarette tobacco. She found the overturned ashtray and called the poison control center right away. They told her to wipe out his mouth in case any tobacco was still there and to wait for EMS, which they would call. She does not know how many cigarette butts Billy swallowed. They were left by dinner guests from the evening before.

In response to the SAMPLE questions, Mrs. Olson tells you that Billy has vomited twice but does not seem to have any other signs or symptoms. You learn that Billy has no allergies, is on no medications, has no past medical history, his last meal was last night's dinner, and there were no significant events leading up to this incident. Billy weighs about 25 pounds (11 kilograms). To conduct the focused physical exam, you open Billy's mouth, but find no more tobacco. You take vital signs and note that his pulse is 112, respirations are 26, skin is still warm, pink, and dry.

After assessing Billy, you call on-line medical direction. He has been notified by the poison control center and advises you to administer one bottle (12.5 grams) of activated charcoal. Billy's mother gets one of his "sipping cups," and you accompany Billy and his mother to the ambulance. You give the activated charcoal en route.

During the trip you perform *ongoing assessment,* repeatedly assessing Billy's vital signs and checking his physical condition. When you arrive at the hospital, Billy is doing well.

How can you know that the patient you encounter at the scene of an emergency call has been poisoned? Family members or bystanders may, of course, report this fact when they call for help. There may also be clues at the scene, such as empty pill bottles or containers of toxic substances. Additionally, the patient's signs and symptoms may indicate poisoning or overdose. After you identify and treat immediately life-threatening problems, such as airway or breathing difficulties, your main assessment task will be to gather information for medical direction, who will guide your care and management of the poisoning or overdose patient.

POISONING

A **poison** is any substance that can harm the body, sometimes seriously enough to create a medical emergency. In the United States there are more than a million cases of poisoning annually. Although some of these result from murder or suicide attempts, most are accidental and involve young children. These accidents usually involve common substances such as medications, petroleum products, cosmetics, and pesticides. In fact, a surprisingly large percentage of chemicals in everyday use contain substances that are poisonous if misused.

We usually think of a poison as some kind of liquid or solid chemical that has been ingested by the poisoning victim. This is often the case, but many living organisms are capable of producing a **toxin,** a substance that is poisonous to humans. For example, some mushrooms and other common plants can be poisonous if eaten. These include some varieties of house plants, including the rubber plant and certain parts of holiday plants such as mistletoe and holly berries. Bacterial contaminants in food may produce toxins, some of which can cause deadly diseases (e.g., botulism).

A great number of substances can be considered poisons, with different people reacting differently to various poisons (Table 21-1). As odd as it may seem, what may be a dangerous poison for one person may have little effect on another person. For most poisonous substances, the reaction is far more serious in the ill and the elderly.

Once on or in the body, poisons can do damage in a variety of ways. A poison may act as a corrosive or irritant, destroying skin and other body tissues. A poisonous gas can act as a suffocating agent, displacing oxygen in the air. Some poisons are systemic poisons, causing harm to the entire body or to an entire body system. These poisons can critically depress or overstimulate the central nervous system, cause vomiting and diarrhea, prevent red blood cells from carrying oxygen, or interfere with the normal biochemical processes in the body. The actual effect and extent of damage is dependent on the nature of the poison, on its concentration, and sometimes on how it enters the body. These factors vary in importance depending on the patient's age, weight, and general health.

Poisons can be classified into four types, according to how they enter the body: ingested, inhaled, absorbed, or injected (Figure 21-1).

TABLE 21-1   Common Poisons

Substance	Signs and Symptoms
acetaminophen	Nausea and vomiting. There may be no signs or symptoms.
acids and alkalis	Burns on or around the lips. Burning in mouth, throat, and abdomen. Vomiting.
antihistamines & cough and cold preparations	Hyperactivity or drowsiness. Rapid pulse, flushed skin, dilated pupils.
aspirin	Delayed signs and symptoms, including ringing in the ears, deep and rapid breathing, bruising.
food poisoning	Different types of food poisoning have different signs and symptoms of varying onset. Most include abdominal pain, nausea, vomiting, and diarrhea, sometimes with fever.
insecticides	Slow pulse, excessive salivation and sweating, nausea, vomiting, diarrhea, difficulty breathing, constricted pupils.
petroleum products	Characteristic odor of breath, clothing, vomitus. If aspiration has occurred, coughing and difficulty breathing.
plants	Wide range of signs and symptoms, ranging from none to nausea and vomiting to cardiac arrest.

- **Ingested poisons** (poisons that are swallowed) can include many common household and industrial chemicals, medications, improperly prepared foods, plant materials, petroleum products, and agricultural products made specifically to control rodents, weeds, insects, and crop diseases.
- **Inhaled poisons** (poisons that are breathed in) take the form of gases, vapors, and sprays. Again, many of these substances are in common use in the home, industry, and agriculture. Such poisons include carbon monoxide (from car exhaust, wood-burning stoves, and furnaces), ammonia, chlorine, insect sprays, and the gases pro-

INHALATION

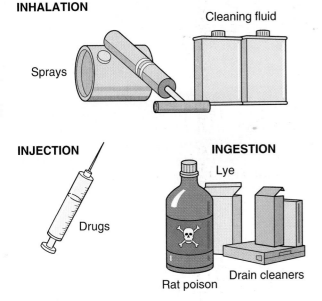

Sprays

Cleaning fluid

INJECTION

Drugs

INGESTION

Lye

Rat poison

Drain cleaners

ABSORPTION

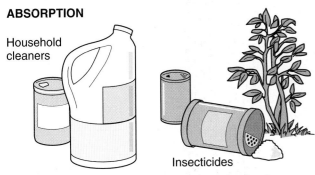

Household cleaners

Insecticides

FIGURE 21-1 How poisons enter the body.

duced from volatile liquid chemicals (*volatile* means "able to change very easily from a liquid into a gas"; many industrial solvents are volatile).

- **Absorbed poisons** (poisons taken into the body through unbroken skin) may or may not damage the skin. Many are corrosives or irritants that will injure the skin and then be slowly absorbed into body tissues and the bloodstream, possibly causing widespread damage. Others are absorbed into the bloodstream without injuring the skin. Examples of these poisons are many insecticides and agricultural chemicals in common use. Contact with a variety of plant materials and certain forms of marine life can lead to skin damage and possible absorption into tissues under the skin.
- **Injected poisons** (poisons inserted through the skin, for example by needle, snake fangs, or insect stinger) will be discussed under Substance Abuse later in this chapter and in Chapter 23, Environmental Emergencies.

Ingested Poisons

Ingested poisons are those that have been swallowed. As in the case of Billy Olson, an ingested poison is often a toxic substance that a curious child has eaten or drunk. In adults, an ingested poison is often a medication on which the patient has accidentally or deliberately overdosed.

Safety Note

Sometimes patients who have ingested poisons will require assisted ventilations. Direct mouth-to-mouth ventilations in such a case are dangerous, not only because of the usual danger of contracting an infectious disease but also because of possible contact with poisonous substances remaining on the patient's lips or in the airway or that may be vomited. Use a pocket face mask with a one-way valve, a bag-valve-mask unit with supplemental oxygen, or positive pressure ventilation when providing ventilations to a patient who is suspected of ingesting a poison.

If intentional poisoning or attempted suicide is suspected, approach the scene with caution and have police backup if indicated.

Patient Assessment—Ingested Poisons

You must gather information quickly in cases of possible ingested poisoning. In order to make the decision about whether activated charcoal is appropriate, your medical director will need certain information.

☐ *What **substance** was involved?* Many products have similar names. It is important to get the exact spelling of the substance. If possible, bring the container to the hospital with the patient. (In Billy Olson's case, of course, there is no container, but samples of the cigarette butts and other contents of the ashtray could be brought along.)

☐ ***When** did the exposure occur?* Some poisons act very quickly and will require immediate treatment. Others may take longer to affect the body and may allow other treatments to be used.

It is sometimes difficult to determine the time of the exposure from family members or witnesses. If you can't get an exact time, determine when the earliest and latest possible times of exposure were. (Billy's mother thinks he ate the cigarette butts within the last hour, after she got him out of bed. She doubts that he came downstairs during the night, but it is possible.)

☐ *How much* *was ingested?* This may be as easy as counting the number of tablets left in a brand new prescription or as difficult as estimating the amount of gasoline spilled on a garage floor. When the amount cannot be estimated reliably, determine the maximum amount that might have been ingested. (Billy's mother does not know how many cigarettes her guests smoked. Billy could have eaten one or a large number.)

☐ *Over* **how long** *a period did the ingestion occur?* Someone who takes certain medication chronically and then overdoses on it may require very different hospital treatment from the patient who has the same overdose but has never taken that medication before. (The Olsons' guests left at midnight. Billy could have gotten out of bed during the night and could have been eating the cigarette butts over a period of up to eight hours.)

☐ *What* **interventions** *have the patient, family, or well-meaning bystanders taken?* Many traditional home remedies for medical problems are harmful, particularly when someone has been exposed to enough of a substance to suffer ill effects. Product labels have been improved over the last few years, but some still contain inaccurate or even dangerous instructions for management of potentially toxic exposures. (Billy's mother called the poison control center immediately. At the poison center's direction, the only action she has taken is to wipe out Billy's mouth.)

☐ *What is the patient's* **estimated weight?** This, in combination with the amount of substance ingested, may be critical in determining the appropriate treatment. (Billy weighs 25 pounds, or 11 kilograms.)

☐ *What* **effects** *is the patient experiencing from the ingestion?* Nausea and vomiting are two of the most common results of poison ingestion, but you may also find altered mental status, abdominal pain, diarrhea, chemical burns around the mouth, and unusual breath odors. (Billy had vomited but exhibited no other signs.)

Emergency Medical Care

To provide the proper emergency care for ingested poisons (Scan 21-1), follow the instructions given to you by medical direction.

Activated Charcoal or Dilution In some cases of ingested poisoning, medical direction will order administration of activated charcoal (Scan 21-2). **Activated charcoal** is not an antidote, but it absorbs many poisons and prevents them from being absorbed by the body. Ordinary charcoal absorbs some substances, but activated charcoal is different because it has been manufactured to have many cracks and crevices. This increases the amount of surface available to bind to poisons (similar to the way corrugated cardboard, if you cut it open, has many more surfaces than you would expect by looking at the smooth outer surface).

Many poisons are absorbed by activated charcoal, but not all. Since there are millions of potential poisons available and the number is always increasing, it makes little sense for the EMT-B to memorize lists of poisons where activated charcoal should not be used. Instead, medical direction (possibly in consultation with a poison control center) will be able to determine whether the use of activated charcoal is appropriate.

There are, however, a few instances the EMT-B should know about where the use of activated charcoal is contraindicated.

- A patient who cannot swallow obviously cannot swallow activated charcoal.
- A patient with altered mental status might choke on activated charcoal and aspirate it into the lungs.
- A patient who has ingested acids or alkalis should not take activated charcoal because the caustic material may have severely damaged the mouth, throat, and esophagus. Activated charcoal cannot help the damage that has already been done, and swallowing it may cause further damage. Examples of such caustic substances are oven cleaners, drain cleaners, toilet bowl cleaners, and lye.
- A patient who has accidentally swallowed while siphoning gasoline should not be given activated charcoal. This patient will be coughing violently and possibly aspirating the gasoline. This patient will be unable to swallow activated charcoal.

Ingested Poisons

FIRST take body substance isolation precautions.

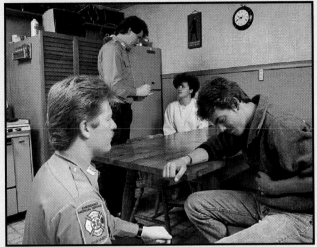

1. Quickly gather information and maintain an open airway.

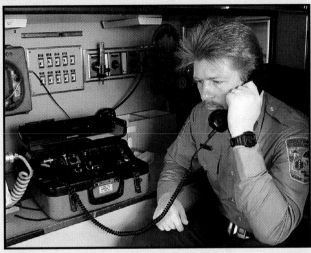

2. Call medical direction on the scene or en route.

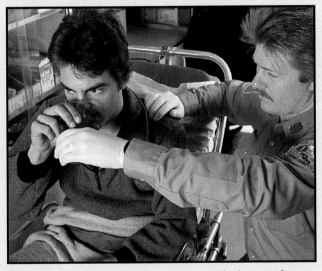

3. If directed, administer activated charcoal.

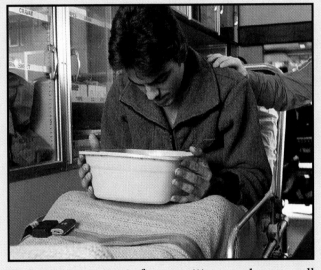

4. Position patient for vomiting and save all vomitus. Have suction equipment ready.

Safety Note: When a patient has ingested a poison, it provides another reason to avoid mouth-to-mouth contact. Provide ventilations through a pocket face mask or other barrier device.

Scan 21-2
Activated Charcoal

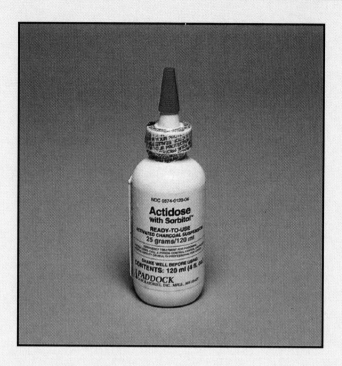

Medication Name
1. Generic: activated charcoal
2. Trade: SuperChar, InstaChar, Actidose, Liqui-Char, and others

Indications
1. Poisoning by mouth

Contraindications
1. Altered mental status
2. Ingestion of acids or alkalis
3. Unable to swallow

Medication form
1. Pre-mixed in water, frequently available in plastic bottle containing 12.5 grams of activated charcoal
2. Powder—should be avoided in field

Dosage
1. Adults and children: 1 gram activated charcoal/kg of body weight
2. Usual adult dose: 25-50 grams
3. Usual pediatric dose: 12.5-25 grams

Administration
1. Consult medical direction.
2. Shake container *thoroughly.*
3. Since medication looks like mud, patient may need to be persuaded to drink it. Providing a covered container and a straw will prevent patient from seeing the medication and so may improve patient compliance.
4. If patient does not drink the medication right away, the charcoal will settle. Shake or stir it again before administering.
5. Record the name, dose, route, and time of administration of the medication.

Actions
1. Activated charcoal binds to certain poisons and prevents them from being absorbed into the body.
2. Not all brands of activated charcoal are the same; some bind much more than others, so consult medical direction about the brand to use.

Side effects
1. black stools
2. Some patients, particularly those who have ingested poisons that cause nausea, may vomit. If patient vomits, repeat the dose once.

Reassessment strategies
1. Be prepared for the patient to vomit or further deteriorate.

Many brands of activated charcoal are on the market, but some have greater surface area than others. Medical direction can guide you in the selection of an appropriate brand.

Occasionally, medical direction will give an order for **dilution** of a poisonous substance. This means an adult patient should drink one to two glasses of water or milk, whichever is ordered. A child should typically be given half to one glass. Dilution with water may slow absorption slightly. Milk may soothe stomach upset. This treatment is frequently advised for patients who, medical direction or poison control determines, do not need transport to a hospital.

Patient Care—Ingested Poisons

Emergency Care Steps

1. Detect and treat immediately life-threatening problems in the initial assessment. Evaluate the need for prompt transport for critical patients.
2. Perform a focused history and physical exam, including SAMPLE history. Use gloved hands to carefully remove any pills, tablets, or fragments from the patient's mouth.
3. Assess baseline vital signs.
4. Consult medical direction. As directed, administer activated charcoal to absorb the poison, or water or milk to dilute it. This can usually be done en route.
5. Transport the patient with all containers, bottles, and labels from the substance.
6. Perform ongoing assessment en route.

In Billy Olson's case, quality care paid off. The nicotine in tobacco is absorbed much better when swallowed than when smoked, so Billy was at risk of having serious complications from nicotine poisoning. In a child his size, three cigarette butts or one whole cigarette has the potential to be lethal. Since you couldn't tell exactly how much tobacco Billy swallowed (which is commonly the case in poisonings), you treated for the worst. Perhaps he didn't swallow enough to get a lethal dose, perhaps he vomited up enough to avoid serious problems, or perhaps the activated charcoal absorbed enough nicotine. You will never know for certain, but one thing you do know is that Billy's mother's prompt action in calling for help and your interventions helped Billy come through the incident successfully.

Infants and Children

It is the nature of infants and children to explore their world—and to get into and often taste whatever they find. Children will swallow substances adults cannot imagine swallowing, including horrible-tasting poisonous substances like bleach or lye. The natural curiosity of children makes them the most frequent victims of accidental poisoning.

It is important to find out an infant's or child's weight, which—in combination with the estimated amount of the poisonous substance that was ingested—will help medical direction determine appropriate treatment.

As an EMT-B, never assume that the infant or child has not ingested a lethal amount of the poison. Because it is usually extremely difficult or impossible to be sure exactly how much the child has taken in, always treat for the worst. Call medical direction, administer the recommended treatments, and transport the child to the hospital.

Inhaled Poisons

On the Scene

You respond to a man who has attempted suicide from exhaust fumes in a garage. Your dispatcher tells you the fire and police departments are also responding.

As you approach the address and *size up the scene,* you note that the fire department and police are already present. You see a house with an attached garage. The garage door is open and firefighters are opening other doors and windows to ventilate the building. You also see two firefighters carrying a man onto the lawn.

As you approach him to begin your *initial assessment,* you get a general impression of an approximately 30-year-old male who is holding his hands to his head. His mental status is awake. He is able to tell you that his name is Tim O'Leary, but he is slow to answer questions and a little confused. He is complaining of a headache. His airway is open and his breathing is adequate. You check his circulation. His radial pulse is rapid and strong, and there is no blood on or around the patient. His skin is pale and sweaty. The priority you assign to this patient is high because of the mechanism of injury and his altered mental status. Your partner prepares a nonrebreather mask and places it on the patient with 15 liters per minute of oxygen as you continue with the assessment.

You begin the *focused history and physical exam* by questioning Tim about his signs and symptoms. He complains of a severe headache, but does not give much more information than that. He tells you that he wishes he had done it right and killed himself. When you ask if he took any pills or tried to hurt himself in any other way, Tim says no. He doesn't want to answer any more questions. A neighbor approaches, who says that she called 911 because she suspected something was wrong. She noticed that a car was running inside the closed garage about 10 minutes ago. When no one answered her knocks on the garage door or the front door, she called for help. Tim has a pulse of 124, BP 140/90, and respirations of 30 and deep. Skin is pale and cool. Pupils are equal and reactive.

Oxygen is the most important part of the treatment for this patient, and you give him as much as you can. You and your partner place him on the stretcher and, with some help from the firefighters at the scene, load him into the ambulance. En route, you perform an *ongoing assessment* every 5 minutes. The patient's vital signs remain about the same, and he is still not interested in talking to you about what happened.

At the hospital, it is discovered that Tim has high levels of carbon monoxide in his blood. He admits that it was a suicide attempt following the loss of a job and a broken romance. He is referred for counseling which, you later learn, is successful in helping him get his life back together. If you had not immediately given him high concentration oxygen, he might have died or suffered brain damage and never had that second chance.

Inhaled poisons are those that are present in the atmosphere and that you, as well as the patient, are at risk of breathing in. Carbon monoxide poisoning is a common problem. Other possible inhaled poisons include chlorine gas (often from swimming pool chemicals), ammonia (often released from household cleaners), sprayed agricultural chemicals and pesticides, and carbon dioxide (from industrial sources).

Safety Note

If you suspect that a patient has inhaled a poison, approach the scene with care. Some EMS systems provide training in the use of protective clothing and self-contained breathing apparatus to be used in a hostile environment (e.g., chlorine gas, ammonia, smoke). Remember that many inhaled poisons can also be absorbed through the skin. Go only where your protective equipment and clothing will allow you to go safely to perform your mission, and only after you have been trained in the use of this equipment. *Do only what you have been trained to do and go only where your protective equipment will allow you to go safely. If you are underequipped or undertrained, get someone there who is properly equipped and trained.*

Patient Assessment—Inhaled Poisons

Gather the following information as quickly as possible.

- [ ] *What **substance** was involved?* Get its exact name.
- [ ] ***When** did the exposure occur?* Estimate as well as you can when the patient was exposed to the poisonous gas by finding out the earliest and latest possible times of exposure.
- [ ] *Over **how long** a period did the exposure occur?* The longer someone is exposed to a poisonous gas, the more poison will probably be absorbed.
- [ ] *What **interventions** has anyone taken?* Did someone remove the patient or ventilate the area right away? When did this happen?
- [ ] *What **effects** is the patient experiencing from the exposure?* Nausea and vomiting are very common in poisoning of all types. With inhaled poisons, find out if the patient is having difficulty breathing, chest pain, coughing, hoarseness, dizziness, headache, confusion, seizures, or altered mental status.

In the case of Tim O'Leary, it was obvious that he had been exposed to carbon monoxide. The interventions included opening the garage windows and doors and getting Tim out onto the lawn. Since Tim is uncommunicative, all you are able to discover about the time and length of his exposure is that the neighbor discovered the problem 10 minutes ago and firefighters arrived to intervene about 2 minutes before your arrival. Tim complained of a headache but did not reveal other symptoms.

Emergency Medical Care

The principal prehospital treatment of inhaled poisoning consists of maintaining the airway and supporting respiration (Scan 21-3). In the case of inhaled poisoning, oxygen is a very

Safety Note: In the presence of hazardous fumes or gases, wear protective clothing and self-contained breathing apparatus or wait for those who are properly trained and equipped to enter the scene and bring the patient out.

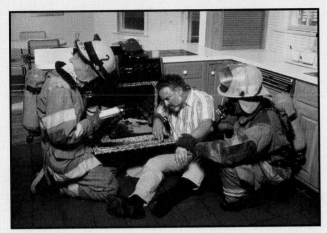

1. Remove patient from source.

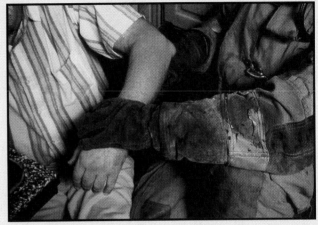

2. Avoid touching contaminated clothing and jewelry.

3. Remember: It is critical to establish and maintain an open airway.

4. Caution: Stay alert for vomiting. Properly position patient and have suction equipment ready.

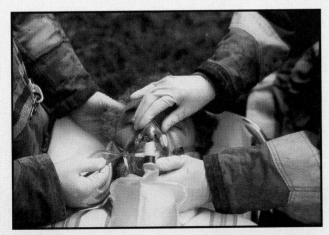

5. Administer a high concentration of oxygen.

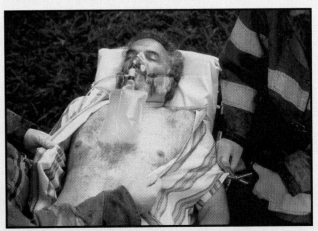

6. Remove contaminated clothing and jewelry.

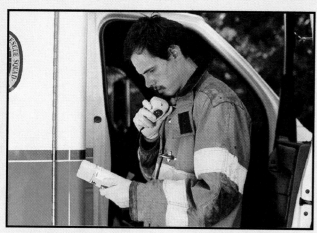

7. Call medical direction. Follow directions.

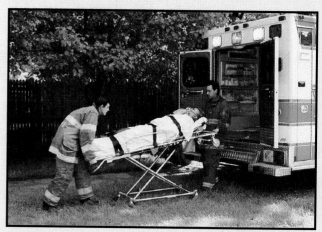

8. Transport as soon as possible.

Warning: If called to the scene of a hazardous material incident, do only what you have been trained to do and what your equipment allows. Be careful to protect other rescuers and assure that the patient has been decontaminated by a hazardous materials response team (see Chapter 32, Overviews, and Appendix C, Hazardous Materials). Remember that inhaled poisons can frequently be absorbed through the skin.

important drug. Some inhaled poisons prevent the blood from transporting oxygen in the normal manner. Some prevent oxygen from getting into the bloodstream in the first place. In either case, the EMT-B's ability to keep the airway open, ventilate as needed, and give high concentration oxygen may make the difference in the survival and quality of life of the patient who has inhaled a poison.

Patient Care—Inhaled Poisons

Emergency Care Steps

1. If the patient is in an unsafe environment, have trained rescuers remove the patient to a safe area. Detect and treat immediately life-threatening problems in the initial assessment. Evaluate the need for prompt transport for critical patients.
2. Perform a focused history and physical exam, including SAMPLE history and vital signs.
3. Administer high concentration oxygen. This is the single most important treatment for inhaled poisoning after the patient's airway is opened.
4. Transport the patient with all containers, bottles, and labels from the substance.
5. Perform ongoing assessment en route.

In Tim O'Leary's case, your prompt administration of high concentration oxygen and immediate transport were of critical importance in a successful outcome.

Carbon Monoxide

Carbon monoxide is one of the most common inhaled poisons, usually associated with motor vehicle exhaust and fire suppression. The number of cases has increased recently because of the carbon monoxide that can accumulate from the use of improperly vented wood-burning stoves and the use of charcoal for heating and indoor cooking in areas without adequate ventilation. Malfunctioning oil, gas, and coal-burning furnaces and stoves can also be sources of carbon monoxide.

Since carbon monoxide is an odorless, colorless, and tasteless gas, you will not be able to directly detect its presence without special equipment. Look for indications of possible carbon monoxide poisoning like wood-burning stoves, doors that lead to a garage, or bedrooms above a garage where motor repair work is in progress, and evidence that suggests the patient has spent a long period of time sitting in an idling motor vehicle. When inhaled, carbon monoxide prevents the normal carrying of oxygen by the red blood cells. Long exposure, even to low levels of the gas, can cause dramatic effects. Death may occur as hypoxia becomes more severe.

The signs and symptoms of carbon monoxide poisoning are deceptive, because they can resemble those of the flu. Specifically, you may see

- headache, especially one described as a band around the head
- dizziness
- breathing difficulty
- nausea
- cyanosis
- altered mental status; in severe cases, unconsciousness may result

Note: There is a commonly accepted idea that a carbon monoxide victim will have cherry red lips. In fact, cherry red skin is NOT typically seen in patients with carbon monoxide poisoning.

You should suspect carbon monoxide poisoning whenever you are treating a patient with vague, flulike symptoms who has been in an enclosed area. This is especially true when a group of people in the same area have similar symptoms. A patient with carbon monoxide poisoning may begin to feel better shortly after being removed from the dangerous environment. It is still very important to continue to administer oxygen and to transport these patients to a hospital. Oxygen is an antidote for carbon monoxide poisoning, but it takes time to "wash out" the carbon monoxide from the patient's bloodstream. These patients need medical evaluation because they can have serious consequences, including neurological deficits, from their exposure.

Absorbed Poisons

On the Scene

The cook at Camp Whoop-It-Up is getting irritated. It is now 10 minutes after 7 in the morning and his kitchen crew is still not in the kitchen. Deciding to use an old remedy for oversleeping, he gets a bottle of ammonia and heads for the bunkhouse where the crew sleeps. He slams open the door, starts yelling about being on time for work, and throws liberal amounts of ammonia around the room. One of the kitchen workers, Gary Wong, is a little faster getting out of bed than his co-workers. Unfortunately, that means he gets some of the ammonia in his eye.

You approach the camp and, **sizing up the scene,** see no dangers or hazards. After you enter the bunkhouse, you notice a smell of ammonia, but the windows are open, fans are blowing, and the odor is not overpowering.

You begin your **initial assessment** as you find a 17-year-old male leaning over the bathroom sink with another teenager helping him rinse his eyes and face. Your general impression is that he is alert and in pain. His mental status, airway, breathing and circulation are all fine. You do not see any immediate reason to assign him a high priority, but you decide to get more information before making a decision.

As you undertake the **focused history and physical exam,** you discover that Gary got splashed in the eye and face by household-strength ammonia (you check the label to be sure it really is ammonia and that it is not industrial strength). He is complaining of a fair amount of pain in his left eye, but irrigation with tap water, which has been going on for 10 minutes, is relieving some of that. When you ask him to stop irrigating for a moment so you can look at his eye and face, you find that the left eye is red and the lids are a little bit swollen. His right eye looks normal. The skin on his face does not look irritated at all. You encourage Gary to continue rinsing his eye.

You now have enough information to confirm that this is not a high priority patient. Gary has a painful injury, but his eye was promptly irrigated. You ask your partner to set up a bag of normal saline or Lactated Ringer's solution so that you can continue to irrigate the patient's eye en route. While your partner does this, you explain to Gary that he should irrigate his eye for another 10 minutes (for a total of 20 minutes) before you take him to the hospital to get further evaluation and treatment.

You continue to irrigate Gary's eye en route to the hospital and do an **ongoing assessment** of his ABCs and vital signs every 15 minutes en route. When you arrive at the emergency department, his eye is feeling a lot better. The emergency department physician examines Gary, determines that his eye is OK, and discharges him with instructions to avoid getting ammonia in his eye again.

Later in the day you find time to drop by Camp Whoop-It-Up to chat with the cook. You strongly encourage him to find another way to wake up his crew.

Absorbed poisons frequently irritate or damage the skin. Some poisons, though, can be absorbed with little or no damage to the skin.

Safety Note

Just as poisonous substances can be absorbed by patients, they can also be absorbed by EMT-Bs. It is critical that the EMT-B take protective measures to prevent exposure to these substances. It may be necessary for firefighters to hose down a patient before the EMT-B touches him.

Patient Assessment—Absorbed Poisons

Gather the following information as quickly as possible.

- [ ] *What* **substance** *was involved?* Get its exact name.
- [ ] **When** *did the exposure occur?*
- [ ] **How much** *of the substance was the patient exposed to? How large an area of skin was the substance on?*
- [ ] *Over* **how long** *a period did the exposure occur? The longer someone's skin is exposed to a poison, the more likely it is to be well absorbed.*
- [ ] *What* **interventions** *has anyone taken? Did someone attempt to wash the substance off the patient? If so, with what? Did anyone attempt to use a chemical to "neutralize" the substance?*
- [ ] *What* **effects** *is the patient experiencing from the exposure?* Common signs and symptoms include a liquid or powder on the patient's skin, burns, itching, irritation, and redness.

When you responded to the Camp Whoop-It-Up incident, you were able to determine that Gary Wong had been splashed with household-strength ammonia at about 7:12 A.M., around 10 minutes before your arrival. The exposure lasted only a few seconds before the boys intervened by helping Gary wash his eye with water. The effects were a reddened eye.

Emergency Medical Care

The most important part of the treatment of a patient with an absorbed poison is to get the poison off the skin or out of the eye (Scan 21-4). The best way to do this is by irrigating the skin or the eye with large amounts of clean water. A garden hose or fire hose can be used to irrigate

Scan 21-4
Absorbed Poisons

 Safety Note: Take care to protect your skin from contact with poisonous substances. Wear protective clothing. If necessary, have firefighters or others who are properly protected hose off the patient before you touch him.

FIRST take body substance isolation precautions.

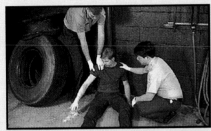

1. Remove patient from source or source from patient. Avoid contaminating yourself with the poison.

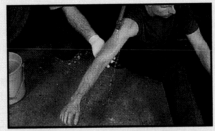

2. Brush powders from the patient. Be careful not to abrade the patient's skin.

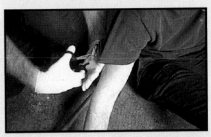

3. Remove contaminated clothing and other articles.

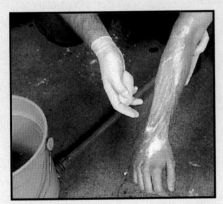

4. Wash with clear water. Call medical direction. Follow directions.

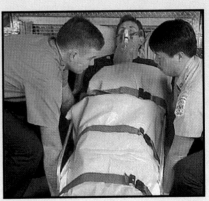

5. Be alert for shock and transport as soon as possible.

Warning: If called to the scene of a hazardous material incident, do only what you have been trained to do and what your equipment allows. Be careful to protect other rescuers and assure that the patient has been decontaminated by a hazardous materials response team (see Chapter 32, Overviews, and Appendix C, Hazardous Materials).

the patient's skin, but care must be taken not to injure the skin further with high pressure.

"Neutralizing" acids or alkalis with solutions such as dilute vinegar or baking soda in water should not be done. When incidents like these occur, such substances are almost never readily available. Even if they were, they would not be appropriate. They have never been shown to help, and there is good reason to believe they would make matters worse. When an acid is mixed with an alkali, it is true that the two may be neutralized. It also true, though, that this reaction produces heat. Skin that has been injured already by an acid or alkali may be further damaged by attempts to neutralize the chemical.

Patient Care—Absorbed Poisons

Emergency Care Steps

1 Detect and treat immediately life-threatening problems in the initial assessment. Evaluate the need for prompt transport of critical patients.

2 Perform a focused history and physical exam, including SAMPLE history and vital signs. This includes removing contaminated clothing while protecting oneself from contamination.

3 Remove the poison by doing one of the following:

- *Powders:* Brush powder off the patient, then continue as for other absorbed poisons.
- *Liquids:* Irrigate with clean water for at least 20 minutes and continue en route if possible.
- *Eyes:* Irrigate with clean water for at least 20 minutes and continue en route if possible.

4 Transport the patient with all containers, bottles, and labels from the substance.

5 Perform ongoing assessment en route.

For Gary Wong, irrigation with water and prompt transport helped assure that the ammonia that was splashed into his eye did no permanent damage.

Prevention

Preventing poisoning is, of course, preferable to having to treat it. The EMT-B's own home and the squad building should be "childproofed" against poisoning by keeping medications and other dangerous substances out of children's reach. The EMT-B can also share poisoning prevention information with children and other members of the public during school visits and community outreach activities.

Documentation Tips—Poisoning

With any kind of poisoning, be sure to gather and document the following kinds of information that medical direction and hospital personnel will need.

1. Route of poisoning—Note whether the poison was ingested, inhaled, or absorbed.
2. Substance—Write down the exact name and spelling of the substance.
3. Amount—Estimate how much of the substance the patient took in or was exposed to. If the exact amount is unknown, note any clues (e.g., *The 1-liter bottle was half empty*). Put witnesses' exact words in quotation marks (e.g., *"There was this funny smell, like nail polish remover."*).
4. Time—Document when the ingestion or exposure took place and over how long a period of time.
5. Interventions—Write down any actions the patient, family members, or bystanders took before you arrived, such as having the patient swallow something or inducing vomiting.
6. Patient's weight—If the poison was ingested, note the patient's body weight. If no one knows, write down your best estimate.
7. Effects of poisoning—Document any effects of the poisoning the patient has experienced (e.g., nausea or vomiting, dizziness, difficulty breathing, altered mental status, itching, burning).
8. Effects of treatment—Document the patient's response to treatments you or others have given.

ALCOHOL AND SUBSTANCE ABUSE

As an EMT-B you will see many patients whose conditions are caused, either directly or indirectly, by alcohol or substance abuse. Although these are often thought of as urban problems, the abuse of alcohol and other drugs crosses all geographic and economic boundaries.

Alcohol Abuse

While many persons consume alcohol without any problems, others occasionally or chronically abuse alcohol. Although alcohol is legal (for adults), it must not be forgotten that alcohol is a drug and has a potent effect on the central nervous system. Emergencies arising from the use of alcohol may be due to the effect of alcohol that has just been consumed, or it may be the result of the cumulative effects of years of alcohol abuse.

EMT-Bs often do not take alcohol abuse patients seriously. This may be partially due to the belligerent or unusual behavior they often exhibit. In addition, frequent calls for intoxicated persons may cause the EMT-B to become callous toward them. The hygiene of many of these patients on the street leaves much to be desired. Nevertheless, as an EMT-B you should provide care for the patient suffering from alcohol abuse the same as for any other patient. Patients who appear intoxicated must be treated with the same respect and dignity as those who are "sober."

Above all, you must not neglect your duty to provide medical care. Not only do alcohol abuse patients often have injuries from accidents and falls, but they are also candidates for many medical emergencies. Chronic drinkers often have derangements in blood sugar levels, poor nutrition, the potential for considerable gastrointestinal bleeding, and other problems. A person can be *both* intoxicated *and* having a heart attack or hypoglycemia. If the patient has ingested alcohol along with other drugs, this can also produce a serious medical emergency. When alcohol is combined with other depressants such as antihistamines and tranquilizers, the effects of alcohol can be more pronounced and, in some cases, can be lethal.

Since EMT-B safety is a critical part of all calls, do not hesitate to ask for police assistance with any patient who appears intoxicated or irrational or exhibits potentially dangerous behavior. The nature of intoxication is such that a passive person may suddenly become aggressive. The EMT-B should always be prepared for this event. (See also Chapter 23, Behavioral Emergencies.)

Keep in mind that, while alcohol *may* be the patient's only problem, there may be another problem present. Conduct a complete assessment to identify any medical emergencies. Remember that diabetes, epilepsy, head injuries, high fevers, hypoxia, and other medical problems may make the patient appear to be intoxicated when he is not. Also look for other injuries. *Do not allow the presence of alcohol or the signs and symptoms of alcohol abuse to override your suspicions of other medical problems or injuries.*

Since getting a SAMPLE history from any patient who appears intoxicated will be difficult and perhaps unreliable, your powers of observation and resourcefulness will be tested. Family members and bystanders may provide important information.

The signs and symptoms of alcohol abuse include those listed below.

Signs and Symptoms of Alcohol Abuse

- [ ] The odor of alcohol on the patient's breath or clothing. By itself, this is not enough to conclude alcohol abuse. Be certain that this odor is not "acetone breath" as with some diabetic emergencies.
- [ ] Swaying and unsteadiness of movement
- [ ] Slurred speech, rambling thought patterns, incoherent words or phrases
- [ ] A flushed appearance to the face, often with the patient sweating and complaining of being warm
- [ ] Nausea or vomiting
- [ ] Poor coordination
- [ ] Slowed reaction time
- [ ] Blurred vision
- [ ] Confusion
- [ ] Hallucinations, visual or auditory ("seeing things" or "hearing things")
- [ ] Lack of memory (blackout)
- [ ] Altered mental status

The alcoholic patient may not be under the influence of alcohol but, instead, may be suffering from alcohol **withdrawal.** This can be a severe reaction occurring when the patient cannot obtain alcohol, is too sick to drink alcohol, or has decided to quit drinking suddenly. The alcohol withdrawal patient may experience seizures or **delirium tremens**

(DTs), a condition characterized by sweating, trembling, anxiety, and hallucinations. In some cases, alcohol withdrawal can be fatal.

Signs of Alcohol Withdrawal

☐ Confusion and restlessness
☐ Atypical behavior, to the point of demonstrating "insane" behavior
☐ Hallucinations
☐ Gross tremor (obvious shaking) of the hands
☐ Profuse sweating
☐ Seizures (common and often very serious)

Warning: Be on the alert for signs, such as depressed vital signs, that the patient has mixed alcohol and drugs. When interviewing the intoxicated patient or the patient suffering from alcohol withdrawal, do not begin by asking the patient if he is taking *drugs*. He may react to this question as if you are gathering evidence of a crime. Ask if any *medications* have been taken while drinking. If necessary, when you are certain that the patient knows you are concerned about his well-being, you can repeat the question using the word "drugs."

Patient Care—Alcohol Abuse

Since these patients often vomit, take body substance isolation precautions, including gloves, mask, and protective eyewear.

Emergency Care Steps

To provide basic care for the intoxicated patient and the patient suffering alcohol withdrawal

1 Stay alert for airway and respiratory problems. Be prepared to perform airway maintenance, suctioning, and positioning of the patient should the patient lose consciousness, seize, or vomit. Help the patient during vomiting so that vomitus will not be aspirated. Have a rigid-tip suction device ready. Provide oxygen and assisted respirations as needed.

2 Be alert for changes in mental status as alcohol is absorbed into the bloodstream. Talk to the patient in an effort to keep him as alert as possible.

3 Monitor vital signs.

4 Treat for shock.

5 Protect the patient from self-injury. Use restraint as authorized by your EMS system. Request assistance from law enforcement if needed.

6 Stay alert for seizures.

7 Transport the patient to a medical facility if indicated.

Note: In some systems, patients under the influence of alcohol who are not suffering from a medical emergency or apparent injury are not transported. They are given over to the police. This may not be wise since some patients having an alcohol-related emergency may die unless they receive additional care. In addition to this, the EMT-Bs may have missed a medical problem or injury. Remember, too, that the patient's condition may worsen as the alcohol continues to be absorbed by his system. Be especially careful of patients with even minor head injuries, since subdural hematoma (see Chapter 28, Injuries to the Head and Spine) is common in alcoholics. If transport is refused or deemed unnecessary, do not leave the patient alone but make sure that he is in the care of a responsible adult. Document this in your prehospital care report. ALL PATIENTS WITH SEIZURES OR DTs MUST BE TRANSPORTED TO A MEDICAL FACILITY AS SOON AS POSSIBLE.

Substance Abuse

Substance abuse is a term that indicates that a chemical substance is being taken for other than therapeutic (medical) reasons. Many of the substances have legitimate purposes when used properly. When these same substances are abused, the results can be devastating.

Individuals who abuse drugs and other chemical substances should be considered to have an illness. They have the right to the same professional emergency care as any other patient.

The most common drugs and chemical substances that are abused and may lead to problems requiring an EMS response can be classified as uppers, downers, narcotics, hallucinogens, and volatile chemicals.

- **Uppers** are stimulants affecting the nervous system to excite the user. Many abusers use these drugs in an attempt to relieve fatigue or to create feelings of well-being. Examples are caffeine, amphetamines, and cocaine. Cocaine may be "snorted," smoked, or injected. Other stimulants are frequently in pill form.

- **Downers** have a depressant effect on the central nervous system. This type of drug may be used as a relaxing agent, sleeping pill, or tranquilizer. Barbiturates are an example, usually in pill or capsule form.
- **Narcotics** are drugs capable of producing stupor or sleep. They are often used to relieve pain and to quiet coughing. Many drugs legitimately used for these purposes (e.g., codeine) are also abused, affecting the nervous system and changing many of the normal activities of the body, often producing an intense state of relaxation or feeling of well-being. Illegal narcotics such as heroin are also commonly abused. Heroin is usually injected into a vein. Other narcotics are in pill form.
- **Hallucinogens** (huh-LOO-sin-uh-jens) such as LSD and PCP are mind-affecting drugs that act on the nervous system to produce an intense state of excitement or a distortion of the user's perceptions. This class of drugs has few legal uses. They are often eaten or dissolved in the mouth and absorbed through the mucous membranes.
- **Volatile chemicals** can give an initial "rush" and then act as a depressant on the central nervous system. Cleaning fluid, glue, model cement, and solutions used to correct typing mistakes are commonly abused volatile chemicals.

Patient Assessment—Substance Abuse

As an EMT-B you will *not* need to know the names of the very many abused drugs or their specific reactions. It is far more important for you to be able to detect possible drug abuse at the overdose level and to relate certain signs to certain types of drugs and drug withdrawal. Table 21-2 provides some of the names of commonly abused drugs. Do not worry about memorizing this list. Read it through so that you can place some of the more familiar drugs into categories in terms of drug type.

The signs and symptoms of substance abuse, dependency, and overdose can vary from patient to patient, even for the same drug or chemical. The problem is made more complex by the fact that many substance abusers take more than one drug or chemical at a time. Often, you will have to carefully combine the information gained from the signs, the symptoms, the scene, the bystanders, and the patient in order to determine that you may dealing with substance abuse. In many cases, you will not be able to identify the substance involved.

When questioning the patient and bystanders, you will get better results if you begin by asking if the patient has been taking any medications. Then, if necessary, ask if the patient has been taking drugs.

Some significant signs and symptoms related to specific types of drugs include those listed below. These are listed for your information in helping you to recognize possible drug abuse in general. Your patient care will not change as a result of this knowledge, but information you can gather about what kind of drug the patient may have been taking will be useful to hospital personnel.

Signs and Symptoms of Drug Abuse

☐ Uppers—Excitement, increased pulse and breathing rates, rapid speech, dry mouth, dilated pupils, sweating, and the complaint of having gone without sleep for long periods. Repeated high doses can produce a "speed run." The patient will be restless, hyperactive, and usually very apprehensive and uncooperative.

☐ Downers—Sluggish, sleepy patient lacking typical coordination of body and speech. Pulse and breathing rates are low, often to the point of a true emergency.

☐ Hallucinogens—Fast pulse rate, dilated pupils, and a flushed face. The patient often "sees" or "hears" things, has little concept of real time, and may not be aware of the true environment. Often what he says makes no sense to the listener. The user may become aggressive or be very timid.

☐ Narcotics—Reduced rate of pulse and rate and depth of breathing, often seen with a lowering of skin temperature. The pupils are constricted, often pinpoint in size. The muscles are relaxed and sweating is profuse. The patient is very sleepy and does not wish to do anything. In overdoses, coma is common. Respiratory arrest or cardiac arrest may develop rapidly.

☐ Volatile chemicals—Dazed or showing temporary loss of contact with reality. The patient may develop coma. The linings of

TABLE 21-2 Commonly Abused Drugs

Uppers	Downers	Narcotics	Mind-Altering Drugs	Volatile Chemicals
AMPHETAMINE (Benzedrine, bennies, pep pills, ups, uppers, cartwheels)	AMOBARBITAL (blue devils, downers, barbs, Amytal)	CODEINE (often in cough syrup)	*Hallucinogenic*	AMYL NITRATE (snappers, poppers)
BIPHETAMINE (bam)	BARBITURATES (downers, dolls, barbs, rainbows)	DEMEROL	DMT	BUTYL NITRATE (locker room, rush)
COCAINE (coke, snow, crack)	CHLORAL HYDRATE (knockout drops, Noctec)	DILAUDID	LSD (acid, sunshine)	CLEANING FLUID (carbon tetrachloride)
DESOXYN (black beauties)	ETHCHLORVYNOL (Placidyl)	FENTANYL (Sublimaze)	MESCALINE (peyote, mesc)	FURNITURE POLISH
DEXTROAMPHET-AMINE (dexies, Dexedrine)	GLUTETHIMIDE (Doriden, goofers)	HEROIN ("H," horse, junk, smack, stuff)	MORNING GLORY SEEDS	GASOLINE
METHAMPHET-AMINE (speed, crank, meth, crystal, diet pills, Methedrine)	METHAQUALONE (Quaalude, ludes, Sopor, sopors)	METHADONE (dolly)	PCP (angel dust, hog, peace pills)	GLUE
METHYLPHENI-DATE (Ritalin)	NONBARBITURATE SEDATIVES (various tranquilizers and sleeping pills: Valium or diazepam, Miltown, Equanil, meprobamate, Thorazine, Compazine, Librium or chlordiazepoxide, reserpine, Tranxene or chlorazepate and other benz-odiazepines)	MORPHINE	PSILOCYBIN (magic mushrooms)	HAIR SPRAY
PRELUDIN		OPIUM (op, poppy)	STP (serenity, tranquillity, peace)	NAIL POLISH REMOVER
		MEPERIDINE (Demerol)		PAINT THINNER
		PAREGORIC (contains opium)	*Nonhallucinogenic*	TYPEWRITING CORRECTION FLUIDS
		TYLENOL WITH CODEINE (1, 2, 3, 4)	HASH	
	PARALDEHYDE		MARIJUANA (grass, pot, tea, wood, dope)	
	PENTOBARBITAL (yellow jackets, barbs, Nembutal)		THC	
	PHENOBARBITAL (goofballs, phennies, barbs)			
	SECOBARBITAL (red devils, barbs, Seconal)			

the nose and mouth may show swollen membranes. The patient may complain of a "funny numb feeling" or "tingling" inside the head. Changes in heart rhythm can occur. This can lead to death.

Warning: When reading the above list, you will have noticed that many of the indications of drug abuse are similar to those for quite a few medical emergencies. As an EMT-B you must never assume drug abuse occurring by itself. You must be on the alert for medical emergencies, injuries, and combinations of drug abuse problems and other emergencies.

Signs and Symptoms of Drug Withdrawal

In addition to the effects of long-term drug use and overdose, you may encounter cases of severe drug withdrawal. Withdrawal occurs when the longterm user of certain drugs such as narcotics, suddenly stops taking the drug. As in reactions to the use of various drugs, withdrawal varies from patient to patient and from drug to drug. In most cases of drug withdrawal, you may see

- [ ] Shaking
- [ ] Anxiety
- [ ] Nausea
- [ ] Confusion and irritability (sometimes retreating from the persons at the scene)
- [ ] Hallucinations (both visual and auditory—"seeing things" or "hearing things")
- [ ] Profuse sweating
- [ ] Increased pulse and breathing rates

Patient Care—Substance Abuse

Your care for the drug abuse patient will be basically the same for all drugs and will not change unless you are so ordered by medical direction. *When providing care for substance abuse patients, you should make certain that you are safe and identify yourself as an EMT-B to the patient and bystanders. Since these patients often vomit, take body substance isolation precautions, including gloves, mask, and protective eyewear.*

The procedures for care may require you to

1. Perform initial assessment. Provide basic life-support measures if required.
2. Be alert for airway problems and inadequate respirations or respiratory arrest. Provide oxygen and assisted ventilations if needed.
3. Treat for shock.
4. Perform a rapid trauma exam or detailed physical exam to assess for signs of injury to all parts of the body. Assess carefully for signs of head injury.
5. Look for gross soft-tissue damage on the extremities resulting from the injection of drugs ("tracks"). Tracks usually appear as darkened or red areas of scar tissue or scabs over veins.
6. Talk to the patient to gain his confidence and to help maintain his level of consciousness. Use his name often, maintain eye contact, and speak directly to the patient.
7. Protect the patient from self-injury and attempting to hurt others. Use restraint as authorized by your EMS system. Request assistance from law enforcement if needed.
8. Transport the patient as soon as possible.

9. Contact medical direction according to local protocols.
10. Perform ongoing assessment with monitoring of vital signs. Stay alert for seizures, and be on guard for vomiting that could obstruct the airway.
11. Continue to reassure the patient throughout all phases of care.

Safety Note

Many drug abusers may appear calm at first and then become violent as time passes. You are always to be on the alert and ready to protect yourself. If the patient creates an unsafe scene and you are not a trained law enforcement officer, GET OUT and find a safe place until the police arrive.

When dealing with drug abuse, you must also protect yourself from the substance itself. Many hallucinogens can be absorbed through the skin and mucous membranes. Intravenous drug users may possess hypodermic syringes which pose a hazard of infectious disease transmission through accidental punctures. Take body substance isolation precautions and follow all infection exposure control procedures. Never touch or taste any suspected illicit substance.

FYI

Topics included in the FYI—"For Your Information"—section are those that go beyond the chapter objectives. The information in this segment is intended to broaden your understanding of the chapter topic but is not essential to an understanding of your job as an EMT-B.

Poison Control Centers

Emergency care in poisoning cases presents special problems for the EMT-B. Signs and symptoms can vary greatly. Some poisons produce a characteristic set of signs and symptoms very quickly, while others are subtle and slow to appear. Poisons that act almost immediately usually produce obvious signs, and the particular poison or its container is often still nearby. Slow-acting poisons can produce effects that mimic an infectious disease or some other medical emergency.

There will be times when you will not know the substance that caused the poisoning. In some of these cases, an expert may be able to tell, based on the combination of signs and symptoms. Even when you know the source of the poison, correct emergency care procedures may still be in question. Ideas about proper care keep changing as more research is done on poisoning. This constant change makes it impossible to print guides and charts for poison control and care that will be up to date when you use them. Although manufacturers have improved the instructions on many container labels, many still have inaccurate or even dangerous advice.

Fortunately, a network of poison control centers exists to provide information and advice to both lay people and health care providers. In most localities, a poison control center can be reached 24 hours a day.

An EMT-B should consult a poison control center only when directed by local protocol. In most cases, EMT-Bs get medical direction from physicians or nurses who are in hospital emergency departments. Unless special arrangements have been made, the poison control center staff does not have the authority to provide on-line medical direction. If the poison control center staff does have the authority to do so, they can tell you what should be done for most cases of poisoning.

If you are permitted to communicate directly with the poison control center in your area, do so by telephone. Even if you have radio contact with your local poison control center, the telephone is the preferred way to communicate. The staff member may need to talk to you for several minutes, far too long a period to monopolize the air waves. The telephone will also allow you to maintain patient confidentiality. Make certain you have memorized the number and/or carry the poison control center number with you into the residence—perhaps pasted inside your kit—so that you don't have to return to the rig to get it.

To help the poison control center staff, gather all of the information you need before you call (see Documentation Tips, above).

Many people have the impression that the poison control center should be called only for cases of ingested poisonings. The center's staff can provide valuable care information for all types of poisoning.

Your community may have special poisoning problems. Not every community is exposed to rattlesnakes, jellyfish, or powerful agricultural chemicals. Many EMS systems have compiled lists of poisoning problems specific for their areas. Check to see if this has been done for the area in which you will be an EMT-B.

Syrup of Ipecac

A traditional treatment for poisoning has been syrup of ipecac. This orally administered drug causes vomiting in most people with just one dose. During recent years, however, it has been used less and less as the use of activated charcoal has increased. Ipecac stimulates both the stomach and the vomiting center in the brain, but it typically takes fifteen to twenty minutes to work. If the first dose had not caused vomiting within twenty to thirty minutes, a second dose was typically given (almost everyone vomits after two doses of ipecac). When vomiting does occur, it results, *on the average*, in removal of less than a third of the stomach contents. Combine the slowness and relative ineffectiveness of syrup of ipecac with the potential for the patient to become drowsy or unconscious in twenty minutes, thus chancing aspiration of vomitus by a non-alert patient, and the disadvantages of ipecac become clear.

Although poison control centers frequently instruct parents of young children in the proper use of syrup of ipecac, activated charcoal is the medication of first choice for health care providers in most poisoning and overdose cases. This is why the national standard EMT-B curriculum now includes the use of activated charcoal and not syrup of ipecac.

Activated Charcoal with Sorbitol

Some EMS systems may direct EMT-Bs to administer an activated charcoal mixture that includes sorbitol, a cathartic. Sorbitol is a rapid-acting laxative which hospital staff frequently administer in order to enhance activated charcoal's ability to prevent absorption of poisons by speeding their passage through the gastrointestinal tract. Because it acts so quickly, sorbitol is not used in most EMS systems, especially those with long transport times.

Antidotes

Many lay people think that every poison has an antidote. The opposite is true. There are only a few genuine antidotes, and they can be used only with a very small number of poisons. Modern treatment of poisonings and overdoses consists primarily of prevention of absorption when possible (e.g., by administration of activated charcoal) and good supportive treatment (e.g., airway maintenance, administration of oxygen, treatment for shock). In a small number of poisonings, advanced treatments are administered in a hospital (e.g., administration of antidotes and dialysis).

Food Poisoning

One way someone can be poisoned is through food that has been handled or cooked improperly. Food poisoning is caused by several different bacteria that grow when exposed to the right conditions. This frequently happens when raw meat, poultry, or fish is left at room temperature before being cooked or the food doesn't reach a high enough temperature to kill the bacteria. Signs and symptoms vary somewhat, depending on the bacteria involved, but frequently include nausea, vomiting, abdominal cramps, diarrhea, and fever.

You can prevent food poisoning at home and at the station by washing hands, utensils, cutting boards, and any surface the food touches before and especially after any contact with raw meat, fish, or poultry (the bacteria can easily be spread to other foods from hands or surfaces); by storing and cooking foods at appropriate temperatures; and by not leaving raw or cooked foods at room temperature for long periods of time.

Smoke Inhalation

Smoke inhalation is a serious problem associated with the scenes of thermal and chemical burns. The smoke from any fire source contains many poisonous substances. Modern building materials and furnishings often contain plastics and other synthetics that release toxic fumes when they burn or are overheated. It is possible for the substances found in smoke to burn the skin, irritate the eyes, injure the airway, cause respiratory arrest, and, in some cases, cause cardiac arrest.

As an EMT-B you will most likely find irritated (reddened, watering) eyes and, of far greater concern, injury of the airway associated with smoke.

Signs of an airway injured by smoke inhalation include

- Difficulty breathing
- Coughing
- Breath that has a "smoky" smell or the odor of chemicals involved at the scene
- Black (carbon) residue in the patient's mouth and nose. Be alert for this residue in any sputum coughed up by the patient.
- Nose hairs singed from super-heated air

Move the patient to a safe area and provide the same care you would provide for any inhaled poison: Assess the patient, administer high concentration oxygen, and transport.

Note: The body's reaction to toxic gases and foreign matter in the airway can often be delayed. Convince all smoke inhalation patients that they must be seen by a physician, even if they are not yet feeling serious effects.

CHAPTER REVIEW

KEY TERMS

You may find it helpful to review the following terms.

absorbed poisons poisons that are taken into the body through unbroken skin.

activated charcoal a substance that absorbs many poisons and prevents them from being absorbed by the body.

delirium tremens (duh-LEER-e-um TREM-uns) **(DTs)** a severe reaction that can be part of alcohol withdrawal, characterized by sweating, trembling, anxiety, and hallucinations. Severe alcohol withdrawal with the DTs can lead to death if untreated.

dilution (di-LU-shun) thinning down or weakening by mixing with something else. Ingested poisons are sometimes diluted by drinking water or milk.

downers depressants, such as barbiturates, that depress the central nervous system, often used to bring on a more relaxed state of mind.

hallucinogens (huh-LOO-sin-uh-jens) mind-affecting or -altering drugs that act on the central nervous system to produce excitement and distortion of perceptions.

ingested poisons poisons that are swallowed.

inhaled poisons poisons that are breathed in.

injected poisons poisons that are inserted through the skin, for example by needle, snake fangs, or insect stinger.

narcotics a class of drugs that affect the nervous system and change many normal body activities. Their legal use is for the relief of pain. Illicit use is to produce an intense state of relaxation.

poison any substance that can harm the body by altering cell structure or functions.

toxin a poisonous substance secreted by bacteria, plants, or animals.

uppers stimulants such as amphetamines that affect the central nervous system to excite the user.

volatile chemicals vaporizing compounds, such as cleaning fluid, that are breathed in by the abuser to produce a "high."

withdrawal referring to alcohol or drug withdrawal in which the patient's body reacts severely when deprived of the abused substance.

SUMMARY

Poisonings and overdoses are frequent causes of medical emergencies. When responding to a poisoning or possible poisoning

1. Perform initial assessment and treat immediately life-threatening problems. Assure an open airway. Administer high concentration oxygen if the poison was inhaled or injected.
2. Perform a focused history and physical exam, including baseline vital signs. Find out if the poison was ingested, inhaled, or absorbed, what substance was involved, how much poison was taken in, when and over how long a period exposure took place, what interventions others have already done, and what effects the patient experienced.

3. Consult medical direction. As directed, administer activated charcoal or water or milk for ingested poisons. Remove the patient who has inhaled a poison from the environment and administer high concentration oxygen; remove poisons from the skin by brushing off or diluting.
4. Transport the patient with all containers, bottles, and labels from the substance.
5. Perform ongoing assessment en route.

Carefully document all information about the poisoning, interventions, and the patient's responses.

REVIEW QUESTIONS

1. What are four ways in which a poison can be taken into the body?
2. What is the sequence of assessment steps in cases of poisoning?
3. What information must you gather in a case of poisoning before contacting medical direction?
4. What are the emergency care steps for ingested poisoning?
5. What are the emergency care steps for inhaled poisoning? for absorbed poisoning?

Application

• A local farmer calls 911, concerned because one of his farm hands has tried to clean up some spilled pesticide powder with his hands. On arrival, you find that the patient insists that he has brushed all the powder off, feels fine, and doesn't need to go to the hospital. As he talks, he continues to make brushing motions at his jeans on which you can see the marks of a powdery residue. How do you manage the situation?

Environmental Emergencies

22

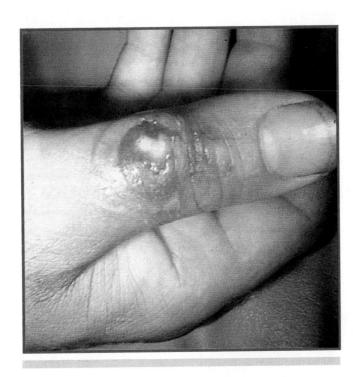

Environmental emergencies can occur in any setting—wilderness, rural, suburban, and urban areas. They include exposure to both heat and cold, near-drownings and other water-related injuries, and bites and stings from insects, spiders, snakes, and marine life. The keys to effective management are recognizing the patient's signs and symptoms and providing prompt and proper emergency care. However, as an EMT-Basic you also must recognize that exposure may not be the only danger to the patient. Environmental emergencies can involve preexisting or cause additional medical problems and injury.

Knowledge and Attitude *At the end of this chapter, you should be able to meet the following objectives.*

1. Describe the various ways that the body loses heat. (pp. 383–384)

2. List the signs and symptoms of exposure to cold. (pp. 384, 386, 388, 389)

3. Explain the steps in providing emergency medical care to a patient exposed to cold. (pp. 386–388, 389–390)

4. List the signs and symptoms of exposure to heat. (pp. 391–392)

5. Explain the steps in providing emergency care to a patient exposed to heat. (pp. 392, 393)

6. Recognize the signs and symptoms of water-related emergencies. (p. 394)

7. Describe the complications of near drowning. (pp. 394–397)

8. Discuss the emergency medical care of bites and stings. (pp. 399–401)

Skills

1. Demonstrate the assessment and emergency medical care of a patient with exposure to cold.

2. Demonstrate the assessment and emergency medical care of a patient with exposure to heat.

3. Demonstrate the assessment and emergency medical care of a near-drowning patient.

4. Demonstrate completing a prehospital care report for patients with environmental emergencies.

On the Scene

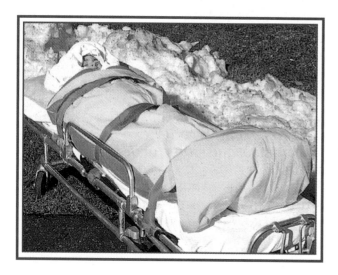

Early one Saturday morning in late November, you respond to a call to the middle fork of the Icicle River where a duck hunter is stranded on a sandbar. As you arrive and begin *sizing up the scene,* you and your partner both pull on leather gloves over your disposable gloves to provide warmth as well as BSI protection. The air temperature is just above freezing. A strong northerly wind blows across the fast-moving river. You are watching the duck hunter, who appears to be an older man, approximately fifty yards away from shore standing in about two feet of water.

Beside you is a distraught citizen. "Don't just stand there, do something!" he shouts. Suddenly he wades into the river. You grab his collar and tell him you won't allow him to become a second patient. Now you are concerned for the safety of the other bystanders. So you explain to them that a law enforcement rescue power boat is due any time. Moments later, the boat pulls up and rescuers carefully place the hunter into the boat.

Meanwhile you learn from witnesses that the hunter fell out of his boat upstream from the sandbar. He has been stranded on the sandbar for at least 30 minutes. Since he is wet and the air temperature is only a bit above freezing, you are concerned about hypothermia. You know generalized cold emergencies are particularly worrisome for elderly patients.

As the boat lands, you begin your *initial assessment.* The man tells you his name is Jim Kyle and he is 72 years old. You tell Mr. Kyle you are an EMT-B and want to help. You see no obvious signs of shivering, so you suspect his condition may be life threatening. He has trouble speaking, but you understand when he tells you he feels only a "little cold." Mr. Kyle does not answer other questions appropriately and responds slowly. Breathing is slow at 8 to 10 breaths per minute, radial pulse is approximately 44 beats per minute. His skin is cool, pale, and dry. You gently have Mr. Kyle recline on your stretcher. Your partner administers oxygen at 15 liters per minute by nonrebreather mask.

You and your partner gently move Mr. Kyle by stretcher to the back of your heated ambulance, careful to keep movement at a minimum. You cut off the patient's wet clothing and remove his hat. You place a blanket over him and towels around his head. You begin immediate transport to the nearest medical facility 15 minutes away.

Since Mr. Kyle is drowsy and confused, you know your *focused history* may not be accurate. During the *physical exam,* you look for signs of deformity, contusions, abrasions, punctures/penetrations, burns, tenderness, lacerations, and swelling. You note his skin is cool. His pulse is 44, respirations 10, and blood pressure 98/48. You perform *ongoing assessment* en route.

When you arrive at the hospital, you communicate the patient's condition, age and sex, chief complaint, present condition, mental status, and your difficulty obtaining a SAMPLE history, baseline vitals, physical exam findings, care given, and response to your care.

Later you find out that Mr. Kyle was, indeed, suffering from severe generalized hypothermia. Doctors are guardedly optimistic about his recovery.

---

*E*xposure to cold temperatures, hot temperatures, and water can cause problems that are subtle or obvious, minor or life-threatening. Basic to understanding environmental emergencies is gaining an understanding of how the human body regulates its own temperature. Doing so can help you recognize and effectively treat the signs and symptoms of excessive heat loss or heat gain—or, simply, getting too cold or getting too hot.

EXPOSURE TO COLD

Generalized Cold Emergencies

How the Body Loses Heat

If the environment is too cold, body heat can be lost faster than it can be generated. The body attempts to adjust by reducing respirations, perspiration, and circulation to the skin—shutting down the avenues by which the body usually gets rid of excess heat. Muscular activity in the form of shivering and the rate at which fuel (food) is burned within the body both increase to produce more heat. At a certain point, however, not enough heat is generated to be available to all parts of the body. This may result in damage to exposed tissues and a general reduction or cessation of body functions.

To prevent or compensate for heat loss, the EMT-B must be aware of the ways in which a body loses heat.

- **Conduction** is the direct transfer of heat from one material to another through direct contact. Heat will flow from the warmer material to the cooler material. Body heat transferred directly into cool air is a problem. But when the body or clothing gets wet, **water chill** is an even greater problem, because water conducts heat away from the body 25 times faster than still air. Mr. Kyle lost body heat directly into the river. Heat loss through conduction can be a major problem when a person is lying on a cold floor or another cold surface. A person who is standing or walking around in cold weather will lose less heat than a person who is lying on the cold ground.
- **Convection** occurs when currents of air or water pass over the body, carrying away heat. The effects of a cold environment are worsened when *moving* water or air surround the body. **Wind chill** is a frequent

problem. The more wind, the greater the heat loss. For example, if it is 10°F with no wind, the body will lose heat, but if there is a 20 mph wind, the amount of heat lost by the body is much greater—the same as if it were minus 25°F. Wind chill was definitely a factor for Mr. Kyle.

- **Radiation** is heat the body sends out in waves. In conduction and convection, heat is "picked up" by the surrounding (still or moving) air or water. In radiation, heat waves or rays are sent out by the body's atoms and molecules as they move and change. If you were in the vacuum of outer space with no air or water around to pick up heat, you would still lose heat by radiating it out into space. Most radiant heat loss occurs from a person's head and neck. Fortunately, Mr. Kyle was wearing a hat, which helped protect him from radiant heat loss. On the stretcher, you helped protect him from radiant heat loss by placing towels around his head.
- **Evaporation** occurs when the body perspires or gets wet. As perspiration on the skin vaporizes, the body experiences a generalized cooling effect. The same effect occurs with evaporation from wet clothing. In Mr. Kyle's condition, very little body heat was lost due to evaporation of perspiration, but much was lost through evaporation from his wet garments.
- **Respiration** causes loss of body heat as a result of exhaled warm air. The amount of

heat loss depends on the outside air temperature as well as the rate and depth of respirations. Due to the cold outside temperature, Mr. Kyle lost considerable body heat simply through breathing.

Generalized Hypothermia

When cooling affects the entire body, a problem known as **hypothermia** (HI-po-THURM-e-ah), or general cooling, develops. Exposure to cold reduces body heat. With time, the body is unable to maintain its proper core (internal) temperature. If allowed to continue, hypothermia leads to death. (See Table 22-1 for a description of the stages of hypothermia.)

Note: *Be aware that hypothermia can develop in temperatures well above freezing.*

Predisposing Factors Patients with injuries, chronic illness, or certain other conditions will show the effects of cold much sooner than healthy persons. These conditions include shock (hypoperfusion), burns, head and spinal-cord injuries, generalized infection, and diabetes and hypoglycemia. Those under the influence of alcohol or other drugs also tend to be affected more rapidly and more severely than others. The unconscious patient lying on the cold ground or other cold surface is especially prone to rapid heat loss through conduction and will tend to have greater cold-related problems than one who is conscious and able to walk around.

TABLE 22-1   Stages of Hypothermia

Core Body Temperature		Symptoms
99°F-96°F	37.0°C-35.5°C	Shivering.
95°F-91°F	35.5°C-32.7°C	Intense shivering. If conscious, patient has difficulty speaking.
90°F-86°F	32.0°C-30.0°C	Shivering decreases and is replaced by strong muscular rigidity. Muscle coordination is affected and erratic or jerky movements are produced. Thinking is less clear, general comprehension is dulled, possible total amnesia. Patient generally is able to maintain the appearance of psychological contact with surroundings.
85°F-81°F	29.4°C-27.2°C	Patient becomes irrational, loses contact with environment, and drifts into stuporous state. Muscular rigidity continues. Pulse and respirations are slow and cardiac arrhythmias may develop.
80°F-78°F	26.6°C-20.5°C	Patient loses consciousness and does not respond to spoken words. Most reflexes cease to function. Heartbeat becomes erratic.

Hypothermia is often an especially serious problem for the aged. The effects of cold temperatures on the elderly are more immediate. During the winter months, many older citizens on small fixed incomes live in unheated rooms or rooms that are kept too cool. Failing body systems, chronic illnesses, poor diets, certain medications, and a lack of exercise may combine with the cold environment to bring about hypothermia.

Infants and Children

Since infants and young children are small with large skin surface areas in relation to their total body mass and little body fat, they are especially prone to hypothermia. Because of their small muscle mass, infants and children don't shiver very much or at all. An infant's or child's inability to shiver effectively is another reason for the susceptibility of the very young to the cold.

Obvious and Subtle Exposure At times, it is obvious that a patient has been exposed to cold and is probably suffering from hypothermia. A patient found lost in a snow bank, for example, has had an obvious exposure.

With other patients, however, exposure is subtle—that is, not so obvious, not the first thing you may think of. Consider, for example, the elderly patient who has fallen during the night and is not discovered until morning. The possibility of a broken hip or other injuries may claim your attention, but if your patient has been on the floor in a cold or cool room all night, he is probably also suffering from hypothermia. The patient trapped in a wrecked auto is probably suffering a variety of injuries caused by the crash, but if the weather is cool and extrication from the vehicle takes awhile, the patient can easily develop hypothermia as well.

Consider the possibility of hypothermia in the following situations when another condition or injury may be more obvious.

- Ethanol (alcohol) ingestion—Has the intoxicated patient passed out on a cold floor or been wandering around outdoors in cool or cold weather?
- Underlying illness—Is the patient suffering from a circulatory disorder or other condition that makes him especially susceptible to cold?
- Overdose or poisoning—Has the patient been lying in a cold garage or on a cold floor? Is he sweating heavily in a cool envi-

ronment with evaporation causing excessive heat loss?
- Major trauma—Has the patient been lying on the ground or trapped in wreckage during cold weather? Is shock (hyoperfusion or inadequate circulation of the blood) preventing parts of the body from being warmed by circulating blood?
- Outdoor resuscitation—While you are performing life-saving procedures such as CPR in an outdoor environment, is your patient also getting too cold? If your patient is a near-drowning victim who has been in the water, has exposure to cool water caused hypothermia?
- Decreased ambient temperature (for example, room temperature)—Is your patient living in a home or apartment that is too cold? Remember that older patients require an ambient temperature that would feel too warm to a younger person. If that patient's environment is slightly cool, even a temperature that might feel quite comfortable to you, consider hypothermia.

Remember that the injured patient is more susceptible to the effects of cold. As an EMT-B you should protect the patient who is in a collision vehicle or is entrapped in other accident debris or wreckage or for any other reason must remain in a cool or cold environment for a period of time. The major course of action is to prevent additional body heat loss. If the patient is entrapped, it may be neither practical nor possible to replace wet clothing, but you can at least create a barrier to the cold with blankets, a salvage cover, an aluminized blanket, a survival blanket, or even articles of clothing. A plastic trash bag can serve as protection from wind and water, and it will help prevent heat loss. Keep in mind that the greatest area of heat loss may be the head. Provide some sort of head covering for the patient.

When the patient's injuries allow, place a blanket between his body and the cold ground. Rotate warm blankets from the heated ambulance to the patient. If the patient will remain trapped in a collision vehicle or other wreckage for a period of time, plug holes in the wreckage with blankets or salvage covers.

Patient Assessment—Hypothermia

For a generalized cold emergency, consider the impact of the following factors: air temperature, wind chill and/or water chill, the patient's age, whether or not the patient's clothing is adequate, health of the patient including underlying illness and existing injuries, how active the patient was during exposure, and whether or not the patient may have used alcohol or drugs.

Signs and Symptoms

The signs and symptoms of hypothermia include the following. Note that decreasing mental status and decreasing motor function both correlate with the degree of hypothermia.

- ☐ Shivering in early stages when core body temperature is above 90°F. In severe cases shivering decreases or is absent.
- ☐ Numbness, or reduced-to-lost sensation to touch
- ☐ Stiff or rigid posture in prolonged cases
- ☐ Drowsiness and/or unwillingness or inability to do even the simplest activities. In prolonged cases, the patient may become irrational, drift into a stuporous state, or actually remove clothing.
- ☐ Rapid breathing and rapid pulse in early stages. Slow to absent breathing and pulse in prolonged cases. Blood pressure may be low to absent.
- ☐ Loss of motor coordination, such as staggering or inability to hold things
- ☐ Joint/muscle stiffness, or muscular rigidity
- ☐ Decreased level of consciousness, or unconsciousness. In extreme cases the patient has a "glassy stare."
- ☐ Cool abdominal skin temperature. (To assess, place the back of your hand inside the clothing and against the patient's abdomen.)
- ☐ Skin may appear red in early stages. In prolonged cases, skin is pale to cyanotic. In most extreme cases, some body parts are stiff and hard (frozen).

Warning: It may be difficult to distinguish between the patient who is alert and responding appropriately and one who is confused and not responding appropriately. During initial assessment, be sure to check an awake patient's orientation to person, place, and time. (Can he tell you his name? where he is? what day it is?) Perform a focused history and physical exam to help you estimate the extent of hypothermia. Assume a case of severe hypothermia if shivering is absent.

Emergency Medical Care

Passive rewarming involves simply covering the patient and taking other steps to prevent further heat loss, allowing the body to rewarm itself. **Active rewarming** includes application of an external heat source to the body. All EMS systems permit passive rewarming. Some EMS systems allow the active rewarming of a hypothermic patient who is alert and responding appropriately. Many do not.

Active rewarming can prove to be a dangerous process if the patient's condition is more serious than believed. If you are allowed to rewarm a patient with hypothermia who is alert and responding appropriately, do not delay transport. Rewarm the patient while en route. *The emergency care steps listed below assume a protocol that permits active rewarming of a patient who is alert and responding appropriately. Follow your local protocols.*

Patient Care—Hypothermic Patient Alert and Responding Appropriately

Emergency Care Steps

For the hypothermic patient who is alert and responding appropriately, proceed with active rewarming.

1. *Remove all of the patient's wet clothing.* Keep the patient dry, dress the patient in dry clothing, or wrap in dry warm blankets. Keep the patient still and handle very gently. Do not allow the patient to walk or exert himself. Do not massage extremities.

2. *During transport, actively rewarm the patient.* Gently apply heat to the patient's body in the form of heat packs, hot water bottles, electric heating pads, warm air, radiated heat, and even your own body heat. *Do not warm the patient too quickly.* Rapid warming will circulate peripherally stagnated cold blood and rapidly cool the vital central areas of the body, possibly causing cardiac arrest. If transport is delayed, move the patient to a warm environment if at all possible.

3. *Provide care for shock. Provide oxygen.* The oxygen should be warmed and humidified, if possible.

4. *Give the alert patient warm liquids slowly.* When warm fluids are given too quickly, circulation patterns change, sending blood away from the core to the skin and extrem-

ities. Do not allow the patient to eat or drink stimulants.

5 *Except in the mildest of cases (shivering), transport the patient.* Continue to provide high concentration oxygen and monitor vital signs. *Never allow a patient to remain in, or return to, a cold environment.*

Take the following precautions when actively rewarming a patient.

■ *Rewarm the patient slowly.* Handle the patient with great care, the same as you would if there were unstabilized cervical-spine injuries.

■ *Use **central rewarming.*** Heat should be applied to the lateral chest, neck, armpits, and groin. You must avoid rewarming the limbs. If they are warmed first, blood will collect in the extremities due to vasodilation (dilation of blood vessels) and cause a fatal form of shock (see Chapter 25, Bleeding and Shock). If you rewarm the trunk and leave the lower extremities exposed, you can control the rewarming process and help prevent most of the problems associated with the procedure.

■ *If transport must be delayed, a warm bath is very helpful,* but you must keep the patient alert enough so that he does not drown. Do not warm the patient too quickly.

■ *Keep the patient at rest.* Do not allow the patient to walk, and avoid rough handling of the patient. Such activity may set off severe heart problems, including ventricular fibrillation. Since the patient's blood is coldest in the extremities, exercise or unnecessary movement could also quickly circulate the cold blood and lower the core body temperature.

Patient Care—Hypothermic Patient Unresponsive or Not Responding Appropriately

A patient who is unresponsive or not responding appropriately has severe hypothermia. For this patient, provide passive rewarming. Do not try to actively rewarm the patient with severe hypothermia. As in the case of Mr. Kyle, remove the patient from the environment and protect him from further heat loss. Active rewarming may cause the patient to develop ventricular fibrillation.

Emergency Care Steps

For the patient with severe hypothermia, you should

1 *Assure an open airway.*

2 *Provide high concentration oxygen that has been passed through a warm water humidifier.* If necessary, the oxygen that has been kept warm in the ambulance passenger compartment can be used. If there is no other choice, oxygen from a cold cylinder may be used.

3 *Wrap the patient in blankets.* If available, use insulating blankets. Handle the patient as gently as possible. Rough handling may cause ventricular fibrillation. Do not allow the patient to eat or drink stimulants. Do not massage extremities.

4 *Transport immediately.*

Patient Care—Extreme Hypothermia

In extreme cases of hypothermia, you will find the patient unconscious, with no discernible vital signs. In extreme hypothermia, the heart rate can slow to less than 10 beats per minute, and the patient will feel very cold to your touch (core body temperature may be below 80°F). Even so, it is possible that the patient is still alive!

Emergency Care Steps

1 *Assess the carotid pulse* for 30-45 seconds. If there is no pulse, start CPR immediately. (If you detect a pulse, do not start CPR.)

2 *Transport immediately.*

Because the hypothermic patient may not reach biological death for over 30 minutes, the staff at the hospital emergency department will not pronounce a patient dead until after he is rewarmed and resuscitative measures applied. This means you cannot assume that a severe hypothermia patient is dead on the basis of body temperature and lack of vital signs. As medical personnel point out, "You're not dead until you're warm and dead!"

Localized Cold Injuries

Cold-related emergencies also can result from **local cooling.** Local cooling injuries are those affecting particular (local) parts of the body.

Localized cold injuries are classified as early or superficial, and late or deep.

Local cooling most commonly affects the ears, nose, face, hands, and the feet and toes. When a part of the body is exposed to intensely cold air or liquid, blood flow to that particular part is limited by the constriction of blood vessels. When this happens, tissues freeze. Ice crystals can form in the skin, and in the most severe cases, gangrene (localized tissue death) can set in and ultimately lead to the loss of the body part.

As you read the following pages, notice how the signs and symptoms of early or superficial cold injuries are progressive. First, the exposed skin reddens in light-skinned individuals, or in dark-skinned individuals the skin color lightens and approaches a blanched (reduced color or whitened) condition. Then, as exposure continues, the skin takes on a gray or white blotchy appearance. Exposed skin surfaces become numb because of reduced circulation. If the freezing process is allowed to continue, all sensation is lost and the skin becomes dead white.

Early or Superficial Local Cold Injury

Early or superficial local cold injuries (sometimes called frostnip) are brought about by direct contact with a cold object or exposure of a body part to cold air. Wind chill and water chill also can be major factors. Tissue damage is minor and the response to care is good. The tip of the nose, the tips of the ears, the upper cheeks, and the fingers (all areas that are usually exposed) are most susceptible to early or superficial local cold injuries. The injury, as its name suggests, is localized with clear demarcation of its limits.

Patient Assessment—Early or Superficial Local Cold Injury

Patients are often unaware of the onset of an early local cold injury until someone indicates that there is something unusual about their skin color.

Signs and Symptoms

☐ The affected area of patients with light skin at first reddens; dark skin lightens. Both then blanch (whiten). Once blanching begins, the color change can take place very quickly.

☐ The affected area feels numb to the patient.

Patient Care—Early or Superficial Local Cold Injury

Emergency Care Steps

Emergency care for early local cold injury is simple.

1 Get the patient out of the cold environment.

2 Warm the affected area.

3 If the injury is to an extremity, splint and cover it. Do not rub or massage, and do not re-expose to the cold.

Usually, the patient can apply warmth from his own bare hands, blow warm air on the site, or if the fingers are involved, hold them in the armpits. During recovery from an early local cold injury, the patient may complain about tingling or burning sensations, which is normal. If the condition does not respond to this simple care, begin to treat for a late or deep local cold injury.

Late or Deep Local Cold Injury

Late or deep local cold injury (also known as frostbite), develops if an early or superficial local cold injury goes untreated (Figure 22-1). In late or deep local cold injury, the skin and subcutaneous layers of the body part are affected. Muscles, bones, deep blood vessels, and organ membranes can become frozen.

Patient Assessment—Late or Deep Local Cold Injury

Signs and Symptoms

☐ In frostbite, the affected area of the skin appears white and waxy. When the condition progresses to actual freezing, the skin turns mottled or blotchy, the color turns from white to grayish yellow and finally to grayish blue. Swelling and blistering may occur.

☐ With frostbite, the affected area feels frozen, but only on the surface. The tissue

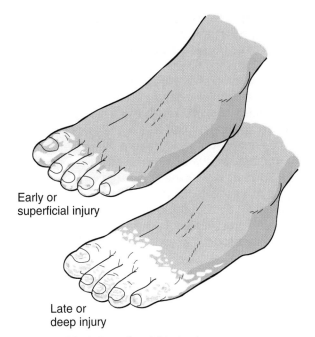

Early or
superficial injury

Late or
deep injury

FIGURE 22-1 Local cold injuries.

below the surface is still soft and has its normal resilience, or "bounce." With freezing, the tissues are not resilient and feel frozen to the touch. (**Note:** Do not squeeze or poke the tissue. The condition of the deeper tissues can be determined by gently feeling the affected area. Do the assessment as if the affected area had a fractured bone.)

Patient Care—Late or Deep Local Cold Injury

Emergency Care Steps

Initial care for late or deep local cold injury—frostbite and freezing—is the same.

1. *Administer high concentration oxygen.*
2. *Transport to a medical facility without delay*, protecting the frostbitten or frozen area by covering it and handling it as gently as possible.
3. *If transport must be delayed, get the patient indoors and keep him warm.* Do not allow the patient to drink alcohol or smoke, because constriction of blood vessels and decreased circulation to the injured tissues may result. Rewarm the frozen part as per local protocol, or request instructions from medical direction.

Important: Never listen to myths and folktales about the care of frostbite. Never rub a frostbitten or frozen area. Never rub snow on a frostbitten or frozen area. There are ice crystals at the capillary level; rubbing the injury site may cause them to seriously damage the already injured tissues. Do not break blisters or massage the injured area. Do not allow the patient to walk on an affected extremity. *Do not thaw a frozen limb if there is any chance it will be refrozen.*

Active Rapid Rewarming of Frozen Parts

Active rewarming of frozen parts is seldom recommended. The chance of permanently injuring frozen tissues with active rewarming is too great. Consider it only if local protocols recommend it, if you are instructed to do so by medical direction, or if transport will be severely delayed and you cannot reach medical direction for instructions. If you are in a situation where you must attempt rewarming without instructions from a physician, follow the procedure described here.

You will need warm water and a container in which you can immerse the entire site of injury without the limb touching the sides or bottom of the container. If you cannot find a suitable container, fashion one from a plastic bag supported by a cardboard box or wooden crate (Figure 22-2). Proceed as follows.

1. Heat water to a temperature between 100°F and 105°F. You should be able to put your finger into the water without experiencing discomfort.
2. Fill the container with the heated water and prepare the injured part by removing clothing, jewelry, bands, or straps.
3. Fully immerse the injured part. Do not allow the injured area to touch the sides or bottom of the container. Do not place any pressure on the affected part. Continuously stir the water. When the water cools below 100°F, remove the affected part and add more warm water. The patient may complain of moderate pain as the affected area rewarms or he may experience some period of intense pain. The presence of pain is usually a good indicator of successful rewarming.
4. If you complete rewarming of the part (it no longer feels frozen and is turning red or blue), gently dry the affected area and apply a dry sterile dressing. Place dry sterile dressings between fingers and toes before

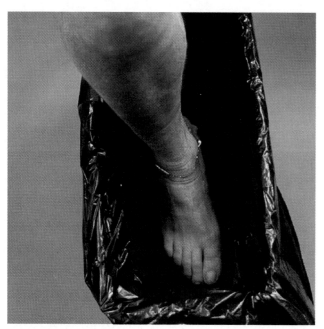

FIGURE 22-2 Rewarming the frozen part.

dressing hands and feet. Next, cover the site with blankets or whatever is available to keep the affected area warm. Do not allow these coverings to come in direct contact with the injured area or to put pressure on the site. It is best if you first build some sort of framework on which the coverings can be placed.

5. Keep the patient at rest. Do not allow the patient to walk if a lower extremity has been frostbitten or frozen.

6. Make certain that you keep the entire patient as warm as possible without overheating. Cover the patient's head with a towel or small blanket to reduce heat loss. Leave the patient's face exposed.

7. Continue to monitor the patient.

8. Assist circulation according to local protocol (some systems recommend rhythmically and carefully raising and lowering the affected limb).

9. Do not allow the limb to refreeze.

10. Transport as soon as possible with the affected limb slightly elevated.

EXPOSURE TO HEAT

On the Scene

It's a warm, humid afternoon in July when you respond to a "woman down" at the charity marathon at the north end of the city park. Runners are crossing the finish line, and your **scene size-up** is as you expect it to be. You see crowds of bystanders and dozens of perspiring runners cooling down. Police and volunteers with orange bibs have control of the scene. As a marathon official directs you to the patient, one of the runners, he tells you that first aid personnel think she has had a heart attack. You and your partner glove up and move quickly toward the patient.

Initial assessment reveals an adult female about 50 years old supine in the shade on the ground under a makeshift tent. First aid personnel tell you the woman staggered, doubled over, and fell down where she is after crossing the finish line. She appears to be drowsy but responds to your voice. Her skin is cool, moist, and pale. Airway is clear, breathing is rapid and shallow, pulse is weak at 120 beats per minute. Your partner administers oxygen by nonrebreather mask at 15 liters per minute. You believe that the patient is suffering from heat exposure, but the possibility of a heart attack cannot be ruled out.

You assign the patient a high priority and move her into the air-conditioned ambulance for immediate transport. As you place the patient on your stretcher, a man runs through the crowd of onlookers and identifies himself as the patient's husband. He tells you the patient's name is Doreen Collin.

"What happened? Doreen is perfectly healthy!" He gives you a **SAMPLE history:** Mrs. Collin takes no medications, has no known allergies or pertinent medical history, and she ate breakfast four hours ago. By this time Mrs. Collin is awake. She denies any pain, has no nausea, but she says she is feeling dizzy. "I should have tried to drink more water," she says. **Physical examination** reveals no signs of trauma and no other signs or symptoms of a heart-related emergency. You take and record her vital signs. Her pulse continues to feel weak at 112 beats per minute, BP is 98/48, respirations rapid and shallow at 34 breaths a minute. Your partner begins to fan Mrs. Collin's skin, and you offer her some water.

You begin your transport to the nearest medical facility, communicating the necessary information to the hospital. En route you perform **ongoing assessment,** monitoring Mrs. Collin's vitals and carefully observing her for any indications of progression to a more serious heat-related condition.

At the hospital, it is confirmed that Mrs. Collin is suffering from heat exposure. After rehydration, cool air, and some rest she fully recovers.

Effects of Heat on the Body

The body generates heat as a result of its constant internal chemical processes. A certain amount of this heat is required to maintain normal body temperature. Any heat that is not needed for temperature maintenance must be lost from the body. If it is not, **hyperthermia** (HI-per-THURM-e-ah), an abnormally high body temperature, will be created. Left unchecked, it will lead to death. Heat and humidity are often associated with hyperthermia.

As you learned earlier in this chapter, heat is lost by the body through the lungs or the skin. Mechanisms of heat loss include *conduction, convection, radiation, evaporation,* and *respiration.* Consider what can happen to the body when it is placed in a hot environment. Air being inhaled is warm, possibly warmer than the air being exhaled. The skin may absorb more heat than it loses. When high humidity is added, the evaporation of perspiration slows. To make things even more difficult, consider all this in an environment that lacks circulating air or a breeze, which would increase convection and evaporative heat loss.

Since evaporative heat loss is reduced in a humid environment, moist heat can produce dramatic body changes in a short time. Moist heat usually tires people quickly, frequently stopping them from harming themselves through overexertion. Dry heat, on the other hand, often deceives people. They continue to work or remain exposed to excess heat far beyond what their bodies can tolerate. This is why you may see problems caused by dry heat exposure more often than those seen in moist heat exposure.

The same rules of care apply to heat emergencies as to any other emergency. You will need to perform the appropriate steps of assessment, remaining alert for problems other than those related to heat. Collapse due to heat exposure, for example, may result in a fall that can fracture bones. Pre-existing conditions such as dehydration, diabetes, fever, fatigue, high blood pressure, heart disease, lung problems, or obesity may hasten or intensify the effects of heat exposure, as will ingestion of alcohol and other drugs. Mrs. Collin's condition was due to dehydration.

Age, diseases, and existing injuries all must be considered when evaluating the patient. The elderly may be affected by poor thermoregulation, prescription medications, and lack of mobility. Newborns and infants also may have poor thermoregulation. Always consider the problem to be greater if the patient is a child or elderly, injured or having a chronic disease.

Heat Emergencies

Patient with Moist, Pale, Normal-to-Cool Skin

Prolonged exposure to excessive heat can create an emergency in which the patient presents with moist pale skin which may feel normal or cool to the touch. The individual perspires heavily, often drinking large quantities of water. As the sweating continues, salts are lost by the body, bringing on painful muscle cramps (sometimes called heat cramps). A person who is actively exercising can lose more than a liter of sweat per hour.

Healthy individuals who have been exposed to excessive heat while working or exercising may experience a form of shock brought about by fluid and salt loss. Mrs. Collin's case is one example of this type of heat emergency. It is also seen among firefighters, construction workers, dock workers, and those employed in poorly ventilated warehouses. It is more of a problem during the summer and reaches a peak during prolonged heat waves. This condition is sometimes known as heat exhaustion.

Patient Assessment—Heat Emergency Patient with Moist, Pale, Normal-to-Cool Skin

Signs and Symptoms

- ☐ Muscular cramps—usually in the legs and abdomen
- ☐ Weakness or exhaustion, sometimes dizziness or periods of faintness
- ☐ Rapid, shallow breathing
- ☐ Weak pulse
- ☐ Moist pale skin which may feel normal to cool
- ☐ Heavy perspiration
- ☐ Loss of consciousness is possible

Patient Care—Heat Emergency Patient with Moist, Pale, Normal-to-Cool Skin

Emergency Care Steps

1. Remove the patient from the hot environment and place in a cool environment (such as the back of an air-conditioned ambulance).
2. Administer oxygen by nonrebreather mask at 15 liters per minute.

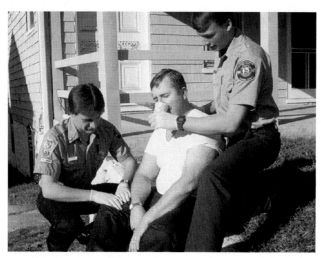

FIGURE 22-3 Give water to the heat-emergency patient, if he has moist, pale, normal to cool skin and if he is responsive and not nauseated.

3 Loosen or remove clothing to cool the patient by fanning without chilling him. Watch for shivering.

4 Put patient in supine position with legs elevated. Keep him at rest.

5 If the patient is responsive and not nauseated, have him drink water (Figure 22-3). If the patient is unresponsive or vomiting, transport to the hospital with patient on his left side.

6 If patient experiences muscular cramps, apply moist towels over cramped muscles.

7 Transport.

Patient with Hot, Dry or Moist Skin

When a person's temperature-regulating mechanisms fail and the body cannot rid itself of excessive heat, you will see a patient with hot, dry, or possibly moist skin. When the skin is hot—whether dry or moist—this is a true emergency. It is a condition that is sometimes known as heat stroke. The problem is compounded when in response to loss of fluid and salt, the patient stops sweating, which prevents heat loss through evaporation. Athletes, laborers, and others who exercise or work in hot environments commonly develop this condition. So do the elderly who live in poorly ventilated apartments without air conditioning, and children left in cars with the windows rolled up.

More cases of patients with hot, dry skin are reported on hot, humid days. However, many cases occur from exposure to dry heat.

Signs and Symptoms

☐ Rapid, shallow breathing
☐ Full and rapid pulse
☐ Generalized weakness
☐ Hot, dry or possibly moist skin
☐ Little or no perspiration
☐ Loss of consciousness or altered mental status
☐ Dilated pupils
☐ Seizures may be seen; no muscle cramps

Patient Care—Heat Emergency Patient with Hot, Dry or Moist Skin

Emergency Care Steps

1 Remove the patient from the hot environment and place in a cool environment (in air-conditioned ambulance with air conditioner running on high).

2 Remove clothing. Apply cool packs to neck, groin, and armpits. Keep the skin wet by applying water by sponge or wet towels. Fan aggressively.

3 Administer oxygen by nonrebreather mask at 15 liters per minute.

4 Transport immediately. Should transport be delayed, find a tub or container, immerse the patient up to the neck in cooled water, and monitor vital signs throughout process.

Infants and Children

For infants or young children, cooling is started using tepid (lukewarm) water. This water can then be replaced with cooler water at the recommendation of medical direction.

Beware of what you are told by some patients. They may not believe heat emergencies are serious. Many simply want to return to work. Nevertheless, conduct a thorough initial assessment, focused history, and physical exam. If you have any doubts, tell the patient why he should be transported and seek his permission. You may have to spend a little time with some patients to gain their confidence.

WATER-RELATED EMERGENCIES

On the Scene

Dispatch sends your unit to an irrigation canal near a corn field. When you arrive you see nothing until you are only a few feet from the banks of the canal. There you see the roof of a pick-up truck a few inches below the water's surface.

During **scene size-up** you approach the fire department rescue personnel who are also on scene. You have been trained in water rescue, and following consultation with them, you agree that the canal's current is safe to enter. As an added precaution, you and members of the rescue team attach safety lines around your waists and slip on personal flotation devices. At this time, you believe there is only one patient, the driver. You pull on your leather gloves and enter the canal.

Even as you approach the vehicle, you start your **initial assessment.** You can see that the driver's compartment is filled with water. You see red hair floating out of a window approximately two feet beneath the water's surface. The cold, murky water makes it impossible to see anything clearly. A drowning is, of course, your immediate impression. Because of the mechanism of injury, you also consider a possible spinal-cord injury.

You move with the team to perform in-line stabilization and removal of the patient from the vehicle with a backboard. You keep the patient's neck rigid and in a straight line with the body's midline. Once the patient's head is above water—he turns out to be a teenage boy—you open the airway with the jaw-thrust maneuver. Next you provide rescue breathing with your pocket mask as other rescuers disentangle the patient's legs. The patient is pulseless. You transport him to the level bank of the canal to start chest compressions. Your partner and a fire department rescuer take over ventilating with a bag-valve-mask and supplemental oxygen. You note no obvious signs of bleeding or traumatic injury.

"How long has he been under water?" someone asks. No one knows the answer, since the truck was discovered already in the canal. Before you can attach the AED, your patient's chest begins to expand slightly. He breathes, and you feel a weak carotid pulse. Maintaining in-line stabilization, you turn the patient on his left side. He vomits. Your partner suctions the patient's airway. As the patient's eyes open, you immobilize him for immediate transport to the hospital. You are almost 40 minutes away. En route, you switch the patient to a nonrebreather mask and administer oxygen at 15 liters per minute.

In the ambulance, you perform a **focused history and physical exam.** During the rapid trauma exam you find no obvious signs of injury. By now the patient is alert, and you begin a SAMPLE history. He tells you his name is Evan Lyndsey and he is 17 years old. He denies any pain, has no allergies, takes no medications, has no pertinent medical history, hasn't eaten anything today. He tells you, "I was just driving way too fast and lost control on a curve." You record vital signs of pulse 96, BP 132/78, and respirations 20. You call the hospital and provide a verbal report of the patient's condition and your estimated time of arrival. You perform a **detailed physical exam,** then **ongoing assessment** every five minutes until arrival.

Evan is a lucky young man. After he gets out of the hospital, he receives follow-up treatment for some respiratory problems caused by water inhalation, but—thanks to the spinal care he received from the team of rescuers—he has no long-term aftereffects from a bruised spinal cord caused by the impact of the crash. He is alive and expecting a full recovery. ∎

Water-Related Accidents

Drowning or near-drowning is the first thing people think of, and usually the first concern, in connection with water-related accidents. However, there are many types of injuries resulting from many types of accidents that can occur on or in the water. Boating, water-skiing, wind surfing, jet-skiing, diving, and scuba-diving accidents can produce fractured bones, bleeding, soft-tissue injuries, and airway obstruction. Even auto collisions can send vehicles or passengers into the water, resulting in any of the injuries usually associated with motor vehicle collisions as well as the complications caused by the presence of water.

Medical problems such as heart attacks can also cause or be caused by water accidents or can simply take place in, on, or near the water. Remember, too, that some water accidents happen far away from pools, lakes, or beaches. Bathtub drownings do occur. Adults, as well as children, can drown in only a few inches of water.

Safety Note

Do not attempt a rescue in which you must enter deep water or swim unless you have been trained to do so and are a very good swimmer. Except for shallow pools and open shallow waters with uniform bottoms, the problems faced in water rescue are too great and too dangerous for the poor swimmer or untrained person to attempt. If this bothers you—having to stand by not being able to help—then take a course in water safety and rescue. Otherwise, if you attempt a deep water or swimming rescue, you will probably become a victim yourself.

Patient Assessment—Water-Related Accidents

Learn to look for the following problems in water-related accident victims.

☐ *Airway obstruction*—This may be from water in the lungs, foreign matter in the airway, or swollen airway tissues (common if the neck is injured in a dive). Spasms along the airway may be present in cases of near-drowning.

☐ *Cardiac arrest*—This is often related to respiratory arrest or occurs before the near-drowning.

☐ *Signs of heart attack*—Through overexertion, the patient may have greater problems than the obvious near-drowning. Some untrained rescuers too quickly conclude that chest pains are due to muscle cramps as a result of swimming.

☐ *Injuries to the head and neck*—These are expected to be found in boating, water-skiing, and diving accidents, but they are also very common in swimming accidents.

☐ *Internal injuries*—While doing the focused physical exam, stay on the alert for musculoskeletal injuries, soft-tissue injuries, and internal bleeding (which may be missed during the first stages of care).

☐ *Generalized cooling, or hypothermia*—The water does not have to be very cold and the length of stay in the water does not have to be very long for hypothermia to occur. In some cases of near-drowning, the patient may have a better chance for survival in cold water.

☐ *Substance abuse*—Alcohol and drug use are closely associated with adolescent and adult drownings. Elevated blood alcohol levels have been found in over 30 per cent of drowning victims. The screening for drug use has not been as extensive as that done for alcohol, but research indicates that drugs are a contributory factor in many water-related accidents.

☐ *Drowning or near-drowning*—The patient may be discovered under or face down in the water. He may be unconscious and without discernible vital signs or may be conscious, breathing, and coughing up water. (Drowning and near-drowning are discussed in detail, below.)

Drowning and Near-Drowning

The process of drowning begins as a person struggles to keep afloat in the water. He gulps in large breaths of air as he thrashes about. When he can no longer keep afloat and starts to submerge, he tries to take and hold one more deep breath. As he does, water may enter the airway. There is a series of coughing and swallowing actions, and the victim involuntarily inhales and swallows more water. As water flows past the epiglottis, it triggers a reflex spasm of the larynx. This spasm seals the airway so effectively that no more than a small amount of water reaches the lungs. Unconsciousness soon results from hypoxia (oxygen starvation).

About 10 per cent of the people who drown die just from the lack of air. In the remaining victims, the person attempts a final respiratory effort and draws water into the lungs, or the spasms subside with the onset of unconsciousness and water freely enters the lungs.

As an EMT-B you should start using the term **near-drowning.** Obviously, if the patient is breathing and coughing up water, he has not drowned but nearly drowned. This is only part of what we mean by near-drowning. In our earlier scenario, Evan was a near-drowning patient. If a patient has "drowned" in lay person's terms, he is not necessarily biologically dead. Resuscitative measures may be able to keep the patient biologically alive long enough for more advanced life support measures to be used to save the patient's life.

Only when sufficient time has passed to render resuscitation useless has **drowning** truly taken place. We now know that some patients in cold water can be resuscitated after 30 minutes or more in cardiac arrest. Once the water temperature falls below 70°F, biological death may be delayed. The colder the water, the better are the patient's chances for survival, unless generalized hypothermia produces lethal complications.

Emergency Care of Near-Drowning Patients

Transport for the near-drowning patient should not be delayed. You may initiate care when the patient is out of the water (already out when you arrive or in the water when you arrive but rescued by others before you initiate care). At other times you may need and be able to initiate care while the patient is still in the water—especially rescue breathing and immobilization for possible spine injuries. As you will recall, this is how Evan was treated. Chest compressions will be effective only after the patient is out of the water.

Safety Note
Unless you are a very good swimmer and trained in water rescue, do not go into the water to save someone. Such training is available from the American Red Cross and the YMCA in the form of water safety and rescue courses.

Rescue Breathing in or out of the Water If needed, rescue breathing should begin without delay. If you can reach the nonbreathing patient in the water, you can provide ventilations as you support him in a semi-supine position. You can continue providing ventilations while the patient is being immobilized and removed from the water. If the patient is already out of the water, you can begin rescue breathing or CPR on the land.

Do not be surprised to find resistance as you ventilate the near-drowning patient. You will probably have to ventilate more forcefully than you would other patients. Remember, you must provide air to the patient's lungs as soon as possible.

A patient with water in the lungs usually has water in the stomach. If there is enough water in the stomach, there will be added resistance to your efforts to provide rescue breathing or CPR ventilations. Since the patient may have spasms along the airway, or swollen tissues in the larynx or trachea, you may find that some of the air you provide will go into the patient's stomach. Remember, the same problem will occur if you do not properly open the airway or if your ventilations are too forceful.

If gastric distention interferes with artificial ventilation, the patient should be placed on his left side. With suction immediately available, the EMT-B should place his hand over the epigastric area of the abdomen and apply firm pressure to relieve the distention. This procedure should only be done if the gastric distention interferes with the ability of the EMT-B to artificially ventilate the patient effectively.

Care for Possible Spinal Injuries in the Water Injuries to the cervical spine are seen with many water-related accidents. Most often, these injuries are received during a dive or when the patient is struck by a boat, skier, or ski, surfer or surfboard. Even though cervical-spine injuries are the most common of the spinal injuries seen in water-related accidents, there can be injury anywhere along the spine.

When a patient is unconscious, you may not be able to detect spinal injuries. In water-related accidents, assume that the unconscious patient has neck and spinal injuries. Should the patient have head injuries, also assume that there are neck and spinal injuries. Keep in mind that a patient found in respiratory or cardiac arrest will need resuscitation started before you can immobilize the neck and spine. Also, realize that you may not be able to carry out a complete assessment for spinal injuries while the patient is in the water. Take care to avoid aggravating spinal injuries, but do not delay basic life support. Do not delay removing the patient from the water if the scene presents an immediate danger. When possible, keep the patient's neck rigid and in a straight line with the body's midline. Use the jaw-thrust maneuver to open the airway.

If the patient with possible spinal injuries is still in the water and you are a good swimmer and able to aid in the rescue, secure the patient to a long spine board before removing him from the water. Assuring the integrity of the spine before removal from the water is critical in preventing permanent neurological damage or paralysis. Steps for this procedure are shown on Scan 22-1. This type of rescue requires special training in the use of the spine board while in the water. This rigid device can "pop up" very easily from below the water surface. Make certain that you know how to control the board and how to work in the water.

Care for Patients Out of the Water In all cases of water-related accidents, assume that the unconscious patient has neck and spinal injuries. If the patient is rescued by others while you wait, or if the patient is out of the water when you arrive, you should

1. Do an initial assessment, protecting the spine as much as possible.

Water Rescue—Possible Spinal Injury

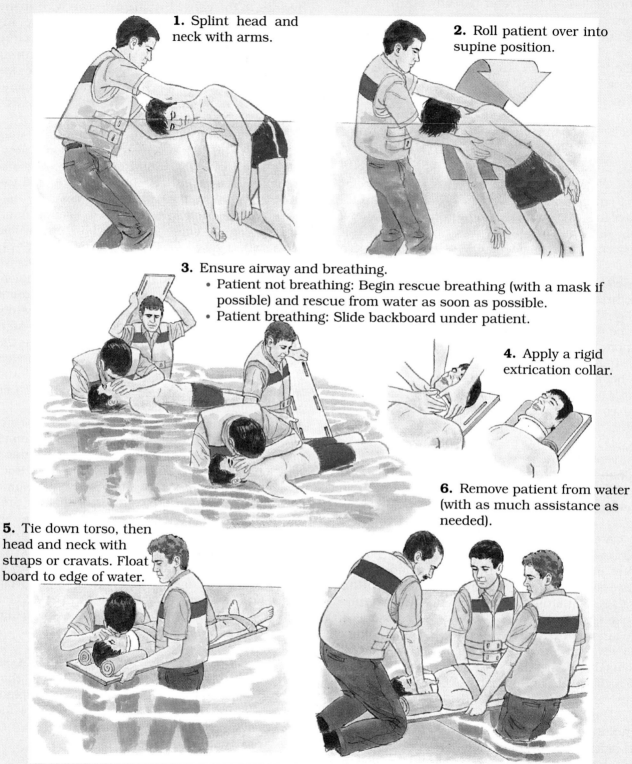

1. Splint head and neck with arms.

2. Roll patient over into supine position.

3. Ensure airway and breathing.
- Patient not breathing: Begin rescue breathing (with a mask if possible) and rescue from water as soon as possible.
- Patient breathing: Slide backboard under patient.

4. Apply a rigid extrication collar.

5. Tie down torso, then head and neck with straps or cravats. Float board to edge of water.

6. Remove patient from water (with as much assistance as needed).

Note: The technique for removing patients from water assuring spine integrity is critical. Interviews of paraplegics whose paralysis resulted from water-related accidents indicate that many were able to tread water after the injury and prior to being improperly removed from the water.

2. Provide rescue breathing or CPR if needed. Protect yourself by using a pocket face mask with a one-way valve or bag-valve-mask unit.

3. Look for and control profuse bleeding. Since the patient's heart rate may have slowed down, take a pulse for 60 seconds in all cold-water rescue situations.

4. Provide care for shock (as described in Chapter 25), administer a high concentration of oxygen, and transport the patient as soon as possible.

5. Continue resuscitative measures throughout transport. Initial and periodic suctioning may be needed.

The near-drowning patient receiving rescue breathing or CPR should be transported as soon as possible. If resuscitation and immediate transport are not required, cover the patient to conserve body heat and complete a focused history and physical exam. Uncover only those areas of the patient's body involved with the stage of the assessment. Care for any problems or injuries detected during the assessment in the order of their priority.

If spinal injury is not suspected, place the patient on his left side to allow water, vomit, and other secretions to drain from upper airway. Suction as needed. When transport is delayed and you believe that the patient can be moved to a warmer place, do so without aggravating any existing injuries. Do not allow the near-drowning patient to walk. Transport the patient.

Information supplied to the dispatcher or to the hospital from the scene and during transport is critical in cases of near-drowning. The hospital emergency department staff needs to know if this is a fresh- or salt-water drowning, if it took place in cold or warm water, and if it is related to a diving accident. You may be asked to transport the patient to a special facility or to a center having a hyperbaric chamber when decompression therapy is needed. (Decompression is discussed later in the "FYI" section of this chapter.)

Diving Accidents

Water-related accidents often involve injuries that occur when individuals attempt dives or enter the water from diving boards. In the majority of these accidents, the patient is a teenager. Basically the same types of injuries are seen in dives taken from diving boards, poolsides, docks, boats, and the shore. The injury may be due to the diver striking the board or some object on or under the water. From great heights, injury may result from impact with the water.

Most diving accidents involve the head and neck, but you will also find injuries to the spine, hands, feet, and ribs in many cases. Any part of the body can be injured depending on the position that the diver is in when he strikes the water or an object. This means that you must perform an initial assessment. You must also perform a focused history and physical exam on all diving accident patients. Do not overlook the fact that a medical emergency may have led to the diving accident.

Emergency care for diving accident patients is the same as for any accident patient, if they are out of the water. Care provided in the water and during removal from the water is the same as for any patient who may have neck and spine injuries. Remember, assume that any unconscious or unresponsive patient has neck and spinal injuries. There may be delayed reactions with patients having spinal injuries. Compression along the spine may cause a patient with no apparent injuries to suddenly exhibit indications of nerve impairment. Often this begins as a numbness or a tingling sensation in the legs.

BITES AND STINGS

On the Scene

Dispatch advises you to respond to the home of an adult female patient who has been bitten by a snake. As you pull up to the residence, pull on gloves, and **size up the scene**—rather nervously scanning the area for snakes—you are greeted by a man. "Hurry," he says as he grabs the handle to open the ambulance door. "My wife's been bitten by a snake."

"When?" you ask.

"Maybe ten minutes or so ago," he responds. Out in the backyard.

Neither he nor his wife can describe the snake, he says, except to say it was small—less than a foot long. You quickly follow him into the house.

The husband goes on to tell you and your partner that he has no idea if the snake was poisonous or not. "We were gardening in the patch overlooking the water—we have a small duck pond back there. We just knelt down. Suddenly I heard a yelp. I turned and saw Anna jump up and a small snake practically fly away through the weeds."

You begin your *initial assessment* as you approach the patient, an approximately 45-year-old woman who is sitting on a chair on the enclosed porch at the back of the house. She is alert but pale and a bit distraught. Her airway is open and respirations are slightly rapid. There is no sign of bleeding nor mechanism of injury. She has her left leg up and resting on a chair, shoes and socks off. You introduce yourself, and she tells you her name is Anna Perrera.

As you begin your *focused history and physical exam,* you notice a slight discoloration on her calf and when you get closer you see a single tiny fang mark. She says there is a growing ache in her lower leg. She cannot tell you any more about the snake. You try to calm her and begin to take a SAMPLE history in a conversational manner.

Mrs. Perrera tells you that she has an allergy to penicillin and though she takes insulin by injection for diabetes, she says she is in good health. Her last meal was breakfast about three hours ago. You take her vital signs, including a pulse at the ankle. Her pulse rate is 96, blood pressure 140/100, and respirations 20 and unlabored. She has no nausea or vomiting. Your partner begins to wash the wound with soap and water as you call medical direction and ask for instructions.

Medical direction tells you to apply constricting bands and transport immediately. You do. En route, your partner applies a splint to the affected leg, and you perform *ongoing assessment* every five minutes to monitor Mrs. Perrera's mental status and vital signs. Though no swelling occurs, you repeatedly check the constricting bands to be sure they do not become too tight.

After your last run of the shift, you ask hospital staff about the patients you brought in today. They tell you Mrs. Perrera's reaction to the bite was minimal. Though it may have been a poisonous snake, it seems that very little if any venom was injected. She will probably be released from the hospital tomorrow morning.

■

Insect Bites and Stings

Insect stings, spider bites, and scorpion stings are typical sources of injected poisons, or **toxins**—substances produced by animals or plants that are poisonous to humans. (**Venom** is a term for a toxin produced by some animals such as snakes, spiders, and certain marine life forms.) Commonly seen insect stings are those of wasps, hornets, bees, and ants. Insect stings and bites are rarely dangerous. However, 5 per

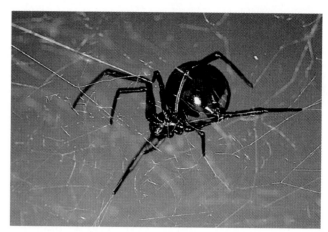

FIGURE 22-4 Black widow spider.

cent of the population of the U. S. will have an allergic reaction, which may result in shock. Those who are hypersensitive develop severe anaphylactic shock that is quickly life threatening (see Chapter 20, Allergies).

All spiders are poisonous, but most species cannot get their fangs through human skin. The black widow spider (Figure 22-4) and the brown recluse, or fiddleback, spider are two that can, and their bites can produce medical emergencies. Almost all brown recluse bites are painless, and patients seldom recall being bitten. The characteristic lesion appears in only 10 per cent of cases, and then only after up to 12 hours (Figure 22-5). EMT-Bs are seldom called to respond

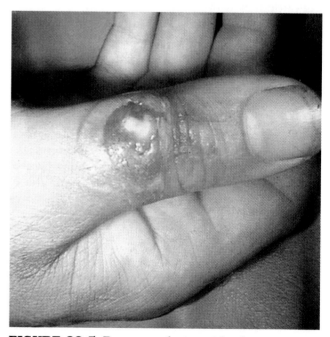

FIGURE 22-5 Brown recluse spider bite.

to a brown recluse bite. Black widow bites cause a more immediate reaction.

Scorpion stings are common in the Southwest U. S. They do not ordinarily cause deaths, but one rare species *(centroroides exilcauda)* is dangerous to humans and can cause serious medical problems in children, including respiratory failure.

Note: Bites and stings belong in the class of injected poisons discussed in Chapter 21, Poisoning and Overdose Emergencies.

Patient Assessment—Insect Bites and Stings

Gather information from the patient, bystanders, and the scene. Find out whatever you can about the insect or other possible source of the poisoning. The signs and symptoms of injected poisoning can include those listed below.

Signs and Symptoms

- [ ] Altered states of awareness
- [ ] Noticeable stings or bites on the skin
- [ ] Puncture marks (especially note the fingers, forearms, toes, and legs)
- [ ] Blotchy skin (mottled skin)
- [ ] Localized pain or itching
- [ ] Numbness in a limb or body part
- [ ] Burning sensations at the site followed by pain spreading throughout the limb
- [ ] Redness
- [ ] Swelling or blistering at the site
- [ ] Weakness or collapse
- [ ] Difficult breathing and abnormal pulse rate
- [ ] Headache and dizziness
- [ ] Chills
- [ ] Fever
- [ ] Nausea and vomiting
- [ ] Muscle cramps, chest tightening, joint pains
- [ ] Excessive saliva formation, profuse sweating
- [ ] Anaphylaxis

Patient Care—Insect Bites and Stings

As an EMT-B you are not expected to be able to identify insects and spiders. Proper identification of these organisms is best left to experts. If the problem has been caused by a creature that is known locally and is not normally dangerous (such as a bee, wasp, or puss caterpillar), the major concern will be anaphylactic shock. If anaphylactic shock does not appear to be a problem, care is usually simple.

If the cause of the bite or sting is unknown, or the organism is unknown, the patient should be seen by a physician. Call medical direction or take the patient to a medical facility and let experts decide on the proper treatment for the patient. If possible, transport the stinging object or organism in a sealed container, taking care not to handle it without proper protection, even if it is dead. If you can accomplish this safely, you may save precious minutes needed to identify the toxin.

Emergency Care Steps

To provide emergency care for injected toxins

1. Treat for shock, even if the patient does not present any of the signs of shock.
2. *Call medical direction.* This should be skipped only if the organism is known and your EMS system has a specific protocol for care.
3. Do not pull out bee and wasp stingers and venom sacs. To do so may inject another dose of venom. Instead, carefully scrape the site using a blade or a card. (Avoid using tweezers or forceps, as these can squeeze venom from the sac into the wound.)
4. Remove jewelry from any affected limbs. This should be done in case the limb swells, which would make removal more difficult later.
5. If local protocol permits and if the wound is on an extremity (not a joint), place constricting bands above and below the sting or bite site. This is done to slow the spread of venom in the lymphatic vessels and superficial veins. The band should be made of ¾ inch to 1-½ inch wide soft rubber or other wide soft material. It should be placed about 2 inches from the wound. The band must be loose enough so that you can slide one finger underneath it. It should not cut off circulation to the limb.

6 Keep the limb immobilized and the patient still to prevent distribution of the poison to other parts of the body. (Note: Some EMS systems recommend placing a cold compress on the wound. Most EMS systems do not use cold for any injected toxin. *Follow local protocol.*)

Remember: Look for medical identification devices that identify persons sensitive to certain stings or bites. Some patients sensitive to stings or bites carry medication to help prevent anaphylactic shock. This situation is described in Chapter 20, Allergies.

Snakebites

Snakebites require special care but are usually not life threatening. Nearly 50,000 people in the U. S. are bitten by snakes each year. Over 8,000 of these cases involve poisonous snakes, but on the average fewer than 10 deaths are reported annually (in the U. S., more people die each year from bee and wasp stings than from snakebites). The signs and symptoms of snakebite poisoning may take several hours to appear. If death does result, it is usually not a rapidly occurring event unless anaphylactic shock develops. Most victims who die survive at least one to two days.

In the U. S. there are two types of poisonous snakes—pit vipers (including rattlesnakes, copperheads, and water moccasins) and coral snakes (Figure 22-6). Up to 25% of pit viper bites and 50% of coral bites are "dry bites" without venom injection, but the venomous bite from a diamondback rattler or coral snake is considered very serious. Since each person reacts differently to snakebite, you should consider the bite from any known poisonous snake or any unidentified snake to be a serious emergency. Staying calm and keeping the patient calm and at rest is critical. Since reaction time is slow, there is time to transport the patient without haste.

Unless you are dealing with a known species of local snake that is not considered poisonous, consider all snakebites to be from poisonous snakes. The patient or bystanders may say that the snake was not poisonous. However, they could be mistaken. The signs and symptoms of snakebite may include the following.

Signs and Symptoms

- ☐ A noticeable bite on the skin. This may appear as nothing more than a discoloration
- ☐ Pain and swelling in the area of the bite. This may be slow to develop, from 30 minutes to several hours
- ☐ Rapid pulse and labored breathing
- ☐ Progressive general weakness
- ☐ Vision problems (dim or blurred)
- ☐ Nausea and vomiting
- ☐ Seizures
- ☐ Drowsiness or unconsciousness

If the dead or captured snake is at the scene, your role as an EMT-B is not to identify the snake, but to transport it in a sealed container along with the patient. Arrange for separate transport of a live specimen. Do not attempt to transport a live snake in the ambulance.

Should you see the live, uncaptured snake, take great care or you may be its next victim. When possible, note its size and coloration. Getting close enough to look for details of the eyes or for a pit between the eye and mouth is foolish. How you classify a snake, whether it is dead or alive, will probably have little to do with subsequent care. The medical center staff will arrange to have an expert classify a captured or dead specimen, and they have protocols to determine care if the snake has not been captured. Unless you

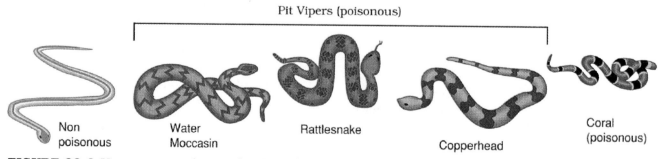

Pit Vipers (poisonous)

Non poisonous   Water Moccasin   Rattlesnake   Copperhead   Coral (poisonous)

FIGURE 22-6 Venomous snakes in the United States.

are an expert in capturing snakes, do not try to catch the snake. Never delay care and transport in order to capture the snake.

Patient Care—Snakebites

Emergency Care Steps

1. *Call medical direction.*
2. Treat for shock and conserve body heat. Keep the patient calm.
3. Locate the fang marks and clean the site with soap and water. There may be only one fang mark.
4. Remove any rings, bracelets, or other constricting items on the bitten extremity.
5. Keep any bitten extremities immobilized—the application of a splint will help. Try to keep the bite at the level of the heart or, when this is not possible, below the level of the heart.
6. Apply light constricting bands above and below the wound if ordered by medical direction. (See more information on constricting bands below.)
7. Transport the patient, carefully monitoring vital signs.

Warning: Do not place an ice bag or cold pack on the bite unless you are directed to do so by a physician or local protocol. Do not cut into the bite and suction or squeeze unless you are directed to do so by a physician. Never suck the venom from the wound using your mouth. Instead, use a suction cup. Suctioning is seldom done.

Apply constricting bands above and below the fang marks. Each band should be about two inches from the wound, but never place the bands on either side of a joint, such as above and below the knee. Since the typical coral snakebite is to a finger or a toe, due to its small mouth, just a single band may be placed above a coral snakebite. If the bite is to a finger, the band can be applied to the wrist.

The purpose of the constricting bands is to restrict the flow of lymph, not of blood. They should be made of ¾ to 1-½ inch wide soft rubber. If only one band is available, place it above the wound (between the wound and the heart). If no bands are available, use a handkerchief or other wide soft material. The bands should be snug but not tight enough to cut off circulation. Monitor for a pulse at the wrist or ankle, depending on the extremity involved. Check to be certain that tissue swelling does not cause the constricting bands to become too tight.

Poisoning from Marine Life

Poisoning from marine life forms can occur in a variety of ways—from eating improperly prepared seafood or poisonous organisms to stings and punctures. Patients who have ingested spoiled, contaminated, or infested seafood may develop anaphylactic shock. They should receive the same care as any patient in anaphylactic shock. During care, you must be prepared for vomiting. Most patients will show the signs of food poisoning. The care for seafood poisoning is the same as for all other food poisonings.

It is extremely rare for someone in the U. S. to eat a poisonous variety of marine life. Creatures such as puffer fish and paralytic shellfish are not readily available. For all cases of suspected poisoning due to ingestion, call your online medical direction or the poison control center as local protocol directs you to. Be prepared for vomiting, convulsions, and respiratory arrest.

Venomous marine life forms producing sting injuries include the jellyfish, the sea nettle, the Portuguese man-of-war, coral, the sea anemone, and the hydra. For most victims, the sting produces pain with few complications. Some patients may show allergic reactions and possibly develop anaphylactic shock. These cases require the same care as rendered for any case of anaphylactic shock. Stings to the face, especially those near or on the lip or eye, require a physician's attention. Swabbing the affected area with rubbing alcohol will reduce the pain of the sting. Be careful not to let the rubbing alcohol get into the patient's mouth or eyes.

Puncture wounds occur when someone steps on or grabs a stingray, sea urchin, spiny catfish, or other form of spiny marine animal. Although it is true that soaking the wound in hot water for 30 minutes will break down the venom, you should not delay transport. Puncture wounds must be treated by a physician and the patient may need an anti tetanus inoculation. Remember, the patient could react to the venom by developing anaphylactic shock.

Documentation Tips—
Environmental Emergencies

In addition to routine observations and measurements related to the patient's signs and symptoms, include the following.

- If the injury is related to exposure to heat, cold, water, or ice, briefly describe environmental conditions. If possible, provide good estimates of measurements, such as temperature and factors relating to wind chill and water chill.
- Ask the patient what caused the emergency. He or she might forget to tell you that the near-drowning was caused by "sudden chest pain" or that the exposure to cold was due to trauma from a fall.
- If the injury is caused by a bite or sting, record the patient's or a bystander's description of the insect or animal. Include size and color if possible.
- Ask the patient or witnesses if the patient lost consciousness. Document all changes in mental status.
- Record vital signs early in the call. Take several sets and record the intervals, so hospital personnel can note the rate of change.

FYI

Topics included in the FYI—"For Your Information"—section are those that go beyond the chapter objectives. The information in this segment is intended to broaden your understanding of the chapter topic but is not essential to an understanding of your job and as EMT-B.

Water Rescues

The following is the order of procedures for a water rescue (Figure 22-7)—most of which can be performed short of going into the water: *reach, throw and tow, row, go.*

- *Reach*—When the patient is responsive and close to shore or poolside, try to *reach* him by holding out an object for him to grab. Then pull him from the water. *Make sure your position is secure.* Line (rope) is considered the best choice. If no line is available, use a branch, fishing rod, oar, stick, or other such object, even a towel, blanket, or article of clothing. If no object is available or you have only one opportunity to grab the person (e.g., in strong currents), position yourself flat on your stomach and extend your hand or leg to the patient (not recommended for the nonswimmer). Again,

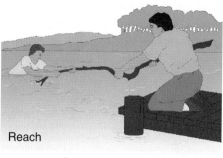
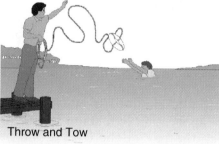
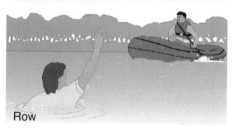

FIGURE 22-7 First try to *reach* and pull the patient from the water. If this fails, *throw* him anything that will float and *tow* him from the water. If this fails, *row* to the patient.

make certain that you are working from a secure position.
- *Throw and Tow*—Should the person be alert but too far away for you to reach and pull from the water, *throw* an object that will float (Figure 22-8). A personal flotation device (PFD or lifejacket) or ring buoy (life preserver) work best. Other buoyant objects include foam cushions, logs, plastic picnic containers, surf boards, flat boards, large beach balls, and plastic toys. Two empty, capped, plastic milk jugs can keep an adult afloat for hours. Inflatable splints can be used if there is nothing at the scene that will float. Once the conscious patient has a flotation device, try to find a way to *tow* him to shore. From a safe position, throw the patient a line or another flotation device attached to a line. If you are a good swimmer and you know how to judge the water, wade out no deeper than waist high, wear a personal flotation device, and have a safety line that is secured on shore.

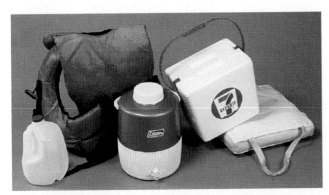

FIGURE 22-8 Throw the patient any object that will float.

- *Row*—When the patient is too far from shore to allow for throwing and towing, or the patient is unresponsive, you may be able to *row* a boat to the patient. Do not attempt this if you cannot swim. Even if you are a good swimmer, wearing a personal flotation device while in the boat is required. In cases in which the patient is conscious, tell him to grab an oar or the stern (rear end) of the boat. You must exercise great care when helping the patient into the boat. This is even more tricky when you are in a canoe. Should the canoe tip over, stay with the canoe and hold onto its bottom and side. Most canoes will stay afloat.
- *Go*—As a last resort, when all other means have failed, you can *go* into the water and swim to the patient. You must be a good swimmer, trained in water rescue and life-saving. Untrained rescuers can become victims themselves.

Scuba Diving Accidents

Scuba (Self-Contained Underwater Breathing Apparatus) diving accidents have increased with the popularity of the sport, especially since many untrained and inexperienced persons are attempting dives. Today, there are more than 2 million people who scuba dive for sport or as part of their industrial or military job. Added to this are a large number who decide to "try it one time," without the benefits of lessons or supervision. Well-trained divers seldom have problems. Those with inadequate training place themselves at great risk.

Scuba diving accidents include all types of body injuries and near-drownings. In many cases, the scuba diving accident was brought about by medical problems that existed prior to the dive. There are two special problems seen in scuba diving accidents. They are air emboli in the diver's blood and the "bends."

Air Embolism

Air embolism—more accurately called *arterial gas embolism* (AGE)—is the result of gases leaving a damaged lung and entering the bloodstream. Severe damage to the lungs may lead to a spontaneous pneumothorax. Air emboli (gas bubbles in the blood) are most often associated with divers who hold their breath because of inadequate training, equipment failure, underwater emergency, or when trying to conserve air during a dive. However, a diver may develop an air embolism in very shallow water (as little as four feet). An automobile collision victim also may suffer an air embolism if, when trapped below water, he takes gulps of air from air pockets held inside the vehicle. When freed, the patient may develop air emboli the same as a scuba diver.

In either case, the onset is rapid, with signs that may include the following.

- Blurred vision
- Chest pains
- Numbness and tingling sensations in the extremities
- Generalized or specific weakness—possible paralysis
- Frothy blood in mouth or nose
- Convulsions
- Rapid lapse into unconsciousness
- Respiratory arrest and cardiac arrest

Decompression Sickness

Decompression sickness is usually caused when a diver comes up too quickly from a deep prolonged dive. The quick ascent causes nitrogen gas to be trapped in the body tissue and then in the patient's bloodstream. Decompression sickness in scuba divers takes from 1 to 48 hours to appear, with about 90% of the cases occurring within 3 hours of the dive. Divers increase the risk of decompression sickness if they fly within 12 hours of a dive. Because of this delay, carefully consider all information gathered from the patient interview and reports from the patient's family and friends. This information may provide the only clues that will allow you to relate the patient's problems to a scuba dive.

The signs and symptoms of decompression sickness include

- Personality changes
- Fatigue
- Deep pain to the muscles and joints (the "bends")
- Itchy blotches or mottling of the skin
- Numbness or paralysis
- Choking
- Coughing
- Labored breathing
- Behavior similar to intoxication (e.g., staggering)
- Chest pains
- Collapse leading to unconsciousness
- Skin rashes that keep changing in appearance (in some cases)

Note: the well-trained scuba diver wears a preplanned dive chart. The chart may provide you with useful information concerning the nature and duration of the dive. This chart must be transported with the patient.

The Diver Alert Network (DAN) was formed to assist rescuers with the care for underwater diving accident patients. The staff, available on a 24-hour basis, can be reached by phoning (919) 684-8111. Collect calls will be accepted for actual emergencies. DAN can give you or your dispatcher information on assessment and care and how to transfer the patient to a hyperbaric trauma care center (one with a special pressure chamber for treatment of such conditions). For non-emergencies, call (919) 684-2948.

For a patient with signs and symptoms of either air embolism or decompression sickness, follow the same emergency care steps.

1. Maintain an open airway.
2. Administer the highest possible concentration of oxygen by nonrebreather mask.
3. Rapidly transport all patients with possible air emboli or decompression sickness.
4. Contact medical direction for specific instructions concerning where to take the patient. You may be sent directly to a hyperbaric trauma center.
5. Keep the patient warm.
6. The patient should be positioned either supine or on either side (Figure 22-9). Continue to monitor the patient. You may have to reposition the patient to ensure an open airway.

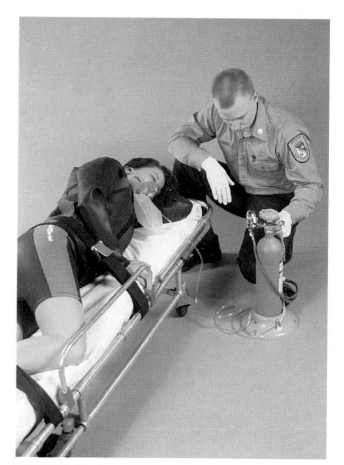

FIGURE 22-9 Position the patient after a scuba diving accident.

Ice Rescues

Every winter many people die who fall through ice while skating or attempting to cross an ice-covered body of water. Often, the ice-related accident scene becomes a multiple-rescue problem as individuals try to reach the victim and also fall through the ice. The number one rule in ice rescue is to protect yourself. Formal ice rescue training is available and needed to assist the EMT-B in making safer ice rescue attempts. A cold-water submersion suit should be worn during any ice rescue attempt.

There are several ways in which you can reach a patient who has fallen through ice.

- Flotation devices can be thrown to the patient.
- A rope in which a loop has been formed can be tossed to the patient. He can put the loop around his body so that he can be pulled onto the ice and away from the danger area.
- A small, flat-bottomed aluminum boat is probably the best device for an ice rescue. It

can be pushed stern (rear end) first by other rescuers and pulled to safety by a rope secured to the bow (front end). The primary rescuer will remain dry and safe should the ice break. The patient can be pulled from the water or allowed to grasp the side of the boat, although he may be unable to grasp or to hold on for long.

- A ladder is an effective tool often used in ice rescue. It can be laid flat and pushed to the patient, then pulled back by an attached rope. The ladder also can serve as a surface on which a rescuer can spread out his weight if he must go onto the ice to reach the patient. The ladder should have a line that can be secured by a rescuer in a safe position. Any rescuer on the ladder should have a safety line.

When attempting to rescue the patient, remember that he may not be able to do much to help in the process. The effects of hypothermia from the cold water may interfere with his mental and physical capabilities in a matter of minutes.

Whenever possible, do not work alone when trying to perform an ice rescue. If you must work alone, do not walk out onto the ice. Never

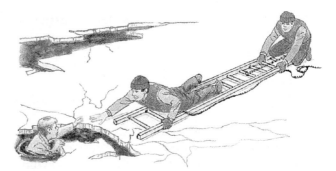

FIGURE 22-10 Safe ice rescue requires team work.

go onto ice that is rapidly breaking. *Never enter the water through a hole in the ice in order to find the victim.* Your best course of action will be to work with others, from a safe ice surface or the shore (Figure 22-10). When there is no other choice, you and your fellow rescuers can elect to form a human chain to reach the patient. However, this is not the safest method to employ, even when all the rescuers are wearing personal flotation devices and using safety lines.

Expect to find injuries to most patients who have fallen through the ice. Treat for hypothermia according to local protocols and treat for any injuries. Transport all patients who have fallen through ice.

CHAPTER REVIEW

KEY TERMS

You may find it helpful to review the following terms.

active rewarming application of an external heat source to rewarm the body of a hypothermic patient. See also *central rewarming.*

air embolism gas bubble in the bloodstream. The plural is *air emboli.* The more accurate term is *arterial gas embolism (AGE).*

central rewarming application of heat to the lateral chest, neck, armpits, and groin of a hypothermic patient. Rewarming of the limbs is avoided to prevent the collection of blood in the extremities and resulting shock.

conduction the direct transfer of heat from one material to another through direct contact.

convection carrying away of heat by currents of air or water or other gases or liquids.

decompression sickness a condition resulting from nitrogen trapped in the body's tissues caused by coming up too quickly from a deep, prolonged dive. A symptom of decompression sickness is "the bends," or deep pain in the muscles and joints.

drowning death caused by changes in the lungs resulting from immersion in water. See also *near-drowning.*

evaporation the change from liquid to gas. When the body perspires or gets wet, evaporation of the perspiration or other liquid into the air has a cooling effect on the body.

hyperthermia (HI-per-THURM-e-ah) an increase in body temperature above normal; life-threatening in its extreme.

hypothermia (HI-po-THURM-e-ah) a generalized cooling that reduces body temperature below normal; life-threatening in its extreme.

local cooling cooling or freezing of particular (local) parts of the body.

near-drowning the condition of having begun to drown. The near-drowning patient may be conscious, unconscious with heartbeat and pulse, or with no heartbeat or pulse but still able to be resuscitated. Only when sufficient time without breathing has passed to render resuscitation useless (sometimes 30 minutes or more if the patient has been in cold water) has drowning truly taken place.

passive rewarming covering a hypothermic patient and taking other steps to prevent further heat loss and help the body rewarm itself.

radiation sending out energy, such as heat, in waves into space.

respiration breathing. During respiration, body heat is lost as warm air is exhaled from the body.

toxins substances produced by animals or plants that are poisonous to humans.

venom a toxin (poison) produced by certain animals such as snakes, spiders, and some marine life forms.

water chill chilling caused by conduction of heat from the body when the body or clothing is wet.

wind chill chilling caused by convection of heat from the body in the presence of air currents.

SUMMARY

Patients suffering from exposure to heat or cold must be removed from the harmful environment as quickly and as safely as possible. Rewarming procedures approved by local protocol should be performed on the cold-exposed patient. Cooling procedures approved by local protocol are necessary for the heat-exposed patient. Immediate resuscitation of the water-related-emergency patient may require quick and persistent intervention. For injection or ingestion of the poisons of insects, spiders, snakes, and marine life, call medical direction and follow local protocol.

REVIEW QUESTIONS

1. Describe when it is appropriate to treat a cold emergency with active rewarming and when you should perform passive rewarming.
2. List five situations in which a patient may be suffering from hypothermia along with another, more obvious medical condition or injury.
3. Name the signs and symptoms of a late or deep localized cold injury.
4. Describe the management of a patient suffering from heat emergency who has moist, pale, and cool skin temperature.
5. Describe the management of a patient suffering from a heat emergency who has hot, dry skin.
6. Describe the proper care for a patient suffering from snakebite.

Application Question

- You are called to respond to an elderly woman who has fallen while walking in the park on a cool fall day. How should you manage assessment and care of this patient?

Behavioral Emergencies

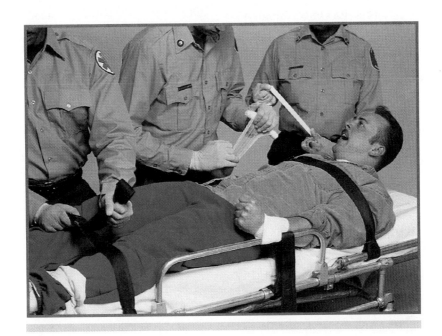

23

As an EMT-Basic you will respond to many emergencies in which the patient is behaving in unexpected and sometimes dangerous ways. The unusual behavior may be the result of stress, physical trauma, or illness, drug and alcohol abuse, or mental illness. Whatever the cause, do not hesitate to request police assistance whenever you feel it is necessary. Local protocol may even require it. Once the scene is secure, you will be able to provide appropriate emergency care.

Objectives

Knowledge and Attitude *At the end of this chapter, you should be able to meet the following objectives.*

1. Define behavioral emergencies. (p. 409)

2. Discuss the general factors that may cause an alteration in a patient's behavior. (pp. 409–410)

3. State the various reasons for psychological crises. (p. 410)

4. Discuss the characteristics of an individual's behavior which suggest that the patient is at risk for suicide. (p. 412)

5. Discuss special medical/legal considerations for managing behavioral emergencies. (p. 415)

6. Discuss the special considerations for assessing a patient with behavioral problems. (pp. 409, 410, 411, 414)

7. Discuss the general principles of an individual's behavior which suggest that he is at risk for violence. (p. 414)

8. Discuss methods to calm behavioral emergency patients. (pp. 409, 410, 411, 416)

9. Explain the rationale for learning how to modify your behavior toward the patient with a behavioral emergency. (pp. 409, 410, 411, 416)

Skills

1. Demonstrate the assessment and emergency medical care of the patient experiencing a behavioral emergency.

2. Demonstrate various techniques to safely restrain a patient with a behavioral problem.

On the Scene

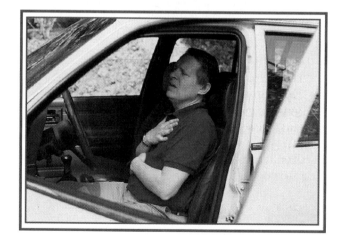

Late one spring afternoon, Ross Ramler runs his car into a tree, and you receive a call to respond to a motor vehicle collision. Dispatch advises you that the police on the scene have requested a patient evaluation for the driver.

When you arrive, pull on disposable gloves, and begin your *scene size-up,* you are met by a uniformed police officer, who says, "I can't figure out what's wrong with the driver. He's conscious, but he won't answer any questions." She assures you that the scene is secure. You observe little if any damage to the vehicle. You approach the patient.

As you begin your *initial assessment,* you have a general impression of a male who appears to be about 40 years old behind the steering wheel, arms across chest, rocking back and forth, and shaking his head from side to side. You see no obvious signs of injury. You calmly introduce yourself and ask what happened. He closes his eyes tightly and begins to cry and shake uncontrollably. "I screwed up. I'm in trouble," he says. Because he is crying and speaking, you believe his airway is adequate. His breathing is deep and within normal limits at approximately 20 per minute. He won't allow you to take his pulse, but you see no signs of bleeding, and his skin is warm, pink, and dry. He is responsive and seems oriented to person, place, and time in spite of his upset emotional state. Your partner explains to Mr. Ramler that he needs to hold his head still because the collision could have injured his spine. Mr. Ramler's response is a pushing-away gesture, and he continues to rock back and forth, making manual immobilization impossible.

"I can see that you're upset," you assure Mr. Ramler. "I'm here to help you if I can. Can you tell me what's wrong?" He shakes his head and continues rocking. You attempt to begin a *focused history and physical exam,* asking OPQRST and SAMPLE questions in a quiet and reassuring tone, but Mr. Ramler refuses to answer. Despite your efforts to calm him, the crying, shaking, and rocking worsen. You are unable to do a physical exam, put a cervical collar on him, or take baseline vital signs.

While uncooperative about being questioned, touched, or examined, Mr. Ramler agrees to be transported to the nearest appropriate facility and does not display any signs of violent behavior that might warrant restraints. En route to the hospital, he continues to cry, shake, and rock and to refuse your requests to do a physical exam. His behavior has not changed since your initial assessment, but you remain alert to the possibility that hostile or aggressive behavior might develop at any time.

You call the receiving facility, identify your unit, and advise them of your estimated time of arrival. You state that you are transporting an approximately 40-year-old male involved in a minor motor vehicle collision who appears to be having a behavioral emergency. You report his current mental status and other essential information. You begin to make notes to document Mr. Ramler's refusal of care, including the names of witnesses: your partner and the police officer at the scene.

Behavioral emergencies can be among the most difficult and stressful that you will handle as an EMT-B. As with Ross Ramler in On the Scene, the patient's behavior often makes it difficult or impossible to do a thorough assessment or perform emergency care. Moreover, the patient's behavior can be erratic and sometimes dangerous to you, himself, or others.

Because of the unpredictable nature of such emergencies, your first priority will always be to ensure your own safety—and then the safety of the patient. Be sure to take all appropriate BSI precautions. Stay calm and help the patient understand that you and other emergency care personnel are trying to help.

RECOGNIZING BEHAVIORAL PROBLEMS

What Is a Behavioral Emergency?

Behavior is defined as the manner in which a person acts. In an emergency, a patient usually behaves in a predictable way. That is, he acts in a way that most other patients have been observed to act under similar circumstances. Based on your training and experience, you will be able to characterize such patients with statements as simple as "the patient is behaving as expected."

A **behavioral emergency** exists when a patient's behavior is not typical for the situation, when the patient's behavior is unacceptable or intolerable to the patient, his family, or the community, or when the patient may harm himself or others. After your initial assessment, check your general impression with family and friends. However, be aware that, while behavioral emergencies may appear to result from a psychological disturbance, they also sometimes result from physical causes. Remember that the following physical conditions may alter a patient's behavior.

- *Low blood sugar,* which may be the cause of rapid onset of erratic or hostile behavior (similar to alcohol intoxication), dizziness and headache, fainting, seizures, sometimes coma, profuse perspiration, hunger, drooling, rapid pulse but normal blood pressure. (See Chapter 19, Diabetes and Altered Mental Status.)
- *Lack of oxygen,* which may cause restlessness and confusion, cyanosis (blue or gray skin), and altered mental status.
- *Inadequate blood to the brain or stroke,* which may cause confusion or dizziness, impaired speech, headache, loss of function or paralysis of extremities on one side of body, nausea and vomiting, and rapid full pulse.
- *Head trauma,* which can cause personality changes ranging from irritability to

irrational behavior, altered mental status, amnesia or confusion, irregular respirations, elevated blood pressure, and decreasing pulse.

- *Mind altering substances,* which may cause highly variable signs and symptoms depending on the substance ingested. (See Chapter 21, Poisoning and Overdose Emergencies)
- *Excessive cold,* which may cause shivering, feelings of numbness, altered mental status, drowsiness, staggering walk, slow breathing, and slow pulse.
- *Excessive heat,* which may cause decreased or complete loss of consciousness. (See Chapter 22, Environmental Emergencies.)

Behavioral emergencies can, of course, be due to psychological causes such as extremes of emotion that may lead to violence or other inappropriate actions. They may also be due to psychiatric problems that result in bizarre thinking and behavior, depression, panic, or agitation. Emergencies involving emotional, psychiatric, suicidal, and aggressive or hostile patients are common types of behavioral or psychological emergencies.

Emotional Emergencies

Emotional emergencies, like all behavioral emergencies, are unpredictable. Be alert for the patient's sudden and unexpected mood changes, which sometimes can signal more aggressive behavior to come. In Ross Ramler's case there was no aggressive activity, yet the potential was always there. Maintain a heightened level of awareness for this possibility. Your job is to try to prevent a behavioral emergency from growing into an unmanageable behavioral crisis.

Patient Assessment—Emotional Emergency

Include in your assessment of mental status the patient's appearance, level of physical activity, speech, and orientation for time, person, and place.

Signs

In an emotional emergency, the patient may

☐ Display emotions beyond what is expected or typical to a point where they interfere with thoughts and behavior.

☐ Seem far more frightened than most patients in a similar situation.

☐ Be unable to calm the excited state after an accident and not calm down during the interview or the beginning of care procedures.

☐ Be unable to respond to people or remain within some bounds of behavioral control.

☐ Show indications of being dangerous to himself or others.

Also, during assessment and care, remember to identify yourself and let the patient know you are there to help. Inform him of what you are doing and ask questions in a calm, reassuring voice. Give the patient a chance to tell you his story without being judgmental. Acknowledge the patient's feelings, and show you are listening by rephrasing or repeating part of what the patient tells you.

Psychiatric Emergencies

On the Scene

One Saturday afternoon you and your partner receive a call to respond to a college football game. You're told there is a 20 year-old-male "acting strange." When you arrive, you put on your disposable gloves. *Scene size-up* reveals one young man screaming at the crowd, which is keeping its distance. Security personnel have isolated and surrounded the patient. Bystanders tell you his name is Jet Nelson.

Your *initial assessment* shows no signs of obvious injury, and your general impression is that Jet is having an emotional or psychiatric emergency. As you slowly approach, he throws himself down and repeatedly bangs his head on the bleacher. Security personnel immediately grab his arms and legs. He begins to cry but offers no resistance.

As you perform a *focused history and physical exam,* Jet tells you he has failed his final exams "because of electrical interference." He talks more and more excitedly as he explains how electrical impulses from transformers near the campus have been interfering with his thoughts and his ability to concentrate on his studies. Your rapid assessment determines tenderness to Jet's forehead where he was banging it on the bleacher. There is no bleeding and no other injuries. His blood pressure is 142/88, pulse 140, respirations 26, and skin is warm, pink, and dry. You decide it's best to get him away from the crowd. You discreetly ask security personnel to accompany you.

Jet agrees to go to the hospital. In transit he permits a **detailed physical exam** but does not answer any more questions. Instead he falls silent and becomes extremely still, staring at a spot on the opposite wall of the ambulance. Your partner calls in the patient's condition, reporting that you are 10 minutes away with an initially "agitated" but now withdrawn 20-year-old male patient who has inflicted some harm to himself (the head-banging) and who appears to be having some kind of psychiatric emergency. Throughout transport you perform **ongoing assessment** of Jet's mental and physical status.

The patient in a psychiatric emergency is far more out of control than the person in an emotional emergency. The patient may have a mental illness, or existing personality problems can worsen through drug use or, in some cases, because of medical illness. Since you are not a doctor or a psychiatrist, you cannot diagnose the patient's mental problem. You only need to rule out a typical stress reaction (which you can help by being calm and reassuring) or an illness or injury (for which you can provide emergency treatment).

When you describe the patient to hospital personnel or in documentation, use descriptive terms such as *excited, fearful, confused, overactive, unpredictable, agitated, aggressive,* and *detached.* Avoid diagnostic terms such as *mentally ill, psychotic, phobic, paranoid, manic, neurotic,* and *schizophrenic.* By all means avoid such terms as *crazy, nuts, wacko, loony,* and other nonprofessional terms.

✋ **Safety Note**

Do not leave a patient who seems to be having an emotional or psychiatric problem alone. Be alert to aggressive or potentially violent behavior, and protect yourself from harm at all times.

Patient Assessment—Psychiatric Emergency

Signs

In a psychiatric emergency, the patient may

☐ Try to hurt himself or others.
☐ Withdraw, no longer responding to people or the environment.
☐ Continue to express rage and hostility.
☐ Continue to cry and express feelings of worthlessness.
☐ Take no action to regain calm.
☐ Allow no one to help.

During assessment, you can help calm the patient by acknowledging that there is a problem. Remind the patient that you are there to help. You may find that it is best to avoid unnecessary physical contact, maintaining a comfortable distance. Encourage the patient to tell you about his troubles, and respond honestly to the patient's questions. Do not "play along" with visual or auditory disturbances the patient might describe. Involve trusted family members or friends to help calm the patient, and be prepared to stay at the scene for a long time.

Potential or Attempted Suicide

On the Scene

You are greeted by the owner at the door of a tavern to which you have been dispatched. The owner thanks you for responding so quickly. He tells you: "I want to close up, but she won't leave." The 30-year-old female who won't leave is Denise Ashley. You have already donned disposable gloves, you **size up the scene,** and decide it is safe to enter. Ms. Ashley is sitting on a bar stool crying. Her head is face down on the counter.

Your **initial assessment** reveals no signs of injury, but you check for evidence of broken glass or sharp objects such as knives or forks. Speaking slowly and calmly, you identify yourself. The patient is crying loudly, so you know her airway is open. Her breathing is adequate, and you see no signs of external bleeding. You ask her what's wrong, but she doesn't answer. You attempt to check her pulse, but she pulls away and tells you to leave her alone. Based on the information you've collected in just a few seconds, you believe there are no immediately life-threatening problems.

You try a **focused history and physical exam.** She refuses to answer any questions. The bartender approaches and tells you she has been upset about her recent divorce and "talking about killing herself." He cannot help you further. At this point, Ms. Ashley allows you to take her vitals—blood pressure 148/88, pulse 144, respirations 24. However, she does not permit you to do a physical exam. You decide the patient should be transported for further evaluation and follow-up. Finally, Ms. Ashley reluctantly agrees to go to the hospital.

You do **ongoing assessment,** continuing to observe her carefully during transit and deciding to remain quiet and let the patient talk if she wishes. Your partner calls in the patient's condition.

Each year in this country, thousands of people commit suicide. Many more suffer both physical and emotional injuries in suicide attempts. Anyone may become suicidal if emotional distress is severe, regardless of gender, age, or ethnic, social, or economic background.

People attempt suicide for many reasons, including depression caused by chemical imbalance, the death of a loved one, financial problems, the end to a love affair, poor health, loss of esteem, divorce, fears of failure, and alcohol and drug abuse. People attempt to end their lives by any one of a variety of methods, often by drug overdose. Less common methods of suicide include hanging, jumping from high places, ingesting poisons, inhaling gas, wrist-cutting, self-mutilation, stabbing, or shooting.

Safety Note

Whenever you are called to care for a patient who has attempted or is about to attempt suicide, *your first concern must be your own safety.*

Patient Assessment—Potential or Attempted Suicide

The following factors can help you assess the patient's risk for suicide.

- [ ] *Threats of suicide,* including discussion about methods of suicide and the actual gathering of potentially dangerous articles (such as pills or weapons).
- [ ] *Depression.* Take seriously a patient's feelings and expressions of despair or suicidal thoughts.
- [ ] *High current or recent stress levels.* If so, take the threat of suicide seriously. Transport the patient.
- [ ] *Previous attempts or suicide threats.* History of self-destructive behavior.
- [ ] *Recent emotional trauma,* such as job loss, loss of a significant relationship, serious illness, arrest, imprisonment.
- [ ] *Age.* High suicide rates occur at ages 15–25 and over age 40.
- [ ] *Alcohol and drug abuse.*

Patient Care—Emotional, Psychiatric, and Potential or Attempted Suicide Emergencies

Patients who are in an emotional, psychiatric, or attempted suicide emergency are cared for in similar ways. In all cases, your personal interaction is key. Try to establish visual and verbal contact with the patient as soon as possible. Avoid arguing. Make no threats, and show no indication of using force.

Remember that you are the first professional to begin both the physical and mental health care of the patient. The more reassurance you can provide for the patient, the easier it will be for the hospital emergency department staff to continue care.

Emergency Care Steps

1. Treatment must begin with scene size-up. Make sure it is safe to approach the patient. If the scene is not safe, request assistance from the police and wait until they have secured the scene. Do not leave the patient alone unless you are at risk of physical harm. Try to talk with the patient from a safe distance until the police arrive. Practice BSI precautions.
2. When the scene is secure, look for and treat life-threatening problems to the extent that the patient will permit it. Seek police assistance in restraining the patient if necessary for care of life-threatening problems.
3. As possible, perform a focused history and physical exam and provide emergency care. Be sure to consider the possibility of head injury, stroke, low blood sugar, drug reactions, high fever, and other such medical emergencies as the cause of the patient's behavior.
4. Perform a detailed physical exam only if it is safe and you suspect the patient may have an injury.
5. Perform on-going assessment. Watch for sudden changes in the patient's behavior and physical condition.
6. Contact the receiving hospital and report on current mental status and other essential information.

Note that a physical exam may be difficult with the emotional or psychiatric patient. You may not be able to proceed beyond the initial assessment phase.

Throughout your interaction with the patient, speak slowly—and patiently await answers to your questions. As you gain the patient's confidence, explain what questions must be answered and what must be done as part of the physical exam and vital sign assessment. Let the patient know that you think it would be best if he goes to the hospital and that you need his cooperation and help. Back off if necessary. If the patient's fear or aggression increases, do not push the issues of the examination or transport. Instead, try to re-establish the conversation and give the patient more time before you again say that going to the hospital is a good idea.

Transport all suicidal patients. Seek police assistance if necessary. Report any attempted suicide or expression of suicidal thoughts to the medical facility, police, or government agency designated by your state law and local protocols.

Aggressive or Hostile Behavior

On the Scene

It's rodeo season, and a certain number of calls to respond to injuries at the arena are predictable—but this call is different. Upon arrival at the scene you and your partner put on your protective eye wear and disposable gloves. **Scene size-up** reveals that it is safe to approach the patient, Reed Jefferson. He is leaning against a fence post, and as you walk toward him, you notice blood over his right eye. The dispatcher has told you he was kicked by a horse.

You introduce yourself. Mr. Jefferson looks at you and says, "What do you want?" You explain who you are and that you were called to help. You begin your **initial assessment** and ask a few questions to determine the patient's mental status. "What do you want?" he keeps repeating. His responses are inappropriate, and he appears increasingly agitated and hostile. Your partner calls for the police. You both back away and wait.

When the police arrive, you attempt a **focused history and physical exam.** Mr. Jefferson yells and begins pacing. You back away so he does not feel trapped. All you can find out from Mr. Jefferson's friends is that he did eat lunch and he began acting in this way only after being kicked.

You consult medical direction. Based on the mechanism of injury and altered mental status, the medical director believes Mr. Jefferson may have a life-threatening injury and requests you to transport as soon as possible. Since Mr. Jefferson continues to be uncooperative and hostile, the police decide to put him under protective custody. As a last resort, your local protocols allow you and the police to restrain and transport Mr. Jefferson. Once he is restrained, you are able to get a cervical collar on him, because the mechanism of injury indicates possible spinal injury, but his thrashing and hostile behavior prevent a physical exam or vital sign assessment.

So the hospital is properly prepared, you advise them of your estimated time of arrival and Mr. Jefferson's current mental status. Later you document the incident and include in the report the names of law enforcement officers at the scene and in the ambulance.

Aggressive or disruptive behavior may be caused by trauma to the brain and nervous system, metabolic disorders, stress, alcohol and other drugs, or psychological disorders. Sometimes you will know that your patient is aggressive from the information you receive from dispatch. Other times the scene may provide quick clues (e.g., drugs, yelling, unclean conditions, broken furniture). Neighbors, family members, or bystanders may tell you that the patient is dangerous or angry or has a history of aggression or combativeness. The patient's stance (tense muscles, fists clenched, or quick irregular movements, for example) or position in the room may give you an early warning of possible violence. On rare occasions, you may start with an apparently calm patient who suddenly turns aggressive.

Safety Note

When a patient acts as if he may hurt himself or others, *your first concern must be your own safety.* Take the following precautions.

- *Do not isolate yourself from your partner or other sources of help.* Make certain that you have an escape route. Do not let the patient come between you and the door. Should a patient become violent, retreat and wait for police assistance.
- *Do not take any action that may be considered threatening by the patient.* To do so may bring about hostile behavior directed against you or others.
- *Always be on the watch for weapons.* Stay out of kitchens. They are filled with dangerous weapons. Stay in a safe area until the police can control the scene.
- *Be alert for sudden changes in the patient's behavior.*

Patient Assessment—Aggressive or Hostile Patient

Your assessment of the aggressive or hostile patient may never go beyond the initial assessment phase. Most of your time may be spent trying to calm these patients and ensuring everyone's safety. An aggressive or hostile patient

- ☐ Responds to people inappropriately
- ☐ Tries to hurt himself or others
- ☐ May have a rapid pulse and breathing
- ☐ Usually displays rapid speech and rapid physical movements
- ☐ May appear anxious, nervous, "panicky"

Patient Care—Aggressive or Hostile Patient

Emergency Care Steps

1. Treatment begins with scene size-up. Make sure it is safe to approach the patient. Request assistance from law enforcement, if necessary. Practice BSI precautions.
2. Seek advice from medical direction if the patient's behavior prevents normal assessment and care procedures.
3. As part of ongoing assessment, watch for sudden changes in the patient's behavior.
4. Seek assistance from law enforcement, as well as from medical direction, if restraint seems necessary.
5. Contact the receiving hospital and report on current mental status and other important information.

GENERAL PRINCIPLES OF CARE FOR BEHAVIORAL EMERGENCIES

Avoiding Unreasonable Force

Reasonable force is the force necessary to keep a patient from injuring himself or others. Reasonableness is determined by looking at all circumstances involved, including the patient's strength and size, type of abnormal behavior, mental status, and available methods of restraint. Understand that you may protect yourself from attack, but otherwise you must avoid actions that can cause injury to the patient.

In addition, in most localities an EMT-B cannot legally restrain a patient, move a patient against his or her will, or force a patient to accept emergency care—even at the family's request. The restraint and forcible moving of patients is within the jurisdiction of law enforcement. The police (and in some areas a physician) can order you to restrain and transport a patient to the appropriate medical facility. However, the physician is not empowered to order you to take action that could place you in danger. If police order restraint and transport, they must assist with these procedures as necessary. Remember to follow local protocol.

Never try to assist in restraining a patient unless there are sufficient personnel to do the job. You must be able to ensure your safety and the safety of the patient. If you help the police or a physician to restrain a patient, make certain that the restraints are humane. Handcuffs and plastic "throwaway" criminal restraints should not be used because of the soft-tissue damage they can inflict. Initially, the police may have to use such restraints. However, in some states they can be replaced with soft restraints such as leather cuffs and belts. If authorized in your state and by local protocol, an ambulance should carry leather cuffs, a waist-size belt, and at least three short belts. Restraints for the wrists and ankles can be made from gauze roller bandages (Figure 23-1.).

Do not remove police restraints until you and the police are certain that soft restraints will hold the patient. To ensure everyone's safety, once they are on remember not to remove soft restraints, even if the patient appears to be acting rationally.

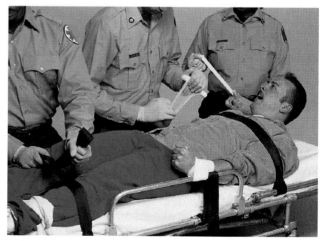

FIGURE 23-1 Gauze bandages may be used as soft restraints.

Follow these guidelines when a patient must be restrained.

- Be sure to have adequate help.
- Plan your activities.
- Estimate the range of motion of the patient's arms and legs and stay beyond range until ready.
- Once the decision to restrain the patient has been reached, act quickly.
- Have one EMT-B talk to and reassure the patient throughout the restraining procedure.
- Approach with four persons, one assigned to each limb, all to act at the same time.
- Secure all four limbs with restraints approved by medical direction.
- Position the patient face up or face down. The position will be dictated by what the restraining process itself permits, the patient's condition (e.g., injuries, breathing problems), and local protocols. Monitor the patient's airway.
- Use multiple straps or other restraints to ensure that the patient is adequately secured. Anticipate that the patient's behavior may turn more violent and be sure that restraint is adequate for this possibility.
- If the patient is spitting on rescuers, place a surgical mask on the patient if he has no breathing difficulty or likelihood of vomiting and if local protocols permit, or have rescuers wear protective masks, eye wear, and clothing.
- Reassess the patient's distal circulation frequently and adjust restraints as safe and necessary if distal circulation is diminished.
- Document the reasons why the patient was restrained and the technique of restraint.
- Use sufficient force, but avoid unnecessary force.

Medical/Legal Considerations

As you have seen in the On the Scenes throughout this chapter, Ross Ramler, Jet Nelson, Denise Ashley, and Reed Jefferson were all reluctant patients. Behavioral emergency patients will frequently resist care and transportation. Your responsibility as an EMT-B is to convince those patients of the need for care. Medical/legal problems are greatly reduced if you can.

A patient who refuses emergency care or transport is a significant medical/legal risk for EMS services and EMT-Bs. You were able to calmly convince Mr. Ramler, Ms. Ashley, and Mr. Nelson of the need for treatment. However, Mr. Jefferson refused treatment and transportation. What should you do when a patient refuses or resists your efforts to provide care?

If, in your judgment, a patient is a threat to himself or others, he may be transported without consent after you contact medical direction. Again know your state laws on treating patients without consent. During these situations you should contact law enforcement and, if necessary and available, community mental health personnel.

When a minor (usually under 18 years of age—check your state laws) refuses treatment or transportation and no consenting adult is present, you should contact law enforcement. If you believe the minor is suffering a life-threatening condition and he refuses treatment, generally it is better to err on the side of treatment than to abandon a patient. Know your state laws and local protocol regarding care, treatment, and transportation of minors.

Emotionally disturbed patients commonly accuse EMT-Bs of sexual misconduct. If possible, EMT-Bs of the same sex as the patient should attend to emergency care. For the aggressive or violent patient, make sure law enforcement officers accompany you to the hospital to protect you and the patient. In the event of a legal problem, they can serve as third party witnesses.

For more information on this topic, see Chapter 3, Medical/Legal and Ethical Issues.

Transport to Appropriate Facility

Your medical protocols or procedures should direct you to the most appropriate medical facility within your community. Not all hospitals are prepared to treat behavioral emergencies.

Documentation Tips—Behavioral Emergencies

Document your actions in your prehospital care report. It is important to include your impressions (e.g., "patient acted in unusual manner," "patient tried to hurt himself"). Include statements that document your belief that the patient might have harmed himself or others had you not provided care. If you suspect use of alcohol or other drugs by the patient, then this too should be documented. Finally, document behavioral emergencies that may be caused by injury or illness.

Note:

Be sure to include in your report the names of law enforcement or other witnesses.

Situational Stress Reactions

Most patients will display emotions such as fear, grief, and anger. These are typical stress reactions at the accident scene and common reactions to serious illness and death. In the vast majority of cases, as you begin to take control of the situation and treat the patient as an individual, personal interaction will inspire confidence in your ability to help. The patient will begin to calm down and may even begin to feel able to cope with the emergency.

Be as unhurried as you can. If you rush the survey and interview, the patient may feel as if the situation is out of control. The patient also may believe that you are concerned about the problem and not about him. Let the patient know that you are there to help. Whenever you care for a patient who is displaying typical stress reactions

- Act in a calm manner, giving the patient time to gain control of emotions.
- Quietly and carefully evaluate the situation.
- Keep your own emotions under control.
- Honestly explain things to the patient.
- Let the patient know that you are listening to what he is saying.
- Stay alert for sudden changes in behavior.

In so doing, you are applying crisis management techniques to help the patient deal with stress. If the patient does not begin to interact with you or calm down, you must assume that there is a problem of a more serious nature, such as an emotional or psychiatric problem, and proceed according to the recommendations for appropriate emergency care procedures that have been described in this chapter.

CHAPTER REVIEW

KEY TERMS

You may find it helpful to review the following terms.

behavior   the manner in which a person acts.

behavioral emergency   when a patient's behavior is not typical for the situation; when the patient's behavior is unacceptable or intolerable to the patient, his family, or the community, or when the patient may harm himself or others.

SUMMARY

As an EMT-Basic you will respond to many behavioral emergencies. Because the treatment for these patients usually requires long-term management, little medical intervention can be done in the acute situation. However, how you interact with the patient during the emergency can make a difference—to the patient and to the medical professionals who take over. On these calls remember that you must assure your own safety, consider the legal ramifications of your actions, and transport the patient in a safe and effective manner to an appropriate facility. Know your local protocols.

1. Name several conditions that can alter a person's mental status and behavior.
2. Describe the signs and symptoms of an emotional or psychiatric emergency.
3. Describe what you can do when scene-size up reveals that it is too dangerous to approach the patient.
4. List several factors that can help you assess the patient's risk for suicide.
5. Research your state law. Then describe the circumstances that must exist for you to treat and transport a minor without consent.
6. List several methods that can help calm the psychiatric emergency patient.

Application

- You are called to respond to an intoxicated minor who is physically aggressive, threatens suicide, and whose parents permit you to treat but not transport. How would you manage this patient?

Obstetrics and Gynecology

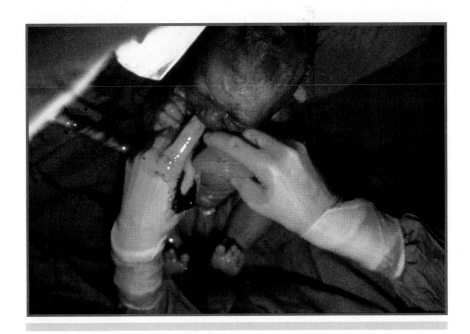

24

Childbirth is a natural process that existed long before there were EMTs. Depending on the area in which you work as an EMT-Basic you may, during your career, be called upon to assist with an out-of-hospital delivery. One of your main responsibilities in this situation will be to help calm the patient and family members through your unruffled professional manner. However, because childbirth is not a common occurrence in the prehospital setting, it might be easy to get flustered and seem uncertain about the procedures you are performing. So it is important that you learn about childbirth and practice the procedures required to assist with delivery, so that if you are ever called upon to assist in a delivery, your skills will contribute to decreased stress and better care of the mother and baby.

Knowledge and Attitude *At the end of this chapter, you should be able to meet the following objectives.*

1. Identify the following structures: uterus, vagina, fetus, placenta, umbilical cord, amniotic sac, perineum. (pp. 422, 434)

2. Identify and explain the use of the contents of an obstetrics kit. (pp. 424–425)

3. Identify predelivery emergencies. (pp. 438–441)

4. State indications of an imminent delivery. (pp. 423–424, 425–426)

5. Differentiate the emergency medical care provided to a patient with predelivery emergencies from a normal delivery. (pp. 438–441)

6. State the steps in the predelivery preparation of the mother. (pp. 426–427)

7. Establish the relationship between body substance isolation and childbirth. (p. 426)

8. State the steps to assist in the delivery. (pp. 427–430)

9. Describe care of the baby as the head appears. (pp. 428–429)

10. Describe how and when to cut the umbilical cord. (pp. 432–433)

11. Discuss the steps in the delivery of the placenta. (pp. 433–434)

12. List the steps in the emergency medical care of the mother post-delivery. (pp. 433–435)

13. Summarize neonatal resuscitation procedures. (pp. 430–432)

14. Describe the procedures for the following abnormal deliveries: breech birth, prolapsed cord, limb presentation. (pp. 435–437)

On the Scene

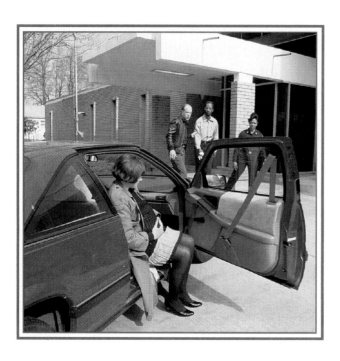

Thirty-three-year-old Deborah Kaczmarek and her husband screech their car to a halt on the fire station ramp. Ed jumps out and explains to the nearest firefighter that Deborah is five days overdue. Her water has broken, and her contractions are very close together. She is sure the baby is going to be born before they can get to the hospital.

You are summoned to the ramp because you are the only EMT-B in the station. You *size up the scene* as you approach the car to begin your *initial assessment.* You immediately form a general impression of a young pregnant woman in the midst of a strong contraction.

You: (Moving to her side and taking hold of her hand) Hello. My name is Bob Holcomb. I'm a firefighter-EMT. What's your name?

Deborah: (Comforted by your touch, but still very anxious.) My name is Deborah Kaczmarek. This baby is coming real soon.

You: OK, Mrs. Kaczmarek. If it does, we'll be ready. (Quickly you start to get the patient's *history.*) Is this your first child?

15. Differentiate the special considerations for multiple births. (p. 437)

16. Describe special considerations of meconium. (pp. 423–424, 429, 438)

17. Describe the special considerations of a premature baby. (pp. 437–438)

18. Discuss the emergency medical care of a patient with a gynecological emergency. (pp. 442–443)

19. Explain the rationale for understanding the implications of treating two patients (mother and baby). (pp. 433–435, 440–441)

Skills

1. Demonstrate the steps to assist in the normal cephalic delivery.

2. Demonstrate necessary care procedures of the fetus as the head appears.

3. Demonstrate infant neonatal procedures.

4. Demonstrate post-delivery care of the infant.

5. Demonstrate how and when to cut the umbilical cord.

6. Attend to the steps in the delivery of the placenta.

7. Demonstrate the post-delivery care of the mother.

8. Demonstrate the procedures for the following abnormal deliveries: vaginal bleeding, breech birth, prolapsed cord, limb presentation.

9. Demonstrate the steps in the emergency medical care of the mother with excessive bleeding.

10. Demonstrate completing a prehospital care report for patients with obstetrical/gynecological emergencies.

Deborah: No. It's going to be my fourth.
You: How far apart are your contractions?
Deborah: About two minutes.

Noting that her contraction is now past, you instruct two of your fellow firefighters to move your patient to a couch in the station and instruct a third firefighter to call the dispatch center to send an ambulance to the station. You grab the obstetrical kit out of the rescue truck's jump kit on your way through the station's bay.

You arrive in the day room and note the firefighters have placed Deborah on the couch and are erecting some screening for privacy as you prepare to begin a *focused physical exam* and check of vital signs. "Mrs. Kaczmarek, I'm going to check to see if the baby might be already pushing out of the birth canal." You put on your gloves, glasses, mask, and gown and prepare to position and drape the patient. When you check the vaginal area, you note that the baby's head is crowning at the vagina. The delivery of Deborah and Ed Kaczmarek's baby girl does not wait for the ambulance to arrive or a trip to the hospital!

B irth is a natural process. The anatomy of the human female and the anatomy of the baby allow for the process to occur with few immediate problems. Nonetheless, EMT-Basics need to know the procedures that can help mother and baby before, during, and after delivery, as well as the techniques that can be employed when complications arise.

THE ANATOMY AND PHYSIOLOGY OF CHILDBIRTH

Pregnancy and Delivery

The developing baby is called a **fetus** (FE-tus). During pregnancy, the fetus grows in its mother's **uterus** (U-ter-us), a muscular organ also called the *womb* (Figure 24-1). When the mother is in labor, the muscles of the uterus contract at ever-shortening intervals and push the baby through the neck of the uterus, known as the **cervix** (SUR-viks). The cervix must dilate some 4 inches during labor to allow the baby's head to pass into the **vagina** (vah-JI-nah), or birth canal, so that delivery can take place.

More than just the fetus develops within the uterus during pregnancy. Attached to the wall of the uterus is a special organ called the **placenta** (plah-SEN-tah). Composed of both maternal and fetal tissues, the placenta serves as an exchange area between mother and fetus. Oxygen and nutrients (and drugs and alcohol) from the mother's bloodstream are carried across the placenta to the fetus. Carbon dioxide and certain other wastes cross from fetal circulation to maternal circulation. Since the placenta is an organ of pregnancy, it is expelled after the baby is born.

The mother's blood does not flow through the body of the fetus. The fetus has its own circulatory system. Blood from the fetus is sent through blood vessels in the **umbilical** (um-BIL-i-kal) **cord** to the placenta where the blood picks up nourishment from the mother, then returns through the umbilical cord to the fetus's body. The umbilical cord, about 1 inch wide and 22 inches long at birth, is fully expelled with the birth of the baby and the delivery of the placenta.

While developing in the uterus, the fetus is enclosed and protected within a thin, membranous "bag of waters" known as the **amniotic** (am-ne-OT-ik) **sac.** This sac contains 1 to 2 quarts of liquid, called amniotic fluid, which allows the fetus to float during development, cushions it from minor injury, and helps maintain a constant fetal body temperature. In the vast majority of cases, the amniotic sac breaks during labor and the fluid gushes from the birth canal. This is a normal condition of childbirth that also provides a natural lubrication to ease the infant's progress through the birth canal.

The nine months of pregnancy are divided into three three-month trimesters. During the first trimester the fetus is being formed. As the fetus remains quite small, there is little uterine growth during this period. After the third month, the uterus grows rapidly, reaching the umbilicus (navel) by the fifth month and the epigastrium (upper abdomen) by the seventh month. Other changes in a woman's body during this time include increased blood volume, increased cardiac output, and increased heart rate. The blood

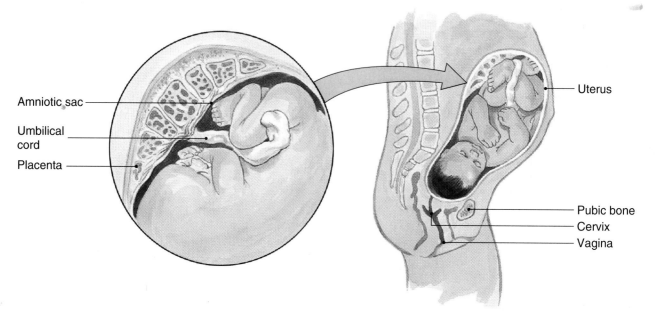

Amniotic sac

Umbilical cord

Placenta

Uterus

Pubic bone

Cervix

Vagina

FIGURE 24-1 The structures of pregnancy.

pressure is usually decreased slightly, and there is slowed digestion. One very important change is a massive increase in vascularity (presence of blood and blood vessels) of the uterus and related structures.

Crowning occurs when the presenting part of the baby first bulges from the vaginal opening. The presenting part is defined as the part of the infant that is first to appear at the vaginal opening during labor. Usually, the presenting part of the baby is the head. The normal head-first birth is called a **cephalic** (se-FAL-ik) **presentation.** If the buttocks or both feet of the baby deliver first, the birth is called a **breech presentation** or breech birth.

Labor

Labor is the entire process of delivery. There are three stages of labor (Figure 24-2).

- First Stage—starts with regular contractions and the thinning and gradual dilation of the cervix and ends when the cervix is fully dilated.
- Second Stage—the time from when the baby enters the birth canal until it is born.
- Third Stage—begins when the baby is born until the **afterbirth** (placenta, umbilical cord, and some tissues from the amniotic sac and the lining of the uterus) is delivered.

The first stage of labor is also called the dilation period. Picture the uterus as a long-neck bottle. In order to expel the contents, the neck of the bottle must be stretched to the size of a wide-mouth jar. Before the cervix can fully dilate, the long neck of the cervix must be shortened and thinned (this process is called effacement) to the wide-mouth-jar shape.

Sometimes several days before the onset of actual labor, uterine muscles begin mild contractions and slight dilation occurs as the cervix begins to thin. When actual labor begins, the contractions of the uterus that occur during the first stage continue the thinning and dilation process, and the infant's head begins to move downward. The cervix gradually shortens and thins enough (wide-mouth-jar shape) to become flush with the vagina or fully open to the birth canal.

The cycle of contractions starts far apart and becomes shorter as birth approaches. Typically, these contractions range from every 30

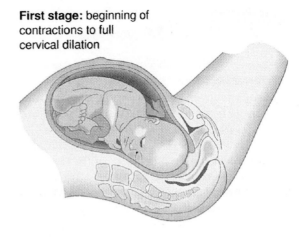

First stage: beginning of contractions to full cervical dilation

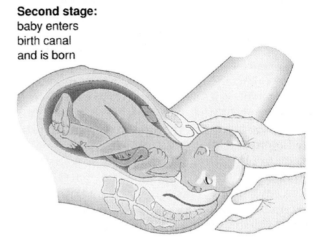

Second stage: baby enters birth canal and is born

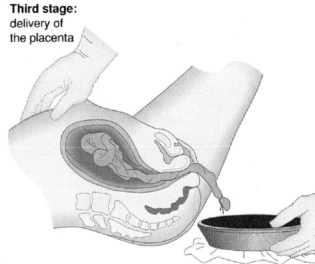

Third stage: delivery of the placenta

FIGURE 24-2 The three stages of labor.

minutes down to 3 minutes apart, or less. Labor pains accompany the contractions.

As the fetus moves downward and the cervix dilates, the amniotic sac usually breaks. Normally, the amniotic fluid is clear. Fluid that is greenish or brownish-yellow in color may be an indication of maternal or fetal distress during labor and is called **meconium staining.** The full dilation of the cervix signals the end of the first stage of labor. Women giving birth for the first time will remain in this first stage for an average of 16 hours. However, some women may remain in this stage for no more than 4 hours, especially if this is not the first child.

There may be a watery, bloody discharge of mucus (not bleeding) associated with the first stage of labor. Part of this initial discharge will be from a mucus plug that was in the cervix. This is usually mixed with blood and is called the "bloody show." It is not necessary to wipe it away. Watery, bloody fluids discharging from the vagina are typical for all three stages of labor.

The second stage of labor begins after the full dilation of the cervix. During this time, contractions become increasingly frequent. Labor pains will become more severe. In the second stage of labor, the cramping and abdominal pains associated with the first stage of labor still may be present, but most women report a major new discomfort, that of feeling they have to move their bowels. This is caused as the baby's body moves and places pressure on the rectum. The moment of birth is nearing, and the EMT-B will have to decide whether to transport or to keep the mother where she is and prepare to assist with delivery.

Labor Pains

The contractions of the uterus produce normal labor pains. Most women report the start of labor pains as an ache in the lower back. As labor progresses, the pain becomes most noticeable in the lower abdomen, with the intensity of pain increasing. The pains come at regular intervals, lasting from 30 seconds to one minute and occur at 2-to-3 minute intervals. When the uterus starts to contract, the pain begins. As the muscles relax, there is relief from the pain. Labor pains may start, stop for a while, then start up again.

As an EMT-B you should time the following characteristics of labor pains.

- Contraction Time, or Duration—the time from the beginning of contraction to when the uterus relaxes (start to end).
- Contraction Interval, or Frequency—the time from the start of one contraction to the beginning of the next (start to start).

When contractions last 30 seconds to one minute and are 2 to 3 minutes apart, delivery of the baby may be imminent.

NORMAL CHILDBIRTH

The Role of the EMT-B

Remember: EMT-Bs do not deliver babies . . . mothers do! Your primary roles will be determining whether the delivery will occur on the scene and, if so, one of helping and *assisting* the mother as she delivers her child.

Equipment and Supplies

Assisting the mother and providing care is much easier if a few basic items are kept as part of the ambulance supplies. You will need a sterile obstetric kit that contains the items required for preparation of the mother, delivery, and initial care of the newborn (Figure 24-3). This kit should include

- Several pairs of sterile surgical gloves to protect from infection
- Towels or sheets for draping the mother
- 1 dozen 2 × 10 (or 4 × 4) gauze pads (sponges) for wiping and drying the baby
- 1 rubber-bulb syringe (3 oz.) to suction the baby's mouth and nostrils
- Cord clamps or hemostats to clamp the umbilical cord (plus extra clamps in case of a multiple birth)
- Umbilical cord tape to tie the cord
- 1 pair of surgical scissors to cut the cord

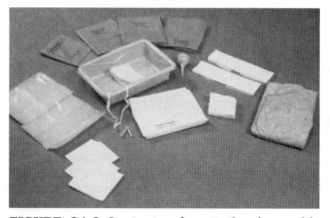

FIGURE 24-3 Contents of a sterile, disposable obstetric kit.

- 1 baby blanket to wrap the baby and keep it warm
- Several individually wrapped sanitary napkins to absorb blood and other fluids
- Plastic bag.

Occasionally, in an off-duty situation, you may need to assist in the delivery of a baby without using a sterile delivery pack. A few simple supplies can be used to assist the mother.

- Clean sheets and towels to drape the mother and wrap the newborn
- Heavy flat twine or new shoelaces to tie the cord (do not use thread, wire, or light string since these may cut through the cord)
- A towel or plastic bag to wrap the placenta after its delivery
- Clean, unused rubber gloves and eye wear. The lack of gloves and eye wear will mean possible exposure to infectious diseases.

The Normal Delivery

Evaluating the Mother

A simple series of questions, an examination for crowning, and determination of vital signs will allow you to make the decision for transport. However, do not let the "urgency" of this decision upset the mother. Your patient needs emotional support at this time. Your calm, professional actions will help her feel more at ease and assure her that the required care will be provided for both her and the unborn child.

Remember: It is best to transport an expecting mother unless, based on your evaluation, you expect delivery within a few minutes.

To begin to evaluate the mother

1. Ask her name and age and expected due date.
2. Ask if this is her first pregnancy. The average time of labor for a woman having her first baby is about 16 to 17 hours. The time in labor is considerably shorter for each subsequent birth.
3. Ask her how long she has been having labor pains, how often she is having pains, and if her "bag of waters" has broken. Ask "Have you had any bleeding or bloody show?" At

this point, with a woman having her first delivery, you may think that you can make a decision about transport. However, you should continue with the evaluation procedure. Also, you should begin to time the frequency and length of the contractions.

4. Ask her if she is straining or if she feels as though she needs to move her bowels. If she says yes, this usually means that the baby has moved into the birth canal and is pressing the vaginal wall against the rectum. Birth will probably occur very soon. The mother may tell you that she can feel the baby trying to move out through her vaginal opening. In such cases, birth is probably very near.
5. Examine the mother for crowning (Figure 24-4). This is a visual inspection to see if there is bulging at the vaginal opening or if the presenting part of the baby is visible. If part of the baby's head or presenting part is visible with each contraction, then birth is imminent.
6. Feel for uterine contractions. You may have to delay this procedure until the patient tells you she is having labor pains. Tell her what you are going to do, then place the palm of your gloved hand on her abdomen, above the navel. This can be done over the top of the patient's clothing. You should be able to feel her uterus and its contraction. All contractions should be timed. Keep track of the duration and frequency of the contractions. The uterus and the tissues between this organ and the skin will feel more rigid as the delivery of the baby nears.
7. Take vital signs at this time if you do not have a partner to do it. Alert the medical

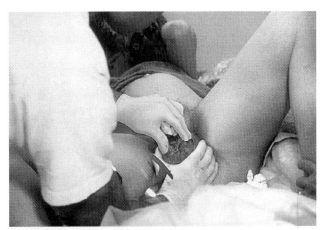

FIGURE 24-4 Crowning of the infant's head occurs in the second stage of labor.

facility staff if the mother's vital signs are abnormal.

Examining for crowning may be embarrassing to the mother, the father, and any required bystanders. For this reason, it is important that you fully explain what you are doing and why. Be certain that you protect the mother from the stares of bystanders. In a polite but firm manner, ask everyone who does not belong at the scene to leave. Carefully help the patient remove enough clothing to allow you an unobstructed view of the vaginal opening.

Remember: A professional appearance coupled with a professional manner instills confidence in patients and bystanders alike.

If this is the woman's first delivery, she is not straining, and there is no crowning, there is little reason why she cannot be transported to a medical facility for delivery. On the other hand, if this is not her first delivery, and she is straining, crying out, and complaining about having to go to the bathroom, birth will probably occur too soon for transport. If the mother is having labor pains from contractions about 2 minutes apart, birth is very near. If you determine that delivery is imminent based on the presence of crowning or other signs, local protocol may require you to contact medical direction for the decision to commit to delivery on the site. If delivery does not occur in 10 minutes, contact medical direction for permission to initiate transport of the mother.

You may find a patient who is afraid of transport because she believes that birth will occur along the way. Assure her that you believe there is enough time before delivery. Let her know that you are trained to assist with the delivery and that the ambulance is well equipped to handle her needs and care for the newborn should she deliver en route. If crowning occurs during transport, stop the ambulance and prepare for delivery.

If your evaluation of the patient leads you to believe that birth is too near at hand for transport, you and your partner should prepare to assist the mother with delivery. Remember, as part of the preparation, the patient will need emotional support.

Remember: Do not allow the mother to go to the bathroom, even though she says that she has to move her bowels. Birth is probably only a few

minutes away. Do not allow the mother to hold her legs together or use any other method to attempt to delay the delivery.

Supine Hypotensive Syndrome

Near the time of birth, the weight of the uterus, coupled with the infant's weight, placenta, and amniotic fluid, approximates 20-24 pounds. When the mother is in a supine position, this heavy mass will tend to compress the inferior vena cava, a major blood vessel, reducing return of blood to the heart and reducing cardiac output. This causes dizziness and a drop in blood pressure, a set of signs and symptoms known as **supine hypotensive syndrome.** The body begins to compensate, when it senses the drop in blood pressure, by contracting the uterine arteries and redirecting blood to the major organs. This can affect the fetus severely.

The drop in blood pressure signals shock, but the method of treating for shock by elevating the legs is not effective in this instance because it does not relieve pressure on the vena cava. To counteract or avoid the possible drop in blood pressure, all third trimester patients should be transported on their left side. A pillow or rolled blanket should be placed behind the back to maintain proper positioning.

Preparing the Mother for Delivery

When your evaluation leads you to believe birth is imminent, you must immediately prepare the mother for delivery. To do so, you should

1. Control the scene so that the mother will have privacy (her coach may remain). If you are not in a private room and transfer to the ambulance is not practical (crowning is present), ask bystanders to leave.
2. In addition to surgical gloves, you and your partner should put on gowns, caps, face masks, and eye protection since there is a high probability of splashing blood during delivery.
3. Place the mother on a bed, sturdy table, or the ambulance stretcher. Elevate the buttocks with blankets or a pillow. Have the mother lie with knees drawn up and spread apart. You will need about 2 feet of work space below the woman's buttocks to place and initially care for the newborn. Having the patient positioned on the stretcher may speed transport if complications arise.

4. Remove any of the patient's clothing or underclothing that obstructs your view of the vaginal opening. Replace your initial non-sterile surgical gloves with sterile gloves from the obstetric kit. Use sterile sheets or sterile towels to cover the mother as shown in Figure 24-5. Clean sheets, clean cloths, towels, or materials such as tablecloths can be used if you do not have an obstetric kit.

5. Position your assistant—your partner, the father, or someone the mother agrees to have assist you—at the mother's head. This person should stay alert to help turn the mother's head should she vomit. As well, this person should provide emotional support to the mother, soothing and encouraging her.

6. Position the obstetric pack on a table or chair. All items must be within easy reach.

Note: If delivery is to take place in an automobile, position the mother flat on the seat. Arrange her legs so that she has one foot resting on the seat and the other foot resting on the floor.

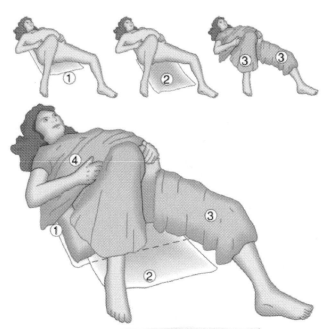

PLACEMENT OF SHEETS OR TOWELS
① One under the buttocks
② One under the vaginal opening
③ One over each thigh
④ One over the abdomen

FIGURE 24-5 Preparing the mother for delivery.

Delivering the Baby

Position yourself in such a way that you have a constant view of the vaginal opening. Be prepared for the baby to come at any moment.

Be prepared for the patient to experience discomfort. Delivering a child is a natural process, but it will be accompanied by pain. Your patient may also have intense feelings of nausea. If this is her first child, she may be very frightened. All these factors may cause your patient to be uncooperative at times. You must remember that the patient is in pain and she may feel ill. She will need emotional support.

During delivery, talk to the mother. Encourage her to relax between contractions. Continue to time her contractions from the beginning of one contraction to the beginning of the next. Encourage her not to strain unless she feels she must. Remind her that her feeling of a pending bowel movement is usually just pressure caused by the baby moving into her birth canal. Encourage her to breathe deeply through her mouth. She may feel better if she pants, although she should be discouraged from breathing rapidly and deeply enough to bring on hyperventilation. If her "bag of waters" breaks, remind her that this is normal.

Note: Unless there are signs of complications, consider the delivery to be normal if there is a cephalic presentation. Observe any unusual color in the amniotic fluid.

The steps for assisting the mother with a normal delivery are

1. Continue to keep someone at the mother's head to provide support, monitor vital signs, and be alert for vomiting. If no one is on hand to help, be alert for vomiting and check vital signs between contractions.

2. Position your gloved hands at the mother's vaginal opening when the baby's head starts to appear. Do not touch the area around the vagina except to assist with the delivery. For legal reasons, it is always preferable for both your protection and the patient's to have your partner present at all times when you are touching a woman's vaginal area.

3. Support the baby's head as it is delivered (Figure 24-6 and Scan 24-1). Place one hand below the baby's head as it is delivered. Spread your fingers evenly around the baby's head, remembering that the skull

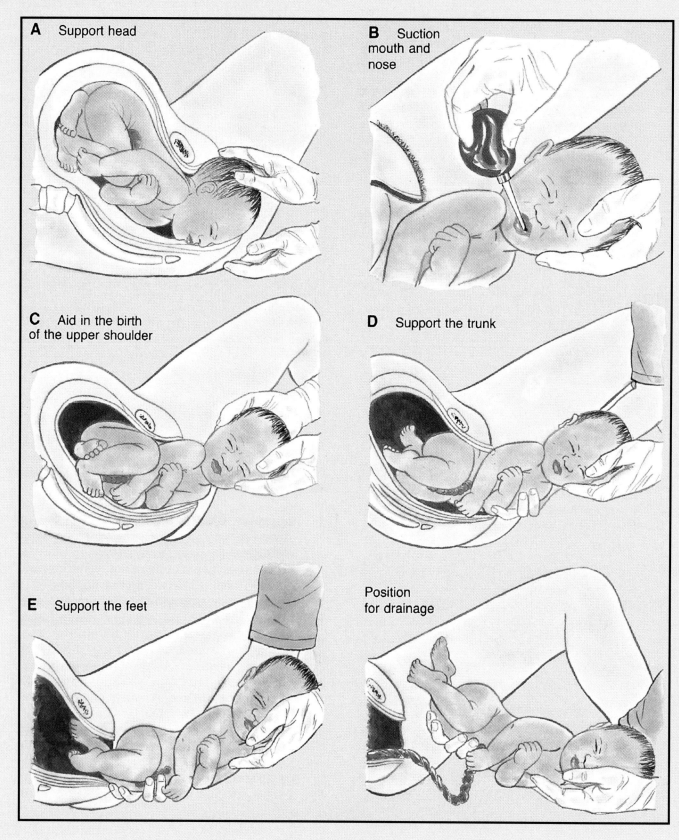

A Support head

B Suction mouth and nose

C Aid in the birth of the upper shoulder

D Support the trunk

E Support the feet

Position for drainage

Note: Assist the mother by supporting the baby throughout the birth process.

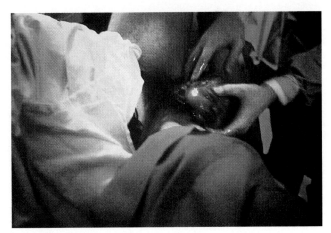

FIGURE 24-6 Delivering the infant's head.

contains "soft spots" or fontanelles. Support the baby's head, but avoid pressure to these soft areas at the top and sides of the skull. A slight, well-distributed pressure may help prevent an explosive delivery. Keeping one hand on the baby's head and using the other hand to hold a sterile towel to support the tissue between the mother's vagina and anus can help prevent tearing of this tissue during delivery of the head. DO NOT PULL ON THE BABY!

4. If the amniotic sac has not broken by the time the baby's head is delivered, use your finger to puncture the membrane. Pull the membranes away from the baby's mouth and nose. The amniotic fluid should be clear. Meconium-stained amniotic fluid is caused by fetal feces (wastes) released during labor, usually because of maternal or fetal stress. If the meconium is aspirated (breathed in) by the fetus, the baby can develop pneumonia or other infections.

5. Once the head delivers, check to see if the umbilical cord is wrapped around the baby's neck. Tell the mother not to push while you check. If she can "pant," or take short quick breaths for just a moment, it may help relieve the urge to push while you check, then gently loosen the cord if necessary. Even though the umbilical cord is very tough, rough handling may cause it to tear. If the cord is wrapped around the baby's neck, try to place two fingers under the cord at the back of the baby's neck. Bring the cord forward, over the baby's upper shoulder and head.

   If you cannot loosen or slip the cord over the baby's head, the baby cannot be delivered. Immediately clamp the cord in two places using the clamps provided in the obstetric kit. Be very careful not to injure the baby. With extreme care, cut the cord between the two clamps. Gently unwrap the ends of the cord from around the baby's neck, and then proceed with the delivery.

6. Check the baby's airway. Most babies are born face down and then rotate to the right or left. Support the baby's head so that it does not touch the mother's anal area. When the entire head of the baby is visible, continue to support the head with one hand and, with the other hand, wipe the mouth and nose with sterile gauze pads. Use the rubber bulb syringe to suction the baby's mouth, then the nose.

   Compress the syringe BEFORE placing it in the baby's mouth. Suction the mouth first, then the nostrils. Carefully insert the tip of the syringe about 1 to 1½ inches into the baby's mouth and release the bulb to allow fluids to be drawn into the syringe. Control the release with your fingers. Withdraw the tip and discharge the syringe's contents onto a towel. Repeat this procedure two or three times in the baby's mouth and once or twice in each nostril. The tip of the syringe should not be inserted more than ½ inch into the baby's nostril.

7. Help deliver the shoulders. The upper shoulder (usually with some delay) will deliver next, followed quickly by the lower shoulder. You must support the baby throughout this entire process. Gently guide the baby's head downward, to assist the mother in delivering the baby's upper shoulder. After the upper shoulder has delivered, if the lower shoulder is slow to deliver, assist the mother by gently guiding the baby's head upward.

8. Support the baby throughout the entire birth process. Remember that newborns are very slippery. As the feet are born, grasp them to assure a good hold on the baby. Once the feet are delivered, lay the baby on its side with its head slightly lower than its body. This is done to allow blood, fluids, and mucus to drain from the mouth and nose. Suction the mouth and nose again with the bulb syringe. Keep the baby at the same level as the mother's vagina until the umbilical cord stops pulsating. Wrap the infant in a warm, dry blanket.

9. Note the exact time of birth.

Caution: Some deliveries are explosive. Do not squeeze the baby, but do provide adequate support. You can prevent an explosive delivery by using one hand to maintain slight pressure on the baby's head, avoiding direct pressure on the infant's soft spot on the skull.

Assessing the Newborn

The vigor of an infant should be assessed as soon as it is born. If you arrive after the birth, it is still your responsibility to make the assessments based on your first observations. Remember, however, that care for the infant and the mother should not be delayed. *The assessment is meant to take place while these other activities are being performed.*

Your EMS system may call for a general or a specific evaluation protocol. A general evaluation usually calls for noting ease of breathing, the heart rate, crying, movement, and skin color. A normal newborn should have a pulse greater than 100/min, be breathing easily, crying (vigorous crying is a good sign), moving its extremities (the more active, the better), and show blue coloration at the hands and feet only. Five minutes later, these signs should still be apparent, with breathing becoming more relaxed. The blue coloration may or may not disappear, but it should not spread to other parts of the body.

To assess the neonate (newborn) you should assess the following.

1. Heart Rate—as determined with a stethoscope over the heart. Count for 30 seconds and multiply by 2. Some newborns can have a normal heart rate as high as 180 beats per minute. This is difficult to count. You are trying to determine if the heart rate is above or below 100 beats per minute. If the rate is below 100, you will then be required to determine if it is below 80 beats per minute.
2. Effort of Breathing—a visual observation of the effort put forth by the baby as it breathes and cries
3. Muscle Tone—a visual observation. Is the newborn limp, or showing some flexion of the extremities, or actively moving its limbs?
4. Irritability (Grimace)—as determined by flicking the infant on the sole of its foot. Is there no response, or some motion and crying, or vigorous motion and crying?
5. Skin Color—noting paleness or cyanosis

Caring for the Newborn

Even with a normal delivery, each step in the care of the baby is essential for its survival. To care for the newborn, you should first place the baby on a sterile sheet on the bed or padded table surface, keeping the baby close to the level of the mother's vagina so that the infant's blood does not transfuse back into the placenta. Do not place the infant on the mother's abdomen at this time (not until after the cord is clamped and cut—see below).

Resuscitation of the Newborn Neonatal resuscitation follows an inverted pyramid (Figure 24-7). As this figure shows, most newborns with abnormal findings on assessment respond to relatively simple maneuvers. Few require CPR or advanced life support measures.

Follow these steps for initial care of the newborn.

1. Clear the baby's airway. Use a bulb syringe, suctioning the mouth first and then the nostrils. It may be necessary to use a sterile gauze pad to clear mucus and blood from around the baby's nose and mouth.

    Note: When the nostrils are suctioned, the baby may gasp or begin breathing and aspirate any meconium, blood, fluids, or mucus from its mouth into its lungs. That is why *it is imperative to suction the mouth before the nostrils.*

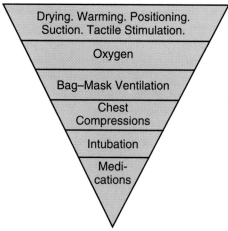

FIGURE 24-7 The inverted pyramid of neonatal resuscitation showing approximate relative frequencies of neonatal resuscitative efforts. Note that a majority of infants respond to simple measures.

2. Keep the baby on its side and again suction the mouth, then the nose with a rubber bulb syringe. If necessary, you can cradle the baby in your arms. However, it is best to keep the baby on the cot or table surface (Figure 24-8).

3. Establish that the baby is breathing. Usually the baby will be breathing on its own by the time you clear the airway. A newborn should begin breathing within 30 seconds. If it is not, then you must "encourage" the baby to breathe (Figure 24-9). Usually, a gentle but vigorous rubbing of the baby's back will promote spontaneous respiration. Should this method fail, snap one of your index fingers against the sole of the baby's foot. Do not hold the baby up by its feet and slap its bottom! Do not become alarmed if the hands and feet of a breathing newborn appear slightly blue. It is not uncommon for this blue color to remain for the first few minutes.

    If assessment of the infant's breathing reveals shallow, slow, or absent respirations, provide artificial ventilations at a rate of 40 to 60 per minute (Figure 24-10). Remember: Provide only small puffs of air to the neonate if using mouth to mask, and small squeezes on the bag if using an infant-sized bag-valve-mask device. Reassess the infant's respiratory efforts after 30 seconds. If there is no change in the effort of breathing, continue with ventilations and reassessment.

4. Assess the infant's heart rate. If the heart rate is less than 100 beats per minute, then provide artificial ventilations at a rate of 40 to 60 per minute. Reassess the heart rate

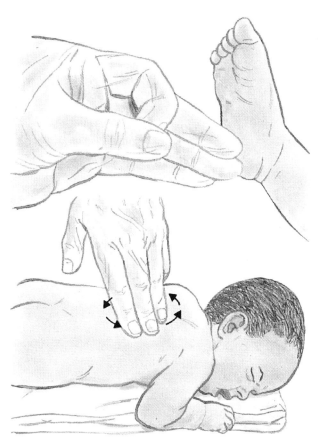

FIGURE 24-9 It may be necessary to stimulate the newborn to breathe.

after 30 seconds. If the heart rate is between 60 and 80 per minute and rising, continue to provide artificial ventilations and reassess again in 30 seconds. If the heart rate on reassessment is less than 60 per minute, or between 60 and 80 per minute and not rising, continue ventilations and initiate chest compressions, as shown in Figure 24-11. Chest compressions in the neonate should be delivered at a rate of 120

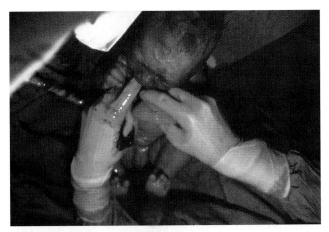

FIGURE 24-8 Suction the mouth, then the nose, of the newborn.

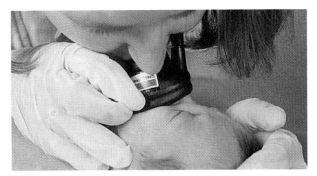

FIGURE 24-10 If assessment of the infant's breathing reveals shallow, slow, or absent respirations, provide artificial ventilations at a rate of 40 to 60 per minute.

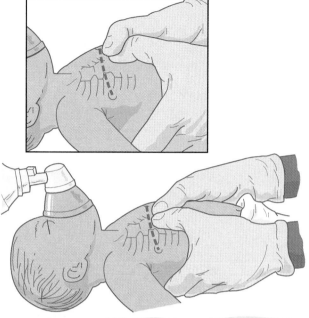

FIGURE 24-11 Chest compressions in the newborn should be delivered at a rate of 120 compressions per minute, midsternum, with two thumbs, fingers supporting the back, at a depth of ½ to ¾ inch.

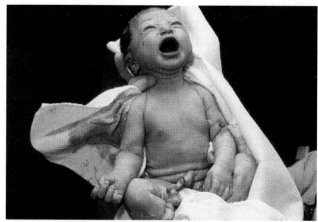

FIGURE 24-12 Placing the infant before clamping the umbilical cord.

compressions per minute, midsternum, with two thumbs, fingers supporting the back. Depth of compression is ½ to ¾ inch. The ratio of compressions to breaths is 3 compressions to 1 breath.

5. If the child has adequate respirations and a pulse rate greater than 100 per minute but exhibits cyanosis of the face and/or torso, provide supplemental oxygen. Oxygen is best delivered at 10-15 liters per minute using oxygen tubing placed close to, but not directly into, the infant's face.

Cutting the Umbilical Cord In a normal birth, the infant must be breathing on its own before you clamp and cut the cord. Before clamping and cutting the cord, palpate the cord with your fingers to make sure it is no longer pulsating. The general procedure for umbilical cord care is as follows.

1. Keep the infant warm. Dry off the baby and wrap it in a baby blanket or infant swaddler, clean towel, or sheet prior to clamping the cord (Figure 24-12). Do not wash the infant. Sometimes the mother may request you to do so, but it is best to leave the protective coating (called the vernix) on the infant until it reaches the medical facility.

2. Use the sterile clamps or umbilical tape found in the obstetric kit. Use extreme care with any tying done to the cord, forming the knot slowly to avoid cutting the cord. Ties should be made using a square knot (right over left, then left over right).

3. Apply one clamp or tie to the cord about 8 to 10 inches from the baby. This leaves enough cord for intravenous lines to be used by paramedics or the staff at the hospital if they are needed.

4. Place a second clamp or tie about 2 to 3 inches closer to the baby. The proximal clamp should be about 4 fingers width from the neonate.

5. Cut the cord between the clamps or knots using sterile surgical scissors (Figure 24-13). Use caution and protect your eyes when cutting the cord as a spurt of blood is very common. Never untie or unclamp a cord once it is cut. The placental end of the cord should be placed on the drape over the mother's legs to avoid contact with expelled blood, feces, and fluids. Examine the fetal end of the cord for bleeding. Do not attempt to adjust the clamp or retie the knot. Should bleeding continue, apply another tie or clamp as close to the original as possible.

6. Be careful when moving the baby so that no trauma is brought to the clamped cord. If the cord does not remain closed off completely, the baby may bleed to death from seemingly little blood loss. In most cases, the cord vessels will collapse and seal themselves.

Warning: Do not tie, clamp, or cut the cord of a baby who is not breathing on its own unless you have to do so to remove the cord from around

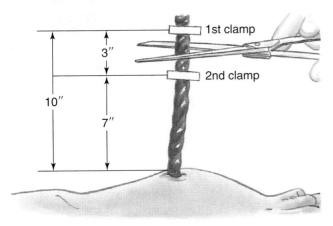

FIGURE 24-13 Cutting the umbilical cord.

the baby's neck during birth, or unless you have to perform CPR on the infant. Do not cut or clamp a cord that is still pulsating.

Keeping the Baby Warm It is critical that the baby be kept warm. Wrap the newborn in an infant swaddler and a warmed blanket or towel and let the mother hold the infant on her abdomen (Figure 24-14). Bubble wrap can also be used. It provides padded protection, warmth (pre-warm it), and allows visual monitoring of the infant. Be sure to cover the infant's head (but not the face). During the delivery of the placenta, have your partner hold the baby unless the mother insists otherwise. Keep the ambulance warm.

Assisting at a Birth When Off Duty If you are assisting at a birth when off duty, you will probably be able to find all the items you need to tie and cut the cord. If no clamps or tying devices are on hand, use clean shoelaces or sim-

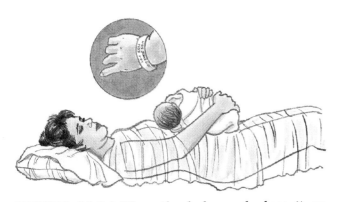

FIGURE 24-14 Wrap the baby and place it on the mother's abdomen. Write the mother's last name and time of delivery on a tape and place it around the baby's wrist. (Do not allow adhesive to contact the baby's skin.)

ilar soft, clean ties. You may delay clamping and tying the cord if the infant will receive this care within 30 minutes. If you tie the cord and believe it will be some time before transport and transfer and don't have sterile scissors, you can soak scissors in alcohol for several minutes and use them to cut the cord. If the baby is still attached to the placenta when the organ is delivered, wrap the placenta in a towel and transport infant and placenta as a unit. The placenta should be placed at the same level as the baby, or slightly higher. Careful monitoring of the baby must be maintained.

Documentation Tips—Recording the Birth

If adhesive tape is available, double face it (put the sticky sides together). Write the mother's last name and the time of delivery on a piece of the tape and loosely secure this tape around the baby's wrist (Figure 24-14). Do not allow the adhesive to come into contact with the baby's skin.

Record, or have your partner record, the exact time of birth (the moment the baby's whole body is out of the birth canal) in accordance with local policy. Usually, this is done on a record of live birth.

Caring for the Mother

Remember that you have two patients to care for: the mother as well as the baby. Care for the mother includes helping her deliver the placenta, controlling vaginal bleeding, and making her as comfortable as possible.

Delivering the Placenta The third stage of labor is the delivery of the placenta with its umbilical cord section, membranes of the amniotic sac, and some of the tissues lining the uterus. (All of these together are known as the afterbirth.) Placental delivery begins with a brief return of the labor pains that stopped when the baby was born. You will notice a lengthening of the cord, which indicates the placenta has separated from the uterus. In most cases, the placenta will be expelled within a few minutes after the baby is born. Although the process may take 30 minutes or longer, avoid the urge to put pressure on the abdomen over the uterus to hasten the delivery of the placenta. If mother and baby are doing well and there are no respiratory problems or significant uncontrolled bleeding, transportation to the hospital can be delayed up to 20 minutes while awaiting delivery of the placenta.

Save all afterbirth tissues (Figure 24-15). The attending physician will want to examine the placenta and other tissues for completeness since any afterbirth tissues remaining in the uterus pose a serious threat of infection and prolonged bleeding to the mother. Try to catch the afterbirth in a container. Place the container in a plastic bag, or wrap it in a towel, paper, or plastic. If no container is available, catch the afterbirth in a towel, paper, or a plastic bag. Label this material "placenta" and include the name of the mother and the time the tissues were expelled.

Remember: If the placenta does not deliver within 20 minutes of the baby's birth, transport the mother and baby to a medical facility without delay.

Note: Some EMS systems recommend transport without waiting for delivery of the placenta. There may be a condition in which the placenta does not separate from the uterine wall and it is important for mother and baby to get to the hospital. You can always stop the ambulance to deliver the placenta if it crowns en route.

Controlling Vaginal Bleeding After Birth

Delivery of the baby and placenta is ALWAYS accompanied by some bleeding from the vagina. Although the blood loss is usually no more than 500 cc, it may be profuse. To control vaginal bleeding after delivery of the baby and placenta (Figure 24-16), you should

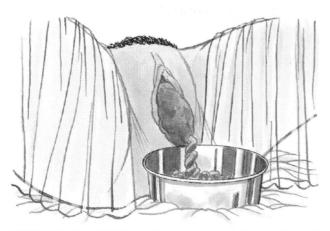

FIGURE 24-15 The placenta must be collected and transported with the mother and baby.

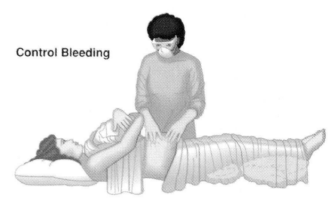

Control Bleeding

FIGURE 24-16 After delivery of the placenta, massaging the uterus helps control vaginal bleeding.

1. Place a sanitary napkin over the mother's vaginal opening. Do not place anything in the vagina.
2. Have the mother lower her legs and keep them together. Tell her that she does not have to "squeeze" her legs together. Elevate her feet.
3. Massaging the uterus will help it contract. This will help control bleeding. Feel the mother's abdomen until you note a "grapefruit-sized" object. This is her uterus. Rub this area lightly with a circular motion. It should contract and become firm, and bleeding should diminish.
4. The mother may want to nurse the baby. This will aid in the contraction of the uterus. Some pediatricians recommend the baby not nurse until a doctor has examined it.

The skin between the vagina and the anus is known as the **perineum.** A tearing of tissue can occur in the perineum at the vaginal opening during the birth process. The mother may feel the discomfort from this torn tissue. Let her know that this is normal and that the problem will be quickly cared for at the medical facility. Treat the torn perineum as a wound. Dress by applying a sanitary napkin and applying some pressure.

Providing Comfort to the Mother Keep contact with the mother throughout the entire birth process and after she has delivered. Your care for the mother does not end when you have completed your duties with the placenta and vaginal bleeding. Take her vital signs frequently. Be aware that she has just undergone a tremendous emotional experience and small acts of kindness will be appreciated and remembered. Childbirth is a rigorous task, and a woman is physically exhausted at the conclusion of delivery. Wiping her face and hands with a damp washcloth and then drying them with a towel will do wonders to refresh her and prepare her for the trip to the hospital. Replacement of blood-soaked sheets and blankets will make that trip more comfortable. Make sure that both she and the baby are warm.

When delivery occurs at home, ask a member of the family or a trusted neighbor to help you clean up. You should clean up whatever disorder EMS care has caused in the house; however, you should not delay transport in order to complete these activities. In some areas, local protocol may have you return to the house after transport in order to complete the clean-up process. If you do, you will have to be accompanied by a member of the family. Be sure to properly dispose of items that have been in contact with blood and other body fluids in a biohazard container.

Remember: Birth is an exciting and joyous event. Talking to the mother and paying attention to her new baby are part of total patient care. A good rule to follow is to treat your patient as you would wish a member of your family to be treated.

CHILDBIRTH COMPLICATIONS

Complications of Delivery

Although most babies are born without difficulty, complications may occur during and after delivery. We have already considered three such complications: the cord around the neck, an unbroken amniotic sac, and infants who need encouragement to breathe. These problems can be handled by simple procedures. However, there are other complications that can threaten the life of both mother and newborn and for which definitive treatment is beyond the EMT-B's level of training. For emergencies such as breech presentation, prolapsed umbilical cord, and limb presentation, you will provide high concentration oxygen and rapid transport to the hospital.

Breech Presentation

Breech presentation is the most common abnormal delivery. It involves a buttocks-first or both-legs-first delivery. The risk of birth trauma to the baby is high in breech deliveries. In addition there is an increased risk of prolapsed cord (see below). In addition, meconium staining often occurs with breech presentations.

Patient Assessment—Breech Presentation

If you evaluate a woman in labor and find the baby's buttocks or both legs presenting, rather than the head presenting, this is a breech presentation. Although breech presentations can spontaneously deliver successfully, the complication rate is high.

Patient Care—Breech Presentation

Emergency Care Steps

1. Initiate rapid transport upon recognition of a breech presentation.
2. Never attempt to deliver the baby by pulling on its legs.
3. Provide high concentration oxygen.
4. Place the mother in a head down position with the pelvis elevated.
5. If the body delivers, support it and prevent an explosive delivery of the head. After delivery, care for the baby, cord, mother, and placenta as in a cephalic delivery.

Prolapsed Umbilical Cord

Sometimes during delivery, the umbilical cord presents first (this is most common in breech births) and the cord is squeezed between the vaginal wall and the head of the baby. The cord is pinched, and oxygen supply to the baby may be totally interrupted. This occurrence is known as a **prolapsed umbilical cord.**

Patient Assessment—Prolapsed Umbilical Cord

If, upon viewing the vaginal area, you see the umbilical cord presenting, the cord is prolapsed.

Patient Care—Prolapsed Umbilical Cord

Emergency Steps

Follow the steps below when the umbilical cord is prolapsed (Figure 24-17).

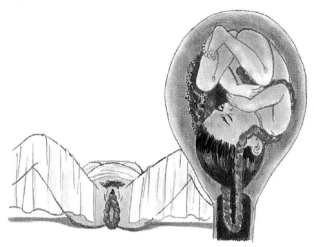

- Elevate hips, administer oxygen and keep warm
- Keep baby's head away from cord
- Do not attempt to push cord back
- Wrap cord in sterile moist towel
- Transport mother to hospital, continuing pressure on baby's head

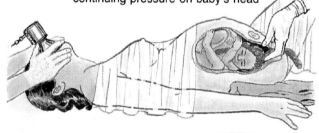

FIGURE 24-17 Prolapsed umbilical cord.

1. Position the mother with her head down and buttocks raised with a blanket or pillow, using gravity to lessen pressure on the birth canal.
2. Provide the mother with a high concentration of oxygen to increase the concentration carried over to the infant.
3. Check the cord for pulses and wrap the exposed cord, using a sterile towel from the obstetric kit. The cord must be kept warm. The best results are obtained if this towel is kept moist with sterile saline and wrapped again with a dry towel to prevent evaporative heat loss.
4. Insert several fingers of a gloved hand into the mother's vagina so that you can gently push up on the baby's head or buttocks to keep pressure off of the cord. You will be pushing up through the cervix. This may be the only chance that the baby has for survival, so continue to push up on the baby until you are relieved by a physician.

You may feel the cord pulsating when pressure is released.

5. Keeping mother, child, and EMT-B as a unit, transport immediately to a medical facility.
6. All patients with prolapsed cords require rapid transport. Have your partner obtain vital signs while en route to the hospital if possible.

Limb Presentation

A **limb presentation** occurs when a limb of an infant protrudes from the vagina. The presenting limb is commonly a foot when the baby is in the breech position. Limb presentations cannot be delivered in the prehospital setting. Rapid transport is essential to the baby's survival.

Patient Assessment—Limb Presentation

When checking for crowning, you may see (Figure 24-18) an arm, a single leg, or an arm and leg together, or a shoulder and an arm. If one or more limbs present, there is often a prolapsed umbilical cord as well.

Patient Care—Limb Presentation

Emergency Care Steps

When you discover a limb presentation

1. If there is a prolapsed cord, follow the same procedures as you would for any delivery involving a prolapsed cord. Remember, you have to keep pushing up on the baby until relieved by a physician. The baby must be kept off of the cord if it is to survive.
2. Transport the mother immediately to a medical facility.
3. Place the mother in a head down position with the pelvis elevated.
4. Administer a high concentration of oxygen.

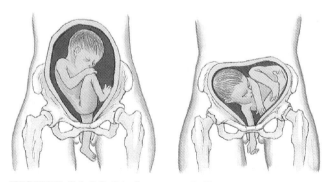

FIGURE 24-18 Limb presentation.

Remember: For a limb presentation, do not try to pull on the limb or replace the limb into the vagina. Do not place your gloved hand into the vagina, unless there is a prolapsed cord.

Multiple Birth

When more than one baby is born during a single delivery, it is called a **multiple birth.** A multiple birth, usually twins, is not considered to be a complication, provided that the deliveries are normal. Twins are generally delivered in the same manner as a single delivery, one birth following the other. However, if a multiple birth is encountered you should have enough personnel and equipment to be prepared for multiple resuscitations. Call for assistance if needed.

Patient Assessment—Multiple Birth

If the mother is under a physician's care, she will probably be aware that she is carrying twins. Without this information, you should consider a multiple birth to be a possibility if the mother's abdomen appears unusually large before delivery, or it remains very large after delivery of one baby. If the birth is multiple, labor contractions will continue and the second baby will be delivered shortly after the first. The second baby may present in a breech position, usually within minutes of the first birth. The placenta or placentas are delivered normally (Figure 24-19).

Patient Care—Multiple Birth

When assisting in the delivery of twins

1. Clamp or tie the cord of the first baby before the second baby is born.
2. The second baby may be born either before or after the placenta is delivered. Assist the mother with the delivery of the second baby.
3. Provide care for the babies, umbilical cords, placenta(s), and the mother as you would in a single-baby delivery.
4. The babies will probably be smaller than in a single birth, so special care should be taken to keep them warm during transport.

When delivering twins, identify the infants as to order of birth (1 and 2 or A and B).

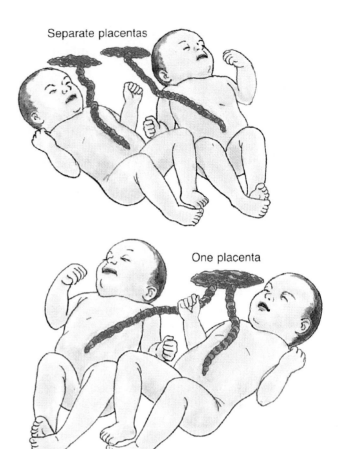

FIGURE 24-19 Multiple births.

Premature Birth

By definition, a **premature infant** is one that weighs less than 5½ pounds at birth, or one that is born before the 37th week of pregnancy.

Patient Assessment—Premature Birth

Since you will probably not be able to weigh the baby, you will have to make a determination as to whether the baby is full-term or premature based on the mother's information and the baby's appearance. By comparison with a normal full-term baby, the head of a premature infant is much larger in proportion to the small, thin, red body.

Patient Care—Premature Birth

Premature babies need special care from the moment of birth. The smaller the baby, the more important is the initial care.

You should take the following steps when providing care for the premature infant (Figure 24-20).

1. *Keep the baby warm.* Premature infants are at great risk of developing hypothermia. Once breathing, the baby should be dried and wrapped snugly in a warm blanket. Additional protection can be provided by an outer wrap of plastic bubble wrap (keep away from the face) or aluminum foil. Premature babies lack fat deposits that would normally keep them warm. Some EMS systems in cold regions are using a plastic or bubble wrap or bag for the infant, covered by a blanket. This helps maintain warmth and allows for easier visual inspection of the clamped cord to check for bleeding. A stockinette cap should be placed on the baby's head to help reduce heat loss.

2. *Keep the airway clear.* Continue to suction fluids from the nose and mouth using a rubber bulb syringe. Keep checking to see if additional suctioning is required.

3. *Provide ventilations and/or chest compressions* as outlined above based upon the baby's pulse and respiratory effort. In some cases resuscitation may not be possible if the baby is extremely premature.

4. *Watch the umbilical cord for bleeding.* Examine the cut end of the cord carefully. If there is any sign of bleeding, even the slightest, apply another clamp or tie closer to the baby's body.

5. *Provide oxygen.* Do not blow a stream of oxygen directly on the baby's face, but arrange for oxygen to flow past the baby's face. If available, use a humidified source of oxygen.

6. *Avoid contamination.* The premature infant is susceptible to infection. Keep it away from other people. Do not breathe on its face.

7. *Transport the infant in a warm ambulance.* The desired temperature is between 90°F and 100°F. Use the ambulance heater to warm the patient compartment prior to transport. In the summer months, the air conditioning should be turned off and all compartment windows should be closed or adjusted to keep the desired temperature.

8. *Call ahead to the emergency department.*

Meconium

Meconium is a result of the fetus defecating (putting out wastes). It is a sign of fetal or maternal distress.

Patient Assessment—Meconium

Meconium stains amniotic fluid greenish or brownish-yellow in color. Infants born with meconium are at increased risk for respiratory problems—especially if aspiration of the meconium occurs at birth.

Patient Care—Meconium

1. To reduce the risk of aspiration, do not stimulate the infant before suctioning the oropharynx.
2. Suction the mouth and then the nose.
3. Maintain an open airway.
4. Provide artificial ventilations and/or chest compression as indicated by effort of breathing and heart rate.
5. Transport as soon as possible.

Predelivery Emergencies

Excessive Prebirth Bleeding

A number of conditions can cause excessive prebirth bleeding late in pregnancy. Whether the vaginal bleeding is associated with abdominal pain or not, the risk to both the mother and the unborn child is great.

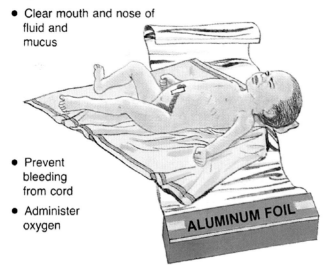

- Keep warm by wrapping in blanket and then in aluminum foil
- Clear mouth and nose of fluid and mucus
- Prevent bleeding from cord
- Administer oxygen

ALUMINUM FOIL

FIGURE 24-20 Premature infants need special care.

One such condition is **placenta previa** (plah-SEN-tah PRE-vi-ah), a condition in which the placenta is formed in an abnormal location (low in the uterus and close to or over the cervical opening) that will not allow for a normal delivery of the fetus. As the cervix dilates, the placenta tears.

Another such condition is **abruptio placentae** (ab-RUPT-si-o plah-SEN-ta), a condition in which the placenta separates from the uterine wall. This can be a partial or a complete abruption. In a complete abruption, the body of the placenta has separated from the uterine wall but the edges remain attached. Blood is trapped between the uterine wall and the placenta. Either placenta previa or abruptio placenta may occur in the third trimester. Both are potentially life threatening to the mother and fetus.

A pregnant woman does not have to be in labor to have excessive bleeding from the vagina. Bleeding in early pregnancy may be due to a miscarriage (see Miscarriage and Abortion later in this chapter). If the bleeding occurs late in pregnancy, it may be due to problems involving the placenta.

Patient Assessment—Excessive Prebirth Bleeding

Signs and Symptoms

☐ The main sign is usually simply profuse bleeding from the vagina.
☐ The mother may or may not experience associated abdominal pain.
☐ During initial assessment, look for signs of shock
☐ Obtain baseline vital signs. A rapid heart beat may indicate significant blood loss

Patient Care—Excessive Prebirth Bleeding

☐ Treatment is based on signs and symptoms. If signs of shock exist, treat with high concentration oxygen and rapid transportation.
☐ Place a sanitary napkin over the vaginal opening. Note the time of napkin placement. DO NOT PLACE ANYTHING IN THE VAGINA. Replace pads as they become soaked, but save all pads to use in evaluating blood loss.
☐ Save all tissue that is passed.

Seizures in Pregnancy

Seizures in pregnancy tend to occur late in pregnancy. The seizures are usually associated with high blood pressure and swelling of the extremities. Seizures in pregnancy pose a serious threat to both the mother and unborn baby.

Patient Assessment—Seizures in Pregnancy

A seizure may be associated with any of the following.

☐ Elevated blood pressure. The risk of abruptio placentae increases with the elevated blood pressure.
☐ Excessive weight gain
☐ Extreme swelling of face, hands, ankles, and feet
☐ Headache

Patient Care—Seizures in Pregnancy

Emergency Care Steps

1. Ensure and maintain an open airway
2. Administer high concentration oxygen
3. Transport patient positioned on her left side
4. Handle gently at all times. Rough handling may induce more seizures
5. Keep her warm, but do not overheat
6. Have suction ready
7. Have a delivery kit ready

Miscarriage and Abortion

For a number of reasons, the fetus and placenta may deliver before the 28th week of pregnancy—generally before the baby can live on its own. This occurrence is an **abortion.** When it happens on its own it is called a **spontaneous abortion;** the common term is **miscarriage.** An **induced abortion** is an abortion that results from deliberate actions taken to stop the pregnancy.

Patient Assessment—Miscarriage and Abortion

Signs and Symptoms

Women having a miscarriage that requires them to seek emergency care generally have

☐ Cramping abdominal pains not unlike those associated with the first stage of labor
☐ Bleeding ranging from moderate to severe
☐ A noticeable discharge of tissue and blood from the vagina

Ask the patient about the starting date of her last menstrual period. If it has been more than 24 weeks, be prepared with a delivery pack. Premature infants may survive if they receive rapid neonatal intensive care.

Patient Care—Miscarriage and Abortion

1. Obtain baseline vital signs.
2. If signs of shock are present, provide a high concentration of oxygen. Treatment should be based on signs and symptoms.
3. Help absorb vaginal bleeding by placing a sanitary napkin over the vaginal opening. Do not pack the vagina.
4. Transport as soon as possible
5. Replace and save all blood-soaked pads.
6. Save all tissues that are expelled. Do not attempt to replace or pull out any tissues that are being expelled through the vagina.
7. Provide emotional support to the mother. Emotional support is very important. When speaking to the patient, her family, or where bystanders may hear you, ALWAYS use the term *miscarriage* instead of *spontaneous abortion*. Most people associate the word *abortion* with an induced abortion, not a miscarriage. It is essential to talk with the patient to gain her confidence and to allow you to provide emotional support.

Trauma in Pregnancy

Obviously the pregnant patient, as any other accident victim, may sustain injury. However, especially during the last two trimesters the uterus and fetus are also subject to injuries when the mother is injured. Injuries to the uterus may be blunt or penetrating. In both cases the greatest danger to mother and baby is hemorrhage (bleeding) and shock.

The most common cause of blunt trauma is automobile collisions, but falls or beatings also account for many injuries. The uterus is well designed to protect the baby. The fetus is inside the uterus, a muscular chamber filled with fluid. The uterus acts as an efficient shock absorber.

Thus most minor trauma to the abdomen, such as a blow or fall, does not harm the fetus.

Automobile collisions are a different story. The magnitude of forces is great. Because of its size and location, the uterus is frequently injured. Sudden blunt trauma to the abdomen during the later months of pregnancy may cause uterine rupture or premature separation of the placenta (abruptio placentae). Other blunt trauma injuries, such as a ruptured spleen or liver, may also occur. Rupture of the diaphragm may occur with blunt trauma during later pregnancy. Multiple trauma with fractures of the pelvis can cause laceration or tearing of the vessels in the pelvis with massive hemorrhage. The common problem with most blunt injuries to the pregnant abdomen or pelvis is massive bleeding and shock.

If a pregnant woman is injured in an accident, such as a motor vehicle collision or a fall, perform a patient assessment and treat her injuries as you would those of any other trauma patient.

Patient Assessment—Trauma in Pregnancy

Follow these patient assessment steps.

☐ During initial assessment and assessment of vital signs, remember the following about the physiology of pregnant women.

- The pregnant patient has a pulse that is 10-15 beats per minute faster than the nonpregnant female. Vital signs may be interpreted as being suggestive of shock when they are normal for the pregnant female.
- A woman in later pregnancy may have a blood volume that is up to 48% higher than her nonpregnant state. With hemorrhage, 30-35% blood loss may occur before otherwise healthy pregnant females exhibit signs or symptoms.
- Although shock is more difficult to assess in the pregnant patient, it is the most likely cause of prehospital death from injury to the uterus.

☐ Question the conscious patient to determine if she has received any blows to the abdomen, pelvis, or back.
☐ Ask the patient if she has had bleeding or rupture of the bag of waters. When in

doubt, examine the vaginal area for bleeding, being certain to provide privacy.

☐ Examine the unconscious patient for abdominal injuries, remembering to consider the mechanism of injury.

Patient Care—Trauma in Pregnancy

Emergency Care Steps

Remember that maintenance of respiration and circulation and the control of bleeding are vital not only to the mother but also to the fetus. A developing fetus is critically dependent on the uninterrupted oxygenated blood supply that enters the placenta. What's good for the mother is good for the baby. Since the mother-to-be may have undetected internal bleeding or the fetus may be injured, provide the following care to the injured mother.

1. Provide resuscitation if necessary.
2. Provide a high concentration of oxygen. (Oxygen requirements of the woman in later pregnancy are 10-20% greater than normal. If in doubt, give oxygen.)
3. Because of slowed digestion and delayed gastric emptying, there is a greater risk the patient will vomit and aspirate. Be ready with suction!
4. Transport as soon as possible. All pregnant women should be transported in the left lateral recumbent position unless a back or neck injury is suspected. If so, first secure the mother to a spine board, then tip board and patient as a unit to the left, relieving pressure on the abdominal organs and vena cava. Support the mother with pillows and folded blankets. Be sure to monitor and record vital signs.
5. Provide emotional support. A pregnant woman who is an accident victim will naturally worry about her unborn child. Remind her that the developing baby is well protected in the uterus. Let her know that she is being transported to a medical facility that can take care of her needs and the needs of the unborn child.

GYNECOLOGICAL EMERGENCIES

There are several emergencies unique to the reproductive systems of non-pregnant women with which you as an EMT-B must be familiar.

Vaginal Bleeding

Vaginal bleeding that is not a result of direct trauma or a women's normal menstrual cycle may indicate a serious gynecological emergency.

Patient Assessment—Vaginal Bleeding

Since it will be impossible for the EMT-B to determine a specific cause of the bleeding, it is important that all women who have vaginal bleeding be treated as though they have a potentially life-threatening condition. This is especially true if the bleeding is associated with abdominal pain.

The most serious complication of vaginal bleeding is hypovolemic shock due to blood loss.

Patient Care—Vaginal Bleeding

Emergency Care Steps

☐ Assure body substance isolation. Wear gloves, gown, protective eye wear and mask as indicated.
☐ Assure an adequate airway
☐ Assess for signs of shock
☐ Administer high concentration oxygen
☐ Transport

Trauma to the External Genitalia

Trauma to a woman's external genitalia can be difficult to care for because of the patient's modesty and the severe pain often involved with such injuries.

Patient Assessment—Trauma to the External Genitalia

Injuries in this area tend to bleed profusely because of the rich blood supply to the area. Injuries to the female external genitalia are frequently the result of straddle-type injuries.

Patient Care—Trauma to the External Genitalia

Emergency Care Steps

1. In sizing up the scene, observe for mechanism of injury.
2. During initial assessment, look for signs of severe blood loss and shock.

3 Control bleeding with direct pressure as you would for any soft-tissue injury. Do not pack the vagina.

4 If signs of shock are present, treat with high concentration oxygen.

5 Maintain a professional attitude.

6 Respect the patient's privacy. Remove unneeded bystanders and expose the patient's body only to the extent necessary to provide appropriate care.

Sexual Assault

Situations where a sexual assault has occurred are always a challenge to the EMT-B. Care of the patient must include both medical and psychological considerations. In addition, law enforcement agencies are also frequently involved.

There is no question that the victim of sexual assault is under tremendous stress. You must be prepared to deal with a wide range of emotions that the patient may exhibit. The best approach is to be nonjudgmental and to maintain a professional but compassionate attitude. It is generally preferable that an EMT-B of the same sex as the patient establish rapport and be the primary provider of emergency care.

Patient Assessment—Sexual Assault

☐ Since you may be entering a potential crime scene, assure that the scene is safe prior to entering. It may be necessary to "stage" your unit near the scene until it is rendered safe by police.

☐ During assessment, identify and treat both the medical and the psychological needs of the patient.

Emergency Care—Sexual Assault

Emergency Care Steps

1 Provide an open airway.

2 Be careful not to disturb potential criminal evidence unless it is absolutely necessary for patient care.

3 Examine the genitals only if severe bleeding is present.

4 Discourage the patient from bathing, voiding, or cleansing any wounds as this may result in loss of important evidence.

5 Fulfill any reporting requirements that are locally mandated

FYI

Topics included in the FYI—"For Your Information"—section are those that go beyond the chapter objectives. The information in this segment is intended to broaden your understanding of the chapter topic but is not essential to an understanding of your job as an EMT-B.

Childbirth and Death

The Stillborn Infant

Some babies die in the womb several hours, days, or even weeks before birth. Such a baby is called **stillborn.**

Patient Assessment—Stillbirth

When a baby has died some time before birth, death is obvious by the presence of blisters, foul odor, skin or tissue deterioration and discoloration, and a softened head. At other times, a baby may be born in pulmonary or cardiac arrest but in otherwise good condition and with the possibility of being resuscitated.

Patient Care—Stillbirth

Emergency Care Steps

1 Stillborn babies who have obviously been dead for some time before birth are not to receive resuscitation.

2 Any other babies who are born in pulmonary or cardiac arrest are to receive basic life support measures.

3 When the baby is alive but death appears to be imminent, prepare to provide life support.

Nothing is quite so sad as a baby born dead or one who dies shortly after birth. It is a tragic moment for the parents and other family members. Your thoughtfulness may provide the distraught parents with comfort.

Do not lie to the mother. Many death-and-dying experts believe that she should be allowed to view her baby if she so desires. Do not stop her from seeing the dead baby if she wants to.

Christian parents may ask you to baptize the baby if death appears likely. This is an acceptable practice for emergency personnel. Regardless of your own religious belief, you should comply with the parents' request. Ask the parents if they know the exact words of baptism for their denomination. Say exactly what they tell you. If they are not sure, simply sprinkle drops of water on the baby's head and say: "I baptize thee in the name of the Father, and of the Son, and of the Holy Spirit."

Needless to say, resuscitative efforts should be continued during and after the baptism and continued until transfer to the hospital. You must keep accurate records of the time of stillbirth and the care rendered for completion of the fetal death certificate. It is a good idea to note if the baby was baptized by EMS personnel.

Accidental Death of a Pregnant Woman

If a woman in advanced pregnancy dies in an accident and you begin CPR on her immediately, there is a chance of saving the life of the infant. CPR must then be continued until an emergency cesarean section can be performed. If CPR is delayed 5 to 10 minutes, chances of saving the baby are fair, while a 25-minute delay reduces the chances to almost zero. Continue CPR on the mother until you are relieved in the emergency department.

CHAPTER REVIEW

KEY TERMS

You may find it helpful to review the following terms.

abortion spontaneous (miscarriage) or induced termination of pregnancy.

abruptio placentae (ab-RUPT-si-o plah-SENT-ta) a condition in which the placenta separates from the uterine wall; a cause of excessive prebirth bleeding.

afterbirth the placenta, membranes of the amniotic sac, part of the umbilical cord, and some tissues from the lining of the uterus that are delivered after the birth of the baby.

amniotic (am-ne-OT-ic) **sac** the "bag of waters" that surrounds the developing fetus.

breech presentation when the baby appears buttocks or both legs first during birth.

cephalic (se-FAL-ik) **presentation** when the baby appears head first during birth. This is the normal presentation.

cervix (SUR-viks) the neck of the uterus at the entrance to the birth canal.

crowning when part of the baby is visible through the vaginal opening.

fetus (FE-tus) the baby as it develops in the womb.

induced abortion expulsion of a fetus as a result of deliberate actions taken to stop the pregnancy.

labor the three stages of the delivery of a baby that begin with the contractions of the uterus and end with the expulsion of the placenta.

limb presentation when an infant's limb protrudes from the vagina before the appearance of any other body part.

meconium staining amniotic fluid that is greenish or brownish-yellow rather than clear; an indication of possible maternal or fetal distress during labor.

miscarriage see *spontaneous abortion.*

multiple birth when more than one baby is born during a single delivery.

perineum (per-i-NE-um) the surface area between the vagina and anus.

placenta (plah-SEN-tah) the organ of pregnancy where exchange of oxygen, foods, and wastes occurs between a mother and fetus.

placenta previa (plah-SEN-tah PRE-vi-ah) a condition in which the placenta is formed in an abnormal location (low in the uterus and close to or over the cervical opening) that will not allow for a normal delivery of the fetus; a cause of excessive prebirth bleeding.

premature infant any newborn weighing less than 5½ pounds or born before the 37th week of pregnancy.

prolapsed umbilical cord when the umbilical cord presents first and is squeezed between the vaginal wall and the baby's head.

spontaneous abortion when the fetus and placenta deliver before the 28th week of pregnancy; commonly called a *miscarriage.*

stillborn   born dead.

supine hypotensive syndrome   dizziness and a drop in blood pressure caused when the mother is in a supine position and the weight of the uterus, infant, placenta, and amniotic fluid compress the inferior vena cava, reducing return of blood to the heart and cardiac output.

umbilical (um-BIL-i-kal) cord   the fetal structure containing the blood vessels that carry blood to and from the placenta.

uterus   (U-ter-us)   the muscular abdominal organ where the fetus develops; the womb.

vagina   (vah-JI-nah)   the birth canal.

SUMMARY

Birth is a natural process that usually takes place without complications. The role of the EMT-B at a birth is generally to provide reassurance and to assist the mother in the delivery of her baby. During the normal delivery, the EMT-B will evaluate the mother to determine if there should be immediate transport to a medical facility or if birth is imminent and will take place at the scene. If birth is to take place at the scene, the EMT-B prepares the mother for delivery, assists in the delivery, assesses the newborn, and cares for the newborn and the mother.

Occasionally there will be some complications to delivery, including breech presentation, prolapsed umbilical cord, limb presentation, multiple birth, premature birth, or meconium staining of the amniotic fluid. There may also be predelivery emergencies (such as excessive bleeding, seizures, abortion, or trauma to the pregnant mother) and gynecological emergencies (such as vaginal bleeding, trauma, or sexual assault) that the EMT-B must be prepared to treat.

REVIEW QUESTIONS

1. Name and describe the anatomical structures of a woman's body that are associated with pregnancy.
2. Describe the three stages of labor.
3. Explain how to evaluate and to prepare the mother for delivery.
4. Name, in the order of the inverted pyramid, the steps that may be taken to resuscitate a newborn infant.
5. Name and describe several possible complications of delivery.
6. Name and describe several possible predelivery emergencies.

Application

- You are called to respond to a pregnant woman who is in labor. During your evaluation, you find that this is the woman's first pregnancy, the baby's head is not yet crowning, and contractions are 10 minutes apart. You ask the mother if she feels she needs to move her bowels, and she says she does not. Do you prepare for delivery at the scene? Or do you transport the mother to the hospital? Explain your reasoning.

Module 5

Trauma

MODULE OVERVIEW

Traumatic injuries are the result of outside forces acting on the body. Falls, automobile collisions, and violence are just a few causes of trauma. Trauma is a major cause of death and disability. This module will prepare you to understand and treat cases of traumatic injury.

One of the major problems associated with trauma is blood loss. The loss of blood, either externally or internally, can cause serious complications, the most serious of which is hypoperfusion, also known as shock. Severe blood loss and shock are life threatening. Chapter 25 deals with these important topics.

Specific injuries and injury patterns are explored throughout the remainder of the module. Soft tissue injuries, which include a wide range of trauma to the skin, underlying tissues, and internal organs, will be the topic of Chapter 26. Injuries to the bones, joints, and muscles, while seldom life threatening, are a frequent cause of emergency calls. They will be covered in Chapter 27. Head and spinal trauma can cause serious physical injury, paralysis, and even death. These injuries and their care are the topic of Chapter 28.

In previous modules, you have studied airway management, assessment, and medical emergencies. This module on trauma will complete the adult emergencies section of the curriculum.

Bleeding and Shock

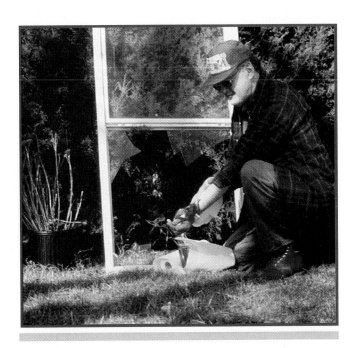

25

Trauma is the leading cause of death in the United States for persons between the ages of 1 and 44. As an EMT-Basic you will be called upon to provide care to victims of traumatic injury. Your identification of serious and potentially serious trauma patients, combined with appropriate care, provides the best chance for the patient to survive these injuries. A vital part of this care is the understanding of the signs, symptoms, and treatment for shock and bleeding.

Objectives

Knowledge and Attitude *At the end of this chapter, you should be able to meet the following objectives.*

1. List the structure and function of the circulatory system. (p. 449)

2. Differentiate between arterial, venous, and capillary bleeding. (pp. 450–451)

3. State methods of emergency medical care of external bleeding. (pp. 452–459)

4. Establish the relationship between body substance isolation and bleeding. (pp. 450, 452, 453, 455)

5. Establish the relationship between airway management and the trauma patient. (pp. 452, 460, 463)

6. Establish the relationship between mechanism of injury and internal bleeding. (pp. 459–460)

7. List the signs of internal bleeding. (p. 460)

8. List the steps in the emergency medical care of the patient with signs and symptoms of internal bleeding. (p. 460)

9. List signs and symptoms of shock (hypoperfusion). (pp. 452, 462)

10. State the steps in the emergency medical care of the patient with signs and symptoms of shock (hypoperfusion). (pp. 463–465)

11. Explain the sense of urgency to transport patients that are bleeding and show signs of shock (hypoperfusion). (p. 463)

Skills

1. Demonstrate direct pressure as a method of emergency medical care of external bleeding.

2. Demonstrate the use of diffuse pressure as a method of emergency medical care of external bleeding.

3. Demonstrate the use of pressure points and tourniquets as a method of emergency medical care of external bleeding.

4. Demonstrate the care of the patient exhibiting signs and symptoms of internal bleeding.

5. Demonstrate the care of the patient exhibiting signs and symptoms of shock (hypoperfusion).

6. Demonstrate completing a prehospital care report for patient with bleeding and/or shock (hypoperfusion).

On the Scene

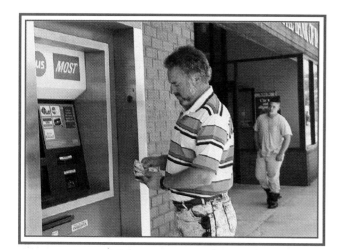

Brian Mitchell stops at an automated teller machine near his house. Rushing to make a dinner meeting, he doesn't notice the man watching him from a short distance away. Immediately after Brian gets his cash, the man dashes in and attempts to steal it. Brian briefly resists and receives a stab wound to his abdomen.

On arrival, you *size up the scene* and see a man lying on the ground with a pool of blood near his abdomen and back. There are three police officers at the scene. One officer motions the ambulance into a specific area to park. In a brief exchange with the officer, you find that the perpetrator has just been apprehended two blocks away. The scene is secure. You note the large pool of blood and instruct your crew members to wear gloves and protective eyewear.

As you begin your *initial assessment,* you observe the patient, a man apparently about 40, with profuse bleeding from an abdominal wound. His eyes were following you as you approached, so you know he is awake. Your general impression of this patient, based on the pool of blood and the chief complaint (stabbing), is one of a potentially serious patient. You crouch beside him.

You: Hello. I'm Lee Friedlander. I'm an Emergency Medical Technician from the ambulance. I see you've been hurt, and I'm here to help you, OK? How do you feel?

Brian: Not good. Am I going to be all right? How bad am I hurt?

As you speak with Brian, you make a mental note of his pale skin color. Since he has spoken clearly, you know his airway is open, and you assess the adequacy of respirations while your partner begins to control the bleeding.

You: (In a calm, reassuring tone) You have a wound in your abdomen, and my partner is putting a dressing and some pressure on it to control the bleeding. I'm going to put an oxygen mask your face. Getting some extra oxygen into your body is important right now. And then we're going to get you to the hospital where they can take good care of you.

Brian: OK. (He clutches fearfully at your hand.)

You start high-flow oxygen through a nonrebreather mask. You note that the patient has a weak radial pulse. You have already noted a pale skin color. You further note that the skin feels cool to the touch. It is apparent that the patient is very anxious.

Recognizing that this patient is rapidly progressing into shock, you decide to transport immediately and perform the rest of your assessment en route. In moments, you have immobilized Brian on a backboard. An ALS squad is located between you and your twenty minute response to the hospital. Radio notification is made for an ALS intercept, and Brian is loaded into the ambulance.

Once under way to the hospital, you ensure control of bleeding and perform the *focused history and physical exam,* then repeat the *initial assessment,* evaluating the ABCs and finding Brian's respirations still adequate and the oxygen flowing properly. You perform a detailed *physical exam* and do not find any additional injuries. You perform *ongoing assessment,* checking vital signs and finding them to be BP 96/52, respirations 28, pulse 116 weak but regular. Brian has breath sounds over both lungs.

The ALS unit is waiting at the designated spot. You brief the ALS personnel as your partner rechecks Brian's status and vitals. Your estimated time of arrival (ETA) to the trauma center is 10 to 12 minutes. There will be several reassessments of the patient during that time. The ALS crew contacts medical direction as the ambulance proceeds to the hospital.

You arrive at the hospital and brief the emergency department staff on your care and findings. They begin to work at a feverish pace. Before long, Brian is wheeled off to surgery. Returning several days later, you speak to the ED physician who coordinated Brian's care. She reports that the patient had a lacerated liver. Your thorough but expeditious care contributed to the fact that Brian survived the incident.

---

*P*rofuse bleeding and the condition called shock are life-threatening conditions that require immediate emergency care. An understanding of blood circulation is basic to understanding and treating both bleeding and shock.

THE CIRCULATORY SYSTEM

The circulatory system, also called the cardiovascular system, is responsible for distribution of blood to all portions of the body. The system contains the heart, the blood vessels, and the blood that flows within the system.

The heart is a muscular organ that lies within the chest. Its job is to pump in a regular, rhythmic fashion to move blood throughout the circulatory system. You learned about the heart and the circulatory system in Chapter 4, The Human Body.

Blood vessels are the means by which blood is transported throughout the body. There are three major types of blood vessels (Figure 25-1). They are

- **Artery**—a blood vessel with thick, muscular walls that carries blood away from the heart

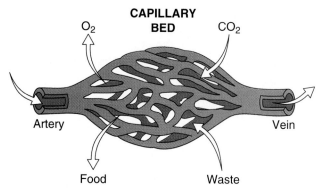

O_2 CO_2

Artery Vein

Food Waste

FIGURE 25-1 The blood vessels.

- **Capillary**—a microscopic blood vessel where oxygen/carbon dioxide and nutrient/waste exchange takes place
- **Vein**—a blood vessel that carries blood back to the heart. A vein contains one-way valves that keep the blood flowing in the proper direction.

As the heart beats, it circulates blood through the arteries into the capillaries where oxygen and nutrients are exchanged for carbon dioxide and waste products. After the blood exits the capillaries it enters the veins to return to the heart and lungs, where the circulation began.

Although they are very small, the capillaries are an important part of the circulatory system. Because the capillaries are where the transfer of oxygen, nutrients, and waste products to and from the cells takes place, it is vital that blood reach each capillary throughout the body. When blood reaches and fills the capillaries, supplying oxygen and nutrients to the cells and tissues, it is called **perfusion.** Without perfusion via the capillaries, oxygen does not reach vital tissues and organs, and dangerous waste products build up in the cells and tissues.

BLEEDING

Bleeding has a devastating effect on perfusion. There is only so much blood to circulate. Once a certain amount of the body's blood volume is lost, perfusion of all capillaries will not occur. The parts of the body that are not perfused will eventually experience tissue death. The brain, nerve cells, and kidneys are especially sensitive to decreased perfusion.

The term **hemorrhage** (HEM-o-rej) means bleeding. Bleeding can be classified as external or internal.

External Bleeding

The use of BSI precautions is essential whenever bleeding is discovered or anticipated. Patients who are bleeding or have open wounds pose a high risk of infection to the EMT-B. Remember that protective gloves must be worn with any bleeding patient. Additionally, protective eyewear will also be required in many cases since the probability of blood spatter reaching the eyes is great. With profuse bleeding, arterial bleeding, or if the patient spits or coughs blood, gowns and masks are required. Even though body substance isolation is designed to prevent any contact with fluids, ALWAYS wash your hands immediately after every call.

In addition to being classified as external or internal, bleeding can be classified as to the type of vessel losing the blood. At the EMT-B level of care, this is done only for external bleeding. External bleeding (Figure 25-2) is classified into three types.

- Arterial Bleeding—the blood loss from an artery. Remember that the artery is the first type of vessel the blood is pumped into as it leaves the heart. Arteries have strong walls that hold blood under high pressure. Therefore, the bleeding from an artery is often rapid, spurting with each heartbeat, and profuse. The blood that comes from an artery is usually bright red.

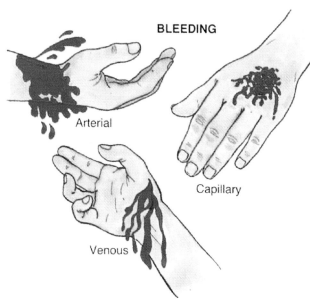

BLEEDING

Arterial

Capillary

Venous

FIGURE 25-2 The three types of external bleeding.

- Venous Bleeding—the loss of blood from a vein. Veins carry blood under lower pressures and return it to the heart. Venous bleeding is usually a steady flow and can be quite heavy. Venous blood is usually dark red or maroon in color.
- Capillary Bleeding—the loss of blood from a capillary. Since capillaries are very small, bleeding from a capillary area, or capillary "bed," is usually slow, often described as "oozing." The color of the blood is red, usually not as bright as arterial blood.

Although the treatments for all types of external bleeding are the same, the type of bleeding (arterial, venous, or capillary) may alert the EMT-B to some additional information. Arterial bleeding is often profuse. Since it is under high pressure, clot formation (which stops bleeding naturally) is difficult. Bleeding control measures may be required during the entire trip to the hospital. Veins sometimes pose special problems. Large veins may suck in debris and air bubbles. This is a serious problem with large veins, such as those in the neck. A bubble of air in the bloodstream, known as an air embolism, may be carried directly to the heart and interfere with or actually stop the heartbeat. The lungs and brain are also sensitive to air emboli.

Capillary bleeding is usually the result of a minor wound or scrape. This type of injury is often associated with contamination of the skin and the chance of infection. Large wounds often have capillary bleeding from the edges in addition to another type of bleeding from a vessel deeper in the wound.

Blood Loss and Patient Condition

Blood loss can range from very minor to fatal. Determining the severity of blood loss and relating this to the patient condition is very important. In an adult, the sudden loss of one liter (1000 cc) of blood is considered serious. In a child, one-half liter (500 cc) is serious. For an infant, who may only have 500 to 800 cc total blood volume, the loss of even 100 cc is serious.

In most patients with minor wounds, blood clots naturally. Some blood vessels may naturally constrict to help reduce blood loss. In patients with more severe wounds, or those with disorders in which blood will not clot naturally, a more severe blood loss may occur. Wounds that are wide or deep may not clot easily.

Although it is difficult to estimate the exact amount of blood lost, it is important that you recognize potentially serious blood loss and the condition of the patient as a result of the blood loss. Severe or uncontrolled blood loss will lead to shock (hypoperfusion) and eventual death. (Shock will be discussed later in this chapter.)

Patient Assessment—External Bleeding

An estimate of the amount of external blood loss is important in terms of predicting possible shock, sorting patients for triage, and identifying bleeding that must be treated during the initial assessment. (Slow bleeding that normally could wait for later treatment may be a priority if it has been steady for a long period of time and the blood loss has become significant.)

Estimating external blood loss may be difficult. Blood may flow to the floor or may be absorbed by furniture, carpeting, or clothing. In any event, it is difficult to make an objective determination of the amount of blood loss. To help form a concept of blood loss, pour a pint of water on the floor next to a fellow student or a manikin. Try soaking an article of clothing with a pint of water and note how much of the article is wet and how wet it feels to your touch. (See also Figure 25-3.)

Since it is difficult to determine the quantity of blood loss, it is important also to observe for other signs of hemorrhage.

Signs

A patient who has experienced significant blood loss will display signs of shock (shock

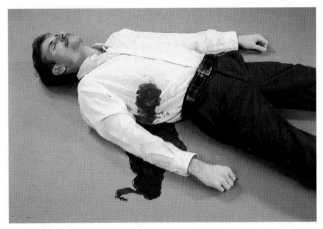

FIGURE 25-3 Estimating external blood loss: ½ liter (approximately 1 pint)

will be discussed later in this chapter). The signs of shock are listed in Table 25-1.

Remember: Regardless of the apparent volume of blood loss, if the patient has any of the indications of shock, then the bleeding must be classified as serious. However, you should not wait for signs of shock to be present before beginning treatment. In fact, *when shock is evident it may be too late!* Any patient with a significant amount (more than a small cut or scrape) of blood loss should cause you to be alert for, and prevent, the development of shock.

TABLE 25-1   Signs of Shock

Signs (in order of appearance)	Description
Altered Mental Status	Altered mental status occurs because the brain is not receiving enough oxygen. The brain is very sensitive to oxygen deficiencies. When it is deprived of oxygen, even slightly, behavioral changes may be noted. These changes may be seen as anxiety, restlessness, and even combativeness.
Pale, Cool, Clammy Skin	When the body senses low blood volume, natural mechanisms take over in an attempt to correct the problem. One of these mechanisms is to divert blood from non-vital areas to be rerouted to vital organs. Blood is quickly directed away from the skin to such organs as the heart and brain, and this results in the loss of color and temperature in the skin. Infants and children may begin to exhibit capillary refill times of greater than two seconds.
Nausea and Vomiting	In the body's continuing effort to keep blood perfusing vital organs, blood is diverted from the digestive system. This causes feelings of nausea and occasional vomiting.
Vital Sign Changes	The first vital signs to change are the pulse and respirations. • *The pulse* will increase in an attempt to pump more blood. As the pulse gradually increases, it becomes weak and thready. • *Respirations* also increase. The respirations will become more shallow and labored as the shock progresses. • Blood pressure is one of the last signs to change. When the blood pressure drops, the patient is clearly in a state of serious, life-threatening shock.

Other signs of shock that you may encounter include thirst, dilated pupils, and in some cases cyanosis (blue color), especially in the lips and nail beds.

Controlling External Bleeding

The control of external bleeding is an important skill. If left uncontrolled, bleeding may lead to shock and death.

Patient Care—External Bleeding

Emergency Care Steps

Care for airway, breathing, and circulation. The major methods used to control external bleeding are (Scan 25-1)

■ Direct pressure
■ Elevation
■ Pressure Points

Applying a tourniquet is a last-resort method of bleeding control. Other methods used to assist in bleeding control are splinting, cold application, and the use of a pneumatic anti-shock garment (PASG). These methods will be discussed below.

In addition to these manual methods of bleeding control, an important treatment for any bleeding patient is

■ Oxygen—Since blood loss reduces perfusion and the supply of oxygen to the tissues, the use of supplemental oxygen is vital. Oxygen should be administered after the bleeding has been controlled. Never delay the manual methods of bleeding control to set up or deliver oxygen to the patient.

Remember: Infection control is a vitally important consideration when you are attempting to control bleeding. Always wear disposable gloves while performing bleeding control, applying dressings, or cleaning up after a bleeding patient. Follow your local infection exposure control plan with regard to disposing of blood-stained sheets and other materials. When there is spurting or possible splashing of blood,

Scan 25-1
Bleeding Control

FIRST take body substance isolation precautions.

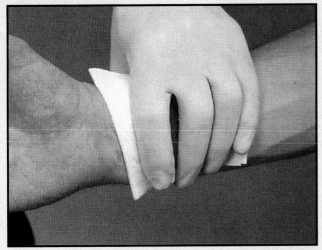

1. Apply direct pressure to the wound. You may cover the wound with a gauze pad. In cases of profuse bleeding, *do not* waste time looking for a pad. Provide pressure directly to the wound with your gloved hand.

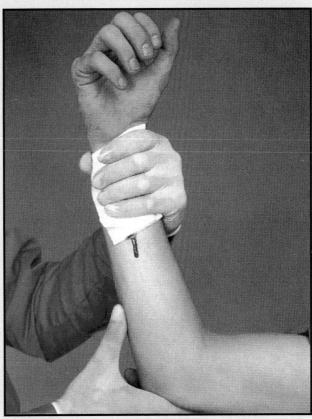

2. Elevate the extremity above the level of the heart.

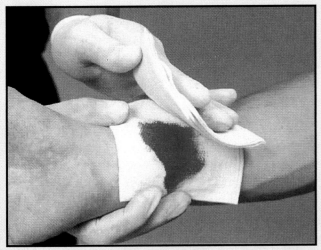

3. Apply a dressing to the wound. If the wound continues to bleed, apply additional dressings.

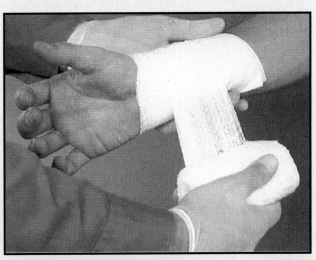

4. Bandage the dressing in place.

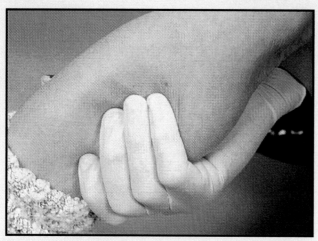

5. If wound still continues to bleed, apply pressure to appropriate arterial pressure point. Press the brachial artery pressure point to control bleeding from the arm.

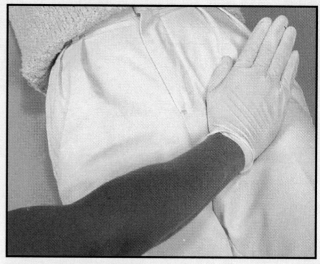

Press the femoral artery to control bleeding from the leg.

wear a mask, goggles or eyeshield, and a protective gown.

Direct Pressure The most acceptable method of controlling external bleeding is by applying pressure directly to the wound (Scan 25-1 and Figure 25-4). Direct pressure can be applied by your gloved hand, by a dressing and your hand, or by a pressure dressing. Always wear protective gloves.

When bleeding is MILD, you should

1. Apply pressure to the wound until the bleeding is controlled. (A clean handkerchief or cloth can be used if a sterile dressing is not immediately available.)
2. Hold pressure firmly on the wound until the bleeding is controlled. Your aim is to control the bleeding and limit additional significant blood loss.
3. Once bleeding is controlled, secure the dressing in place with bandaging.
4. Never remove a dressing once it is in place. To do so may restart bleeding or cause additional injury to the site. Apply another dressing on top of the blood-soaked one and hold them both in place. Continue the pressure until bleeding is controlled or until you deliver the patient to the staff of a medical facility.

If bleeding is PROFUSE, you should

1. Not waste time trying to find a dressing (Figure 25-4).

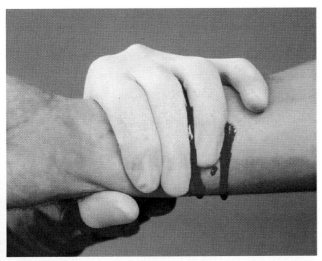

FIGURE 25-4 In cases of profuse bleeding, do not waste time hunting for a dressing.

2. Place your gloved hand directly on the wound and exert firm pressure.
3. Keep applying steady, firm pressure until the bleeding is controlled.
4. Once bleeding is controlled, bandage a dressing firmly in place to form a pressure dressing.

A **pressure dressing** can be applied to establish enough direct pressure to control most bleeding. Several sterile gauze pad dressings are placed on the wound. A bulky dressing is placed over the gauze pads. An effective bulky dressing for a severely bleeding wound is the combined, or universal, dressing. Sanitary napkins also can be used. The dressings should be held in place with a self-adhering roller bandage wrapped tightly over the dressing and above and below the wound site. Enough pressure must be created to control the bleeding.

Note: After controlling the bleeding from an extremity using a pressure dressing, check for a distal pulse to be certain that the dressing has not restricted blood flow in the treated limb. If you do not feel a pulse, you may have to adjust the pressure to reestablish circulation. Frequent checks of the distal pulse should continue throughout your care for the patient. In some cases, the severing of a major artery will stop the circulation needed to produce a pulse.

The dressings should not be removed once they are applied. If bleeding continues, more pressure can be added using the palm of your gloved hand, or a tighter bandage can be applied. In some cases, you may have to create more bulk by adding dressings. In rare cases, you may have to remove a blood-soaked bulky bandage leaving the initial dressing in place so that bleeding can be controlled by direct pressure.

A variety of dressings can be used in emergency situations. Some of these are shown in Figure 25-5.

Be aware that, in certain areas of the body, you may be unable to apply an effective pressure dressing, for example when bleeding is from the armpit. You may have to maintain pressure by holding your gloved hand directly over the wound. Even though you may be contaminating the wound, the risk of uncontrolled bleeding far outweighs that of possible infection.

Remember: Direct pressure is usually the quickest and most efficient means of controlling external bleeding.

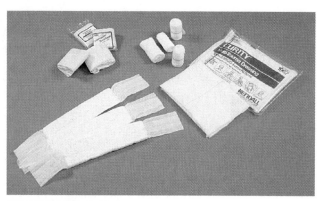

FIGURE 25-5 Dressings.

Elevation This method is used along with direct pressure (Scan 25-1). When an injured extremity is elevated so that the wound is above the level of the heart, gravity helps to reduce blood pressure, thus slowing bleeding. This method should not be used if there are possible musculoskeletal injuries to the extremity, objects impaled in the extremity, or possible spinal injury. To use elevation, you should

1. Apply direct pressure to the site of bleeding.
2. Elevate the injured extremity. If the forearm is bleeding, simply elevate the forearm. You do not have to elevate the entire limb.

Pressure Points If direct pressure or direct pressure and elevation fail, your next approach may be the use of pressure points (Figure 25-6). A **pressure point** is a site where a main artery lies near the surface of the body and directly over a bone (these correspond well to pulse sites). Four sites (two on each side) are used to control profuse bleeding in field emergency care. These sites are the

- **Brachial** (BRAY-ke-al) **artery**—for bleeding from the upper limb
- **Femoral** (FEM-o-ral) **artery**—for bleeding from the lower limb

The use of pressure points requires skill. Unless you know the exact location of the point and how much pressure to apply, the pressure point technique is of no use.

Remember: Pressure point techniques are to be used only after direct pressure or direct pressure and elevation have failed to control the bleeding.

Following are guidelines for controlling bleeding from the extremities using pressure points.

- *Bleeding from the Upper Extremity*—Apply pressure to a point over the brachial artery (Scan 25-1). To find the artery, hold the patient's arm out at a right angle to his body, with the palm facing up. (If it is not possible to raise the arm this far, do the best you can without forcing the arm or aggra-

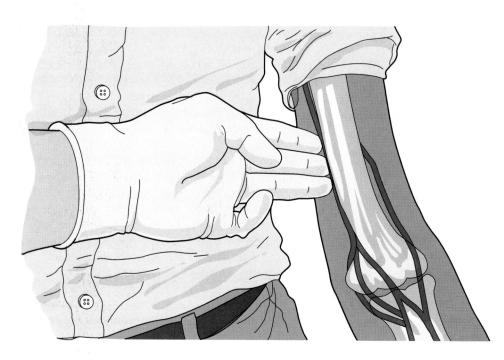

FIGURE 25-6 The use of pressure points can stop profuse bleeding from an arm or leg.

vating an injury.) Find the groove between the biceps muscle and the arm bone (humerus), about midway between the elbow and the armpit. Cradle the upper arm in the palm of your hand and position your fingers into this medial groove. You can now compress the brachial artery against the underlying bone by pressing your finger into this groove. If pressure is properly applied, you will not be able to feel a radial pulse. If the wound is to the distal end of the limb, bleeding may not be effectively controlled by this method. This is because blood is being sent to this region from many smaller arteries that have branched off of the major arteries in the limb.

- *Bleeding from the Lower Extremity*—Apply pressure to a point over the femoral artery (Scan 25-1). Locate this artery on the medial side of the thigh where it joins the lower trunk. You should be able to feel pulsations at a point just below the groin. Place the heel of your hand over the site and exert pressure downward toward the bone until it is obvious that the bleeding has been controlled. You will need more pressure than that applied for the brachial artery pressure point. Considerable force must be exerted if the patient is very muscular or obese. If pressure is properly applied, a distal pulse cannot be felt. As discussed above for the upper extremity, this method may not control bleeding for distal wounds.

Tourniquet A **tourniquet** (TURN-i-ket) is a device that constricts all blood flow to and from an extremity. THIS PROCEDURE IS A LAST RESORT, used only when other methods to control life-threatening bleeding have failed. Experienced EMT-Bs realize that the use of a tourniquet is a "life or limb" situation. The use of the tourniquet will stop the life-threatening bleeding, but it sometimes results in the loss of the limb the tourniquet is applied to.

Fortunately, when direct pressure and pressure dressings, elevation, and pressure points are used effectively, tourniquets are rarely needed.

Clean-edged amputations often do not require the application of a tourniquet. This is because many of the injured blood vessels seal shut as a result of spasms produced in their muscular walls (vasospasms). Bulky pressure dressings are very effective in controlling the bleeding associated with this type of injury.

Rough-edged amputations, usually produced by crushing or tearing injuries, often bleed freely since the nature of the injury does not allow for effective vasospasms. This type of amputation may cause more persistent bleeding that may require a tourniquet to control. However, never apply a tourniquet before trying direct pressure, elevation, and pressure points first.

Tourniquets are used only for wounds of the extremities. Do not apply a tourniquet directly over the knee or elbow. The tourniquet should be made of a wide material, preferably 4 inches in width and 6 to 8 layers thick. There are commercially made tourniquets, or a makeshift device may be made from a cravat or other wide, soft material. Among the items that should never be used as a tourniquet are ropes, wires, and other narrow items that may cut into the skin.

Once a tourniquet is in place, it should not be removed or loosened unless ordered by medical direction. Loosening of the tourniquet may dislodge clots and cause bleeding to resume. This will add to the blood loss that occurred prior to tourniquet application and almost certainly cause severe shock. Another complication of tourniquet removal or loosening is tourniquet shock. Severely injured tissues release harmful substances that gather below the level of the tourniquet. If the tourniquet is loosened or released, these substances may be released in high concentrations to the rest of the body. If you keep the tourniquet in place, the patient has a better chance of survival, even if it means the loss of a limb.

Remember: The tourniquet is only to be used as a last resort. The device itself should be made of a wide material that will not cut into a patient's skin. The devices are only to be used on extremities but not directly over a joint. Once a tourniquet has been applied, it should not be loosened or removed in the field.

While you are applying a tourniquet, you may have another rescuer apply direct pressure and pressure point techniques. This may slow the bleeding and reduce blood loss until the tourniquet is in place. To apply a tourniquet, you should (Figure 25-7)

1. Select a place between the heart and the wound, as close as possible to, but not even with, the edge of the wound. This should be within 2 inches of the wound. If the wound is on a joint, apply the tourniquet above the joint (toward the heart).

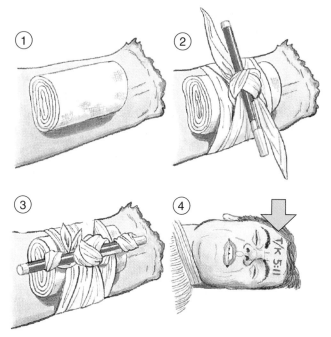

FIGURE 25-7 Application of a tourniquet.

2. Place a pad made from a dressing (a roll of gauze bandage) or a folded handkerchief over the main supplying artery before applying the constricting band. This will help protect the site and will apply additional pressure over the artery.

3. If a commercial tourniquet is used, carefully place it around the limb at the site and pull the free end of the band through the buckle or friction catch and draw this end tightly over the pad. You should tighten the tourniquet to the point where bleeding is controlled. Do not tighten the tourniquet beyond this point.

   If you are using cravats or other pieces of material, carefully slip the material around the injured limb and tie a knot with the ends of the tourniquet. The knot should be over the pad. A stick, rod, or similar device should be inserted into the knot and used to tighten the tourniquet. Turn the device until bleeding is controlled. Do not tighten beyond this point. Tape or tie the tightening device in place. KEEP THE TOURNIQUET IN PLACE. DO NOT LOOSEN.

4. Attach a notation to the patient to indicate that a tourniquet has been applied and the time of application. Note the location of the tourniquet and the time it was applied on your prehospital care report. Make certain that you do not cover the extremity to which the tourniquet has been applied.

This is done for the visual monitoring of the effectiveness of the tourniquet and to ensure that the tourniquet does not go unnoticed.

It is the EMT-B's responsibility to advise the emergency department staff of the application of a tourniquet. Even if this is done via radio, it must also be done in person at the hospital.

There may be instances in which you arrive at a scene and find that bystanders have applied a tourniquet. Most EMS systems have standard operating procedures that must be followed in such cases. Sometimes bystanders apply tourniquets thinking that this is a proper procedure for all bleeding. If the EMT-B can determine that the bleeding was not severe and may be controllable by means other than a tourniquet and that the tourniquet has not been in place for long, and if your local EMS guidelines permit, the tourniquet may be released while someone applies direct pressure to the wound site. Follow your local EMS guidelines. If in doubt, radio for medical direction.

Blood Pressure Cuff This device can be applied as a tourniquet to control apparently life-threatening arterial bleeding from an extremity. The cuff is placed above the wound (between the wound and the heart) and inflated to the pressure required to control the bleeding. This is usually in the 150-mm Hg range for persons with normal blood pressure. A dressing and bandage is secured after the bleeding is controlled. The cuff can safely be left inflated for up to 30 minutes or more; however, it must be closely monitored to make certain that cuff pressure is not lost.

Splinting The splinting of musculoskeletal injuries will be covered in Chapter 27. Often when an injured extremity is splinted, bleeding associated with the injury may be controlled (Figure 25-8). This occurs when the sharp ends of broken bones are stabilized, preventing additional damage to blood vessels at the injury site.

Inflatable splints, also called air splints, are sometimes used to help control internal and external bleeding from an extremity, even when there is no suspected bone or joint injury. They may be useful when a severe laceration extends over the length of the extremity. The pressure produced by the splint is a form of direct pressure.

Since these splints are inflated by mouth, there is a limit to the amount of pressure produced. The pressure may not be sufficient to

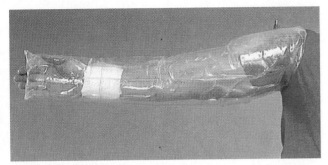

FIGURE 25-8 Inflatable splints are sometimes used to help control internal and external bleeding from an extremity, even when there is no other suspected injury.

control arterial bleeding and may even make it worse. However, these devices can be helpful in maintaining pressure after other manual methods have already controlled bleeding.

Cold Application   The application of ice or cold packs to an injury has been done for centuries. Cold minimizes swelling and reduces bleeding by constricting blood vessels. It does not, by itself, control bleeding, but it may be useful in combination with other techniques. Cold application can also help reduce the pain of the injury that caused the bleeding.

Ice or cold packs should never be applied directly to the skin. Prolonged contact may actually cause frostbite. Wrap the ice pack in a cloth or towel before placing it against the skin, and do not leave it there for more than 20 minutes at a time.

Pneumatic Anti-Shock Garment (PASG)   Although the use of anti-shock garments is controversial, many experts agree that they are useful for controlling bleeding from areas the garment covers. Refer to your local protocols for information on how your EMS system uses anti-shock garments. The PASG will be discussed in Chapter 27, Musculoskeletal Injuries.

Other Situations Involving Bleeding

While bleeding is usually the result of some type of direct trauma, there are other situations in which you may encounter bleeding.

Head Injury   Injuries such as a fractured skull may cause bleeding or the loss of a clear fluid from the ears or nose. This blood or fluid loss is not due to trauma to the ears or nose directly. It is a secondary problem as a result of the skull fracture. In this case, the bleeding or clear fluid should not be stopped. Use a sterile gauze pad to collect the drainage.

Nosebleed   Nosebleeds (epistaxis) may be caused by direct trauma. Occasionally, there are other, primarily medical, causes for the nosebleed. High blood pressure can cause nosebleeds. In a patient who exhibits a nosebleed with no apparent trauma, consider high blood pressure as a cause. Other causes may be sinus or respiratory infections, or nose picking.

To stop a nosebleed

1.   Have the patient get into a sitting position, leaning forward.
2.   Apply direct pressure by pinching nostrils.
3.   Keep the patient calm.
4.   If the patient becomes unconscious or is unable to maintain his own airway for any reason, turn on side and be prepared to provide suction and other airway maintenance techniques.

Internal Bleeding

Internal bleeding, as implied by the name, is bleeding that occurs inside the body. This type of bleeding is serious for several reasons.

- There are many internal organs and large blood vessels under the skin. Damage to one of these structures can result in the loss of a large quantity of blood in a very short period of time.
- The blood loss is hidden. External bleeding is easy to identify. This is not the case with internal bleeding. A person can bleed to death without ever spilling a drop of blood outside of the body.
- Severe blood loss may occur even from injury to the extremities. A fractured femur can be the site of enough blood loss to cause severe shock.

Patient Assessment—Internal Bleeding

Since internal bleeding may not be obvious, it is up to you, as an EMT-B, to identify patients who may have internal bleeding. This is done by performing a thorough history and physical exam with special attention to mechanism of injury.

If the patient has a mechanism of injury that suggests internal bleeding, consider that patient as having internal bleeding and treat accordingly. Treatment for internal injuries will not cause harm. Not treating these injuries may have serious consequences.

Blunt trauma is a leading cause of internal injuries. Mechanisms of blunt trauma which may cause internal injuries include

- ☐ Falls
- ☐ Motor vehicle or motorcycle crashes
- ☐ Auto-pedestrian collisions
- ☐ Blast injuries

Penetrating trauma may also cause internal injuries. Examples of mechanism of injury that are caused by penetrating trauma include

- ☐ Gunshot wounds
- ☐ Knife wounds and stabbings
- ☐ Impaled objects

Signs

Specific signs of internal bleeding may be present in patients that you encounter. Many of the signs and symptoms seen are those of shock, which has developed as a result of the uncontrolled internal bleeding. These are *late* signs and indicate that a serious condition has already developed. Do not wait for signs of internal injuries or shock to develop to treat the patient. Signs of internal bleeding are

- ☐ Injuries to the surface of the body that indicate underlying injury
- ☐ Bruises (Figure 25-9), swelling, or pain over vital organs (especially in the chest and abdomen)

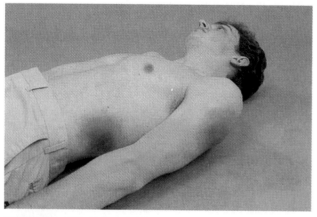

FIGURE 25-9 Bruising is one sign of internal bleeding.

- ☐ Painful, swollen, and deformed extremities
- ☐ Bleeding from the mouth, rectum, vagina, or other body orifice
- ☐ Tender, rigid, or distended abdomen
- ☐ Vomiting a coffee ground-like substance or bright red vomitus
- ☐ Dark, tarry stools, or bright red blood in stool
- ☐ Signs and symptoms of shock. (See Table 25-1). These are late signs, occurring after internal bleeding has already caused significant blood loss.

Patient Care—Internal Bleeding

Care for the patient with internal bleeding centers around the prevention and treatment of shock. As with any patient, airway, breathing, and circulation are the first priority. Since a patient with internal bleeding may deteriorate rapidly, monitor the ABCs often. Be prepared to assist ventilations, or provide CPR as needed.

1. Maintain ABCs and provide support as needed.
2. Administer high concentration oxygen by nonrebreather mask (if this was not already done in the initial assessment phase of care).
3. Control any external bleeding. If internal bleeding is suspected in an extremity, apply a splint.
4. Provide prompt transport to an appropriate facility for any patient with suspected internal bleeding. While emergency care steps are important, the patient requires care at a hospital and possible emergency surgery. Since this cannot be performed in the field, prompt transport is required.

SHOCK

Shock, also known as **hypoperfusion** or **hypoperfusion syndrome,** is the inability of the body to supply (perfuse) cells with oxygen and nutrients. (*Hypo* means "less than"; *hypoperfusion* means "less-than-adequate perfusion.") Hypoperfusion also causes the inadequate removal of waste products from the cells. Shock, if not treated, results in death.

Causes of Shock

The heart and the blood vessels make up the *vascular container*, the system that contains the body's blood. To function properly, this container must be filled with blood, which must be efficiently pumped by the heart. The failure of perfusion that causes shock happens when the vascular container is not filled.

Three elements of the vascular system—the heart, the blood, and the blood vessels—can be related to the failure to keep the vascular container full and the consequent development of shock.

- The Heart—If the heart fails to pump blood efficiently enough to keep the vascular container filled, shock will develop.
- The Blood—There must be enough blood to fill the vascular container. A serious loss of blood will lead to shock.
- The Blood Vessels—The vascular container must not be too large for the volume of blood. Dilation (expansion) of some blood vessels—without sufficient constriction (shrinking or contraction) of other blood vessels to compensate—can cause shock.

If there is a failure of any of these three factors—the pumping of the heart, the supply of blood, or the dilation and compensatory constriction of the blood vessels—perfusion of the brain, lungs, and other body organs will not be adequate.

Understanding the role of the blood vessels in the development of shock is important. Blood vessels can change their diameter. If an area of the body requires more blood because it is doing more work, the vessels in that area dilate as needed to allow greater flow. At the same time, another area of the body that does not require the extra blood flow may constrict its vessels to reduce the blood flow in that area and help keep the overall system filled with blood. For example, if you are running, blood flow to the muscles increases through dilated arteries. At the same time, blood flow to the stomach and intestines lessens because vessels supplying these organs have constricted.

If all the vessels in the body dilated at once, there would not be nearly enough blood to fill the entire system, causing circulation to fail. Whenever too many vessels dilate to allow for adequate perfusion (filling the capillaries), shock develops.

As shock develops, the failure of any one part of the vascular system can create problems in the other parts. For example, if blood is being lost through bleeding, the heart rate will increase in an effort to circulate blood to all the vital tissues. This action causes more blood to be lost. Immediately, the body will react to this additional blood loss by again increasing the heart rate. This process will continue until it leads to the death of the patient.

At the onset of shock, the body tries to adjust to the loss of blood, improper heart activity, or the dilation of too many blood vessels. However, at a certain point in some types of shock, enough blood has been lost so that the system is no longer filled, no matter how hard the heart pumps or how much the blood vessels constrict. In other cases of shock, the heart becomes too inefficient in circulating blood and perfusion fails. There are also cases in which there is no loss of blood volume and the heart is performing properly, but too many vessels are dilated. For these cases, there is too much volume (capacity) in the system to be filled by the available blood.

Regardless of the mechanism, shock is the failure of the cardiovascular system to provide sufficient blood and oxygen to all the vital tissues of the body.

Remember: Shock may develop (1) if the heart fails as a pump, or (2) blood volume is lost, or (3) blood vessels dilate to create a vascular container capacity too great to be filled by the available blood.

Hypovolemic shock (or **hemorrhagic shock**), is caused by a low blood volume. Traumatic injury with resulting bleeding—either external, internal or both—is the most common cause of shock.

Fainting is an example of temporary hypoperfusion when the blood vessels suddenly dilate. A sudden emotional reaction or frightening experience occasionally causes a person to pass out. The person obviously hasn't been bleeding. Suddenly, as a result of the emotional reaction, the body dilated too many blood vessels at the same time causing a temporary lack of perfusion to the brain. Once the person falls to the ground, blood is able to perfuse the brain more readily and the patient rapidly regains consciousness. Other, more serious causes include severe nervous system reaction to illness or injury.

Shock may also be caused by problems with the heart. If the heart does not beat properly, blood will not be circulated to the body. This is another cause of poor perfusion. There is an adequate blood volume and good control over the blood vessels, but the pump is not functioning properly. Persons having a heart attack may sustain damage to the wall of the heart. It is not able to contract as forcefully as it once did. This causes reduced output, leading to shock.

As you can see, shock can actually be caused by many factors within the body. Fortunately, the treatment for most types of shock is the same regardless of the cause.

Patient Assessment—Shock

The signs and symptoms for shock are the same no matter what the cause of shock. The symptoms follow a logical progression as shock develops and then worsens (Table 25-1 and Figure 25-10). The signs and symptoms, in order of appearance, are as follows (this may vary slightly from patient to patient). A brief reason for each sign or symptom is given.

☐ Altered Mental Status—This occurs because the brain is not receiving enough oxygen. The brain is very sensitive to oxygen deficiencies. When it is deprived of oxygen, even slightly, behavioral changes may be noted. These changes may be seen as anxiety, restlessness, and even combativeness.

☐ Pale, Cool, Clammy Skin—When the body senses low blood volume, natural mechanisms take over in an attempt to correct the problem. One of these mechanisms is to divert blood from non-vital areas to be rerouted to vital organs. Blood is quickly directed away from the skin to such organs as the heart and brain, and this results in the loss of color and temperature in the skin. Infants and children may begin to exhibit capillary refill times of greater than two seconds.

☐ Nausea and Vomiting—In the body's continuing effort to keep blood perfusing vital organs, blood is diverted from the digestive system. This causes feelings of nausea and occasional vomiting.

☐ Vital Sign Changes—The first vital signs to change are the pulse and respirations.

- The *pulse* will increase in an attempt to pump more blood. As the pulse gradually increases, it becomes weak and thready.
- *Respirations* also increase. The respirations will become more shallow and labored as the shock progresses.
- *Blood pressure* is one of the last signs to change. When the blood pressure drops, the patient is clearly in a state of serious, life-threatening shock.

☐ Other Signs—Others signs of shock that you may encounter include thirst, dilated pupils, and in some cases cyanosis (blue color), especially in the lips and nail beds.

Infants and Children

Infants and children can maintain their blood pressure until more than half of their blood volume is gone. By the time their blood pressure drops, they are near death. Additionally, children and infants have less blood volume in reserve. *This means that shock must be considered and cared for early—without waiting for the appearance of the signs of shock—in all children and infants with bleeding or traumatic injury.*

You may have noticed, above, that the body has mechanisms that attempt to compensate for the loss of blood and lack of perfusion. You may hear the term **compensated shock.** This means that the patient is developing shock but the body

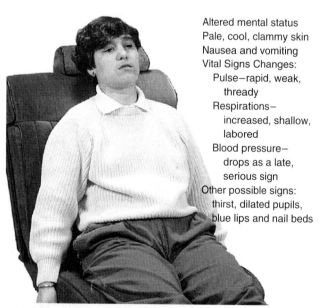

Altered mental status
Pale, cool, clammy skin
Nausea and vomiting
Vital Signs Changes:
    Pulse—rapid, weak, thready
    Respirations—increased, shallow, labored
    Blood pressure—drops as a late, serious sign
Other possible signs:
    thirst, dilated pupils, blue lips and nail beds

FIGURE 25-10 Signs and symptoms of shock.

has been able to maintain perfusion. Some signs may be evident, such as elevated heart rate, but the patient does not appear "shocky." This is one reason that full patient assessments and considering the mechanism of injury are so important. If you wait for the blood pressure to drop or signs of shock to become obvious, *it is too late.*

Decompensated shock occurs when the body can no longer compensate for the low blood volume or lack of perfusion. The late signs and symptoms such as decreasing blood pressure become evident.

Emergency Care for Shock

The principles of care for shock include airway maintenance and oxygen administration, attempting to stop what is causing the shock (external bleeding), and measures to attempt to maintain perfusion.

As important as the treatments you will provide as an EMT-B is *recognizing shock and initiating immediate transport.* There is a term in trauma care called the **"golden hour,"** which refers to the optimum limit of one hour between time of injury and surgery at the hospital. Survival rates are best if surgery takes place within the golden hour. The goal of shock and trauma care is to provide immediate transportation from the scene to the hospital so the patient can be seen in the emergency department and moved to surgery within one hour from the time of injury.

In EMS there is a **"platinum ten minutes,"** which refers to an optimum limit of ten minutes (excluding extrication time) at the scene with a serious trauma patient in order for the patient to receive surgery within the golden hour after time of injury. In order for the patient to get to surgery within the hour, scene procedures must be kept to a minimum. In patients in whom there are signs of shock, or a mechanism of injury that makes internal injuries seem possible, some elements of assessment and care must be done en route to the hospital. Many parts of our care may be more beneficial to the patient if they are performed en route to the hospital to prevent delay at the scene.

Recall Brian Mitchell, your On the Scene patient from the beginning of this chapter. His injuries were serious and shock was developing. Realizing this, you and your partner took appropriate actions including immediate transport. If too much time had been spent on the scene doing in-depth assessments and care, valuable minutes of the golden hour would have ticked away.

The need for immediate transport should never take the place of adequate care. ABCs must be assessed and spinal precautions must be taken before attempting to move any patient who may have a spine injury. It is important to complete the initial assessment to determine the patient priority and the focused history and physical exam for a trauma patient, immobilize the spine, and move to the ambulance. The detailed physical exam may be performed en route to the hospital. No harm has been done to the patient and you have begun the trip to the hospital as soon as possible. Always drive safely and responsibly to the hospital no matter how serious your patient may be.

Patient Care—Shock

The emergency care steps for shock (Scan 25-2) are as follows.

1. Maintain an open airway and assure the adequacy of respirations. Administer high concentration oxygen by nonrebreather mask if the patient is breathing adequately. Assist ventilations and perform CPR if it becomes necessary.
2. Control any external bleeding.
3. Apply and inflate the pneumatic anti-shock garment (PASG) if approved or ordered by local medical direction. The PASG is usually indicated for bleeding in areas covered by the suit, pelvic injury, and some abdominal trauma. In some areas, the suit is contraindicated (not to be used) when there are chest injuries.
4. Elevate the legs 8 to 12 inches. Do this only if there are no signs of injury to the legs, hips, or pelvis. This also should be avoided with spinal injuries and injury to the chest or abdomen or extremities or when using PASG. In these cases leave the patient supine.
5. Splint any suspected bone or joint injuries. In patients with shock, this should be done en route to the hospital. Do not take time to splint multiple injuries and waste valuable parts of the golden hour. If there are suspected injuries, place the patient on a backboard. This will serve to splint the whole body until further care can be given.
6. Keep the patient warm. Cover the patient with a blanket if the patient is in a cold or cool environment.
7. Transport the patient immediately. Notify the hospital of your impending arrival.

Shock Management

FIRST take body substance isolation precautions.

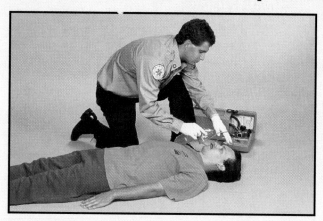

1. Maintain an open airway. Give high concentration oxygen by nonrebreather mask. Control external bleeding. Assist ventilations and perform CPR as necessary.

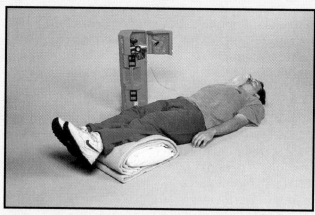

2. Properly position the patient. If there is no serious injury, usually position the patient supine with legs elevated 8 to 12 inches.

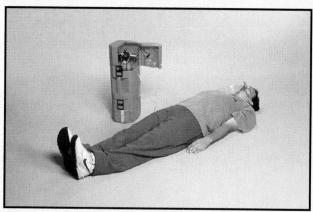

3. If there is any possibility of serious injuries to head, neck, spine, chest, abdomen, pelvis, hip, or extremities, position patient supine with NO elevation of extremities.

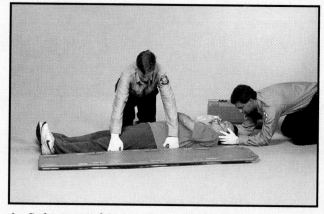

4. Splinting of bone and joint injuries can help control shock but should be done en route. Meanwhile, placing the patient on a spine board will have the effect of splinting the whole body.

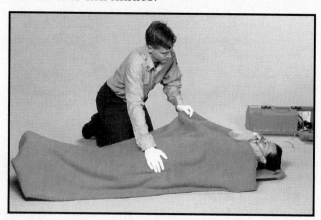

5. Protect the patient from heat loss.

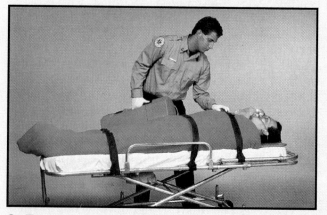

6. Transport immediately.

Provide information on the patient's injuries and current condition. Contact medical direction if necessary while en route. If there is an ALS agency available and your transport or extrication time may be extended, call for their assistance for the special interventions they are trained to perform.

> **Documentation Tips—Bleeding and Shock**
>
> In "painting a picture" of your patient in the narrative portion of the prehospital care report, be sure to describe significant things you saw at the scene that hospital personnel did not see, such as the mechanism of injury (an important clue to internal injuries and bleeding) and your best estimate or description of the amount of external blood loss.
>
> Assess vital signs early and reassess and record frequently. Remember, however, that vital sign changes such as a drop in blood pressure are *late* signs of shock. Be sure to pay special attention to mental status and the color, temperature, and condition of the skin. Changes in mental status and skin are *early* signs of shock and should be carefully documented.

FYI

Topics included in the FYI—"For Your Information"—section are those that go beyond the chapter objectives. The information in this segment is intended to broaden your understanding of the chapter topic but is not essential to an understanding of your job as an EMT-B.

Functions of Blood

While blood was discussed in the main portion of the chapter, there are several other functions of blood that were not mentioned. Some of these functions include

- Transportation of Gases—to carry oxygen from the lungs to the tissues and to carry carbon dioxide from the tissues to the lungs
- Nutrition—to carry food substances from the intestine or storage tissues (fatty tissue, the liver, and muscle cells) to the rest of the body tissues

- Excretion—to carry wastes away from the tissues to the organs of excretion (kidneys, lungs, and liver)
- Protection—to defend against disease-causing organisms by engulfing and digesting them, or by producing antibodies against them (immunity)
- Regulation—to carry hormones, water, salt, and other chemicals that control the functions of organs and glands. The regulation of body temperature is aided by the blood, which carries excessive body heat to the lungs and skin surface.

Types of Shock

Shock may accompany many emergency situations; thus treatment for it is included in emergency care procedures for virtually every serious injury and medical problem. Information provided below about these different types of shock are to expand your understanding of the condition. The treatment for most types of shock is identical.

- Hypovolemic (HI-po-vo-LE-mik) Shock—caused by the loss of blood or other body fluids. When shock develops due to blood loss or loss of plasma (a liquid that is a component of the blood), this form of hypovolemic shock is called hemorrhagic (HEM-or-AJ-ik) shock. Dehydration due to diarrhea, vomiting, or heavy perspiration can also lead to the development of hypovolemic shock.
- Cardiogenic (KAR-di-o-JEN-ic) Shock—caused by the heart failing to pump blood adequately to all vital parts of the body
- Neurogenic (NU-ro-JEN-ic) Shock—caused by the failure of the nervous system to control the diameter of blood vessels (seen with spinal cord injury). Once the blood vessels are dilated, there is not enough blood in circulation to fill this new volume, causing shock.
- Anaphylactic (AN-ah-fi-LAK-tik) Shock—a life-threatening reaction of the body to a substance to which the patient is extremely allergic. (Anaphylactic reactions were discussed in Chapter 20, Allergies.)
- Septic Shock—caused by severe infection. Toxins are released into the bloodstream and cause blood vessels to dilate, increasing the volume of the circulatory system beyond functional limits. In addition, plas-

ma is lost through vessel walls, causing a loss in blood volume. This type of shock is seldom seen by the EMT-B in the field since the patient is usually hospitalized before it occurs.

The most common form of serious shock associated with injury is the form of hypovolemic shock known as hemorrhagic shock (think of the word hemorrhage, meaning "bleeding"), due to the loss of blood. Bleeding can be external or internal. In addition to the loss of whole blood, enough plasma may also be lost to result in a severe drop in blood volume. This may be the case with burns and crushing injuries. A pre-existing condition of dehydration will hasten the reaction. Be alert to this in areas of high temperatures, such as warehouses and factories. This also can be a problem if the patient was sweating profusely prior to injury, as in sports and hunting accidents. Certain strenuous work situations, such as those of dock workers and steel workers, may cause enough body fluid loss prior to the accident to quicken the effects of blood loss.

Cardiogenic shock is usually brought about by injury to a heart valve or a heart attack. Many diseases, if allowed to go untreated, may eventually do enough heart damage to cause cardiogenic shock. Be on the alert for low blood pressure, edema (swelling) of the ankles, and the signs of heart failure (see Chapter 18, Cardiac Emergencies).

In neurogenic shock due to nerve paralysis caused by spinal cord injuries, there is no actual loss of blood but rather a dilation of blood vessels that increases the volume of the circulatory system beyond the point where it can be filled. Blood can no longer adequately fill the entire system and pools in the blood vessels in certain areas of the body.

CHAPTER REVIEW

KEY TERMS

You may find it helpful to review the following terms.

artery a blood vessel with thick, muscular walls that carries blood away from the heart.
brachial (BRAY-ke-al) **artery** the major artery of the upper arm.
capillary a microscopic blood vessel where oxygen/carbon dioxide and nutrient/waste exchange takes place.
compensated shock when the patient is developing shock but the body is still able to maintain perfusion. See *shock*.
decompensated shock occurs when the body can no longer compensate for low blood volume or lack of perfusion. Late signs such as decreasing blood pressure become evident. See *shock*.
femoral (FEM-or-al) **artery** the major artery supplying the thigh.
golden hour refers to the optimum limit of one hour between time of injury and surgery at the hospital. Survival rates are best if surgery takes place within the "golden hour." See also *platinum ten minutes*.
hemorrhage (HEM-o-rej) bleeding.

hemorrhagic (HEM-or-AJ-ik) **shock** shock resulting from blood loss.
hypoperfusion (HI-po-per-FEW-zhun) See *shock*.
hypoperfusion syndrome hypoperfusion. See *shock*.
hypovolemic (HI-po-vo-LE-mik) **shock** shock resulting from blood or fluid loss.
perfusion when blood reaches and fills the capillaries, supplying cells and tissues with oxygen and nutrients.
platinum ten minutes refers to an optimum limit of ten minutes at the scene with a serious trauma patient in order for the patient to receive surgery within an hour after time of injury. See *golden hour*.
pressure dressing a bulky dressing held in position with a tightly wrapped bandage to apply pressure to help control bleeding.
pressure point a site where a main artery lies near the surface of the body and directly over a bone. Pressure on such a point can stop distal bleeding (bleeding that is farther from the heart than the pressure point).
shock also known as *hypoperfusion* or *hypo-*

perfusion syndrome. The inability of the body adequately to circulate blood to the body's cells to supply (perfuse) the cells with oxygen and nutrients. A life-threatening condition. See also *compensated shock; decompensated shock; hemorrhagic shock; hypovolemic shock.*

tourniquet (TURN-i-ket) a device that constricts all blood flow to and from an extremity.
vein a blood vessel that carries blood back to the heart. A vein contains one-way valves that keep the blood flowing in the proper direction.

SUMMARY

Traumatic injuries may not be the most common calls you will respond to as an EMT-B, but they can be the most challenging. An understanding of the circulatory system is basic to an understanding of both bleeding and shock, two potentially life-threatening conditions often present when there are traumatic injuries.

Blood loss may be external or internal. The main procedures for controlling external blood loss are direct pressure, elevation, and the use of pressure points. (Remember that it is essential to take BSI precautions whenever you anticipate the possibility of coming into contact with blood.) Treatment for internal bleeding centers around the prevention and treatment of shock.

The mechanism of injury is very important in determining potential injury to a patient. Since the signs and symptoms of shock may not be evident early in the call, treating the patient based on the mechanism of injury may be life-saving.

Shock is a condition in which there is reduced perfusion to the tissues of the body. The body tries to compensate for this by shunting blood from the skin and digestive system and routing it to vital organs such as the brain and heart. These compensatory mechanisms can only work for so long. Once the body can no longer maintain perfusion to vital organs, signs of severe shock develop. Shock is usually first seen in a patient as restlessness or anxiety develops, the skin becomes pale, and eventually the pulse and respirations increase. Finally, the patient's blood pressure begins to drop.

Treatment for shock includes oxygen administration, airway maintenance, and preventing further progression of the shock. One of the most important treatments is immediate transport to the hospital so the patient can be given surgery and other care that can only be provided in the hospital.

REVIEW QUESTIONS

1. Describe what you would expect to see in arterial, venous, and capillary bleeding.
2. List the patient care steps in bleeding control.
3. Define *perfusion.*
4. List the signs and symptoms of shock. Which would you expect to see early? Which are late signs?
5. List the emergency care steps for treating a patient with shock.

Application

- A patient has been involved in a motor vehicle accident. There is considerable damage to his vehicle. The steering column and wheel are badly bent. He complains of a "sore chest." The patient's vital signs are pulse 116, respirations 20, blood pressure 106/70. Would you expect and treat for shock? Why or why not?

Soft Tissue Injuries

26

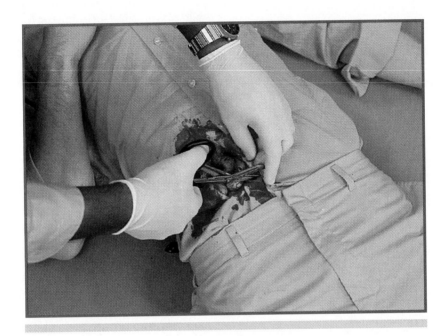

Injuries to the soft-tissues of the body are frequent calls for the EMT-B. These injuries may range from minor scrapes and bruises to life-threatening injuries to the chest and abdomen. It is the responsibility of the EMT-B to identify and treat each of these injuries skillfully and professionally. Many soft tissue injuries are open wounds, which may be very upsetting to the patient. Your emotional care and demeanor will mean a great deal. Overall, the assessment and care of the patient with soft tissue injury will be a challenging part of your responsibilities as an EMT-B.

Objectives

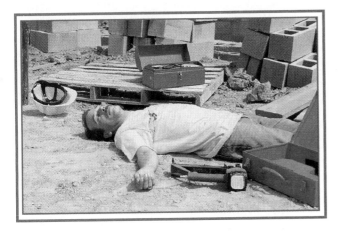

Tom Jansen has been in the construction business for many years. At the end of a work shift, he is packing his equipment and comes to the nail gun. This "gun" is used to shoot nails deep into wood. Unfortunately, while storing the gun, Tom accidentally triggers the device. A large nail is sent forcefully into his chest. A co-worker hears the groan and goes to Tom's aid. Another worker calls 911.

You arrive and *size up the scene* to assure safety. Another worker has already moved and properly stored the nail gun. There are no structural or other hazards from the construction site. As you put on gloves and protective eyewear, the co-worker explains the force behind the nail-gun. You make a mental note of the mechanism of injury and move toward Tom.

As you begin your *initial assessment,* you see that Tom is awake. He appears anxious. His color is pale and his respirations are labored. This is obvious even without trying to conduct an exam. Your general impression of this patient, based on his color, respiratory difficulty, and mechanism of injury is one of a critically injured patient. You greet Tom and he is able to respond. He is able to answer questions and seems alert. You observe a ripped portion of his T-shirt where a nail protrudes about an inch from his chest. You hear a sucking noise and observe bubbles near the wound. You cut away the shirt, seal the wound, and stabilize the nail with two gloved fingers on each side of the nail. Your partner places Tom on a nonrebreather oxygen mask at 15 lpm. He radios for ALS assistance and prepares an occlusive dressing for immediate treatment of this life-threatening injury.

After the chest wound is sealed and the nail stabilized, you begin the *focused history and physical exam* for a trauma patient. Meanwhile, your partner gets the stretcher to expedite transport. Tom did not fall or suffer any further injuries that you can detect during the rapid trauma exam. Tom is otherwise healthy and you obtain no significant information from the SAMPLE history. His vital signs are blood pressure 100/78, pulse 104, respirations 24. The nail is in the left side of his chest, and there are slightly decreased lung sounds on that side. His skin is pale, cool, and clammy. His pupils are normal.

You and your partner transfer Tom to the stretcher and move him to the ambulance. While en route, you conduct a *detailed physical exam* without further findings.

As part of an *ongoing assessment,* vitals are rechecked. Tom's blood pressure is now 96/70, pulse 128, respirations are 30. You radio your findings to the trauma center and the ALS unit. When you meet the ALS unit, a paramedic joins the crew and the trip to the hospital resumes.

Tom spends a short time in the emergency department and is wheeled off to surgery even before you get a chance to restock your equipment. Your treatments, and scene time of less than ten minutes, have given him a chance to survive this serious injury.

---

*I*njuries to the body can be classified as musculoskeletal (bone and joint) injuries and injuries to the soft tissues. Musculoskeletal injuries will be covered in Chapters 27 and 28. In this chapter, soft tissue injuries will be described.

THE SOFT TISSUES

The soft tissues of the body include the skin, fatty tissues, muscles, blood vessels, fibrous tissues, membranes (tissues that line or cover organs), glands, and nerves (Figure 26-1). The

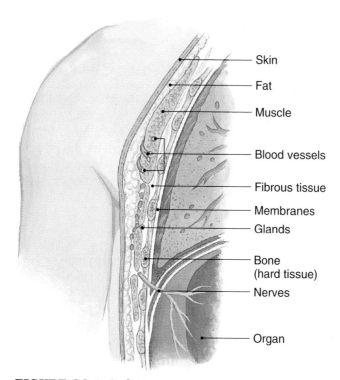

FIGURE 26-1 Soft tissues.

teeth, bones, and cartilage are considered hard tissues.

The most obvious soft tissue injuries involve the skin (Figure 26-2). Most people do not think of the skin as a body organ, but it is. In fact, it is the largest organ of the human body. The major functions of the skin include

- Protection—The skin serves as a barrier to keep out microorganisms (germs), debris, and unwanted chemicals. Underlying tissues and organs are protected from environmental contact.
- Water Balance—The skin helps prevent water loss and stops environmental water from entering the body. This helps preserve the chemical balance of body fluids and tissues.
- Temperature Regulation—Blood vessels in the skin can dilate (increase in diameter) to carry more blood to the skin, allowing heat to radiate from the body. When the body needs to conserve heat, these vessels constrict (decrease in diameter) to prevent heat

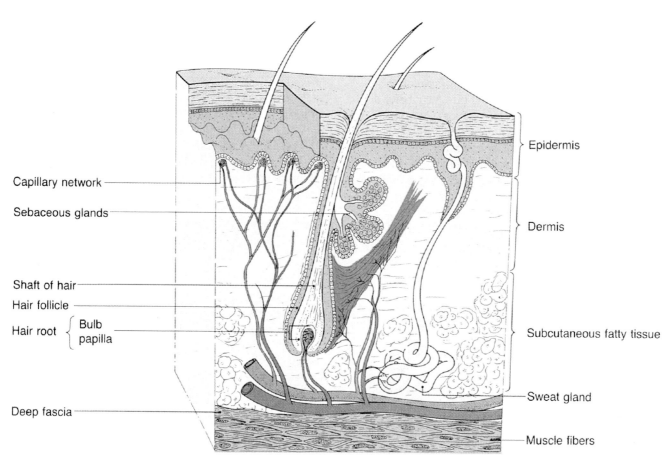

FIGURE 26-2 The skin.

loss. The sweat glands found in the skin produce perspiration, which will evaporate and help cool the body. The fat that is part of the skin serves as a thermal insulator.

- Excretion—Salts, carbon dioxide, and excess water can be released through the skin.
- Shock (impact) Absorption—The skin and its layers of fat help protect the underlying organs from minor impacts and pressures.

The skin has three major layers: the epidermis, the dermis, and the subcutaneous layer.

The outer layer of the skin is called the **epidermis** (ep-i-DER-mis). The outermost epidermis is composed of dead cells, which are rubbed off or sloughed off and are replaced. The pigment granules of the skin and living cells are found deeper in the epidermis. The cells of the innermost portion are actively dividing, replacing the dead cells of the outer layers. The epidermis contains no blood vessels or nerves. Except for certain types of burns and injuries due to cold, injuries of the epidermis present few problems in EMT-B-level care.

The layer of skin below the epidermis is the **dermis** (DER-mis). This layer is rich with blood vessels, nerves, and specialized structures such as sweat glands, sebaceous (oil) glands, and hair follicles. Specialized nerve endings in the dermis are involved with the senses of touch, cold, heat, and pain. Once the dermis is opened to the outside world, contamination and infection become major problems. Such wounds can be serious, accompanied by profuse bleeding and intense pain.

The layers of fat and soft tissue below the dermis are called the **subcutaneous** (SUB-ku-TAY-ne-us) **layers.** Shock absorption and insulation are major functions of this layer. Again, there are the problems of tissue and bloodstream contamination, bleeding, and pain when these layers re injured.

SOFT TIS UE INJURIES

Soft tissue injuries are generally classified as closed wounds or open wounds.

Closed Wounds

A **closed wound** is an internal injury; that is, there is no open pathway from the outside to the injured site. These wounds usually result from the impact of a blunt object. Although the skin itself may not be broken, there may be extensively crushed tissues beneath it. Closed wounds can be simple bruises, internal lacerations (cuts), and internal punctures caused by fractured bones, crushing forces, or the rupture (bursting open) of internal organs (Figure 26-3). Internal bleeding can range from minor to life threatening. As an EMT-B, you should always consider the possibility of closed soft tissue injuries when there are swollen, painful deformities and a mechanism of blunt trauma.

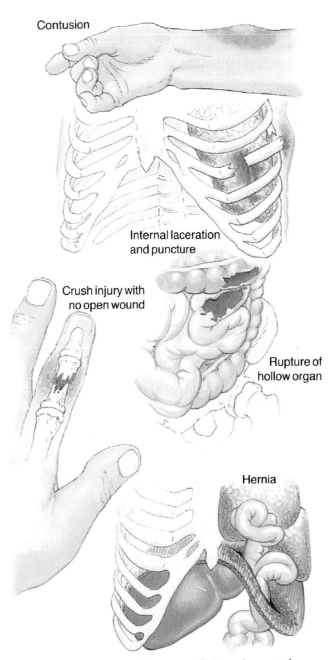

Contusion

Internal laceration and puncture

Crush injury with no open wound

Rupture of hollow organ

Hernia

FIGURE 26-3 Classification of closed wounds.

Contusions

A **contusion** (kun-TU-zhun) is a bruise (Figure 26-4). The epidermis remains intact, but cells and blood vessels in the dermis are damaged. A variable amount of bleeding occurs at the time of injury and may continue for a few hours after the trauma. There is pain, swelling, and discoloration at the wound site. Swelling and discoloration may occur immediately or may be delayed as much as 24 to 48 hours. The swelling is caused by a collection of blood under the skin or in the damaged tissues.

Blood almost always collects at the injury site. This results in a **hematoma** (hem-ah-TO-mah). A hematoma differs from a contusion in that hematomas involve a larger amount of tissue damage, including damage to larger blood vessels with greater blood loss. As much as one liter of blood may be lost in a hematoma.

Crush Injuries

Force can be transmitted from the body's exterior to its internal structures, even when the skin remains intact and even in cases in which the only indication of injury is a simple bruise. This force can cause the internal organs to be crushed or to rupture and bleed internally. Such an injury is called a **crush injury.** Solid organs such as the liver and spleen normally contain considerable amounts of blood. When crushed, they bleed severely and cause shock. Contents of

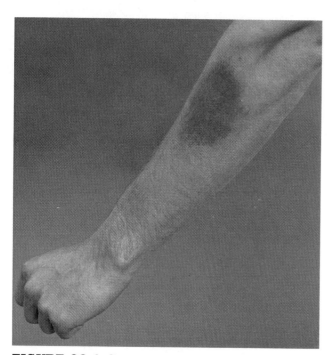

FIGURE 26-4 Contusions are the most common form of closed wounds.

TABLE 26-1 Contusions (Bruises) as Signs of Soft Tissue Injury

Sign	Indicates
Large bruise or bruised areas directly over body organs such as the spleen, liver, or kidneys	Possible injury to underlying organs
Swelling or deformity at site of bruise	Possible underlying fracture
Contusion on the head or neck	Possible injury to the cervical spine or brain. Search for blood in the mouth, nose, and ears.
Bruise on the trunk or signs of damage to the ribs or sternum	Possible chest injury. Determine if the patient is coughing up frothy red blood, which may indicate a punctured lung, and assess for difficult breathing. Use your stethoscope to listen for equal air entry and any unusual breath sounds.
Bruise on the abdomen	Possible injury to the abdominal organs. Look to see if the patient has vomited. If so, is there any substance in the vomitus that looks like coffee grounds (partially digested blood)? Palpate to detect if patient's abdomen is rigid or tender.

Note: Treatment for internal bleeding was discussed in Chapter 25, Bleeding and Shock. Treatment of head, chest, and abdominal injuries is discussed in this chapter.

hollow organs, such as digested food or urine, can leak into the body cavities, causing severe inflammation and tissue damage.

Emergency Care for Closed Wounds

Contusions are the most frequently encountered closed wounds. Most simple bruises will not require emergency care in the field. However, bruising may also be a sign of internal injury and bleeding.

Patient Assessment—Closed Wounds

Signs

A bruise may be an indication of internal injuries and related internal bleeding. Each of the signs listed in Table 26-1 indicates possible serious internal injuries requiring special care.

Emergency Care Steps

1. Take appropriate body substance isolation precautions.
2. Manage the patient's airway, breathing and circulation. Apply high concentration oxygen by nonrebreather mask. (Figure 26-5).
3. MANAGE AS IF THERE IS INTERNAL BLEEDING, AND CARE FOR SHOCK if you believe that there is a possibility of internal injuries.
4. Splint extremities that are painful, swollen, or deformed.
5. Stay alert for the patient to vomit.
6. Continue to monitor the patient for the development of shock and transport as soon as possible.

Open Wounds

An **open wound** is an injury in which the skin is interrupted, or broken, exposing the tissues underneath. The cause of the interruption can come from the outside, as a laceration, or from the inside when a fractured bone end tears outward through the skin.

Abrasions

The classification of **abrasion** (ab-RAY-zhun) includes simple scrapes and scratches in which the outer layer of the skin is damaged but all the layers are not penetrated (Figure 26-6). Skinned elbows and knees, "road rash," "mat burns," "rug burns," and "brush burns" are examples of abrasions. There may be no detectable bleeding or only the minor ooze of blood from capillary beds. The patient may be experiencing great pain, even though the injury is minor. Because of dirt ground into the skin, the opportunity for infection is great with this type of injury.

Lacerations

A **laceration** (las-er-AY-shun) is a cut. It may be smooth (Figure 26-7) or jagged (Figure 26-8). This type of wound is often caused by an object having a sharp edge, such as a razor blade, broken glass, or a jagged piece of metal. However, a laceration can also result from a severe blow or impact with a blunt object. If the laceration has rough edges, they may tend to fall together and obstruct the view as you try to determine the wound depth. It is usually impossible to look at the outside of a laceration and determine the

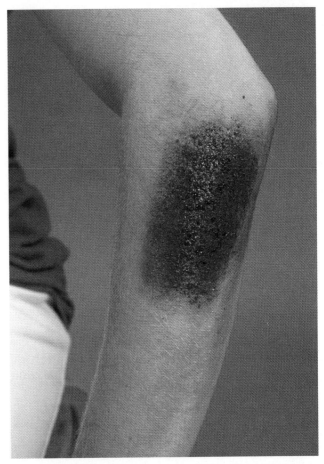

FIGURE 26-6 Abrasions are the least serious form of open wound.

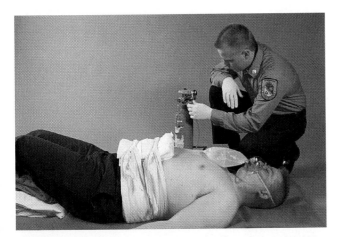

FIGURE 26-5 Administer a high concentration of oxygen and care for shock.

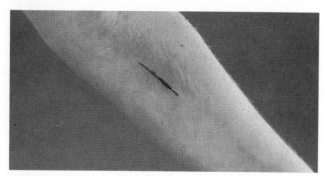

FIGURE 26-7 Some lacerations have smooth edges.

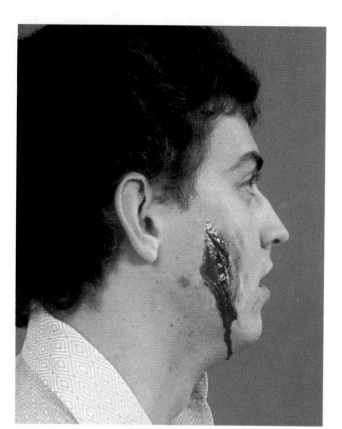

FIGURE 26-8 Some lacerations have jagged edges.

extent of the damage to underlying tissues. If significant blood vessels have been torn, bleeding will be considerable. Sometimes the bleeding is partially controlled when blood vessels are stretched and torn. This is due to the natural retraction and restriction of the cut ends that aid in rapid clot formation.

Punctures

When a sharp, pointed object passes through the skin or other tissue, a **puncture wound** has occurred. Typically, puncture wounds are caused by objects such as nails, ice picks, splinters, or knives. Often, there is no severe external bleeding problem, but internal bleeding may be profuse. Contamination must always be viewed as serious. There are two types of puncture wounds. A **penetrating puncture wound** can be shallow or deep (Figure 26-9). In either case, tissues and blood vessels are injured. A **perforating puncture wound** has both an entrance wound and an exit wound (Figure 26-10). The object causing the injury passes

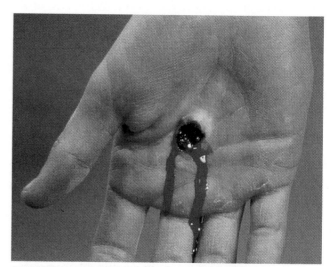

FIGURE 26-9 A penetrating puncture wound.

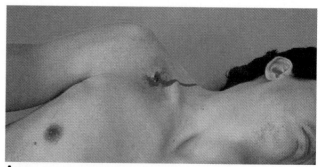

A.

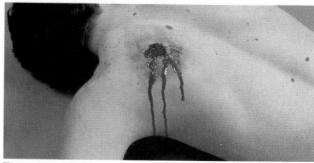

B.

FIGURE 26-10 A perforating puncture wound has an entrance and an exit.

through the body and out to create an exit wound. In many cases, the exit wound is more serious than the entrance wound. A "through-and-through" gunshot wound is an example of a perforating puncture wound.

Avulsions

In an **avulsion** (a-VUL-shun), flaps of skin and tissues are torn loose or pulled off completely (Figure 26-11). When the tip of the nose is cut or torn off, this is an avulsion. The same applies to the external ear. A degloving avulsion occurs when the hand is caught in a roller. In this type of accident, the skin is stripped off like a glove. An eye pulled from its socket (extruded) is a form of avulsion. The term avulsed is used in reporting the wound, as in "an avulsed eye," or "an avulsed ear."

Amputations

The extremities are sometimes subject to **amputation** (am-pyu-TAY-shun). The fingers (Figure 26-12), toes, hands, feet, or limbs are completely

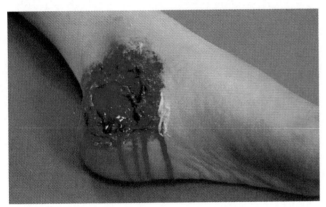

FIGURE 26-11 Avulsed skin.

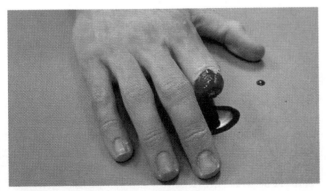

FIGURE 26-12 An amputation.

cut through or torn off. Jagged skin and bone edges can be observed. There may be massive bleeding; however, the force that amputates a limb may close off torn blood vessels, limiting the amount of bleeding. Often, blood vessels collapse or retract and curl closed to limit the bleeding from the wound site.

Crush Injuries

A crush injury can result when an extremity is caught between heavy items, such as pieces of machinery, resulting in a painful, swollen, and deformed extremity. Blood vessels, nerves and muscles are involved and swelling may be a major problem with resulting loss of blood supply distally. Bones are fractured and may protrude through the wound site. Soft tissues and internal organs can be crushed to produce both profuse external and internal bleeding (Figure 26-13). Patients who are pinned under heavy objects may suffer "tourniquet shock" (see Chapter 25, Bleeding and Shock) when the object is removed and toxins that have built up behind the blockage are suddenly released into the bloodstream. Sometimes, external bleeding may be mild or totally absent.

Emergency Care for Open Wounds

Open wounds require strict attention to body substance isolation procedures. In addition to wearing protective gloves, a gown and protective eyewear may also be required. Remember to properly dispose of all soiled materials and wash your hands after each call.

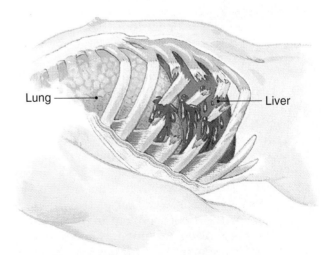

FIGURE 26-13 Both soft tissues and internal organs are damaged in crush injuries.

Patient Assessment—Open Wounds

Airway, breathing, circulation, and severe bleeding are identified and treated in the initial assessment. Once the initial assessment and the appropriate physical examination have been completed, care for the individual wounds begins.

Patient Care—Open Wounds

Care for open wounds is as follows.

1. *Expose the wound.* Clothing that covers a soft tissue injury must be lifted, cut, or split away. For some articles of clothing, this is best done with scissors or a seam cutter. Do not attempt to remove clothing in the usual manner. To do so may aggravate existing injuries and cause additional damage and pain.
2. *Clean the wound surface.* Do not try to pick out embedded particles and debris from the wound. Simply remove large pieces of foreign matter from its surface. When possible, use a piece of sterile dressing to brush away large debris from the surface while protecting from contact with your soiled gloves. Do not spend much time cleaning the wound. Control of bleeding is the priority.
3. *Control bleeding.* Start with direct pressure or direct pressure and elevation. When necessary, employ pressure point procedures. Remember, a tourniquet is used only as a last resort (see Chapter 25, Bleeding and Shock).
4. *Care for shock.* For all serious wounds, care for shock, including the administration of a high concentration of oxygen (see Chapter 25, Bleeding and Shock).
5. *Prevent further contamination.* Use a sterile dressing, if possible. When none is available, use the cleanest cloth material at the scene.
6. *Bandage the dressing in place after bleeding has been controlled.* If an extremity is involved, check for a distal pulse to make certain that circulation has not been interrupted by the application of a tight bandage. With the exception of a pressure dressing, bleeding must be controlled before bandaging is started. Periodically recheck the bandage to make certain that bleeding has not restarted.
7. *Keep the patient lying still.* Any patient movement will increase circulation and could restart bleeding.
8. *Reassure the patient.* This will help ease the patient's emotional response and perhaps lower his pulse rate and blood pressure. In some cases this may help to reduce the bleeding rate. Also, a patient who feels reassured will usually be more willing to lie still, reducing the chances of restarting controlled bleeding.

Emergency care steps specific to various kinds of open wounds are detailed below.

Treating Abrasions and Lacerations

In treating abrasions, care should be provided to reduce wound contamination. Bleeding from a long, deep laceration may be difficult to control, but direct pressure over a dressing usually works well. The air-inflated splint can be useful in the management of this type of wound when it is applied over the top of a dressing. Do not pull apart the edges of a laceration in an effort to see into the wound.

Most lacerations can be cared for by bandaging a dressing in place. Some EMS systems recommend using a butterfly bandage for minor lacerations. A gauze dressing should be bandaged over the butterfly strip.

Note: Do not underestimate the effects of a laceration. When evaluating a distal pulse, also check for sensory and motor function distal to the injury. The patient may need stitches, plastic surgery, or a tetanus shot at the hospital. So do not put on butterfly bandages and leave the patient at the scene. A serious infection or scarring can result.

Treating Puncture Wounds

Use caution when caring for puncture wounds. An object that appears to be embedded only in the skin may actually go all the way to the bone. In such cases, it is possible that the patient may not have any serious pain. Even an apparently moderate puncture wound may cause extensive internal injury with serious internal bleeding. What appears at first to be a simple, shallow puncture wound may be only part of the problem. There also could be a severe exit wound that requires immediate care, so be sure to search for one.

Gunshot wounds are puncture wounds that can fracture bones and cause extensive soft tissue and organ injury. The seriousness of the wound cannot be determined by the caliber of the bullet or the point of entry and exit. The bullet may have tumbled through tissues, been deflected off a bone, fragmented, or exploded inside the body. All bullet wounds are considered to be serious. If the bullet has penetrated the body, you must assume that there is considerable internal injury. Close-range shootings often have burns around the entry wound. Air guns fired at close range can cause serious damage by injecting air into the tissues.

When caring for a patient with a moderate or serious puncture wound

1. Reassure the alert patient. Such wounds are frightening to the patient.
2. Search for an exit wound when there is a gunshot wound. Control of bleeding and adequate wound treatment require care of both the entry and the exit wounds.
3. Assess the need for basic life support measures whenever there is a gunshot wound. Care for shock, administering oxygen at a high concentration.
4. Immobilize the patient's spine when the head, neck, or torso is involved.

Treating Impaled Objects

As an EMT-B you may have to care for patients with puncture wounds containing impaled objects (Figure 26-14). The object may be a knife, a fence post or guard rail, a shard of glass, or even a wooden stick, piercing any part of the body. Even though it is rare, you may be confronted with a long impaled object that must be shortened before care can begin or transport is possible. In such cases, contact the emergency department physician for specific directions. Usually, someone must hold the object, keeping it very stable, while you gently saw it through at the desired length. A fine-toothed saw with rigid blade support (e.g., a hack saw or reciprocating saw) should be used.

In general, when caring for a patient with a puncture wound involving an impaled object

1. *DO NOT REMOVE THE IMPALED OBJECT.* The object may be plugging bleeding from a major artery while it is in place, so to remove it may cause severe bleeding when the pressure is released. Removal of the object may cause further injury to nerves, muscles, and other soft tissues.
2. *Expose the wound area.* Cut away clothing to make the wound site accessible. Take great care not to disturb the object. Do not attempt to lift clothing over the object; you may accidentally move it. Long impaled objects may have to be stabilized by hand during the exposure, bleeding control, and dressing steps.
3. *Control profuse bleeding by direct pressure if possible.* **Caution:** Position your gloved hands on either side of the object and exert pressure downward. Do not put pressure on the object. This pressure must be applied with great care if the object has a cutting edge, such as a knife or a shard of glass; otherwise, you may cause additional injury to the patient. Be careful not to injure your hands or damage your latex gloves.
4. *Stabilize the impaled object with a bulky dressing.* While you continue to stabilize the object and control bleeding, have another trained rescuer place several layers of bulky dressing around the injury site so that the dressings surround the object on all sides. Manual stabilization must con-

A.

B.

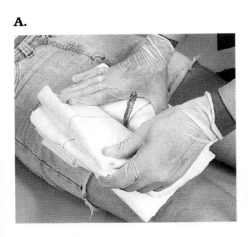
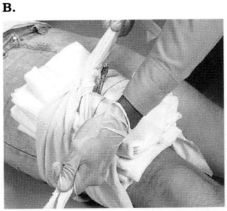

FIGURE 26-14 Impaled objects. A. Expose the wound and control bleeding. B. Stabilize the impaled object.

tinue until the stabilizing dressings are secured in place.

The second EMT-B will begin by placing folded universal pads, sanitary napkins, or some other bulky dressing material on opposite sides of the object. For long or large objects, folded towels, blankets, or pillows may have to be used in place of dressing pads. Remove your hands from under the pads. Place them on top and apply pressure as each layer is placed in position. The next layer of pads should be placed on opposite sides of the object, perpendicular to the first layer. Continue this process until as much of the object as possible has been stabilized.

Once bandaged in place, the dressings will stabilize the object and exert downward pressure on bleeding vessels. Keep in mind that there is a limited amount of time that can be given to impaled object stabilization. Stay in contact with the medical director for directions and recommendations.

5. *Hold the dressings in place.* Adhesive strips may hold the dressings in place; however, blood around the wound site, sweat, and body movements may not allow you to use tape. Triangular bandages folded into strips (cravats) can be applied, tying one above and one below the impaled object. The cravats should be wide (no less than four inches in width once folded). A thin rigid splint can be used to push the cravats under the patient's back when they are needed to care for objects impaled in the trunk of the body.

6. *Care for shock and provide oxygen at the highest possible concentration.* When appropriate, the administration of oxygen and the covering of the patient to conserve body heat should be done as soon as possible. When working by yourself, these may have to be delayed while you attempt to control bleeding.

7. *Keep the patient at rest and provide emotional support.* Position the patient for minimum stress. If possible, immobilize the affected area, for example with a splint or a spine board.

8. *Carefully transport the patient as soon as possible.* Avoid any movement that may jar, loosen, or dislodge the object. If the object was removed by bystanders before you arrived, bring it to the hospital for examination by a physician.

9. *Reassure the patient throughout all aspects of care.* An alert patient with an impaled object is usually very frightened.

Impaled objects to the cheek and eye pose special problems in treatment for the EMT-B.

Impaled Object in the Cheek A dangerous situation exists when the cheek has been penetrated by a foreign object. First, the object may go into the oral cavity and immediately become a possible airway obstruction, or it may stay impaled in the cheek wall to work its way free and enter the oral cavity later. Second, when the cheek wall is perforated, bleeding into the mouth and throat may be profuse and interfere with breathing, or it may make the patient nauseated and induce vomiting. Simple external wound care will not stop the flow of blood into the mouth.

If you find a patient with an object impaled in the cheek, you should (Figure 26-15)

1. *Gently examine both the external cheek and the inside of the mouth.* Use your penlight and look into the patient's mouth. If need be, carefully use your gloved fingers to probe the inside cheek to determine if the object has passed through the cheek wall. This is best done with a dressing pad used to protect your fingers.

2. *If you find perforation and you can SEE BOTH ENDS of the object, carefully REMOVE THE IMPALED OBJECT by pulling it out in the direction that it entered the cheek.* If this cannot be done easily, leave the object in place. Do not twist the object.

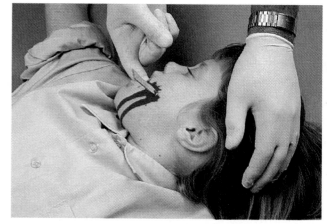

FIGURE 26-15 Procedure for removing an object impaled in the cheek.

3. If you find perforation but the tip of the object is also IMPALED INTO A DEEPER STRUCTURE (e.g., the palate), STABILIZE THE OBJECT. Do not try to remove it.

4. *Make certain that you position the patient's head to allow for drainage* (the possibility of spinal injuries may require you to immobilize the head, neck, and spine first, then tilt the patient and the spine board as a unit). Keep in mind that an object penetrating the cheek wall also may have broken teeth or dentures, creating the potential danger for airway obstruction.

5. *Once the object is removed or stabilized, be prepared to suction as necessary. Monitor the patient's airway.*

6. *Dress the outside of the wound* using a pressure dressing and bandage or apply a sterile dressing and use direct hand pressure to control the bleeding.

7. *Provide oxygen and care for shock.* You may have to use a nasal cannula if constant suctioning is required. If any dressing materials are placed in the patient's mouth, use of standard face masks can be dangerous unless you leave 3 to 4 inches of the dressing outside of the patient's mouth.

Puncture Wound to the Eye or Object Impaled in the Eye Use loose dressings for puncture wounds with no impaled objects. If you find an object impaled in the eye, you should (Figure 26-16)

1. *Place a roll of 3-inch gauze bandage or folded 4 x 4s on either side of the object, along the vertical axis of the head.* These rolls should be placed so that they stabilize the object.

2. *Fit a disposable paper drinking cup or paper cone over the impaled object and allow it to come to rest on the dressing rolls. Do not allow it to touch the object.* This will offer rigid protection and will call attention to the patient's problem.

3. *Have another rescuer stabilize the dressings and cup while you secure them in place with self-adherent roller bandage or with a wrapping of gauze. Do not secure the bandage over top of the cup.*

4. *The uninjured eye should be dressed and bandaged to reduce eye movements.*

5. *Provide oxygen and care for shock.*

6. *Continue to reassure the patient and provide emotional support.*

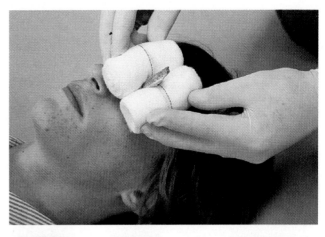

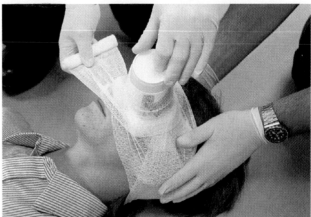

FIGURE 26-16 Managing a patient with an object impaled in the eye.

The above method can also be used as a pressure dressing to control bleeding in the area of the eye.

An alternative to the above method calls for the rescuer to make a thick dressing with several layers of sterile gauze pads or universal dressings (Figure 26-17). A hole is cut in the center of this pad, approximately the size of the impaled object. The rescuer then carefully passes this dressing over the impaled object and positions the pad so that the impaled object is centered in the opening. The rest of the procedure remains the same as previously described. If your EMS system has you use this technique, remember that you must take great care not to touch the object as the dressing is set in place.

Treating Avulsions

Emergency care for avulsions requires the application of large, bulky pressure dressings. In addition, you should make every effort to preserve any avulsed parts and transport them to

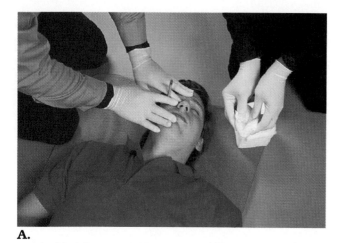

A.

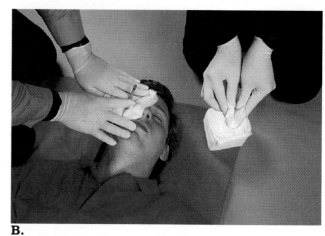

B.

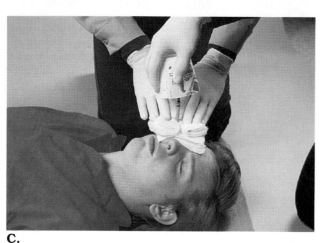

C.

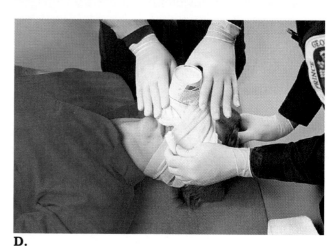

D.

FIGURE 26-17 Alternative method of care for lacerated eyelid or injury to the eyeball. A. 4 × 4 sterile pads. B. Fold 2 or 3 sterile pads and cut a half moon in the fold. C. Open gauze pad and place over injury. Cut and add pads as needed. Place cup on pads. D. Secure with roller bandage.

the medical facility along with the patient. It may be possible to surgically restore the part or use it for skin grafts.

In cases in which flaps of skin have been torn loose but not off

1. *Clean the wound surface.*
2. *Fold the skin back to its normal position* as gently as possible.
3. *Control bleeding and dress the wound* using bulky pressure dressings.

Should skin or another body part be torn from the body

1. *Control bleeding and dress the wound* using a bulky pressure dressing.
2. *Save the avulsed part* by wrapping it in a dry sterile gauze dressing secured in place by self-adherent roller bandage and placing the wrapped part in a plastic bag, plastic wrap, or aluminum foil, in accordance with local protocol. If none of these items is available at the scene, wrap the avulsed part in a lint-free, dry sterile dressing. (Some research suggests that the sterile wrap should be soaked in sterile saline to make a moist dressing. Follow local protocols.) Make certain that you label the part, noting what it is and the patient's name, date, and time the part was wrapped and bagged. Your records should show the approximate time of the avulsion.

3. *Keep the avulsed part as cool as possible, without freezing.* Place the wrapped and bagged part in a cooler or any other available container so that it is on top of a cold pack or a SEALED bag of ice (do not use dry ice). Do not immerse the avulsed part in ice, cooled water, or saline. Label the container the same as the label used for the saved part.

Remember: Serious avulsions can be frightening. You must reassure the patient.

Note: The care of avulsed tissues is directed by local protocols, often written to match the reimplantation procedures of the hospitals in your EMS system. Some EMS systems prefer that the dressing used to wrap the avulsed part be moistened with normal sterile saline (sterile distilled water is not recommended). This saline must be from a fresh sterile source. Keep in mind that once a sterile source of saline has been opened it is no longer considered sterile. Take great care if you use this method, since the saline may carry microorganisms from your gloved hand through the dressing to the avulsed part.

Treating Amputations

As in other external bleeding situations, the most effective method to control bleeding is a snug pressure dressing.

1. Place the pressure dressing over the stump.
2. Use pressure point techniques to control bleeding.
3. A tourniquet should not be applied unless other methods used to control bleeding have failed. Never complete a partial amputation.
4. When possible, wrap the amputated part in a sterile dressing and secure the dressing material in place with self-adhesive gauze bandage. Wrap or bag the amputated part in plastic, label it, and transport the part with the patient. The amputated part should be kept cool in the same manner as an avulsed part.
5. Do not immerse the amputated part directly in water or saline. It can be sealed in a plastic bag and the bag placed in a bedpan with water kept cool by cold packs. Do not let the amputated part come in direct contact with ice or it may freeze.

Wounds to the Neck

Due to the fact that large arteries and veins lie close to the surface of the neck, the potential for serious bleeding from an open wound is great. In addition to the severe bleeding, the possibility of an **air embolus** (air bubble) being sucked in through a vein is also great. An air embolism can be carried to the heart and interfere with the heartbeat or actually cause cardiac arrest. The treatment of neck veins is aimed at stopping bleeding and preventing an embolus from entering the circulation.

Patient Assessment—Open Neck Wound

Signs

An injury that has severed a major artery or vein of the neck will produce these signs.

- ☐ Arterial bleeding will be profuse, with bright red blood spurting from the wound.
- ☐ Venous bleeding can be profuse with dark red to maroon-colored blood flowing steadily from the wound.

Patient Care—Open Neck Wound

Emergency Care Steps

1. Assure an open airway
2. Place your gloved hand over the wound.
3. Apply an occlusive dressing to the wound (Scan 26-1). The dressing should be a thick material that will not be sucked into the wound and must extend two inches past the sides of the wound.
4. Place a dressing over the occlusive dressing.
5. Apply pressure as needed to stop the bleeding. Use caution so you do not compress both carotid arteries at once.
6. Once bleeding has stopped, bandage the dressing in place. Use caution not to restrict the airway or the arteries and veins of the neck.
7. If the mechanism of injury could have caused cervical injury, immobilize the spine.

Chest Injuries

The chest can be injured in a number of ways, including

- Blunt Trauma—A blow to the chest can fracture the ribs, the sternum, and the costal (rib) cartilages. Whole sections of the chest may collapse. With severe blunt trauma, the lungs and airway can be damaged and the great vessels (aorta and venae cavae) and the heart may be seriously injured.
- Penetrating Objects—Bullets, knives, pieces of metal or glass, steel rods, pipes, and various other objects can penetrate the chest

Open Neck Wound—Occlusive Dressing

FIRST take body substance isolation precautions.

Dressing must be heavy plastic, sized to be 2 inches larger in diameter than wound site.

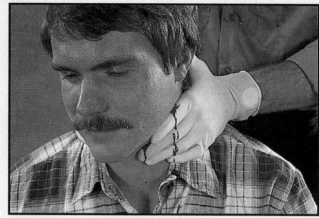

1. Do not delay! Place your gloved palm over the wound.

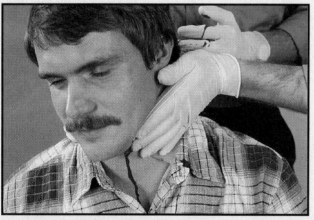

2. Occlusive dressing is placed over wound site.

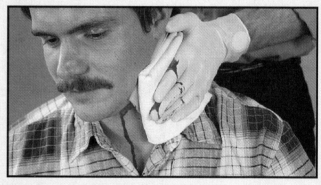

3. A dressing is placed over the occlusive dressing. (A roll of gauze can be placed between the trachea and the dressing to help keep pressure off the airway.)

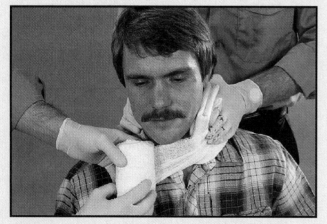

4. Start a figure-eight, bringing bandage over dressing.

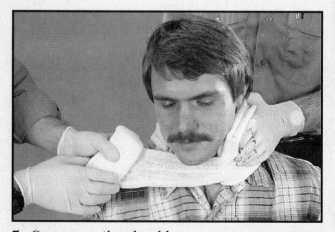

5. Cross over the shoulder.

Note: For demonstration purposes, the patient is upright.

wall, damaging internal organs and impairing respiration.

- Compression—This is a severe form of blunt trauma in which the chest is rapidly compressed, as when the driver of a motor vehicle pitches forward after a head-on collision and strikes his chest on the steering column. The heart can be severely squeezed, the lungs can be ruptured, and the sternum and ribs can be fractured.

Chest injuries are classified as *open* or *closed.*

- Open—When the skin is broken, the patient has an open wound. However, the term *open chest wound* usually means that the chest wall is penetrated, as, for example, by a bullet or a knife blade. An object can pass through the wall from the outside, or a fractured and displaced rib can penetrate the chest wall from within. The heart, lungs, and great vessels can be injured at the same time the chest wall is penetrated. It may be difficult to tell if the chest cavity has been penetrated by looking at the wound. Do not open the wound to determine its depth. Specific signs (see below) will indicate possible open chest injury.

- Closed—The skin is not broken with a closed chest injury, leading many people to think that the damage done is not serious. However, such injuries, sustained through blunt trauma and compression injuries, can cause contusions and lacerations of the heart, lungs, and great vessels.

Open Chest Wounds

An open wound to the chest occurs when an object tears or punctures the chest wall, opening the chest cavity to the atmosphere. *You must consider all open wounds to the chest to be life threatening.*

Open chest wounds are usually puncture wounds, classified as penetrating or perforating. A penetrating puncture wound is one that penetrates the chest wall once; a perforating puncture wound has both an entrance and an exit wound as, for example, many gunshot wounds. An object producing a wound may remain impaled in the chest, or the wound may be completely open.

When air enters the chest cavity, a serious wound has occurred. The air can enter through an external wound, or the air may come out of a punctured lung, or both (Figure 26-18). The delicate pressure balance within the chest cavity is

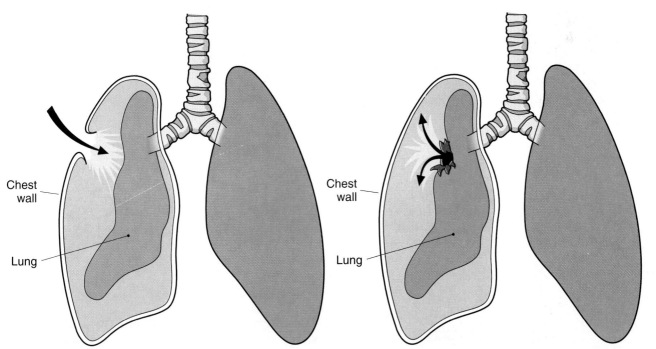

FIGURE 26-18 Air can enter the chest cavity through a wound to the chest wall or from a punctured lung, or both.

destroyed. This causes the lung on the injured side to collapse.

Patient Assessment—Open Chest Wounds

The term **sucking chest wound** is used when the chest cavity is open to the atmosphere. Each time the patient breathes, air can be sucked into the opening. This patient will develop severe difficulty breathing.

Signs

☐ A wound to the chest
☐ There may or may not be the characteristic sucking sound associated with an open chest wound.
☐ The patient may be gasping for air.

Be aware that the object that penetrated the chest wall may have seriously damaged a lung, major blood vessel, or the heart itself.

Patient Care—Open Chest Wounds

An open chest wound is a TRUE EMERGENCY that requires rapid initial care and immediate transport to a medical facility.

Emergency Care Steps

1 Maintain an open airway. Provide basic life support if necessary.
2 Seal the open chest wound as quickly as possible. If need be, use your gloved hand. Do not delay sealing the wound to find an occlusive dressing.
3 Apply an occlusive dressing to seal the wound. When possible, the occlusive dressing should be at least two inches wider than the wound. If there is an exit wound in the chest, apply an occlusive dressing over this wound too.

There are two methods now in use. One approach, recommended in many local protocols, calls for taping the occlusive dressing in place, leaving a corner or one side of the dressing unsealed (Figure 26-19). As the patient inhales, the dressing will seal the wound. As the patient exhales, the free corner or edge will act as a flutter valve to release air that is trapped in the chest cavity.

A more traditional approach, still recommended in many local protocols, calls for sealing all four edges (Figure 26-20),

On inspiration, dressing seals wound, preventing air entry

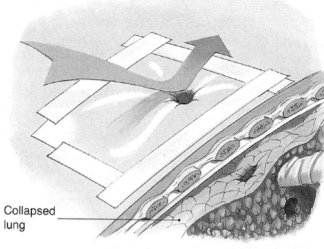

Collapsed lung

Expiration allows trapped air to escape through untaped section of dressing

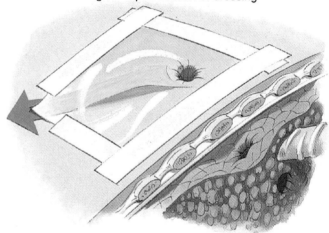

FIGURE 26-19 Creating a flutter valve to allow air to escape from the chest cavity.

the last edge being sealed when the patient forcefully exhales. If the seal is effective, respirations will be partially stabilized.

Follow local protocols as to the preferred type of dressing.
4 Administer a high concentration of oxygen.
5 Care for shock.
6 Transport as soon as possible. Unless other injuries prevent you from doing so, keep the patient positioned on the injured side. This allows the uninjured lung to expand without restriction.

Complications of Open Chest Wounds Occlusive dressings are important treatments for open chest wounds. Occasionally, however, this treatment may cause the patient's condition to

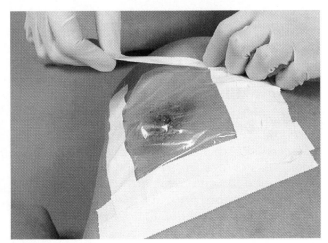

FIGURE 26-20 Sealing all four edges of an occlusive dressing.

worsen because air becomes trapped in the chest cavity. This trapped air causes the uninjured lung, the great blood vessels, and the heart to be compressed, severely affecting oxygen distribution and the heart's ability to pump. This condition may also be caused by a lung that punctures from the inside with no wound open to the outside.

If a patient has a penetrating chest wound with a punctured lung, air will enter the chest cavity through the open wound in the chest wall and through the opening in the lung (Figure 26-21). If you seal off the chest wall opening, air will still flow from the punctured lung into the cavity with each breath. The air will not be able to escape and pressure will build in the cavity. This causes compression of the unaffected lung and the heart. This is a serious emergency.

Open chest wound with punctured lung

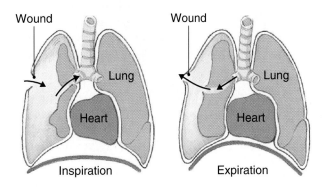

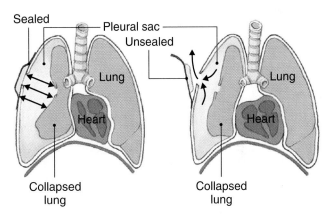

Sealing wound can cause increase in pressure within thoracic (chest) cavity.

If patient's condition declines after sealing puncture wound, open the seal immediately.

FIGURE 26-21 Open chest wound with punctured lung.

☐ Head, neck, and shoulders appearing dark blue or purple

Patient Assessment—Open Chest Wound Complications

Signs

There are several signs of complication for open chest wounds.

☐ Increasing respiratory difficulty
☐ Indications of developing shock, including rapid, weak pulse, cyanosis, and low blood pressure due to decreased cardiac output
☐ Distended neck veins
☐ Tracheal deviation to the uninjured side
☐ Uneven chest wall movement
☐ Reduction of breathing sounds heard in the affected side of the chest (listen with stethoscope)

Patient Care—Open Chest Wound Complications

Emergency Care Steps

1️⃣ The complications of treatment for open chest injuries are the reason why some medical authorities now recommend the flutter-valve occlusive dressing instead of the traditional occlusive dressing. If, instead, your local protocols recommend that you treat a sucking chest wound with a traditional dressing sealed on all four sides and you find that the patient worsens rapidly, you will have to lift a corner of the seal to let air escape. (The patient should respond almost immediately as pressure is released around the heart, great blood vessels, and uninjured lung.) Then you must reseal the wound and monitor the patient. You may have to unseal and reseal the wound again, continuing this process throughout care and transport.

Remember: Once the chest wound is sealed, you must continue to monitor the patient and stay alert for complications. Even if you use a flutter valve, you still must monitor the patient for this condition. The free corner of the dressing may stick to the chest or the dressing may be drawn into the wound, causing the valve to fail.

2 Monitor the patient, making certain that the airway is open.

3 Be prepared to suction blood from the oral cavity.

4 Administer high concentration oxygen.

5 Call ahead to alert the emergency department staff.

Note: Household plastic wrap is not thick enough to make an effective occlusive dressing for open chest wounds. If no other source for an occlusive dressing is available, this wrap can be used, but it must be folded several times to be of the proper thickness. Even then, it may fail. Most ambulances carry sterile disposable items that are wrapped in plastic. The inside surface of the plastic is sterile. If you do not have an occlusive dressing, use one of these wrappers or an IV bag. If there is no other choice, aluminum foil can be used to make the seal. Be careful, however; foil edges may lacerate skin and may tear when lifted to release pressure.

Note: You may have to maintain hand pressure over the occlusive dressing en route to the hospital. The plastic dressings normally used are semipermeable and slowly allow air to enter. The tape also may not stick well to bloody skin or to skin that is sweaty from shock.

Documentation Tips—Open Chest Wounds

With an open chest wound, be sure to document the patient's response to treatment. After application of the occlusive dressing, record any changes—whether improvements

or deteriorations—in respiratory difficulty, breathing sounds, chest wall movement, color, and signs of shock.

Abdominal Injuries

Abdominal injuries can be open or closed, with closed injury usually due to blunt trauma. Internal bleeding can be severe if organs and major blood vessels are lacerated or ruptured. Very serious and painful reactions can occur when the hollow organs are ruptured and their contents leak into the abdominal cavity. Penetrating wounds to the abdomen can be caused by objects such as knives, ice picks, arrows, and the broken glass and twisted metal of vehicular collisions and structural accidents. Very serious perforating wounds can be caused by bullets a (Figure 26-22), even when the bullet is small caliber.

Patient Assessment—Abdominal Injuries

Although some persons believe otherwise, gunshot wounds without exit wounds can cause serious abdominal damage, just as those with exit wounds do. Another misconception about bullet wounds is that internal damage can be assessed easily. On the contrary, any projectile entering the body can be deflected, or it can explode and send out

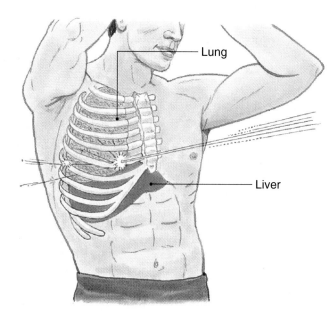

FIGURE 26-22 The damage done by gunshot wounds cannot be fully assessed in field emergency care.

pieces in many directions. Do not believe that only the structures directly under the entrance wound have been injured. Also, keep in mind that the pathway of a bullet between entrance wound and exit wound is seldom a straight line.

Complicating the problem even more is the fact that penetrating abdominal wounds can be associated with wounds in adjacent areas of the body. For example, a bullet can enter the chest cavity, pierce the diaphragm, and cause widespread damage in the abdomen. A complete patient survey is essential in determining the probable extent of injuries.

Remember: Always check for an exit wound.

Signs and Symptoms

The signs of abdominal injury can include

- [ ] Obvious lacerations and puncture wounds to the abdomen
- [ ] Lacerations and puncture wounds to the pelvis and middle and lower back or chest wounds near the diaphragm
- [ ] Indications of blunt trauma, such as a large bruised area or an intense bruise on the abdomen
- [ ] Indications of developing shock, including restlessness; pale, cool, and clammy skin; rapid shallow breathing,; a rapid pulse; and low blood pressure. (Sometimes patients with abdominal injury who are in extreme pain show an initial elevated blood pressure.)
- [ ] Coughing up or vomiting blood—The vomitus may contain a substance that looks like coffee grounds (partially digested blood).
- [ ] Rigid and/or tender abdomen—The patient tries to protect the abdomen (guarded abdomen).
- [ ] Distended abdomen
- [ ] The patient tries to lie very still, with the legs drawn up in an effort to reduce the tension on the abdominal muscles.

The symptoms of abdominal injury can include

- [ ] Pain, often starting as mild pain then rapidly becoming intolerable

- [ ] Cramps
- [ ] Nausea
- [ ] Weakness
- [ ] Thirst

Patient Care—Abdominal Injuries

Some emergency care steps apply to both closed and open abdominal injuries. Some additional care steps are necessary for open abdominal injuries.

Emergency Care Steps

For both closed and open abdominal injuries

1. Stay alert for vomiting and keep an open airway.
2. Place the patient on his back, legs flexed at the knees, to reduce pain by relaxing abdominal muscles.
3. Administer a high concentration of oxygen.
4. Care for shock.
5. Apply anti-shock garments if indicated and local protocols recommend
6. Give nothing to the patient by mouth. This may induce vomiting or pass through open wounds in the esophagus, stomach, or intestine and enter the abdominal cavity.
7. Constantly monitor vital signs.
8. Transport as soon as possible.

In addition, for open abdominal injuries

1. Control external bleeding and dress all open wounds.
2. Do not touch or try to replace any eviscerated, or exposed, organs (Figure 26-23). Apply a sterile dressing moistened with sterile saline over the wound site before you apply an occlusive dressing. Cover exposed organs with an occlusive dressing and maintain warmth by placing layers of bulky dressing or a lint-free towel over the occlusive dressing. (**Warning:** Do not use aluminum foil. Aluminum foil occlusive dressings have been found to cut eviscerated organs.)
3. Do not remove any impaled objects. Stabilize impaled objects with bulky dressings that are bandaged in place. Leave the patient's legs in the position in which you found them to avoid muscular movement that may move the impaled object.

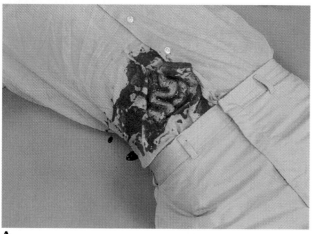

A.

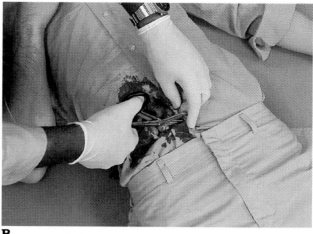

B.

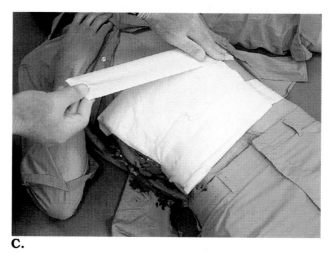

C.

FIGURE 26-23 A. Open abdominal wound with evisceration. B. Cut away clothing from wound. Apply a sterile saline-soaked dressing. Apply an occlusive dressing over the moist dressing if local protocols recommend. C. Cover the dressed wound to maintain warmth. Secure covering with tape or cravats tied above and below position of exposed organ.

Protruding Organs

Open wounds of the abdomen may be so large and deep that organs protrude through the wound opening. This is known as an **evisceration** (e-vis-er-AY-shun). In such cases

1. Administer high concentration oxygen as soon as possible.
2. Care for shock, positioning the patient to provide for a clear airway and minimum stress to the wound site.
3. Do not touch or try to replace the organ.
4. Expose the wound site, cutting away clothing. Do not attempt to pull away any article or piece of clothing that does not lift off easily.
5. Flex the patient's uninjured legs at the hips

and knees, if possible, to reduce tension on the abdominal muscles.

6. Apply a sterile, lint-free dressing that is soaked with sterile saline. The dressing should extend at least two inches beyond the wound edges or the edges of the exposed organ.
7. Create an occlusive dressing. Tape the dressing in place, sealing the edges. This will help prevent the loss of moisture from the internal organs, membranes, and tissues.
8. Apply a thick dressing pad or clean towel over the top of the first dressing. This will help to prevent heat loss. Hold this in place with cravats.
9. Apply an anti-shock garment and inflate

the leg sections if appropriate and local protocols permit. (Do not inflate the garment on the eviscerated organs).

10. Reassure the patient through all steps of care.

Burns

Most people think of burns as injuries to the skin; but burns can do much more. Burn injuries often involve structures below the skin, including muscles, bones, nerves, and blood vessels. Burns can injure the eyes beyond repair. Respiratory system structures can be damaged, producing airway obstruction due to tissue swelling, even respiratory failure and respiratory arrest. In addition to the physical damage caused by burns, patients often suffer emotional and psychological problems that begin at the emergency scene and may last a lifetime.

When caring for a burn patient, always think beyond the burn. For example, a medical emergency or accident may have led to the burn. The patient may have had a heart attack while smoking a cigarette, and the unattended cigarette caused a fire. During the patient assessment, the EMT-B should detect the heart problem even though the burn may be the most obvious injury. Conversely, a fire or burn may cause or aggravate another injury or medical condition. Someone trying to escape a fire may fall and suffer spinal damage and fractures. The EMT-B should detect not only the burn but the spinal damage and fractures as well.

Remember: The patient assessment should never be neglected in order to go immediately to burn care procedures.

Classifying and Evaluating Burns

The process of patient assessment, when there are burns, involves classifying, then evaluating, the burns.

Patient Assessment—Burns

Burns can be classified and evaluated in three ways.

☐ By agent and source
☐ By degree
☐ By severity

All are important in deciding the urgency and the kind of emergency care the burn requires. These classifications are discussed in detail below.

Agent and Source Burns can be classified according to the agent causing the burn (e.g., chemicals or electricity). Noting the source of the burn (e.g., dry lime or AC current) can make the classification more specific. You should report the agent and also, when practical, the source of the agent (Table 26-2). For example, a burn can be reported as "chemical burns from contact with dry lime."

Never assume the agent or source of the burn. What may appear to be a thermal burn could be from radiation. You may find minor thermal burns on the patient's face and forget to consider light burns to the eyes. Always gather information from your observations of the scene, bystanders' reports, and the patient interview.

Depth of the Burn Burns involving the skin are classified as superficial, partial-thickness burns, and full-thickness burns. Partial-thickness burns can involve the epidermis, or the epidermis and upper dermis, but they do not include burns that pass through the dermis to damage underlying tissues. A full-thickness burn will pass through epidermis and dermis, causing injury to the subcutaneous layers. Superficial, partial- and full-thickness burns may also be described using an evaluation system employing the term degree, with burns involving the skin classified as first-, second-, or

TABLE 26-2 Agents and Sources of Burns

Agents	Sources
Thermal	Including flame; radiation; excessive heat from fire, steam, hot liquids, hot objects
Chemicals	Including various acids, bases, caustics
Electricity	Including AC current, DC current, lightning
Light (typically involving the eyes)	Including intense light sources, ultraviolet light (includes sunlight)
Radiation	Usually from nuclear sources; ultraviolet light can also be considered to be a source of radiation burns

third-degree (Figure 26-24 and Scan 26-2). The least serious burn is the first-degree burn.

- **Superficial Burn**—a burn that involves only the epidermis (the outer layer of the skin). It is characterized by reddening of the skin and perhaps some swelling. An example is a sunburn. The patient will usually complain about pain (sometimes severe) at the site. The burn will heal of its own accord, without scarring. Burns such as this are also called first-degree burns.
- **Partial-Thickness Burn**—a burn in which the epidermis is burned through and the dermis (the second layer of the skin) is damaged, but the burn does not pass through to underlying tissues. There will be deep intense pain, noticeable reddening, blisters, and a mottled (spotted) appearance to the skin. Burns of this type cause swelling and blistering for 48 hours after the injury as plasma and tissue fluids are released and rise to the top layer of skin. When treated with reasonable care, partial-

thickness burns will heal themselves, producing very little scarring. Partial thickness burns are also called second degree burns.
- **Full-Thickness Burn**—a burn in which all the layers of the skin are damaged. Some full-thickness burns are difficult to tell from partial-thickness; however, there are usually areas that are charred black or brown or areas that are dry and white. The patient may complain of severe pain, or if enough nerves have been damaged, he may not feel any pain at all (except at the periphery of the burn where adjoining partial-thickness burns may be causing pain). This type of burn may require skin grafting. As these burns heal, dense scars form. Full thickness burns damage all layers of the skin and additionally may damage subcutaneous tissue, muscle, bone, and underlying organs. These burns are sometimes called third degree burns.

Severity When determining the severity of a burn, consider the following factors.

- **Agent or Source of the Burn**—The agent or source of the burn can be significant in terms of patient assessment. A burn caused by electrical current may cause small areas of skin injury, but pose a great risk of severe internal injuries. Chemical burns are of special concern since the chemical may remain on the skin and continue to burn for hours or even days, eventually entering the bloodstream. This is sometimes the case with certain alkaline chemicals.
- **Body Regions Burned**—Any burn to the face is of special concern since it may involve injury to the airway or the eyes. The hands and feet also are areas of special concern because scarring may cause loss of movement of fingers or toes. Special care is required to reduce aggravation to these injury sites when moving the patient and to prevent the damaged tissues from sticking to one another. When the groin, genitalia, buttocks, or medial thighs are burned, the chances for bacterial contamination present problems that can be far more serious than the initial damage to the tissues.

  Circumferential burns (burns that encircle the body or a body part) can be very serious because they constrict the skin and, when they occur to an extremity, they can interrupt circulation to the distal tissues. The burn healing process can be

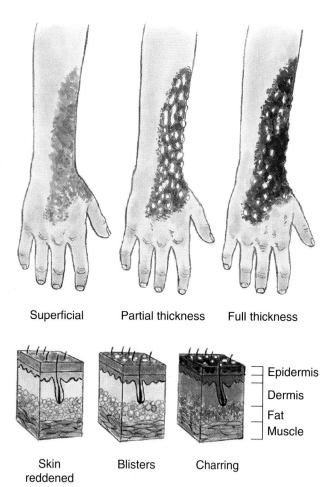

Superficial   Partial thickness   Full thickness

Epidermis
Dermis
Fat
Muscle

Skin reddened   Blisters   Charring

FIGURE 26-24 Burns are classified by depth.

Care for Thermal Burns

FIRST take body substance isolation precautions.

STOP THE BURNING PROCESS!

1. Flame—Wet down, smother, then remove clothing.
   Semi-solid (grease, tar, wax)—Cool with water . . . do **not** remove substance.
2. Ensure an open airway. Assess breathing.
3. Look for airway injury: soot deposits, burnt nasal hair, and facial burns.
4. Complete the initial assessment.
5. Treat for shock. Provide a high concentration of oxygen. Treat serious injuries.

6. Evaluate burns ⟵ Depth / Rule of Nines or Rule of Palm / Severity   Decide if special transport is needed.

Remove clothing if necessary.

Type of Burn	Tissue Burned			Color Changes	Pain	Blisters
	Outer Layer of Skin	2nd Layer of Skin	Tissue Below Skin			
Superficial	Yes	No	No	Red	Yes	No
Partial Thichness	Yes	Yes	No	Deep red	Yes	Yes
Full Thickness	Yes	Yes	Yes	Charred black or white	Yes/No	Yes/No

7. **Do not** clear debris. Remove clothing and jewelry.
8. Wrap with dry sterile dressing.
9A. Burns to hands or toes—Remove rings or jewelry that may constrict with swelling. Separate digits with sterile gauze pads.
9B. Burns to the eyes—Do not open eyelids if burned. Be certain burn is thermal, not chemical. Apply sterile gauze pads to **both** eyes to prevent sympathetic movement of injured eye if only one eye is burned. If burn is chemical, flush eyes for 20 minutes en route to hospital.

FOLLOW LOCAL BURN CENTER PROTOCOL, AND TRANSPORT ALL BURN PATIENTS AS SOON AS POSSIBLE.

very complicated with circumferential burns. This is particularly true when the burns occur to joints, the chest, and the abdomen where the encircling scarring tends to limit normal functions.

- **Depth of Burn**—The depth of the burn is important. In partial thickness and full thickness burns, the outer layer of the skin is penetrated. This can lead to contamination of exposed tissues and the invasion of the circulatory system by harmful chemicals and microorganisms.
- **Extent of Burn Area**—It is important that you be able to estimate roughly the extent of the burn area. The amount of skin surface involved can be calculated quickly by using the **"Rule of Nines"** (Figure 26-25). For an adult, each of the following areas represents 9% of the body surface: the head and neck, each upper extremity, the chest, the abdomen, the upper back, the lower back and buttocks, the front of each lower extremity, and the back of each lower extremity. These make up 99% of the body's surface. The remaining 1% is assigned to the genital region.

The percentages are modified for infants and young children, whose heads are much larger in relationship to the rest of the body than adults' heads are. The infant's or young child's head and neck are counted as 18%; each upper extremity, 9%; the chest and abdomen, 18%; the entire back, 18%; each lower extremity, 14%; and the genital region, 1%. (This adds up to 101%, but it is only used to give a rough determination. Some systems count each lower limb as 13.5% to achieve an even 100%.)

An alternative way to estimate the extent of a burn is the **"Rule of Palm,"** which uses the patient's hand to approximate the surface area. The rule of palm can be applied to any patient—infant, child, or adult. Since the palm of the hand equals about 1% of the body's surface area, mentally compare the patient's palm with the size of the burn to estimate its extent (for example, a burn the size of five palms = 5% of the body). The rule of palm may be easier to apply to smaller or localized burns, the rule of nines to larger or more widespread burns.

- **Age of the Patient**—Age is a major factor in burn cases. Infants, children under age 5, and adults over age 55 have the most severe body reactions to burns as well as different healing patterns than other age groups. Burn intensity and body area

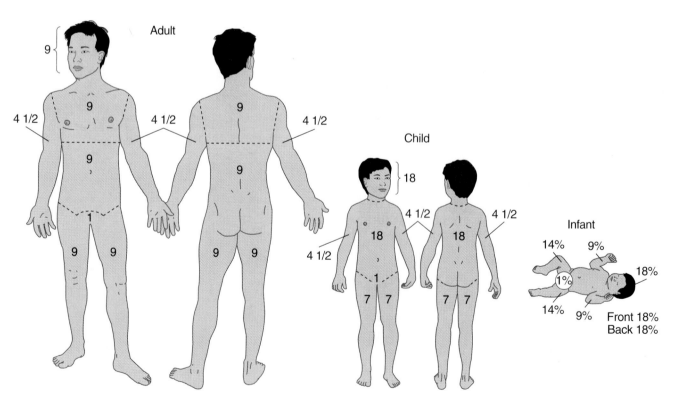

FIGURE 26-25 The Rule of Nines.

involvement that would be classified as minor to moderate for a young adult may be fatal for the infant or an aged person. The infant and young child have a surface area that is much greater in proportion to the total body size when compared with the older child and adult. This factor means that a burn will produce a greater body fluid loss for the patient under age 5. In late adulthood, the body's ability to cope with injury is reduced by aging tissues and failing body systems. The ability of tissues to heal from any injury is lessened and the time of healing is increased. **Note:** An adult's reactions to a burn and the complications associated with burn injury healing increase significantly after age 35.

- **Other Patient Illnesses and Injuries—** Obviously, a patient with existing respiratory illnesses will be especially vulnerable to exposure to heated air or chemical vapors. Likewise, the stress of a fire or other environmental emergency will be of particular concern for patients with heart disease. Patients with respiratory ailments, heart disease, or diabetes will react more severely to burn damage. What may be a minor burn for a healthy adult could be of major significance to a patient with an existing medical condition. Similarly, the stress of a burn added to other injuries sustained during the emergency may lead to shock or other life-threatening problems that would not have resulted from the non-burn injuries or the burn alone.

Note: All burns are to be treated as more serious if accompanied by other injuries or medical problems. If you discover that the patient is hypotensive, always assume that he has other serious injuries. Attempt to determine the patient's problem through standard assessment techniques.

Classifying Severity Burns must be classified as to severity to determine the order of care, type of care, and order of transport and to supply the emergency department with as much information as possible. In some cases, the severity of the burn may determine if the patient is to be taken directly to a hospital with special burn care facilities. The following classification can be used.

Minor Burns

- Full-thickness-burns involving less than 2% of the body surface, excluding face, hands, feet, genitalia, or respiratory tract
- Partial-thickness burns that involve less than 15% of the body surface

Moderate Burns

- Full-thickness burns that involve 2% to 10% of the body surface, excluding face, hands, feet, genitalia, or respiratory tract
- Partial-thickness burns that involve 15% to 30% of the body surface
- Superficial burns that involve more than 50% of the body surface

Critical Burns

- All burns complicated by injuries of the respiratory tract, other soft tissue injuries, and injuries of the bones
- Partial- or full-thickness burns involving the face, hands, feet, genitalia, or respiratory tract
- Full-thickness burns involving more than 10% of the body surface
- Partial-thickness burns involving more than 30% of the body surface
- Burns complicated by painful, swollen, or deformed extremities
- Burns which by classification are moderate, but appear in a person less than 5 or greater than 55
- Circumferential burns

Infants and Children

Burns pose greater risks to infants and children. This is because their body surface area is greater in relation to their total body size. This results in greater fluid and heat loss than would be found in an adult patient. Infants have a higher risk of shock, airway problems, and hypothermia from burns. Additionally classification of burns (severity) differs in patients less than five:

- Any partial thickness burn of less than 10% is considered a minor burn.
- Any partial thickness burn of 10 to 20% is considered a moderate burn in a child.
- Full thickness burns or partial thickness burns of more than 20% are to be considered critical burns in the child.

When a child has been burned, consider the possibility of child abuse.

Emergency Care for Burns

There are special approaches to the care of thermal burns, general chemical burns, and chemical burns to the eyes, as described below.

Patient Care—Thermal Burns

As an EMT-B you will have to care for thermal burns caused by scalding liquids, steam, contact with hot objects, flames, and flaming liquids and gases. On rare occasions, you may be called to care for sunburn, which can be severe when involving infants and young children. These patients may also have other heat-related injuries.

Emergency Care Steps

The steps for basic care of thermal burns are set forth in Scan 26-2.

Currently, dry sterile dressings are recommended by the national EMT-B curriculum for all burns. The standing orders for burn care are the decision of your EMS Medical Director and the regional EMS system.

An example of varying protocols: Some EMS systems state that all third-degree burns are to be wrapped with dry sterile dressing or a burn sheet, while some burn centers recommend moist dressings for partial-thickness burns to 9% or less of the body and dry dressings for more severe cases. The latter protocol is now being adopted by most EMS systems.

Note: EMT-Bs must manage burns correctly until the patient can be transferred to the care of the staff of a medical facility. Never apply ointments, sprays, or butter (to do so would trap the heat against the burn site and the hospital staff would just have to scrape it off the burn surface). Do not break blisters. Do not apply ice to any burn (it can cause tissue damage). Keep the burn site clean to prevent infection. Keep the patient warm, as the temperature regulation function of the skin may be affected by the burn.

Safety Note

Do not attempt to rescue persons trapped by fire unless you are trained to do so and have the equipment and personnel required. The simple act of opening a door might cost you your life. In some fires, opening a door or window may greatly intensify the fire or even cause an explosion.

Patient Care—Chemical Burns

Chemical burns require immediate care. It is hoped that people at the scene will begin this care before you arrive. At many industrial sites, workers and First Responders are trained to provide initial care for accidents involving the chemicals in use. Most major industries have emergency deluge-type safety showers to wash dangerous chemicals from the body. This will not always be the case. Be prepared for situations in which nothing has been done and there is no running water near the scene.

Emergency Care Steps

1. The primary care procedure is to WASH AWAY the chemical with flowing water. If a dry chemical is involved, brush away as much of the chemical as possible and then flush the skin. Simply wetting the burn site is not enough. Continuous flooding of the affected area is required, using a copious but gentle flow of water. Avoid hard sprays that may damage badly burned tissues (Figure 26-26). Continue to wash the area for at least 20 minutes, and continue the process en route to the hospital. Remove contaminated clothing, shoes, socks, and jewelry from the patient AS YOU APPLY THE WASH.

Note: Do not contaminate skin that has not been in contact with the chemical.

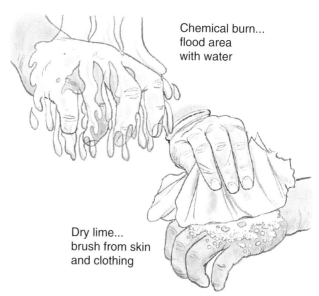

Chemical burn... flood area with water

Dry lime... brush from skin and clothing

FIGURE 26-26 Emergency care of chemical burns.

Warning: Protect yourself during the washing process. Wear vinyl or latex gloves and protective eyewear and control the wash to avoid splashing.

2 Apply a sterile dressing or burn sheet.
3 Treat for shock.
4 Transport.

When possible, find out the exact chemical or mixture of chemicals involved in the accident. Be on the alert for delayed reactions that may cause renewed pain or interfere with the patient's ability to breathe. Should the patient complain of increased burning or irritation, wash the burned areas again with flowing water for several minutes.

Safety Note
Some scenes where chemical burns have taken place can be very hazardous. Always evaluate the scene. There may be large pools of dangerous chemicals around the patient. Acids could be spurting from containers. Toxic fumes may be present. If the scene will place you in danger, do not attempt a rescue unless you have been trained for such a situation and have the needed equipment and personnel at the scene.

Patient Care—Chemical Burns to the Eyes

A corrosive chemical can burn the globe of a person's eye before he can react and close the eyelid. Even with the lid shut, chemicals can seep through onto the globe.

Emergency Care Steps

To care for chemical burns to the eye (Figure 26-27), you should

1 IMMEDIATELY flood the eyes with water. Often the burn will involve areas of the face as well as the eye. When this is the case, you will have to flood the entire area. Avoid washing chemicals back into the eye or into an unaffected eye.
2 Keep running water from a faucet, low pressure hose, bucket, cup, bottle, rubber bulb syringe, IV setup, or other such source flowing into the burned eye. The flow should be from the medial (nasal) corner of the eye to the lateral corner. Since the patient's natural reaction will be to

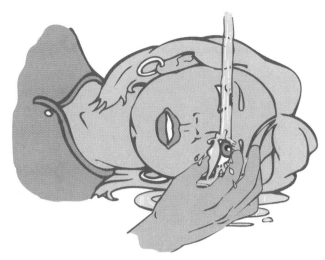

FIGURE 26-27 Care of chemical burns to the eyes.

keep the eyes tightly shut, you may have to hold the eyelids open.
3 Start transport and continue washing the eye for at least 20 minutes or until arrival at the medical facility.
4 After washing the eye, cover both eyes with moistened pads.
5 Wash the patient's eyes for 5 more minutes if he begins to complain about renewed burning sensations or irritation.

Warning: Do not use neutralizers such as vinegar or baking soda in a patient's eyes.

Electrical Injuries

Electric current, including lightning, can cause severe damage to the body. The skin is burned where the energy enters the body and where it flows into a ground. Along the path of this flow, tissues are damaged due to heat. In addition, significant chemical changes take place in the nerves, heart, and muscles, and body processes are disrupted or may completely shut down.

Safety Note
The scenes of injuries due to electricity are often very hazardous. Assume that the source of electricity is still active unless a qualified person tells you that the power has been turned off. Do not attempt a rescue unless you have been trained to do so and have the necessary equipment and personnel. For information about electrical hazards at the scene of a vehicle collision, see Chapter 31.

Signs and Symptoms

The victim of an electrical accident may have any or all of the following signs and symptoms (Figure 26-28).

- ☐ Burns where the energy enters and exits the body
- ☐ Disrupted nerve pathways displayed as paralysis
- ☐ Muscle tenderness, with or without muscular twitching
- ☐ Respiratory difficulties or respiratory arrest
- ☐ Irregular heartbeat or cardiac arrest
- ☐ Elevated blood pressure or low blood pressure with the signs and symptoms of shock
- ☐ Restlessness or irritability if conscious, or loss of consciousness
- ☐ Visual difficulties
- ☐ Fractured bones and dislocations from severe muscle contractions or from falling. This can include the spinal column.
- ☐ Seizures (in severe cases)

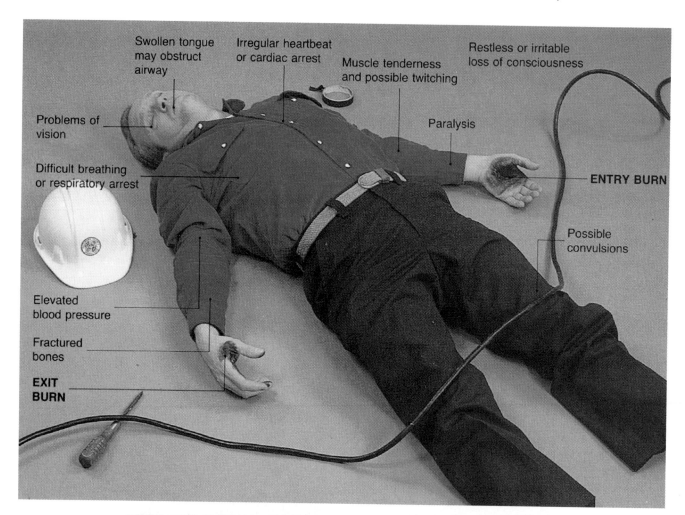

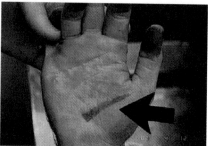

Electrical burn—contact with source

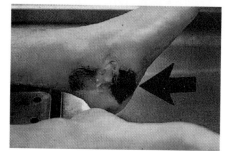

Electrical burn—exit

FIGURE 26-28 Injuries due to electrical shock.

Emergency Care Steps

1. **Warning:** Make certain that you and the patient are in a SAFE ZONE (not in contact with any electrical source and outside the area where downed or broken wires or other sources of electricity can reach you).
2. Provide airway care (remembering that electrical shock may cause severe swelling along the airway).
3. Provide basic cardiac life support as required. Since cardiac rhythm disturbances are common, be prepared to perform defibrillation if necessary.
4. Care for shock and administer high concentration oxygen.
5. Care for spinal injuries, head injuries, and severe fractures.
6. Evaluate electrical burns, looking for at least two external burn sites: contact with the energy source and contact with a ground.
7. Cool the burn areas and smoldering clothing the same as you would for a flame burn.
8. Apply dry sterile dressings to the burn sites.
9. Transport as soon as possible. Some problems have a slow onset. If there are burns, there also may be more serious hidden problems. In any case of electrical shock, heart problems may develop.

Remember: The major problem caused by electrical shock is usually not the burn. Respiratory and cardiac arrest are real possibilities. Be prepared to provide basic cardiac life support measures with automated defibrillation.

Documentation Tips—
Burns and Electrical Injuries

In the narrative portion of your prehospital care report, be sure to include things you have observed at the scene that hospital personnel will not be able to see. For example, note the source and agent of the burn, such as "thermal burns from hot radiator," or "chemical burns from contact with hydrochloric acid" or "electrical burns from contact with household AC current."

If possible, note the exact chemical or mixture of chemicals involved in a chemical burn. If safe for you to do so, copy exact information from a label or describe the container of the chemical if it is too large or unsafe to bring along to the hospital.

Dressing and Bandaging

Most cases of open wound care require the application of dressings and bandages (Scan 26-3). The basic dressing and bandaging skills described below can be applied to most open wounds.

Dressings and Bandages

To start with, you should know the following definitions (Figure 26-29).

- **Dressing**—Any material applied to a wound in an effort to control bleeding and prevent further contamination. Dressings should be sterile.
- **Bandage**—Any material used to hold a dressing in place. Bandages need not be sterile.

Warning: Be certain to wear disposable gloves and other barrier devices to avoid contact with the patient's blood and body fluids and follow infection control procedures.

Various dressings are carried in emergency care kits. These dressings should be sterile, meaning that all microorganisms and spores that can grow into active organisms have been killed. Dressings also should be aseptic, meaning that all dirt and foreign debris have been removed. In emergency situations, when commercially prepared dressings are not available, clean cloth, towels, sheets, handkerchiefs, and other similar materials may be suitable alternatives.

The most popular dressings are individually wrapped sterile gauze pads, typically 4 inches square. A variety of sizes are available, referred to according to size in inches, such as 2 by 2s, 4 by 4s, 5 by 9s, and 8 by 10s.

Large bulky dressings, such as the multitrauma or **universal dressing,** are available when bulk is required for profuse bleeding or

Scan 26-3
Examples of General Dressing and Bandaging

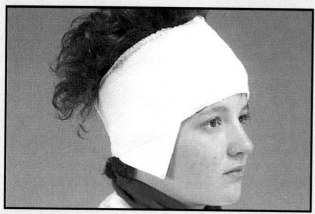

FOREHEAD (NO SKULL INJURY) OR EAR Place dressing and secure with self-adherent roller bandage.

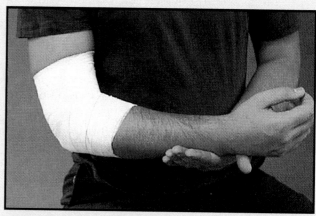

ELBOW OR KNEE Place dressing and secure with cravat or roller bandage. Apply roller bandage in figure 8 pattern.

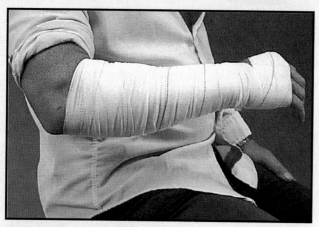

FOREARM OR LEG Place dressing and secure with roller bandage, distal to proximal. Better protection is offered if palm or sole is wrapped.

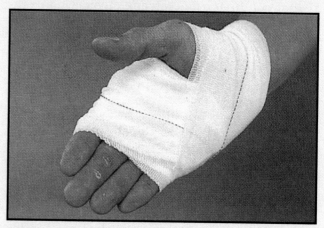

HAND Place dressing, wrap with roller bandages, and secure at wrist. When possible, bandage in position of function.

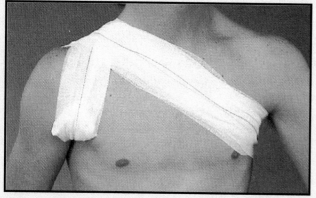

SHOULDER Place dressing and secure with figure 8 of cravat or roller dressing. Pad under knot if cravat is used.

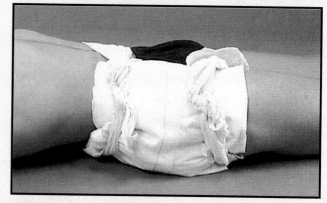

HIP Place bandage and large dressing to cover hip. Secure with first cravat around waist and second cravat around thigh on injured side.

Note: Always leave fingertips or toes showing to assess circulation.

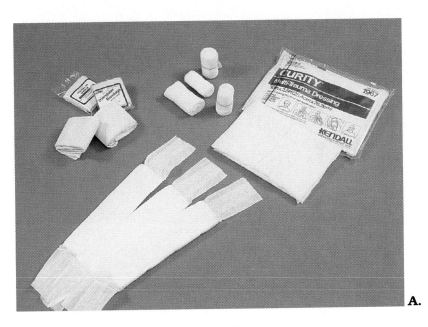
A.

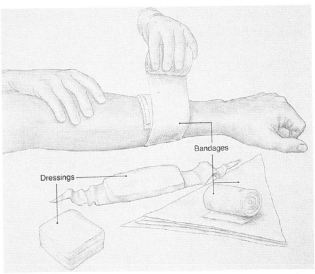

Dressings

Bandages

B.

FIGURE 26-29 A. Materials used for dressings and bandages. B. Dressings cover wounds, while bandages hold dressings in place.

when a large wound must be covered. These dressings are especially useful for stabilizing impaled objects. Sanitary napkins can sometimes be used in place of the standard bulky dressings. Although not sterile, they are separately wrapped and have very clean surfaces (do not apply any adhesive surface of the napkin directly to the wound). Of course, bulky dressings can be made by building up layers of gauze pads.

A pressure dressing is used to control bleeding. Gauze pads are placed on the wound and a bulky dressing is placed over the pads. A self-adherent roller bandage is wrapped tightly over the dressing and above and below the wound. Distal pulse must be checked and frequently rechecked, and you may need to readjust the pressure to ensure distal circulation.

The **occlusive dressing** is used when it is necessary to form an airtight seal. This is done when caring for open wounds to the abdomen, for external bleeding from large neck veins, and for open wounds to the chest. Sterile, commercially prepared occlusive dressings are available in two different forms. There are plastic wrap and petroleum gel-impregnated gauze occlusive dressings. Local protocols vary as to which form to use. Nonsterile wrap and foil also can be used in emergency situations. In emergencies, EMT-Bs have been known to fashion occlusive dressings from plastic credit cards, plastic bags, aluminum foil wrappers, and defibrillator pads.

Warning: Some EMS Systems report that aluminum foil has caused lacerations of exposed abdominal organs.

Large dressings are sometimes needed in emergency care. Sterile, disposable burn sheets are commercially available. Bed sheets can be sterilized and kept in plastic wrappers to be later used as dressings. These sheets can make effective burn dressings or may be used in some cases to cover exposed abdominal organs.

Bandages are provided in a wide variety of types. The preferred bandage is the self-adherent, form-fitting roller bandage (Figure 26-30). It eliminates the need to know many specialized bandaging techniques developed for use with ordinary gauze roller bandages.

Dressings can be secured using adhering or nonadhering gauze roller bandage, triangular bandages, strips of adhesive tape, or an air splint. In a situation where one of these is not available, you can use strips of cloth, handkerchiefs, and other such materials. Elastic bandages that are used in the general care of strains and sprains should not be used to hold dressings in place. They can become constricting bands, interfering with circulation. This is very likely to occur as the tissues around the wound site begin to swell after the elastic bandage is in place.

Patient Care—Dressing Open Wounds

Emergency Care Steps

The following rules apply to the general dressing of wounds (Figure 26-31).

1. *Expose the wound.* Cut away any clothing so the entire wound is exposed.
2. *Use sterile or very clean materials.* Avoid touching the dressing in the area that will come into contact with the wound. Grasp the dressing by the corner, taking it directly from its protective pack, and place it on the wound.
3. *Cover the entire wound.* The entire surface of the wound and the immediate surrounding areas should be covered.
4. *Control bleeding.* With the exception of the pressure dressing, a dressing should not be bandaged into place if it has not controlled the bleeding. You should continue to apply dressings and pressure as needed for the proper control of bleeding.
5. *Do not remove dressings.* Once a dressing has been applied to a wound, it must remain in place. Bleeding may restart and tissues at the wound site may be injured if the dressing is removed. If the bleeding

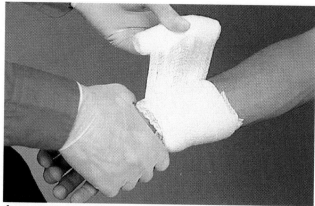

A.

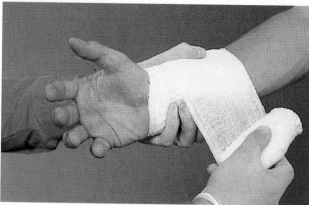

B.

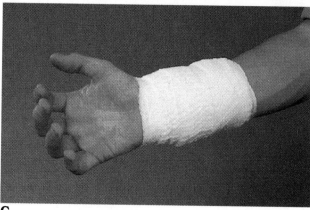

C.

FIGURE 26-30 Applying a self-adherent roller bandage: A. Secure with several overlying wraps. B. Overlap the bandage, keeping it snug. C. Cut and tape or tie into place.

continues, put new dressings over the blood-soaked ones.

There is an exception to the rule prohibiting the removal of dressings. If a bulky bandage has become blood-soaked, it may be necessary to remove the bandage so that direct pressure can be reestablished or a new bulky bandage can be

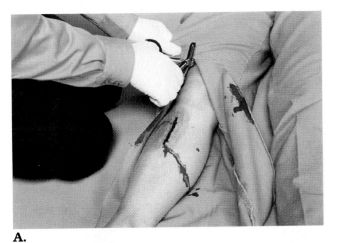

A.

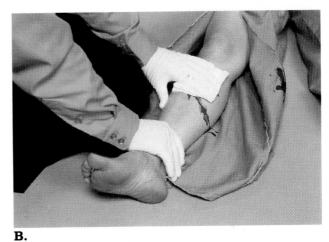

B.

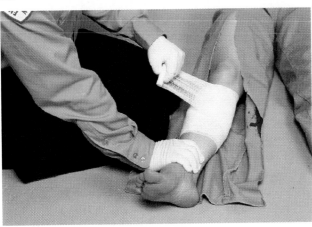

C.

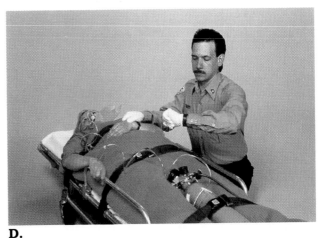

D.

FIGURE 26-31 Care for open wounds. A. Expose wound. B. Apply direct pressure. C. Bandage wound. D. Keep patient at rest.

added and a pressure dressing created. Protection for the wound site is better maintained if one or more simple gauze dressing pads are placed over the top of the injured tissues prior to the placement of the bulky bandage. This will allow for the removal of a bulky bandage without disturbing the wound.

Remember: Do not remove the dressings that lie in contact with the wound, as you may disturb the clots that have formed. Doing so may cause the bleeding to start again.

Patient Care—Bandaging Open Wounds

Emergency Care Steps

The following rules apply to general bandaging (Figure 26-31).

1 *Do not bandage too tightly.* All dressings should be held snugly in place, but they must not restrict the blood supply to the affected part.

2 *Do not bandage too loosely.* Hold the dressing by bandaging snugly, so the dressing does not move around or slip from the wound. Loose bandaging is a common error in emergency care.

3 *Do not leave loose ends.* Any loose ends of gauze, tape, or cloth may get caught on objects when the patient is moved.

4 *Do not cover the tips of fingers and toes.* When bandaging the extremities, leave the fingers and toes exposed whenever possible to observe skin color changes that indicate a change in circulation and to allow for easier neurologic reassessment. Pain, pale or blue-colored skin, cold skin, numbness, and tingling are all indications that a bandage may be too tight. If the fingers or toes are burned, they will have to be covered.

5 *Cover all edges of the dressing.* This will

help to reduce additional contamination. The exception is found in the procedures for open chest wounds (see earlier in this chapter).

There are two special problems that occur when bandaging an extremity. First, point pressure can occur if you apply the bandage around a very small area. It is best to wrap a large area of the extremity, ensuring a steady, uniform pressure. Apply the bandage from the smaller diameter of the limb to the larger diameter (distal to proximal) to help ensure proper pressure and contact. Second, the joints of the extremity have to be considered. You can bandage across a joint, but do not bend the limb once the bandage is in place. To do so may restrict circulation, loosen the dressing and bandage, or both. In some cases, it may be necessary to apply an inflatable or rigid splint, or to use a sling and swathe to prevent movement of the joint. Problems with tourniquet application were discussed in Chapter 25, Bleeding and Shock.

FYI

Topics included in the FYI—"For Your Information"—section are those that go beyond the chapter objectives. The information in this segment is intended to broaden your understanding of the chapter topic but is not essential to an understanding of your job as an EMT-B.

Chest Injury Complications

In trauma to the chest, the lungs, heart, and great blood vessels can be injured. Such injuries can result in serious complications, including pneumothorax, tension pneumothorax, hemothorax, hemopneumothorax, cardiac tamponade, and traumatic asphyxia.

Pneumothorax and Tension Pneumothorax

Pneumothorax (NU-mo-THOR-aks) occurs when the lung collapses within the chest cavity. It frequently occurs as a result of an open chest wound. Air entering the chest cavity can be deadly to a patient. One of the most serious conditions that can result from chest wounds is a *tension pneumothorax.*

Tension pneumothorax is a complication that may be found after application of an occlu-

sive dressing. This condition may also be seen with closed injuries to the chest. The lung may be punctured by a broken rib or other cause. If there is no opening from outside the chest, or if the opening has been completely sealed by an occlusive dressing that was taped down on all four sides, the air that leaks from the lung has no avenue of escape. It builds up in the chest cavity and puts pressure on the heart, the great blood vessels, and the unaffected lung, reducing cardiac output and the ability of the lungs to oxygenate the blood.

Patient Assessment—Pneumothorax and Tension Pneumothorax

Patient assessment for pneumothorax and tension pneumothorax were discussed earlier in this chapter under Open Chest Wounds.

Hemothorax and Hemopneumothorax

You may also hear the term *hemothorax* (HE-mo-THOR-aks). Hemothorax is a condition in which the chest cavity fills with blood. With *hemopneumothorax* (HE-mo-NU-mo-THOR-aks), the chest cavity fills with both blood and air.

It is easy to compare these two complications with pneumothorax (Figure 26-32) if you remember that *pneumo* means "air" and *hemo* means "blood." In pneumothorax, there was a buildup of air in the thorax. In hemothorax and hemopneumothorax, blood creates or adds to the pressure buildup.

In hemothorax, lacerations within the chest cavity can be produced by penetrating objects or fractured ribs. Blood will flow into the space around the lung, the lung may collapse, and the patient will experience a loss of blood leading to shock. Hemopneumothorax is a combination of blood and air, usually producing the same results: a collapsed lung and loss of blood leading to shock.

Patient Assessment—Hemothorax and Hemopneumothorax

Signs

☐ Hemothorax and hemopneumothorax usually present the same signs as pneumothorax, including gasping for breath and a possible sucking wound.
☐ In addition, the patient may cough up frothy red blood, or flecks of blood may appear on the lips.

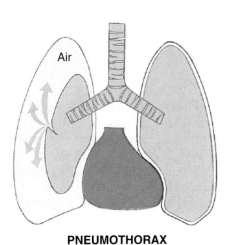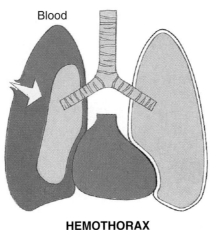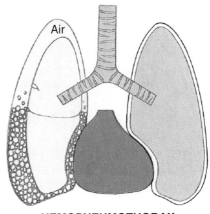

| PNEUMOTHORAX | HEMOTHORAX | HEMOPNEUMOTHORAX |

FIGURE 26-32 Conditions produced by chest injuries.

Traumatic Asphyxia

Traumatic asphyxia (traw-MAT-ik a-SFIKS-e-ah) is a group of signs and symptoms that can be associated with sudden compression of the chest. When this occurs, the sternum and the ribs exert severe pressure on the heart and lungs, forcing blood out of the right atrium up into the jugular veins in the neck.

Patient Assessment—Traumatic Asphyxia

Signs

The signs of traumatic asphyxia are shown in Figure 26-33. Although signs may be most apparent on the head and neck, it is the associated chest injuries that can rapidly be fatal. This is a TRUE EMERGENCY.

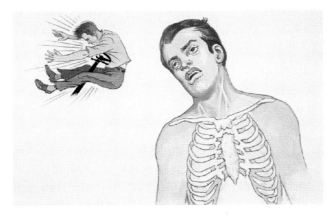

- Distended neck veins
- Head, neck, and shoulders appear dark blue or purple
- Eyes may be bloodshot and bulging
- Tongue and lips may appear swollen and cyanotic
- Chest deformity may be present

FIGURE 26-33 Signs of traumatic asphyxia.

Cardiac Tamponade

When a penetrating or blunt injury to the heart causes blood to flow into the surrounding pericardial sac, the condition produced is *cardiac tamponade* (KAR-de-ak TAM-po-NOD). The heart's unyielding sac fills with blood and compresses the chambers of the heart to a point where they will no longer fill adequately, backing up blood into the veins.

Patient Assessment—Cardiac Tamponade

Signs

- ☐ Distended neck veins
- ☐ Very weak pulse
- ☐ Low blood pressure
- ☐ Steadily decreasing pulse pressure. Pulse pressure is the difference between systolic and diastolic readings. When the two readings approach each other (systolic falling, diastolic rising or unchanging), it is a reliable sign of serious chest cavity injury. A pulse pressure below 15 mm HG is critical.

Cardiac tamponade is life threatening, a TRUE EMERGENCY.

Patient Care—Chest Injury Complications

The treatment for any type of penetrating injury to the chest is the same.

1. Maintain an open airway.
2. Follow local protocols as to the preferred type of dressing for any open wound.
3. Administer a high concentration of oxygen.

4 Care for shock.
5 Transport as soon as possible.

Care of Specific Chemical Burns

Some special chemical burn situations require specific care procedures.

Patient Care—Specific Chemical Burns

Emergency Care Steps

☐ *Mixed or Strong Acids or Unidentified Substances*—Many of the chemicals used in industrial processes are mixed acids. Their combined action can be immediate and severe. The pain produced from the initial chemical burn may mask any pain being caused by renewed burning due to small concentrations left on the skin. When the chemical is a strong acid (e.g., hydrochloric acid or sulfuric acid), a combination of acids, or an unknown, play it safe and continue washing even after the patient claims he is no longer experiencing pain.

☐ *Dry Lime*—If dry lime is the burn agent, do not wash the burn site with water. To do so will create a corrosive liquid. Brush the dry lime from the patient's skin, hair, and clothing. Make certain that you do not contaminate the eyes or airway. Use water only after the lime has been brushed from the body, contaminated clothing and jewelry have been removed, and the process of washing can be done quickly and continuously with running water.

☐ *Carbolic Acid (Phenol)*—Carbolic acid does not mix with water. When available, use alcohol for the initial wash of unbroken skin, followed by a long steady wash with water. (Follow local protocols.)

☐ *Sulfuric Acid*—Heat is produced when water is added to concentrated sulfuric acid, but it is still preferable to wash rather than leave contaminant on the skin.

☐ *Hydrofluoric Acid*—Hydrofluoric acid is used for etching glass and in many other manufacturing processes. Burns from this acid may be delayed, so treat all patients who may have come into contact with the chemical, even if burns are not in evidence. Flood with water if burning sensations are severe on your arrival, immediately begin the water wash. Do not delay care and transport to find neutralizing agents. (Follow local protocols.)

☐ *Inhaled Vapors*—Whenever a patient is exposed to a caustic chemical and may have inhaled the vapors, provide a high concentration of oxygen (humidified, if available) and transport as soon as possible. This is very important when the chemical is an acid that is known to vaporize at standard environmental temperatures (e.g., hydrochloric acid or sulfuric acid).

CHAPTER REVIEW

KEY TERMS

You may find it helpful to review the following terms.

abrasion (ab-RAY-zhun)   a scratch or scrape.

air embolus (EM-bo-lus)   a bubble of air in the bloodstream.

amputation (am-pyu-TAY-shun)   the surgical removal or traumatic severing of a body part, usually an extremity.

avulsion (ah-VUL-shun)   the tearing away or tearing off of a piece or flap of skin or other soft tissue. This term also may be used for an eye pulled from its socket or a tooth dislodged from its socket.

bandage   any material used to hold a dressing in place.

closed wound   an internal injury with no open pathway from the outside.

contusion (Kun-TU-zhun)   a bruise.

crush injury   An injury caused when force is transmitted from the body's exterior to its internal structures. Bones can be broken, muscles, nerves and tissues damaged, and internal organs ruptured, causing internal bleeding.

dermis (DER-mis)   the inner (second) layer of the skin found beneath the epidermis. It is rich in blood vessels and nerves.

dressing any material (preferably sterile) used to cover a wound that will help control bleeding and help prevent additional contamination.

epidermis (ep-i-DER-mis) the outer layer of the skin.

evisceration (e-vis-er-AY-shun) an intestine or other internal organ protruding through a wound in the abdomen.

full-thickness burn a burn in which all the layers of the skin are damaged. There are usually areas that are charred black or areas that are dry and white. Also called a third-degree burn.

hematoma (hem-ah-TO-mah) a swelling caused by the collection of blood under the skin or in damaged tissues as a result of an injured or broken blood vessel.

laceration (las-er-AY-shun) a cut.

occlusive dressing any dressing that forms an airtight seal.

open wound an injury in which the skin is interrupted, exposing the tissue beneath.

partial-thickness burn a burn in which the epidermis (first layer of skin) is burned through and the dermis (second layer) is damaged. Burns of this type cause reddening, blistering, and a mottled appearance. Also called a second degree burn.

puncture wound an open wound that tears through the skin and destroys underlying tissues. A **penetrating puncture wound** can be shallow or deep. A **perforating puncture wound** has both an entrance and an exit wound.

Rule of Nines a method for estimating the extent of a burn. For an adult, each of the following areas represents 9% of the body surface: the head and neck, each upper extremity, the chest, the abdomen, the upper back, the lower back and buttocks, the front of each lower extremity, and the back of each lower extremity. The remaining 1% is assigned to the genital region. For an infant or child the percentages are modified so that 18% is assigned to the head, 14% to each lower extremity.

Rule of Palm a method for estimating the extent of a burn. The palm of the patient's hand, which equals about 1% of the body's surface area, is compared with the patient's burn to estimate its size.

subcutaneous (SUB-ku-TAY-ne-us) **layers** the layers of fat and soft tissues found below the dermis.

sucking chest wound an open chest wound in which air is "sucked" into the chest cavity.

superficial burn a burn that involves only the epidermis, the outer layer of the skin. It is characterized by reddening of the skin and perhaps some swelling. An example is a sunburn. Also called a first-degree burn.

universal dressing a bulky dressing.

SUMMARY

Injuries to the soft tissues of the body are common calls for the EMT-B. Soft tissue injuries may be closed (internal, with no pathway to the outside) or open (an injury in which the skin is interrupted, exposing the tissues below). An open chest or abdominal wound is considered to be one that penetrates not only the skin but the chest or abdominal wall to expose internal organs. Closed injuries include contusions (bruises), hematomas, and crush injuries. Open wounds include abrasions, lacerations, punctures, avulsions, amputations, and crush injuries. Open neck, chest, and abdominal wounds are life-threatening. For open wounds, expose the wound, control bleeding, and prevent further contamination. For an open neck, chest, or abdominal wound apply an occlusive dressing. For both open and closed injuries, take appropriate BSI precautions, note the mechanism of injury, protect the patient's airway and breathing, administer high concentration oxygen by nonrebreather mask, treat for shock, and transport.

Burn severity is determined by considering the source of the burn, body regions burned, depth of burn (superficial, partial thickness, and full thickness), extent of burn (by Rule of Nines or Rule of Palm), age of patient (children under 5 and adults over 55 react most severely), and other patient illnesses or injuries. Care for burns includes stopping the burning process (water for a thermal burn, brushing away chemicals), covering a thermal burn with a dry sterile dressing, flushing a chemical burn with sterile water, protection of the airway, administration of oxygen, treatment for shock, and transport.

For treatment of electrical injuries, be sure that you and the patient are in a safe zone away from possible contact with electrical sources. Protect airway, breathing, and circulation. Be prepared to care for respiratory or cardiac arrest. Treat for shock, care for burns, and transport.

REVIEW QUESTIONS

1. List three types of closed soft tissue injury.
2. List four types of open soft tissue injury.
3. Describe the care for an open wound to the chest.
4. Describe the care for impaled objects in the eye.
5. Explain when you would remove an object impaled in the cheek and when you would, instead, stabilize an object impaled in the cheek.
6. Describe the three classifications (depths) of burns.
7. Differentiate between a dressing and a bandage.
8. List the qualities and purpose of an effective bandage. How could you tell if a bandage were improperly applied?

Application

- Tom Jansen, the patient from the On the Scene for this chapter, has suddenly begun to deteriorate. He is having extreme difficulty in breathing and his color has worsened. Breath sounds have become almost totally absent on the side with the impaled nail. What complication might you suspect is causing his worsening condition? How could this be corrected?

Musculoskeletal Injuries

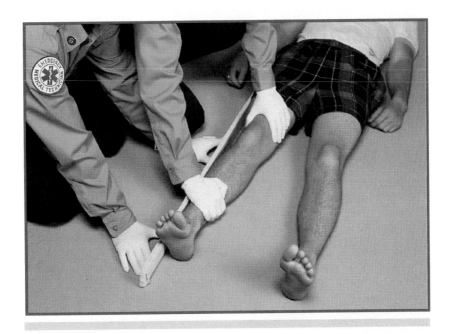

27

Musculoskeletal injuries are among the most common complaints encountered by the EMT-Basic. Although such injuries are usually not life threatening, most can result in permanent disability if improperly treated. Proper identification and emergency care of musculoskeletal injuries is crucial in reducing pain, preventing further injury, and minimizing damage to nerves, arteries, and other soft tissues.

Knowledge and Attitude *At the end of this chapter, you should be able to meet the following objectives.*

1. Describe the function of the muscular system. (pp. 511–512, 516)

2. Describe the function of the skeletal system. (pp. 511–516)

3. List the major bones or bone groupings of the spinal column, the thorax, the upper extremities, and the lower extremities. (pp. 512, 514, 515)

4. Differentiate between an open and a closed painful, swollen, deformed extremity. (p. 518)

5. State the reasons for splinting. (p. 519)

6. List the general rules of splinting. (pp. 520–521)

On the Scene

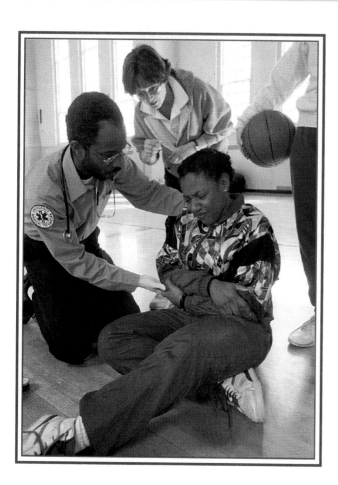

During tryouts at the college, freshman Joanne McGurk is having a great time on the basketball court. She's taking turns with her classmates jumping high and easing balls into the hoop. Several of them are good for the women's team, and as the excitement grows, so do the fancy moves. In what turns out to be her last jump of the season, Joanne leaps for a rebound and collides with another player. They both hit the court pretty hard, but Joanne falls on her outstretched hand, hears a crack, and feels sudden pain. The other player is OK. However, it only takes a second for everyone to realize that Joanne is hurt. The coach stays with Joanne and sends a student to call for help.

When you and your partner arrive, *scene size-up* reveals the patient sitting on the floor in center court of the college gym. She's holding her injured arm close to her chest, and the coach is trying to comfort her. On the edges of the court, the assistant coach is dispersing a small crowd. Access is otherwise clear, and you approach the patient.

During your *initial assessment,* you form a general impression of an alert young adult female, guarding her swollen and slightly discolored forearm. Your partner applies manual stabilization to Joanne's head. You determine that her airway, breathing, and circulation are all normal, with no visible bleeding, so she is not a high priority for immediate transport.

As your partner continues manual stabilization, you begin the *focused history and physical exam* by examining the obviously injured arm. The mechanism of injury suggests that there may be injuries along the path of the force. If great enough,

7. List the complications of splinting. (pp. 521–522)

8. List the emergency medical care for a patient with a painful, swollen, deformed extremity. (pp. 519–555)

9. Explain the rationale for splinting at the scene versus load and go. (pp. 519, 520)

10. Explain the rationale for immobilization of the painful, swollen, deformed extremity. (p. 519)

Skills

1. Demonstrate the emergency medical care of a patient with a painful, swollen, deformed extremity.

2. Demonstrate completing a prehospital care report for patients with musculoskeletal injuries.

the energy could have been transmitted to Joanne's elbow, humerus, shoulder, or even her neck. You already know from the discoloration in the arm that there is damage to the soft tissues. She has no other apparent injuries.

You apply a cervical collar and your partner takes her vital signs. As you begin splinting the arm, you take a SAMPLE history. Joanne reports she hasn't lost consciousness and denies any other pain. She denies having any allergies, being on medication, or having any pertinent past medical history. Her last meal was at 1200, and it's now 1600 hours. She describes the events that led to her fall and injury.

You and your partner have decided to apply a padded rigid splint that extends from above the elbow past the fingertips. "Joanne, we are going to have to move your arm in order to apply the splint. It will hurt when I move it, but it will feel much better when we're done," you explain. You establish that Joanne has good pulses in her hand, senses your touch, and wiggles her fingers. Then with one hand at her elbow and one at her wrist, you provide gentle tension until the splint is positioned and secured. You confirm that she still has good pulses and motor and sensory function, so you apply a sling and swathe.

Inside the ambulance you perform a **detailed physical exam,** during which you find no further injuries or problems. She has no other obvious injuries. **Ongoing assessment** assures that her vital signs are still normal, the splint, sling, and swathe are still correctly applied, and distal function in Joanne's arm is still good.

In the hospital emergency department Joanne is diagnosed as having a closed fracture of the radius and ulna. An orthopedic surgeon applies a cast. Joanne spends the rest of the basketball season watching from the sidelines and planning to try out for the team again next year.

Musculoskeletal injuries can be very dramatic, and you will provide emergency care for them often. However, to do so properly and effectively in the field, you must make an effort to follow your emergency care routine. Always check for and treat life-threatening conditions first. Then as appropriate splint the injured extremity to reduce pain, prevent further injury, and minimize permanent damage.

THE MUSCULOSKELETAL SYSTEM

The musculoskeletal system is composed of all the **muscles, bones,** and **joints** of the body, as well as **tendons, ligaments,** and **cartilage.** As an EMT-B you do not need to know every structure found in the body. However, you will need to remember how complex the structures are and how damage may be done to soft tissues in case of injury. See Figures 27-1 through 27-5. You should also review the musculoskeletal system in Chapter 4, The Human Body. In this chapter, we will pay special attention to the **extremities**—the portions of the skeleton that include the clavicles, scapulae, arms, wrists, and hands (upper extremities) and the pelvis, thighs, legs, ankles, and feet (lower extremities).

The Anatomy of Bone

Generally, bones are classified according to their appearance (Figure 27-6)—long, short, flat, and irregular. The bones found in the arm and thigh are examples of long bones. The major short bones of the body are in the hands and feet. Among the flat bones are the sternum, shoulder

The Skeleton

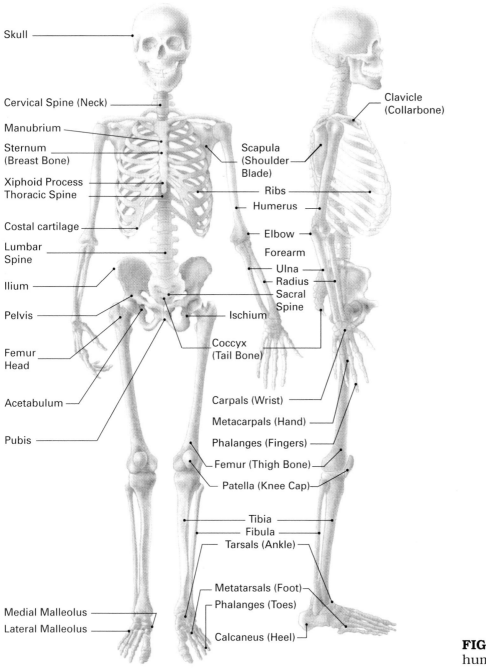

Skull

Cervical Spine (Neck)

Manubrium

Sternum (Breast Bone)

Xiphoid Process
Thoracic Spine

Costal cartilage

Lumbar Spine

Ilium

Pelvis

Femur Head

Acetabulum

Pubis

Medial Malleolus

Lateral Malleolus

Clavicle (Collarbone)

Scapula (Shoulder Blade)

Ribs

Humerus

Elbow

Forearm

Ulna

Radius

Sacral Spine

Ischium

Coccyx (Tail Bone)

Carpals (Wrist)

Metacarpals (Hand)

Phalanges (Fingers)

Femur (Thigh Bone)

Patella (Knee Cap)

Tibia

Fibula

Tarsals (Ankle)

Metatarsals (Foot)

Phalanges (Toes)

Calcaneus (Heel)

FIGURE 27-1 The human skeleton.

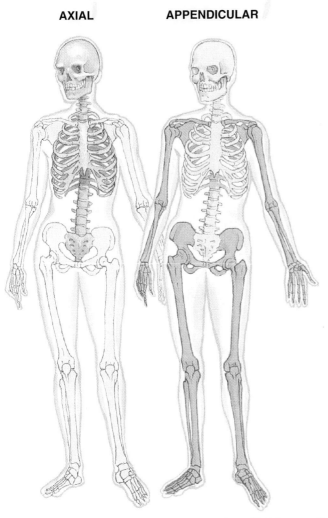

AXIAL **APPENDICULAR**

FIGURE 27-2 There are two major divisions of the human skeleton.

blades, and ribs. The vertebrae of the spinal column are examples of irregular bones.

The outward appearance of a typical long bone creates the impression that it is a simple, rigid structure made of the same material throughout. Actually, it is quite complex. Most people are aware that bone contains calcium, which helps to make it very hard. Bone also contains protein fibers that make it somewhat flexible. The strength of our bones is a combination of this hardness and flexibility. As we age, less protein is formed in the bones, less calcium is stored, and as a result, bones become brittle and **fracture** (break) more easily.

Bones are covered by a strong, white, fibrous material called the *periosteum* (per-e-OS-te-um). Blood vessels and nerves pass through this membrane as they enter and leave the bone.

When bone is exposed as a result of injury, the periosteum becomes visible. You may see fragments of bones and foreign objects on this covering, but do not remove them. If they have pierced the periosteum, the objects may be held firmly in place and offer a great resistance to any pulling or sweeping efforts. In addition, you will not be able to tell if the object has entered the bone or is impaled in an underlying blood vessel or nerve.

The *shafts* of bones appear to be straight, but each bone has its own unique curvature. When the end of a bone is involved in forming a ball-and-socket joint, it will be rounded to allow for rotational movement. This rounded end is called the *head* of the bone. It is connected to the shaft by the *neck*. Bone marrow is contained in the center of bones.

The Self-Healing Nature of Bone

The first effects of an injury to bone are swelling of soft tissue and the formation of a blood clot in the area of the fracture. Both the swelling and the clotting are due to the destruction of blood vessels in the periosteum and the bone, and to loss of blood from adjacent damaged vessels.

Interruption of the blood supply causes death to the cells at the injury site. Cells a little farther from the fracture remain intact and within a few hours begin to divide rapidly. They soon grow together to form a mass of tissue that completely surrounds the fracture site. New bone is generated from this mass to eventually heal the damaged bone. The whole process can take weeks or months, depending on the bone that has been fractured, the type of fracture, and the health and age of the patient.

It is therefore very important for a broken bone to be immobilized quickly and remain immobilized to heal properly. Should the fractured bone be mishandled early in care, more soft tissue may be damaged, which would require a longer period for the formation of a tissue mass and replacement of bone. If the bone ends are disturbed during regeneration, proper healing will not take place and a permanent disability may result. In children the majority of growth of a long bone occurs in the area known as the *growth plate,* which is near the ends of the shaft. If a fracture in this area is not properly handled, the child may grow up with one limb shorter than the other.

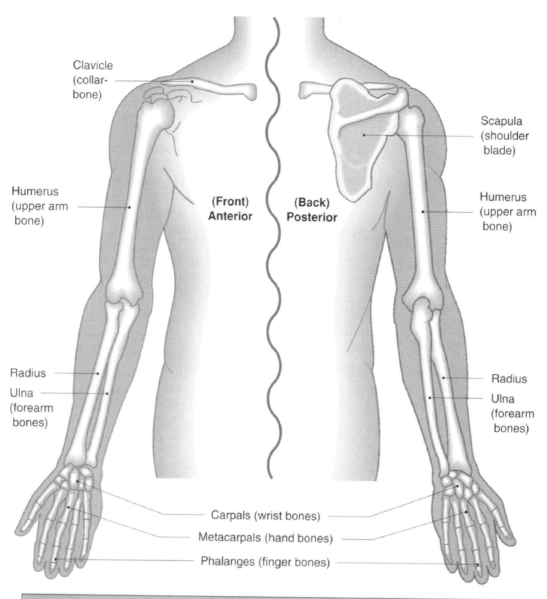

Clavicle
(collar-
bone)

Humerus
(upper arm
bone)

Radius
Ulna
(forearm
bones)

(Front)
Anterior

(Back)
Posterior

Scapula
(shoulder
blade)

Humerus
(upper arm
bone)

Radius
Ulna
(forearm
bones)

Carpals (wrist bones)

Metacarpals (hand bones)

Phalanges (finger bones)

THE UPPER EXTREMITIES

COMMON NAME	ANATOMICAL NAME
Shoulder girdle	Pectoral girdle (pek-TOR-al): clavicle, scapula, and head of humerus
Collarbone (1/side)	Clavicle (KLAV-i-kul)
Shoulder blade (1/side)	Scapula (SKAP-u-lah)
Arm bone (1/limb, from shoulder to elbow)	Humerus (HU-mer-us)
Forearm bones (2/limb, from elbow to wrist: 1/medial, 1/lateral)	Ulna (UL-nah)– medial Radius (RAY-de-us)– lateral
Wrist bones (8/wrist)	Carpals (KAR-pals)
Hand bones (5/palm, palm bones)	Metacarpals (meta-KAR-pals)
Finger bones (14/hand)	Phalanges (fah-LAN-jez)

FIGURE 27-3 Bones of the upper extremities.

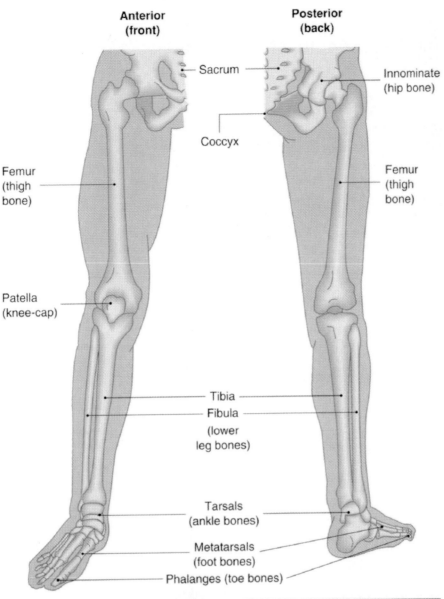

Anterior (front)

Sacrum

Femur (thigh bone)

Patella (knee-cap)

Tibia

Fibula (lower leg bones)

Tarsals (ankle bones)

Metatarsals (foot bones)

Phalanges (toe bones)

Posterior (back)

Innominate (hip bone)

Coccyx

Femur (thigh bone)

THE LOWER EXTREMITIES

COMMON NAMES	ANATOMICAL NAMES
Pelvic girdle (pelvis or hips)	Innominate on each side made up of the fused ilium, ischium, and pubis bones, as well as sacrum and coccyx posteriorly
Thigh bone (1/limb)	Femur (FE-mer)
Kneecap (1/limb)	Patella (pah-TEL-lah)
Leg bones (shin bones, 2/leg, 1 medial, 1 lateral)	Tibia (TIB-e-ah) – medial
	Fibula (FIB-yo-lah) – lateral
Ankle bones (7/foot)	Tarsals (TAR-sals)
Foot bones (5/foot)	Metatarsals (meta-TAR-sals)
Toe bones (14/foot. some people have two bones in their little toe, others may have three)	Phalanges (Fah-LAN-jez)

FIGURE 27-4 Bones of the lower extremities.

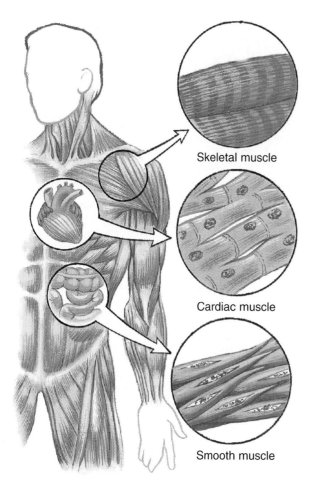

Skeletal muscle

Cardiac muscle

Smooth muscle

FIGURE 27-5 There are three types of muscle in the human body.

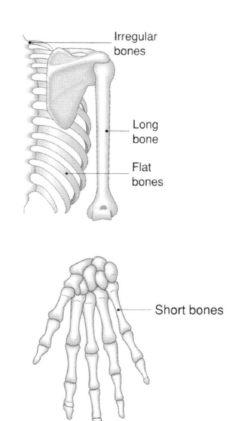

Irregular bones

Long bone

Flat bones

Short bones

FIGURE 27-6 Bones are classified by shape.

GENERAL GUIDELINES FOR EMERGENCY CARE

Mechanisms of Musculoskeletal Injury

There are basically three types of mechanisms that cause musculoskeletal injuries: direct force, indirect force, and twisting force (Figure 27-7). An example of direct force is a person being struck by an automobile, causing crushed tissue and fractures. Joanne's injury, in On the Scene, was caused by indirect forces, which moved from the point of impact (her hand) to break the bones in her forearm. Twisting or rotational forces can cause stretching or tearing of muscles and ligaments, as well as broken bones.

While it may be easy to see how direct forces cause injuries, indirect force can be just as powerful. For example, a well known injury pattern occurs when people fall from heights and land on their feet. While the direct forces cause injuries to the feet and ankles, the indi-rect forces usually cause injuries to the knees, femurs, pelvis, and spinal column.

In fact, most injuries to the upper extremities are caused by forces applied to an outstretched arm. In the course of a fall the person reaches out with an arm in an effort to "break the fall" and in doing so often breaks the radius, ulna, or clavicle, or dislocates the shoulder.

Painful, Swollen, or Deformed (PSD) Extremity

Unless there is very obvious deformity, it is not possible or even important for you to decide if a patient's injury is a fracture, dislocation, sprain, or severe bruise. Most patients simply present with pain, swelling, and—sometimes—deformity. It would take an X ray or other imaging process to diagnose the injury precisely. So in the field the worst must be assumed, and patients with a painful, swollen, or deformed (PSD) extremity should be treated as though they have a fracture.

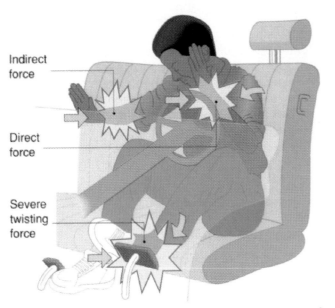

FIGURE 27-7 There are three basic types of mechanisms of musculoskeletal injury.

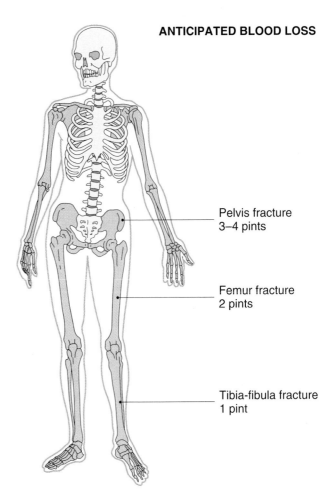

Pelvis fracture
3–4 pints

Femur fracture
2 pints

Tibia-fibula fracture
1 pint

FIGURE 27-8 Bones bleed. There may be considerable blood loss even from an uncomplicated closed injury.

While most fractures are not life threatening, you must remember that bones are living tissue. Even in simple uncomplicated fractures, bones bleed. For example, a simple closed tibia-fibula fracture typically causes 1 pint of blood loss. Fractures of the femur typically cause a 2-pint blood loss, and pelvic fractures cause a 3- to 4-pint loss. (See Figure 27-8.)

In World War I, the battlefield death rate from closed fracture of the femur was about 80% from complications such as blood loss. Two surgeons noticed that large muscle groups in the thigh go into spasms (contract, or shrink), forcing the broken femoral ends to override each other, injuring the blood vessels. To correct the problem, they invented the **traction splint,** a splint that applies constant pull along the length of the leg to help stabilize the fractured bone and reduce muscle spasms. With early application of the traction splint, the mortality rate from femur fractures dropped to under 20%.

Remember—splinting painful, swollen, deformed (PSD) extremities can prevent additional blood loss, pain, and complications from nerve and blood vessel injury. Therefore, treat for the worst (a fracture) and immobilize. Physicians in the hospital emergency department will diagnose the actual injury, using medical imaging techniques such as the X ray.

While it is not important for you to attempt to diagnose the underlying problem, it may be helpful for you to know the terminology health professionals use to define various types of musculoskeletal injuries.

- *Fracture*—any break in a bone. Fractures can be open or closed (Figure 27-9). They are also classified by the way a bone is broken, such as *comminuted* if broken in several places, or *greenstick* if the break is incomplete, or *angulated* if the broken bone is bent at an angle.
- *Dislocation*—the disruption or "coming apart" of a joint. In order for a joint to dislocate, the soft tissue of the joint capsule and ligaments must be stretched beyond the normal range of motion and torn.
- *Sprain*—the stretching and tearing of soft tissues such as muscles and ligaments. The term *sprain* is most commonly associated with joint injuries.

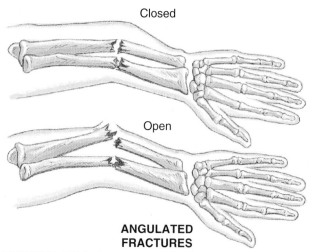

Closed

Open

ANGULATED
FRACTURES

FIGURE 27-9 Injuries to the bones may be open or closed. A broken bone may be angulated (bent).

A **closed painful, swollen, deformed extremity** is one in which the skin is not broken. An **open, painful, swollen, deformed extremity** is one in which the skin has been broken or torn through from the inside by the injured bone or from the outside by something that has caused a penetrating wound with associated injury to the bone. An open PSD is a serious situation because of the increased likelihood of infection. While many closed injuries can be handled simply in the hospital emergency department, all patients with open fractures require surgery. *Proper splinting and prehospital care of musculoskeletal injuries help prevent closed injuries from becoming open ones.*

Assessment of Musculoskeletal Injuries

Examination involves your senses and the skills of inspection (looking), palpation (feeling) and auscultation (listening). One of the basic principles of assessment is that it is difficult to do a proper examination on patients when they are fully clothed. However, it often is difficult, impractical, or inadvisable to completely disrobe or cut away a patient's clothing due to weather, patient modesty, or patient refusal. A good rule of thumb is cut or remove clothing according to the environment and severity of the situation.

In cases of severe extremity trauma, injuries can be very obvious. However, when *treating trauma patients, your first priority must be to rapidly identify and treat life-threatening conditions in order of risk to the patient.* Do not let a grotesque but relatively minor extremity injury sidetrack you. Once the initial assessment and focused examination have ruled out obvious life-threatening airway, breathing, or circulation problems and injuries to the head, spine, chest, and abdomen, then your attention can be focused on musculoskeletal injuries to the extremities.

Patient Assessment—Musculoskeletal Injuries

Signs and Symptoms

☐ *Pain and tenderness*—The PSD extremity patient experiences pain when the injured part is moved and when it is touched. Generally a patient will hold the injured part still, or guard it, in an effort to minimize pain. When examining a conscious patient, ask him to point to the specific location of pain if possible. Then, avoiding that location, carefully examine the injured part to assess if there are any other painful or injured areas. With unresponsive patients, suspicion of injury must be based on other physical findings.

☐ *Deformity or angulation*—The force of trauma causes bones to fracture and become deformed or angulated out of anatomical position (Figure 27-9). Note that with joint injuries, sometimes the deformity is subtle. When in doubt, look at the uninjured side and compare it to the injured one.

☐ *Grating, or* **crepitus** (KREP-i-tus)—This is a sound or feeling caused by broken bone ends rubbing together. It can be painful for the patient. *Never intentionally cause crepitus.* The patient may report grating noises or sensations that occurred prior to your arrival and examination.

☐ *Swelling*—When bones break and soft tissue is torn, bleeding occurs and causes swelling that may increase the proportions of a deformity. Rings, watches, and other jewelry can easily constrict and injure underlying tissue. Therefore, they should be slid or cut off as soon as possible if swelling is likely to occur.

☐ *Bruising*—Ecchymosis, or large black-and-blue discoloration of the skin, indicates an underlying injury that may be hours or days old. Obvious bruises indicate the need for splinting.

Exposed bone ends—Bone ends protruding through the skin indicate a fracture and the need for splinting. Again, the more gruesome the appearance of the extremity, the greater the temptation to treat that injury first. Remember to care for life-threatening injuries first. Extremity injuries usually do not kill patients.

Joints locked into position—When joints are dislocated, they may lock into normal or abnormal anatomical positions. Joint injuries must usually be splinted as found.

Nerve and blood vessel compromise—Examine for pulses, sensation, and movement distal to the injury site. This must be accomplished *before* and *after* splinting. Check for nerve injury by asking the patient if he can sense your touch and can move all fingers or toes. Any problem of sensation or movement must be noted. Then feel for pulses in the wrist (radial) or ankle (dorsalis pedis or posterior tibial). Obviously, to accurately examine for sensation, movement, and pulses, the patient's gloves and footwear must be removed.

Patient Care—Musculoskeletal Injuries

Emergency Care Steps

1. Take and maintain appropriate BSI precautions.

2. Perform the initial assessment. Remember, do not get distracted from your initial assessment and priority determination because of grotesque and painful extremity injuries. While they may be painful and cause disability, such injuries are rarely fatal. Manually stabilize the head. Be sure the patient's airway is open and stays open. Make sure the patient is breathing and that breathing is adequate. Provide oxygen and assist ventilations as necessary. Assess pulses and skin color. Control bleeding and manage shock. Determine patient priority; that is, check to see if the patient is unstable with high priority problems or if the patient is stable with one isolated injury. During the rapid trauma exam, apply a cervical collar if spine injury is suspected.

3. After life-threatening conditions have been addressed, all patients with a PSD extremity must be splinted. For a low-priority (stable) patient, splint individual injuries before transport. For a high-priority (unsta-

ble) patient, immobilize the whole body on a long spine board, then "load and go."

4. If appropriate, cover open wounds with sterile dressings, elevate the extremity, and apply a cold pack to the area to help reduce swelling.

If initial assessment reveals the patient is unstable, then management of extremity injuries becomes a low priority. An unstable patient with "load and go" problems must have the ABCs managed and the entire body splinted or immobilized on a long spine board. Do not take time to splint each injury individually. It is not in the patient's best interest to waste the "Golden Hour" treating minor injuries and delivering a perfectly packaged but unsavable patient to the hospital.

Splinting

Emergency care for all painful, swollen, or deformed extremities is splinting. *For any splint to be effective, it must immobilize adjacent joints and bone ends.* Effective splinting minimizes the movement of disrupted joints and broken bone ends, and it decreases the patient's pain. It helps prevent additional injury to soft tissue such as nerves, arteries, veins, and muscles. It can prevent a closed fracture from becoming an open fracture, a much more serious condition, and it can help to minimize blood loss. In the case of the spine, splinting on a backboard prevents injury to the spinal cord and helps to prevent permanent paralysis.

Realignment of the Deformed Extremity

The object of realignment (straightening) is to assist in restoring effective circulation to the PSD extremity and to fit it into a splint. Some injuries such as Colles fractures of the wrist (see Scan 27-7) may be completely splintable because they are only slightly deformed. In this case the only reason to attempt realignment would be to restore circulation to the hand if it appeared to be cyanotic or lacked pulses.

The thought of realigning an angulated injury can be a frightening one. However, remember these points.

- If the extremity is not realigned, the splint may be ineffective, causing increased pain and possible further injury (including an open fracture) during transportation.

- If the extremity is not realigned, the chance of nerves, arteries, and veins being compromised increases. When distal circulation is compromised or shut down, tissues beyond the injury become starved for oxygen and die.
- Pain is only increased for a moment during realignment under traction. Pain is reduced by effective splinting.

Due to the size and weight of extremities, attempting to splint one in the deformed position is usually futile and only increases the chance of its becoming an open fracture. When angulated injuries to the tibia or fibula, femur, radius or ulna, and humerus cannot be fit into a rigid splint, realign the bone. Also realign a long bone when the distal extremity is cyanotic or lacks pulses, indicating compromised circulation.

The general guidelines for realigning an extremity are as follows (Figure 27-10).

1. One EMT-B grasps the distal extremity while a partner places one hand above and below the injury site.
2. The partner supports the site while the first EMT-B pulls gentle **manual traction** in the direction of the long axis of the extremity. If resistance is felt or if it appears that bone ends will come through the skin, stop realignment and splint the extremity in the position found.
3. If no resistance is felt, maintain gentle traction until the extremity is properly splinted.

Generally, injuries to joints should be splinted in the position found unless the distal extremity is cyanotic or lacks pulses. If so, an attempt should be made to align the joint to a neutral anatomical position using gentle traction, provided that no resistance is felt.

The Art of Splinting

Effective splinting may require you to use some ingenuity. Even though you carry different types of splinting devices, many situations will require you to improvise. In a pinch, you can use pillows or rolled blankets as soft splints. For rigid splints you can use a piece of lumber, cardboard, a rolled newspaper, an umbrella, a cane, a broom handle, a catcher's shin guard, or a tongue depressor for a finger. Bystanders can often rummage through their car trunk and find something suitable. Regardless of the method of

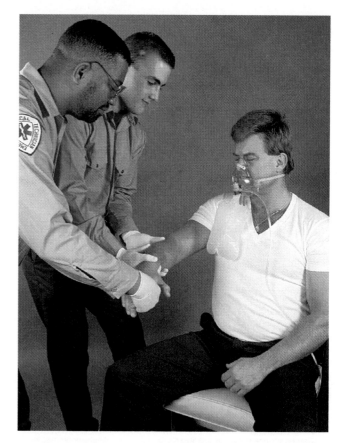

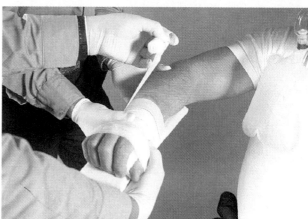

FIGURE 27-10 General procedure for realigning an injured extremity.

splinting, the following basic principles must be kept in mind.

- A splint must immobilize adjacent joints (joints above and below the injury) and bone ends (the site itself).
- The method of splinting is always dictated by the severity of the patient's condition and the priority for transport. If the patient is a high priority for "load and go" transport, choose a fast method of splinting. If the

patient is a low priority for transport, choose a slower-but-better splinting method.

- The methods of splinting from slowest to fastest are: each site is individually splinted (slowest but best); the limb is secured to the torso or an uninjured leg (a bit faster, but second choice to individual splints); and the entire body is secured to a spine board (fastest, but only better than no splint at all).

Splints carried on EMS units come in three basic types: rigid splints, formable splints, and traction splints (Figure 27-11). *Rigid splints* require the limb be moved to anatomical position. They tend to provide the greatest support and are ideally used to splint long bone injuries. Examples are cardboard, wood, pneumatic splints such as air splints and vacuum splints, and the pneumatic anti-shock garment. *Formable splints* are capable of being molded to different angles and generally allow for considerable movement. They are most commonly used to immobilize joint injuries in the position found. Examples are pillow and blanket splints. *Traction splints* are used specifically for femur fractures.

Regardless of the method of splinting, general rules that apply to all types of immobilization are as follows.

- Before moving the injured extremity, expose the area and control any bleeding.
- Because complications of musculoskeletal injury include nerve and blood vessel injury, examine for and record <u>m</u>otor ability, <u>s</u>ensory response, and <u>c</u>irculation (MSC) before and after splinting.

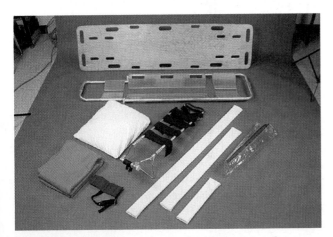

FIGURE 27-11 Splints and accessories for musculoskeletal injuries.

- Align long bone injuries to anatomical position under gentle traction if severe deformity exists or distal circulation is compromised.
- No attempt should be made to push protruding bones back into place. However, when realigning deformed open injuries, they may slip back into position under traction.
- Splints must immobilize adjacent joints and the injury site. In order for splints to be effective, they must keep the injury site and the joints above and below still.
- Splint patients before moving them to a stretcher or other location, if possible. A good rule of thumb is "least handling causes least damage." Sometimes patients must be extricated from where they are before ideal splinting techniques can occur. Attempt to immobilize the extremity as well as you can (for example, prior to extrication, the injured extremity might be immobilized to the uninjured one).
- If the patient is unstable, do not waste time with splinting. Care for life-threatening problems first. You can align the injuries in anatomical position and immobilize the whole body to a long spine board.
- Many rigid splints do not conform to body curves and allow too much movement of the limb. Pad the voids, or spaces between the body part and the splint, to increase patient comfort and ensure proper immobilization.

Documentation Tip—Realigning an Extremity

When realigning an open PSD extremity, be sure to make a note on the prehospital care report—and verbally report to the emergency department staff—if bone ends initially protruded from the open wound and slipped back into position, and out of sight, during realignment.

Hazards of Splinting

By far the most serious hazard of splinting is "splinting someone to death": splinting before life-threatening conditions are addressed or spending time splinting a high-priority patient instead of immediately getting the patient into the ambulance and to the hospital. Always assure airway, breathing, and circulation before going on to care for other injuries. Remember, the method of splinting is always dictated by the severity of the patient's condition and by the priority for transportation.

Other hazards include improper or inadequate splinting. If a splint is applied too tightly, it can compress soft tissue and injure nerves, blood vessels, and muscles. If it is applied too loosely or inappropriately, it will allow so much movement that further soft tissue injury or an open fracture may occur. In addition, because rescue workers may be insecure about realigning a deformed injury, they may attempt to splint it in a deformed position and actually do more harm than good. Remember, it can be very difficult to splint deformed injuries in long bones well enough to prevent excessive movement.

Splinting Long Bone and Joint Injuries

Before you start the splinting process you will need to select a splint appropriate to the severity of the patient's condition and method of transportation. Remember that most upper extremity injuries can be immobilized with a sling and swathe in the sitting patient. A supine patient's upper extremities can be immobilized to the patient's side. Be sure to have cravats, padding, and roller bandages immediately at hand.

The splinting of joints usually requires considerable ingenuity. In most cases formable splints are required to splint the extremity in the position it is found. If the distal extremity is pulseless or cyanotic, an attempt should be made to align it to anatomical position using gentle traction. As with long bone splinting, get all of your equipment ready before starting the splinting process.

To splint long bone or joint injuries, follow these guidelines (Scans 27-1 and 27-2).

1. Take BSI precautions and expose the area to be splinted, if possible.
2. Manually stabilize the injury site. This can be done either by you or by a helper.
3. Assess motor ability, sensory response, and circulation (MSC). See if the patient can feel your touch distal to the injury. Ask the patient to wiggle the fingers or toes. Then check for pulses.
4. Realign the injury if deformed or if the distal extremity is cyanotic or pulseless. **Note:** Attempt to realign an injured joint *only* if the distal extremity is pulseless or cyanotic.
5. Measure or adjust the splint and move it into position under the limb. Maintain

manual stabilization or traction during positioning and until the splinting procedure is complete.
6. Apply and secure the splint to immobilize adjacent joints and injury site.
7. Reassess the MSC distal to the injury.

The application of splints to specific types of injuries will be discussed later in this chapter.

The Traction Splint

The exception to the general guidelines for splinting long bone and joint injuries is splinting injuries to the femur. The major problem with femur fractures is the tendency for the large muscle groups of the thigh (quadriceps and hamstrings) to go into spasm, forcing the bone ends to override each other, causing pain and further soft-tissue injury. A traction splint counteracts the muscle spasms and greatly reduces the pain.

Traction splints come in two basic varieties: unipolar and bipolar. Examples of a bipolar splint is the half-ring splint, Hare, and Fernotrac (Scans 27-9 and 27-10). Examples of the unipolar splint are the Sager (Scan 27-11) and Kendrick traction splints.

One of the most common questions is "How much traction should I pull?" An answer commonly given is "Pull enough traction to give the patient some relief from the pain." This answer can be misleading. When the thigh muscles begin to spasm and the bones begin to override, the patient is in real pain. When manual or mechanical traction is applied, you are pulling against a muscle spasm and that hurts too. Most patients do not begin to feel relief with the traction splint until it has been applied for several minutes and the muscle spasm begins to subside. (With the Sager splint, traction can be measured. The amount of traction applied should be roughly 10% of the patient's body weight and not exceed 15 pounds.) With a bipolar splint, firm traction should be applied to align the limb. Exert and maintain a firm pull to prevent bones from continuing to override.

No traction splint applied in the field pulls true traction. All exert "counter traction." The splint pulls on an ankle hitch and the splint frame is anchored against the pelvis. Once anchored, a pull is felt on the leg. With bipolar splints, any movement of the pelvis off the ground causes a shifting of the splint and loss of traction. Unipolar splints, such as the Sager, are

Scan 27-1
Immobilizing a Long Bone

FIRST take body substance isolation precautions.

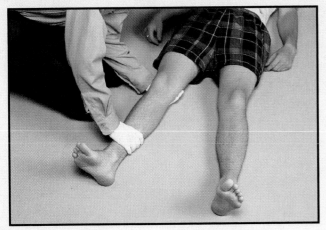

1. Direct application of manual stabilization.

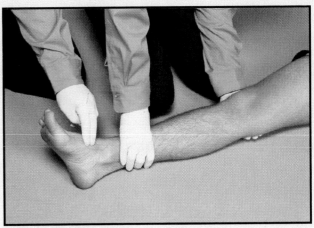

2. Assess distal motor ability, sensory response, and circulation (MSC).

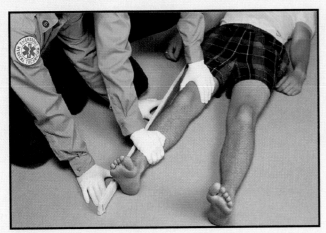

3. Measure splint. It should extend several inches beyond joints above and below injury.

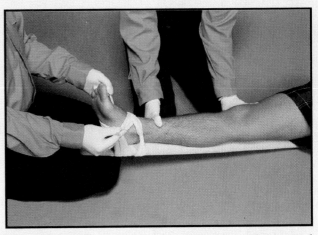

4. Apply splint and immobilize joints above and below injury.

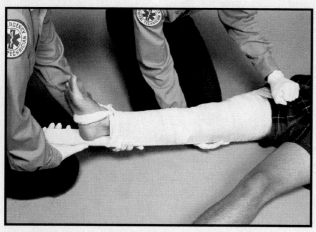

5. Secure the entire injured extremity.

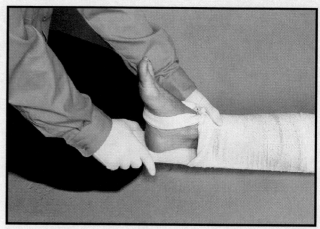

6.a. Secure foot in position of function as shown . . .

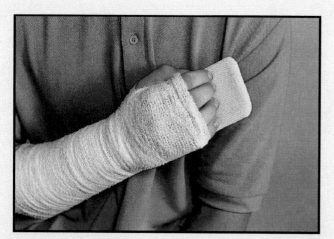

6.b. . . . or if splinting an arm, secure hand in position of function. This is the position the hand would be in if the patient were holding a palm-sized ball. A roll of bandage can be placed in the patient's hand to help maintain the position of function.

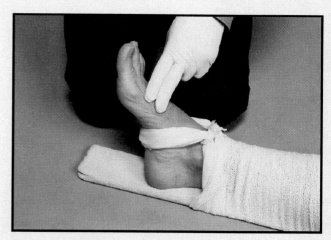

7. Reassess distal MSC function.

Immobilizing a Joint

FIRST take body substance isolation precautions.

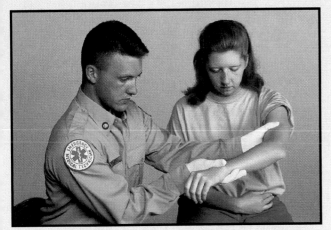

1. Direct application of manual stabilization.

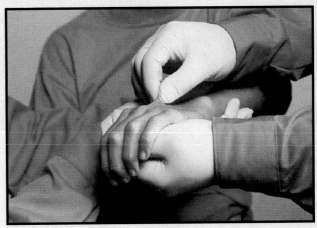

2. Assess distal motor ability, sensory response, and circulation (MSC).

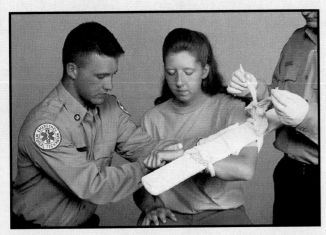

3. Select proper splint material. Immobilize site of injury and bones above and below.

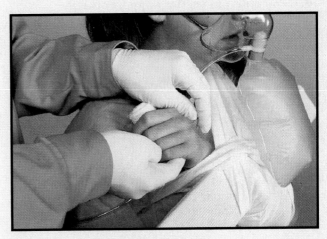

4. Reassess distal MSC function.

anchored against the pubis between the legs and are less apt to shift during patient movement and cause a loss of traction.

The indications for a traction splint are a painful, swollen, deformed (PSD) mid-thigh with no joint or lower leg injury. A traction splint is contraindicated if there is a pelvis, hip, or knee injury, if there is an avulsion or partial amputation where traction could separate the extremity, or if there is injury to the lower third of the leg which would interfere with the ankle hitch.

General guidelines for the application of a traction splint are as follows (Scan 27-3).

1. Take BSI precautions and expose the area to be splinted if possible.
2. Manually stabilize the leg and apply manual traction.
3. Assess motor ability, sensory response, and circulation (MSC). See if the patient can feel your touch distal to the injury. Ask the patient to wiggle the toes. Then check for pulses.
4. Adjust the splint to the proper length, and position it at or under the injured leg.
5. Apply the proximal securing device (ischial strap).
6. Apply the distal securing device (ankle hitch).
7. Apply mechanical traction.
8. Position and secure support straps.
9. Re-evaluate the proximal and distal securing devices, and reassess the MSC distal to the injury.
10. Secure the patient's torso and the traction splint to a long spine board to immobilize the hip and to prevent movement of the splint.

Whenever possible, three rescuers should be used to apply a traction splint. This allows one rescuer to support the injury site when the limb is lifted to position the traction splint.

Note: Most of the traction splints in use today require that the patient's shoe be removed for proper traction splinting. With some older splints, the patient's shoe may remain in place if neurologic and pulse assessment is possible, if the shoe will not prevent the ankle hitch from being properly placed, and if the shoe will not slip off after mechanical traction (tension) is applied.

Application of specific types of traction splints will be discussed later in this chapter.

EMERGENCY CARE OF SPECIFIC INJURIES

The specific injuries described in this section are usually identified as fractures or dislocations. Remember, however, that you do not need to determine the exact nature of an injury to an extremity. You will splint or immobilize any painful, swollen, or deformed extremity. Specific techniques are discussed below.

Upper Extremity Injuries

Shoulder Girdle Injuries

Patient Assessment—Shoulder Girdle Injuries

Signs and Symptoms

☐ Pain in the shoulder may indicate several types of injury. Look for specific signs.
☐ A dropped shoulder, with the patient holding the arm of his injured side against the chest, often indicates a fracture of the clavicle (Figure 27-12).

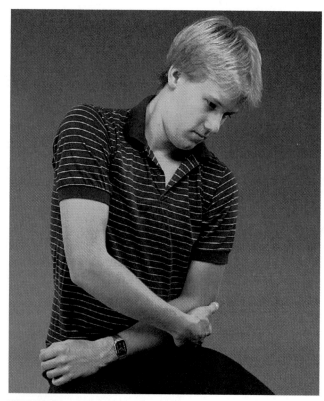

FIGURE 27-12 A fractured clavicle may be noted by a "dropped" shoulder.

Traction Splinting

FIRST take body substance isolation precautions.

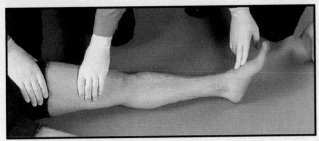

1. Direct manual stabilization of injured leg. Assess distal motor ability, sensory response, and circulation (MSC).

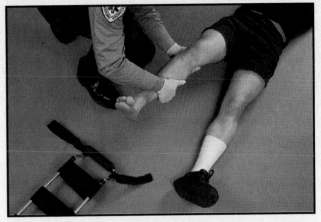

2. Direct application of manual traction.

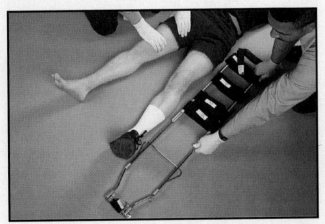

3. Adjust and position splint at injured leg.

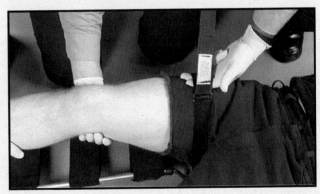

4. Apply proximal securing device (e.g., ischial strap).

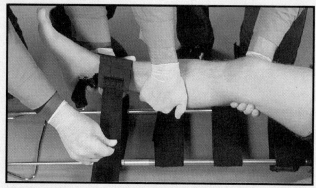

5. Apply distal securing device (e.g., ankle hitch).

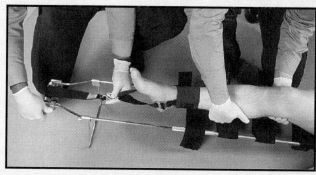

6. Apply mechanical traction.

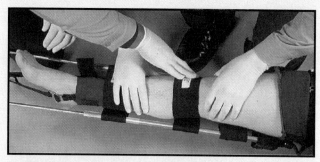

7. Position and secure support straps.

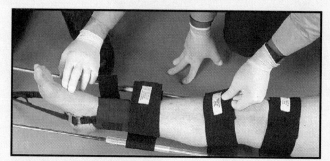

8. Reassess distal MSC.

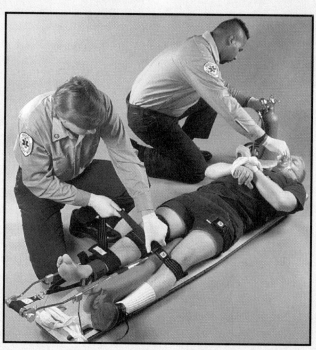

9. Secure patient's torso and traction splint to long board for transport.

A severe blow to the back over the scapula may cause a fracture of that bone. (All the bones of the shoulder girdle can be felt except the scapula. Only the superior ridge of the scapula, called its spine, can be easily palpated. Injury to the scapula is rare but must be considered if there are indications of a severe blow at the site of this bone.)

Check the entire shoulder girdle. Check for deformity where the clavicle attaches to the sternum. Feel for deformity where the clavicle joins the scapula. Feel and look along the entire clavicle for deformity. Note if the head of the humerus can be felt or moves in front of the shoulder. This is a sign of possible anterior dislocation. This displacement also may be due to a fracture.

Patient Care—Shoulder Girdle Injuries

Emergency Care Steps

1. Check for distal motor, sensory, and circulatory function (MSC). If distal function is impaired, immobilize and transport as soon as possible, notifying the receiving facility.
2. It is not practical to use a rigid splint for injuries to the clavicle, scapula, or the head of the humerus. Use a sling and swathe (Scan 27-4). If there is possible cervical-spine injury, do not tie a sling around the patient's neck.
3. If there is evidence of a possible anterior dislocation of the head of the humerus (the bone head is pushed toward the front of the body), place a thin pillow between the patient's arm and chest before applying the sling and swathe.
4. Do not attempt to straighten or reduce any dislocations.
5. Recheck distal MSC function.

Note: Sometimes a dislocated shoulder will reduce itself ("pop back into place"). When this happens, you should check for a distal pulse and nerve function. Apply a sling and swathe and transport the patient. The patient must be seen by a physician. Be certain to note the self-reduction on the report form and to report the event to the emergency department staff.

Scans 27-5 through 27-8—contain additional information on emergency care for injuries to the upper extremities.

Lower Extremity Injuries

Injuries to the Pelvis

Fractures of the pelvis may occur with falls, in motor vehicle collisions, or when a person is crushed by being squeezed between two objects. Pelvic fractures may be the result of direct or indirect force.

Patient Assessment—Pelvic Injuries

Warning: Indications of pelvic fractures mean that there may be serious damage to internal organs, blood vessels, and nerves. Internal bleeding may be profuse and lead to shock. Any force strong enough to fracture the pelvis also can cause injury to the spine.

Signs and Symptoms

☐ Complaint of pain in pelvis, hips, groin, or back. This may be the only indication, but it is significant if the mechanism of injury indicates possible fracture. Usually, obvious deformity is associated with the pain.
☐ Painful reaction when pressure is applied to the iliac crests (wings of the pelvis) or to the pubic bones.
☐ Patient complains that he cannot lift his legs when lying on his back. (Do not test for this, but do check for sensation.)
☐ The foot on the injured side may turn outward (lateral rotation). This also may indicate a hip fracture.
☐ The patient has an unexplained pressure on the urinary bladder and the feeling of having to void the bladder.

Patient Care—Pelvic Injuries

Note: It may be very difficult to tell a fractured pelvis from a fracture to the upper femur. When there is doubt, care for the patient as if there is a pelvic fracture to protect blood vessels and nerves associated with the joint. Remember, there may be spinal injuries.

Emergency Care Steps

1. Move the patient as little as possible. Any emergency move should be done so that the patient moves as a unit. Never lift the patient with the pelvis unsupported. *Warning: do not use a log roll to move a patient with a suspected pelvic fracture.*

Scan 27-4
Sling and Swathe

A sling is a triangular bandage used to support the shoulder and arm. Once the patient's arm is placed in a sling, a swathe can be used to hold the arm against the side of the chest. Commercial slings are available. Velcro straps can be used to form a swathe. Use whatever materials you have on hand, provided they will not cut into the patient.

Note: Assess distal motor ability, sensory response, and circulation (pulse) both before and after immobilizing or splinting an extremity.

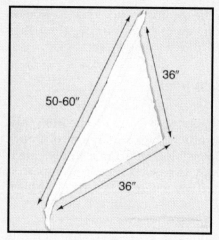

1. The sling should be in the shape of a triangle.

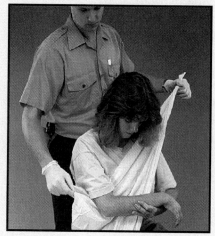

2. Position the sling over the top of the patient's chest as shown. Fold the patient's injured arm across the chest.

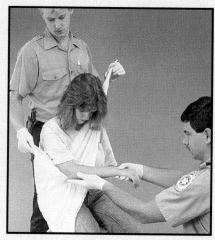

3. If the patient cannot hold his arm, have someone assist until you tie the sling.

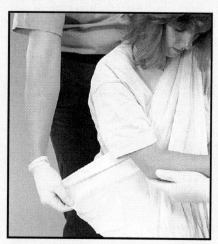

4. One point of the triangle should extend behind the elbow on the injured side.

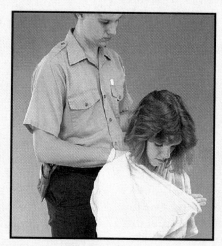

5. Take the bottom point of the triangle and bring this end up over the patient's arm. When you are finished, this point should be taken over the top of the patient's injured shoulder.

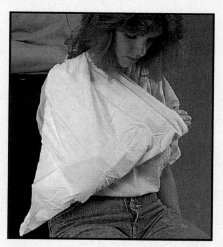

6. Draw up on the ends of the sling so that the patient's hand is about four inches above the elbow (exceptions are discussed later).

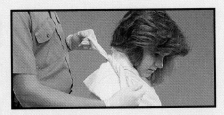

7. Tie the two ends of the sling together, making sure that the knot does not press against the back of the patient's neck. The area can be padded with bulky dressings or sanitary napkins.

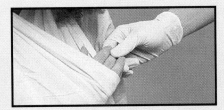

8. Leave the patient's fingertips exposed to permit check of motor and sensory function and circulation.

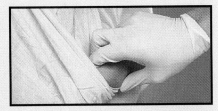

9. Check motor and sensory function. Check for radial pulse. If the pulse has been lost, take off the sling and repeat the procedure. Repeat sling procedure if necessary.

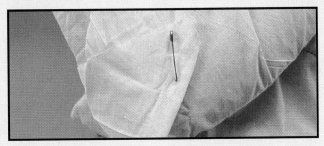

10A. Take hold of the point of material at the patient's elbow and fold it forward, pinning it to the front of the sling. This forms a pocket for the patient's elbow.

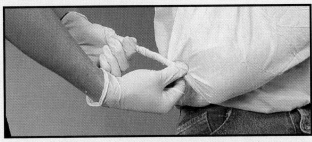

10B. If you do not have a pin, twist the excess material and tie a knot in the point.

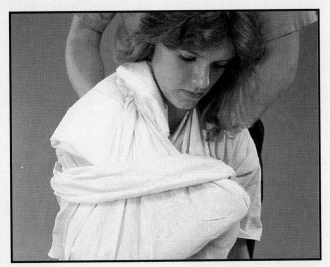

11. A swathe can be formed from a second piece of triangular material. This swathe is tied around the chest and the injured arm, over the sling. Do not place this swathe over the patient's arm on the uninjured side.

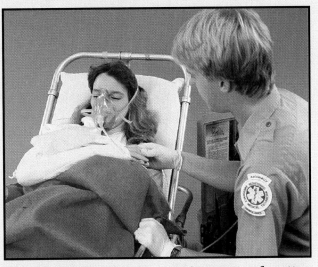

12. Assess distal motor and sensory function and circulation. Treat for shock. Provide a high concentration of oxygen. Take vital signs. Perform detailed and ongoing assessments as appropriate.

Note: If the patient has a cervical spine injury, do not tie sling around neck.

Injuries to the Humerus—Soft Splinting

Note: Assess distal motor ability, sensory response, and circulation (pulse) both before and after immobilizing or splinting an extremity.

Signs: Injury to the humerus can take place at the proximal end (shoulder), along the shaft of the bone, or at the distal end (elbow). Deformity is the key sign used to detect fractures to this bone in any of these locations; however, assess for all signs of skeletal injury. Follow the rules and procedures for care of an injured extremity.

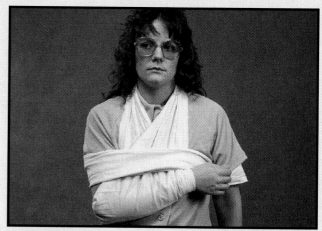

1. Fracture at proximal end. Gently apply a sling and swathe. If you have only enough material for a swathe, bind the patient's upper arm to his body, taking great care not to cut off circulation to the forearm.

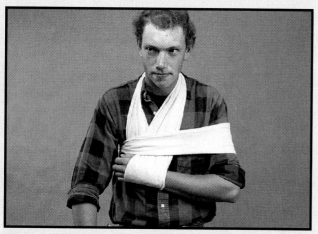

2. Fracture of the shaft. Use rigid splints whenever possible; otherwise, gently apply a sling and swathe. The sling should be modified so that it supports the wrist only.

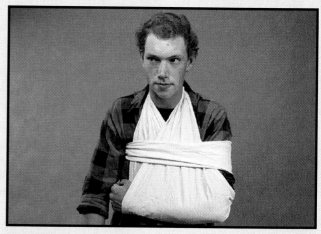

3. Fracture at distal end. Gently apply a full sling and swathe. Do not draw the hand upward to a position above the elbow. Instead, keep elbow flexion as close to a 90° angle as possible.

Warning: Before applying a sling and swathe to care for injuries to the humerus, check for distal motor and sensory function and circulation. If you do not feel a pulse, attempt to straighten any slight angulation if the patient has a closed fracture (follow local protocol). Otherwise, prepare for immediate immobilizaion and transport. Should straightening of the angulation fail to restore the pulse or function, splint with a medium board splint, keeping the forearm extended. If there is no sign of circulation or sensory or motor function, you will have to attempt a second splinting. If this fails to restore distal function, transport immediately. Do not try to straighten angulation of the humerus if there are any signs of fracture or dislocation of the shoulder or elbow.

Arm and Elbow Injuries

Note: Assess distal motor ability, sensory response, and circulation (pulse) both before and after immobilizing or splinting an extremity.

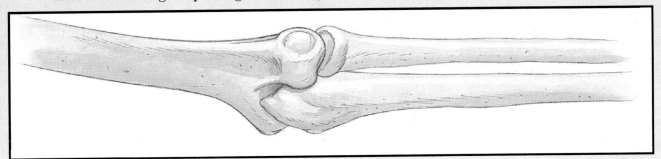

The elbow is a joint and not a bone. It is composed of the distal humerus and the proximal ulna and radius, forming a hinge joint. You will have to decide if the injury is truly to the elbow. Deformity and sensitivity will direct you to the injury site.

Care: If there is a distal pulse, the dislocated elbow should be immobilized in the position in which it is found. The joint has too many nerves and blood vessels to risk movement. When a distal pulse is absent, make one attempt to slightly reposition the limb after contacting medical direction. Do not force the limb into anatomical position.

Elbow in or Returned to Bent Position

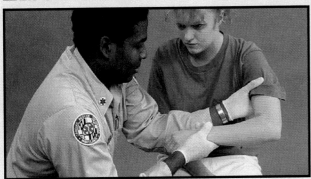

1. Move limb only if necessary for splinting or if pulse is absent. **Do not** continue if you meet resistance or significantly increase the pain.

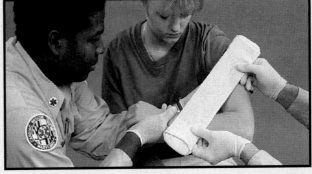

2. Use a padded board splint that will extend 2 to 6 inches beyond the arm and wrist when placed diagonally.

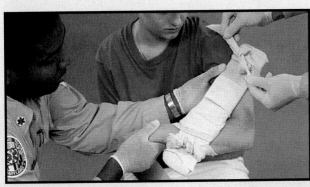

3. Place the splint so it is just proximal to the elbow and to the wrist. Use cravats to secure to the forearm, then the arm.

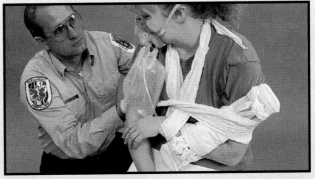

4. A wrist sling can be applied to support the limb; keep the elbow exposed. Apply a swathe if possible.

Elbow in a Straight Position

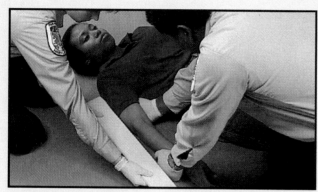

1. Assess distal motor and sensory function and circulation (pulse).

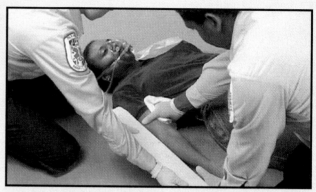

2. Use a padded board splint that extends from under the armpit to a point past the fingertips. Pad the armpit.

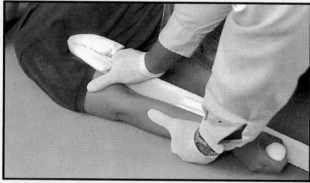

3. Place a roll of bandages in the patient's hand to help maintain position of function. Place padded side of board against medial side of limb. Pad all voids.

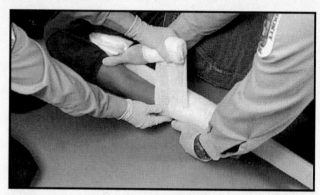

4. Secure the splint. Leave fingertips exposed.

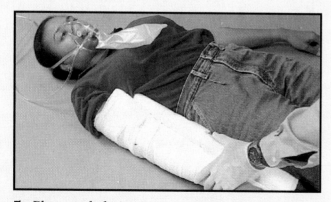

5. Place pads between patient's side and splint.

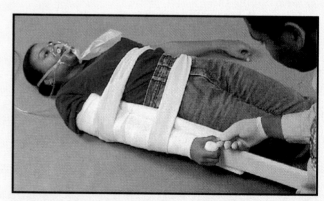

6. Secure splinted limb to body with two cravats. Avoid placing over suspected injury site. Reassess distal motor, sensory, and circulatory function.

534

Injuries to the Forearm, Wrist, and Hand

Note: Assess distal motor ability, sensory response, and circulation (pulse) both before and after immobilizing or splinting an extremity.

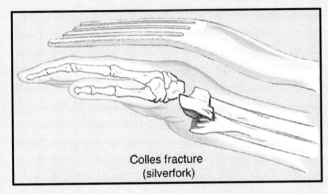

Colles fracture
(silverfork)

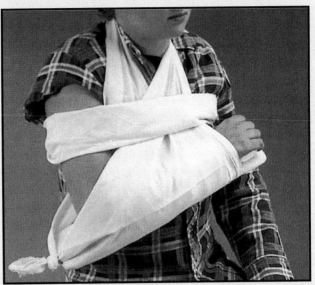

SIGNS:

- Forearm—deformity and tenderness. If only one bone bone is broken, deformity may be minor or absent.
- Wrist—deformity and tenderness, with the possibility of a Colles (KOL-ez) fracture that gives a "silverfork" appearance to the wrist.
- Hand—deformity and pain. Dislocated fingers are obvious.

CARE: Injuries occurring to the forearm, wrist, or hand can be splinted using a padded rigid splint that extends from the elbow past the fingertips. The patient's elbow, forearm, wrist, and hand all need the support of the splint. Tension must be provided throughout the splinting. A roll of bandage should be placed in the hand to ensure the position of function. After rigid splinting, apply a sling and swathe.

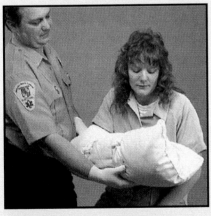

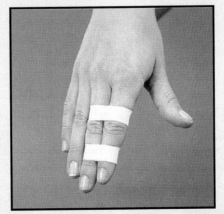

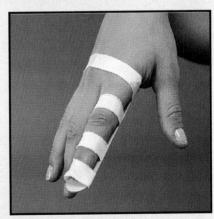

ALTERNATIVE CARE: Injuries to the hand and wrist can be cared for with soft splinting by placing a roll of bandage in the hand to maintain position of function, then tying the forearm, wrist, and hand into the fold of one pillow or between two pillows. An injured finger can be taped to an adjacent uninjured finger or splinted with a tongue depressor. Some emergency department physicians prefer that care be limited to a wrap of soft bandages. **DO NOT** try to "pop" dislocated fingers back into place.

Air-Inflated Splints

Note: Assess distal motor ability, sensory response, and circulation (pulse) both before and after immobilizing or splinting an extremity.

Warning: Air-inflated splints may leak. When applied in cold weather, an inflatable splint will expand when the patient is moved to a warmer place. Variations in pressure also occur if the patient is moved to a different altitude. Frequently monitor the pressure in the splint with your fingertip. Air-inflated splints may stick to the patient's skin in hot weather.

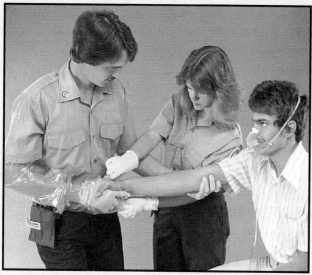

1. Slide the inflated splint up your forearm, well above the wrist. Use this same hand to grasp the hand of the patient's injured limb as though you were going to shake hands and apply steady tension.

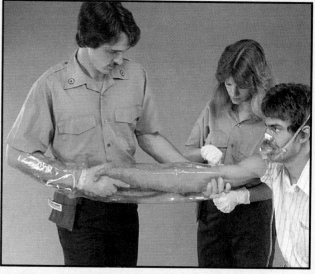

2. While you support his arm, your partner gently slides the splint over your hand and onto the patient's injured limb. The lower edge of the splint should be just above his knuckles. Make sure the splint is free of wrinkles.

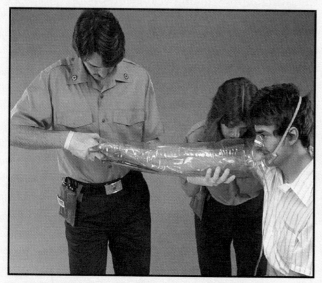

3. Continue to support the arm while your partner inflates the splint by mouth to a point where you can make a slight dent in the plastic when you press it with your thumb.

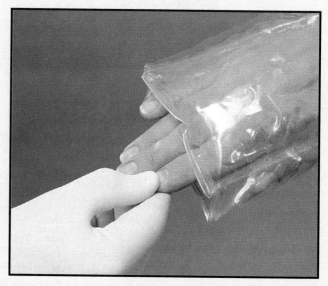

4. Continue to assess distal motor and sensory function and circulation.

2. Determine MSC function distal to the injury site.

3. Straighten the patient's lower limbs into the anatomical position if there are no injuries to the hip joints and lower limbs and if it is possible to do so without meeting resistance or causing excessive pain.

4. Prevent additional injury to the pelvis by stabilizing the lower limbs. Place a folded blanket between the patient's legs, from the groin to the feet, and bind them together with wide cravats. Thin rigid splints can be used to push the cravats under the patient. The cravats can then be adjusted for proper placement at the upper thigh, above the knee, below the knee, and above the ankle.

5. Assume that there are spinal injuries. Immobilize the patient on a long spine board (Figure 27-13). When securing the patient, avoid placing the straps or ties over the pelvic area.

6. Reassess distal MSC function.

7. Care for shock, providing a high concentration of oxygen.

8. Transport the patient as soon as possible.

9. Monitor vital signs.

Some EMS systems use the anti-shock garment for a patient with a possible pelvic fracture. If your local protocols call for this, place the garment on the spine board prior to moving the patient onto the board (Scan 27-18). When pelvic fracture is a possibility, always be alert for shock and possible injuries to internal organs.

Once the patient is in the ambulance and prepared for transport, the EMT-B in some EMS systems is allowed to make adjustments to improve patient comfort and reduce muscle spasms of the abdomen and lower limb. This can be done by gently flexing the patient's legs and placing a pillow under the knees. If you are allowed to follow this protocol, be extremely careful not to move the spine, since the patient may have associated spinal injuries.

Injuries to the Hip

Patient Assessment—Hip Dislocation

A hip dislocation (Figure 27-14) occurs when the head of the femur is pulled or pushed from its pelvic socket. It is difficult to tell a hip dislocation from a fracture to the proximal femur. Conscious patients will complain of intense pain with both types of injury. Patients who have had a surgical replacement of the hip joint are at increased risk of hip dislocation.

Signs and Symptoms

☐ *Anterior hip dislocation*—The patient's entire lower limb is rotated outward and the hip is usually flexed.

☐ *Posterior hip dislocation* (most common)— The patient's leg is rotated inward, the hip is flexed, and the knee is bent. The foot may hang loose (foot drop), and the patient is unable to flex the foot or lift the toes. Often, there is a lack of sensation in the limb. These signs indicate possible damage, caused by the dislocated femoral head, to the sciatic (si-AT-ik) nerve, the major nerve that extends from the lower spine to the posterior thigh. This injury often occurs when a person's knees strike the dashboard during a motor vehicle collision.

Patient Care—Hip Dislocation

Emergency Care Steps

1. Check for distal MSC function.

2. Move patient onto a long spine board. Some systems use a scoop-style stretcher. When this device is used, the limb should be immobilized (see Step 3).

3. Immobilize the limb with pillows or rolled blankets.

4. Secure the patient to the long spine board with straps or cravats.

5. Reassess distal MSC function. *If there is a pulse or sensory or motor problem, notify medical directon and transport immediately.*

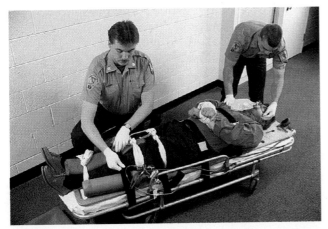

FIGURE 27-13 Immobilizing a patient with hip or pelvis injury on a long spine board.

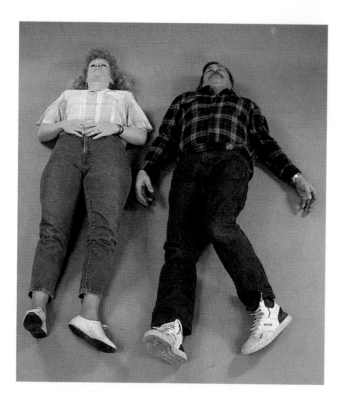

If the head of the femur slides or pops back into place, note this on the patient form and report the event to the hospital emergency department staff so that the previous dislocation does not go unnoticed.

Note: If you find a painful, swollen, or deformed thigh and the leg is flexed and will not straighten, the patient may also have a dislocated hip or a fractured femur.

Documentation Tip—
Correction of a Dislocation

Remember: If a shoulder or hip dislocation corrects itself ("pops back into place") spontaneously, be sure to note this on the prehospital care report—and verbally report it to the emergency department staff.

Patient Assessment—Hip Fractures

A hip fracture is a fracture to the uppermost portion of the femur, not to the pelvis. The fracture can occur to the femoral head, the femoral neck, or at the proximal end of the femur just below the neck of the bone. Direct force (motor vehicle collision) and twisting forces (falls) can cause a hip fracture. Elderly people are more susceptible to this type of injury because of brittle bones or bones weakened by disease.

Signs and Symptoms

- ☐ Pain is localized, but some patients complain of pain in the knee.
- ☐ Sometimes the patient is sensitive to pressure exerted on the lateral prominence of the hip (greater trochanter).
- ☐ Surrounding tissues are discolored. This may be delayed.
- ☐ Swelling may be evident.
- ☐ Patient is unable to move limb while on his back.
- ☐ Patient complains about being unable to stand.
- ☐ Foot on injured side usually turns outward; however, it may rotate inward (rarely).
- ☐ Injured limb may appear shorter.

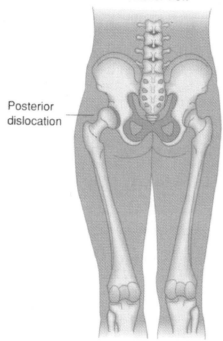

Posterior view

Posterior
dislocation

FIGURE 27-14 Signs of anterior and posterior hip dislocation.

6 Care for shock, providing a high concentration of oxygen.

7 Transport carefully, monitor vital signs, and continue to check for nerve and circulation impairment.

Patient Care—Hip Fractures

Be certain to check for distal MSC function before and after splinting and during transport. The patient should be managed for shock and receive oxygen at a high concentration. It is recommended that the patient be placed on a long spine board or orthopedic stretcher after splinting.

Emergency Care Steps

One of the following methods can be used to stabilize a hip fracture.

- [ ] *Bind the legs together*—Place a folded blanket between the patient's legs and bind the legs together with wide straps, Velcro-equipped straps, or wide cravats. Carefully place the patient on a long spine board and use pillows to support the lower limbs. Secure the patient to the board. An orthopedic stretcher can be used in place of the long spine board.
- [ ] *Padded boards*—Use thin splints to push cravats or straps under the patient at the natural voids (e.g., small of the back and back of the knees) and readjust them so that they will pass across the chest, the abdomen just below the belt, below the crotch, above and below the knee, and at the ankle. Splint with two long padded boards. Ideally, one should be long enough to extend from the patient's armpit to beyond the foot. The other should be long enough to extend from the crotch to beyond the foot. Cushion with padding in the armpit and crotch and pad all voids created at the ankle and knee. Secure the boards with the cravats or straps (Figure 27-15).
- [ ] Apply an anti-shock garment if local protocols indicate.

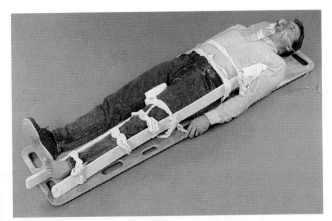

FIGURE 27-15 Long board splinting for a fractured hip (padded splint).

Injuries to the Femoral Shaft

Patient Assessment—Femoral Shaft Fractures

Because the femur is a large, strong bone, considerable force is necessary to cause a fracture of the femoral shaft. As noted earlier, the thigh's large muscle mass can complicate femoral fractures. Muscle contractions can cause bone ends to ride over each other or to recede from an open fracture wound. You must check for the signs of an open fracture and never assume that a wound on the thigh is of external origin.

Signs and Symptoms

- [ ] Pain, often intense
- [ ] Often there will be an open fracture with deformity and sometimes with the end of the bone protruding through the wound. When the injury is a closed fracture, there will be deformity with possible severe angulation.
- [ ] The injured limb may appear to be shortened because the contraction of the thigh muscles caused the bone ends to override each other.

Infants and Children

Traction splint thigh injuries in children using appropriately-sized splints. Warning: Studies of mechanisms of injury indicate that infants and children with fractured femurs often have injury to internal organs.

Patient Care—Femoral Shaft Fractures

In addition to splinting the fractured bone, you must attempt to control serious bleeding from deep thigh arteries. This can be difficult because of the barrier of the thigh's muscle mass.

Emergency Care Steps

1. Control bleeding by applying direct pressure (avoiding the possible fracture site) forcefully enough to overcome the barrier of muscle mass. The femoral artery pressure point may be used.
2. As soon as possible, manage the patient for shock and provide a high concentration of oxygen.

3 Check distal MSC function.
4 Apply a traction splint. If a traction splint is not available, bind the legs together after placing them in the anatomical position.
5 Recheck distal MSC function.

See Scans 27-3 and 27-9 through 27-11 for application of specific types of traction splints.

Warning: The traction splint should not be applied if you suspect that there may be additional injuries or fractures to the area of the knee or tibia/fibula of the same limb.

An anti-shock garment may be used (if local protocols permit) if there are multiple leg fractures. It is not, however, a good splint for the lower leg since it does not immobilize the ankle.

Injuries to the Knee

The knee is a joint and not a single bone. Fractures can occur to the distal femur, to the proximal tibia and fibula, and to the patella (kneecap).

Patient Assessment—Knee Injuries

What may appear to be a dislocation may prove to be a fracture or a combined fracture and dislocation. Even if you believe that the patient has suffered a dislocated patella and the kneecap has repositioned itself, realize that other damage may be hidden. Whether the patient has a fracture, dislocation, sprain, or strain, always manage as if there is a fracture and transport.

Signs and Symptoms
- Pain and tenderness
- Swelling
- Deformity with obvious swelling

Do not confuse a knee dislocation with a patella dislocation. The patella can become displaced by ligament damage when the lower leg and knee are twisted, as in a skiing or racquetball accident. A knee dislocation occurs when the tibia itself is forced either anteriorly or posteriorly in relation to the distal femur. Always check for a distal pulse, since the dislocated knee joint can compress the popliteal artery and stop the major blood supply to the lower leg. If there is no pulse, this is a *true emergency*. Con-tact medical direction for permission to gently move the lower leg anteriorly to allow for a pulse, and transport immediately.

Once splinting is done, monitor the patient. If there is a loss of distal pulse, a loss of sensation, or if the foot becomes discolored (white, mottled, or blue) and turns cold, transport the patient without delay. Notify medical direction while en route.

Patient Care—Knee Injuries

There are two general methods of immobilizing the knee—one if the knee is bent, the other if it is straight.

Emergency Care Steps
- *Knee Bent*—Check distal MSC function. Immobilize in the position in which the leg is found. Tie two padded board splints to the thigh and above the ankle so that the knee is held in position. A pillow can be used to support the leg. Recheck distal MSC function. (See Scans 27-12 and 27-13.)
- *Knee Straight or Returned to Anatomical Position*—Check distal MSC function. Immobilize with two padded board splints or a single padded splint. When using two padded boards, one medial and one lateral offer the best support. Remember to pad the voids created at the knee and ankle. Recheck distal MSC function (See Scans 27-14 and 27-15.)

Injuries to the Tibia or Fibula

Patient Assessment—Tibia/Fibula Injuries

Signs and Symptoms
- Pain and tenderness
- Swelling
- Possible deformity (You might expect to see a deformity of the lower leg when the tibia or fibula is fractured. However, such deformity is often absent.)

Patient Care—Tibia/Fibula Injuries

Immobilizing the leg by application of a splint may also help to relieve pain and control bleeding.

The Fernotrac Traction Splint—
Preparing the Splint

Note: Assess distal motor ability, sensory response, and circulation (pulse) both before and after immobilizing or splinting an extremity.

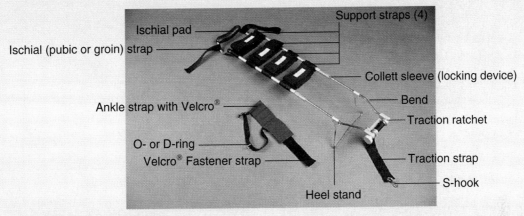

1. The Fernotrac Traction Splint

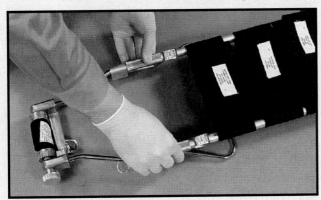

2. Loosen sleeve locking device.

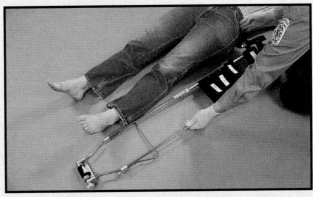

3. Place next to uninjured leg—ischial pad next to iliac crest.

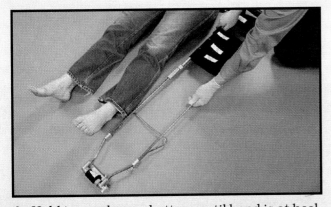

4. Hold top and move bottom until bend is at heel.

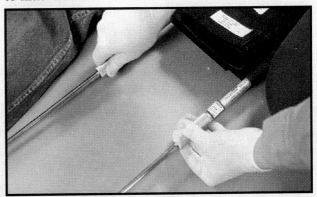

5. Lock sleeve.

Note: Some splints in use are measured by placing the ring at the level of the bony prominence that can be felt in the middle of each buttock (ischial tuberosity) and the distal end of the splint placed 8 to 10 inches beyond the foot.

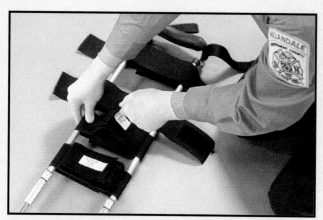

6. Open support straps.

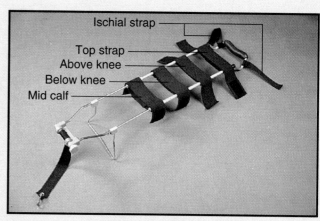

7. Place straps under splint.

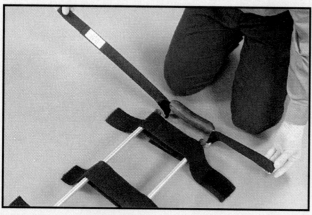

8. Release ischial strap. Attached ends should be next to ischial pad.

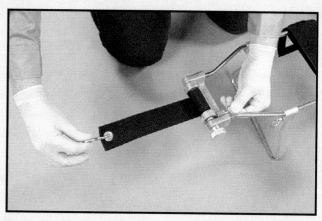

9. Pull release ring on ratchet and. . .

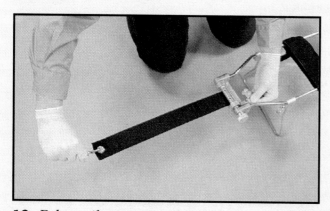

10. Release the traction strap.

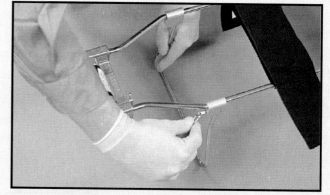

11. Extend and position heel stand after splint is in position under patient.

Note: Traction splints vary depending on the manufacturer. Learn to use the equipment supplied in your area and keep up to date with new equipment as it is approved for use.

Note: Assess distal motor ability, sensory response, and circulation (pulse) both before and after immobilizing or splinting an extremity.

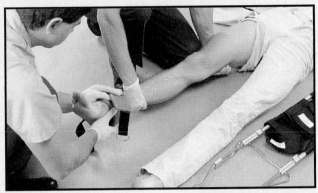

1. Some systems attach the ankle hitch prior to applying manual traction (tension). EMT-B 1 should apply the hitch while EMT-B 2 stabilizes the limb.

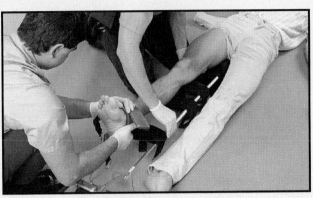

2a. While EMT-B 1 applies manual traction (tension), EMT-B 2 can position the splint.

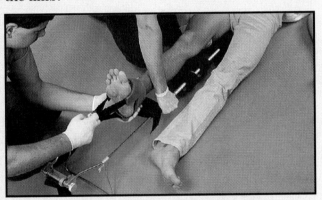

2b. Some systems allow manual traction to be applied by grasping the D-ring and ankle.

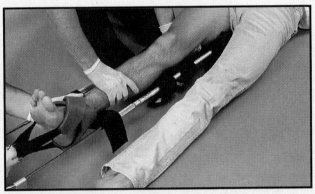

3. EMT-B 1 maintains manual traction (tension) and lowers the limb onto the cradles of the splint.

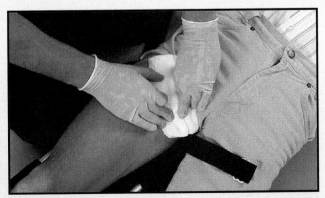

4. While EMT-B 1 maintains manual traction, EMT-B 2 applies padding to the groin area before securing the ischial strap. **Note:** Some EMS systems do not apply padding in order to reduce slippage.

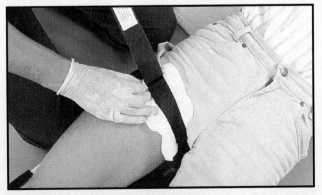

5. EMT-B 2 secures the ischial strap, connects the ankle hitch to the windlass, tightens the ratchet to equal manual traction (tension), and secures the cradle straps.

The Sager Traction Splint

Note: Assess distal motor ability, sensory response, and circulation (pulse) both before and after immobilizing or splinting an extremity.

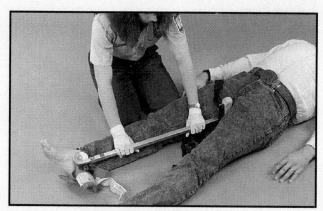

1. Splint will be placed medially.

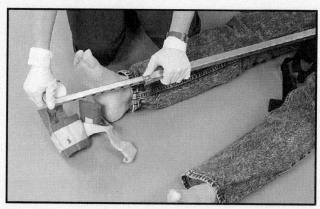

2. Length should be from groin to 4 inches past heel. Unlock to slide.

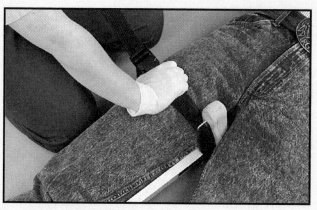

3. Secure thigh strap.

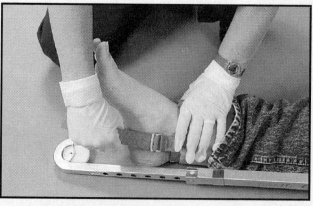

4. Wrap ankle harness above ankle (malleoli) and secure under heel.

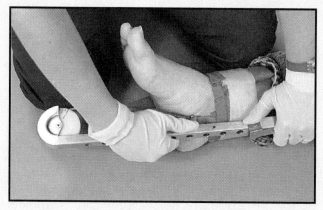

5. Release lock and extend splint to achieve desired traction (in pounds on pulley wheel).

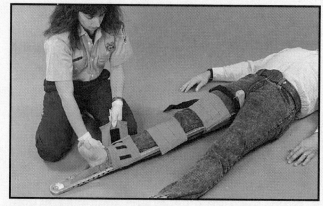

6. Secure straps at thigh, lower thigh and knee, and lower leg. Strap ankles and feet together. Secure to spine board.

Knee Injuries—Knee Bent—
Two Splint Method

Note: Assess distal motor ability, sensory response, and circulation (pulse) both before and after immobilizing or splinting an extremity.

If there is a distal pulse and nerve function, or the limb cannot be straightened without meeting resistance or causing severe pain, knee injuries should be splinted with the knee in the position in which it is found.

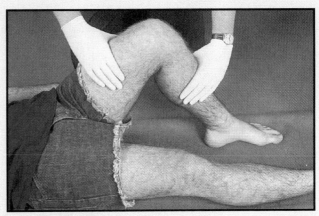

1. One EMT-B stabilizes the knee above and below the injury site as shown

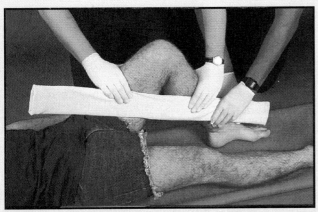

2. The splints should be equal and extend 6-12 inches beyond the mid thigh and mid calf.

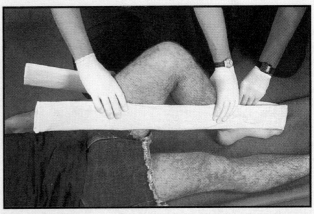

3. Place padded side of splints next to extremity.

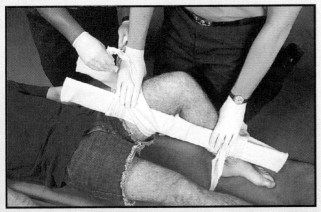

4. Place a cravat through the knee void and tie the boards together.

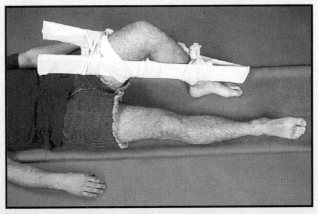

5. Using a figure eight, secure one cravat to the ankle and the boards, secure the second cravat to the thigh and the boards.

The Ankle Hitch

Note: Assess distal motor ability, sensory response, and circulation (pulse) both before and after immobilizing or splinting an extremity.

The ankle hitch can be used with a single padded board splint to immobilize injured knees and legs. It is made with a 3-inch wide cravat.

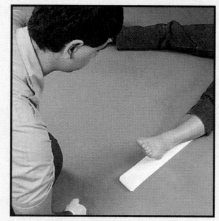

1. Kneel at distal end of limb.

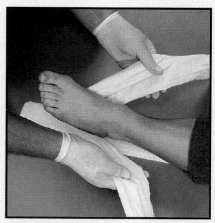

2. Center cravat in arch.

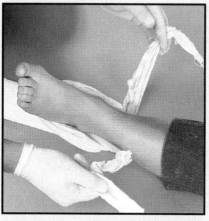

3. Place cravat along sides of foot and cross cravat behind ankle.

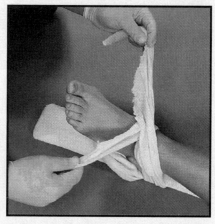

4. Cross cravat ends over top of ankle.

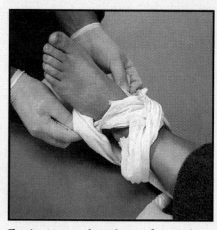

5. A stirrup has been formed.

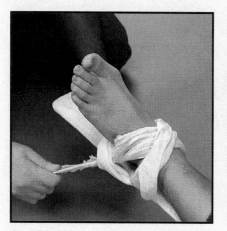

6. Thread ends through stirrup.

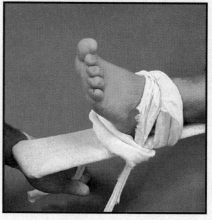

7. Pull ends downward to tighten.

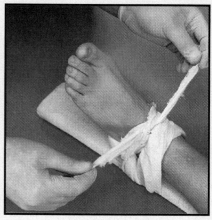

8. Pull upward and tie over ankle wrap.

546

Scan 27-14
Knee Injuries—Knee Straight— Single Splint Method

Note: Assess distal motor ability, sensory response, and circulation (pulse) both before and after immobilizing or splinting an extremity.

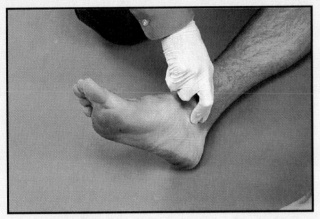

1. Assess distal motor and sensory function and circulation (pulse).

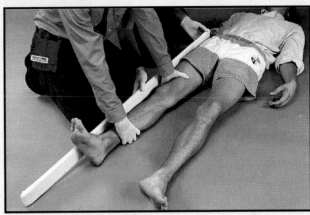

2. Use a padded board splint that extends from buttocks to 4 inches beyond heel.

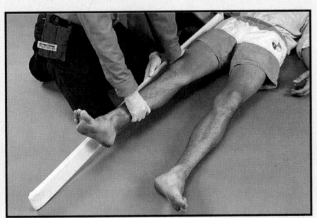

3. Stabilize and lift the limb.

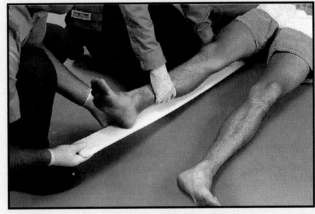

4. Place splint along posterior of limb.

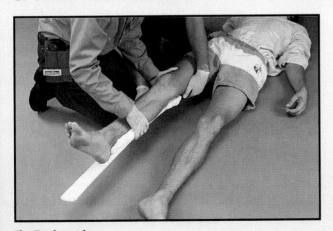

5. Pad voids.

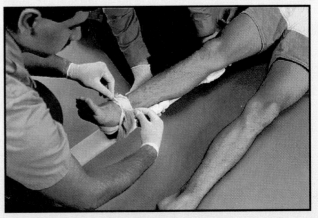

6. Apply an ankle hitch (see Scan 27-13).

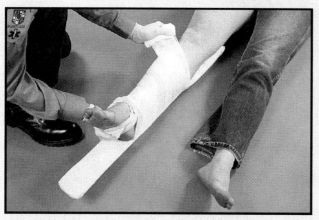

7. Use a 6-inch self-adhering roller bandage or use cravats.

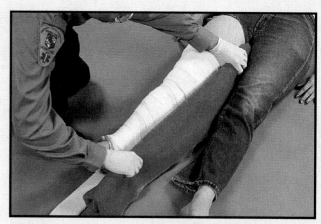

8. Place folded blanket between legs, groin to feet.

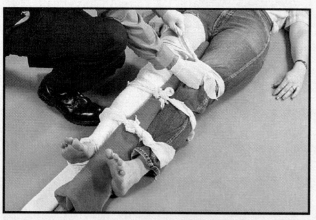

9. Tie thighs, calves, and ankles together; knot over uninjured limb.

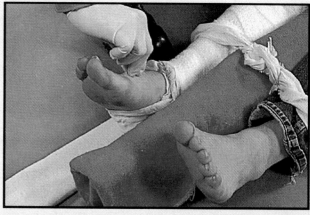

10. Reassess distal motor and sensory function and circulation (pulse).

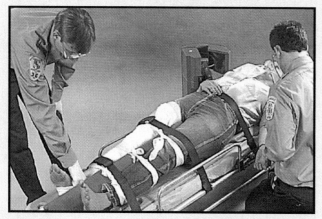

11. Care for shock and continue to provide a high concentration of oxygen.

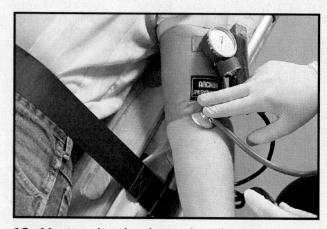

12. Monitor distal pulse and vital signs.

Knee Injuries—Knee Straight or Returned to Anatomical Position—Two Splint Method

Note: Assess distal motor ability, sensory response, and circulation (pulse) both before and after immobilizing or splinting an extremity.

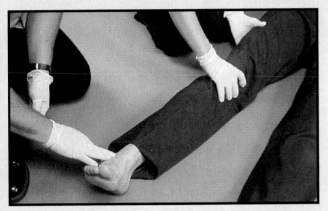

1. Assess distal motor and sensory function and circulation (pulse).

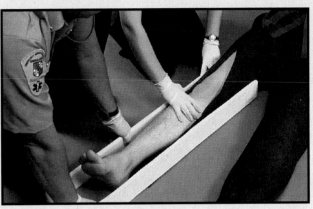

2. Padded board splints, medial from groin, lateral from iliac crest, both to 4 inches beyond foot.

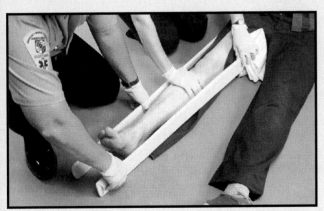

3. Stabilize the limb and pad groin.

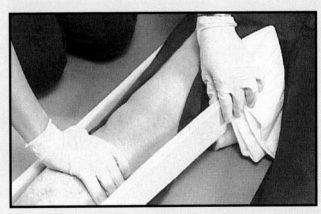

4. Position splints.

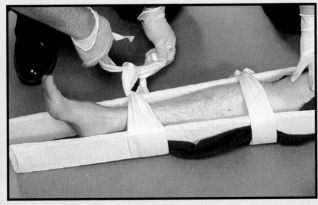

5. Secure splints at thigh, above and below knee, and at mid calf. Pad voids.

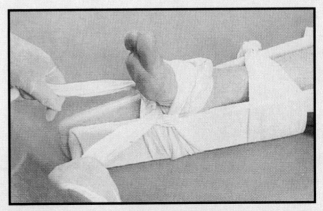

6. Cross and tie two cravats at the ankle or hitch the ankle.

Reassess distal function, care for shock, and provide high concentration oxygen.

Emergency Care Steps

1. Care for shock. Consider administering a high concentration of oxygen.
2. Check distal MSC function.
3. Splint using one of the methods described below.

   Air-inflated splint—Apply an air-inflated splint (Figure 27-16). Slide the uninflated splint over your hand and gather it in place until the lower edge clears your wrist. Grasp the patient's foot with one hand and his leg just above the injury site using your free hand. While maintaining manual traction, have your partner slide the splint over your hand and onto the injured leg. Your partner must make sure that the splint is relatively wrinkle free and that it covers the injury site. Continue to maintain traction while your partner inflates the splint. Test to see if you can cause a slight dent in the plastic with fingertip pressure. Remember to check periodically to see that the pressure in the splint has remained adequate and has not decreased or increased.

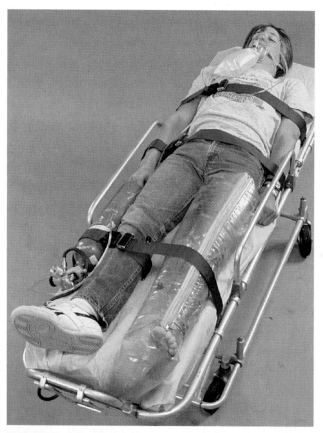

FIGURE 27-16 Using an air-inflated splint for lower leg fractures.

Two splint method—You can immobilize the fracture using two rigid board splints (Scan 27-16).

Single splint with ankle hitch—A single splint with an ankle hitch can be applied (Scan 27-17).

4. Recheck distal MSC function.

Injuries to the Ankle and Foot

Sprains (torn ligaments) and fractures are the most common musculoskeletal injuries to the ankle and foot. It is often difficult to distinguish between them, so always treat for a fracture.

Patient Assessment—Ankle and Foot Injuries

Signs and Symptoms

☐ Pain
☐ Swelling
☐ Possible deformity

Patient Care—Ankle and Foot Injuries

Long splints, extending from above the knee to beyond the foot, can be used. However, soft splinting is an effective, rapid method and is recommended for most patients (Figure 27-17). To soft splint, you should follow the steps described below.

Emergency Care Steps

1. Assess distal MSC function.
2. Stabilize the limb. Remove the patient's shoe if possible, but only if it removes easily and can be done with no movement to the ankle.
3. Lift the limb, but do not apply manual traction (tension).
4. Place three cravats on the floor under the ankle. Then place a pillow lengthwise under the ankle on top of the cravats. The pillow should extend six inches beyond the foot.
5. Gently lower the limb onto the pillow, taking care not to change the position of the ankle. Stabilize by tying the cravats, and adjust them so they are at the top of the pillow, midway, and at the heel.
6. Tie the pillow to the ankle and foot.
7. Tie a fourth cravat loosely at the arch of the foot.

Leg Injuries—Two Splint Method

Note: Assess distal motor ability, sensory response, and circulation (pulse) both before and after immobilizing or splinting an extremity.

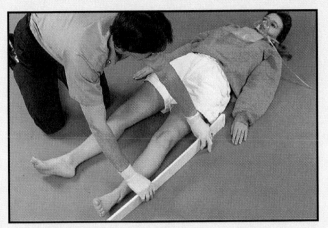

1. Measure splint. It should extend above the knee and below the ankle.

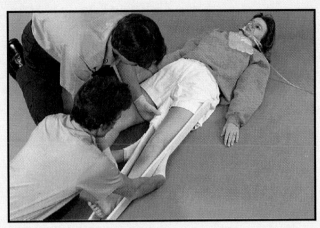

2. Apply manual traction (tension) and place one splint medially and one laterally. Padding is toward the leg.

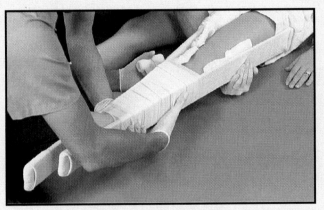

3. Secure splints, padding voids.

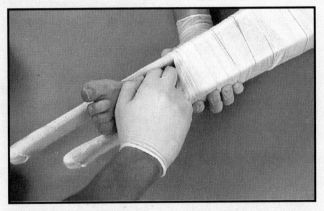

4. Reassess distal motor and sensory function and circulation (pulse).

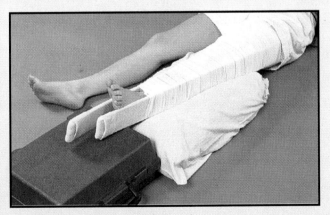

5. Elevate, once immobilized.

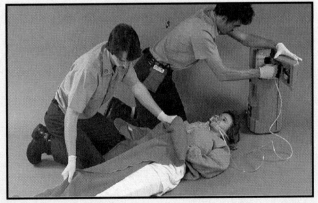

6. Treat for shock and administer high concentration oxygen. Transport on a long spine board.

Leg Injuries—Single Splint Method

Note: Assess distal motor ability, sensory response, and circulation (pulse) both before and after immobilizing or splinting an extremity.

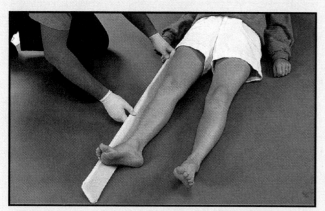

1. Measure splint. It should extend from mid thigh to 4 inches below ankle.

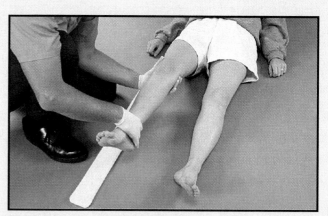

2. Apply manual traction (tension) and lift limb 10 inches off ground.

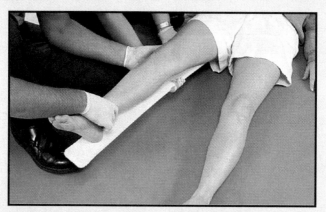

3. Place splint along the posterior of the limb, from mid thigh.

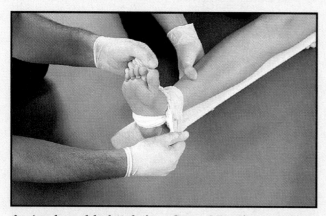

4. Apply ankle hitch (see Scan 27-13).

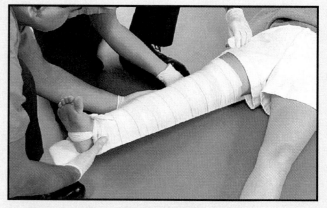

5. Secure splint to leg.

Note: Reassess distal motor and sensory function and circulation (pulse). Elevate the injured limb, care for shock, and continue to administer a high concentration of oxygen.

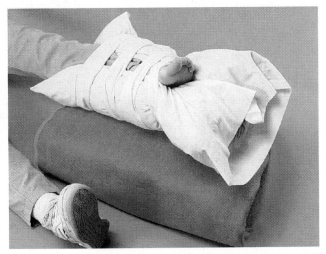

FIGURE 27-17 Pillow splinting an injured ankle.

8 Elevate with a second pillow or blanket. Reassess distal pulse and nerve function.

9 Care for shock if needed.

10 An ice pack can be applied to the injury site to reduce bleeding and swelling. Do not apply the ice pack directly to the skin.

Note that a commercial splint with a foot and leg that extends above the knee may be better than a pillow since it will immobilize the knee, the joint adjacent to the ankle.

Documentation Tip—PSD Extremities

When caring for a painful, swollen, deformed extremity, always check and record distal motor, sensory, and circulation function both before and after splinting. If the hospital staff discovers that MSC function is impaired, they will need to know if this occurred before splinting, as a possible result of splinting, or did not occur until after the patient was at the hospital. Documenting this information not only contributes to good patient care but can also protect you from charges that the function of the limb was impaired by incorrect splinting or other prehospital procedures.

Applying an Anti-Shock Garment

Anti-shock garments are used both to control shock and for splinting pelvic, hip, femoral, and multiple leg fractures. They are strongly indicated for use with a pelvic fracture with hypotension (blood pressure below 90).

An anti-shock garment is to be applied in accordance with local protocols. In many localities, application requires an order from a physician. The procedure for application of the garment is shown in Scan 27-18.

There are three major types of anti-shock garments in use. The plain garment does not have any pressure gauges. The one-gauge garment measures individual pressures, one compartment at a time. The three-gauge garment has a pressure gauge for each compartment.

The patient's clothing should not be left on under the garment. The removal of the patient's lower outer garments improves the application of the garment and allows for the easier insertion of a urinary catheter at a later time. If this is not possible, then remove the patient's belt and any sharp objects found in the pockets before applying the garment. Since transport will be required, the anti-shock garment should be placed on the patient-carrying device before the patient.

Note:

Vital signs are to be taken before applying an anti-shock garment and should be monitored EVERY 5 MINUTES thereafter.

Removing an Anti-Shock Garment

The garment should be removed only when a physician is present and

- The physician orders the removal of the garment.
- Intravenous correction of volume loss has begun.
- Vital signs have just been monitored and recorded, noting that the patient is stable.
- An operating room is available.

Application of an Anti-Shock Garment

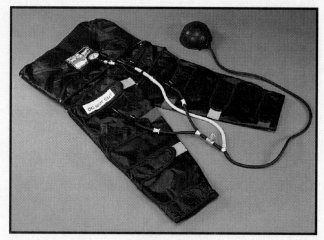

Adult garment and inflation pump.

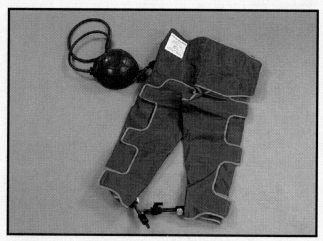

Pediatric garment.

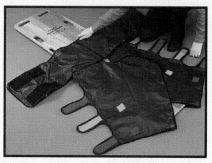

1. Unfold the garment and lay it flat on a backboard. It should be smoothed of wrinkles.

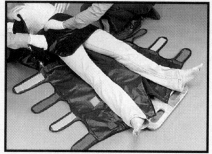

2. Log roll the patient onto the garment, or slip it under him. The upper edge of the garment must be just below the rib cage.

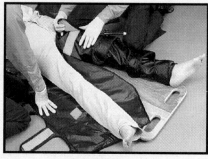

3. Enclose the left leg, securing the Velcro straps.

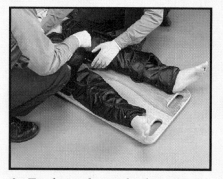

4. Enclose the right leg, securing the Velcro straps.

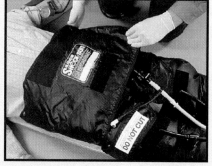

5. Enclose the abdomen and pelvis, securing the Velcro straps.

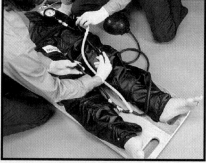

6. Check the tubes leading to the compartments and the pump.

Note: Patient's clothing remains on for demonstration purposes. In actual use, clothing should be removed. Anti-shock garment can be placed over traction splint.

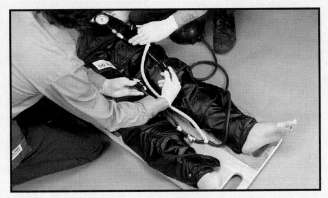

7. Open the stopcocks to the legs and close the abdominal compartment stopcock.

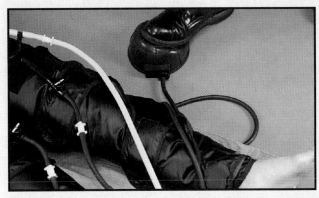

8. Use the pump to inflate the lower compartments simultaneously, or the required lower extremity compartment. Inflate until air exhausts through the relief valves, the Velcro makes a crackling noise, or the patient's systolic blood pressure is stable at 90 mm Hg or higher.

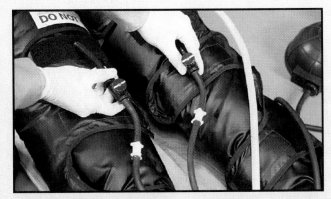

9. Close the stopcocks.

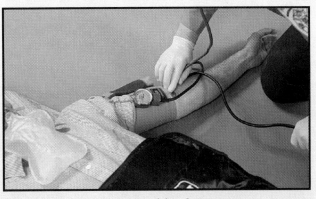

10. Check the patient's blood pressure.

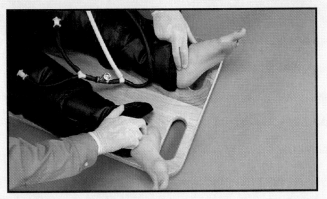

11. Check both lower extremities for a distal pulse.

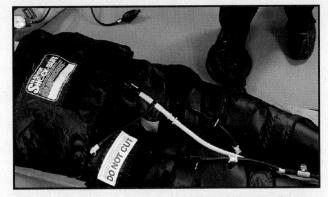

12. If BP is below 90, open the abdominal stopcock and inflate abdominal compartment. Close stopcock.

Note: Monitor and record vital signs every 5 minutes. If the garment loses pressure, add air as needed. Some protocols call for the inflation of all three compartments of the garment simultaneously.

You may find it helpful to review the following terms.

bones hard but flexible living structures that provide support for the body and protection to vital organs. Types of bones are long, short, flat, and irregular. The typical long bone has a cylindrical *shaft* and a rounded end or *head*, which is connected to the shaft by the *neck*.

cartilage tough tissue that covers the joint ends of bones and helps to form certain body parts such as the ear.

closed painful, swollen, or deformed extremity an injury to an extremity with no associated opening in the skin.

crepitus (KREP-i-tus) a grating sensation or sound made when fractured bone ends rub together.

extremities (ex-TREM-i-teez) the portions of the skeleton that include the clavicles, scapulae, arms, wrists, and hands (upper extremities) and the pelvis, thighs, legs, ankles, and feet (lower extremities).

fracture (FRAK-cher) any break in a bone.

joints places where bones articulate, or meet.

ligaments tissues that connect bone to bone.

manual traction the process of applying tension to straighten and realign a fractured limb before splinting. Also *tension.*

muscles tissues or fibers that cause movement of body organs and parts.

open painful, swollen, or deformed extremity an extremity injury in which the skin has been broken or torn through from the inside by an injured bone or from the outside by something that has caused a penetrating wound with associated injury to the bone.

tendons tissues that connect muscle to bone.

traction splint a special splint that applies constant pull along the length of a lower extremity to help stabilize the fractured bone and to reduce muscle spasms in limb. Traction splints are used primarily on femoral shaft fractures.

Injuries to bones and joints require splinting prior to the movement of the patient. If life-threatening injuries exist, address them first and, if patient is a high priority for transport, immobilize the whole patient on a long spine board. When time permits, proper splinting of a bone or joint injury can prevent further damage to soft tissues, organs, nerves, and muscles, and it can keep a closed injury from becoming an open one. It also can help to control the pain and bleeding associated with the injury, and prevent permanent damage or disability.

1. Describe the basic anatomy of bone.
2. Identify the signs and symptoms of musculoskeletal injury.
3. Describe basic emergency care for painful, swollen, deformed extremities, including general guidelines for splinting injured long bones and joints.
4. Explain why angulated deformed injuries to the long bones should be realigned to anatomical position.
5. List the basic principles of splinting.
6. Describe the hazards of splinting.
7. Describe the basic types of splints.

Application

- A hiker drives his boot under an old tree root and is tossed head over heels down the slope of a small hill. When he finally comes to rest, his left leg is bent below the knee at an unusual angle. Your initial assessment shows an alert adult male, guarding a grossly deformed left leg. He hasn't lost consciousness and has no other pain. You find he has a strong radial pulse, normal skin, and no bleeding. How should you proceed?

Injuries to the Head and Spine

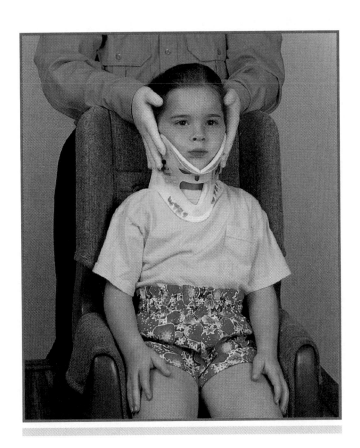

28

You have probably noticed that throughout the earlier chapters of this book there have been many cautions about special stabilization, airway, and immobilization procedures for patients with possible injuries to the head and spine. This is because injuries to the head and spine are extremely serious and may result in severe permanent disability or death if missed during your assessment or improperly treated. Second only to proper assessment and care for the ABCs, proper assessment and care for head and spinal injuries will be your most important responsibility as an EMT-B.

Objectives

6. Demonstrate securing a patient to a long spine board.

7. Demonstrate using the short board immobilization technique.

8. Demonstrate the procedure for rapid extrication.

9. Demonstrate preferred methods for stabilization of a helmet.

10. Demonstrate helmet removal techniques.

11. Demonstrate alternative methods for stabilization of a helmet.

12. Demonstrate completing a prehospital care report for patients with head and spinal injuries.

On the Scene

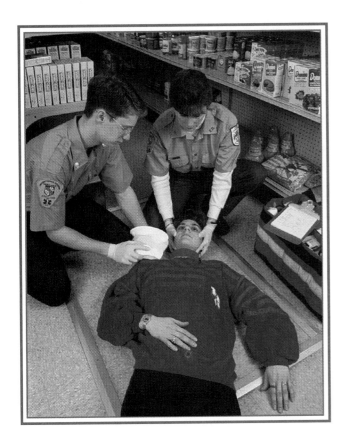

Nineteen-year-old Linda Ruiz works at the local convenience store. Her parents were worried about her taking a job where she would be working alone, but Linda argued that it was a way to earn money for college. It turns out Linda's parents were right. Early one morning, someone strikes Linda on the back of the head with an object she never saw coming.

The robber scoops out the cash drawer and escapes just minutes before a patron stops in and finds Linda lying unconscious on the floor between shelves. Fighting panic, the patron phones 911. Your ambulance service receives the call as "unknown injuries from an assault." You arrive at the scene to find the police already there. As you *size up the scene,* a sergeant explains what has happened and assures you that the scene has been secured. You pull on disposable gloves and enter the store.

As you approach to begin your *initial assessment,* you get a general impression of a young woman who is now conscious but still lying supine on the floor where a police-officer first responder has advised her to remain. She has manually stabilized Linda's head pending your arrival. Your partner takes over manual stabilization as you introduce yourself.

You: Hi. We're emergency medical technicians from the ambulance. We're here to help you. I'm Stacy Barnes. What's your name?
Linda: Linda Ruiz.
You: What happened, Linda?
Linda: I must have gotten hit over the head with something. Real hard.
You: Did you pass out?

Linda: I guess so. The police officer says I was unconscious when she got here. But I don't even remember getting hit. This man asked me to find something for him on the shelf. I turned my back to hunt for what he wanted, and the next thing I know I'm on the floor looking up at the officer.

You: Is this a day when you usually work? What day is today?

Linda: Today? Is it Saturday?

From her responses, it is obvious that Linda is alert and oriented to person and place but not time (it's Tuesday, not Saturday) and that her airway and breathing are OK. As your partner maintains manual stabilization, you continue talking reassuringly with Linda while you check her pulse, which is strong and slightly rapid, and her skin, which remains warm, pink, and dry. There is no evidence of blood loss.

You begin your *focused history and physical exam* for a trauma patient with a rapid trauma exam. Checking Linda's head, you discover a painful swelling on the right side but no bleeding. As soon as you have checked her neck, you measure and apply a cervical collar before completing the physical exam. Examination of her extremities reveals obvious weakness in her left arm and leg. When you log roll her to check her posterior body, the police officer helps by sliding the spine board under her so you can roll her onto the board and immobilize her. You find no injuries other than the bump on her head. Your partner takes vital signs, finding them all within normal ranges, as you get a SAMPLE history and check vital signs. Then you load Linda into the ambulance for transport to the hospital, performing a *detailed physical exam* and *ongoing assessment* en route.

A week later you learn that Linda suffered no permanent injuries, but her parents have talked her out of returning to work at the store. Her college money will have to be earned some other way!

■

When studying injuries to the head and the spine, it is first necessary to review and expand your knowledge of the anatomy of the nervous and skeletal systems. In this chapter, we will consider the skull, the vertebral column, and the close relationship of the skeletal system to the nervous system. Then you will study the mechanisms and kinds of injuries that can occur to the skull and spine, the signs and symptoms of such injuries, and emergency care.

THE NERVOUS AND SKELETAL SYSTEMS

Below are brief summaries of information about the nervous system, head, and spine. For more complete information, review Chapter 4, The Human Body.

The Nervous System

The major components of the **nervous system** are the brain and the spinal cord. The nervous system provides the overall control of thought, sensations, and motor functions of all parts of the body. The skeletal system provides support and protection. The skull protects the brain, while the bones of the spine protect the spinal cord. Whenever there is an injury to the skull or the spine, suspect possible nervous system damage as well.

The nervous system (Figure 28-1) is divided into two sub-systems: the central nervous system and the peripheral nervous system. The **central nervous system** consists of the brain and the spinal cord. The **peripheral nervous system** includes the pairs of nerves that enter and exit the spinal cord between each pair of vertebrae and the twelve pairs of cranial nerves that travel from the brain without passing through the spinal cord.

Messages sent from the body to the brain are carried by sensory nerves. The nerves sending messages from the brain to the muscles are called motor nerves. These nerves are responsible for voluntary motion. They control voluntary movements, those we consciously control, such as walking or grasping. When nerves exit the brain to go down the spinal cord, they cross over to the opposite side of the body. This is why an injury to the left side of the brain may produce effects such as weakness or lack of sensation on the right side of the body. That is why Linda Ruiz, your patient in On the Scene, exhibited weakness in her left arm and leg when her head injury was on the right side.

Some nerves control involuntary functions—those we do not consciously control—including heartbeat, breathing, and digestion. These nerves are part of the **autonomic nervous system** (autonomic is another way of saying automatic).

The brain is the master organ of life. Messages from all over the body are received by the brain, which decides how to respond to changing

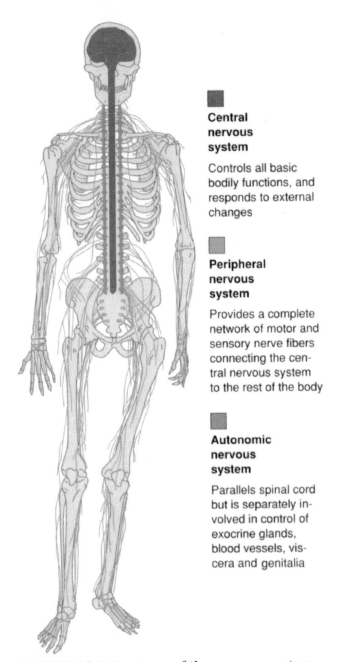

Central nervous system

Controls all basic bodily functions, and responds to external changes

Peripheral nervous system

Provides a complete network of motor and sensory nerve fibers connecting the central nervous system to the rest of the body

Autonomic nervous system

Parallels spinal cord but is separately involved in control of exocrine glands, blood vessels, viscera and genitalia

FIGURE 28-1 Anatomy of the nervous system.

conditions both inside and outside the body. The brain sends messages to the muscles so that we can move, or to a particular organ so that it will carry out a desired function (e.g., it may tell the adrenal gland to dump epinephrine into the blood stream, which speeds up the heart rate). Any major skull injury can damage the brain, causing vital body functions to fail.

The spinal cord is a relay between most of the body and the brain. A large number of the messages to and from the brain are sent through the spinal cord. Damage to the cord can isolate a part of the body from the brain. Function of this part can be lost, possibly forever.

The healing power of nerve tissue is limited. This is especiallly true in certain areas. If nerve tissue in the brain or spinal cord is damaged, to a certain extent function is lost and cannot be restored. As an EMT-B your initial care will often prevent additional damage to the brain, spinal cord, and major nerves of the body.

The Anatomy of the Head

The skull is made up of the **cranium** and the facial bones (Figure 28-2). The cranium forms the forehead (frontal), top (parietal), back (occipital), and upper sides (temporal) of the skull. The **cranial floor** is the inferior wall of the brain case, the bony floor beneath the brain. The cranial bones are fused together to form immovable joints.

There are fourteen irregularly shaped bones forming the face. The facial bones are fused into immovable joints, except for the **mandible.** It joins on each side of the cranium with a **temporal bone** to form the **temporomandibular joint.** This joint is sometimes referred to as the TM joint.

The upper jaw is made up of two fused bones called the **maxillae.** Each is known as a *maxilla.* The upper third, or bridge, of the nose

The Skull: Cranium and Face

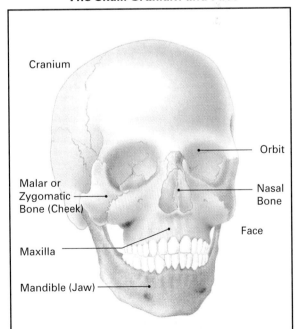

FIGURE 28-2 The skull: cranium and face.

contains two **nasal bones.** There is a cheek bone on each side of the skull. The cheek bone can be called the **malar** or the *zygomatic* bone. The malars and the maxillae form a portion of the **orbits** (sockets) of the eyes.

The brain is held in place within the skull. The spinal cord exits the base of the brain and leaves the skull through a large hole where the spinal column is attached. The brain is bathed in a fluid called **cerebrospinal fluid (CSF).** This fluid also circulates down the spine around the spinal cord.

Anatomy of the Spine

The spine is actually 33 separate irregularly shaped bones, called **vertebrae** (singular *vertebra*), which sit one on top of another to form the spinal column. Each vertebra has a **spinous process,** which is a bony bump you can palpate on a patient's back. Every vertebra has a hollow space like the hole in a donut. These hollow spaces form a channel that runs the length of the spinal column and contains the spinal cord, which is cushioned by the cerebrospinal fluid. The vertebrae are divided into five areas (shown in Figure 28-3)—from top to bottom: the 7 cervical (in the neck), the 12 thoracic (to which the ribs attach), the 5 lumbar (mid back), the 5 sacral (lower back) and 4 coccygeal (in the coccyx, or tailbone). Both the sacral and coccygeal

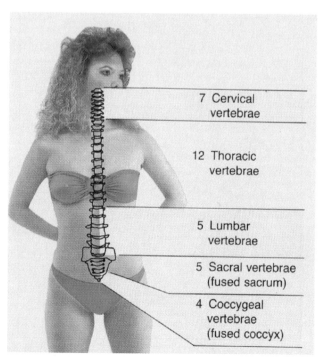

7 Cervical vertebrae

12 Thoracic vertebrae

5 Lumbar vertebrae

5 Sacral vertebrae (fused sacrum)

4 Coccygeal vertebrae (fused coccyx)

FIGURE 28-3 The divisions of the spinal column.

vertebrae are fused together, forming the posterior portion of the pelvis.

INJURIES TO THE BRAIN AND SKULL

Scalp Injuries

The scalp has many blood vessels, so any scalp injury may bleed profusely. Control bleeding with direct pressure and dress and bandage as described in Chapter 26, Soft Tissue Injuries. Be careful about applying direct pressure when the scalp injury covers a possible skull injury. Do not apply pressure if the injury site shows bone fragments or depression of the bone or if the brain is exposed. Instead, use a loose gauze dressing.

Skull Injuries

Skull injuries include fractures to the cranium and fractures to the face. If severe enough, these injuries can include direct and indirect injuries to the brain.

Skull injuries can be either open or closed. The words *open* and *closed* refer to the skull bones. When the bones of the cranium are fractured, and the scalp overlying the fracture is lacerated, the patient has an *open head injury.* In other cases, there may be a laceration of the scalp; however, if the cranium is intact, or free of fractures, the term *closed head injury* is used. In practice, it may not be possible for the EMT-B to determine if a head injury is open or closed. It is safest for you to assume that there may be an open head injury beneath any contusion or laceration of the scalp.

Brain Injuries

Brain injuries can be classified as direct or indirect. *Direct injuries* can occur in open head injuries, with the brain being lacerated, punctured, or bruised by the broken bones of the skull, by bone fragments, or by foreign objects. *Indirect injuries* occur in cases of closed head injuries and certain types of open head injuries. In an indirect injury, the shock of impact against the skull is transferred to the brain. Indirect injuries to the brain include concussions and contusions.

Note: The signs and symptoms of possible injury to the skull or brain should alert you to the strong additional possibility of cervical spine injury.

Patient Assessment—Skull Fractures and Brain Injuries

The signs of skull fracture and of brain injury are very similar. You should consider the possibility of a skull fracture or brain injury whenever you note any of the signs or symptoms listed below (Figure 28-4).

Signs

☐ *Visible bone fragments* and perhaps even bits of brain tissue are the most obvious signs of skull fracture, but the majority of skull fractures do not produce these signs.

☐ *Altered mental status.* Check mental status by using the AVPU scale (alert, response to verbal stimulus, response to painful stimulus, unresponsive). If alert, check for orientation to person, place, and time.

☐ *Deep laceration or severe bruise or hematoma* to the scalp or forehead. Do not probe into the wound or separate the wound opening to determine wound depth.

☐ *Depressions or deformity of the skull,* large swellings ("goose eggs"), or anything that looks unusual about the shape of the cranium

☐ Any *severe pain* at the site of a head injury. Pain may be a symptom of skull injury. Do not palpate the injury site with your finger tips as you may push bone fragments into the injury. Pain may range from a headache to severe discomfort.

☐ *"Battle's sign,"* (a bruise behind the ear)

☐ *Pupils unequal or unreactive to light*

☐ *"Raccoon eyes,"* (black eyes or discoloration of the soft tissues under both eyes)

☐ *One eye appears to be sunken*

☐ *Bleeding from the ears and/or nose*

☐ *Clear fluid flowing* from the ears and/or the nose

☐ *Personality change,* ranging from irritable to irrational behavior (a major sign)

☐ *Increased blood pressure and decreased pulse rate* (Cushing's syndrome)

☐ *Irregular breathing patterns*

☐ *Temperature increase* (late sign due to inflammation, infection, or damage to temperature-regulating centers)

☐ *Blurred or multiple image vision* in one or both eyes

☐ *Impaired hearing* or ringing in the ears

☐ *Equilibrium problems.* The patient may be unable to stand still with his eyes closed or may stumble when attempting to walk. (Do not test for this.)

☐ *Forceful or projectile vomiting*

☐ *Posturing.* When painful stimulus is applied, the patient may exhibit *neurological posturing* such as: flexes the arms and wrists and extends the legs and feet (called decorticate posture) or extends the arms with the shoulders rotated inward and the wrists flexed, legs extended (decerebrate posture). These postures may also be assumed spontaneously, without painful stimulus.

☐ *Paralysis or disability on one side of the body*

☐ *Seizures*

☐ *Deteriorating vital signs*

Note: *Shock is generally not a sign of head injury, except in infants.* There simply is not enough room in the adult skull to permit enough bleeding to cause shock. If there is head injury with shock, look for indications of blood loss somewhere else on the body.

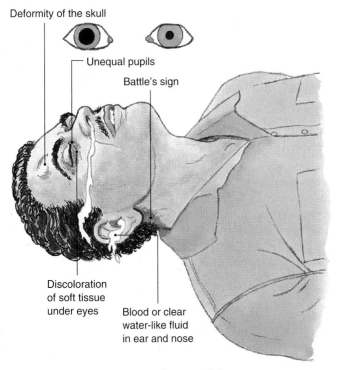

Deformity of the skull

Unequal pupils

Battle's sign

Discoloration of soft tissue under eyes

Blood or clear water-like fluid in ear and nose

FIGURE 28-4 Signs of cranial fracture.

With so many factors to consider, determining possible skull or brain injury based on the signs of such injury, as listed above, can be very difficult. Therefore, assume skull or brain injury when the mechanism of injury and the location of the injury site indicate a possible head injury.

Note: Some of the signs of brain injury can cause an untrained person to assume that a patient with a brain injury is intoxicated from alcohol or abusing other drugs. Never assume intoxication or drug abuse without assessment.

Patient Care—Skull Fractures and Brain Injuries

Emergency Care Steps

1. *Take appropriate body substance isolation (BSI) precautions.*

2. *Assume a neck or spine injury in your initial assessment and use the jaw-thrust maneuver to open and maintain the airway.* Have someone provide manual in-line stabilization of the patient's head. For the unconscious patient, an oropharyngeal airway should be inserted. This must be done without hyperextending the neck. Have suctioning equipment ready for immediate use since these patients are prone to vomiting.

3. *Monitor the conscious patient for changes in breathing.* Provide artificial ventilations if breathing is inadequate.

4. *Apply a rigid collar and immobilize the neck and spine and, if appropriate, determine the method of extrication,* either normal or rapid (see later in this chapter).

5. *Administer high concentration oxygen by nonrebreather mask and evaluate the need for artificial ventilations with supplemental oxygen.* This is critical should there be any brain damage. In some areas, if the patient shows signs of a brain injury (e.g., increased blood pressure with decreased pulse, altered level of consciousness) then EMT-Bs are instructed to hyperventilate the patient with oxygen-assisted ventilations (bag-valve mask or positive pressure) at the rate of 25+ per minute rather than the usual 12 ventilations per minute. The hyperventilation will help reduce brain tissue swelling by lowering carbon dioxide levels and raising oxygen levels. Follow your local protocol.

6. *Control bleeding.* Do not apply pressure if the injury site shows bone fragments or depression of the bone or if the brain is exposed. Do not attempt to stop the flow of blood or cerebrospinal fluid from the ears or the nose. If the skull is fractured, you may increase intracranial pressure and may also increase the risk of infection. Instead, use a loose gauze dressing.

7. *Keep the patient at rest.* This can be a critical factor.

8. *Talk to the conscious patient, providing emotional support.* Ask the patient questions so that he will have to concentrate. This procedure will help you to detect changes in the patient's mental status.

9. *Dress and bandage open wounds.* Stabilize any penetrating objects. (Do not remove any objects or fragments of bone.)

10. *Manage the patient for shock* even if shock is not present, to prevent shock from developing. Avoid overheating.

11. *Be prepared for vomiting.* It may be necessary to turn the long backboard on its side to allow the patient's airway to drain if he vomits, so make sure the patient is securely immobilized and that a suction unit is ready for use.

12. *Transport the patient promptly.*

13. *Monitor vital signs every five minutes* en route to the hospital.

If you are not certain as to the severity of the patient's injuries, if there is evidence of cervical spine injury, or if the patient with a head injury is unconscious, then a rigid cervical collar must be applied and the patient positioned on a long spine board. With the entire head, neck, and body rigidly immobilized, the patient may be rotated into a lateral recumbent position so that blood and mucus can drain freely. If the patient vomits, as brain-injured patients are likely to do, the vomitus is less likely to cause an airway obstruction or be aspirated (breathed into the lungs). Some patients with a head injury will vomit without warning. Many vomit without first experiencing nausea. If injuries prevent such positioning, constant monitoring and frequent suctioning are required.

Cranial Injuries With Impaled Objects

If there is an object impaled in the patient's cranium, do not remove it. Instead, stabilize the object in place with bulky dressings. (See information on stabilizing impaled objects in Chapter 26, Soft Tissue Injuries.) This, plus care in handling, minimizes accidental movement of the object during the remainder of care and transport.

In some situations you may be confronted with a patient whose skull has been impaled by a long object. This can make transporting the patient impossible until the object is cut or shortened. Pad around the object with bulky dressings, then carefully (and rigidly) stabilize the object on both sides of where the cut will be made. Cutting should be done with a tool that will not cause the object to move or vibrate when it is finally severed. Often, a hand hacksaw with a fine tooth blade is the best tool to use because it can be carefully controlled and produces only a small amount of heat. In any case in which you may have to cut a long impaled object, call and seek advice from medical direction or the emergency department physician.

Injuries to the Face and Jaw

Facial fractures are usually produced by an impact, as when a child is struck in the face by a baseball bat or when someone is thrown against the windshield during a motor vehicle crash. Bone fragments may lodge in the back of the throat, causing airway obstruction. Blood, blood clots, dislodged teeth, or a separated palate also may cause partial or total airway obstruction. Signs of a facial fracture are shown in Figure 28-5.

The mandible is subject to dislocation as well as to fracture. As with any facial injury, there may be pain, discoloration, swelling, and facial distortion. In addition, when the mandible

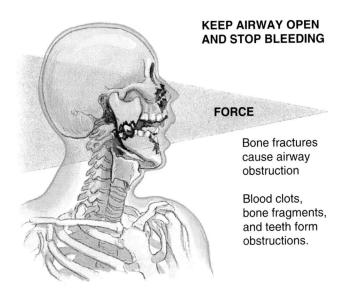

KEEP AIRWAY OPEN AND STOP BLEEDING

FORCE

Bone fractures cause airway obstruction

Blood clots, bone fragments, and teeth form obstructions.

FIGURE 28-6 Complications of facial fracture.

is injured or dislocated, the patient may be unable to move the lower jaw or have difficulty speaking. There may be an improper alignment of the upper and lower teeth and bleeding around the teeth.

The primary concern for emergency care of facial fractures or jaw injuries is the state of the patient's airway (Figure 28-6). Be prepared to suction to remove debris and blood from the airway. Because of the possibility of spinal injury, use the jaw-thrust maneuver to open and maintain the airway. Using BSI precautions, control profuse bleeding. (See Chapter 26, Soft Tissue Injuries, for care of an object impaled in the cheek.) Apply a rigid collar and immobilize the patient on a spine board. If possible, position the patient for drainage from the mouth. Care for shock.

Remember: The face is part of the skull. When there is a suspected facial fracture from a blow of sufficient force, there may also be brain injury. Treat this patient as you would for any patient with a suspected skull or brain injury.

Nontraumatic Brain Injuries

Many of the signs of brain injury may be caused by an internal brain event such as a hemorrhage or blood clot. (See the information on stroke in Chapter 19, Diabetes and Altered Mental Status). The signs of nontraumatic (not caused by external trauma) brain injury will be the same as those for a traumatic injury, except that there will be no evidence of trauma nor mechanism of injury.

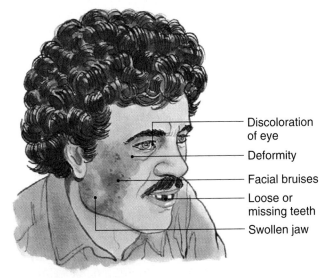

— Discoloration of eye

— Deformity

— Facial bruises

— Loose or missing teeth

— Swollen jaw

FIGURE 28-5 Signs of facial fracture.

INJURIES TO THE SPINE

Injuries to the spine must always be considered when you find serious injury to the body. Remember that spinal injury can be associated with head, neck, and back injuries. Do not overlook the possibility of spinal injury when dealing with chest, abdominal, and pelvic injuries. Even injuries to the upper and lower extremities can be associated with forces intense enough also to produce spinal injury.

Failure to complete an initial assessment and focused trauma exam and decide the most appropriate immobilization method could lead to a spine-injured patient being further injured or to an unsavable patient with a "picture perfect" spinal immobilization that took too much time to complete at the scene, delaying transport to the hospital. As an EMT-B, you should "uptriage," or overtreat, patients with potential spinal injuries because you cannot rule out a spinal injury in the field and because the costs in terms of pain, suffering, disability, and dollars are very high when a spine-injured patient is unintentionally made worse by failure to immobilize his spine.

Injuries to the spinal column include fractures, with and without bone displacement, dislocations, ligament sprains, and disk injury, including compression. The vertebral column may be injured without damage to the spinal cord or spinal nerves. For example, a fractured coccyx is below the level of the spinal cord. Ligament sprains are relatively simple injuries. However, when displaced fractures and dislocations occur, the cord, disk, and spinal nerves may be severely injured. Serious contusions and lacerations, accompanied by pressure-producing swelling, can take place. The entire column can become unstable, leading to cord compression that may produce paralysis or death.

Mechanisms of Injury

There is a simple rule you can follow. If the mechanism of injury exerts great force on the upper body (Figure 28-7) or if there is any soft tissue damage to the head, face, or neck due to trauma (e.g., from being thrown against a dashboard), you should then assume that there is a possible cervical spine injury. Any blunt trauma above the clavicles may damage the cervical spine.

Some parts of the spine are more susceptible to injury than others. Because they are somewhat splinted by the attached ribs, the seg-

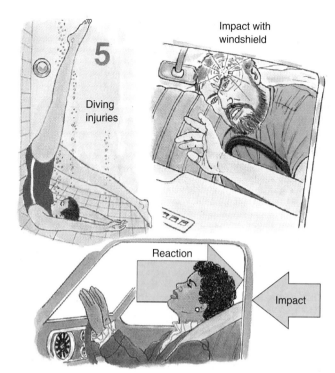

FIGURE 28-7 Mechanisms of injury to the upper body.

ments of the thoracic spine are not usually damaged except in the most violent accidents or in gunshot wounds. The pelvic-sacral spine attachment helps to protect the sacrum in the same way. On the other hand, the cervical and lumbar vertebrae are susceptible to injury because they are not supported by other bony structures.

The spine is most often injured by compression or excessive flexion, extension, or rotation from falls, diving accidents, and motor vehicle collisions. EMS workers often injure their spine by not adhering to the proper techniques of lifting (discussed in Chapter 6, Lifting and Moving), causing lateral bending or disk injuries. When the spine is excessively pulled, it can cause what is referred to as a distraction injury. This is the mechanism that occurs in a hanging, which injures the spine. Years ago rescuers were taught to pull traction on the neck of an injured patient sitting in an automobile. This actually had the potential to cause injury, so today EMT-Bs are taught to manually stabilize the head and neck, or basically hold it still.

You should maintain a high degree of suspicion of a potential spine injury when your patient is a victim of a motor vehicle or motorcycle collision, was struck by a vehicle, fell to the ground, received blunt injury to the spine or above the clavicles, sustained penetrating trauma to the head, neck or torso, was involved in a diving accident, was found hanging by his neck, or was found unconscious due to trauma.

The adult skull weighs more than 17 pounds, and it rests on a very small area of the cervical spine (sometimes described as like a pumpkin on a broom handle). Motor vehicle collisions produce violent whiplash injuries because of the speed and sudden deceleration of the vehicle. When a vehicle strikes another vehicle or a fixed object head on, the neck can whip quickly back and forth. The vehicle decelerates abruptly, but the head continues to travel forward at the same rate of speed that the vehicle was traveling, even though the body is held by seat restraints. This neck movement may exceed the normal range of motion. Virtually the same thing occurs when the vehicle is struck from behind.

A fall can produce spinal injury when the victim strikes an object, the ground, or the floor. The force generated during a fall may be enough to fracture, crush, or dislocate vertebrae. Cases of needless disability have been reported when head injuries or other injuries were noted and cared for but spinal injuries were overlooked.

Today more and more people are participating in sports of all kinds: roller-blading, bicycling, surfing, rock climbing, and others too numerous to mention. Many sports accidents can cause spinal injury. A sledding or skiing accident may hurl a person into a tree or other fixed object, twisting or compressing the spinal column. There may be no open wound or fracture of an extremity, or signs of injury may be hidden by bulky clothing. As a result, improper care may be rendered as the victim with a possible spinal injury is placed on a stretcher without adequate examination and immobilization.

Diving accidents often produce injury to the cervical spine. When the diver strikes the diving board, the side or bottom of the pool, or an underwater object, the head can be severely forced beyond its normal limits of motion (flexion, extension, or compression). Cervical vertebrae may be fractured or dislocated, ligaments may be severely sprained, and the spinal cord may be compressed or otherwise traumatized in the cervical region and at other spots along the cord.

Football and other contact sports can cause accidents severe enough to produce spinal injury. Spear tackling, using the head, has been outlawed in grade schools and high schools for a number of years due to the incidence of cervical compression fractures. Whenever a game involves player contact or falling to the ground, be on the alert for spinal injury.

Any violent or falling accident can produce spinal injury. As a rule of thumb, assume that any fall three times the patient's height or with enough force to cause open fractures to the ankles will also be accompanied by a spine injury. The most common causes of spinal cord injury are motor vehicle collisions, fractured spines in the elderly (often caused by falls, or spontaneous fractures of brittle bones that, in turn, cause falls), diving accidents, and gunshot wounds. You must do a complete assessment of the patient. You should assume that all unconscious trauma patients have spinal injury. Whenever you are in doubt, assume that there are spinal injuries and immobilize the torso and the head and neck.

Patient Assessment—Spinal Injury

Signs and Symptoms of Spinal Injury

- [ ] *Paralysis of the Extremities*—PARALYSIS OF THE EXTREMITIES IS PROBABLY THE MOST RELIABLE SIGN OF SPINAL CORD INJURY IN CONSCIOUS PATIENTS.
- [ ] *Pain without movement*—The pain is not always constant and may occur anywhere from the top of the head to the buttocks. Pain in the leg is common for certain types of injury to the lower spinal cord and vertebral column. Other painful injuries can mask this symptom of spinal injury.
- [ ] *Pain with movement*—The patient normally tries to lie perfectly still to prevent pain on movement. You should not request the patient to move just to determine if pain is present. However, if the patient complains of pain in the neck or back experienced with voluntary movements, you must consider this to be a symptom of possible spinal injury. Spine pain with movement in apparently uninjured shoulders and legs is a good indicator of possible spinal injury.
- [ ] *Tenderness anywhere along the spine*—Gentle palpation of the injury site, when accessible, may reveal point tenderness.

The above are reliable indicators of possible spinal injury in the conscious patient. If any one of these is present, you have sufficient reason to immobilize the patient. If immediate immobilization is not possible, use extreme care in handling the patient. In the field, it is not possible to rule out spinal injury even in cases in which the patient has no pain and is able to move his limbs. The mechanism of injury alone may be the deciding factor. Additional signs of spinal injury may include

☐ *Impaired Breathing*—Neck injury can impair nerve function to the chest muscles. Watch the patient breathe. If there is only a slight movement of the abdomen, with little or no movement of the chest, it is safe to assume that the patient is breathing with the diaphragm alone (diaphragmatic breathing). This is also true if there is a reversal of normal breathing patterns with the rib cage collapsing on inspiration, rising on expiration. Panting due to respiratory insufficiency may develop. Damage to the nerves that control the movement of the rib cage can prevent this. The nerve that controls the diaphragm is located high in the cervical area and is often unharmed, but the intercostal nerves that control the chest muscles are often damaged in cervical and thoracic injuries. As a result, when the diaphragm moves downward to pull in air, the ribs, instead of expanding, collapse; when the diaphragm relaxes and air is expelled, the rib cage rises—the opposite of the normal pattern. This is characteristic of spinal cord injury. Check abdominal movement from the side by placing your hand on the patient's abdomen and looking for reversed movements during respiration.

☐ *Deformity*—The removal of clothing to check the back for deformity of the spine is not recommended. OBVIOUS SPINAL DEFORMITIES ARE RARE. However, if you note a gap between the spinous processes (bony extensions) of the vertebrae or if you can feel a broken spinous process, you must consider the patient to have serious spinal injuries. It is also possible to feel tight muscles in spasm.

☐ *Priapism*—Persistent erection of the penis is a sign of spinal injury affecting nerves to the external genitalia.

☐ *Posturing*—In some cases of spinal injury, motor nerve pathways to the muscles that extend the arm can be interrupted, but those that lead to the muscles that bend the elbow and lift the arm remain functional. The patient may be found on his back, with the arms extended above the head, which may indicate a cervical spine injury. Arms flexed across the chest or extended along the sides with wrists flexed also signals spinal injury.

☐ *Loss of Bowel or Bladder Control*—Loss of bowel or bladder control may indicate spinal injury.

☐ *Nerve Impairment to the Extremities*—The patient may have loss of use, weakness, numbness, tingling, or loss of feeling in the upper and/or lower extremities—especially below the suspected level of the injury.

☐ *Severe Spinal Shock*—This may occur even when there are no indications of external or internal bleeding. It can be caused by the failure of the nervous system to control the diameter of blood vessels (neurogenic shock). The pulse rate may be normal because the message to "speed up" the heart may never have gotten to the heart due to the cord injury.

☐ *Soft Tissue Injuries Associated with Trauma*—Traumatic soft tissue injuries to the head and neck may signal injury of the cervical spine; traumatic soft tissue injuries to the shoulders, back, or abdomen may signal injury of the thoracic or lumbar spine; traumatic soft tissue injuries to the lower extremities may signal injury of the lumbar or sacral spine.

Remember: The ability to walk, move the extremities, or feel sensation, or a lack of pain in the spinal area, does not rule out the possibility of spinal column or spinal cord injury.

Assessment Strategies

When you suspect a spinal injury, use the following assessment strategies.

Responsive Patient

☐ Ascertain the mechanism of injury
☐ Ask these questions (tell the patient not to move while answering):

1. What happened?
2. Where does it hurt? Does your neck or back hurt?
3. Can you move your hands and feet?
4. Can you feel me touching (lightly) your fingers? your toes?
5. Do you feel "pins and needles" (tingling) in your legs? anywhere?

☐ Inspect for contusions, deformities, lacerations, punctures, penetrations, swelling.

☐ Palpate for tendernesss or deformity.

☐ Assess equality of strength in the extremities by checking hand grip or pushing against the patient's hands and feet.

Unresponsive patient

☐ Ascertain from bystanders the mechanism of injury and information about the patient's mental status prior to your arrival.

☐ Inspect for contusions, deformities, lacerations, punctures, penetrations, swelling.

☐ Palpate for area of tenderness (some unresponsive patients will withdraw from or react to pain) or deformity.

Note: Do not waste much time trying to rule out spinal injury in an unresponsive patient. If there is a mechanism of injury associated with spinal injury, immobilize the patient and treat as if there is a spinal injury.

Patient Care—Spinal Injury

Regardless of where the apparent spinal injury is located on the cord, care is the same. First take body substance isolation precautions and do the initial assessment and focused trauma exam. Determine the patient's priority since this will be important in deciding how to immobilize him (Figure 28-8).

Emergency Care Steps

For all patients with possible spinal injury, and for all accident victims when there is doubt as to the extent of injury, first take BSI precautions, and then

1. *Provide manual in-line stabilization for the head and neck during the initial assessment. Continue to maintain manual stabilization.* Place the head in a neutral in-line position unless the patient complains of pain or the head is not easily moved into that position. If that is the case, steady the head in the position found. Maintain constant stabilization until the patient is properly secured to a backboard.

2. *Assess airway, breathing, and circulation.* If necessary, open and control the airway with the jaw-thrust maneuver, maintaining in-line stabilization of the head.

3. *In your focused trauma exam, assess the head and neck. Then apply a rigid cervical collar.* Make sure the collar is properly sized. A wrong-size collar may do more

harm than good by hyperextending the neck if too large or allowing flexion of the neck if too small. Also make sure the collar is not applied so as to obstruct the airway. Maintain manual stabilization even after the collar is in place until the patient is secured to a backboard, since no collar completely restricts motion. For an infant or child, be sure to use a pediatric-sized collar. If you don't have the right pediatric size, use a rolled towel, maintaining manual support of the infant's or child's head.

4. *Quickly assess sensory and motor function in all four extremities* if the patient is responsive.

5. *Based on the patient's priority apply the appropriate spinal immobilization device at the appropriate speed* (see Figure 28-8). The following Scans are provided to demonstrate the proper procedure to use based upon the condition of the patient and the position in which the patient is found:

- Scan 28-1 Immobilization of a seated patient using a KED
- Scan 28-2 Rapid extrication
- Scan 28-3 The 4-person log roll
- Scan 28-4 Placing the supine patient on a long backboard
- Scan 28-5 Rapid takedown of the standing patient
- Scan 28-6 Helmet removal from injured patient
- Scan 28-7 Child safety seat immobilization
- Scan 28-8 Rapid extrication from a child safety seat

6. *If the patient has paralysis or weakness of the extremities, administer high concentration oxygen via nonrebreather mask and evaluate the need for artificial ventilations with supplemental oxygen.* This is critical should there be any cord damage.

7. *Reassess sensory and motor function in all four extremities* if the patient is responsive.

IMMOBILIZATION ISSUES

Tips for Applying a Cervical Collar

Cervical spine immobilization devices, or extrication collars, have come a long way since the early days of EMS. Originally ambulance person-

EXTRICATION AND IMMOBILIZATION PROCEDURE DECISIONS

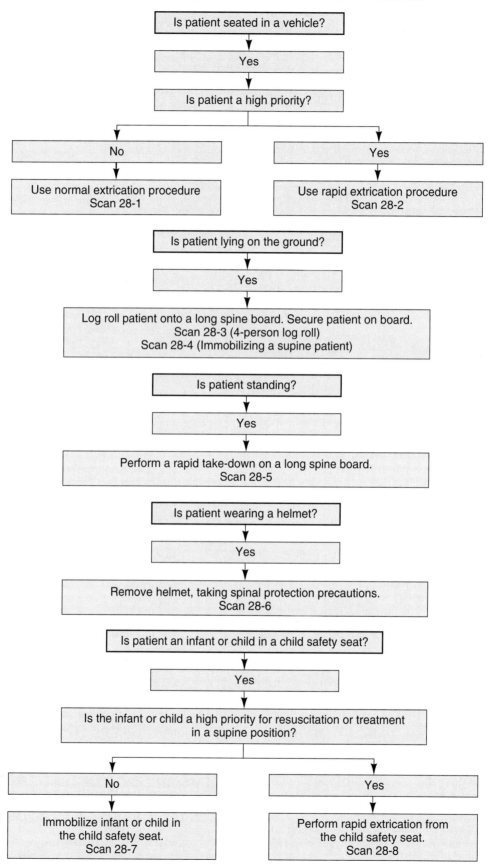

FIGURE 28-8 Choose appropriate extrication and immobilization procedures.

nel would borrow soft collars from the hospital emergency department. Unfortunately most early ambulance personnel did not realize that the only collars used in emergency departments were put on patients who had been X-rayed and, who it was clear, had no fracture or dislocation. The collar was merely a tool to remind them not to move their necks to allow the muscle strain to heal. Patients with fractures were admitted and placed in traction. These soft collars, or "neck warmers," had no place in the field!

The collars of today are rigid and designed to limit flexion, extension, and lateral movement when combined with an immobilization device such as a long backboard or a vest-style device. Even though there have been marked improvements in collars, there is still no collar that completely eliminates movement of the spine. For this reason when applying a collar you should always maintain the neck and head in a neutral position in alignment with the rest of the body.

You may want to review the information on manual stabilization in Chapter 9, The Initial Assessment and the information and scan on cervical collar sizing and application in Chapter 10, The Focused History and Physical Exam—Trauma Patient.

Tips for Immobilizing a Seated Patient

When a patient is found in a sitting position, you will need to decide if he is a high priority or low priority. If the patient is stable and a low priority, the normal procedure for spinal immobilization is used as shown in Scan 28-1. In such situations, where time is not of the essence, the patient must be secured to a short spine board or extrication vest that will immobilize the head, neck, and torso until the patient can be transferred to a long spine board or other full body immobilization device.

In high priority situations when there is not enough time to apply a short board or extrication vest—or if the patient must be moved rapidly because of dangers at the scene, or if he must be moved rapidly to provide access to other potentially more seriously injured patients—the technique used is to immobilize the patient manually while moving him onto the long spine board. This is called the Rapid Extrication Technique and is shown in Scan 28-2.

The normal extrication technique is as follows: The patient's head and neck are manually stabilized during the initial assessment. Then

after the head and neck are assessed in the focused trauma exam, a rigid collar is applied. Then the patient is secured to the short spine board or extrication vest.

A short spine board is just a shortened version of a long spine board. It is the original extrication device and has been used for many years. It is used less frequently now, not because of loss of popularity among users, but by necessity. Today's automobiles have fewer bench-type seats and more bucket-type seats whose contoured backs do not accommodate a flat board. Also, the conventional short spine board is often too wide and too high to be used effectively in a small car.

A vest-style extrication device is a flexible piece of equipment useful for immobilizing patients with possible injury to the cervical spine. It can be used when the patient is found in a bucket seat, in a short compact car seat, in a seat with a contoured back, or in a confined space. It is also useful when the short spine board cannot be inserted into a car because of obstructions. A number of commercial vest-style extrication devices such as the Kendrick Extrication Device (KED) (Figure 28-9), Kansas Backboard, XP-1, LSP Vest, are available. You should use the devices approved by your EMS system.

A particular sequence must be followed in all applications, whether of a short spine board or a flexible extrication device. You must secure the torso first and the head last. This approach offers greater stability throughout the strapping process and may help prevent compression of the cervical spine. If the patient has suffered abdominal injuries or displays diaphragmatic breathing that prevents adequate securing of the torso, the torso straps will still be needed but

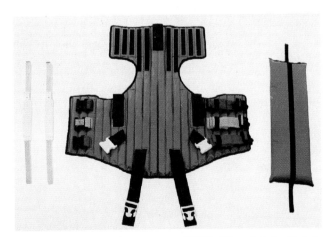

FIGURE 28-9 The Ferno KED (Kendrick Extrication Device).

Spinal Immobilization of a Seated Patient

FIRST take body substance isolation precautions.

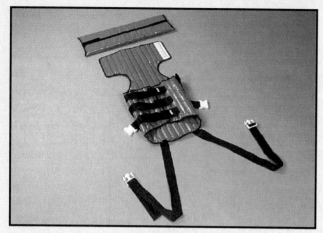

1. Select immobilization device.

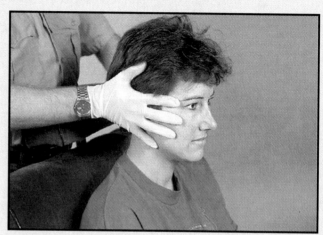

2. Manually immobilize patient's head in neutral, in-line position.

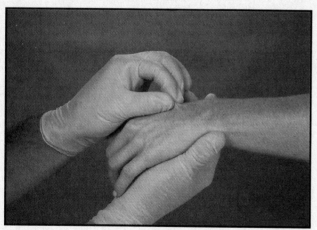

3. Assess distal motor and sensory function and circulation.

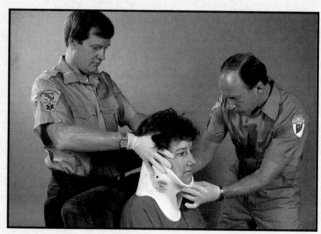

4. Apply appropriate size extrication collar.

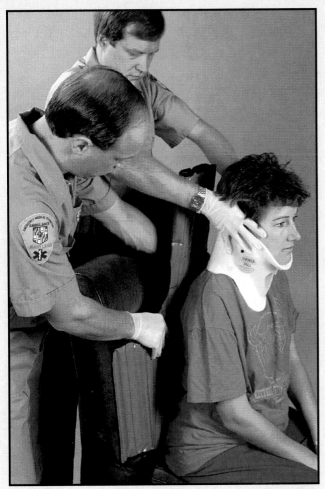

5. Position immobilization device behind patient.

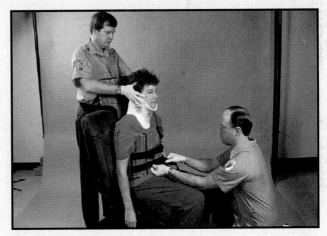

6. Secure device to patient's torso.

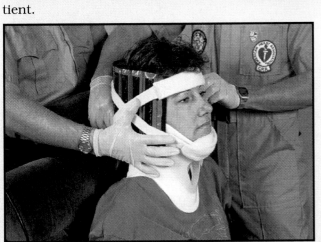

7. Evaluate and pad behind patient's head as necessary. Secure patient's head to device.

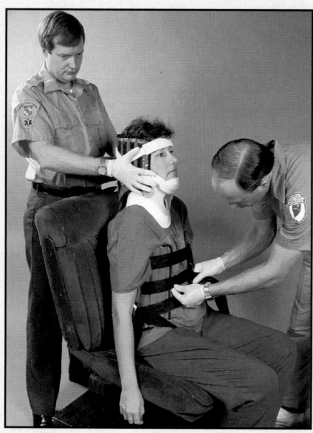

8. Evaluate and adjust straps. They must be tight enough so device does not move excessively up, down, left, or right—not so tight as to restrict patient's breathing.

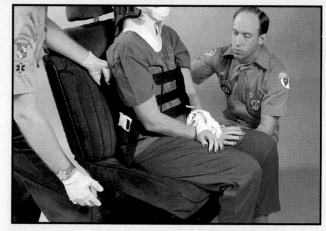

9. As needed, secure patient's wrists and legs and transfer the patient to the long board.

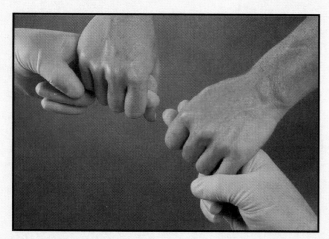

10. Reassess distal motor and sensory function and circulation.

Rapid Extrication Procedure—
For High Priority Patients Only

Note: In the photos, the roof of the vehicle has been removed to allow for easier illustration of the positions of the EMT-Bs. In most cases, this procedure will be done and should be practiced with the roof intact.

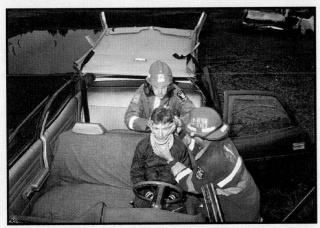

1. Manually stabilize the patient's head and neck and have a second EMT-B apply a cervical collar.

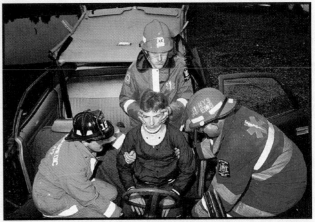

2. At the direction of the EMT-B stabilizing the head and neck, two EMT-Bs each lift the patient by his armpits and buttocks/thighs just enough for a bystander or additional rescuer to slide a long spine board between the patient and the vehicle seat.

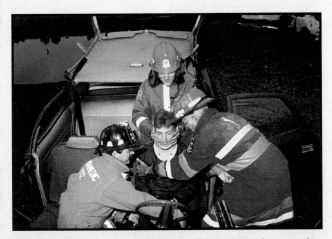

3. The EMT-Bs reposition their hands so the EMT-B on the front seat inside the vehicle holds the patient's legs and pelvis while the EMT-B outside the vehicle holds the upper chest and arms.

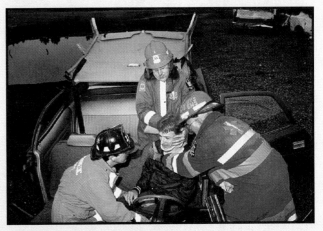

4. At the direction of the EMT-B holding the head and neck, carefully turn the patient a quarter turn so his back is facing the side door of the vehicle.

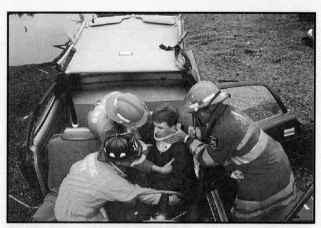

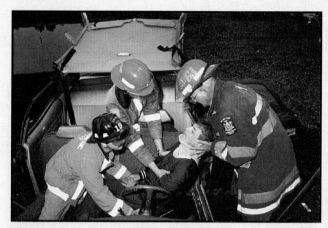

5. The EMT-B who was holding the pelvis temporarily holds the chest so the EMT-B who was holding the chest can take over head and neck stabilization. The EMT-B in the back seat can then reach over the seat and assist with the chest, and the EMT-B inside on the front seat can move his hands back to the pelvis.

6. At the direction of the EMT-B at the head and neck, gently lower the patient to the spine board. **Note:** Sometimes it may be necessary to move the patient inside the vehicle a few inches so there is ample room to lay him down without touching the upper door opening.

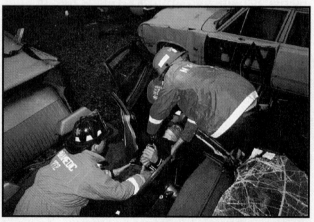

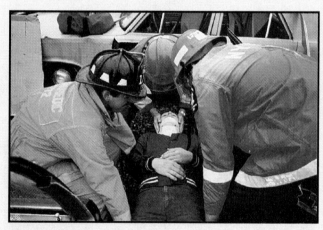

7. As a bystander or additional rescuer holds the end of the spine board, the EMT-Bs slide the patient to the head end of the board.

8. Quickly apply straps to the patient's chest, pelvis, and legs and remove the patient to a stretcher or the ground, under the direction of the EMT-B stabilizing the head and neck. **Note:** Since the patient's head is not yet fully immobilized (it is only being manually held stable by the EMT-B and collar), DO NOT walk more than a few steps with the patient. Once on stable ground or the stretcher, apply a head immobilizer or blanket roll and wide tape.

Note: The rapid extrication procedure is only for critical or unstable high-priority patients who must be moved in less time than would be required to apply a short spine board or extrication vest inside the vehicle before moving the patient to the long spine board. The normal extrication procedure is shown in Scan 28-1.

care must be taken so as not to interfere with breathing.

There are a number of special considerations when applying a short board to the patient.

- Any assessment or reassessment of the back, shoulder blades, arms, or collarbones must be done before the device is placed against the patient.
- The EMT-B applying the board must angle it to fit between, without striking or jarring, the arms of the rescuer who is stabilizing the head from behind the patient.
- To provide full cervical support, the uppermost holes must be level with the patient's shoulders. The base of the board should not extend past the coccyx.
- Never place a chin cup or chin strap on the patient. Such devices may prevent the patient from opening his mouth if he has to vomit.
- When applying the first strap to secure the torso, you must not apply the strap too tightly. This could aggravate existing abdominal injury or limit respirations for the diaphragmatic breathing patient.
- Some short spine boards have buckles with release mechanisms that can be accidentally loosened during patient transfer operations. This is especially true of "quick-release" buckles. These buckles must be taped closed after the final adjustment of the straps.
- Do not pad between collar and board. To do so will create a pivot point that may cause the hyperextension of the cervical spine when the head is secured. Instead, padding should be placed at the occipital region, but only enough to fill any void. This will help

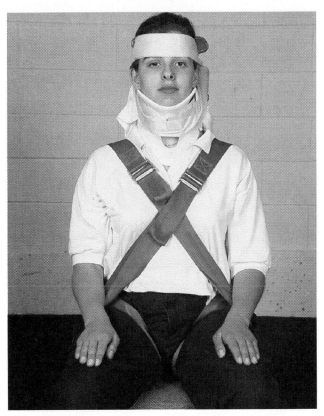

FIGURE 28-11 The seated patient, "packaged."

keep the head in a neutral position. Often if the shoulders are rolled back to the board, the head will come back to the board enough that padding isn't even needed. Never use excessive padding behind the head, because once the patient is removed from the vehicle he will be placed in a supine position. At that point the shoulders will fall back but the head will not be able to due to the excessive padding. This will place the patient in a position of flexion and not a neutral position which is not desired during immobilization.
- Follow the instructions of the manufacturer of the device you are using.
- The placement of straps for the short spine board is a little complex. (See Figure 28-10.) After applying the short spine board, the packaging of the patient will be completed as shown in Figure 28-11.

Tips for Applying a Long Backboard

The following tips relate to immobilization of the supine patient.

- You will need to log roll the patient to apply the long backboard (Scan 28-3 and Scan

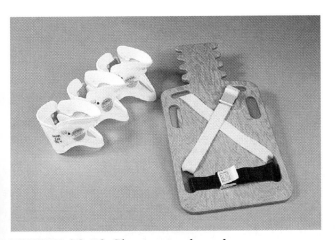

FIGURE 28-10 Short spine board.

The Four-Rescuer Log Roll

FIRST take body substance isolation precautions.

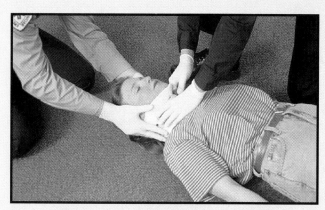

1. Stabilize the head and apply a rigid collar.

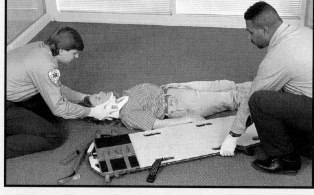

2. Place the board parallel to the patient.

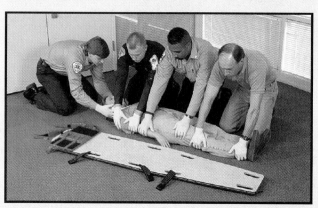

3. Three rescuers will kneel at the patient's side opposite the board, leaving room to roll the patient toward them. Place one rescuer at the shoulder, one at the waist, and one at the knee. One EMT-B will continue to stabilize the head. The rescuers will reach across the patient and take proper hand placement before the roll.

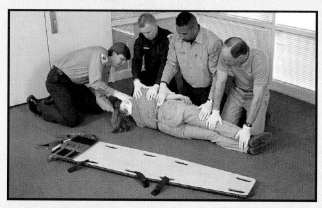

4. The EMT-B at the head and neck will direct the others to roll the patient as a unit.

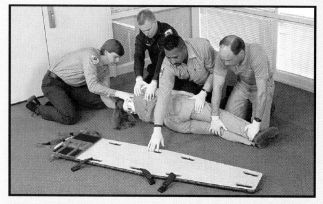

5. The EMT-B at the patient's waist will grip the spine board and pull it into position against the patient. (This can be done by a fifth rescuer.)

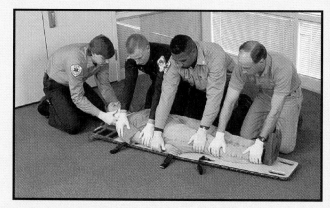

6. Roll the patient onto the board.

Scan 28-4
Spinal Immobilization of a Supine Patient

FIRST take body substance isolation precautions.

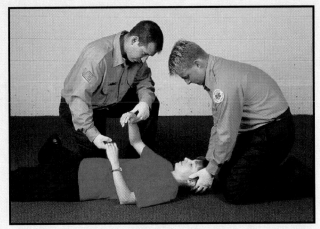

1. Place head in neutral, in-line position and maintain manual immobilization of head. Assess distal motor and sensory function and circulation.

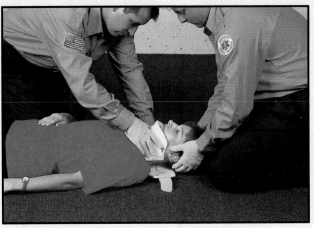

2. Apply appropriate size cervical collar.

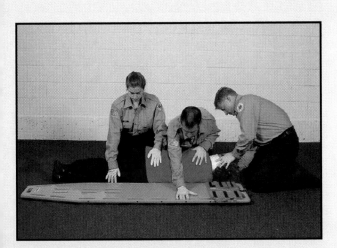

3. Position immobilization device.

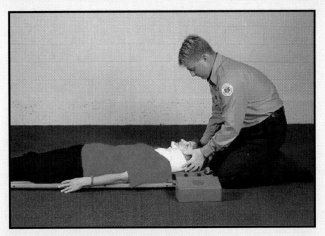

4. Move patient onto device without compromising integrity of spine. (Apply padding to voids between torso and board as necessary.)

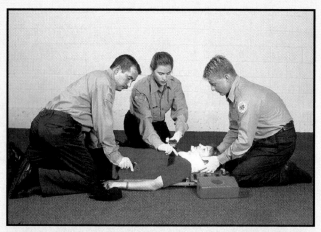

5. Immobilize patient's torso to the board.

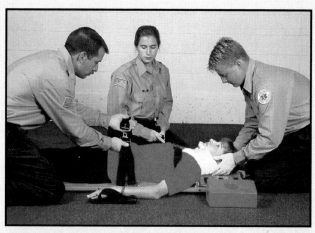

6. Secure torso straps.

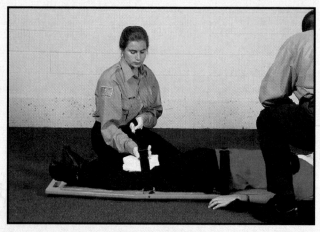

7. Secure patient's legs to board.

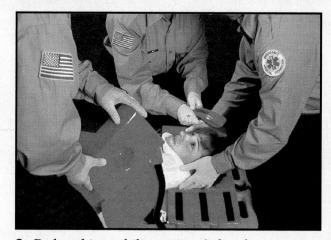

8. Pad and immobilize patient's head.

Reassess distal motor and sensory function and circulation.

28-4). This procedure must be done carefully, keeping the spine in alignment. Quickly assess the posterior body before rolling the patient back onto the board. Whenever a move is done involving neck stabilization, the EMT-B holding the neck calls for the move ("We will turn on three: One . . . two . . . three").

- Pad voids between the patient's head and torso and the board. Be careful not to cause extra movement or to move the patient's spine out of alignment.
- When immobilizing a six-year-old-or-younger child it will be necessary to provide padding beneath the shoulder blades to compensate for the large head, and padding from shoulders to toes as needed to establish a neutral position.
- When a patient is secured to a long spine board, the head is secured last. This can be made easier by using a backboard with Velcro straps (Figure 28-12) or speed clip straps (Figure 28-13).
- Additional immobilization for the head and neck can be provided with light foam-filled cushions, a commercial head immobilization device (such as the Ferno Washington head immobilizer, or Bashaw CID, or the Laerdal Head Bed), or a blanket roll. If used, these are applied after securing the patient's body to the long backboard. Secure the head with 3-inch hypoallergenic adhesive tape. The tape offers support, especially if the patient and board are to be tilted to allow for drainage. However, blood on the patient's skin and hair may make using tape impractical. You should learn to use cravats or self-adhering roller bandages

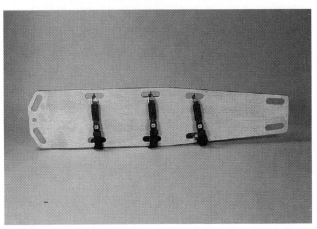

FIGURE 28-13 Long spine board with quick-hook straps.

as a backup method. Do not tape or tie the cravats across the patient's eyes.
- If the patient is a full-term pregnant woman, after immobilizing on the back board you will need to prop the board on its side to minimize the effect of the uterus compressing the vena cava and causing hypotension and dizziness.
- Unless the spine board has specific directions for straps intended to criss-cross the shoulder and chest area, it is best to strap across the upper chest including the arms, the pelvis excluding the hands, and the thighs. If the patient will need to be stood up to carry him out of a tight building, up a basement stairwell, or down a small elevator, make sure the chest strap is secure under the axillae (arm pits) and tight on the thighs so the patient does not shift on the board.
- If you do not carry a pediatric long spine immobilization device, then practice immobilizing children using adult equipment and lots of towels or blankets to pad around the child. EMT-Bs are usually very good at improvising. In this case, however, the first time you improvise should be in the classroom so you will be quick in the field!
- If your service transports to a helicopter, make sure that your backboard fits. There are some restrictions on the size or taper of the long backboard, depending on the helicopter's loading configuration, so find this out ahead of time.
- For a water rescue or diving injury there are various specialty back boards such as the Miller board (Figure 28-14) that are designed to float up beneath the patient and use Velcro closures for ease of application.

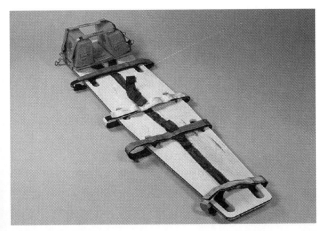

FIGURE 28-12 Long spine board with head immobilization and strapping devices.

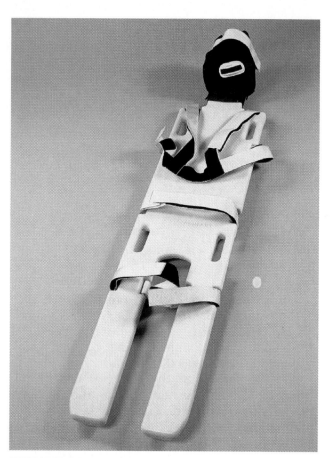

FIGURE 28-14 Miller board.

Tips for Dealing With a Standing Patient

When you approach a vehicle and see the tell-tale sign of a spider-web-cracked windshield, you know whoever sat behind that crack needs full spinal immobilization. Sometimes this patient is up and walking around at the collision scene. He still has the potential for a spine injury but may not have dislocated the fracture or ligament injury site yet. It would be dangerous to have him sit down or lie down on your long backboard, so instead use a backboard to carefully but rapidly take him down to the supine position without compromising his spine. Some EMS providers advocate strapping the patient onto the long board while the patient is standing. However, this is often not practical in the field. (It works in the classroom because the simulated patients are not in shock, intoxicated, head injured, combative, or just dizzy!)

The easiest technique to use is the rapid takedown, which like all skills in this text should be demonstrated by a qualified instructor and practiced in the classroom setting prior to using

in the field. The procedure takes three EMT-Bs, a set of collars, and a long backboard. It is shown in Scan 28-5.

Patient Found Wearing a Helmet

Helmets are worn in many sporting events and by many motorcycle riders. The sporting helmets are typically open in the front, making it easier to access the patient's airway than with a motorcycle helmet, which has a shield and often a full face section that is not removable. Facial, neck, and spinal injury care and airway management may call for the removal of the helmet, especially if the helmet will prevent you from reaching the patient's mouth or nose if resuscitation efforts are needed. If the helmet is left on, protection shields can be lifted and face guards can be cut away. If the face guard is to be cut, one EMT-B must steady the patient's head and neck with manual stabilization. The other EMT-B should snap off the guard or unscrew it.

Do not attempt to remove a helmet if doing so causes increased pain, or if the helmet proves difficult to remove, unless there is a possible airway obstruction or ventilatory assistance must be provided.

The indications for leaving the helmet in place include the following.

1. A helmet with a snug fit that provides little or no movement of the patient's head within the helmet.
2. Absolutely no impending airway or breathing problems nor any reason to resuscitate or hyperventilate the patient.
3. Removal would cause further injury to the patient.
4. Proper spinal immobilization can be done with the helmet in place.
5. There is no interference with the EMT-B's ability to assess and reassess airway or breathing.

The indications for removing the helmet would include the following.

1. Helmet interferes with ability to assess and manage airway and breathing.
2. Helmet is improperly fitted, allowing for excessive head movement within the helmet.
3. Helmet interferes with immobilization.
4. Cardiac arrest.

Scan 28-5
Rapid Takedown of a Standing Patient

FIRST take body substance isolation precautions.

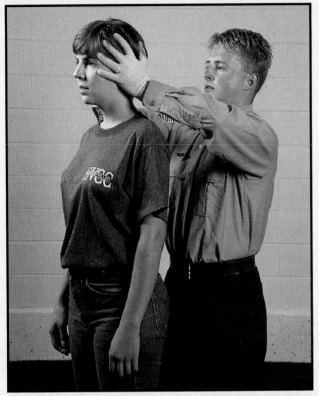

1. Position your tallest crew member (EMT-Basic A) behind patient and hold manual in-line stabilization of the head and neck. This person's hands will not leave the patient's head until entire procedure is complete and head is secured to the long spine board.

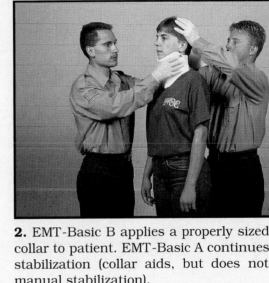

2. EMT-Basic B applies a properly sized cervical collar to patient. EMT-Basic A continues manual stabilization (collar aids, but does not replace manual stabilization).

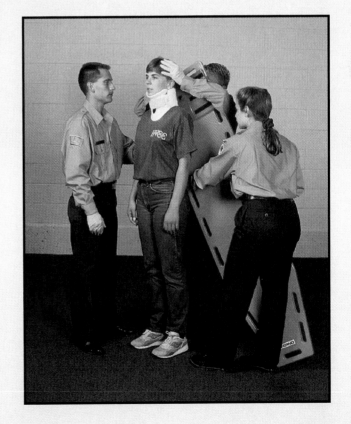

3. EMT-Basic A continues manual stabilization as EMT-Basic B positions a long spine board behind the patient, being careful not to disturb EMT-Basic A's manual stabilization of patient's head. It will help if EMT-Basic A spreads elbows to give EMT-Basic B more room to maneuver the spine board.

583

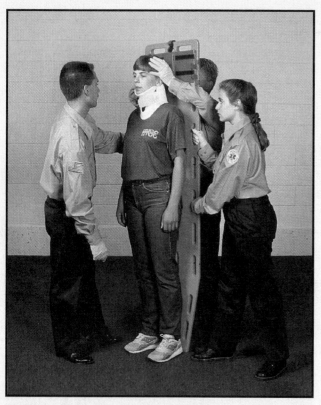

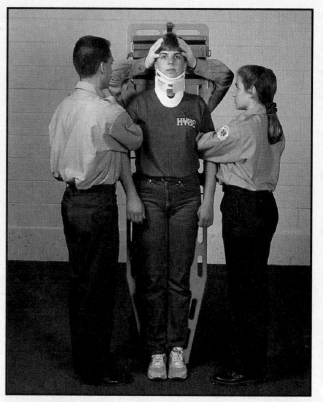

4. EMT-Basic A continues manual stabilization. EMT-Basic B looks at the spine board from the front of the patient and does any necessary repositioning to be sure it is centered behind the patient.

5. EMT-Basic A continues manual stabilization. EMT-Basic B and a third rescuer or helper reach arm that is nearest patient under patient's armpits and grasp the spine board. (Once the board is tilted down, patient will actually be temporarily suspended by armpits.) To keep patient's arms secure, they use other hand to grasp patient's arm just above elbow and hold it against patient's body.

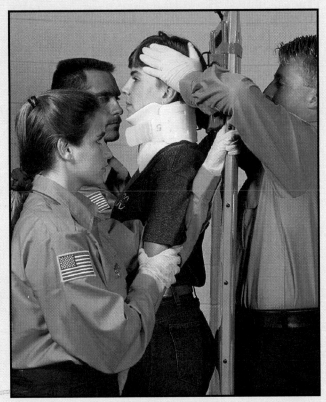

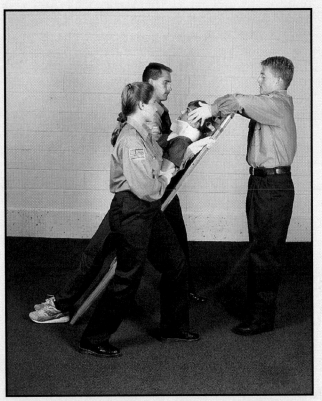

6. EMT-Basic B and third rescuer, when reaching under patient's armpits, must grasp a handhold on the spine board at patient's armpit level or higher.

7. EMT-Basic A continues manual stabilization. EMT-Basic B and third rescuer maintain their grasp on the spine board and patient. EMT-Basic A explains to patient what is going to happen, then gives signal to begin slowly tilting board and patient backward to lower to the ground. As board is lowered, EMT-Basic A walks backward and crouches, keeping up with the board as it is lowered. As patient is lowered, EMT-Basic A must allow patient's head to slowly move back to the neutral position against the board. EMT-Basic A must accomplish all this without holding back or slowing the lowering of the board. EMT-Basic A may need to rotate somewhat so that once the board is almost flat he or she is holding the head down on the board. *Once patient's head comes in contact with the board, it must not be allowed to leave the board, to avoid flexing the neck.* The job of the two persons doing the lowering is to control it so that it is slow and even on both sides. They should also move into a squatting position as they lower the board to avoid injuring their backs.

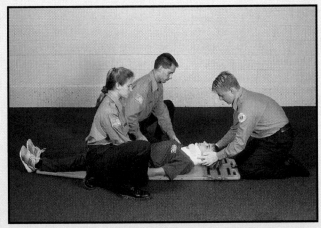

EMT-Basic A continues manual in-line stabilization throughout the procedure.

Many EMS providers put the controversy of removal versus non-removal into the following perspective: If your child's neck were injured in a football accident, would you want the trainer and the EMT-B to work together carefully to remove the helmet at the scene, or would you prefer this be left to emergency department personnel who probably will not have the help of the trainer nor the benefit of lots of practice in the helmet removal technique?

Note: If a football player is wearing shoulder pads, you should either remove the pads or pad behind the head to make up for the fact that his shoulders are off the ground. This will prevent the head from falling into a hyperextended position when the helmet is removed and the head is slowly lowered to the ground.

When a helmet must be removed, it is a two-rescuer procedure, as shown in Scan 28-6.

Infants and Children

Occasionally, EMT-Bs are confronted at a motor vehicle collision with an infant or young child who was riding in a child safety seat. Placing a child in a supine position with the legs elevated, as you will need to do if you are going to tip the seat backwards and move the child onto a spine board, places a great deal of pressure on the abdominal organs and diaphragm, making respiration difficult. So, provided the patient is not in need of immediate resuscitative measures, or for any other reason needs to be placed in the supine position, it makes sense to let the child remain sitting upright and use the child safety seat as an immobilization device. The key decision on when to immobilize the child in the seat versus rapidly removing the child from the seat onto a spine board is based upon the patient's priority and the need to place in a supine position. The procedure for immobilization in the child safety seat is described in Scan 28-7 and the procedure for rapid extrication from the car seat is shown in Scan 28-8.

Documentation Tips— Injuries to the Head and Spine

In documenting a possible head or spine injury, it is critical to note whether the patient lost consciousness, even if only briefly. If the patient did not lose consciousness, be sure to document that fact as a pertinent negative.

Also be sure to document carefully the patient's mental status. If responsive, note his orientation to person, place, and time. Carefully document any changes in the patient's mental status throughout assessment, treatment, and transport.

FYI

Topics included in the FYI—"For Your Information"—section are those that go beyond the chapter objectives. The information in this segment is intended to broaden your understanding of the chapter topic but is not essential to an understanding of your job as an EMT-B.

More about Brain Injuries

The brain may be subject to several kinds of injuries.

A **concussion** (Figure 28-15) may be so mild that the patient is unaware of the injury. When a person strikes his head in a fall, or is struck by a blunt object, a certain amount of the force is transferred through the skull to the brain. Usually there is no detectable damage to the brain and the patient may or may not become unconscious. Most patients with a concussion will feel a little "groggy" after receiving a blow to the head. Headache is common. If there is a loss of consciousness, it usually lasts only a short time and does not tend to recur. There may also simply be a period of altered mental status where bystanders state after the collision the patient, "just sat there staring off into space for a few minutes." Some loss of memory (amnesia) of the events surrounding the accident is fairly common. A common saying is that the fighter didn't see the punch that did him in. Actually, he probably did see the punch but forgot that moment due to the amnesia from a concussion. Long-term memory loss associated with concussion is rare.

A bruised brain, or **contusion** (Figure 28-15), can occur with closed head injuries, when the force of the blow is great enough to rupture blood vessels found on the surface of, or deep within, the brain. A contusion is often caused by acceleration/deceleration injuries in which the brain hits the inside of the skull on acceleration, bounces off the opposite side on deceleration, and rebounds to strike the first side of the skull again. When the bruising of the brain occurs on the side of the injury, it is called a *coup*; when it

Helmet Removal from Injured Patient

1

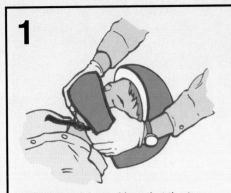

EMT-Basic A is positioned at the top of the patient's head and maintains manual stabilization with two hands holding the helmet stable while the finger tips hold the lower jaw.

2

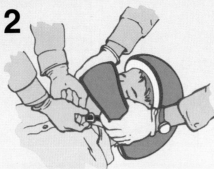

EMT-Basic B opens, cuts, or removes the chin strap.

3

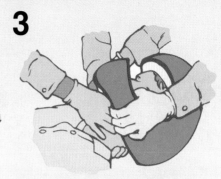

EMT-Basic B then places one hand on the patient's mandible and, using the other hand, reaches in behind the neck and applies stabilization at the occipital region. Using the combination of the hand in front of the chin and the hand behind the neck, this EMT-Basic should be able to hold the head very secure. *If the patient has glasses on, they should be removed now, prior to removal of the helmet.*

4

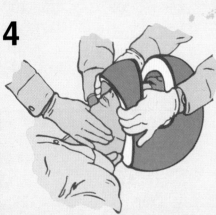

EMT-Basic A can now release manual stabilization and slowly remove the helmet. The lower sides, or ear cups, of the helmet will have to be gently pulled out to clear the ears.

5

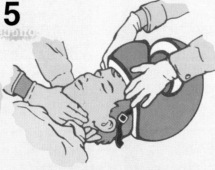

The helmet should come off straight without tilting it backwards, which could cause unnecessary flexion of the neck. If it is a full-face helmet, it may be necessary to tilt the helmet backwards just a bit to clear the nose with the chin guard. EMT-Basic B should be prepared to take the full weight of the head without allowing the head to move as the helmet is removed.

6

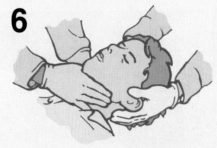

EMT-Basic A, after removing the helmet, re-establishes manual stabilization and maintains an open airway by using the jaw-thrust.

7

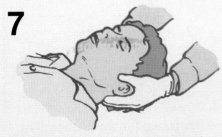

EMT-Basic B can now release manual stabilization and apply an extrication collar. The patient should then be fully assessed, and torso, then head, secured to a long spine board.

Note: If the patient has shoulder pads and you are removing a football helmet, remember to pad behind the head to keep it aligned with the padded shoulders.

From John E. Campbell, M.D., and Alabama Chapter, American College of Emergency Physicians, *BTLS Basic Prehospital Trauma Care*, The Brady Company, 1988.

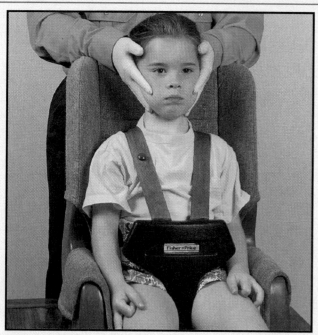

1. EMT-Basic A stabilizes car seat in upright position, applies manual head/neck stabilization. . . . .

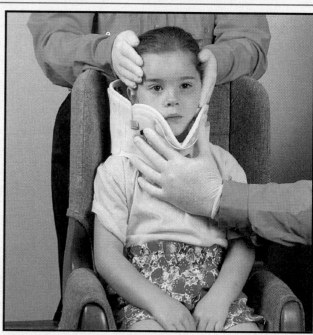

. . . as EMT-Basic B prepares equipment, then applies cervical collar, or improvises with rolled hand towel for the newborn or infant.

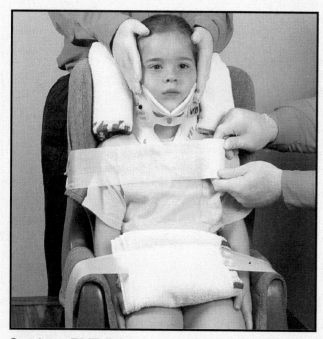

2. As EMT-Basic A maintains manual head/neck stabilization, EMT-Basic B places small blanket or towel on child's lap, then straps or uses wide tape to secure pelvis and chest area to seat.

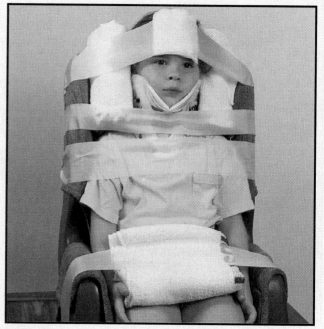

3. EMT-Basic A maintains manual head/neck stabilization as patient and seat are carried to ambulance and strapped onto stretcher with stretcher head raised. EMT-Basic B places a towel roll on both sides of head to fill voids, tapes forehead in place, then tapes across collar or maxilla. (Avoid taping chin, which would place pressure on child's neck.)

Rapid Extrication from a Child Safety Seat

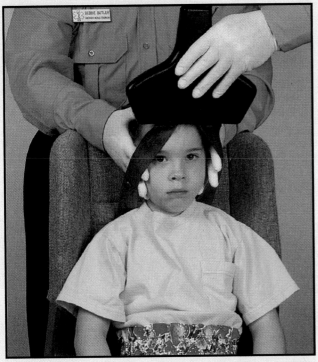

1. EMT-Basic A stabilizes car seat in upright position, applies manual head/neck stabilization as EMT-Basic B prepares equipment, then loosens or cuts the seat straps and raises the front guard.

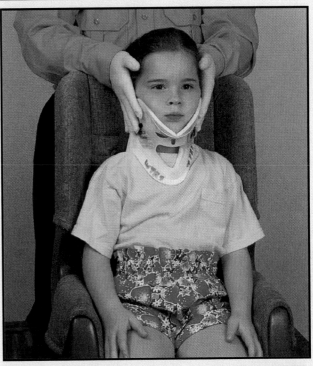

2. Cervical collar is applied to patient as EMT-Basic A maintains manual stabilization of the head and neck.

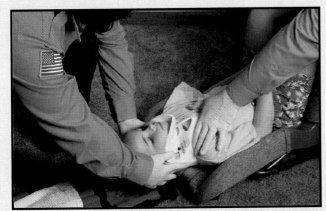

3. As EMT-Basic A maintains manual head/neck stabilization, EMT-Basic B places child safety seat on center of backboard and slowly tilts it into supine position. EMT-Bs are careful not to let child slide out of chair. For child with large head, place a towel under area where shoulders will eventually be placed on the board to prevent head from tilting forward.

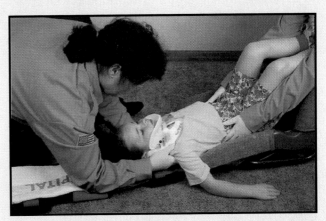

4. EMT-Basic A maintains manual head/neck stabilization and calls for a coordinated long axis move onto backboard.

589

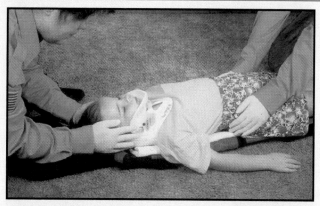

EMT-Basic A maintains manual head/neck stabilization as move onto board is completed, child's shoulders over the folded towel.

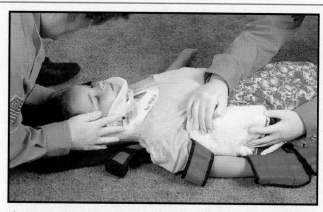

5. EMT-Basic A maintains manual head/neck stabilization as EMT-Basic B places rolled towels or blankets on both sides of patient.

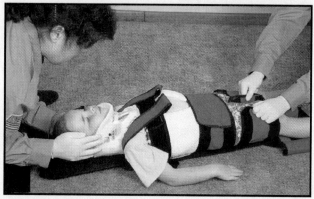

6. EMT-Basic A maintains manual stabilization as EMT-Basic B straps or tapes patient to board at level of upper chest, pelvis, and lower legs. DO NOT STRAP ACROSS ABDOMEN.

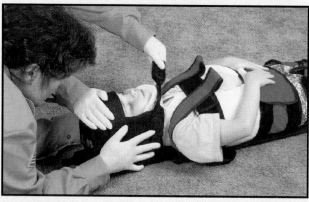

7. EMT-Basic A maintains manual head/neck stabilization as EMT-Basic B places rolled towels on both sides of head, then tapes head securely in place across forehead and maxilla or cervical collar. DO NOT TAPE ACROSS CHIN TO AVOID PRESSURE ON NECK.

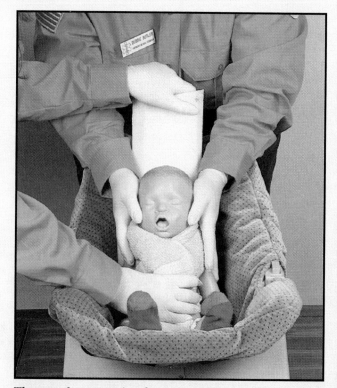

The newborn and infant procedure is exactly the same as for a child, except that an armboard is inserted behind the child in Step Two. If the infant is very small, the armboard may actually be used as the spine board.

A. CONCUSSION

- Mild injury usually with no detectable brain damage
- May have brief loss of consciousness
- Headache, grogginess, and short term memory loss common

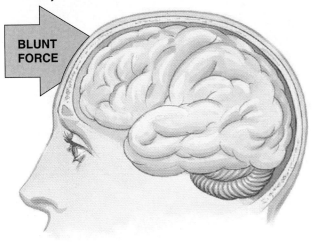

CONTUSION

- Unconsciousness or decreased level of consciousness
- Bruising or rupturing of brain tissue

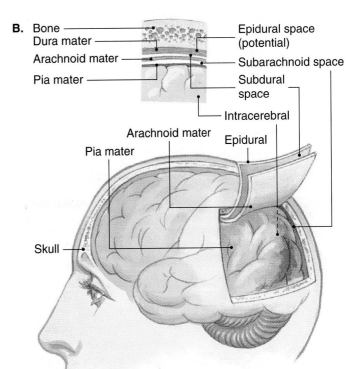

FIGURE 28-15 A. Closed head injuries. B. The meninges.

CRANIAL HEMATOMAS

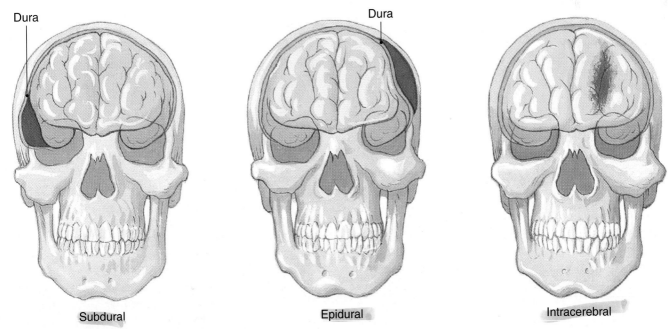

FIGURE 28-16 Hematomas within the cranium.

occurs on the side opposite the injury it is called a *contrecoup*.

A laceration, or cut, to the brain can occur from the same forces that might cause a contusion, when a blow causes the brain to strike the inside of the skull. The inner skull has many sharp, bony ridges that can lacerate a moving brain. A laceration or a puncture wound also can occur to the brain as a result of a penetrating or perforating injury of the cranium.

A **hematoma** is a collection of blood within the skull or the brain (Figure 28-16). A *subdural hematoma* is a collection of blood between the brain and its protective covering, the dura. An *epidural hematoma* is blood between the dura and the skull. An *intracerebral hematoma* occurs when blood pools within the brain itself.

Head injury is made worse by several problems. There is limited room for expansion inside the hard skull. When a hematoma develops, pressure inside the skull increases, making it difficult for normal blood flow to enter the head. To meet this challenge the blood pressure is forced to increase. As a result of decreased blood flow, the brain becomes starved for oxygen and high in waste carbon dioxide, causing even more swelling. Finally, serious head injury causes decreased respiratory effort, which further increases oxygen starvation and swelling in the brain.

Assessing Mental Status

All patients having head injury or suspected brain damage must be carefully monitored and reassessed during transport. Be prepared in case the patient has a seizure. Keep a constant watch over the patient. What you observe and report can have a great bearing on the initial actions taken by the emergency department staff. The early signs of deterioration are subtle changes in mental status that may be overlooked if you are not watching for them.

Since a number of observations concerning mental status have to be made at relatively close intervals, some EMS agencies use the Glasgow Coma Scale (GCS) in addition to AVPU for ongoing neurological assessment as well as triage. Some systems would immediately transport a patient with a GCS score of 8 or less directly to the trauma center if they are within 30 minutes transport time. You should become familiar with the GCS if it is used in your system (Figure 28-17). When using this score, remember to consider the following.

GLASGOW COMA SCALE

Eye Opening	Spontaneous	4
	To Voice	3
	To Pain	2
	None	1
Verbal Response	Oriented	5
	Confused	4
	Inappropriate Words	3
	Incomprehensible Sounds	2
	None	1
Motor Response	Obeys Command	6
	Localizes Pain	5
	Withdraw (pain)	4
	Flexion (pain)	3
	Extension (pain)	2
	None	1
Glasgow Coma Score Total		

TOTAL GLASGOW COMA SCALE POINTS	
14-15=5	CONVERSION = APPROXIMATELY ONE-THIRD TOTAL VALUE
11-13=4	
8-10=3	
5-7=2	
3-4=1	

Neurologic Assessment	

FIGURE 28-17 The Glasgow Coma Scale.

- Note if there are eye injuries or injuries to the face that prevent the patient from opening the eyes. If the injuries are more than minor ones, do not ask the patient to open his eyes.
- Spontaneous eye opening means that the patient has the eyes open without your having to do anything. If his eyes are closed, then you should say, "Open your eyes" to see if the patient will obey this command. Try a normal level of voice. If this fails, shout the command. Should the patient's eyes remain closed, apply an accepted painful stimulus (e.g., pinch a toe, scratch the palm or sole, rub the sternum).

- When evaluating the patient's verbal responses, use the following criteria.

  1. Oriented—The patient, once aroused, can tell you who he is, where he is, and the day of the week. A person who can answer all three of these questions appropriately is said to be alert on the AVPU scale.
  2. Confused—The patient cannot answer the above questions, but he can speak in phrases and sentences.
  3. Inappropriate words—The patient says or shouts a word or several words at a time. Usually this requires physical stimulation. The words do not fit the situation or a particular question. Often, the patient curses.
  4. Incomprehensible sounds—The patient responds with mumbling, moans, or groans.
  5. No verbal response—Repeated stimulation, verbal and physical, does not cause the patient to speak or make any sounds.

- The following are the criteria used to evaluate motor response.

  1. Obeys command—The patient must be able to understand your instruction and carry out the request. For example, you can ask (when appropriate) for the patient to hold up two fingers.
  2. Localizes pain—Should the patient fail to respond to your commands, apply pressure to one of the nail beds for 5 seconds or firm pressure to the sternum. Note if the patient attempts to remove your hand. Do not apply pressure over an injury site. Do not apply pressure to the sternum if the patient is experiencing difficulty breathing.
  3. Withdraws—after painful stimulation. Note if the elbow flexes, he moves slowly, there is the appearance of stiffness, he holds his forearm and hand against the body, or the limbs on one side of the body appear to be paralyzed (hemiplegic position).
  4. Posturing—after painful stimulation. Note if the legs and arms extend, there is apparent stiffness with these moves, and if there is an internal rotation of the shoulder and forearm.

CHAPTER REVIEW

KEY TERMS

You may find it helpful to review the following terms.

autonomic nervous system controls involuntary functions.

central nervous system the brain and the spinal cord.

cerebrospinal (SAIR-uh-bro-SPI-nal) **fluid (CSF)** the fluid that surrounds the brain and spinal cord.

concussion mild closed head injury without detectable damage to the brain. Complete recovery is usually expected.

contusion in brain injuries, a bruised brain caused when the force of a blow to the head is great enough to rupture blood vessels.

cranial (KRAY-ne-al) **floor** the inferior wall of the brain case; the bony floor beneath the brain.

cranium (KRAY-ne-um) the bony structure making up the forehead, top, back, and upper sides of the skull.

hematoma (HE-mah-TO-mah) in a head injury, a collection of blood within the skull or brain.

malar (MAY-lar) the cheek bone, also called the zygomatic bone.

mandible (MAN-di-bl) the lower jaw bone.

maxillae (mak-SIL-e) the two fused bones forming the upper jaw.

nasal (NAY-zul) **bones** the bones that form the upper third, or bridge, of the nose.

nervous system provides overall control of thought, sensation, and the voluntary and involuntary motor functions of the body. The major components of the nervous system are the brain and the spinal cord. See also *central nervous system; peripheral nervous system.*

orbits the bony structures around the eyes; the eye sockets.

peripheral nervous system the nerves that enter and exit the spinal cord between the vertebrae and the twelve pairs of cranial nerves that travel between the brain and organs without passing through the spinal cord.

spinous (SPI-nus) **process** the bony bump on a vertebra.

temporal (TEM-po-ral) **bone** bone that forms part of the side of the skull and floor of the cranial cavity. There is a right and a left temporal bone.

temporomandibular (TEM-po-ro-mand-DIB-yuh-lar) **joint** the movable joint formed between the mandible and the temporal bone, also called the TM joint.

vertebrae (VERT-uh-bray) the bones of the spinal column (singular *vertebra*).

SUMMARY

It is important to maintain a high index of suspicion for head or spine injury whenever there is a relevant mechanism of injury. When there is a head injury, assume a brain injury as well as a spine injury. Provide high concentration oxygen, immobilize, and transport.

Assume a spine injury whenever there is a mechanism of injury of sufficient force or an injury to the head, neck, or upper body. Provide manual stabilization of the head and neck and apply a cervical collar, continuing manual stabilization until the patient is fully immobilized on a long spine board.

In the event of a suspected head or spine injury, ascertain if there has been a loss of consciousness, however brief, and carefully assess the patient's mental status, including orientation to person, place, and time. Monitor and document any changes in the patient's mental status.

REVIEW QUESTIONS

1. Name the two components of the nervous system and discuss their functions.
2. List five signs of a brain injury and explain why mechanism of injury is important in determining possible brain injury.
3. Describe the appropriate emergency treatment of a patient with possible head or brain injury.
4. List five mechanisms of injury that would support suspicion of a spine injury.
5. Describe the appropriate emergency care for a patient with a possible spine injury.

Application

- You are called to the scene of a motor vehicle collision. After assuring scene safety and taking BSI precautions, you approach the car, which has struck a bridge abutment, and note a deformed steering wheel. The driver's side door is open and, out in the middle of the bridge, you see a person you presume to be the driver wandering erratically toward the opposite side of the bridge. How should you proceed?

Module 6

Infants and Children

IN THIS MODULE
Chapter 29   Infants and Children

MODULE OVERVIEW

Emergencies involving infants and children, or pediatric emergencies, pose special problems for the EMT-Basic. Calls for infants and children are much less common than those for adult patients. When you arrive at the scene, there is an additional emotional component to treating a critically ill or injured child.

Children often have the same medical problems as adults. They develop shock, allergic reactions, seizures, and other conditions, just as adults do. The difference in treating pediatric patients often lies in understanding the differences in their anatomy, physiology, mental development, and psychology. Throughout this textbook, you have noticed a frequent feature titled "Infants and Children," pointing out special aspects of pediatric care for the medical emergencies and injuries that were discussed in those chapters.

In this module, you will explore these special aspects of pediatric care in more depth and will learn about assessing the infant or child patient, about care of the infant and child airway, and about some of the medical conditions and injury patterns that are more common or more critical for infants and children than for adults.

Infants and Children

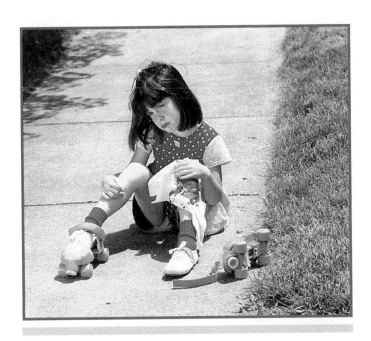

Emergencies involving children can be the most difficult for the EMT-B. We all react more intensely to the troubles of infants and children and consider them to be special patients. We would like to be able to stop the pain and discomfort and correct all the problems. But it is necessary to control our emotions so we are not overwhelmed by the cries of pain, fearful looks, or the unnerving silence of the child who normally should be crying. To treat infants and children effectively, you will need to know something about the special characteristics of children and the illnesses and injuries to which they are prone.

Objectives

Knowledge and Attitude *At the end of this chapter, you should be able to meet the following objectives.*

1. Identify the developmental considerations for the following age groups: (p. 600)
   • infants
   • toddlers
   • preschool
   • school age
   • adolescent

2. Describe differences in anatomy and physiology of the infant, child, and adult patient. (pp. 601–603)

3. Differentiate the response of the ill or injured infant or child (age specific) from that of an adult. (pp. 600–603)

4. Indicate various causes of respiratory emergencies. (pp. 615, 626–627)

5. Differentiate between respiratory distress and respiratory failure. (pp. 615–616)

6. List the steps in the management of foreign body airway obstruction. (pp. 614–615)

7. Summarize emergency medical care strategies for respiratory distress and respiratory failure. (pp. 615–616)

8. Identify the signs and symptoms of shock (hypoperfusion) in the infant and child patient. (pp. 618–619)

9. Describe the methods of determining end organ perfusion in the infant and child patient. (pp. 610, 612)

10. State the usual cause of cardiac arrest in infants and children versus adults. (p. 616)

11. List the common causes of seizures in the infant and child patient. (p. 616)

On the Scene

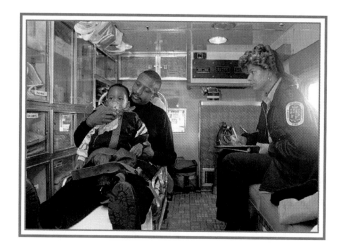

Three-year-old Danny Martin has a high fever. His father—who is taking over parenting responsibilities while his wife is out of town—noticed the fever as he was getting his little boy ready for bed. When Mr. Martin looked in on his son later, he found him sitting on the edge of his bed. Danny's fever had risen to 103°F. His ribs were heaving, as if he was having to work hard to breathe. Mr. Martin was frightened and called 911.

You **size up the scene,** a quiet home, and pull on gloves as Mr. Martin rushes over to meet you and bring you into the house. Your **initial assessment** begins as soon as you reach Danny's bedroom doorway. From across the room, you can see that the child is in respiratory distress, leaning forward, working hard to breathe, and drooling. Danny's father is nervous, and Danny can see that. You involve Mr. Martin by asking him to prepare clothes to bring with Danny and to introduce you to his child.

You: Hi, Danny. My name is Carmen. I'm here to help you because your daddy tells me you don't feel well. (You pause a moment to observe his reaction and

12. Describe the management of seizures in the infant and child patient. (pp. 616–617)

13. Differentiate between the injury patterns in adults, infants, and children. (pp. 620–621)

14. Discuss the field management of the infant and child trauma patient. (p. 621)

15. Summarize the indicators of possible child abuse and neglect. (pp. 622–624)

16. Describe the medical legal responsibilities in suspected child abuse. (pp. 624–625)

17. Recognize the need for EMT-Basic debriefing following a difficult infant or child transport. (p. 626)

18. Explain the rationale for having knowledge and skills appropriate for dealing with the infant and child patient. (pp. 597, 600)

19. Attend to the feelings of the family when dealing with an ill or injured infant or child. (p. 608)

20. Understand the provider's own response (emotional) to caring for infants or children. (pp. 597, 626)

Skills

1. Demonstrate the techniques of foreign body airway obstruction removal in the infant.

2. Demonstrate the techniques of foreign body airway obstruction removal in the child.

3. Demonstrate the assessment of the infant and child.

4. Demonstrate bag-valve-mask artificial ventilations for the infant.

5. Demonstrate bag-valve-mask artificial ventilations for the child.

6. Demonstrate oxygen delivery for the infant and child.

continue.) It looks like you're having some trouble breathing. I'll bet that's scary. You're a pretty brave guy!

Danny: (Nods his head yes but does not look at you. He seems more concerned with his breathing than with your presence in the room.)

You: Your daddy is going to carry you outside. We're going to take a ride in the ambulance to go see the doctor and help you feel better.

You have noted that there is no mechanism of injury and no sign of bleeding. Capillary refill is all right, but Danny's lips are slightly blue. His obvious breathing distress makes him a high priority for immediate transport. The rest of the assessment process can take place en route.

You enlist Danny's father to carry him outside to minimize the stress of moving to the ambulance, which could make his condition worse. Once in the ambulance, Danny is allowed to sit on his father's lap. You prepare a pediatric nonrebreather mask and give

it to Mr. Martin. Danny is afraid of the mask but tolerates his father holding it just in front of him so the oxygen can "blow by" his face. You prepare a pediatric bag-valve mask and suction, just in case.

The receiving hospital is alerted to expect Danny's arrival and made aware of his condition. During the ride to the hospital, you perform a *focused history and physical exam,* getting a SAMPLE history from Danny's father, by reassessing Danny's airway and breathing, and taking and recording vital signs. You perform an *ongoing assessment* every five minutes until you reach the hospital with continuing attention to Danny's airway and breathing.

At the hospital, you transfer Danny and his father to the emergency department staff. When you check back the next day, you learn that Danny's mother arrived during the night. Danny is suffering from a serious condition, epiglottitis, but is expected to recover. His father's prompt call to 911 and your speed in transporting him to the hospital are probably responsible for saving Danny's life.

The principles of managing the pediatric patient are similar to those for an injured or ill adult. Yet, children are not just little adults, and the EMT-B must be aware of differences between the pediatric and adult patient in order to provide effective care. In addition, when your patient is an infant or child, you must usually provide support to parents and other family members or friends.

DEFINING THE PEDIATRIC PATIENT

Medical practice considers a child to be in the pediatric category up to the age of 15. However, children often are treated by their pediatrician until they leave home for college, get married, or live on their own. For basic life support (rescue breathing and CPR), the American Heart Association defines an infant as birth to 1 year, a child as 1 to 8 years, and an adult as anyone over 8. These age ranges do not always apply to the care of children in other medical or trauma cases. In general emergency care, the following age categories are more useful to keep in mind.

- Newborns and infants: birth to 1 year
- Toddlers: 1 to 3 years
- Preschool: 3 to 6 years
- School age: 6 to 12 years
- Adolescent: 12 to 18 years

There will be calls when it will not be possible to get the age of the patient and you will have to

TABLE 29-1 Developmental Characteristics of Infants and Children

Age Group	Characteristics	Assessment and Care Strategies
Newborns and infants— birth to 1 year	• Infants do not like to be separated from their parents. • There is minimal stranger anxiety. • Infants are used to being undressed but like to feel warm, physically and emotionally. • The younger infant follows movement with his eyes. • The older infant is more active, developing a personality. • They do not want to be "suffocated" by an oxygen mask.	• Have the parent hold the infant while you examine him. • Be sure to keep them warm—warm your hands and stethoscope before touching the infant. • It may be best to observe their breathing from a distance, noting the rise and fall of the chest, the level of activity, and their color. • Examine the heart and lungs first and the head last. This is perceived as less threatening to the infant and therefore less likely to start them crying. • A pediatric nonrebreather mask may be held near the face to provide "blow-by" oxygen.
Toddlers—1 to 3 years	• Toddlers do not like to be touched or separated from their parents. • Toddlers may believe that their illness is a punishment for being bad. • Unlike infants, they do not like having their clothing removed. • They frighten easily, overreact, have a fear of needles, pain. • Toddlers may understand more than they communicate. • They begin to assert their independence. • They do not want to be "suffocated" by an oxygen mask.	• Have a parent hold the child while you examine him. • Assure the child that he was not bad. • Remove an article of clothing, examine, and then replace the clothing. • Examine in a trunk-to-head approach to build confidence. (Touching the head first may be frightening.) • Explain what you are going to do in terms the toddler can understand (taking the blood pressure becomes a squeeze or a hug on the arm). • Offer the comfort of a favorite toy. • Consider giving the toddler a choice: "Do you want me to look at your belly or your chest first?" • A pediatric nonrebreather mask may be held near the face to provide "blow-by" oxygen.

guess at the age, based on the child's physical size and emotional reactions.

Developmental Characteristics

Each age group has its own general characteristics of psychology and personality that will affect the way you assess and care for the patient. These are outlined in Table 29-1.

Key Anatomy and Physiology Differences

Infants and children differ from adults not only in psychology but also in anatomy and physiology. (Review Chapter 4, The Human Body, focusing on the special characteristics described for infants and children.) Understanding some of

these differences will help you do a better job of assessing and caring for these young patients. Key differences have to do with the head, airway and respiratory system, chest and abdomen, body surface, and blood volume.

Head

The child's head is proportionately larger and heavier than the adult's until about the age of 4. The implication for emergency care is that you should suspect head injury whenever there is a mechanism of injury because a child is likely to be propelled forward head first.

Infants up until about a year or 18 months of age will have a "soft spot" or anterior fontanelle, which is flat and soft while the child is quiet. The fontanelle is just anterior to the center of the skull. A sunken fontanelle may

Age Group	Characteristics	Assessment and Care Strategies
Preschool—3 to 6 years	• Preschoolers do not like to be touched or separated from their parents. • They are modest and do not like their clothing removed. • Preschoolers may believe that their illness is a punishment for being bad. • Preschoolers have a fear of blood, pain, and permanent injury. • They are curious, communicative, and can be cooperative. • They do not want to be "suffocated" by an oxygen mask.	• Have a parent hold the child while you examine him. • Respect their modesty. Remove an article of clothing, examine, and then replace the clothing. • Have a calm, confident, reassuring, respectful manner. • Be sure to offer explanations about what you are doing. • Allow the child the responsibility of giving the history. • Explain as you examine. • A pediatric nonrebreather mask may be held near the face to provide "blow-by" oxygen.
School age—6 to 12 years	• This age group cooperates but likes their opinions heard. • They fear blood, pain, disfigurement, and permanent injury. • School age children are modest and do not like their bodies exposed.	• Allow the child the responsibility of giving the history. • Explain as you examine. • Present a confident, calm, respectful manner. • Respect their modesty.
Adolescent—12 to 18 years	• Adolescents want to be treated as adults. • Adolescents generally feel that they are indestructible but may have fears of permanent injury and disfigurement. • Adolescents vary in their emotional and physical development and may not be comfortable with their changing bodies.	• Although they wish to be treated as adults, they may need as much support as children. • Present a confident, calm, respectful manner. • Be sure to explain what you are doing. • Respect their modesty. You may consider assessing them away from their parents. Have the physical exam done by an EMT-B of the same sex as the patient if possible.

indicate dehydration. A bulging fontanelle may indicate elevated intracranial pressure. One time when a bulging fontanelle may be normal is when the infant is crying.

Airway and Respiratory System

The infant's and child's neck muscles are immature and airway structures narrow and less rigid than an adult's. There are several special characteristics of the infant and child airway (Figure 29-1).

- The mouth and nose are smaller and more easily obstructed than in adults.
- In infants and children the tongue takes up more space proportionately in the mouth than in adults.
- Newborns and infants are obligate nose breathers. This means that they will not know to open their mouths to breathe when the nose becomes obstructed.
- The trachea (windpipe) is softer and more flexible in infants and children.
- The trachea is narrower and is easily obstructed by swelling or foreign objects.
- The chest wall is softer, and infants and children tend to depend more on their diaphragms for breathing.

These differences in respiratory anatomy pose several implications for the emergency treatment you provide to an infant or a child.

- Because infants are obligate nose breathers, be sure to suction secretions from the nose as needed to help the patient breathe.
- Hyperextension or flexion of the neck (tipping the head too far back or letting it fall forward) may result in airway obstruction. A folded towel under the shoulders of a supine infant or young child will help to keep the airway in a neutral in-line position. (Figure 29-2)
- "Blind" finger sweeps are not performed when trying to clear airway obstruction in an infant or child because your finger might force the obstruction back and wedge it in the narrow trachea.

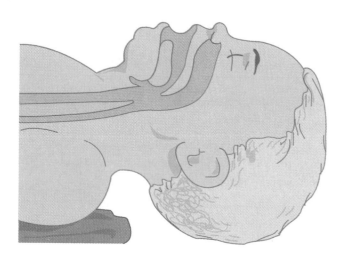

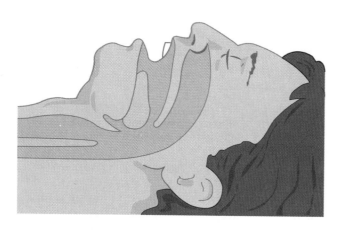

Chest and Abdomen

The less developed and more elastic chest structures of an infant or child make labored or distressed breathing obvious from a distance. The muscles above the sternum and between the ribs, and the ribs themselves, will pull inward when breathing is labored. Infants and young children are abdominal breathers, using their diaphragms for breathing more than adults. Watch the abdomen as well as the chest to evaluate breathing.

In addition, the fact that musculoskeletal structures of the chest and abdomen are less well developed means that the vital organs are not as well protected from injury as those of adults.

FIGURE 29-1 Adult and child airways compared.

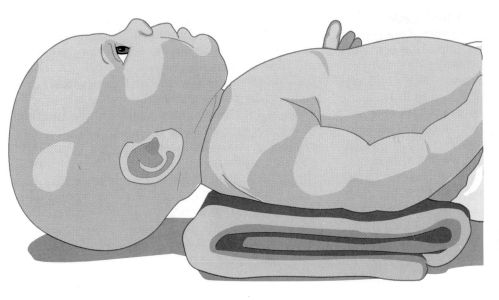

FIGURE 29-2 Use a folded towel to keep the infant's or young child's airway aligned.

Body Surface

A child's body surface area is larger in proportion to their body mass, making them more prone to heat loss through the skin. This makes infants and children more vulnerable to hypothermia (see Chapter 22, Environmental Emergencies). They must be kept covered and warm.

Because an infant's and child's head, body, and extremities are proportioned differently from an adult's (the head being larger, for example), the extent of a burn is estimated differently for a child, using a special child or infant "Rule of Nines," as was described in Chapter 26, Soft Tissue Injuries.

Blood Volume

As you would expect, the blood volume of a pediatric patient is less than the blood volume of an adult. A newborn doesn't have enough blood to fill a 12-ounce soda can, and an 8-year-old has only about 2 liters of blood. Therefore, a blood loss that might be considered moderate in an adult can be life threatening for a child.

AIRWAY AND OXYGEN THERAPY

As with the adult patient, keeping the airway open, supporting breathing, and providing adequate oxygen are critical for the infant or child patient. At this point, you may want to review the information from your basic life support course as reviewed in Basic Life Support: Airway, Rescue Breathing, and CPR at the end of this book. You should also review Chapter 7, Airway Manage-

ment, and Chapter 17, Respiratory Emergencies. Each of these segments includes special information about infant and child patients.

Maintaining an Open Airway

Just as with an adult, it is important to position the child's head and neck to align and open the airway. As mentioned above, it is important not to hyperextend or to permit flexion of a child's neck. The child's head should be positioned in a more neutral position than an adult's, because of the danger of closing the airway when the neck is hyperextended. Remember to place a folded towel under the shoulders of a young infant or child as necessary to keep the airway aligned. (Figures 29-1 and 29-2).To achieve the proper position, perform a head-tilt, chin-lift if there is no trauma, a jaw-thrust with spinal immobilization if trauma is suspected. Review the head-tilt, chin-lift and jaw-thrust maneuvers in Chapter 7, Airway Management.

Be prepared to suction the airway as needed. Use suction catheters that are sized for infant and child patients. Do not touch the back of the patient's throat, as this may activate the gag reflex, causing vomiting. It is also possible to stimulate the vagus nerve in the back of the throat, which can slow the heart rate. Do not suction for more than a few seconds at a time as cutting off the body's oxygen supply is especially dangerous to infants and children, causing cardiac arrest more quickly than in adults. You may hyperventilate the patient (provide artificial ventilations at a faster-than-normal rate) before and after suctioning. Review suctioning procedures in Chapter 7, Airway Management.

To clear complete obstructions of the airway by foreign objects, for infants less than 1 year old alternate back blows and chest thrusts (Figure 29-3) and use finger sweeps to remove visible objects (no blind sweeps). For children older than 1 year, provide abdominal thrusts and finger sweeps to remove visible objects. Review the procedures for clearing airway obstructions in Basic Life Support: Airway, Rescue Breathing, and CPR at the end of this book. These procedures are summarized in Table 29-2.

As with adults, the tongues of infants and children are likely to fall back into and block the airway. In fact, this is even more likely with infants and children because their tongues are proportionately larger in size. If the patient is unconscious and does not have a gag reflex, you may insert an oropharyngeal airway to prevent the tongue from blocking the airway. To insert an oropharyngeal airway, insert a tongue depressor to the base of the tongue. Push down against the tongue while lifting the jaw upward. Then insert the oropharyngeal airway. An important difference to note is that when an oropharyngeal airway is inserted in an adult, it is inserted with the tip pointing toward the roof of the mouth, then rotated 180 degrees into position. *For an infant or child, the oropharyngeal airway is inserted with tip pointing toward the tongue and throat, in the same position it will be in after insertion* (Figure 29-4).

Providing Supplemental Oxygen and Ventilations

As for adults, high-concentration oxygen should be administered to children in respiratory distress or with inadequate respirations or with possible shock. *Hypoxia is the underlying reason for many of the most serious medical problems with children. Inadequate oxygen will have immediate effects on the heart rate and the brain, as shown by a slowed heart rate and an altered mental status.*

However, infants and young children are often afraid of an oxygen mask. For these patients, try a "blow-by" technique. Have a parent hold the oxygen tubing or the pediatric nonrebreather mask 2 inches from the patient's face so the oxygen will pass over the face and be inhaled. Some children respond well when the tubing is pushed through the bottom of a paper cup, especially if the cup is colorful or has a picture drawn inside it. Hand the cup to the child. Infants and young children instinctively explore new things by bringing them up to their mouths. As the patient handles and explores the cup, he will breathe in the oxygen (Figure 29-5). Do not use a Styrofoam cup. Styrofoam will flake and the particles can be swallowed.

Artificial ventilations should be provided at the rate of 20 per minute (one every 3 seconds) for an infant or child. Use a pediatric-size pocket face mask or a bag-valve-mask unit in the correct infant or child size. Follow these guidelines when ventilating the infant or child patient.

- Avoid breathing too hard through the pocket face mask or excessive bag pressure and volume. Use only enough to make the chest rise.

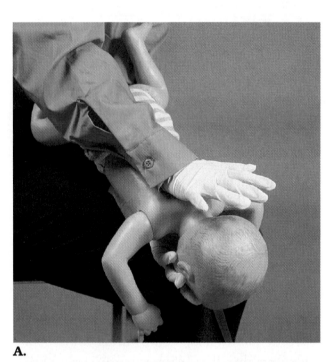

A.

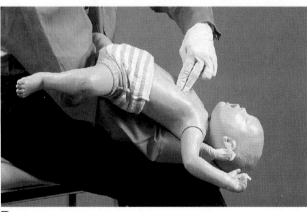

B.

FIGURE 29-3 For a complete airway obstruction in an infant, alternate A. back blows and B. chest thrusts.

TABLE 29-2 Airway Clearance Sequences

	Child over 8	*Child 1 to 8*	*Infant*
Age	8 yrs and older	1-8 yrs	birth-1 yr
Conscious	Ask, "Are you choking?" Perform Heimlich maneuvers.	Ask, "Are you choking?" Perform series of 5 Heimlich maneuvers.	Observe signs of choking (small objects or food, wheezing, agitation, blue color, not breathing). Series of: 5 back blows. 5 chest thrusts.
Loses consciousness during procedure	Assist patient to floor. If alone, call for help, then . . . Open airway with tongue-jaw lift. Perform finger sweeps. Attempt to ventilate. If unsuccessful, reposition head and attempt to ventilate again. If unsuccessful, perform Heimlich maneuver. (Repeat as needed.)	Assist patient to floor. Open airway with tongue-jaw lift. Remove visible objects (NO blind sweeps). Attempt to ventilate. If unsuccessful, reposition head and attempt to ventilate again. If unsuccessful, perform Heimlich maneuver. (Repeat as needed.) After 1 minute, call for help if alone.	Open airway with tongue-jaw lift. Remove visible objects (NO blind sweeps). Attempt to ventilate. If unsuccessful, reposition head and attempt to ventilate again. If unsuccessful, perform 5 back blows and 5 chest thrusts. (Repeat as needed.) After 1 minute, call for help if alone.
Unconscious when found	Establish unresponsiveness. If alone, call for help, then . . . Open airway. Attempt to ventilate. If unsuccessful, reposition head and attempt to ventilate again. If unsuccessful, 5 Heimlich maneuvers. Finger sweeps. (Repeat as needed.)	Establish unresponsiveness. Open airway. Attempt to ventilate. If unsuccessful, reposition head and attempt to ventilate again. If unsuccessful, Perform Heimlich maneuver up to 5 times. Remove visible objects (NO blind sweeps). (Repeat as needed.) After 1 minute, call for help if alone.	Establish unresponsiveness. Open airway. Attempt to ventilate. If unsuccessful, reposition head and attempt to ventilate again. If unsuccessful, 5 back blows and 5 chest thrusts. Remove visible objects (NO blind sweeps). (Repeat as needed.) After 1 minute, call for help if alone.

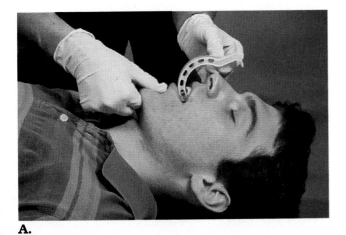

A.

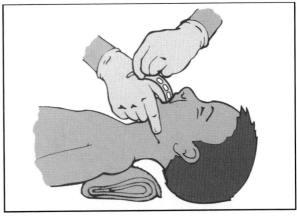

B.

FIGURE 29-4 A. In an adult, the airway is inserted with the tip pointing to the roof of the mouth, then rotated into position. B. In an infant or child, the airway is inserted with the tip pointing toward the tongue and throat, in the same position it will be in after insertion.

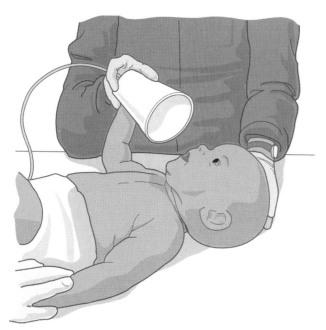

FIGURE 29-5 You can deliver oxygen by the blow-by method.

- Use properly sized face masks to assure a good mask seal.
- Flow-restricted, oxygen-powered ventilation devices are contraindicated in infants and children.
- If ventilation is not successful in raising the patient's chest, perform procedures for clearing an obstructed airway, then try to ventilate again.

Review the procedures for artificial ventilation in Basic Life Support: Airway, Rescue Breathing, and CPR at the end of this book. These procedures are summarized in Table 29-3.

INTERACTING WITH THE PEDIATRIC PATIENT

You will not be able to interview infants, and most toddlers are poor communicators. However, the parents or the care providers who called for help can usually provide a history of the small child's illness or injury.

At the other end of the pediatric age range, adolescents should be able to tell you exactly how they feel and what happened. However, tact may be required to get information from an adolescent who is embarrassed, intimidated by the attention, or trying to hide the fact that he was doing something wrong.

In between are preschoolers and school-age children. Preschoolers can usually be interviewed if you take your time and keep your language simple. School-age children will be able to describe more clearly how they feel and what happened. They will talk with you honestly, but may feel that the injury or illness is a punishment for something they did. They must be reassured and told it's all right to feel this way or to cry. If parents, teachers, or care-providers are at the scene, talk with them but do not exclude the child. Seeing that familiar adults are being included gains the child's confidence if you follow up by talking directly to the child. If the parents are injured, you may not be able to get information from them, and the child needs to know that someone is caring for his or her parent as well.

All patients have some degree of fear at the emergency scene. Infants and children are usually more fearful than adults because they lack

TABLE 29-3 Artificial Ventilation and Clearing the Airway

	Child over 8	Child 1 to 8	Infant
Age	8 yrs and older	1-8 yrs	birth-1 yr
Initial ventilation	1½ to 2 sec.	1 to 1½ sec	1 to 1½ sec
Ventilation rate	10–12 breaths/min.	20 breaths/min.	20 breaths/min.
Obstructed Airway—Conscious	abdominal thrusts	abdominal thrusts	alternate 5 back blows with 5 chest thrusts
Obstructed Airway—Unconscious	5 abdominal thrusts finger sweep, ventilate	5 abdominal thrusts remove visible objects, ventilate	5 back blows 5 chest thrusts, remove visible objects, ventilate
Working alone: when to call for help	After establishing unresponsiveness—before beginning resuscitation	After establishing unresponsiveness and 1 minute of resuscitation	After establishing unresponsiveness and 1 minute of resuscitation

experience with illness and injury. In addition to this, children are easily frightened by the unknown. Since so many details of the emergency scene are unknowns, it is easy to see why emergencies can be scary for children. The elements associated with the emergency (pain, noise, bright lights, cold) can set off a panic reaction in infants.

At an emergency, if the child feels he does not understand you, or believes that you do not understand in return, fear will increase. If the child is to communicate, he must remain calm. Putting the child at ease is a very important part of the care you must provide. Some children, when stressed, will act like a younger child. This is called regression.

Any problems faced by the child will be intensified if the parents are not at the scene. Children find security by interacting with their parents when facing new problems or emergencies. Asking for mom or dad may be the child's first priority, even above that of having your help.

When dealing with pediatric patients you should

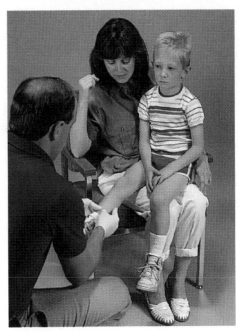

FIGURE 29-6 Kneel or sit at the child's eye level.

1. Identify yourself simply by saying "Hi, I'm Pat. What's your name?"
2. Let the child know that someone will call his or her parents.
3. Determine if there are life-threatening problems and treat immediately. If there are no problems of this nature, continue the patient survey and interview at a relaxed pace. Fearful children cannot take the pressure of a rapidly paced assessment and "meaningless" questions fired at them by a stranger.
4. Let the child have any nearby toy that he may want.
5. Kneel or sit at the child's eye level (Figure 29-6). Assure that bright light is not directly behind you and shining into the child's eyes.
6. SMILE. This is a familiar sign from adults that reassures children.
7. Touch the child or hold his hand or foot. Young children sometimes like to have their toes played with. A child who does not wish to be touched will let you know. Do not force the issue; smile and provide comfort through your conversation.
8. Do not use any equipment on the child without explaining what you will do with it. Many children fear the medical items that are so familiar to the EMT-B, thinking they

will cause pain. Always tell the child what you are going to do as you take vital signs and do a physical exam. Do not try to explain the entire procedure at once. Instead, explain each step as you do it. Use simple language and remember that children tend to take things literally. If you tell a young child you are going to "take your pulse," he may think you are going to take something away from him. Instead say, "I'm going to hold your wrist for a minute." If the child is older, explain why.

9. Let the child see your face and make eye contact without staring at the child. (Staring makes children uncomfortable.) Speak directly to the child, making a special effort to speak clearly and slowly in words he can understand. Be sure the child can hear you.
10. Stop occasionally to find out if the child understands. Never assume the child understood you, but find out by asking questions if the child is old enough to respond.
11. NEVER LIE TO THE CHILD. Tell him or her when the examination may hurt. If the child asks if he is sick or hurt, be honest, but be sure to add that you are there to help and will not leave. Let the child know that other people also will be helping.

SUPPORTING THE PARENTS OR OTHER CARE PROVIDERS

Parents may react in one of several ways when their child suffers a sudden life-threatening injury or illness. Their first reaction may be one of denial or shock. Some parents will react by crying, screaming, or becoming angry. Another common reaction is self-blame and guilt. In all of these instances, be calm, reassuring, and supportive. Use simple language to explain what has happened and what is being done to and for their child.

In some cases, an hysterical parent may interfere with your care of the child. This is a natural reaction to protect the child from further harm. Usually you can persuade the parent to assist you by holding the child's hand, giving you a medical history, or comforting the child. If, however, the parent is out of control and cannot or will not cooperate, have a friend or relative remove the parent from the scene.

At this point it should be noted that not all children live with two parents in a traditional nuclear family. The child may have a single parent or may be living with a grandparent or other relative or even with someone who is not related to the child. Whoever the child's full-time caretaker or guardian is, that person is likely to have the same emotional responses in an emergency as any parent. The EMT-B should be sensitive to the fact that the child may or may not call this person "Mommy" or "Daddy" and may be upset if asked where his or her mother or father is. Tact is often required to find out who is responsible for the child and what the child calls that person. Keep this in mind as you read the rest of the chapter in which we will use "parent" or "mom and dad" to stand for any person or persons who act as parent, guardian, or principal caretaker to the child.

You need to gain the confidence and establish emotional control of all the people around the scene in order to be able to treat the child effectively. Your interactions with the child will show everyone present your concern, and the manner in which you provide care will show your professionalism.

In general, involving the parent in the care of the child helps both the child and the parent. The most effective method may be to have the parent hold the child in a position of comfort in the parent's lap, if appropriate, during assessment and treatment procedures (Figure 29-7).

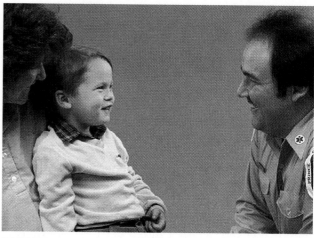

FIGURE 29-7 Have the parent hold the child in a position of comfort to involve the parent and soothe the child.

Offer as much emotional support as possible to the parent. *However, never forget that your patient is the child, not the parent. Do not allow communication with the parent to distract you from care of the child.*

ASSESSMENT

The steps of assessment are the same for the pediatric patient as they are for the adult patient. Below, certain special concerns for the pediatric patient during assessment are discussed.

Scene Size-up and Safety

When entering the area where there is a pediatric patient, enter slowly and make some important observations. The first is to determine if the scene is safe. Even though it is a rare occurrence, sometimes there may be a risk from violence or abusive behavior, possibly directed toward the child. Look around carefully for any mechanism of injury.

Body substance isolation precautions must be taken for the usual reasons. Additionally, be aware that ordinary childhood diseases can be devastating when contracted as an adult.

Initial Assessment

A great deal of information can and should be gathered from the doorway, before you approach and possibly upset the patient. From across the room, you can gain a general impression of the child. First decide: Is the child well or sick? The child's general appearance and behavior will usually provide the answer. As soon as you saw Danny, your patient in On the Scene, and saw his labored respirations, you knew that he was a sick child who would need immediate transport.

A child who is alertly watching your approach, squirming and able to talk with you, vigorously crying, obviously has an open airway, is breathing, and has a pulse and blood pressure. If the child is silent, appears to be sleeping deeply, or is unresponsive, the child's airway, breathing, and circulation must be assessed immediately.

Forming a General Impression

As you approach and form your general impression, making the following observations.

- Mental status—The well child is alert. The sick child may be drowsy, inattentive, or sleeping.
- Effort of breathing—The well child's breathing should be unlabored. The sick child will be making a visible effort to breathe, including flared nostrils, and muscle and rib contractions.
- Skin color—A sick child may be pale, cyanotic, or flushed.
- Quality of cry or speech—In general, a strong cry or normal speech indicate a well child with good air exchange. The child who can speak only in short sentences or grunts has significant respiratory distress.
- Interaction with the environment or others—The healthy child exhibits normal behavior for his age. He moves around, plays, is attentive, establishes eye contact, and interacts with his parents. The sick child may be silent, listless, or unconscious.
- Emotional state—The well child's emotional state is appropriate to the situation. Crying may be his normal response to pain or fear. A withdrawn child or one who is emotionally flat is probably a sick child.
- Response to you—A well child may be interested in you or afraid of you. A sick child will give little attention to a stranger. (Remember that Danny, in On the Scene, was more interested in his breathing difficulty than in answering questions.)
- Tone and body position—A sick child may be limp with poor muscle tone. Pediatric patients with respiratory distress often assume characteristic positions that seem to help them breathe. (Danny was sitting on the edge of his bed, leaning forward.)

Assessing Mental Status

Use the AVPU method of assessing mental status, taking the child's age and development into account. You may need to shout to elicit a response to verbal stimulus. Tap or pinch the patient to test for response to painful stimulus. *Never shake an infant or child.*

Assessing the Airway

Consider not only whether the airway is open but whether it is endangered. A depressed mental status, secretions, blood, vomitus, foreign bodies, face or neck trauma, and lower respiratory infections may all compromise the airway. *Be careful not to hyperextend the child's neck. Do not attempt to manipulate the airway of the child with suspected lower airway infection (see below).*

Assessing Breathing

First assess if the patient is breathing or not. If the patient is not breathing or is breathing inadequately, provide artificial ventilations with supplemental oxygen. If the patient is experiencing respiratory distress, provide high concentration oxygen by pediatric nonrebreather mask.

To assess breathing, observe the following.

- Chest expansion—present and equal on both sides of the chest
- Effort of breathing—Watch for nasal flaring when the patient inhales, retractions or "pulling in" of the sternum and ribs with inhalation.
- Sounds of breathing—Listen for stridor, crowing, or other noisy respirations. Breath sounds should be present and equal on both sides of the chest. Note the presence of grunting at the end of expiration, a worrisome sign.
- Breathing rate—Normal respiratory rates for infants and children are 12 to 20 per minute in an adolescent, 15 to 30 per minute in a child, 25 to 50 per minute in an infant. *Breathing that is either faster or slower than normal is inadequate* and requires artificial ventilation as well as oxygen.
- Color—Cyanosis (blue color) indicates that the patient is not getting enough oxygen.

Assessing Circulation

As with an adult, check for normal warm, pink, and dry skin and pulse as indications of adequate circulation and perfusion. For basic life support, check the carotid pulse in a child, the brachial or femoral pulse in an infant. In infants and children, check capillary refill. When you press on the nail bed or press the top of a hand or foot, the area will turn white. If circulation is adequate, the normal pink color will return in less than 2 seconds, or in less time than it takes to say "capillary refill." Check for and control any blood loss.

Identifying Priority Patients

A patient who is a high priority for immediate transport is one who

- Gives a poor general impression
- Is unresponsive or listless
- Has a compromised airway
- Is in respiratory arrest or has inadequate breathing or respiratory distress
- Has a possibility of shock
- Has uncontrolled bleeding

Focused History and Physical Exam

At times, the child may be the only source of a history. He may be at school or another place where medical records are not kept or where adults who know his medical history are not present. Get as much history as you can from the child by asking simple questions that cannot be answered merely yes or no. A child who cannot tell you where it hurts can usually point to the area.

Perform a focused history and physical exam for a medical patient, a rapid trauma exam for a trauma patient, as you would for an adult. Explain to the awake child what you are doing, and do the exam in trunk-to-head order to avoid frightening the child.

Take and record vital signs, assessing blood pressure only in children older than 3, using an appropriate-size cuff. See Table 29-4 for pediatric vital sign normal ranges.

Detailed Physical Exam

The EMT-B normally performs the physical examination or body survey in head-to-toe order; but on alert infants and small children this is reversed. Starting with the toes or trunk and working your way toward the head will let the child get used to you and your touch before you, who after all are a stranger, attempt to touch them around the head and face. Playing with infants' feet often puts them at ease.

Unless there are possible injuries that indicate that the child should not be moved, the child should be held on the parent's lap during the physical exam. Many EMS teams carry clean toys that can be given to the child during the physical exam. They can provide comfort to the child and allow you to explain the survey by using the toy as model. Point to an area on the toy to show the child where you must touch during the survey and where you will bandage when you need to provide emergency care. This type of one-to-one communication also helps build parent and bystander confidence, letting them know that a professional, compassionate EMT-B is caring for the child. (If you use a toy, then give it to the child to keep.)

Most young children will suffer no embarrassment when clothing is removed or repositioned during the exam. Nonetheless, protect the child from the stares of onlookers. Many children around the age of 5 to 8 go through a stage of intense modesty. You may have to keep explaining why you must remove certain articles of clothing. Many parents, teachers, and day care personnel teach children that strangers should not remove their clothing or touch them. The children that you examine may not understand your intentions and may resist. Some children may become upset because they feel you are taking something away from them. Take your time and do not rush children into accepting all that is happening. Remember that children lose body heat rapidly, so if you expose them, quickly cover them with a blanket.

The young adolescent is often worried about the changes occurring to his or her body and uncertain if these changes are "normal." Handling the clothing of a teenager of the opposite sex can be awkward for the EMT-B as well as for the patient. In most cases, a simple description of the survey will set the patient at ease. However, you should make sure that both the adolescent and the parents understand what you are going to do and why it must be done. When possible, have the exam conducted by or in the presence of an EMT-B of the same sex as the patient. However, do not delay patient evaluation and care because you or the patient may be embarrassed. As a professional, you must put such feelings aside and act in a manner that will

TABLE 29-4 Normal Vital Sign Ranges, Infants and Children

Normal Pulse Rate (beats per minute, at rest)	
Newborn	120 to 160
Infant 0-5 months	90 to 140
Infant 6-12 months	80 to 140
Toddler 1-3 years	80 to 130
Preschooler 3-5 years	80 to 120
School age 6-10 years	70 to 110
Adolescent 11-14 years	60 to 105

Normal Respiration Rates (breaths per minute, at rest)	
Newborn	30 to 50
Infant 0-5 months	25 to 40
Infant 6-12 months	20 to 30
Toddler 1-3 years	20 to 30
Preschooler 3-5 years	20 to 30
School age 6-10 years	15 to 30
Adolescent 11-14 years	12 to 20

Blood Pressure Normal Ranges		
	Systolic Approx. 80 plus 2 x age	Diastolic Approx. ⅔ Systolic
Preschooler 3-5 years	average 99 (78 to 116)	average 65
School age 6-10 years	average 105 (80 to 122)	average 57
Adolescent 11-14 years	average 115 (94-140)	average 59

Notes: A high pulse in an infant or child is not as great a concern as a low pulse. A low pulse (heart rate) may indicate imminent cardiac arrest (stoppage of heart function). Blood pressure is usually not taken on a child under 3 years. In cases of blood loss or shock, a child's blood pressure will remain within normal limits until near the end, then fall swiftly.

allow the patient to relax and understand that there is no need for embarrassment.

The survey of an infant or child is done to look for the same signs of injury and illness as in the case of the adult patient. However, you should take special care with the following (Figure 29-8).

- Head—Do not apply pressure to the "soft spots" (fontanelles) of an infant. The skin over the anterior fontanelle is normally level with the skull, or slightly sunken, and may bulge naturally when the infant cries. Meningitis and head trauma cause the fontanelle to bulge due to increased intracranial pressure. Accidents involving infants and children can often produce head injuries.
- Nose and Ears—Look for blood and clear fluids from the nose and ears. Suspect skull fractures if present. Children are nose breathers and mucus or blood clot obstruction will make it hard for them to breathe.
- Neck—Children are more vulnerable to spinal cord injuries than adults. The head is proportionately larger and heavier than an adult's and has less support because muscles and bone structure are less developed. In medical emergencies, the neck may be sore, stiff, or swollen.
- Airway—Keep the infant's head in the neutral position and the child's head in the neutral-plus or sniffing position (chin thrust forward to maintain an open airway). If there is no suspicion of spinal injury, place a flat, folded towel under the shoulders to get the appropriate airway opening. Children's airways are more pliable and smaller than an adult's. Hyperextension or hyperflexion may close off the airway. For

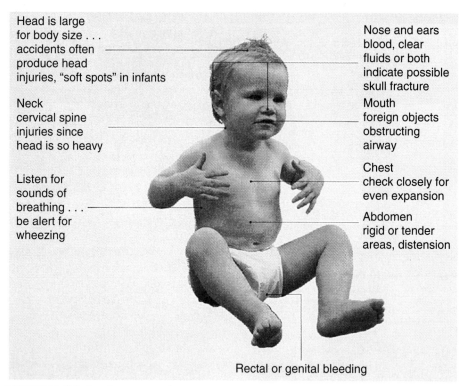

Head is large for body size . . . accidents often produce head injuries, "soft spots" in infants

Neck cervical spine injuries since head is so heavy

Listen for sounds of breathing . . . be alert for wheezing

Nose and ears blood, clear fluids or both indicate possible skull fracture

Mouth foreign objects obstructing airway

Chest check closely for even expansion

Abdomen rigid or tender areas, distension

Rectal or genital bleeding

FIGURE 29-8 The special areas to consider during assessment of the infant or child.

medical respiratory problems, the child may want to sit up.

- Chest—Listen closely for even air entry and the sounds of breathing on both sides of the chest. Be alert for wheezes and other noises. Check for symmetry, bruising, paradoxical movement, and retraction of the sternum or the muscles between the ribs. Remember that a child's soft ribs may not break, but there may be underlying injuries to the organs within the chest.
- Abdomen—Note any rigid or tender areas and distention. Because a child's abdominal organs (especially the spleen and liver) are large in relation to the size of the abdominal cavity, and because there is little protection offered by the still-undeveloped abdominal muscles, these organs are more susceptible to trauma than an adult's. Any injury that impedes the movement of the diaphragm will compromise a young child's breathing, as most children 8 years of age or younger are abdominal breathers.
- Pelvis—Check for stability of the pelvic girdle and bleeding or bloody discharge from the genital area.
- Extremities—Perform a neurological assessment with capillary refill and distal motor, sensory, and pulse check. With an infant or

young child you do not have to press on a nail bed. You can quickly check capillary refill by squeezing a hand or foot, forearm or lower leg. Check for painful, swollen, and deformed injury sites. (The bones of an infant or child are more pliable so they bend, splinter, and buckle before they fracture.)

Ongoing Assessment

Pediatric patients are dynamic—constantly changing. Continual assessment is essential to good patient care. A rule of thumb for infants and children is: *Don't take your eyes off them for a minute!*

As time permits, the following should be done. In some cases where the patient is seriously ill or traumatized, maintaining the airway and supporting ventilations will keep the EMT-B from performing a detailed physical exam and a complete history.

1. Reassess mental status
2. Maintain open airway
3. Monitor breathing
4. Reassess pulse

5. Monitor skin color, temperature, and moisture
6. Reassess vital signs

   - every 5 minutes in unstable patients
   - every 15 minutes in stable patients

7. Assure that all appropriate care and treatment are being given.

Additional Concerns During Assessment

Fever

Above-normal body temperature is one of the most important signs of an existing or impending acute illness. Fever usually accompanies simple virus infections and ear aches as well as such childhood diseases as measles, mumps, chicken pox, mononucleosis, pneumonia, epiglottitis, and meningitis. The fever also may be due to heat exposure, any infection, or some other noninfectious disease problem.

Never regard a fever as unimportant. Parents may have an opinion about what they believe may be the problem, but the EMT-B is not qualified to diagnose or determine what is likely to happen over the next few hours. Fever with a rash is a sign of a potentially serious condition.

Use relative skin temperature as a sign. Generally oral or rectal temperatures are not taken in the prehospital setting unless permitted by local medical direction. Either a skin thermometer or information provided by the parents should be used for determining the patient's temperature. A high relative skin temperature is always enough reason to transport and seek medical opinion.

- Any child 1 to 5 years old with a temperature above 103°F must be evaluated at the hospital.
- Any child from 5 to 12 with a body temperature above 102°F must be evaluated at the hospital.
- When in doubt, transport.

Be aware that a mild fever can quickly turn into a high fever that may indicate a serious, if not life-threatening, problem. If the infant or child feels very warm to hot to the touch, then prepare the patient for transport.

Children can tolerate a high temperature, and only a small percent will have a seizure due to fever (febrile seizure). It is the rapid rise in temperature rather than the temperature itself that causes seizures. Should you find an infant or child with high fever

- Remove the child's clothing, but do not allow him or her to be exposed to conditions that may bring on sudden chills (hypothermia). If the child objects, let the patient keep on light clothing or underwear.
- If the condition is a result of heat exposure, and if local protocols permit, cover the child with a towel soaked in tepid water. This will cool the child quickly.
- Monitor for shivering and avoid hypothermia. This may develop quickly in children. If shivering develops, stop the cooling activities and cover the child with a light blanket.
- If local protocols permit, give the child fluids by mouth or allow him or her to suck on chipped ice. This may not prevent dehydration but will increase comfort.
- Transport all children who have suffered a seizure as quickly as possible, protecting the patient from temperature extremes.

There are also some "do nots" in treating an infant or child with fever.

- Do not submerge the child in cold water, or cover with a towel soaked in ice water (which can cause hypothermia rapidly).
- DO NOT USE RUBBING ALCOHOL TO COOL THE PATIENT (IT CAN BE ABSORBED IN TOXIC AMOUNTS AND IS A FIRE HAZARD).

Hypothermia

Hypothermia is always a concern with the pediatric patient. It is important when providing care to a pediatric patient that the patient is kept warm. Attention should be paid to covering the head when hypothermia is a concern as the head is a major area of heat loss.

Because children have a large surface area in proportion to their body mass, exposure to cool weather and water can easily result in hypothermia, or cooling of the body temperature, a condition that in extreme cases is life-threatening. (You learned about hypothermia in Chapter 22, Environmental Emergencies.) Other causes of hypothermia in children include ingestion of alcohol or drugs that dilate peripheral vessels and cause loss of body heat; metabolic problems such as hypoglycemia; brain disorders that interfere with temperature regulation; severe infection or sepsis; and shock.

Like adults, children lose heat more readily if their clothes are wet, if they are exposed to wind, or if they are submerged in cold water. The child's body attempts to compensate for a decrease in body temperature, but as these compensatory functions begin to fail, the core body temperature drops.

Field care for children is the same as for adults. Cover the patient to avoid further loss of body heat. Consult medical direction for advice on active rewarming by application of hot water bottles or other heat sources to the body if the patient is awake and responding appropriately. Avoid rough handling and inserting anything in the mouth as these actions may cause ventricular fibrillation or cardiac arrest in the severely hypothermic child. Suction very gently if suctioning is necessary, being alert to the possibility of cardiac arrest.

Diarrhea and Vomiting

Diarrhea and vomiting are common in childhood illness. Both diarrhea and vomiting can cause dehydration that worsens whatever other condition the child may have and may lead to life-threatening shock. Infants are more susceptible to the effects of dehydration because, compared to adults, a greater percentage of their body proportion is water and their fluid maintenance needs are greater.

For any pediatric patient with diarrhea or vomiting

1. Monitor the airway and be prepared to provide oral suctioning.
2. Monitor breathing and provide oxygen.
3. If signs of shock are present, contact medical direction immediately and transport.
4. If your protocols or medical direction permits, offer the child sips of clear liquids or chipped ice as the child can tolerate without vomiting.
5. Save a sample of vomitus and rectal discharge (e.g., a soiled diaper).

TREATMENT SUMMARIES— MEDICAL

Airway Obstructions

Infants and children are naturally curious. They explore their environment and often put things in their mouths. They can easily choke on foreign objects as well as on a piece of food.

An airway obstruction can be partial or complete. With many partial obstructions, the child is still able to breathe and get enough oxygen. With other partial obstructions or with complete obstruction of the airway, the supply of air is cut off to a significant extent or completely. The assessment and care summaries below detail how to assess if an obstruction is partial or complete and how to manage an obstruction.

Patient Assessment—Partial Airway Obstruction

Signs

- [ ] Noisy breathing (stridor, crowing)
- [ ] Retractions of the muscles, ribs, sternum when inhaling
- [ ] Skin is still pink
- [ ] Peripheral perfusion is satisfactory (capillary refill under 2 seconds)
- [ ] Still alert, not unconscious

Patient Care—Partial Airway Obstruction

Emergency Care Steps

1. Allow the child to assume a position of comfort, sitting up, not lying down. Assist an infant or younger child into a sitting position. Allow child to sit on parent's lap.
2. Offer high concentration oxygen by pediatric nonrebreather mask or blow-by technique.
3. Transport.
4. Do not agitate the child. Do a limited exam. Do not assess blood pressure.

Patient Assessment—Complete Airway Obstruction or Partial Obstruction with No Crying or Speaking and Cyanosis

The obstruction may be complete, or a partial obstruction may be severe enough to prevent adequate intake of oxygen.

Signs

- [ ] Cyanosis.
- [ ] Child's cough becomes ineffective. Child cannot cry or speak.
- [ ] Increased respiratory difficulty accompanied by stridor or respiratory arrest.
- [ ] Altered mental status or child has lost or loses consciousness.

Emergency Care Steps

1. Perform airway clearing techniques (abdominal thrusts for a child, back blows and chest thrusts for an infant, as described earlier in this chapter. (See Figure 29-3 and Table 29-2).

2. Attempt artificial ventilations with a bag-valve-mask unit, pediatric size for a good seal, and supplemental oxygen, as described earlier in this chapter. (See Table 29-3.)

Respiratory Disorders

Differentiating Airway Obstruction from Respiratory Disease

In infants and children, it is especially important to try to distinguish between an upper airway obstruction and a lower airway disease. Many of the signs of an airway obstruction are the same as the signs of lower airway respiratory disease, since respiratory infection or disease will also often swell and obstruct the passages of the airway.

With some of these diseases, it is dangerous to perform finger sweeps or to place a tongue depressor or any other instrument in the patient's mouth or pharynx because this may set off spasms along the airway. Do not attempt to clear the airway of a foreign obstruction unless it is clear that this is the problem—the child has been observed ingesting a foreign object or the signs of such ingestion are clear.

Transport as quickly as possible if you see the following signs of a lower respiratory problem.

- Wheezing
- Breathing effort on exhalation
- Rapid breathing without any stridor (harsh, high-pitched sound)

Respiratory Distress

There are a number of lower respiratory diseases or disorders an infant or child may have that will cause respiratory distress, including serious ones like epiglottitis, and less serious ones like a cold. It is not easy to determine which respiratory problem the child may have. Many signs and symptoms are similar, and age ranges for occurrence overlap.

As an EMT-B, you will not have time, nor is it necessary, to decide what respiratory disorder a child is suffering from. Instead, follow the guidelines below for recognizing and managing respiratory distress. It is especially important to recognize the signs of *early* respiratory distress and treat it before it advances to a life-threatening stage or to respiratory arrest.

Gather information quickly from the parents and do a rapid assessment of the child. Do not put a tongue depressor in the child's mouth to examine the airway. This may cause spasms that can totally obstruct the airway. Rely on any of the following signs of early respiratory distress (Figure 29-9).

Signs

- Nasal flaring
- Retraction of the muscles above, below, and between the sternum and ribs
- Use of abdominal muscles
- Stridor (high-pitched, harsh sound)
- Audible wheezing
- Grunting
- Breathing rate greater than 60

In addition to the above signs of early respiratory distress, watch for these additional signs.

- Cyanosis
- Decreased muscle tone
- Poor peripheral perfusion (capillary refill greater than 2 seconds)
- Altered mental status

Emergency Care Steps

PROVIDE OXYGEN TO ALL CHILDREN WITH RESPIRATORY EMERGENCIES.

For children in early respiratory distress

- Provide oxygen by pediatric nonrebreather mask or blow-by technique.

For children in severe respiratory distress (those with respiratory distress and altered mental status, cyanosis even when oxygen is

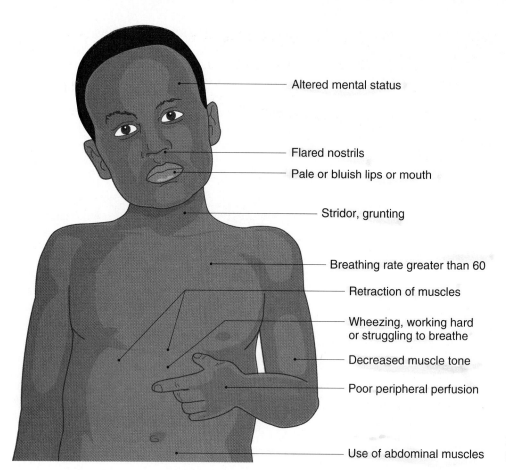

Altered mental status

Flared nostrils

Pale or bluish lips or mouth

Stridor, grunting

Breathing rate greater than 60

Retraction of muscles

Wheezing, working hard or struggling to breathe

Decreased muscle tone

Poor peripheral perfusion

Use of abdominal muscles

FIGURE 29-9 Signs of respiratory distress.

administered, poor muscle tone, or inadequate breathing)

▣ Provide assisted ventilations with pediatric bag-valve mask and supplemental oxygen.

For children in respiratory arrest

▣ Provide assisted ventilations with pediatric bag-valve mask and supplemental oxygen.

ALL RESPIRATORY DISORDERS IN CHILDREN MUST BE TAKEN SERIOUSLY. RESPIRATORY DISEASE IS THE PRIMARY CAUSE OF CARDIAC ARREST NOT DUE TO TRAUMA. If you treat the respiratory system, the heart will also respond. The EMT-B's primary concern when caring for infants and children with respiratory problems, whether medical or trauma related, is to establish and maintain an open airway. About one-third of all pediatric trauma deaths are related to airway mismanagement.

Seizures

High fever, epilepsy, infections, poisoning, hypoglycemia, trauma including head injury, or de-

creased levels of oxygen can bring on seizures. Some seizures in children are idiopathic; that is, they have no known cause. They may be brief or prolonged. They are rarely life threatening in children who have them frequently. However, SEIZURES, INCLUDING THOSE CAUSED BY FEVER, SHOULD BE CONSIDERED LIFE-THREATENING BY THE EMT-B.

Usually, you will arrive after the convulsion has passed.

Patient Assessment—Seizures

Interview the patient as well as family members and bystanders who saw the convulsion. Ask them if the child has a history of seizures. Ask

☐ Has the child had prior seizures?
☐ If yes, is this the child's normal seizure pattern? (How long did the seizure last? What part of the body was seizing?)
☐ Has the child had a fever?
☐ Has the child taken any anti-seizure medication? Other medication?

Assess the child for symptoms and signs of illness or injury, taking care to note any injuries sustained during the convulsion. All infants and children who have undergone a seizure require medical evaluation. The seizure itself may not be serious but it may be a sign of an underlying condition. Be aware that seizures may be caused by a head injury.

Emergency Care Steps

If the patient has a seizure in your presence, possibly during transport, provide the following care.

1. Maintain an open airway; do not insert an oropharyngeal airway or bitestick.
2. Position the patient on his side if there is no possibility of spinal injury.
3. Be alert for vomiting. Suction as needed.
4. Provide oxygen. If in respiratory arrest provide artificial ventilations with supplemental oxygen.
5. Transport.
6. Monitor for inadequate breathing and/or altered mental status, which may occur following a seizure.

Altered Mental Status

Altered mental status may be caused by a variety of conditions, including hypoglycemia, poisoning, infection, head injury, decreased oxygen levels, shock (hypoperfusion), or the aftermath of a seizure.

Assessment of the patient with altered mental status focuses on life-threatening problems discovered during the initial assessment.

☐ Be alert for a mechanism of injury that may have caused the altered mental status, such as head or spinal injury.
☐ Be alert for shock (hypoperfusion).
☐ Look for evidence of poisoning by ingested, inhaled, or absorbed substances.
☐ Attempt to quickly obtain a history of any seizure disorder or diabetes.

Emergency Care Steps

1. Assure an open airway. Be prepared to suction.
2. Protect the spine while managing the airway if a head injury or other trauma is present.
3. Administer high concentration oxygen by pediatric nonrebreather mask or blow-by technique. Be prepared to perform artificial ventilations by pediatric bag-valve mask with supplemental oxygen.
4. Treat for shock.
5. Transport.

Poisoning

Children are often the victims of accidental poisoning, often resulting from the ingestion of household products or medications. Poisons can quickly depress the respiratory system and cause respiratory arrest and also can cause life-threatening conditions of the circulatory and nervous systems. The airway and gastrointestinal track can also be burned by corrosive substances on ingestion and with subsequent vomiting.

Review Chapter 21, Poisoning and Overdose Emergencies, for information on ingested, inhaled, absorbed, and injected poisons. This information applies to children as well as to adults. There are some special types of poisonings not often associated with adult patients that are common to children. These special cases include

☐ Aspirin Poisoning—Look for hyperventilation, vomiting, and sweating. The skin may feel hot. Severe cases cause seizures, coma, or shock.
☐ Acetaminophen Poisoning—Many medications have this compound, including Tylenol, Comtrex, Bancap, Excedrin P.M., and Datril. The child may be restless (early) or drowsy. Nausea, vomiting, and heavy perspiration may occur. Loss of consciousness is possible.
☐ Lead Poisoning—This usually comes from ingesting chips of lead-based paint. It is often chronic (building up over a long

time). Look for nausea with abdominal pain and vomiting. Muscle cramps, headache, muscle weakness, and irritability are often present.

☐ Iron Poisoning—Iron compounds such as ferrous sulfate are found in some vitamin tablets and liquids. As little as one gram of ferrous sulfate can be lethal to a child. Within 30 minutes to several hours, the child will show nausea and bloody vomiting, often accompanied by bloody diarrhea. Typically the child will develop shock, but this may be delayed for up to 24 hours as the child appears to be getting better.

☐ Petroleum Product Poisoning—The patient will usually be vomiting with coughing or choking. In most cases, you will smell the distinctive odor of a petroleum distillate (e.g., gasoline, kerosene, heating fuel).

☐ Cyanide—Such seemingly innocent items as apple seeds contain cyanide.

Patient Care—Poisoning

Emergency Care Steps

For a responsive patient

1. Contact medical direction.
2. Consider the need to administer activated charcoal.
3. Provide oxygen.
4. Transport.
5. Continue to monitor the patient. He may become unresponsive.

For an unresponsive patient

1. Assure an open airway.
2. Provide oxygen.
3. Be prepared to provide artificial ventilation.
4. Call medical direction.
5. Transport.
6. Rule out trauma as a cause of altered mental status.

Shock

Shock is another term for hypoperfusion, or the inadequate circulation of blood and oxygen throughout the body. The physiological causes of shock were discussed in Chapter 26, Bleeding and Shock.

One common cause of shock in adults—a failure of heart function or of the cardiovascular system—is rare in infants and children. Common causes of shock in infants and children include

- Diarrhea and dehydration
- Trauma
- Vomiting
- Blood loss
- Infection
- Abdominal injuries.

Less common causes include

- Allergic reactions
- Poisoning
- Cardiac events (rare)

It is important to remember the low blood volume of an infant or child, as discussed earlier in this chapter. Shock can develop in the small child who has a laceration to the scalp (with its many blood vessels), or in the three-year old who loses as little as a cup of blood.

The most important thing to understand about shock in infants and children is that their bodies are able to compensate for it for a long time. Then the compensating mechanisms fail and decompensated shock develops very rapidly. This means that a child may appear to be fine, then "go sour" in a hurry. This is in contrast to the adult patient in whom decompensated shock develops earlier and more gradually, making it easier to assess and treat than in a child.

The definitive care for shock takes place at the hospital. Since infants and children are prone to go into decompensated shock so suddenly, IT IS IMPORTANT NOT TO WAIT FOR SIGNS OF DECOMPENSATED SHOCK TO DEVELOP. Instead, in any situation in which shock is a possibility, provide oxygen (which provides extra oxygen to poorly perfused tissues and helps keep up heart function) and transport as quickly as possible.

The signs and emergency treatment of shock (Figure 29-10) are detailed below.

Patient Assessment—Shock

Signs

☐ Rapid respiratory rate
☐ Pale, cool, clammy skin
☐ Weak or absent peripheral pulses
☐ Delayed capillary refill
☐ Decreased urine output (Ask parents about diaper wetting; look at diaper)
☐ Mental status changes
☐ Absence of tears, even when crying

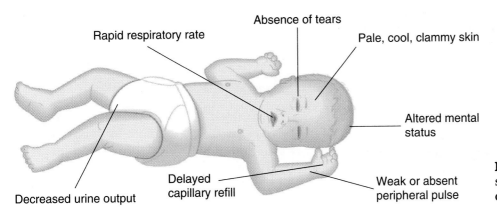

SIGNS OF SHOCK IN A CHILD

Rapid respiratory rate

Absence of tears

Pale, cool, clammy skin

Altered mental status

Decreased urine output

Delayed capillary refill

Weak or absent peripheral pulse

FIGURE 29-10 Signs of shock in an infant or child.

Patient Care—Shock

Emergency Care Steps

1. Assure an open airway.
2. Provide high concentration oxygen. Be prepared to artificially ventilate.
3. Manage bleeding, if present.
4. Elevate legs if there is no trauma.
5. Keep warm.
6. Transport immediately. Perform any additional assessment and treatments en route, if time permits.

Near-Drowning

Near-drowning means that a patient has been submerged in water and is either still alive or is clinically dead (without breathing or heartbeat) but not biologically dead (brain cells are still alive). Patients who have been submerged in cold water have been revived 30 minutes or more after submersion. Review the information on near-drowning in Chapter 22, Environmental Emergencies.

When treating a near-drowning patient, follow these guidelines.

- Provide artificial ventilation or CPR as necessary. This is your first treatment priority.
- Protect the airway. Suction if necessary.
- Consider the possibility of trauma as a cause or result of the submersion incident (for example, injury from a dive).
- Consider the possibility of hypothermia, especially if the patient has been in cool or cold water.
- Consider possible ingestion of alcohol as a cause of the near-drowning, especially in adolescents.

- Consider the possibility of "secondary drowning syndrome"—deterioration after normal breathing resumes, minutes to hours after the event. Transport all near-drowning patients to the hospital, even if they seem to have recovered.

Sudden Infant Death Syndrome

In the United States, sudden infant death syndrome (SIDS)—the sudden unexplained death during sleep of an apparently healthy baby in its first year of life—occurs to between 6,500 and 7,500 babies each year. These babies were usually receiving proper care and frequently have passed physical examinations within days of their sudden death. Many possible causes have been investigated but are not well understood. The problem is not caused by external methods of suffocation or by vomiting or choking. The problem may possibly be related to nerve cell development in the brain or the tissue chemistry of the respiratory system or the heart. Some relationships have been drawn to family history of SIDS and respiratory problems, but there is still no accepted reason why these babies die.

When asleep, the typical SIDS patient will show periods of cardiac slowdown and temporary cessation of breathing known as *sleep apnea*. Eventually, the infant will stop breathing and will not start again on its own. Unless reached in time, the episode can be fatal. The baby's condition is most commonly discovered in the early morning when the parents go to wake the baby.

It is not up to you, as an EMT-B, to diagnose SIDS. All you or the parents will know is that the baby is in respiratory and cardiac

CHAPTER 29 Infants and Children **619**

arrest. You will treat the baby as you would any patient in this condition:

1. Unless there is rigor mortis (stiffening of the body after death), provide resuscitation and transport to the hospital. Let the pronouncement of death come from hospital personnel, not from you.

2. Be certain that the parents receive emotional support and that they believe that everything possible is being done for the child at the scene and during transport.

Parents who lose a child to SIDS often suffer intense guilt feelings from the moment they find the child. Whether or not the parents express such guilt, remind them that SIDS occurs to apparently healthy babies who are receiving the best of parental care. Do not speak with a suspicious tone or ask inappropriate questions. Do not be embarrassed to express your sorrow for their loss, but be sure to do so only after a physician has officially informed them of the child's death.

TREATMENT SUMMARIES— TRAUMA

Trauma is the number one cause of death in infants and children. Nearly half of all pediatric traumatic deaths result from motor vehicles, followed by drowning, burns, firearms, and falls. Blunt trauma far exceeds penetrating trauma in infants and children. Much trauma to infants and children occurs because they are curious and learning about their environment. Exploring often leads to injury from accidental falls or things falling on them, burns, entrapment, crushing, and other mechanisms of injury.

This section will discuss assessment and management of accidental trauma as well as the trauma caused by child abuse.

When providing emergency care for the injured child, always tell him what you are going to do before you do it. If the child cries, let him know this is all right and you know he is trying to be brave, but everyone gets scared when hurt. Carry brightly colored adhesive bandages to hold dressings in place, and let the child know these are especially for him as a reward for bravery. You can carry along other small rewards like sheets of peel-off stickers. (Be sure the rewards are not small items that can be swallowed.)

Pediatric Trauma Considerations

Injury management is basically the same for children as for adults. However, their anatomical and physiological differences cause children to have different patterns of injury.

During motor vehicle collisions

- Unrestrained child passengers (those without seatbelts or restraint in a child safety seat) tend to have head and neck injuries.
- Restrained passengers may have abdominal and lower spine injuries.

Children who are struck by autos while bicycle riding often have head, spinal, and abdominal injuries. The child who has been struck by a vehicle may present with the following triad of injuries:

- Head injury, and . . .
- Abdominal injury with possible internal bleeding, and . . .
- Lower extremity injury (possibly a fractured femur)

Other common injuries include diving injuries with associated head and neck injury, sports injuries, which also often involve the head and neck, and injuries from child abuse.

You will need to have a good understanding of pediatric anatomic and physiologic characteristics as they relate to trauma in order to deliver expert emergency care. These include features of the head, chest, abdomen, and extremities, as described below.

- Head—Recall that the head is proportionately larger and heavier in the small child. This leads to head injury when the head is propelled forward in an accident. This is often combined with internal injuries. Suspect internal injuries whenever a child with a head injury presents with shock, since head injury itself is seldom a cause of shock. Respiratory arrest is a common secondary effect of head injury, so be alert to this possibility. Although the most frequent sign of head injury is an altered mental status, nausea and vomiting also often occur.

The most important common cause of hypoxia in the unconscious head-injury patient is the tongue falling back and blocking the airway. Use the jaw-thrust maneuver to reposition the tongue and open the airway.

An error to avoid in caring for the child head-injury patient is using sandbags to stabilize the head. Should the patient begin to vomit, the backboard will need to be turned on its side, and the weight of the heavy sandbag on the child's head may cause further injury.

- Chest—The less-developed respiratory muscles of the chest and the more elastic ribs make the pediatric chest more easily deformed. The immature respiratory muscles may tire easily and cannot maintain rapid respiratory rates for long. The more elastic ribs rarely fracture; however there is more likely to be injury to the structures beneath the ribs. You must suspect internal chest injuries when the mechanism of injury is significant, despite the absence of external signs of chest injury.

- Abdomen—Infants and young children are abdominal breathers, using their diaphragms for breathing. Thus they may not have significant movement of their chests while breathing. Watch the abdomen to evaluate breathing. In addition, other abdominal muscles are immature and therefore provide less protection to internal organs than do adult abdominal muscles.

  The abdomen can be a site of "hidden" injuries. You must suspect an internal abdominal injury when the patient deteriorates even without evidence of external injury. In addition, air in the stomach can distend the abdomen and interfere with artificial ventilation. This may also lead to vomiting. Be prepared to suction the patient.

- Extremities—Despite the more flexible bones in the pediatric patient, their extremity injuries are managed the same way as extremity injuries in adults.

Other Pediatric Trauma Considerations

Pneumatic Anti-Shock Garments

In some EMS systems, pneumatic anti-shock garments (PASG), may be employed for the treatment of shock and bleeding in pediatric patients (see Chapter 27, Musculoskeletal Injuries). Some general principles for their use in pediatric patients include the following.

- Use them only if they fit the patient. Never place the infant in one leg of an adult garment.

- Do not inflate the abdominal compartment. This may compromise breathing.
- PASG are indicated for the treatment of the pediatric trauma patient with signs of severe hypoperfusion and pelvic instability.

Burns

Burns are a common pediatric injury. Review the information on burns in Chapter 26, Soft Tissue Injuries. Especially review Figure 26-25 illustrating the Rule of Nines as it applies to estimating the extent of burns in children and infants.

Follow these guidelines when managing patients with burns.

- Identify candidates for transportation to burn centers. Local protocols should guide your determination.
- Cover the burn with sterile dressings. Nonadherent dressings are the best, but sterile sheets may be used.

Moist dressings should be used with caution in the pediatric patient. Remember that the child's body surface area is larger proportionately to their body mass, making them more prone to heat loss. Burned patients who become hypothermic have a higher death rate. You must keep the infant or child covered to prevent a drop in body temperature.

Emergency Care of the Trauma Patient

Emergency care steps for the pediatric trauma patient should include the following.

1. Assure an open airway. Use the modified jaw-thrust maneuver.
2. Suction as necessary, using a large bore suction catheter.
3. Provide high concentration oxygen.
4. Ventilate with a bag-valve mask as needed.
5. Provide spinal immobilization.
6. Transport immediately.
7. Continue to reassess en route.
8. Assess and treat other injuries en route if time permits.

Review Chapter 28, Injuries to the Head and Spine, on how to immobilize an infant or child who is in a child safety seat.

CHILD ABUSE AND NEGLECT

At one time, people thought child abuse was a rare phenomenon; but it is a complex social and health problem that seems increasingly common. The number of known child abuse cases is large but may be even larger than the statistics indicate. Experts believe that for every abused child seen by the emergency or family physician, there are many more unreported cases who never receive care.

Child abusers are mothers, fathers, sisters, brothers, grandparents, stepparents, baby-sitters and other care givers, white-collar workers, blue-collar workers, and those who are unemployed, rich, or poor. There is no distinction as to race, creed, or ethnic or economic background. There is no such person as a "typical" child abuser. In other words, ANYONE could be a child abuser, and the abuse can continue with increasing severity until death results.

Child abuse can take several different forms, often occurring in combination. These forms include

- Psychological (emotional) abuse
- Neglect
- Physical abuse
- Sexual abuse

A child's psychological problems and pathologic behavior are difficult to trace back to specific abuse, and this is not typically a problem directly in the realm of the EMT-B. What constitutes neglect is a serious legal question. As a child goes without proper food, shelter, clothing, supervision, treatment of injuries and illnesses, a safe environment, and love, the effects surely will be seen, but seldom is this the major part of an emergency response. Physical and sexual abuse are the problems likely to be seen by EMT-Bs. However, if signs of neglect are observed in the course of a call, they should be reported to the proper authorities.

Physical and Sexual Abuse

The best way to describe the types of injuries that can be inflicted in child physical abuse cases is to say, "If it can happen to the body, it has been done by a child abuser." Physically abused children—often called "battered" children—are those who are beaten with fists, hair brushes, straps, electric cords, pool cues, razor straps, bottles, broom handles, baseball bats, pots and pans, and almost any object that can be used as a weapon. Included in this group are children who are intentionally burned by hot water, steam, open flames, cigarettes, and other thermal sources. Battered children also include those who are severely shaken, thrown into their cribs or down steps, pushed out of windows and over railings, and even pushed from moving cars. The horror grows as we find children who are shot, stabbed, electrocuted, and suffocated.

The problems of sexual abuse range from adults exposing themselves to children to sexual intercourse or sexual torture. Many of the cases that get reported are for adults exposing themselves to children. Cases in which there is physical injury done to the child also are usually reported. The cases in between, especially those in which emotional injury or minor physical injury were done, are usually not reported, and therefore are difficult to estimate.

Patient Assessment—Physical Abuse

Signs

In child physical abuse cases, you will find

- ☐ Slap marks, bruises, abrasions, lacerations, and incisions of all sizes and with shapes matching the item used. You may see wide welts from belts, in a looped shape from cords, or in the shape of a hand from slapping. You may find swollen limbs, split lips, black eyes, and loose or broken teeth. Often the injuries are to the back, legs, and arms. The injuries may be in various stages of healing, as evidenced by different-colored bruises.
- ☐ Broken bones are common and all types of fractures are possible. Many battered children have multiple fractures, often in various stages of healing, or have fracture-associated complications.
- ☐ Head injuries are common, with concussions and skull fractures being reported. Closed head injuries occur to many infants and small children who have been severely shaken.
- ☐ Abdominal injuries include ruptured spleens, livers and lungs lacerated by broken ribs, internal bleeding from blunt trauma and punching, and lacerated and avulsed genitalia.
- ☐ Bite marks may be present showing the teeth size and pattern of the adult mouth.

Burn marks that are small and round from cigarettes; "glove" or "stocking" burn marks from dipping in hot water; burns on buttocks and legs (creases behind the knees and at the thighs are protected when flexed); and demarcation burns in the shape of an iron, stove burner, or other hot utensil are frequently found.

Indications of shaking an infant include a bulging fontanelle due to increased intracranial pressure from the bleeding of torn blood vessels in the brain, unconsciousness, and typical signs and symptoms of head and brain injury. Injuries to the central nervous system from "the shaken baby syndrome" are the most lethal child abuse injuries.

There are times when you will treat an injured child and never think that he has been abused. The child relates well with the parents and there appears to be a strong bond between them. However, there are certain indications that abuse may be occurring in or outside the home, with the family feeling they must not admit to the problem. Be on the alert for

Repeated responses to provide care for the same child or children in a family. Remember that in areas with many hospitals you may see the child more frequently than any one hospital.

Indications of past injuries. This is why you must do a physical examination and why you must remove articles of clothing. Pay special attention to the back and buttocks of the child.

Poorly healing wounds or improperly healed fractures. It is extremely rare for a child to receive a fracture, be given proper orthopedic care, and then show angulations and large "bumps" and "knots" of bone at the "healed" injury site.

Indications of past burns or fresh bilateral burns. Children seldom put both hands on a hot object or touch the same hot object again (true, some do . . . this is only an indication, not proof). Some types of burns are almost always linked to child abuse, such as cigarette burns to the body and burns to the buttocks and lower extremities that result from the child being dipped in hot water.

Many different types of injuries to both sides or the front and back of the body.

This gains even more importance if the adults on the scene keep insisting that the child "falls a lot."

Fear on the part of the child to tell you how the injury occurred. The child may seem to expect no comfort from the parents and may have little or no apparent reaction to pain.

The parent or care giver at the scene who does not wish to leave you alone with the child, tells conflicting or changing stories, overwhelms you with explanations of the cause of the injury, or faults the child may rouse your suspicions and cause you to assess the situation more carefully.

Pay attention to the adults as you treat the child.

Do they seem inappropriately unconcerned about the child?

Do they have trouble controlling anger?

Do you feel that at any moment there may be an emotional explosion?

Do any of the adults appear to be in a deep state of depression?

Are there indications of alcohol or drug abuse?

Do any of the adults speak of suicide or seeking mercy for their unhappy children?

Parents or care givers who have called for help for the injured child may be reluctant to assist you with history of the injury and may even refuse transport. Take note of any parent who refuses to have their child sent to the nearest hospital or to a hospital where the child has been seen many times. This may indicate a fear of the staff remembering or seeing a record of past injuries that suggest possible abuse. (You can't transport without parental consent; however, you may be able to convince the parents the child needs to be seen by a doctor because of certain signs and symptoms that are "difficult to determine" in the field.) Be the child's advocate, but do not accuse the parent.

Patient Assessment—Sexual Abuse

Do your physical assessment and rearrange or remove clothing only as necessary to determine and treat injuries. This will help preserve evidence where possible. Examine the genitalia only if there is obvious injury or the child tells you of a recent injury. The child may be hysterical, frightened, or withdrawn and unable to give you a history of the incident. Be calm and as reassuring as possible.

Signs

- ☐ Obvious results of sexual assault, including burns or wounds to the genitalia
- ☐ Any unexplained genital injury such as bruising, lacerations, or bloody discharge from genital orifices (openings)
- ☐ Seminal fluid on the body or clothes or other discharges associated with sexually transmitted diseases
- ☐ In rare cases, the child may tell you that he was sexually assaulted.

Remain professional and control your emotions. Do not allow the child to become embarrassed. Do not say anything that may make the child believe that he is to blame for the sexual assault (many believe that they are). Tell the child that the people at the hospital will help and that he is not to be embarrassed.

Patient Care—Physical or Sexual Abuse

Emergency Care Steps

1. Dress and provide other appropriate care for injuries as necessary.
2. Preserve evidence of sexual abuse if it is suspected
   - Discourage the child from going to the bathroom (for both defecation and urination).
   - Give nothing to the patient by mouth.
   - Do not have the child wash or change clothes.
3. Transport the child.

Note: You must plainly and clearly report to the medical staff any of your findings or suspicions that there has been physical or sexual abuse.

The Role of the EMT-B

Remember that you are charged with providing emergency care for an injured child. You are not a physician trained to detect abuse, a police officer, court investigator, social worker, judge, or one-person jury.

Gather information from the parents or care giver away from the child without expression of disbelief or judgment. Talk with the child separately about how the injury occurred. As you

assess the patient and provide appropriate care, control your emotions and hold back accusations. Do not indicate to the parents or other adults at the scene that you suspect child abuse. Do not ask the child if he has been abused. To do so when others are around could produce stress too great for the injured child to handle.

If you are suspicious about the mechanism of injury, transport the child even though the severity of injury may not warrant such action. Have the parents or care giver follow you to the hospital to keep them separate if necessary.

ALWAYS report your suspicions to the emergency department staff and in accordance with local policies. Every medical facility should take action to see if your fears are well founded. If you fear that the medical staff has not taken you seriously, then you must report your suspicions to the juvenile authorities of the local police department. In some states, EMT-Bs are mandatory reporters; that is, they are required by law to report suspicions of child abuse. Be familiar with your state laws. Even if reporting possible child abuse is not a legal requirement in your state, it is a professional obligation.

Documentation Tip—Child Abuse

Keep accurate records of possible child abuse. State all your objective findings, but do not conclude that there is abuse. Draw a picture to indicate the size and location of all the child's injuries. Do not assume the cause of an injury (e.g., a cigarette burn). Instead, provide a detailed description of the injury site.

Maintain patient and family confidentiality. You cannot name the child or the family or give any details concerning the family to anyone other than the medical staff, the police, or your superior officer. Follow department requirements and state laws in reporting the problem.

Past responses can be checked and future responses noted in case a pattern develops to indicate possible abuse. However, even when talking to your partner, the hospital staff, the police, and your superiors, use the terms "suspicious" and "possible." Do not call someone a child abuser. If you break confidentiality, you could be sued. Keep in mind that the courts can deal harshly with those who provide patient care and then violate the confidentiality of the patient, the family, and the home. Keep in mind that rumors about abuse may, in the long run, cause mental or physical harm to your child patient.

It may be difficult, but keep in mind that the parent or care giver needs help also. Your actions, response, and concern directed toward the suspected abuser can help them recognize their problem and may encourage them to seek therapy and rehabilitation. Also bear in mind that your suspicions may be unfounded. Not every injury to a child is the result of child abuse. Suspicions should be aroused not by individual injuries but by the patterns of injuries and behavior that have been discussed above.

INFANTS AND CHILDREN WITH SPECIAL NEEDS

Over the years, medical expertise has improved significantly, allowing many children who would formerly have died to live. The group of children with special needs includes

- Premature infants with lung disease
- Infants and children with heart disease
- Infants and children with neurological disease
- Children with chronic disease or altered function from birth

Often these children are able to live at home with their parents. This means that you may receive calls to care for children who have complicated medical problems and are dependent on various technologies. The children's parents will be familiar with the various devices and can serve as a valuable resource. Some of the more common devices you might find include tracheostomy tubes, home artificial ventilators, central intravenous lines, gastrostomy tubes and gastric feeding, and shunts.

Tracheostomy Tubes

Tracheostomy tubes are tubes that have been placed into the child's trachea to create an open airway. They are often used when a child has been on a ventilator for a prolonged time. Although there are various types of tubes, the potential complications are identical. You may be called to help when there is

- Obstruction
- Bleeding from the tube or around the tube
- An air leak around the tube

- An infection
- A dislodged tube

Your emergency care will consist of

- Maintaining an open airway
- Suctioning the tube as needed
- Allowing the patient to remain in a position of comfort, perhaps on the parent's lap
- Transporting the patient to the hospital

Home Artificial Ventilators

Artificial ventilators in the home are becoming more common. The parents will be trained in its use but will call EMS when there is trouble. Regardless of the problem, your emergency care will include

- Maintaining an open airway
- Artificially ventilating with a bag-valve mask with oxygen
- Transporting the patient

Central Intravenous Lines

Central lines are intravenous lines that are placed close to the heart. Unlike most peripheral IV lines, central lines may be left in place for long-term use. Possible complications of central lines are

- Infection
- Bleeding
- Clotting-off of the line
- Cracked line

Your emergency care will include

- Applying pressure if there is bleeding
- Transporting the patient

Gastrostomy Tubes and Gastric Feeding

Gastrostomy tubes are tubes placed through the abdominal wall directly into the stomach. These are used when a patient is not able to be fed orally. The most dangerous potential problem involves respiratory distress. The emergency care will include

- Being alert for altered mental status in diabetic patients. They may become hypoglycemic quickly when unable to eat.

- Assuring an open airway
- Suctioning the airway as needed
- Providing oxygen if needed
- Transporting the patient in either a sitting position or lying on the right side with the head elevated to reduce the risk of aspiration

Shunts

A shunt is a drainage device that runs from the brain to the abdomen to relieve excess cerebrospinal fluid. There will be a reservoir on the side of the skull. Should the shunt malfunction, pressure inside the skull will rise, causing an altered mental status. An altered mental status may also be caused by an infection. These patients are prone to respiratory arrest. Your emergency care will include

- Maintaining an open airway
- Ventilating with a bag-valve mask and high concentration oxygen if needed
- Transporting the patient

THE EMT-B'S RESPONSE TO PEDIATRIC EMERGENCIES

We have discussed many types of pediatric illnesses and injuries and their emergency care. Our focus has been on the patient. Now we will look at the psychological responses of the EMT-B.

It is well known that pediatric calls can be among the most stressful for the EMT-B, even when they are uneventful. EMT-Bs who have children often identify their patients with their own children. Other EMT-Bs have no experience with children and feel anxiety about communicating with them and treating them—even about estimating their ages. However, the skills of communicating with and treating children can be learned and applied. Often the EMT-B who starts out "knowing nothing about children" turns out to have a real knack for dealing with them.

Most of the care of children consists of applying what you have learned about the care of adult patients with knowledge of the key differences in developmental characteristics, anatomy, and physiology of children.

Often the most serious stresses an EMT-B faces result from pediatric calls that involve a very sick, injured, or abused child, or a child who has died or who dies during or after emergency care. Such calls are, fortunately, rare, and can be prepared for with advance training.

When you have had an experience like this, talk with other EMT-Bs. If your squad or service has a counselor, see this person for advice. You may think that you can handle the stress or sorrow by yourself, but experienced EMT-Bs know better. Unless you resolve the impact of stressful events the problems created will compound, and could lead to "burn out." Contact your local Critical Incident Stress Debriefing (CISD) team for assistance after incidents such as these.

FYI

Topics included in the FYI—"For Your Information"—section are those that go beyond the chapter objectives. The information in this segment is intended to broaden your understanding of the chapter topic but is not essential to an understanding of your job as an EMT-B.

Among the diseases that children sometimes suffer are croup, epiglottitis, and meningitis.

Croup and Epiglottitis

Croup (KROOP) is a group of viral illnesses that cause inflammation of the larynx, trachea, and bronchi (Figure 29-11). It is typically an illness of children 6 months to about 4 years of age that often occurs at night. This problem sometimes follows a cold or other respiratory infection. Tissues in the airway (particularly the upper airway) become swollen and restrict the passage of air.

Patient Assessment—Croup

Signs

During the day, the child usually will have

☐ Mild fever
☐ Some hoarseness

At night, the child's condition will worsen and he or she will develop

☐ A loud "seal bark" cough
☐ Difficulty breathing
☐ Signs of respiratory distress including nasal flaring, retraction of the muscles between the ribs, tugging at the throat

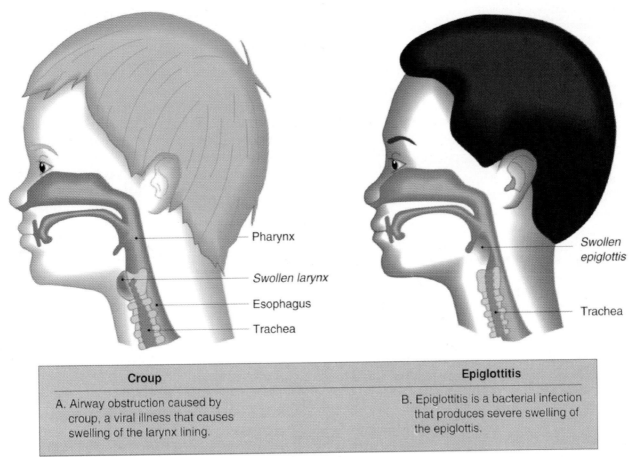

Croup

A. Airway obstruction caused by croup, a viral illness that causes swelling of the larynx lining.

Pharynx
Swollen larynx
Esophagus
Trachea

Epiglottitis

B. Epiglottitis is a bacterial infection that produces severe swelling of the epiglottis.

Swollen epiglottis
Trachea

FIGURE 29-11 Comparing the airway in croup and epiglottitis.

☐ Restlessness
☐ Paleness with cyanosis

Patient Care—Croup

Emergency Care Steps

1 Place the patient in a position of comfort (usually sitting up).
2 Administer high concentration oxygen. When possible, this should be from a humidified source.
3 Walking to the ambulance in the cool night air may provide relief as the cool air reduces the edema in the airway tissues.
4 Do not delay transport unless ordered to do so by medical direction.

Epiglottitis (ep-i-glo-TI-tis) is most commonly caused by a bacterial infection that produces swelling of the epiglottis and partial airway obstruction (Figure 29-11). The typical patient will be between 3 and 7 years old.

Patient Assessment—Epiglottitis

Signs

☐ A sudden onset of high fever
☐ Painful swallowing (the child often will drool to avoid swallowing)
☐ The patient will assume a "tripod" position, sitting upright and leaning forward with the chin thrust outward (sniffing position) and the mouth wide open in an effort to maintain a wide airway opening.
☐ The patient will sit very still, but the muscles will work hard to breathe, and the child can tire quickly from the effort.
☐ The child appears more generally ill than with croup.

Note: All cases of epiglottitis must be considered to be life threatening, no matter how early the detection.

Patient Care—Epiglottitis

Emergency Care Steps

1. Immediately transport the child, sitting on the parent's lap. This is a TRUE EMERGENCY.
2. Provide high concentration oxygen from a humidified source. Do not increase the child's anxiety. If he or she resists the mask, let the parent hold it in front of the child's face.
3. Constantly monitor the child for respiratory distress or arrest and be ready to resuscitate.
4. DO NOT PLACE ANYTHING INTO THE CHILD'S MOUTH, including a thermometer, tongue blade, or oral airway. To do so may set off spasms along the upper airway that will totally obstruct the airway.

Note: The child will not want to lie down and you should not force him to do so. The child must be handled gently, since rough handling and stress could lead to a total airway obstruction from spasms of the larynx and swelling tissues.

Meningitis

Meningitis (men-in-JI-tis) is caused by either a bacterial or a viral infection of the lining of the brain and spinal cord (the meninges). The majority of meningitis cases occur between the ages of 1 month and 5 years.

Patient Assessment—Meningitis

Signs and Symptoms

- ☐ High fever
- ☐ Lethargy
- ☐ Irritability
- ☐ Headache
- ☐ Stiff neck
- ☐ Sensitivity to light
- ☐ In infants, the fontanelles may be bulging unless the child is dehydrated.
- ☐ Movement is painful and the child does not want to be touched or held.
- ☐ Sudden excitement may cause seizures.
- ☐ A rash may be present in the bacterial type infection.

Patient Care—Meningitis

It is most important to carefully take appropriate body substance isolation precautions.

Emergency Care Steps

1. Monitor airway, breathing, circulation, and vital signs.
2. Provide high concentration oxygen by non-rebreather mask.
3. Ventilate with a bag-valve mask with supplemental oxygen if necessary.
4. Provide CPR if necessary.
5. Be alert for seizures.
6. Transport immediately. This is a TRUE EMERGENCY. Do not delay.

Safety Note

All EMS personnel should immediately get a follow-up evaluation by a physician after any call where meningitis is suspected.

CHAPTER REVIEW

SUMMARY

For the most part, treatment for the illnesses and injuries of infants and children is like the treatment for adults. However, children do have some special developmental characteristics and characteristics of anatomy and physiology. To treat infants and children effectively, you will need to know something about these special characteristics of children and the illnesses and injuries to which infants and children are prone.

1. Describe key differences in the anatomy and physiology of infants and children with regard to

   - the head
   - the airway and respiratory system
   - the chest
   - the abdomen
   - the body surface
   - blood volume

2. Describe how each of the differences you named for question 1, above, will affect your assessment or treatment of the infant or child patient.

3. Describe ways of calming and interacting effectively with the infant or child patient. With the parent or care giver.

4. Explain some of the elements of a general impression of the infant or child patient that you can form "from the doorway"—before you approach the patient.

5. Explain how to differentiate between an upper airway obstruction and a lower airway disease or disorder. Explain how and why the two should be treated differently.

6. Explain the main steps of emergency treatment for any infant or child trauma patient.

7. Explain how suspicion of child abuse should or should not affect the care you provide for an infant or child patient. Explain how you are expected to report such suspicions in your state or local system.

Application

- You are called to respond to a sick child. As you come down the hall toward the apartment door, you hear crying and loud voices. When you enter the apartment, you see a toddler sitting on the kitchen floor bleeding from what appears to be a severely cut hand. Several adults—parents and aunts and uncles—are milling about, extremely upset, with everyone talking and arguing at the top of their lungs and no one actually tending to the child. The adults are yelling and crying and so is the patient. How should you manage the situation?

Module 7

Operations

IN THIS MODULE

MODULE OVERVIEW

In previous modules you have learned about the assessment and care of adult and pediatric patients. This module deals with nonmedical operations and organization for the day-to-day conduct of your job as an EMT-Basic as well as for certain special situations.

Chapter 30 will lead you through the sequence of tasks you will perform before, during, and after an ambulance call—from the moment you report for duty at the beginning of your shift until the ambulance is back in quarters at the end of the last call of your day.

In Chapter 31, you will learn how access is gained to entrapped patients and about your role as an EMT-B at the scene of a vehicle collision.

In every other chapter of this textbook, you have learned how to act as an EMT-B in dealing with a single patient or the occupants of a single vehicle. Chapter 32 will cover multiple-casualty incidents—those that may involve large numbers of patients—including emergencies that involve the leakage of hazardous materials onto surfaces or into the atmosphere.

This is the final required module of the EMT-Basic course.

Ambulance Operations

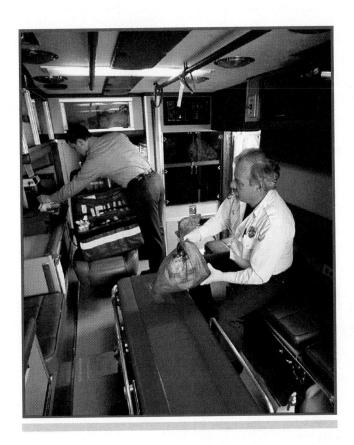

By this time in your EMT-Basic course you have learned most of the prehospital assessment and treatment that you will learn until you actually begin riding on an ambulance gaining field experience. This chapter covers the "nuts and bolts" of an ambulance call.

Objectives

On the Scene

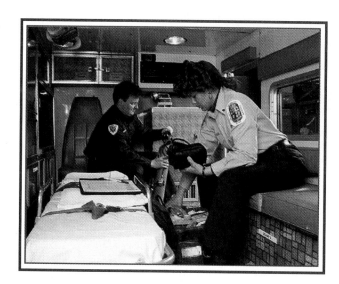

06:00 seems a little earlier than usual this particular morning. At the change of shifts for your ambulance squad, the two crews converse as they usually do. It's been a quiet night . . . only one minor call. As the night crew is about to leave, one of them says, "The rig should be in pretty good shape. We didn't use anything last night."

After pouring a cup of coffee, you and your more experienced partner head for the garage.

Your partner: Sounds like the rig is in pretty good shape. But let's check it over and then grab some breakfast.
You: You go ahead. I had a bite before I left home. I'll check the rig.
Your partner: Thanks, but let's do it together . . . and then we'll have a couple of those donuts I picked up on the way in.
You: Fair enough.

While checking the rig, you find a few important things missing. The portable oxygen tank is empty, and there are no nonrebreather masks on board. Checking the ambulance turns out to have been a good idea, because before you and your partner can get to those donuts, a cardiac call comes in. If you

6. Discuss "Due Regard For Safety of All Others" while operating an emergency vehicle. (p. 664)

7. State what information is essential in order to respond to a call. (pp. 642–643)

8. Discuss various situations that may affect response to a call. (pp. 646–647)

9. Differentiate between the various methods of moving a patient to the unit based upon injury or illness. (pp. 649–651)

10. Apply the components of the essential patient information in a written report. (pp. 651, 652, 654)

11. Summarize the importance of preparing the unit for the next response. (p. 654)

12. Identify what is essential for completion of a call. (pp. 654–661)

13. Distinguish among the terms cleaning, disinfection, high-level disinfection, and sterilization. (pp. 657–660)

14. Describe how to clean or disinfect items following patient care. (p. 660)

15. Explain the rationale for appropriate report of patient information. (pp. 651, 652, 654)

16. Explain the rationale for having the unit prepared to respond. (p. 654)

and your partner hadn't been careful to check the ambulance, the implications could have been severe!

Cleaning, restocking, and maintaining the ambulance are not, by far, the most exciting parts of EMS, but the possible consequences of not doing these tasks properly are too grim to contemplate. Imagine not having oxygen at a cardiac call, or finding a patient hemorrhaging and not having materials for a pressure bandage, or disposable gloves, mask, and eye wear for infection control! You're glad you ignored the night crew's assurances and restocked the ambulance this morning. You know it won't be the last time you'll be glad you took this part of your job seriously.

Your responsibilities as an EMT-B may differ somewhat depending on the type of service you join. However most of the non-medical operational responsibilities can be broken into the following five phases.

- Preparing for the ambulance call
- Receiving and responding to a call
- Transferring the patient to the ambulance
- Transporting the patient to the hospital
- Terminating the call.

PREPARING FOR THE AMBULANCE CALL

The modern ambulance has come a long way from its primitive beginnings. It is far more than just a vehicle for transporting a patient to the hospital. Today's ambulance is a well-equipped and efficiently organized mobile pre-hospital emergency department and communications unit.

The U. S. Department of Transportation has issued specifications for Type I, Type II, and

Type III ambulances. Because of the extra equipment placed on ambulances in the 1990s for specialty rescue, advanced life support, and hazardous materials operations, the gross vehicle weight has been easily exceeded in some communities. This has made way for the introduction of a medium-duty truck chassis built for rugged durability and large storage and work areas (Figure 30-1). As patient needs and mandates evolve, the standards for ambulances will also continue to evolve.

Ambulance Supplies and Equipment

An ambulance is just another truck if it does not have the proper equipment for patient care and transportation. Following are lists of supplies and equipment that should be carried in an ambulance. The lists are based on recommendations of the American College of Surgeons and various ambulance services.

Basic Supplies for Infection Control and Patient Comfort and Protection

The following supplies should be carried in the ambulance.

- Two pillows
- Four pillow cases
- Two spare sheets
- Four blankets
- Six disposable emesis bags or basins
- Two boxes of facial tissues
- Disposable bedpan, urinal, and toilet paper
- A package of drinking cups
- One package of wet wipes
- Four liters of sterile water or saline
- Four soft restraining devices (upper and lower extremities)
- Packages of large and small red biohazard bags for waste or severed parts
- A package of large yellow bags for used linens or garbage (or otherwise color-coded or labeled according to your service's Exposure Control Plan)
- EPA-registered, intermediate-level disinfectant (which destroys mycobacterium tuberculosis)
- EPA-registered, low-level disinfectant such as Lysol
- An empty plastic spray bottle with lines at the 1:100 levels, a plastic bottle of water, and a plastic bottle of bleach for cleaning

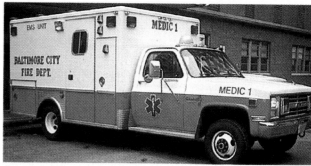

A.

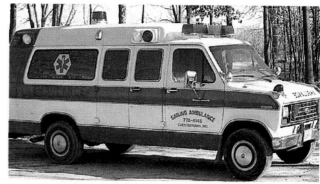

B.

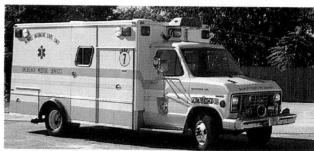

C.

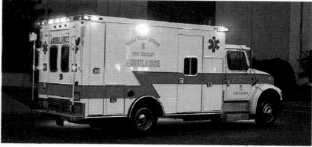

D.

FIGURE 30-1 A. Type I ambulance. B. Type II ambulance. C. Type III ambulance. D. Medium-duty ambulance.

up blood spills (Measure a fresh mixture of 1 part bleach to 100 parts water each day as needed)
- Eye shields or other protective eye wear for each crew member

- Sharps container for the vehicle (and the ALS unit) and the drug box if an ALS Unit
- Disposable latex, vinyl, or other synthetic gloves: a box of each size
- HEPA mask for each crew member

Initial and Focused Assessment Equipment

Portable kits or first-in kits come in all shapes and sizes with either hard cases or soft bags. When designing a first-in kit, keep in mind the steps of the initial assessment and the focused medical or trauma exam, which are aimed at detection and immediate treatment of life-threatening conditions and assessment of vital signs. Include supplies for

- *Airway*—airways, suction, infection control, personal protective equipment; if permitted for EMT-B use by local protocols, equipment for adult and pediatric orotracheal
- *Breathing*—stethoscope, pocket mask with one way valve, bag-valve mask, oxygen, oxygen delivery devices
- *Circulation*—blood pressure cuff, bandages and dressings, occlusive dressings, pneumatic anti-shock garment, AED (automated external defibrillator)
- *Neck and spine stabilization*—set of rigid cervical collars
- *Exposure*—scissors and blankets to expose and deal with exposure
- *Vital signs*
  — Sphygmomanometer kit with separate cuffs for average-sized and obese adults as well as child sizes
  — An adult and a pediatric stethoscope
  — Thermometer and a hypothermia thermometer that goes down to at least 82 degrees Fahrenheit
  — A penlight
  — A portable pulse oximeter with adult and child finger probes (optional)

Equipment for Transfer of Patient

The following carrying devices should be included.

- The wheeled ambulance stretcher is designed so that a sick or injured person can be transported in the sitting, supine, or Trendelenberg positions. Also called a cot or gurney, the wheeled stretcher should have a number of features. It should be adjustable in height and have detachable supports for intravenous fluid containers. Restraining devices should be provided so that a patient can be prevented from falling off the stretcher or sliding past the foot end or head end.
- A Reeves stretcher for carrying a patient who must lie supine down stairs when a cot is too heavy or wide
- A folding stair chair for moving patients down stairs in a sitting position
- A scoop stretcher, also called an orthopedic stretcher, for picking up patients found in tight spaces with a minimum of movement
- A Stokes or basket stretcher for long-distance carries, high-angle, or off-the-road rescues.
- A child safety seat (optional) for transporting infants and small children in the ambulance

Equipment for Airway Maintenance, Ventilation, and Resuscitation

A number of devices should be carried for maintaining an open airway and assisting breathing.

- Oropharyngeal airways in sizes suitable for adults, children, and infants
- Soft rubber nasopharyngeal airways in sizes 14 through 30
- Two pocket face masks with one-way valves and filters for times when ventilation is necessary or when you are the only person ventilating a patient who does not have an endotracheal tube inserted
- Three manually operated, self-refilling bag-valve-mask units (one infant, one child and one adult) capable of delivering 100% oxygen to a patient by the addition of a reservoir. Masks of various sizes should be designed to ensure a tight face seal and should have an air cushion. The masks should be clear so that you can see vomitus and the clouding caused by exhalations during breathing.

Oxygen Therapy and Suction Equipment

It is recommended that an ambulance be provided with two oxygen supply systems (one fixed and one portable) so that oxygen can be supplied to two patients simultaneously.

- The fixed oxygen delivery system supplies oxygen to a patient within the ambulance. A typical installation consists of a minimum 3,000-liter reservoir, a two-stage regulator, and the necessary yokes, reducing valve, non-gravity-type flowmeter. The oxygen delivery tubes, transparent masks, and controls should all be located within easy reach when you are sitting at the patient's head. The system should be capable of delivering at least 15 liters of oxygen per minute, and the system must be adaptable to the bag-valve-mask units carried on the ambulance.
- Two portable oxygen delivery systems that have a capacity of at least 350 liters. Each system should have a regulator capable of delivering at least 15 liters of oxygen per minute. Many ambulances are equipped with multiple function regulators that can be used for liter flow oxygen, suctioning, and positive pressure ventilation.
- Spare D, E, or jumbo D oxygen cylinders with a current hydrostat test date seal imprinted in the tank
- Six adult and four pediatric nonrebreather masks
- Six adult and four pediatric nasal cannulas
- A flow-restricted, oxygen-powered ventilation device
- An automatic transport ventilator (ATV—optional)
- A plastic comic cup for administering blow-by oxygen to a child
- The fixed suction system should be sufficient to provide an air flow of over 30 liters per minute at the end of the delivery tube. A vacuum of at least 300 mmHg should be reached within 4 seconds after the suction tube is clamped. The suction should be controllable. The installed system should have a large-diameter, nonkinking tube fitted with a rigid tip. There should be a spare nonbreakable, disposable suction bottle, and a container of water for rinsing the suction tubes. There should be an assortment of sterile catheters. The suction system should be capable of being used by you as you are seated at the head of the patient.
- The portable suction unit can be one of the many models powered by battery, hand or foot action, oxygen, or compressed air. The unit should be fitted with a nonkinking tube as well as a large-bore Yankauer tip.

Equipment for Assisting with Cardiac Resuscitation

The following equipment for assisting with cardiopulmonary resuscitation and defibrillation should be carried on the ambulance.

- Short or long spine board to provide rigid support during CPR efforts
- An AED
- The mechanical CPR compressor (e.g., Thumper)—especially helpful for doing CPR for services with transports over 15 minutes to the hospital (optional)

Supplies and Equipment for the Immobilization of Suspected Bone Injuries

A well-equipped ambulance carries a variety of devices that can be used to immobilize painful, swollen, or deformed extremities and suspected spine injuries.

- Adult and pediatric traction splints (e.g., Sager or Hare) for the immobilization of a painful, swollen, or deformed thigh
- A number of padded board splints for the immobilization of upper and lower extremities. Recommended are two 3 × 54-inch splints, two 3 × 36-inch splints, and two 3 × 15-inch splints.
- A variety of splints: air-inflatable splints, vacuum splints, wire ladder splints, cardboard splints, soft rubberized splints with aluminum stays and Velcro fasteners, padded aluminum (SAM) splints, and splints that are inflated with cryogenic (cold) gas
- A number of tongue depressors to use to immobilize broken fingers
- Triangular bandages for use with splints and for making slings and swathes
- Several rolls of self-adhering roller bandage for securing the various splints
- 6 chemical cold packs for use on painful, swollen, or deformed extremities
- Two long spine boards for full-body immobilization, preferably with speed clips or Velcro straps. The long spine board can also be used for patient transfer
- Rigid cervical collars in a variety of adult and child sizes
- A KED, XP1, Kansas Board, or LSP board for seated persons who have possible spinal injuries

- Six 9-foot-by-2-inch web straps with aircraft-style buckles or D-rings for securing patients to carrying devices
- Head immobilizer device such as the Headbed, Bashaw CID, Ferno Head Immobilizer, or a rolled blanket

Supplies for Wound Care and Treatment of Shock

A variety of the following dressings and bandaging materials should be carried on the ambulance.

- Sterile gauze pads (2 × 2 inches and 4 × 4 inches)
- 5 × 9 inch combine dressings
- Sterile universal dressings (multi-trauma dressing) approximately 10 × 36 inches
- Self-adhering roller bandages in 4 and 6 inch width × 5 yards
- Occlusive dressings (Vaseline gauze) for the sealing of sucking chest wounds and eviscerations
- Aluminum foil (sterilized in separate package) for various uses such as occlusive dressing and also to maintain body heat or to form an oxygen tent for a newborn infant
- Sterile burn sheets or prepackaged burn kit
- Adhesive strip bandages for minor wound care (1 × 3/4 inch and 1 × 1/2 inch), individually packaged
- Hypoallergenic adhesive tape (1 and 3 inch rolls)
- Large safety pins for the securing of slings and swathes
- Bandage scissors
- Pneumatic anti-shock garments (PASG). These should be in sizes for adults and children.
- Aluminum blankets (survival blankets) for maintaining body heat

Supplies for Childbirth

A sterile childbirth kit should be carried. In some areas, ambulances carry kits provided by local medical facilities. In other areas, ambulances are provided with commercially available disposable obstetric kits that should contain the following.

- Several pairs of sterile surgical gloves
- Four umbilical cord clamps or umbilical tape

- One pair of sterile surgical scissors
- A rubber bulb syringe (3 oz.)
- Twelve 4 × 4 inch gauze pads
- Four pairs of sterile disposable gloves
- Five towels
- A baby blanket (receiving blanket)
- Infant swaddler
- Sanitary napkins
- Two large plastic bags
- Two stockinette infant caps

In addition, an ambulance should be provided with items that you can wear to minimize contamination of or by the mother and baby during and after childbirth.

- Two surgical gowns
- Two surgical caps
- Two surgical masks
- Two pairs of goggles or eye shields

Supplies, Equipment, and Medications for the Treatment of Acute Poisoning, Snakebite, Chemical Burns, and Diabetic Emergencies

A number of poison control kits are available from emergency care equipment suppliers. Whether purchased intact or hand-made, a poison control kit should include these items.

- Drinking water that can be used to dilute poisons
- Activated charcoal
- Paper cups and other equipment for oral administration
- Equipment for irrigating a patient's eyes or skin with sterile water
- Constriction bands for snakebites
- Instant Glucose paste

Special Equipment for Paramedics and Physicians

Depending on state laws and your medical director, some ambulances are provided with locked kits of supplies and equipment that can be used by paramedics or physicians, especially in rural areas. This equipment may include supplies for

- Endotracheal intubation, orotracheal and endotracheal suctioning, and pediatric nasogastric intubation (In some areas EMT-Bs will be trained to perform these proce-

dures. See elective Chapter 33, Advanced Airway Management)
- Chest decompression
- Drug administration
- Advanced airways such as the esophageal obturator airway (EOA), esophageal gastric tube airway (EGTA), Combitube® airway, or pharyngo-tracheal lumen airway (PtL®)
- Cricothyrotomy
- Cardiac monitoring and defibrillation
- Supplies for medication administration
  — Epinephrine pens
  — Nitroglycerin pills
  — An inhaled bronchodilator

Miscellaneous and Safety Equipment

Ambulances should also be provided with personal protective equipment for you, equipment for warning, signaling and lighting, hazard control devices, and tools for gaining access and disentanglements, including

- The U. S. D.O.T. *Emergency Response Guidebook*
- Binoculars
- Clipboard, prehospital care reports (PCRs), and other documentation forms
- Ring cutter
- Portable radio
- Multiple casualty incident management logs
- Triage tags and destination logs
- Command vests
- Tarps in red, green, black and yellow for MCI field treatment areas
- Disposable Tyvek jumpsuits (optional)
- Flares
- Jumper cables
- Set of turnout gear (coat, helmet, protective eye wear, gloves) for each crew member
- Large floodlight/spotlight
- Concentrated Gatorade and a cooler for rehabilitation sector (optional)
- Self-contained breathing apparatus (SCBA—optional)
- Spring loaded center punch
- Glas-Master or flat head axe
- Small sledge hammer, prybar, Biel tool, and other tools for gaining access
- Wheel chocks
- Utility rope
- Stuffed animal for child patients

When you have an opportunity, compare the items listed in this chapter with the inventory of your ambulance. Learn where each item

is stored so that you can reach it quickly in any emergency situation. Learn what every item is for and when it should be used. If the item is a mechanical device, learn not only what it is for and when it should be used but also how it works and how it should be maintained.

Ensuring That the Ambulance is Ready for Service

The most modern well-equipped ambulance is not worth the room it takes up in the garage unless it is ready to respond at the time of an emergency. A state of readiness results from a planned preventive maintenance program that includes periodic servicing. Oil should be changed regularly, tires should be rotated, the vehicle should be lubricated, and so on.

Let us say that you and your partner have just reported for duty. As soon as it is practical, speak with the crew going off duty. Learn whether they experienced any problems with either the ambulance or its equipment during their shift. Make a thorough bumper-to-bumper inspection of the ambulance. Use the checklist provided by your service to do this.

Ambulance Inspection, Engine Off

Following are inspection steps that can be taken while the ambulance is in quarters.

1. Inspect the body of the vehicle. Look for damage that could interfere with safe operation. A crumpled fender, for example, may prevent the front wheels from turning the maximum distance.
2. Inspect the wheels and tires. The tires take a beating in normal operation. At collision scenes they may contact shards of glass and sharp pieces of metal and other debris. Check for damage or worn wheel rims and tire sidewalls. Check the tread depth. Use a pressure gauge to ensure that all tires are properly inflated. Don't forget to inspect the inside rear tires.
3. Inspect windows and mirrors. Look for broken glass and loose or missing parts. See that mirrors are clean and properly adjusted for maximum visibility.
4. Check the operation of every door and latches and locks.
5. Inspect the components of the cooling system. (**Warning**: Allow the engine to cool before removing any pressure caps.) Check

the level of the coolant. Inspect the cooling system hoses for leaks and cracks.

6. Check the level of the other vehicle fluids, including the engine oil and the brake, power steering, and transmission fluids.

7. Check the battery. If the battery has removable fill caps, check the level of the fluid. If the battery is the sealed type, determine its condition by checking the indicator port. Inspect the battery cable connections for tightness and signs of corrosion.

8. Inspect the interior surfaces and upholstery for damage and cleanliness.

9. Check the windows for operation. See that the interior surface of each window is clean.

10. Test the horn.

11. Test the siren for the full range of operations.

12. Check the seat belts. Examine each belt to see that it is not damaged. Pull each belt from its storage spool to ensure that the retractor mechanisms work. Buckle each belt to ensure that latches work properly.

13. Adjust the seat for comfort and optimum steering wheel and pedal operation.

14. Check the fuel level. An ambulance should be refueled after each call whenever practical.

Ambulance Inspection, Engine On

The next steps require you to start the engine. Pull the ambulance from quarters if engine exhaust fumes will be a problem. Set the parking brake, put the transmission in "park," and have your partner chock the wheels before undertaking the following steps.

1. Check the dash-mounted indicators to see if any light remains on to indicate a possible problem with oil pressure, engine temperature, or the vehicle's electrical system.

2. Check dash mounted gauges for proper operation.

3. Depress the brake pedal. Note whether pedal travel seems correct or excessive. Check air pressure as needed.

4. Test the parking brake. Move the transmission level to a drive position. Replace the level to the "park" position as soon as you are sure that the parking brake is holding.

5. Turn the steering wheel from side to side.

6. Check the operation of the windshield wipers and washers. The glass should be wiped clean each time the blade moves.

7. Turn on the vehicle's warning lights. Have your partner walk around the ambulance and check each flashing and revolving light for operation. Turn off the warning lights.

8. Turn on the other vehicle lights. Have your partner walk around the ambulance again, this time checking the headlights (high and low beams), turn signals, four-way flashers, brake lights, side and rear scene illumination lights, and box marker lights.

9. Check the operation of the heating and air-conditioning equipment. While you check the operation of the equipment in the driver's compartment, have your partner check the equipment in the patient compartment. This is also a good time for your partner to check the onboard suction if the engine is running.

10. Operate the communications equipment. Test portable as well as fixed radios and any radio-telephone communications.

Return the ambulance to quarters, and while you are backing up, have your partner note whether the backup alarm is operating (if the vehicle is so equipped).

Inspection of Patient Compartment Supplies and Equipment

Shut off the engine and complete your inspection by checking the patient compartment and all exterior cabinets.

1. Check the interior of the patient compartment. Look for damage to the interior surfaces and upholstery. Be certain that any needed decontamination has been completed and that the compartment is clean.

2. Check treatment supplies and equipment and rescue equipment. See that an item-by-item inspection of everything carried on the ambulance is done, with findings recorded on the inspection report.

Not only should items be identified during the ambulance inspection, they should also be checked for completeness, condition, and operation. The pressure of oxygen cylinders should be checked. Air splints should be inflated and examined for leaks. Oxygen and ventilation equipment should be tested for proper operation. Rescue tools should be examined for rust and dirt that may prevent them from working properly. Battery-powered devices should be operated to ensure that the batteries have a proper charge. Some equipment may require additional testing, for example the AED (see checklist in Chapter 18, Cardiac Emergencies).

When you are finished with your inspection of the ambulance and its equipment, complete the inspection report. Correct any deficiencies. Replace missing items. Make your supervisor aware of any deficiencies that cannot be immediately corrected.

Finally, clean the unit if necessary for infection control and appearance. Maintaining the ambulance's appearance enhances your organization's image in the public's eye. People who take pride in their work, show it by taking pride in the appearance of their ambulance.

RECEIVING AND RESPONDING TO A CALL

In many areas of the country, a person needs only to dial the universal number, 911, to access a community's ambulance service, fire department, or police department, 24 hours a day. A trained Emergency Medical Dispatcher (EMD) records information from callers, decides which service is needed, and alerts that service to respond. (Always say "nine-one-one" when talking to community or school groups. Children can't find "eleven" on the phone dial or key pad.)

The Role of the Emergency Medical Dispatcher

Many cities and communication centers have implemented training and certification of Emergency Medical Dispatchers (EMDs), based upon the medical priority card system, which originated in 1979 through the leadership of Jeffrey Clawson, M.D. An EMD is trained to perform the following tasks.

- To interrogate the caller and assign a priority to the call
- To provide prearrival medical instructions to callers and information to crews
- To dispatch and coordinate EMS resources
- To coordinate with other public safety agencies

When answering a call for help, the EMD must obtain as much information as possible about the situation that may help the responding crew. The questions the EMD should ask are

1. *What is the exact location of the patient?* The EMD must ask for the house or building number and the apartment number, if any. It is important to ask the street name with the direction designator (e.g., North, East), the nearest cross street, the name of the development or subdivision, and the exact location of the emergency.

2. *What is your call-back number? Stay on the line. Do not hang up until I (the EMD) tell you to.* In life-threatening situations, the EMD will offer instruction to the caller, after the units have been dispatched, that the caller or others on the scene should follow until the units arrive. It is also important for the caller to stay on the line in case a question arises about the location that was given.

3. *What's the problem?* This will provide the chief complaint. It will help the EMD decide which line of questioning to follow and the priority of the response to send.

4. *How old is the patient?* Most ambulances are set up to respond to the scene with a pediatric kit if the patient is a child rather than an adult. If pre-arrival CPR instructions are given, it will be necessary to distinguish between an infant, a child, and an adult.

5. *What's the patient's sex?* (if not obvious from caller's voice or information)

6. *Is the patient conscious?* An unconscious patient is a higher response priority.

7. *Is the patient breathing?* If the patient is conscious and breathing, the EMD will often ask many additional questions relative to the chief complaint to determine the appropriate level of response, for example first response, paramedics, or ambulance responding COLD (at normal speed—sometimes called Priority 3) or HOT (an emergency, lights-and-siren mode—sometimes called Priority 1). If the patient is not breathing, or the caller is not sure, the EMD will dispatch the maximum response and begin the appropriate pre-arrival instructions for a non-breathing patient, which may also involve telephone CPR if the patient is pulseless.

If the call is for a traffic collision, a series of key questions must be asked to help determine the priority and amount of response. With good interrogation of the caller, it may be possible for the EMD to appropriately dispatch one unit HOT and backup units COLD, which in turn will help prevent emergency vehicle collisions.

1. *How many and what kinds of vehicles are involved?* The EMD should determine, if possible, how many vehicles are involved in the collision and if they are cars, trucks or buses. Any injury resulting from a collision involving a bicycle, motorcycle, or pedestrian versus an automobile should receive the highest priority of response because of the mechanisms of injury involved. If the EMD learns that a truck is involved, he will try to determine if it is a vehicle which may be carrying a hazardous load.

2. *How many persons do you think are injured?* When the EMD learns from the caller that five people have been injured, then he may send two or three ambulances at the same time. Time, and perhaps lives, may be saved by knowing precisely the number of people injured in a vehicle collision.

3. *Do the victims appear trapped?* It may be necessary to dispatch a rescue unit also.

4. *What is the exact location of the collision?* You should be able to learn a street address or the name of the nearest cross street. If the collision has occurred in a rural or wilderness area, the EMD must try to pinpoint the location by asking questions about the nearest landmark visible from the caller's point of view (e.g. mileposts, water towers, large silos, or radio antennas). If the caller cannot pinpoint his location, the telephone company should be able to provide the location of the phone.

Next, the EMD should attempt to learn something about the scene by asking the caller additional questions. If the EMD learns that all lanes of a road leading to the collision scene are blocked, for example, operators can select alternative response routes.

5. *Is traffic moving?*
6. *How many lanes are open?*
7. *How far is traffic backed up?*
8. *Are any of the vehicles on fire?*
9. *Are any of the vehicles leaking fuel?*
10. *Are any electrical wires down?*
11. *Do any of the vehicles appear unstable? Is any vehicle on its side or top?*

12. *Does a truck appear to be carrying a hazardous cargo?*

This is how an EMD might dispatch an ambulance to the location of an injured person.

MEDCOM to Ambulance 621 and Medic 620, respond priority one to a 60-year-old unconscious male with breathing difficulty. The location is the Community Center at 1653 Central Ave. with Locust Park on the cross. Time now is 1645 hours.

The EMD will repeat the message to minimize any question as to its content and assure the ambulance has received the call.

Operating the Ambulance

If you will be driving an ambulance even occasionally, you should attend—or may be mandated to attend—an emergency vehicle operator training program that has both classroom and in-vehicle road sessions.

Being a Safe Ambulance Operator

To be a safe ambulance operator, you must

- Be physically fit. You should not have any impairment that prevents you from operating the ambulance, nor should you have any medical condition that might disable you while driving.
- Be mentally fit, with your emotions under control. Driving an ambulance is not a job for someone who gets turned on by lights and sirens!
- Be able to perform under stress.
- Have a positive attitude about your ability as a driver but not be an overly confident risk taker.
- Be tolerant of other drivers. Always keep in mind that people react differently when they see an emergency vehicle. Accept and tolerate the bad habits of other drivers without flying into a rage.
- Never drive while under the influence of alcohol, "recreational" drugs such as cocaine, medicines such as antihistamines, "pep pills," or tranquilizers.
- Never drive with a restricted license.
- Always wear your glasses or contact lenses if required for driving.

- Evaluate your ability to drive based on personal stress, illness, fatigue, or sleepiness.

Understanding the Law

Every state has statutes that regulate the operation of emergency vehicles. Although the wording of the laws may vary, the intent of the laws is essentially the same. Emergency vehicle operators are generally granted certain exemptions with regard to speed, parking, passage through traffic signals, and direction of travel. However, the laws also clearly state that *if an emergency vehicle operator does not drive with due regard for the safety of others, he must be prepared to pay the consequences for his actions—consequences such as tickets, law suits, or even time in jail.*

Following are some points usually included in typical state laws regulating the operation of ambulances.

- An ambulance operator must have a valid driver's license and may be required to have completed a training program.
- Privileges granted under the law to the operators of ambulances apply when the vehicle is responding to an emergency or is involved in the emergency transport of a sick or injured person. When the ambulance is not on an emergency call, the laws that apply to the operation of non-emergency vehicles also apply to the ambulance.
- Even though certain privileges are granted during an emergency, the exemptions granted do not provide immunity to the operator in cases of reckless driving or disregard for the safety of others.
- Privileges granted during emergency situations apply only if the operator used warning devices in the manner prescribed by law.

Most statutes allow emergency vehicle operators to

- Park the vehicle anywhere so long as it does not damage personal property or endanger lives.
- Proceed past red stop signals, flashing red stop signals, and stop signs. Some states require that emergency vehicle operators come to a full stop, then proceed with caution. Other states require only that an operator slow down and proceed with caution.

- Exceed the posted speed limit as long as life and property are not endangered.
- Pass other vehicles in designated no-passing zones after properly signaling, ensuring that the way is clear, and taking precautions to avoid endangering life and property. This does not include passing a school bus with its red lights blinking. Wait for the bus driver to clear the children and then turn off the red lights.
- With proper caution and signals, disregard regulations that govern direction of travel and turning in specific directions.

Should you ever become involved in an ambulance collision, the laws will be interpreted by the court based upon two key issues. *Did you use due regard for the safety of others?* and *Was it a true emergency?*

The requirement of due regard actually sets a higher standard for drivers of emergency vehicles than for the rest of the driving public. This is why it is not uncommon for there to be an investigation by the district attorney or grand jury, as well as your ambulance service, following a collision.

Most states reserve the emergency mode of operation for a true emergency, defined as one in which the best information you have available to you is that there is a possibility of loss of life or limb. When dispatched to a call, there is often not much information to go on, so a "collision" will get an emergency response. However, once you arrive and find that your patient is stable with no life-threatening injuries or conditions, it is no longer a true emergency. A lights-and-siren, high-speed response to the hospital in such a situation would be ruled illegal in most states.

The exemptions described here are just examples of those often granted to ambulance operators. Do not assume that they are granted in your state. Obtain a copy of your state's motor vehicle rules and regulations and study them carefully.

Using the Warning Devices

Safe emergency vehicle operation can be achieved only when the proper use of warning devices is coupled with sound emergency and defensive driving practices. It is important to note that studies have shown that other drivers do not see or hear your ambulance until it is within 50 to 100 feet of their vehicle. So never let the lights and siren give you a false sense of security.

The Siren   Although the siren is the most commonly used audible warning device, it is also the most misused. Consider the effects that sirens have on other motorists, patients in ambulances, and ambulance operators themselves.

- Motorists are less inclined to give way to ambulances when sirens are continually sounded. Many feel that the right-of-way privileges granted to ambulances by law are being abused when sirens are sounded.
- The continuous sound of a siren may cause a sick or injured person to suffer increased fear and anxiety, and his condition may worsen as stress builds up.
- Ambulance operators themselves are affected by the continuous sound of a siren. Tests have shown that inexperienced ambulance operators tend to increase their driving speeds from 10 to 15 miles per hour while continually sounding the siren. In some reported cases, operators using a siren were unable to negotiate curves that they could pass through easily when not sounding the siren. Sirens also affect hearing, especially if used for long periods of time with the siren speaker over the cab. The best placement for the speaker is in the grille of the vehicle.

Many states have laws that regulate the use of audible warning signals, and where there are no such statutes, ambulance organizations usually create their own operating procedures or policies. If your organization does not, you may find some of the following suggestions helpful when you think it necessary to use the siren during an ambulance call.

- *Use the siren sparingly, and only when you must.* Some states require the use of the siren at all times when the ambulance is responding in the emergency mode. Other states require it only when the operator is exercising any of the exemptions discussed above.
- *Never assume that all motorists will hear your signal.* Buildings, trees, and dense shrubbery may block siren sounds. Soundproofing keeps outside noises from entering vehicles, and radios or tape systems also decrease the likelihood that an outside sound will be heard.
- *Always assume that some motorists will hear your siren but ignore it.*
- *Be prepared for the erratic maneuvers of other drivers.* Some drivers panic when they hear a siren.
- *Do not pull up close to a vehicle and then sound your siren.* Such action may cause the driver to jam on his brakes so quickly that you will be unable to stop in time. Use the horn when you are close to a vehicle ahead.
- *Never use the siren indiscriminately, and never use it to scare someone.*

The Horn   The horn is standard equipment on all ambulances. Experienced operators find that in many cases the judicious use of the horn clears traffic as quickly as the siren. The guidelines for using a siren apply to the ambulance's horn as well.

Visual Warning Devices   Whenever the ambulance is on the road, night or day, the headlights should be on. This increases the visibility of the vehicle to other drivers. In some states headlights are now required of all vehicles in low visibility conditions or whenever the window wipers are in use. Alternating flashing headlights should be used only if they are attached to secondary head lamps. In most states it is illegal to drive at night with one headlight out.

Probably the most useful light is the one in the front vehicle hood. This is easily seen in the rearview mirror of another driver to get his attention if your siren has not yet alerted him. The lights on the front bumper in the grille are generally mounted too low to be effective. The large box lights found in the outermost corners of the box, or modular, should blink in tandem, or unison, rather than wigwagging or alternating. This helps the vehicle that is approaching from a distance identify the full size of your vehicle.

There is a lot of controversy about the use of strobes on ambulances. When planning the lighting package of an ambulance, check the research before making your decision. In general, it is wisest for the package to combine single beam bulbs and strobes rather than just one type of lighting system.

Four-way flashers and directional signals should not be used as emergency lights. This is very confusing to the public, as well as being illegal in some states. Drivers expect a vehicle with four-way flashers on to be traveling at a very slow speed. Additionally, the flashers disrupt the function of the directional signals.

When the ambulance is in the emergency response mode, either responding to the scene or responding to the hospital with a high priority patient, all the emergency lights should be used. The vehicle should be easily seen from 360 degrees.

In some communities, fire department ambulances still follow an old tradition of using their emergency lights when returning to the station. However, the practice of keeping emergency lights on is very confusing to the public. Don't be surprised if other drivers do not pull over when you are on an emergency run if they constantly see your ambulance with emergency lights on.

SAVE THE USE OF LIGHTS AND SIREN FOR LIFE– OR LIMB–THREATENING EMERGENCIES.

Speed and Safety

You are often told to drive slowly and carefully. At this point you may be inclined to say something like, "How will I ever get a seriously ill or injured person to a hospital if I poke along?" We are not suggesting that you "poke along." But do drive with these facts in mind.

- Excessive speed increases the probability of a collision.
- Speed increases stopping distance and so reduces the chance of avoiding a hazardous situation.

Remember that the laws in most states excuse you from obeying certain traffic laws only in a true emergency and only with due regard for the safety of others. Except in these circumstances, obey speed limits, stoplights and signs, yield signs, and other laws and posted limits. Approach intersections with caution, avoid sudden turns, and always properly signal lane changes and turns.

Be sure that the ambulance driver and all passengers wear seat belts whenever the ambulance is in motion.

Escorted or Multiple-Vehicle Responses

When the police provide an escort for an ambulance, there are additional hazards. Too often, the inexperienced ambulance operator follows the escort vehicle too closely and is unable to stop when the lead vehicle(s) make an emergency stop. Also, the inexperienced operator may assume that other drivers know his vehicle is following the escort. In fact, other drivers will often pull out in front of the ambulance just after the escort vehicle passes.

Because of the dangers involved with escorts, most EMS systems recommend no escorts unless the operator is not familiar with the location of the patient (or hospital) and must be given assistance from the police.

In cases of multiple-vehicle responses, the dangers can be the same as those generated by escorted responses, especially when the responding vehicles travel in the same direction, close together.

In multiple-vehicle responses, a great danger also exists when two vehicles approach the same intersection at the same time. Not only may they fail to yield for each other; other drivers may yield for the first vehicle but not the second. Obviously, great care must be used at intersections during multiple-vehicle responses.

Factors That Affect Response

Most ambulance collisions take place in seemingly safe conditions. A New York State study, based on 18 years of ambulance-collision statistics, shows that the typical ambulance collision happens on a dry road (60%) with clear weather (55%) during daylight hours (67%) in an intersection (72%). During this period there were 5,782 ambulance collisions which involved 7,267 injuries and 48 fatalities! Additionally, an ambulance response can be affected by several factors.

- *Day of the Week*—Weekdays are usually the days of heaviest traffic flow because people are commuting to and from work. In resort areas, weekend traffic may be heavier than weekday traffic.
- *Time of Day*—In major employment centers, traffic over major arteries tends to be heavy in all directions during commuter hours.
- *Weather*—Adverse weather conditions reduce driving speeds and thus increase response times. A heavy snowfall can temporarily prevent any response at all. Be careful to lengthen your following distance whenever there is decreased road grip due to inclement weather.

- *Road Maintenance and Construction*—The movement of vehicles can be seriously impeded by road construction and maintenance activities. Be aware of the road construction in your district and plan responses accordingly.
- *Railroads*—There are still more than a quarter-million grade crossings in the United States with many opportunities for traffic to be blocked by long, slow-moving freight trains. In some communities there actually needs to be a secondary response system on the other side of train tracks that split the town in half.
- *Bridges and Tunnels*—Traffic over bridges and through tunnels slows during rush hours. Collisions—including ambulance collisions—tend to occur when drivers forget that bridges freeze before roadways.
- *Schools and School Buses*—The reduced speed limits in force during school hours slow the flow of vehicles. An emergency vehicle should never pass a stopped school bus with its red lights flashing. Wait for the school bus driver to signal you to proceed by turning off the lights. In addition, emergency vehicles attract children, who often venture out into the street to see them. The operator of every emergency vehicle should slow down when approaching a school or playground. Obey the directions given by school crossing guards.

Selecting an Alternative Route

When it appears that an ambulance will be delayed in reaching a sick or injured person because of the above or other factors, the operator should consider taking an alternative route or requesting the response of another ambulance. You should plan for times when changing conditions affect response. Obtain detailed maps of your service area. On the maps, indicate usually troublesome traffic spots such as schools, bridges, tunnels, railroad grade crossings, and heavily congested areas. Also indicate temporary problems such as road and building construction sites and long- and short-term detours. Using another color, indicate alternative routes to areas where normal routes are often blocked. Indicate snow routes, and so on.

Hang one map in quarters and place another map in the ambulance. Then when you must travel past a problem area in response to an urgent call, you will be able to select an alternative route that will get you to your destination quickly and safely.

Positioning the Ambulance at the Scene of a Vehicle Collision

When responding to the scene of a vehicle collision, be sure to take all steps to size up the scene—assessing scene safety and establishing a danger zone—as described in Chapter 8, Scene Size-Up. Park at least 100 feet from the wreckage and on the same level and upwind to avoid any escaping hazardous liquids or fumes.

Park in front of the wreckage if you are the first emergency vehicle on the scene so that your warning lights can warn other approaching motorists before flares and other warning signals can be placed. If the scene has been secured when you arrive, park the ambulance beyond the wreckage to prevent having your expensive ambulance struck by oncoming traffic (see Scan 30-1).

Studies have been done that show that red revolving beacons attract drunk or tired drivers. Consider pulling off the road, turning off your headlights, and using just amber rear sealed beam blinkers that blink in tandem or unison to identify the size of your vehicle. Once the ambulance is parked, set its parking brake and firmly wedge wheel chocks under the tires in such a way that forward movement will be retarded if the ambulance is struck.

Before approaching the scene, be sure to perform a scene size-up and take all necessary body substance isolation and hazardous materials precautions.

TRANSFERRING THE PATIENT TO THE AMBULANCE

On most ambulance runs you will be able to reach a sick or injured person without difficulty, assess his condition, carry out emergency care procedures where he lies, and then transfer him to the ambulance. At times, dangers at the scene or the priority of the patient will dictate moving the patient before assessment and emergency treatments can be completed. Emergency and non-emergency patient moves were discussed in Chapter 6, Lifting and Moving Patients.

Parking the Ambulance

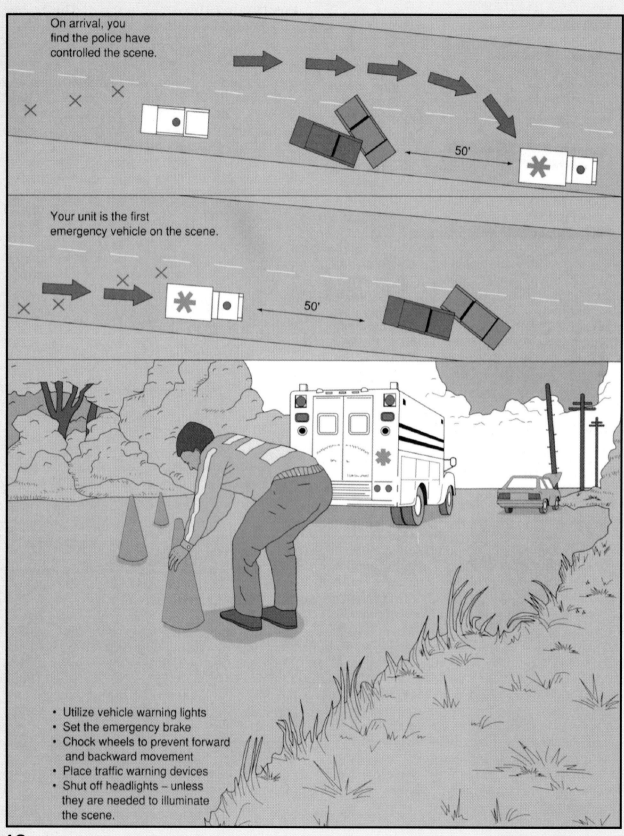

On arrival, you find the police have controlled the scene.

50'

Your unit is the first emergency vehicle on the scene.

50'

- Utilize vehicle warning lights
- Set the emergency brake
- Chock wheels to prevent forward and backward movement
- Place traffic warning devices
- Shut off headlights – unless they are needed to illuminate the scene.

When a spinal injury is suspected, the patient's head must be manually stabilized, a cervical collar must be applied, and the patient must be immobilized on a spine board. These techniques were discussed in Chapter 9, The Initial Assessment, Chapter 10, The Focused History and Physical Exam—Trauma Patient, and Chapter 28, Injuries to the Head and Spine.

Transfer to the ambulance is accomplished in four steps, regardless of the complexity of the operation.

1. Selecting the proper patient-carrying device
2. Packaging the patient for transfer
3. Moving the patient to the ambulance
4. Loading the patient into the ambulance

The wheeled ambulance stretcher is the most commonly used device for transferring the patient to the ambulance. This and other patient-carrying devices were listed above under ambulance equipment and discussed in Chapter 6, Lifting and Moving Patients.

Packaging refers to the sequence of operations required to ready the patient to be moved and to combine the patient and the patient-carrying device into a unit ready for transfer. A sick or injured patient must be packaged so that his condition is not aggravated. Necessary care for wounds and other injuries should be completed, impaled objects must be stabilized, and all dressings and splints must be checked before the patient is placed on the patient-carrying device. The properly packaged patient is covered and secured to the patient-carrying device.

Do not waste time packaging a badly traumatized patient. Whenever a patient is categorized as high priority, transport quickly. A neatly packaged corpse has not received optimal care.

Covering a patient helps to maintain body temperature, prevents exposure to the elements, and helps assure privacy (Figure 30-2). A single blanket or perhaps just a sheet may be all that is required in warm weather. A sheet and blankets should be used in cold weather. When practical, cuff the blankets under the patient's chin, with the top sheet outside. Do not leave sheets and blankets hanging loose. Tuck them under the mattress at the foot and sides of the stretcher. In wet weather, a plastic cover should be placed over the blankets during transfer. This can be removed once in the ambulance to prevent the patient from overheating. In cold or wet weather cover the patient's head, leaving the face exposed.

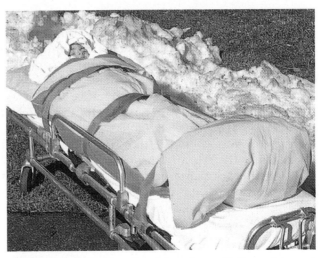

FIGURE 30-2 A patient "packaged" for cold, wet conditions.

A patient-carrying device should have a minimum of three straps for holding the patient securely to the device. The first strap should be at the chest level, the second at the hip or waist level, and the third on the lower extremities. Sometimes there is a fourth strap used if two are crossed at the chest.

All patients, including those receiving CPR, must be secured to the patient-carrying device before you attempt to transfer them to the ambulance.

If your patient is not on a carrying device such as a spine board but is just on the ambulance stretcher, some states, as a matter of policy, require shoulder harnesses that secure the patient to the stretcher to prevent him from sliding forward in case of a short stop.

TRANSPORTING THE PATIENT TO THE HOSPITAL

Activities during transport include far more than just driving the patient to the hospital. A series of tasks must be undertaken from the time a patient is loaded into the ambulance until he is handed over to emergency department personnel.

Preparing the Patient for Transport

The following activities may be required to prepare the patient for transport once he is in the ambulance.

- *Perform ongoing assessment.* Make sure that a conscious patient is breathing without difficulty once you have positioned him on the stretcher. If the patient is unconscious with an airway in place, make sure he has an adequate air exchange once you have moved him into position for transport.
- *Secure the stretcher in place in the ambulance.* Always ensure that the patient is safe during the trip to the hospital. Before closing the door, and certainly before signaling the ambulance operator to move, make sure that the cot is securely in place.

    Patient compartments are equipped with a locking device that prevents the wheeled ambulance stretcher from moving about while the ambulance is in motion. Failure to fully engage the locking device at both ends of the stretcher can have disastrous consequences once the ambulance is in motion.
- *Position and secure the patient.* During transfer to the ambulance, the patient must be firmly secured to a stretcher. This does not mean, however, that he must be transported to the hospital in that position. Positioning in the ambulance should be dictated by the nature of his illness or injury.
    - If he was not transferred to the ambulance in that position, shift an unconscious patient who has no potential spine injury, or one with an altered level of consciousness, into a position on his side that will promote maintenance of an open airway and the drainage of fluids.
    - Remember that the head and foot ends of the ambulance stretcher can be raised. A patient with breathing difficulty and no possibility of spinal injury may be more comfortable being transported in a sitting position. A patient in shock can be transported with the legs raised 8 to 12 inches.
    - A patient with potential spinal injury must remain immobilized on the long spine board, patient and board together being secured to the stretcher. If resuscitation is required, he must remain supine with constant monitoring of the airway and suctioning equipment ready. If resuscitation is not required, the unresponsive patient and spine board can be rotated as a unit and the board propped on the stretcher so that the patient is on his side for drainage of fluids and vomitus from the mouth.
    - Adjust the security straps. Security straps applied when a patient is being prepared for transfer to the ambulance may tighten unnecessarily by the time he is loaded into the patient compartment. Adjust straps so they still hold the patient safely in place but are not so tight that they interfere with circulation or respiration or cause pain.
- *Prepare for respiratory or cardiac complications.* If the patient is likely to develop cardiac arrest, position a short spine board or CPR board underneath the mattress prior to starting on the trip to the hospital. Then, if he does go into arrest, there will be no need to locate and position the board. Riding on a hard board may not be comfortable for a patient, but it is better that he suffer temporary discomfort than permanent injury or even death from delayed resuscitation efforts.
- *Loosen constricting clothing.* Clothing may interfere with circulation and breathing. Loosen ties and belts and open any clothing around the neck. Straighten clothing that is bunched under safety straps. Remember that clothing bunched at the crotch may be painful to the patient. Before you do anything to rearrange the clothing of a patient, however, tell him or her what you are going to do and why.
- *Check bandages.* Even properly applied bandages can loosen during transfer to the ambulance. Check each bandage to see that it is secure. Do not consider the problem of a loosened bandage lightly. Severe bleeding can resume when the pressure from a bandage is removed from a dressing, and if the wound site is covered with a sheet or blanket, bleeding may go unnoticed until the patient develops shock or is delivered to the hospital.
- *Check splints.* Immobilizing devices can also loosen during transfer to the ambulance. Inspect the bandages or cravats that hold board splints in place. Test air splints with your fingertip to see that they have remained properly inflated. Inspect traction devices to ensure that proper traction is still maintained. Check the splinted limb for distal motor and sensory function and circulation, and capillary refilling in infants and children. Remember that the safe

adjustment of splinting devices is virtually impossible when an ambulance is pitching about during the trip to a hospital, so complete this step before the ambulance moves unless immediate transport is required.

- *Load a relative or friend who must accompany the patient.* Consider the following guidelines if your service does not prohibit the transportation of a relative or friend with a sick or injured person: First, encourage the person to seek alternative transportation, if such is available. If there is just no other way the relative or friend can get to the hospital, allow him to ride in the passenger's seat in the operator's compartment—not in the patient's compartment where he may interfere with your activities. Make certain the person buckles his seat belt. If an uninjured child must come along, bring the family's child car seat and use it.
- *Load personal effects.* If a purse, briefcase, overnight bag, or other personal item is to accompany the patient, make sure it is properly secured in the ambulance. If you load personal effects at the scene of a vehicle collision, be sure to tell a police officer what you are taking. Follow the policies and fill out the forms, if any, required by your local system for safeguarding of personal effects.
- *Reassure the patient.* Apprehension often mounts in a sick or injured person after he is loaded in an ambulance. Not only is he held down by straps in a strange, confined space, but he may also be suddenly separated from family members and friends. Say a few kind words and offer a reassuring hand in a compassionate manner.

When you are satisfied that the patient is ready for transportation, signal the operator to begin the trip to the hospital. If this is a high priority patient, most of the preparation steps—loosening clothing, checking bandages and splints, reassuring the patient, even vital signs—can be done en route rather than delaying transport.

Infants and Children

Remember that a toy such as a stuffed teddy bear can do much to calm a frightened child. Many ambulance units carry a sanitized, soft or padded brightly colored toy in a compartment just for these occasions. It is

difficult at best to get information from a young child whose parents may have been injured and transported in another ambulance. Small children don't, as a rule, carry identification and you are a complete stranger in a hostile environment.

The crash scene, confusion, noise, injuries, possible pain, disappearance of a parent, EMT-Bs caring for injuries and gathering information all create a terrifying experience for a child. A female EMT-B or police officer may be helpful. Sometimes young children feel more comfortable talking to a woman. A smile and calm reassuring tone of voice are something that cannot be learned from a textbook, and they may be the most critical care needed by the frightened child.

Caring For The Patient en Route

At least one EMT-B in the patient compartment is minimum staffing for the ambulance—two is preferred.

Seldom will you be able to merely ride along with your patient. You may have to undertake a number of activities on the way to the hospital.

- *Notify the EMD that you are departing the scene.*
- *Continue to provide emergency care as required.* If life-support efforts were initiated prior to loading the patient into the ambulance, they must be continued during transportation to the hospital. Maintain an open airway, resuscitate, administer to the patient's needs, provide emotional support, and do whatever else is required, including updating your findings from the initial patient assessment effort.
- *Compile additional patient information.* If the patient is conscious and emergency care efforts will not be compromised, record patient information. Compiling information during the trip to the hospital serves two purposes. First, it allows you to complete your report. Second, supplying information temporarily takes your patient's mind off his problems. Remember, however, that this is not an interrogation session. Ask your questions in an informal manner.
- *Perform ongoing assessment and continue monitoring vital signs.* Keep in mind that changes in vital signs indicate a change in a patient's condition. For example, an unexplained increase in pulse rate may sig-

nify deepening shock. Record vital signs on your report form and be prepared to relate changes in vital signs to an emergency department staff member as soon as you reach the medical facility. Reassess vital signs every 5 minutes for an unstable patient, every 15 minutes for a stable patient.

- *Notify the receiving facility.* Transmit patient information and provide your estimated time of arrival and other information as discussed in Chapter 14, Communications.
- *Recheck bandages and splints.* Even though you checked bandages after loading the patient into the ambulance, check them again while in transit.
- *Collect vomitus if the patient becomes nauseated.* If he is not already in position, arrange the patient so that the chance of his aspirating vomitus is minimized. Be prepared to apply suction. Place an emesis basin or bag by his mouth. When he has finished vomiting, place a towel over the container and deliver it to emergency department personnel when you hand over the patient. Examination of the vomitus may be important to treatment, especially in cases of poisoning. Wear a mask, protective eye wear, and disposable gloves if your patient is vomiting.
- *Talk to the patient, but control your emotions.* Continued conversation is often soothing to a frightened patient.
- *Advise the ambulance operator of changing conditions.* No one likes a "back seat driver." However, there will be times when you must ask the ambulance operator to adjust speed or alter his driving technique to suit the needs of your patient. On the one hand, if what began as a routine transport develops into an emergency call, you may have to ask the operator to accelerate. On the other hand, if you think that swaying because of high speeds and uneven streets is detrimental to a patient's condition, have the operator slow down or take an alternative route.

   While the operator of an ambulance is responsible for his vehicle and the passengers carried in it, it is your responsibility to care for sick and injured persons; thus the operator should drive the ambulance according to your suggestions. The decision on use of lights and siren should always be made with the medical condition of the patient in mind.

- *If cardiac arrest develops, have the operator stop the ambulance while you apply and operate the AED.* Signal the operator to start up again once you have completed the shock sequence or determined that the patient does not have a shockable rhythm. Make certain that the emergency department is made aware of the arrest. If you routinely position a rigid device between the back of high-risk patients and the cot mattress, you have only to drop the cot back to a horizontal position and start CPR. If not, you must position an object like a short spine board or CPR board so that chest compression efforts will be effective.

   If the patient remains pulseless despite the AED, begin CPR. Local protocols may mandate intercept by an advanced-life-support team.

   You may want the ambulance operator to assist you with CPR or use of the AED while additional resources come to your aid. Use your judgment on this.

TRANSFERRING THE PATIENT TO THE EMERGENCY DEPARTMENT STAFF

The following are steps that you should take to see that the transfer of a patient to the care of emergency department personnel is accomplished smoothly and without incident. Brief as it may be, the transfer is a crucial step during which your primary concern must be the continuation of patient care activities. The steps of the transfer are illustrated in Scan 30-2.

- *In a routine admissions situation or when an illness or injury is not life-threatening, check first to see what is to be done with the patient.*

   If emergency department activity is particularly hectic, it might be better to leave your patient in the relative security and comfort of the ambulance while your operator determines where he is to be taken. Otherwise the patient may be subjected to distressing sights and sounds and perhaps be in the way. (If you do this, make sure an EMT-B remains with the patient at all times.) UNDER NO CIRCUMSTANCES SHOULD YOU SIMPLY WHEEL A NON-EMERGENCY PATIENT INTO A HOSPITAL, PLACE HIM IN A BED, AND LEAVE HIM!

Scan 30-2
Transferring the Patient

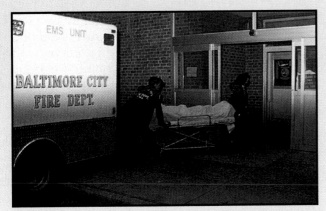

1. Transfer the patient as soon as possible. Stay with the patient until transfer is complete.

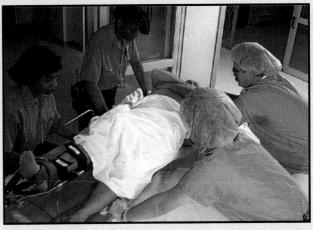

2. Assist the emergency department staff as required.

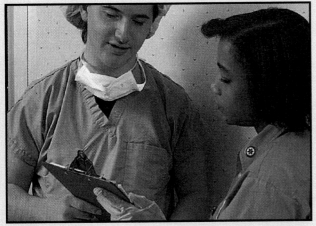

3. Transfer patient information as a verbal report and in a written prehospital care report.

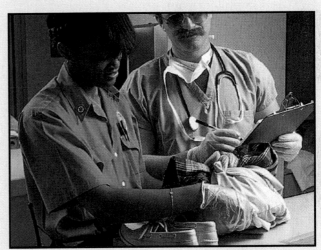

4. Transfer the patient's personal effects.

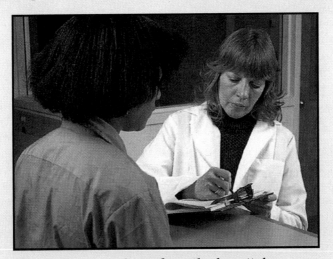

5. Obtain your release from the hospital.

This is an important point. Unless you transfer care of your patient directly to a member of the hospital staff, you may be open to a charge of abandonment.

Keep in mind that staff members may be treating other seriously ill and injured persons, so suppress any urge to demand attention for your patient. Simply continue emergency care measures until someone can assume responsibility for the patient. When properly directed, transfer the patient to a hospital stretcher. Transfer to the hospital stretcher was discussed in Chapter 6, Lifting and Moving.

- *Assist emergency department staff as required and provide a verbal report.* Stress any changes in the condition of the patient that you have observed.
- *As soon as you are free from patient care activities, prepare the prehospital care report.* Remember the job is not over till the paperwork is complete! Find a "quiet" spot and complete your prehospital care report. Preparation of a PCR was discussed in Chapter 15, Documentation.
- *Transfer the patient's personal effects.* If a patient's valuables or other personal effects were entrusted to your care, transfer them to a responsible emergency department staff member. Some services have policies that involve obtaining a written receipt from emergency department personnel as protection from a charge of theft.
- *Obtain your release from the hospital.* This task is not as formal as it sounds. Simply ask the emergency department nurse or physician if your services are still needed. In rural areas where not all hospital services are available, it may be necessary to transfer a seriously ill or injured person to another medical facility. If you leave and have to be recalled, valuable time will be lost.

TERMINATING THE CALL

An ambulance run is not really over until the personnel and equipment that comprise the prehospital emergency care delivery system are ready for the next response.

The functions of EMT-Bs in this final phase of activity include more than just changing the stretcher linen and cleaning the ambulance. A number of tasks must be accomplished at the hospital, during the return to quarters, and after arrival at the station.

At the Hospital

While still at the hospital, the ambulance crew should begin making the ambulance ready to respond to another call. Time, equipment, and space limitations sometimes preclude vigorous cleaning of the ambulance while it is parked at the hospital. However, you should make every effort to quickly prepare the vehicle for the next patient (Scan 30-3).

1. Quickly clean the patient compartment while wearing heavy duty rubber dishwashing-style gloves. Follow biohazard disposal procedures according to your agency's exposure control plan. Examples of biohazards are contaminated dressings and used suction catheters.

   - Clean up blood, vomitus, and other body fluids that may have soiled the floor. Wipe down any equipment that has been splashed. Place disposable towels used to clean up blood or body fluids directly in a red bag.
   - Remove and dispose of trash such as bandage wrappings, open but unused dressings, and similar items.
   - Sweep away caked dirt that may have been tracked into the patient compartment. When the weather is inclement, sponge up water and mud from the floor.
   - Bag dirty linens or blankets to be appropriately laundered.
   - Use a deodorizer to neutralize odors of vomit, urine, and feces. Various sprays and concentrates are available for this purpose.

2. Prepare respiratory equipment for service.

   - Clean and disinfect nondisposable, used bag-valve-mask units and other reusable parts of respiratory-assist and inhalation-therapy devices to keep them from becoming reservoirs of infectious agents that can easily contaminate the next patient. Disinfect the suction unit.
   - Place used disposable items in a plastic bag and seal it. Replace the items with similar ones carried in the ambulance as spares.

Scan 30-3
Actions That Can Be Taken at the Hospital

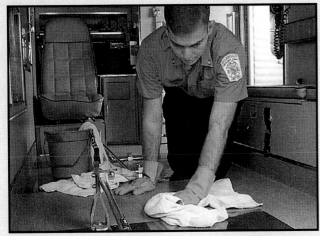

1. Clean the ambulance interior as required.

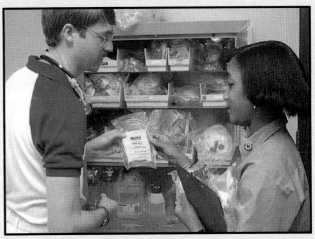

2. Replace respiratory equipment as required.

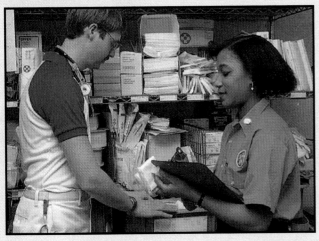

3. Replace expendable items per local policies.

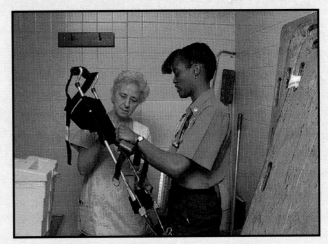

4. Exchange equipment per local policies.

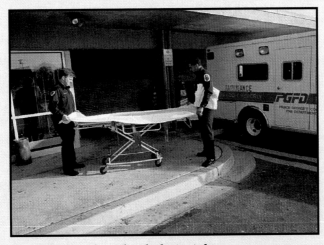

5. Make up the wheeled stretcher.

3. Replace expendable items.

- If you have a supply replacement agreement with the hospital, replace expendable items from the hospital storerooms on a one-for-one basis—items such as sterile dressings, bandaging materials, towels, disposable oxygen masks, disposable gloves, sterile water, and oral airways.
- Do not abuse this exchange program. Keep in mind that the constant abuse of a supplies-replacement program usually leads to its discontinuation. At the very least, abuse places a strain on ambulance-hospital relations.

4. Exchange equipment according to your local policy.

- Exchange items such as splints and spine boards. Several benefits are associated with an equipment exchange program: there is no need to subject patients to injury-aggravating movements just to recover equipment, crews are not delayed at the hospital, and ambulances can return to quarters fully equipped for the next response.
- When equipment is available for exchange, quickly inspect it for completeness and operability. Parts are sometimes lost or broken when an immobilizing device is removed from a patient.
- If you do find that a piece of equipment is broken or incomplete, notify someone in authority so the device can be repaired or replaced.

5. Make up the ambulance cot. The following procedure is one of many that can be used to make up a wheeled ambulance stretcher.

- Raise the stretcher to the high-level position, if possible; this makes the procedure easier. The stretcher should be flat with the side rails lowered and straps unfastened.
- Remove unsoiled blankets and pillow and place them on a clean surface.
- Remove all soiled linen and place it in the designated receptacle.
- Clean the mattress surface with an appropriate EPA-approved, low-level disinfectant unless there is visible blood, which should be cleaned up using a 1:100 bleach/water solution.
- Turn the mattress over; rotation adds to the life of the mattress.
- Center the bottom sheet on the mattress and open it fully. If a full-sized bed sheet is used, first fold it lengthwise.
- Tuck the sheet under each end of the mattress; form square corners and then tuck under each side.
- Place a disposable pad, if one is used, on the center of the mattress.
- Fully open the blanket. If a second blanket is used, open it fully and match it to the first blanket. This task should be done with an EMT-B at each end of the stretcher.
- Open a top sheet in the same way, placing it on top of the blanket. Fold the blanket(s) and top sheet together lengthwise to match the width of the stretcher; fold one side first, then the other.
- Tuck the foot of the folded blanket(s) and sheet under the foot of the mattress.
- Tuck the head of the folded blanket(s) and sheet under the head of the mattress.
- Place the slip-covered pillow lengthwise at the head of the mattress and secure it with a strap.
- Buckle the safety straps and tuck in excess straps.
- Raise the side rails and foot rest.

The stretcher is now ready for the next patient. It must be reemphasized that this is one of many techniques for preparing a wheeled ambulance stretcher for service. Whatever the method, it should meet the following objectives.

- Preparation for the next call should be done as soon and as quickly as possible.
- All linens, blankets, and pouches should be stored neatly on the stretcher.
- All linen and blankets should be folded or tucked so that they will be contained within the stretcher frame.
- The cot must be replaced in the ambulance.
- Any nondisposable patient care items should be replaced.
- A check should be made for equipment left in the hospital.

Note: A neatly prepared stretcher inspires the patient's confidence. Don't use stained linen, even though it might be clean. Always make the presentation of your stretcher a matter of personal and professional pride!

En Route to Quarters

Emphasis should be on a safe return. An ambulance operator may practice every suggestion for safe vehicle operation while en route to the hospital and then totally disregard those suggestions during the return to quarters. Defensive driving must be a full-time effort. Don't forget that the driver and all passengers must wear seat belts.

1. *Radio the EMD that you are returning to quarters and that you are available (or not available) for service.* Valuable time is lost if an EMD has to locate and alert a back-up ambulance when he does not know that a ready-for-service unit is on the road. Be sure that you notify the EMD if you stop and leave the ambulance unattended for any reason during the return to quarters.
2. *Air the ambulance if necessary.* If the patient just delivered to the hospital has an airborne communicable disease, or if it was not possible to neutralize disagreeable odors while at the hospital, make the return trip with the windows of the patient compartment partially open, weather permitting. If the unit has sealed windows, use the air-conditioning or ventilating system (do not set on recirculate) to air the patient compartment out.
3. *Refuel the ambulance.* Local policy usually dictates the frequency with which an ambulance is refueled. Some services require the operator to refuel after each call regardless of the distance traveled. In other services the policy is to refuel when the gauge reaches a certain level. At any rate, the fuel should be at such a level that the ambulance can respond to an emergency and then to the hospital without fear of running out.

In Quarters

When you return to quarters, there are a number of activities that need to be completed before the ambulance can be placed in service and before it is ready for another call (Scan 30-4).

With the emphasis today on protection from infectious diseases, you need to take every precaution to protect yourself. It is essential that you follow your service's exposure control plan, as discussed in detail in Appendix B, Infectious Diseases. Always wear gloves when handling contaminated linen, cleaning the equipment, handling the respiratory equipment and cleaning the ambulance interior (where there may be many hidden nooks and crannies where the patient's blood or body fluids could be).

Once in quarters, you are ready to complete cleaning and disinfecting chores. Consult Scan 30-5 for the levels of reprocessing to be used for equipment.

1. Place contaminated linens in a biohazard container, noncontaminated linens in a regular hamper.
2. As necessary, clean any equipment that touched the patient. Brush stretcher covers and other rubber, vinyl, and canvas materials clean, then wash them with soap and water.
3. Clean and sanitize used nondisposable respiratory-assist and inhalation therapy equipment in the following manner:

   - Disassemble the equipment so that all surfaces are exposed.
   - Fill a large plastic container with the cleaning solution outlined in your service's infection control plan.
   - Soak the items for 10 minutes, or as directed by the manufacturer.
   - Clean the inner and outer surfaces with a suitable brush. Inner surfaces can be cleaned with a small bottle brush, while outer surfaces can be cleaned with a hand or nail brush. Make sure all encrusted matter is removed.
   - Rinse the items with tap water.
   - Soak the items in an EPA approved germicidal solution. An inhalation therapist at a local hospital can suggest a germicide suitable for respiratory equipment. Follow directions for dilution, safe handling, and soaking time. Rubber gloves are recommended when using some germicides.
   - After the prescribed soaking period, hang the equipment in a well-ventilated clean area and allow it to dry for 12 to 24 hours.

4. Clean and sanitize the patient compartment. Use an EPA-approved germicide to clean any fixed equipment or surfaces contacted by the patients body fluids.

Termination of Activities in Quarters

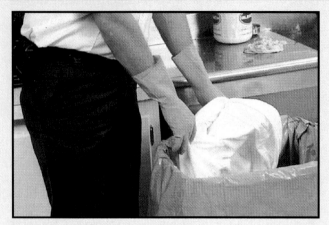

1. Place contaminated linens in a biohazard container, noncontaminated linens in a regular hamper.

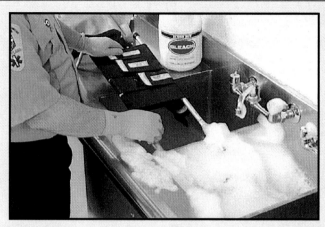

2. Remove and clean patient care equipment as required.

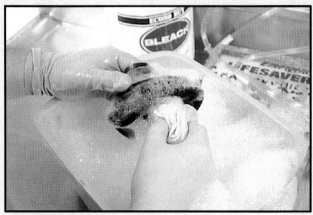

3. Clean and sanitize respiratory equipment as required.

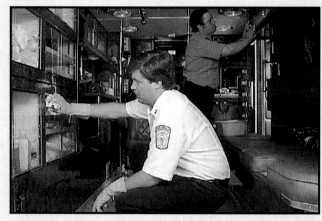

4. Clean and sanitize the ambulance interior as required. Any devices or surfaces that have come into contact with a patient's blood or other body fluids must be cleaned with germicide.

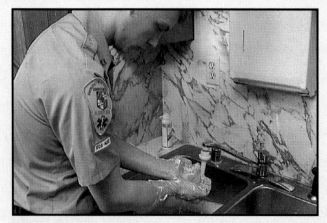

5. Wash thoroughly. Change soiled clothing. If exposed to a communicable disease, you should do this first.

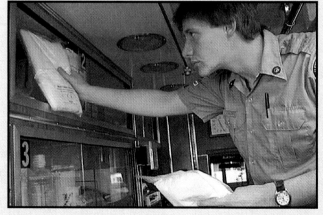

6. Replace expendable items as required.

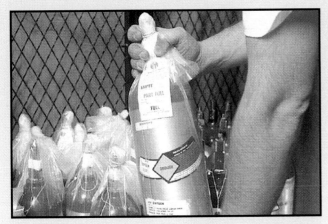

7. Always replace oxygen cylinders as necessary.

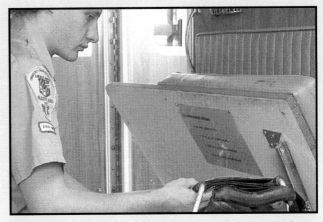

8. Replace patient care equipment as needed.

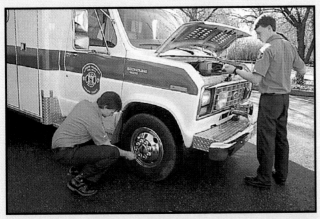

9. Maintain the ambulance as required. Report problems that will take the vehicle out of service.

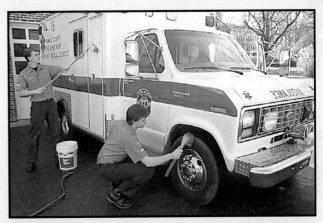

10. Clean the ambulance exterior as needed.

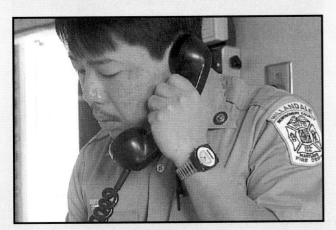

11. Report the unit ready for service.

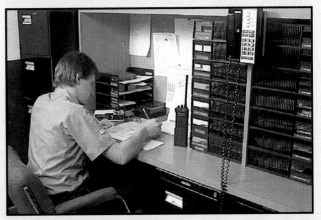

12. Complete any unfinished report forms as soon as possible.

Cleaning and Disinfecting Equipment

There are four levels of cleaning and disinfecting.

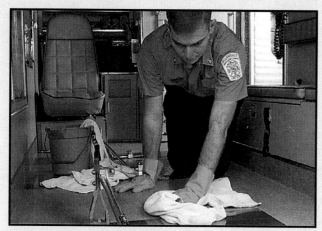

1. A **low-level disinfectant** approved by the U. S. Environmental Protection Agency, for example a commercial product such as Lysol, will clean and kill germs on ambulance floors and walls.

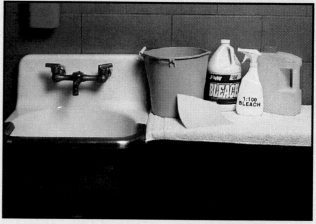

2. An **intermediate-level disinfectant,** such as a mixture of 1:100 bleach-to-water can be used to clean and kill germs on equipment surfaces.

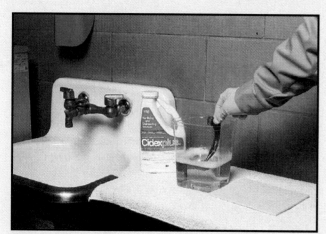

3. A **high-level disinfectant,** such as Cidex Plus, will destroy all forms of microbial life except high numbers of bacterial spores.

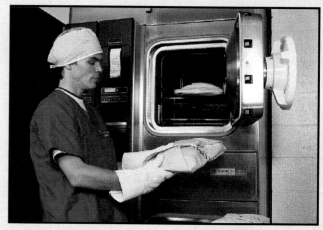

4. Sterilization is required to destroy all possible sources of infection on equipment that will be used invasively.

5. Prepare yourself for service.

   - Wash thoroughly, paying attention to the areas under your fingernails. Remember that contaminants can collect there and become a source of infection not only to you but also to the persons whom you touch.
   - Change soiled clothes. Clean contaminated clothing as soon as possible, especially if you were exposed to someone with a communicable disease. It is a good policy to bring a spare uniform to work, and each EMS agency should have a washer and dryer. It is against OSHA regulations for blood- or body-fluid-soiled clothes to be taken home to be washed.

6. Replace expendable items with items from the unit's storeroom.
7. Replace or refill oxygen cylinders in accordance with your service's procedures.
8. Replace patient care equipment.
9. Carry out post-operation vehicle maintenance procedures as required. If you find something wrong with the vehicle, correct the problem or make someone in authority aware of it.
10. Clean the vehicle. A clean exterior lends a professional appearance to an ambulance. Check the vehicle for broken lights, glass and body damage, door operation, and other parts that may need repair or replacement.
11. Complete any unfinished report forms as soon as possible.
12. Report the unit ready for service.

AIR RESCUE

In some circumstances, it is best for a patient to be transported by an air rescue helicopter or fixed-wing aircraft. The following are some considerations for use of this kind of transport. Since geographic and other circumstances and the availability of such transport will vary in different localities, follow your local protocols.

When to Call for Air Rescue

Air rescue may be required for any of the following reasons.

- Operational Reasons—To speed transport to a distant trauma center or other special facility, or when extrication of a high priority patient is prolonged and air rescue can speed transport, or when a patient must be rescued from a remote location that can only be reached by helicopter. Follow local protocols.
- Medical Reasons—The patient is high priority for rapid transport, e.g., is in shock, has a head injury with altered mental status, chest trauma with respiratory distress, penetrating injuries to the body cavity, amputations, extensive burns, or a serious mechanism of injury. Cardiac arrest patients are usually not transported by air rescue unless hypothermic. Follow local protocols.

How to Call for Air Rescue

Air rescue may be called for by any law enforcement, fire, or EMS command officer at the scene of an incident, or you may radio dispatch for advice if you think such a service is needed. When calling an air rescue service, give your name and callback number, your agency name, the nature of the situation, the exact location including crossroads and major landmarks, and the exact location of a safe landing zone (see below). Follow local protocols.

How to Set up a Landing Zone

A helicopter requires a landing zone approximately 100-by-100 feet (approximately 30 large steps on each side) on ground with less than an 8-degree slope. The landing zone and approach should be clear of wires, towers, vehicles, people, and loose objects (Figure 30-3). The landing zone should be marked with one flare in an upwind position. No lights should be directed toward the helicopter or the landing zone. Keep emergency red lights on.

Describe the landing zone to the air rescue service.

- Terrain—"The landing zone is located on top of a hill." "The landing zone is located in a valley."
- Major Landmarks—"There is a river (major highway, factory, water tower) to the north (or other direction) of the landing zone."

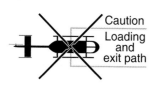

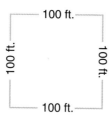

FIGURE 30-3 The air rescue helicopter landing zone.

- Estimated Distance to Nearest Town—"The landing zone is approximately 12 miles from Centerville."
- Other Pertinent Information—"There are wires on the east side of the landing zone."

"There is a deep ditch to the west." "Winds are out of the north-northeast at about 10 mph."

How to Approach a Helicopter

Do not approach a helicopter unless escorted by the helicopter crew. Allow the helicopter crew to direct the loading on board of the patient. Stay clear of the tail rotor at all times. Keep all traffic and vehicles 100 feet or more distant from the helicopter. Do not smoke within 100 feet of the helicopter. Be aware of the danger areas around helicopters, as shown in Scan 30-6.

CHAPTER REVIEW

SUMMARY

There are 5 phases to ambulance operations.

- Preparing for the call—Make sure that all required equipment and supplies are on board, in good repair or operating order, and properly stored. Inspect the ambulance itself to make sure that it is ready for service.
- Receiving and responding to the call—Receive call information from the EMD (Emergency Medical Dispatcher). Operate the ambulance safely. Understand the laws of your state and locality with regard to operation in an emergency situation, and always operate the ambulance with due regard for the safety of others. Park the ambulance outside the danger zone at a vehicle collision site.
- Transferring the patient to the ambulance—Select a patient-carrying device suitable for the patient's injuries or medical condition. Make sure that the patient is properly packaged and secured to the device. Assure that the stretcher is secured within the ambulance before the ambulance begins to move.

- Transporting the patient to the hospital—Perform and document ongoing assessment, needed treatments, and patient's condition. Notify dispatch, and transmit information to the receiving facility.
- Transferring the patient to the emergency department staff—Do not leave the patient until emergency department personnel have taken over his care. Assist in transferring the patient to the hospital stretcher. Give a verbal report to emergency department personnel. Complete your prehospital care report. Transfer the patient's personal effects. Obtain your release from hospital personnel.

At the conclusion of the call, make up the ambulance stretcher, clean and restock the ambulance, and make sure that it is in good order for the next call.

On some occasions your service may request that an air rescue service transport the patient. Be aware of procedures for requesting this service, for setting up a landing zone, and for safety procedures around a helicopter.

Danger Areas around Helicopters

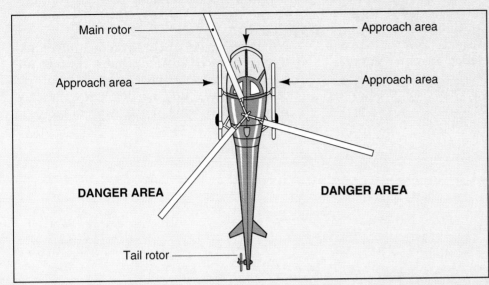

Main rotor

Approach area

Approach area

Approach area

DANGER AREA

DANGER AREA

Tail rotor

A. The area around the tail rotor is extremely dangerous. A spinning rotor cannot be seen.

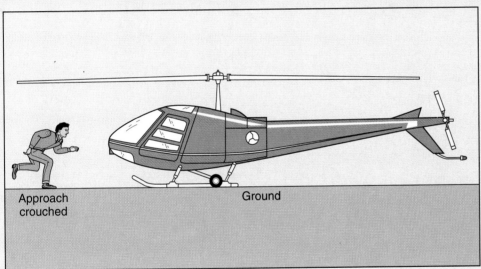

Approach crouched

Ground

B. A sudden gust of wind can cause the main rotor of a helicopter to dip to a point as close as 4 feet from the ground. Always approach a helicopter in a crouch when the rotor is moving.

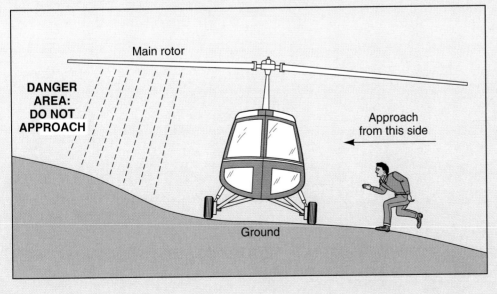

Main rotor

DANGER AREA: DO NOT APPROACH

Approach from this side

Ground

C. Approach the aircraft from the downhill side when a helicopter is parked on a hillside.

1. List five categories of equipment and supplies that should be carried on an ambulance.
2. Describe the laws (those described in this chapter or your local or state laws) with regard to operation of an ambulance in an emergency. Describe considerations for safe operation of an ambulance in emergency and nonemergency situations.
3. Describe the steps that must be followed in transferring a patient to an ambulance; for care of the patient en route; for transfer-ring a patient to emergency department personnel.
4. Describe the steps that should be followed when air rescue is required.

Application

- What equipment should you include in a kit that you carry to the scene? How should the equipment be positioned so that you can reach urgently needed items quickly? What special items, if any, should be in the kit to meet local needs?

Gaining Access

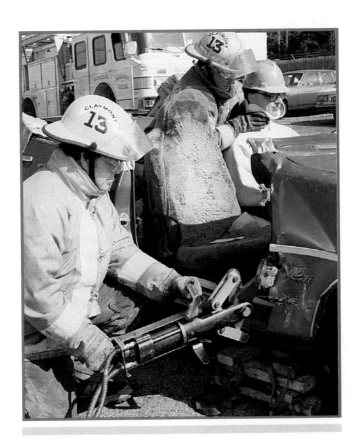

31

As an EMT-B, you will usually have no trouble reaching your patient. You will walk into a home, for example, and find your patient lying on a sofa. At times, however, a patient may not be so easy to get to. He may be lost on a remote mountainside, trapped in the debris of an explosion, or—the most common situation—pinned inside a vehicle. In such a situation, someone must rescue the patient, perhaps disentangling him from machinery or rubble, before emergency care can begin or be completed. Although, as an EMT-B, you will not usually be responsible for extrication and rescue, it is important to understand how the process is done, how it may affect the patient, and what is the earliest point in the process that you can get to the patient to begin care.

Knowledge and Attitude *At the end of this chapter, you should be able to meet the following objectives.*

1. Describe the purpose of extrication. (p. 667)

2. Discuss the role of the EMT-Basic in extrication. (pp. 667, 685)

3. Identify what equipment for personal safety is required for the EMT-Basic. (pp. 669–670)

4. Define the fundamental components of extrication. (p. 667)

5. State the steps that should be taken to protect the patient during extrication. (p. 670)

6. Evaluate various methods of gaining access to the patient. (pp. 679–685)

7. Distinguish between simple and complex access. (p. 679)

On the Scene

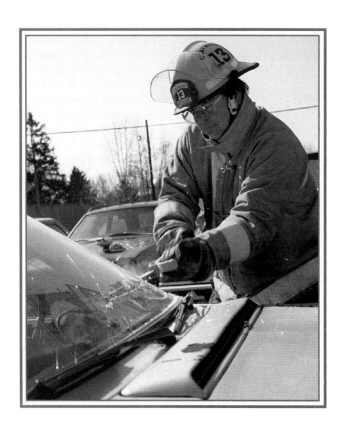

One sunny summer afternoon, a drunk driver runs a stop sign, strikes Nancy Sanchez's car, and keeps on going. The sound of colliding metal startles neighbors for several blocks. Your area's 911 dispatch center receives numerous calls for a "bad accident," and police, EMS, and fire-rescue units are simultaneously dispatched. Initial units arrive at the "T-bone" intersection and report a woman trapped inside a vehicle.

Your ambulance arrives at the scene amidst the other emergency apparatus. A firefighter from the first-response engine confirms a woman is trapped inside a car. You survey the scene, the vehicle, and—through the windshield—Mrs. Sanchez inside.

You: This patient appears to be unconscious with potential injuries. We have to get her out of there fast.
Fire Command: Let's get the roof off and you can do a rapid extrication vertically.

Wearing protective clothing, you gain access through a window to begin manual stabilization and initial assessment of Mrs. Sanchez, while a member of the fire rescue team begins to cut out the windshield in preparation for cutting through the posts and removing the roof. You and your partner will conduct a rapid extrication of the patient as soon as the roof is out of the way.

With the combined efforts of the EMS and fire services, Nancy Sanchez is quickly extricated and transported to a waiting trauma center in time for surgeons to save her life.

There are at least ten types of specialty rescue teams that may be available in various communities. Each specialty requires a significant amount of additional training over and above your EMT-Basic course. These specialties include vehicle rescue, water rescue, ice rescue, high angle rescue, hazardous materials response, trench rescue, dive rescue, back country or wilderness rescue, farm rescue, and confined space rescue. Training that is available in each of these specialties often depends on the types of emergency responses that might be required in your community. If there is a gorge in the area, there often is a high angle team. If there is a river with low-head dams running through your district, a water rescue team would be appropriate.

In this chapter the focus will be the role of the EMT-B at a vehicle collision where extrication of the patient is required, since this is the most common type of rescue across the United States.

VEHICLE RESCUE

Extrication is the process by which entrapped patients are rescued from vehicles, buildings, tunnels, or other places. There are ten phases of the extrication or rescue process that you, as an EMT-B, should understand.

1. Preparing for the Rescue
2. Sizing up the situation
3. Recognizing and managing hazards
4. Stabilizing the vehicle prior to entering
5. Gaining access to the patient
6. Providing initial patient assessment and a rapid trauma exam
7. Disentangling the patient
8. Immobilizing and extricating the patient from the vehicle
9. Providing a detailed physical exam, ongoing assessment, treatment, and transport to the most appropriate hospital
10. Terminating the rescue

Every step of this process needs input from you, the EMT-B, acting as an advocate for the patient's medical needs. Attention to safety must be your highest priority—to help minimize the potential for injury to yourself, the other rescuers, or any additional injury to your patient. Although you may never personally perform dis-

entanglement, since in many communities this is accomplished by a fire department rescue squad, it is important for you to understand the process so you can keep your patient informed and anticipate any dangerous steps in the extrication action plan.

You have already learned about some of the ten phases of the extrication process. You will learn about others in this chapter, as the chart below explains.

You have read or will read about . . .	in . . .
Phases 1-5 and 7	This chapter
Phases 2 and 3	Chapter 8, Scene Size-up
Phase 6	Chapter 9, The Initial Assessment
	Chapter 10, The Focused History and Physical Exam—Trauma
Phase 8	Chapter 28, Injuries to the Head and Spine
Phase 9	Chapter 12, The Detailed Physical Exam
	Chapter 13, Ongoing Assessment
Phase 10	Chapter 30, Ambulance Operations

Preparing for the Rescue

Vehicle rescue prior to the mid 1960s is best described as crude. So-called "rescue" trucks were usually small walk-in step vans that carried more equipment for fire suppression and salvage than for rescue. The inventory of rescue equipment might have included some long pry bars, a few lengths of utility rope, a minimal hand tool kit, shovels and brooms, and—if the rescue unit was progressive—a 4-ton hydraulic jack kit. Proper protective clothing and gear for rescue personnel were similarly lacking. Personnel were poorly trained for rescue and, more often than not, victims were simply pulled through openings created by the collision.

Modern rescue is a far more sophisticated process. It requires preparation that is a combination of training, practice, and the right protective gear and tools. As discussed above, training and practice for specific types of rescue, including vehicle rescue, will be above and beyond your EMT-B course. Availability of such training will depend to a great extent on the kinds of rescues most likely to be required in your area. The kinds of protective gear and tools that should be available for vehicle rescue will be discussed throughout this chapter.

Sizing Up the Situation

As you arrive on the scene of a collision, it is important to have a keen eye, because the first thing you need to do is evaluate hazards and calculate the need for additional BLS (basic life support—EMT-B level) or ALS (advanced life support—paramedic level) backup, police, fire, or specialty rescue response, or services such as a power company representative. Quickly determine how many patients are involved, their priority, and the mechanisms of injury. If you think additional ambulances will be needed, call for them right away. You can always cancel them if they are not actually needed.

An important part of scene size-up is determining the extent of the patient's entrapment and the most appropriate means of getting the patient out. As soon as possible, evaluate if the patient is high or low priority. During size-up, you must be able to "read" a collision vehicle and develop a plan of action based on your knowledge of rescue operations and your estimate of the patient's condition and priority. During all of this you will keep in mind that the most seriously injured patients have, at a maximum, a "golden hour" from the time of the injury until surgery at the hospital to control internal bleeding and other life-threatening conditions. Beyond the golden hour, survival rates diminish drastically. As the patient advocate on the scene, you must plan how you can begin emergency care and initiate transport as rapidly as possible.

A low priority patient can wait for rescue personnel to force open the doors, then remove the roof and/or displace the front end of the vehicle. For such a patient, there is time to do a short spine board or vest immobilization, then carefully transfer the patient to the stretcher using the long board, as described in Chapter 28. If the patient is a high priority, it may make more sense to use the rapid extrication technique, also described in Chapter 28, whether for a vertical removal through the opened roof or for a horizontal removal through a doorway. The principles of spinal immobilization remain the same whether the patient is low or high priority, but the requirements for speed of removal will dictate the specific technique you use.

During the size-up, check to see if the vehicle is equipped with air bags. A car with an air bag has a large, rectangular steering wheel hub.

Special steps should be followed if the air bag has not deployed (see "Step Three: Disentangle Occupants by Displacing the Front End" later in this chapter). If the air bag has deployed, observers may have noticed "smoke" inside the vehicle during deployment. This is actually not smoke but dust from the cornstarch or talcum used to lubricate the bag as well as from the seal and particles from within the bag. The powder may contain sodium hydroxide, which can irritate the skin. For this reason, it will be important to wear protective gloves and eye wear when you gain access to the passenger compartment and to protect the patients from getting additional dust in their eyes or wounds. Air bag manufacturers recommend that the EMT-B move the bag and examine the steering wheel, which may reveal if the patient struck the wheel with enough energy to damage it.

Recognizing and Managing Hazards

In some rural areas, fire departments have no rescue capabilities, and ambulance services are called upon to carry out vehicle rescue on their own. In areas where rescue and fire units are available, the ambulance may nevertheless arrive at the scene first. In this situation, time and lives can be saved if the EMT-Bs—after sizing up the situation and calling for the appropriate additional help—are able to recognize and initiate hazard management, at least until personnel with more expertise arrive.

Hazards at a collision scene can range from nuisances—such as broken glass and debris, a slippery road, inclement weather, or darkness—to severe threats to safety—such as downed wires, spilled fuel, or fire. Also during size-up, watch out for loaded bumpers. Most cars are equipped with 5-mile-per-hour bumpers designed to absorb low-speed front and rear end collision damage. If the bumpers were involved in the collision, you may notice that the bumper shock absorber system is compressed, or "loaded." Never stand in front of a loaded bumper. If it springs out and strikes your knees, it will mostly likely break your legs. Some rescue teams are trained to unload the shock absorber or to chain it to prevent an uncontrolled release.

Traffic and spectators can become hazards if they are not controlled. A number of EMT-Bs have been killed at the scenes of collisions by oncoming traffic when drivers were watching the collision and not the EMT-B crossing—or working near or in—the street.

As explained below, some collision-related hazards must be managed, if not eliminated, before any attempt is made to reach injured persons in damaged vehicles.

Safeguarding Yourself from Hazards

Collision sites can be dangerous workplaces. Jagged edges, flying glass, and fire are only a few of the hazards you may need to deal with. Remember that you are no good to your patient and crew if you become a patient yourself. It is vital that you take the time to properly protect yourself before engaging in any rescue activities.

The unsafe act that contributes most to collision scene injuries is failure to wear protective gear during rescue operations. Many of the following human factors can increase the potential for an EMT-B to be injured at a collision site.

- A careless attitude toward personal safety
- Lack of skill in tool use
- Physical problems that impede strenuous effort

Unsafe and improper acts also cause injuries.

- Failure to eliminate or control hazards
- Failure to select the proper tool for the task
- Using unsafe tools
- Failure to recognize mechanisms of injury and unsafe surroundings
- Lifting heavy objects improperly
- Deactivating safety devices designed to prevent injury
- Failure to wear highly visible outer clothing, especially when exposed to highway traffic

Figure 31-1 shows two EMT-Bs dressed for collision scene operations. The EMT-B on the left is dressed for a wide range of hazard management and extrication operations. At a collision scene any personnel who are allowed to work in the "inner circle," that is the area immediately around and including the vehicle, should wear full protective gear to avoid being injured. The EMT-B on the right is dressed for situations where hazards are minimal.

Learn the value of protective gear, get your own if your service doesn't provide it (most states require it on ambulances), and use it! Consider reviewing the following National Fire Protection Association standards when purchasing protective gear and uniforms: NFPA 1972 (Helmets for Structural Firefighting), NFPA 1973

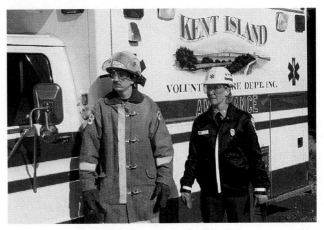

FIGURE 31-1 Two EMT-Bs dressed for vehicle operations.

(Gloves for Structural Firefighting), and NFPA 1975 (Station/Work Uniforms).

Following are descriptions of personal protective gear that EMT-Bs should use during rescue operations.

Headgear Good head protection is essential. Trendy baseball caps, uniform hats, and wool watch caps do little except protect against sunlight, identify the wearer as a member of an emergency service, or keep the head warm. Plastic "bump caps" worn by butchers and warehouse workers also do not provide adequate protection.

One good piece of headgear that does offer adequate protection is the rescue helmet. The model illustrated in Figure 31-1 does not have the firefighter's helmet rear brim, which can be awkward in tight spaces, although many EMT-Bs do prefer and use firefighters' helmets.

All helmets should be brightly colored with reflective stripes and lettering to make the wearer visible both day and night, and the Star of Life on each side to identify the wearer as an EMS provider. The level of training should also be indicated to make scene management easier when many EMS and rescue units are on hand.

Eye Protection Eye protection is vital. Hinged plastic helmet shields do not provide adequate protection; flying particles can strike the eyes from underneath or from the side. Protection is best provided by safety goggles with a soft vinyl frame that conforms to the face and indirect venting to keep them fog-free, or safety glasses with large lenses and side shields.

Hand Protection Because EMT-Bs stick their hands into all sorts of unfriendly places, every

EMT-B should have optimal hand protection. Good protection is afforded by wearing disposable latex, vinyl, or other synthetic gloves underneath either firefighter's gloves or leather gloves.

Firefighter's gloves will protect an EMT-B's hands from a variety of sharp, hot, cold, and dangerous surfaces. They are bulky, but can be worn in most rescue situations. If greater dexterity is needed, intermediate weight leather gloves can be worn. Fabric garden or work gloves are too thin to offer adequate protection.

Body Protection An EMT-B will often protect head, eyes, and hands and leave the body virtually unprotected. Light shirts or nylon jackets should never be allowed inside the inner circle because they do little to protect from jagged metal, broken glass, or flash fires. Good upper body protection is offered by wearing either a short or midlength turnout coat that meets Occupational Safety and Health Administration (OSHA) requirements. A heavy-duty EMS or rescue jacket can be used to protect you from weather and minor injury. As with helmets, bright colors and reflective material will help make your jacket more visible.

Good lower body protection can be provided by wearing either turnout pants with cuffs wide enough to pull over work shoes or fire-resistant trousers or jumpsuits. Serious consideration should be given to wearing high-top, steel toe, work shoes with extended tops to protect the ankles.

Safeguarding Your Patient from Hazards

When your patients have been injured in a collision, it is your responsibility to see to it that further injuries are not inflicted during the rescue operation. You can minimize the chance of such additional injuries by shielding the patient and exercising care. The following items can be used to protect the patient from heat, cold, flying particles, and other hazards.

- An aluminized rescue blanket offers protection from weather and, to a degree, from flying particles. A paper blanket does not afford this protection; it merely hides the patient's view of the debris that is about to strike him.
- A lightweight vinyl-coated paper tarpaulin can protect from weather.
- A wool blanket should be used to protect from cold. Cover the wool blanket with an aluminized blanket or a salvage cover

whenever glass must be broken near a patient, since glass particles are just about impossible to remove from wool blankets.
- Short and long spine boards can shield a patient from contact with tools and debris.
- Hard hats, safety goggles, industrial hearing protectors, disposable dust masks, and thermal masks (in cold weather—and unless the patient has airway or breathing problems or is on oxygen) will protect a patient's head, eyes, ears, and respiratory passages.

Managing Traffic Hazards

Collisions almost always produce traffic problems. Often the wreckage blocks lanes of traffic. Even if it doesn't, backups are caused when curious drivers slow down to "rubberneck," or stare at the scene. Rescuers, firefighters, and police usually handle traffic control; but what if the ambulance EMT-Bs are responding alone or ahead of other emergency service units?

Obviously, personal safety, rescue, and emergency care have priority. However, an ambulance crew should still initiate basic traffic control, channeling vehicles past the scene. Remember to be extremely watchful and careful when you work to control traffic to be sure that you are not struck by an approaching or passing vehicle.

Your ambulance with its warning lights will serve as the first form of traffic control; however, you should position other warning devices as soon as possible. Bad weather, darkness, vegetation, and curved or hilly roadways may keep approaching motorists from seeing your ambulance soon enough to stop safely.

Using Flares for Traffic Control Although some argue that flares are unsafe, when used properly they are still a good device for warning motorists of dangerous conditions. Moreover, several dozen flares can be carried behind the front seat of an ambulance, while battery-powered flashing lights—an alternative to flares—take up valuable compartment space.

Scan 31-1 shows the proper positioning of flares at collision scenes, including a straight road, a curved road, and a hill. Keep in mind that the stopping distance for large trucks is much greater than for cars. When the road carries truck traffic, extend the flare strings beyond the distances shown.

Remember these points when you place flares.

Positioning Flares to Control Traffic

Posted speed (mph)	Stopping distance for that speed*		Posted speed (in feet)		Distance of the farthest warning device
20 mph	50 feet	+	20 feet	=	70 feet
30 mph	75 feet	+	30 feet	=	105 feet
40 mph	125 feet	+	40 feet	=	165 feet
50 mph	175 feet	+	50 feet	=	225 feet
60 mph	275 feet	+	60 feet	=	335 feet
70 mph	375 feet	+	70 feet	=	445 feet

A. Flares are positioned according to a formula that includes the stopping distance for the posted speed plus a margin of safety.

*Distances are given for passenger cars.

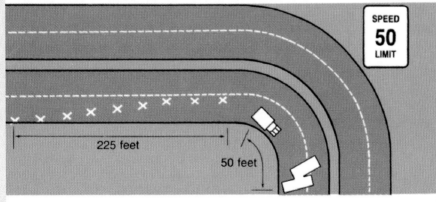

B. Flares positioned on a straight road. Approaching vehicles are moved into the correct lane before they reach the edge of the danger zone.

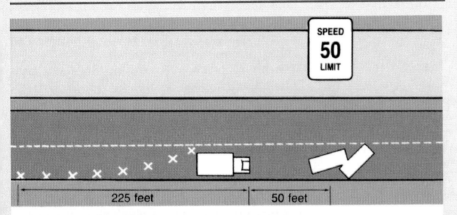

C. Flares positioned ahead of a curved section of road. The start of the curve is considered to be the edge of the danger zone.

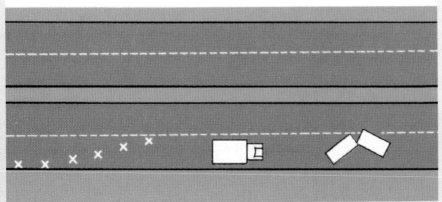

D. Flares positioned on a hill. The flares slow approaching vehicles and make them turn into the correct lane before they reach the top of the hill.

1. Look for and avoid spilled fuel, dry vegetation, and other combustibles before you ignite and position flares, especially at a road edge.
2. Do not throw flares out of moving vehicles.
3. Position a few flares at the edge of the danger zone as soon as the ambulance is parked. They will supplement the ambulance warning lights.
4. Take a handful of flares and walk (carefully) toward oncoming traffic.
5. Position the flares every 10 feet, if possible, to channel vehicles into an unblocked lane. (Don't turn your back to traffic while placing flares.)
6. If the collision has occurred on a two-lane road, position flares in both directions.
7. Never use a flare as a traffic wand; flares can spew molten phosphorous, which can cause third degree burns to the skin.

Controlling Spectators

Spectators do more than just create problems for passing motorists. If allowed to wander freely, they will close in on the wreckage just to get a better view. They may get so close that they interfere with rescue and emergency care efforts.

Rescue squads, police, and fire units have personnel and equipment for crowd control; ambulances usually do not. However, an EMT-B can usually initiate some crowd-control measures. If local policies permit it, ask for assistance from one or more responsible-looking bystanders. Ask the persons you recruit to keep the spectators away from the danger zone. Give them a roll of barricade tape if you have one. Be sure not to put the recruited personnel in unsafe positions such as near spilled fuel or an unstable vehicle.

Coping with Electrical Hazards

Electricity poses many dangers at vehicle collision scenes. When there is an electrical hazard, establish a danger zone and a safe zone (see Chapter 8, Scan 8-2, Establishing the Danger Zone). The danger zone should only be entered by individuals responsible for controlling the hazard, such as power company personnel or specialty rescue. The safe zone should be sufficiently far away to assure that an arcing or moving wire could not possibly injure any of the rescue personnel or bystanders.

Keep the safety points below in mind. Many have to do with taking precautions around con-

ductors. A conductor is a wire or any other object or material that will carry electricity.

- High voltages are not as uncommon on roadside utility poles as people often think. In some areas, wood poles support conductors of as much as 500,000 volts.
- Assume that the entire area is extremely dangerous. Conductors may have touched and energized any part of the system, including electrical, telephone, cable television, and other wires supported by the utility pole, guy wires, ground wires, the pole itself, the ground surrounding the pole, and nearby guard rails and fences. Assume that severed or displaced conductors may be touching and energizing every wire and conductor at the highest voltage present. Dead wires may be re-energized at any moment. Energized conductors may arc to the ground.
- Ordinary protective clothing does not protect against electrocution.

Remembering these points and the following procedures may keep you alive at the scene of a collision where unconfined electricity is a hazard.

Broken Utility Pole with Wires Down A broken utility pole with wires down is very dangerous. You probably cannot work safely in the area until a power company representative assures you that the power is off and the scene is safe.

If you discover that a utility pole is broken and wires are down

1. Park the ambulance outside the danger zone.
2. Before you leave the ambulance, be sure that no portion of the vehicle, including the radio antenna, is contacting any sagging conductors.
3. Order spectators and nonessential emergency service personnel from the danger zone. Use perimeter tape to set a large safety zone.
4. Discourage occupants of the collision vehicle from leaving the wreckage.
5. Prohibit traffic flow through the danger zone.
6. Determine the number of the nearest pole you can safely approach, and ask your dispatcher to advise the power company of the pole number and location.

7. Do not attempt to move downed wires. Metal implements will, of course, conduct electricity, but even implements that may not appear to be conductive, such as tools with wood handles or natural fiber ropes, may have a high moisture content that will conduct electricity and may cause a well-intentioned rescuer to become electrocuted.
8. Stand in a safe place until the power company cuts the wires or disconnects the power.

Be especially careful when approaching a collision located in a dark area such as a rural roadside at night. As you walk from the ambulance, sweep the area ahead of you, to each side and overhead, with the beam of a powerful hand light. An energized conductor may be dangling just at head level. If you discover that a wire is down, leave the area immediately and notify the power company.

Sometimes, especially in wet weather, a phenomenon known as ground gradient may provide your first clue that a wire is down. Voltage is greatest at the point where a conductor touches the ground, then diminishes with distance from the point of contact. That distance may be several inches or many feet. Being able to recognize and respond properly to energized ground can save your life.

Stop your approach immediately if you feel a tingling sensation in your legs and lower torso. This sensation means that you are on energized ground. Current is entering one foot, passing through your lower body, and exiting through your other foot. If you continue on, you risk being electrocuted!

Turn 180 degrees and take one of two escape measures. Hop to a safe place on one foot. Or shuffle away from the danger area with both feet together, allowing no break in contact between your two feet or between your feet and the ground. Either technique helps prevent your body from completing a circuit with energized ground, which can cause electrocution. (A circuit is a circular path for electrical flow, such as up one leg, down the other, and through the ground. Hopping on one leg or keeping your feet together creates a straight path rather than a circular circuit, which may prevent electrocution.)

Broken Utility Pole with Wires Intact Even if wires are intact, a broken utility pole is still dangerous. Wires that are still holding up the pole can break at any time, dropping pole and wires onto the scene. If you arrive to find such a situation

1. Park the ambulance outside the danger zone.
2. Notify your dispatcher of the situation.
3. Stay outside the danger zone until power company representatives can de-energize the conductors and stabilize the pole.
4. Keep spectators and other emergency service personnel out of the danger zone.

Damaged Pad-Mounted Transformer When electrical cables run underground, the transformer may be mounted on a pad above ground. When an above-ground pad-mounted electrical transformer is struck and damaged, it poses a serious threat. In such a situation

1. Request an immediate power company response.
2. Do not touch either the transformer case or a vehicle touching it, and warn other emergency service personnel not to.
3. Stand in a safe place until the power company de-energizes the transformer.
4. Keep spectators out of the danger zone.

Coping with Vehicle Fires

When you find a vehicle on fire, always request the response of firefighting apparatus. Do not assume that someone else has called the fire department. In fact, an engine should always stand by at a vehicle rescue.

Extinguishing a vehicle fire is the responsibility of persons who are trained and equipped for the job: firefighters. Nonetheless, there are some measures that trained EMT-Bs can take when they arrive before fire units (Scan 31-2).

For small fires, a 15- or 20-pound class A:B:C dry chemical fire extinguisher can extinguish virtually anything that may be burning in a vehicle, including upholstery, fuel, and electrical components. Only burning magnesium and other flammable metals cannot be extinguished by an A:B:C extinguisher. Before you try to put out a fire always put on a full set of protective gear.

Fire in the Engine Compartment If the hood is fully open, stand close to an A-post (front roof-supporting post) of the vehicle and, if possible, with your back to the wind to guard against the

Extinguishing Fires in Collision Vehicles

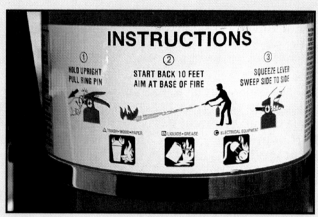

A. Markings that identify an extinguisher that can be used for Class A, B, and C fires.

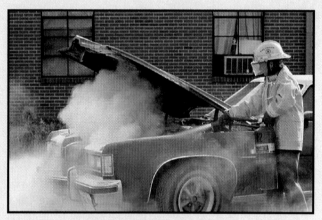

B. Extinguishing a fire in the engine compartment when the hood is fully open.

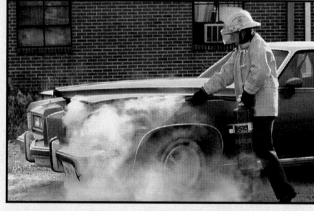

C. Extinguishing a fire in the engine compartment when the hood is partially open.

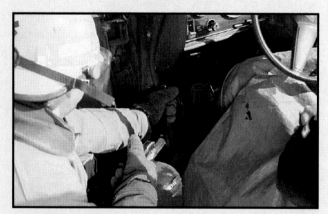

D. Extinguishing a fire under the dash. Care must be taken not to fill the vehicle's interior with a cloud of agent.

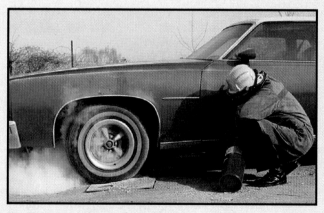

E. Extinguishing fuel burning under a vehicle. Flames are swept away from the vehicle.

agent blowing back into your face or entering the passenger compartment. (Dry chemical extinguishing agent irritates respiratory passages and may contaminate open wounds.) Then sweep the extinguisher across the base of the fire with short bursts. Use no more than necessary to extinguish the fire. You will need what is left if there is a subsequent flare-up.

If the hood is open to the safety latch, do not raise the hood further. This will help to restrict air flow and deprive the fire of oxygen. Then direct the agent through any opening to the engine compartment: between hood and fender, around the grill, under a wheel well, or through a broken head lamp assembly. Again, use no more agent than is needed.

If the hood is closed tight, let the fire burn under the closed hood, leaving its extinguishment to the fire department, and continue to get the patients out of the vehicle. The firewall should protect the passenger area long enough to get the patients out of the vehicle, using emergency moves.

Fire in the Passenger Compartment or Trunk

If the fire is under the dash or in upholstery or other combustibles, carefully apply the agent directly to the burning material. Apply sparingly to avoid creating a cloud of powder that may be harmful to occupants. If there is fire in the trunk, as with fire under a closed hood, leave extinguishment to the fire department and continue working to get patients out of the vehicle.

Fire under the Vehicle

Using a portable unit to extinguish burning fuel under a vehicle may be an exercise in futility when the spill is large. But when people are trapped in the vehicle, you may feel you must try. Attempt to sweep the flames from under the passenger compartment as you apply the agent. If you do extinguish the fire, be sure that sources of ignition are then kept away. The vehicle's own catalytic converter (usually found in the area under the front passenger's feet) can be an ignition source since its temperature can reach over 1000 degrees.

Truck Fires

An A:B:C extinguisher can also be used to combat truck fires. Be aware, however, that burning truck tires are especially dangerous. Flames can quickly spread to the body of the vehicle and its cargo, or the tires can blow apart when heated by fire. NEVER stand directly in front of a truck wheel when there is a fire; approach from a 45-degree angle.

At times you will find that fuel is leaking from a damaged vehicle but is not on fire. *If you discover that a fuel tank is leaking, call for fire department response.* The decision to continue the rescue effort should be governed by your perception of the danger. You should not be expected to continue rescue operations if gasoline is pooled under the vehicle or flowing toward a source of ignition. Warn spectators away from flowing fuel to minimize possible sources of ignition. Do not use flares near spilled fuel or in the path of flowing fuel. Watch where you park your vehicle, as your ambulance's catalytic converter can easily ignite spilled fuel or other combustibles.

Coping with a Vehicle's Electrical System

Many rescue units routinely disable the electrical system of every collision vehicle by cutting a battery cable. This was a reasonable practice years ago when vehicles had more combustible materials and when wiring did not have self-extinguishing insulation. Today, however, the situation is different. Unless gasoline is pooled under a vehicle or undeployed air bags need to be disabled, cutting the battery out of the electrical system may not only be a waste of time, it may actually hinder the rescue operation.

Remember that many cars have electrically powered door locks, window operators, and seat adjustment mechanisms. Being able to lower a window rather than breaking it eliminates the likelihood of spraying occupants with glass. Being able to operate door locks may eliminate the need to force doors open. And being able to operate a powered seat will create space in front of an injured driver.

If there is reason to disrupt the electrical system, disconnect the ground cable from the battery. In this way, you will not be likely to produce a spark that can drop onto spilled fuel or ignite battery gases. Such a spark can be created when the positive cable is pulled away from the battery terminal, or when a tool touches a metal component while in contact with the positive terminal or cable.

Stabilizing a Vehicle

Unstable collision vehicles pose a hazard to rescuers and patients alike. Scan 31-3 shows methods for stabilizing a vehicle on its wheels, a vehicle on its side, and a vehicle on its roof.

Stabilizing Collision Vehicles with Cribbing

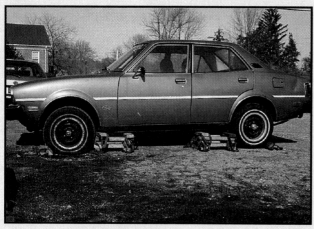

A. A car on its wheels can be stabilized by placing cribbing under the rocker panels to minimize rescuer-produced movements that may be harmful to the occupants. Deflate the vehicle's tires for maximum stability.

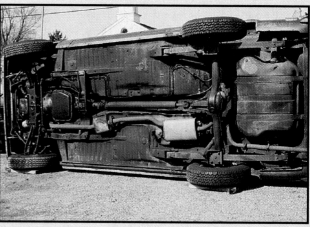

B. A car on its side can be stabilized by placing cribbing under the wheels, moving the car to the vertical poisition, and then . . .

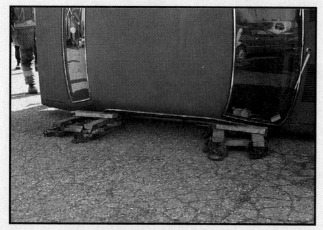

C. . . . placing cribbing under the A- and C-posts. Stabilizing in this manner allows EMTs to pull the roof down to expose the entire interior of the car.

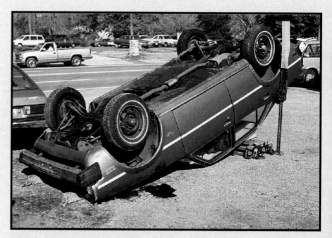

D. An overturned car can be stabilized by placing jacks and/or cribbing under the trunk, under the hood, or at both locations, depending on the position of the vehicle.

Rescuers often fail to stabilize a collision vehicle because it appears to be stable. Rather than taking the chance of incorrectly "reading" a collision vehicle's stability—and having the vehicle move during rescue with disastrous results—you should consider any collision vehicle from which patients need to be extricated to be unstable and act accordingly.

If your ambulance is equipped with stabilization equipment, you should attend a formal vehicle rescue course that includes basic stabilization procedures taught by a qualified instructor. If the ambulance is not equipped for stabilization procedures, or if you are not trained, stand by until a rescue unit has stabilized the vehicle, even if roof posts are intact and the vehicle appears to be stable.

The information on vehicle stabilization that follows is intended only to help you, as an EMT-B, understand the process that trained personnel will be following. It is not a substitute for formal training in stabilization procedures.

A Vehicle on Its Wheels

A collision vehicle that is upright on four inflated tires looks stable. However, it is easily rocked up and down, side to side, and back and forth as rescuers climb into and over it. These motions can seriously aggravate occupants' injuries. First, if rescuers have access to the inside of the vehicle, they should make sure the engine is turned off, the vehicle is in park, the keys are removed from the ignition, and the parking brake is set. Using three step chocks, one on each side and a third under the front or back of the vehicle, is the best method of stabilizing a vehicle on its wheels.

Then all the tires should be deflated. This can be accomplished by simply pulling the valve stems from their casing with pliers. A police officer should be told that this has been done so investigators will not think that the tires are flat as a result of the collision.

A listing of the equipment that can be carried to accomplish vehicle stabilization and gaining access is listed in Table 31-1. If the ambulance is not equipped with step chocks, a degree of stabilization can be accomplished by placing wheel chocks or 2 × 4-inch cribbing in front of and behind two tires on the same side.

If a car has rolled over several times and come to rest on its wheels, the roof may be crushed and access through windows precluded. The roof may need to be raised with heavy-duty

TABLE 31-1 Supplies and Equipment for Vehicle Stabilization and Gaining Access

Quantity	Item
10	2 × 4 × 18-inch cribbing
10	4 × 4 × 18-inch cribbing
4	step chocks
6	wood wedges
2	vehicle wheel chocks
100 feet	nylon ½-inch utility rope
2	Hi-lift heavy duty jacks
1	"Door-and-window kit" with hand tools such as...
	1 pair battery pliers
	1 12-inch adjustable wrench
	1 3- or 4-pound drilling hammer
	1 spring-loaded center punch
	2 hacksaws with spare blades
	1 10-inch locking-type pliers
	1 10-inch water-pump pliers
	several 12- to 15-inch flat pry bars
	1 8-inch flat blade screwdriver
	1 12-inch flat blade screwdriver
	1 spray container of power steering fluid as a lubricant
1	flat-head ax
1	glas-Master windshield saw
1	combination forcible entry tool such as a Halligan or a Biel tool
500 feet	perimeter tape

jacks before doors can be opened or the roof removed.

A Vehicle on Its Side

When a vehicle is on its side, spectators will often attempt to push it back onto its wheels. They fail to realize that this movement may injure, or more severely injure, occupants of the vehicle. Instead, the vehicle should be stabilized on its side. If the vehicle is on its side, do not attempt to gain access before it is stabilized using ropes, hi-lift jacks, and/or cribbing. While a car on its side may appear stable, simply climbing onto one side in an attempt to open a door may cause the vehicle to drop onto its roof or wheels. Moreover, you can be trapped under the vehicle when it topples.

A person who will act as a safety guide can be placed at each end of the vehicle to "feel" the movement of the vehicle and quickly warn the rescuers placing cribbing, jacks, or ropes to get back if the vehicle begins to fall over. Some services will deploy two ropes looped around the same wheel in both directions so that personnel can temporarily hold the vehicle stable while jacks and/or cribbing are placed. There are many ways to stabilize a vehicle on its side, from using manpower alone to using hydraulic rams and pneumatic jacks. The objective is to increase the number of contacts with the ground to make the vehicle on its side more stable.

Safety Note

When placing cribbing, NEVER kneel down. Always squat, staying on both feet so you can quickly move away from the vehicle if you have to.

Once the vehicle is stabilized, if a door must be opened, tie it in the fully open position before you try to crawl inside.

A Vehicle on Its Roof

If the vehicle is resting on its roof, roof posts are intact, and the vehicle appears stable, it may be tempting to try to reach the vehicle's occupants by gaining access through window or door openings—immediately, and without stabilizing the vehicle. However, if the posts collapse, as is often the case when the windshield integrity has been broken, the vehicle may come crashing down and injure the EMT-B who is attempting to climb into the vehicle or who has an arm in a window opening. You must wait to gain access until the rescue crew has stabilized the vehicle. This is usually accomplished by building a box crib with 4 x 4s under the vehicle.

A vehicle on its roof is likely to be in one of four positions:

- Horizontal, with the roof crushed flat against the body of the vehicle and both the trunk lid and hood contacting the ground
- Horizontal, resting entirely on the roof, with space between the hood and the ground and space between the trunk lid and the ground
- Front end down, with the front edge of the hood contacting the ground and the rear of the car supported by the C-posts (rear posts)
- Front end up, with the trunk lid contacting the ground and much of the weight of the vehicle supported by the A-posts (front posts)

If the vehicle is tilted with the engine, which is the heaviest part of the vehicle, on the ground and the trunk in the air, it can often be stabi-

lized by using two step chocks upside down under the trunk.

When the roof is crushed flat against the body, as when all the roof posts have collapsed, the car is essentially a steel box resting on the ground with the occupants completely trapped inside. Unless the vehicle is on a hill or perched precariously on debris or another vehicle, this is the one time when stabilization is unnecessary: The structure is rigid. In such a situation it will, of course, be impossible to gain access through a window, door, or the roof. However, it may be possible to cut through the floor pan and have an EMT-B either crawl inside, if the opening is big enough or the EMT-B small enough, or to reach through the opening to touch and offer emotional support to the occupants until rescue personnel can lift or open the vehicle.

If the vehicle is unstable and cannot be safely approached by an EMT-B, get as close as you safely can so you can talk or signal to the occupants to reassure them that help is on its way and begin getting an idea of their condition.

Remember that when the vehicle is found in one of the positions described above, it should be considered unstable and must be stabilized by trained personnel prior to entry by an EMT-B.

Gaining Access

The National Highway Safety Act of 1966 required states to improve prehospital emergency care capabilities. It was recognized that EMS personnel could not do much for collision victims who could not be extricated from vehicles in time for live-saving efforts to be effective. So vehicle rescue training courses were developed, and bigger and better-equipped rescue units were placed in service.

Training courses began to prepare EMS personnel for a wide range of collision scene rescue activities aimed at gaining access to patients: unlocking and unlatching doors with commercially available and homemade tools, removing windshields intact, using hydraulic rescue tools to open vehicle doors one at a time, and so on.

Problems did not start to plague the rescue services until the mid 1980s. Suddenly extrications were taking longer, powerful rescue tools did not seem to be working properly, and procedures that had worked well for years were no longer successful. The reason for this apparent backslide? Improved vehicle construction. For example, the Nader pin (named for Ralph Nader, the consumer advocate who lobbied for the device), is a case-hardened pin in an automobile door. In a collision, the cams in the door locks grasp the pin to keep the door from flying open. Prior to the Nader pin, rescue personnel could open a door with a crowbar. Subsequently, rescuers had to start using a hydraulic spreader to peel the cams off the pins. Safety features designed to keep occupants inside wrecked vehicles were keeping rescuers out! Each new safety improvement to vehicles created a new challenge to rescue personnel.

Vehicle rescue training was becoming a complicated business, and rescuers were being asked to learn dozens of techniques, some of which could be used only on certain models of cars. The need for effective but simplified procedures became evident. The next few pages will describe a three-step procedure that has been developed to meet this need.

Simple Access

First remember that, as an EMT-B, your responsibility is not the rescue of the vehicle but the rescue of the patient. You will usually assume that an occupant or occupants of the vehicle have sustained life-threatening injuries, and that at least one EMT-B needs to gain quick access to the patient, even while rescuers are working to gain a more wide-open access, create exitways, and disentangle occupants.

After the vehicle is stable enough for you to approach it safely, check to see if a door can be opened or if an occupant of the vehicle can roll down a window or unlock a door. (Try Before You Pry!) Such ordinary ways of getting into the vehicle are known as simple access.

Complex Access

If simple access fails, you may need to use tools or special equipment to break a window and gain access even while the rescue crew is dismantling the vehicle for extrication of the occupants. When tools or equipment are used for this purpose, the process is known as complex access.

All automotive glass is one of two types: laminated or tempered. Windshields and some side and rear van and truck windows are laminated safety glass—two sheets of plate glass bonded to a sheet of tough plastic like a glass-and-plastic sandwich. Most passenger car side and rear windows are tempered glass. They are very resilient, but when they do break, rather than shattering into sharp fragments they break into small, rounded pieces.

You will usually try to gain access through a side or rear window as far as possible from the passengers. Use a center punch against a lower corner to break the glass. Punch out finger holds in the top of the window and use your gloved fingers to pull fragments away from the window.

A flathead ax is usually required to break through a windshield. This can also be done very quickly using a Glas-Master saw (Figure 31-2). A windshield is usually not broken to gain access, but the rescue squad may need to remove it if they plan to displace the dash or steering column or remove the roof. Before the windshield is broken, passengers should be covered with aluminized rescue blankets or tarps, if possible.

Once an entry point is gained, at least one EMT-B, who is properly dressed, should crawl inside the vehicle and immediately begin the initial assessment and rapid trauma exam as well as manual cervical stabilization. Don't forget to explain what is going on and provide emotional support to the patient by talking and reassuring him that everything that can be done for him is being done. Access points are usually much smaller holes than those that patients are taken out of. Do not be tempted to pull a patient out of an access hole prior to spinal immobilization, as you have learned in Chapter 28, Injuries to the Head and Spine.

Disentanglement: A Three-Part Action Plan

In most instances EMT-Bs will not be directly involved in disentanglement other than acting as the patient's advocate and being the EMT-B

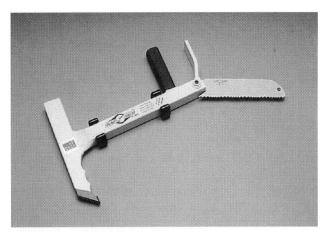

FIGURE 31-2 A Glas-Master saw can aid in windshield removal.

inside the vehicle. However, it is helpful to understand the plan for complex access that may be used by rescue personnel to free the trapped patient. Following is a description of a three-part procedure that can be accomplished by fire, rescue, and EMS personnel with the appropriate equipment. The procedure is not vehicle specific; that is, it can be used on virtually any car or truck. The procedure does not include a lot of techniques that require special equipment. Personnel can be trained in a short course. And, most important to EMS personnel, there is no need to fill several compartments of the ambulance with rescue equipment.

Step One: Gain Access by Disposing of the Roof

For more than 20 years, emergency service personnel have been trained to carry out a progression of procedures to reach the occupants of a wrecked vehicle: first try the doors; if that fails, unlock and unlatch the doors by nondestructive or destructive means; when all else fails, gain access through window openings. This multi-part procedure is time-consuming and requires a number of tools.

A quicker and far more efficient procedure is to dispose of the roof of a collision vehicle as soon as hazards have been controlled and the vehicle is stable. Disposing of the roof has three benefits.

- It makes the entire interior of the vehicle accessible. EMS personnel can stand beside or climb into the vehicle and pursue emergency care efforts while rescuers carry out disentanglement procedures.
- It creates a large exitway through which an occupant can be quickly removed when he has a life-threatening injury or when fire or another hazard is threatening the operation.
- It provides fresh air and helps cool off the patient when heat is a problem.

Scan 31-4 illustrates the procedure for folding a collision vehicle's roof back like the roof of a convertible. While this is the most commonly used procedure, it is not the only way to dispose of a roof. A roof can be folded forward after cutting both C- and B-posts (rear and middle posts), folded to either side after cutting the posts of the opposite side, or removed altogether after severing all of the roof posts. Lacking a hydraulic rescue tool, you can accomplish all of these procedures with ordinary hacksaws and a spray container of lubricant.

Step Two: Create Exitways by Displacing Doors and Roof Posts

When rapid vertical extrication through the opened roof is not indicated, the next step is to open doors and displace roof posts. The benefits of this step are that EMS personnel can kneel beside the vehicle while carrying out patient care and immobilization procedures, and the immobilized patients can be easily rotated onto a long spine board. Scan 31-5 shows a team of rescuers using a combination hydraulic rescue tool to open doors that cannot be unlatched and pulled open in the usual manner, as when doors are damaged or locks and latches jammed.

Step Three: Disentangle Occupants by Displacing the Front End

Most vehicle rescue training courses include procedures for displacing or removing seats, dash assemblies, steering wheels, steering columns, and pedals. A quicker and more efficient way to disentangle an injured driver and/or passenger from these mechanisms of entrapment is to displace the entire front end of the vehicle. While the task sounds difficult, it is not. Scan 31-6 illustrates the procedure for displacing the front end of a passenger car with a combination hydraulic rescue tool. A dash displacement can also be accomplished with heavy duty jacks and hacksaws.

If the steering wheel hub is large and rectangular, the car probably has an air bag or bags (the passenger-side bag being in the glove compartment). If the bags have not deployed, they are not likely to deploy now unless extrication involves displacing the dash or steering wheel. If such displacement is to be done, air bag manufacturers recommend following these steps.

1. Avoid placing your body or objects against an air bag module or in its path of deployment.
2. Disconnect the battery cables.
3. Do not displace or cut the steering column until the system has been fully deactivated.
4. Do not cut or drill into an air bag module.
5. Do not apply heat in the area of the steering wheel hub.

Must the three-part procedure just described be used for all extrication operations? Must the three procedures always be accomplished in the same order? Must all three procedures always be used? Not at all. In some cases, it may be necessary only to force a door open to reach a single patient and create an exitway for

Disposing of the Roof of a Car

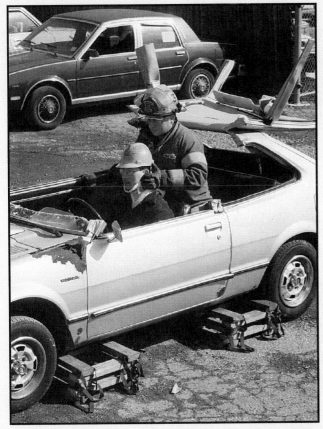

A. The traditional procedure for disposing of the roof is to sever the A- and B-posts, cut through the roof rails just ahead of the C-posts, and fold the roof back like the roof of a convertible. It is necessary either to remove or to cut the windshield, depending on the need for working space.

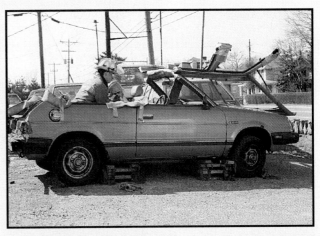

B. Folding the roof forward can be accomplished quickly when the C-posts are narrow. The roof is hinged either on the top or the bottom of the windshield, depending on the need for working space.

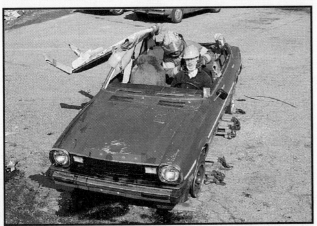

C. When a car has only one occupant, the roof can be folded to one side after severing the A-, B-, and C-posts of the opposite side.

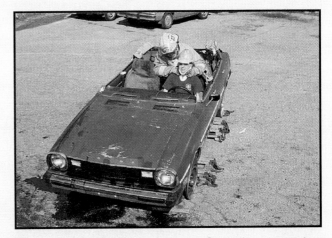

D. When a car has narrow C-posts, removing the roof altogether provides maximum working space.

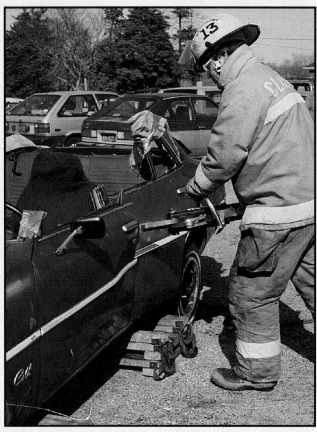

A. A collision vehicle's doors can be opened quickly with a hydraulic rescue tool. Doors can be opened at the latch or by breaking the hinges.

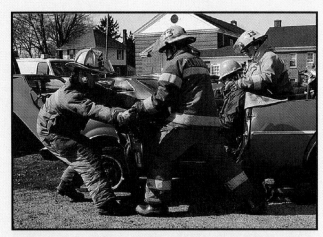

B. Once the front door has been opened, it can be moved beyond the normal range of motion by simply pushing on it. Seldom is there a need for removing a front door.

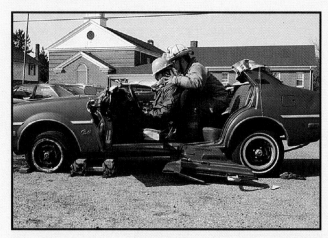

C. When the front doors of a four-door car have been opened at the latch side, the roof post and rear door can be pulled down simultaneously to expose the entire side of the vehicle.

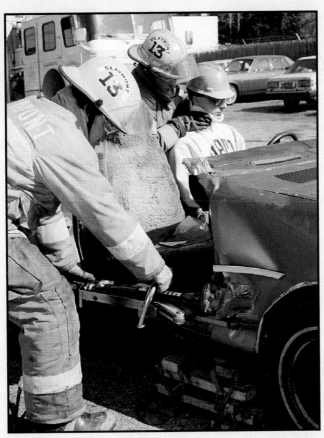

A. Relief cuts are made at the junction of the A-post with the rocker panel, and in the A-post between the door hinges.

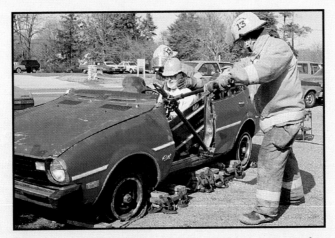

B. Heavy duty jacks can be used to pivot the front end of the vehicle away from the relief cuts.

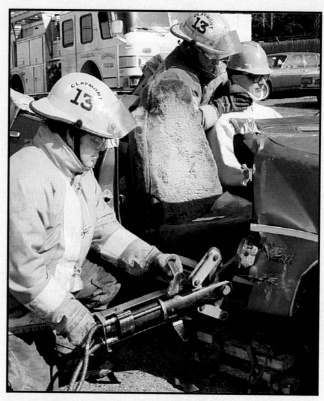

C. The combination hydraulic tool can be used in the spreading mode to displace the front end.

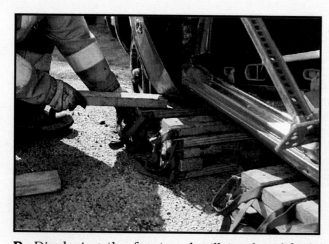

D. Displacing the front end will tend to lift the vehicle from the cribs. Cribbing must be added to the front cribs to prevent destabilization.

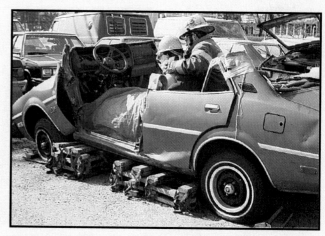

E. Displacing the front end creates working space by moving a number of mechanisms of entrapment away from front seat occupants.

his removal. In other cases, it may be prudent to open doors before disposing of the roof. In still other situations, there may not be a need to displace the front end of a collision vehicle.

The extent to which you, as an EMT-B, will participate in vehicle rescue procedures depends on the role your EMS unit plays in vehicle rescue and whether or not your ambulance arrives ahead of fire and rescue units. The main purpose for the EMT-B to know extrication procedures is to incorporate them into the patient care plan.

CHAPTER REVIEW

SUMMARY

As an EMT-B, you will not usually be responsible for vehicle or other kinds of rescue and extrication unless you undertake special training. However, it is important to understand how the process is done, how it may affect the patient, and how you can gain early access to the patient to begin care. Vehicle extrication or rescue includes 10 phases: preparing for the rescue, sizing up the situation, recognizing and managing hazards, stabilizing the vehicle, gaining access to the patient, providing initial assessment and a rapid trauma exam, disentangling the patient, immobilizing and extricating the patient, providing ongoing assessment and transport, and terminating the rescue.

REVIEW QUESTIONS

1. Explain the role of the EMT-B in the size-up of a motor vehicle collision.
2. Discuss what the EMT-B should do upon arrival at a collision if a power pole is broken in half and the lines are down in the street.
3. Explain whom you should call for assistance in your community if, on size-up of a collision, you observe a truck turned on its side and leaking fuel.
4. Discuss ways to stabilize a vehicle that is resting on its wheels, a vehicle that is resting on its side, and a vehicle that is resting on its roof.

5. Explain the difference between simple access and complex access to a patient in a vehicle.

Application
- With knowledge of your own community, which of the ten types of rescue specialty teams are needed and who provides the service?
- After considering safety of yourself and others, what should be your primary goal at the scene of a vehicle collision?

Overviews

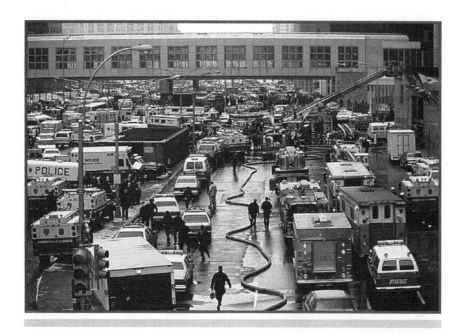

32

As an EMT-Basic, you will respond to scenes that require expertise beyond your training. Such incidents may involve hazardous materials or the challenge of multiple patients. Most communities have a plan that details how to meet the needs of such incidents. Your responsibility is to become familiar with those plans and the roles EMS, fire, law enforcement, and other agencies play.

Objectives

On the Scene

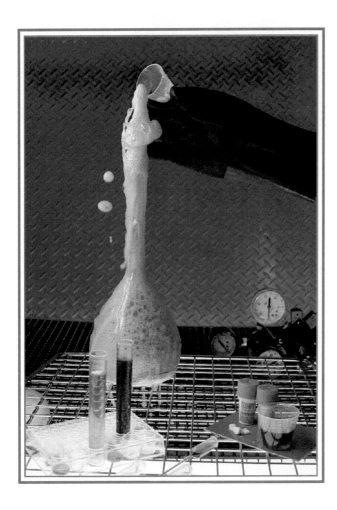

Twenty students are at work in the chemistry lab at Jefferson High School when an explosion takes place. Since you are the first EMS unit to arrive and the most senior EMT-B present, you are designated the EMS command officer. The fire command officer, who is also acting as Incident Commander, advises you that there are approximately ten injured students who have apparently inhaled the unknown gas. Three of them also have injuries from the blast. He advises you that the north parking lot and the softball field are upwind of the accident.

You radio a report to the EMS dispatcher. "Dispatcher, this is EMS Command. I am declaring a multiple-casualty incident. I will need seven additional ambulances to start. Have the responding ambulances stage in the north parking lot. The triage area will be set up on the softball field."

You determine the danger and safe zones, and your partner takes the MCI and jump kits and begins triage. You put on the triage officer bib. Just then the Incident commander informs you that they are about to make entry to the lab to try to find the other victims. He also identifies the decontamination area for you.

"I'll call for our disaster van with extra supplies," you tell him. "Have you spoken with the teacher to get an idea of what chemicals are involved?"

"We're doing it now," he responds. "Parents are starting to show up. The police and the school will deal with them."

You immediately go to the staging area to make sure it is clear for EMS resources and to assign and coordinate EMS personnel as they arrive. When an EMS worker of higher rank takes over EMS command, you proceed with your new assignment—help with patient care, packaging, and transport.

at the scene of a hazardous materials situation. (p. 692)

5. Break down the steps to approaching a hazardous situation. (pp. 690–692)

6. Discuss the various environmental hazards that affect EMS. (pp. 689–690)

7. Describe the criteria for a multiple-casualty situation. (p. 693)

8. Evaluate the role of the EMT-Basic in the multiple-casualty situation. (pp. 693–694)

9. Summarize the components of basic triage. (pp. 694–696)

10. Define the role of the EMT-Basic in a disaster operation. (pp. 694–697)

11. Describe basic concepts of incident management. (pp. 693–694)

12. Explain the methods for preventing contamination of self, equipment, and facilities. (pp. 690–692)

13. Review the local mass casualty incident plan. (p. 693)

Skills

1. Given a scenario of a mass casualty incident, perform triage.

You have already learned how to deal with many situations in which an individual patient needs emergency care. However, you also need to know what to do if you are called to the scene of an explosion, an airline crash, a multiple vehicle pile-up, an earthquake, or other situation in which there may be many real or potential victims. Even though you are not trained to deal with all the complexities of such emergencies, you must be able to recognize them and call for the appropriate assistance.

HAZARDOUS MATERIALS

According to the U.S. Department of Transportation (DOT), a **hazardous material** is "any substance or material in a form which poses an unreasonable risk to health, safety, and property when transported in commerce." One of the undesirable aspects of our modern world is the growing number of such materials (Table 32-1). Hazardous materials are used for the manufacture of products and can also be the waste products of manufacturing. Even though safety procedures have been established and are followed for the most part, accidents involving hazardous materials do occur. Hazardous materials accidents are especially likely to take place at factories, along railroads, and on local, state, and federal highways.

Warning: Do not attempt a rescue when an accident involves hazardous materials unless you have been trained to do so, have the proper equipment, and have the personnel necessary to ensure a safe scene. Many excellent courses are offered in hazardous materials. As an EMT-B you would do well to take such a course as part of your continuing education. You should follow the guidelines set by the U. S. Department of Transportation, the Occupational Safety and Health Administration (OSHA 1910.120), and

TABLE 32-1 Examples of Hazardous Materials

Material	Possible Hazard
Benzene (benzol)	Toxic vapors; can be absorbed through the skin; destroys bone marrow
Benzoyl peroxide	Fire and explosion
Carbon Tetrachloride	Damages internal organs
Cyclohexane	Explosive; eye and throat irritant
Diethyl ether	Flammable and can be explosive; irritant to eyes and respiratory tract; can cause drowsiness or unconsciousness
Ethyl acetate	Irritates eyes and respiratory tract
Ethylene dichloride	Strong irritant
Heptane	Respiratory irritant
Hydrochloric acid	Respiratory irritant; exposure to high concentration of vapors can produce pulmonary edema; can damage skin and eyes
Hydrofluoric acid	Vapors can cause pulmonary edema and severe eye burns; vapors and liquid can burn skin; vapors can be lethal; possible delayed reactions
Hydrogen cyanide	Highly flammable; toxic through inhalation or absorption
Methyl isobutyl ketone	Irritates eyes and mucous membranes
Methylene chloride	Damages eyes
Nitric acid	Produces a toxic gas (nitrogen dioxide); skin irritant; can cause self-ignition of cellulose products (e.g., sawdust).
Organochloride (Chlordane, DDT, Dieldrin, Lindane, Methoxychlor)	Irritates eyes and skin; fumes and smoke toxic
Perchloroethylene	Toxic if inhaled or swallowed
Silicon tetrachloride	Water-reactive to form toxic hydrogen chloride fumes
Tetrahydrofuram (THF)	Damages eyes and mucous membranes
Toluol (toluene)	Toxic vapors; can cause organ damage
Vinyl chloride	Flammable and explosive; listed as a carcinogen

the National Fire Protection Association (NFPA 479), as well as your community's emergency response plan for hazardous materials.

As an EMT-B you will be highly skilled in emergency care. However, without specialized training, you are still a lay person when it comes to hazardous materials. Special training is required to understand hazardous materials, to work at the scene of incidents involving these materials, and to render the scene safe. You cannot judge the state of a container or the probability of explosion without the benefit of such training. Do not believe that you can use safety equipment unless you are trained in the care, field testing, and actual use of the equipment. With hazardous materials accidents, you may be able to do nothing more than stay a safe distance away from the scene until expert help arrives.

At the Scene

As a responding EMT-B, you may be the first to recognize that a hazardous materials situation exists. For example, you may answer a call to a business where four employees are ill after being in the warehouse. When there are multiple medical victims, think "hazmat."

Your primary concerns at the scene of a hazardous materials incident are your safety and the safety of your crew, the patient, and the public. Should you arrive first at the scene of a hazardous materials accident, establish a "danger zone" and a "safe zone." Keep all people out of the danger zone, and try to convince them to leave the immediate area. Stay in the safe zone until expert help arrives and makes other areas safe to enter.

The safe zone should be on the same level as, and upwind from, the hazardous materials accident site. Avoid being downhill in case there are flowing liquids or gases that are burning or otherwise unsafe. Avoid low-lying areas in case fumes are escaping and hanging close to the ground. Avoid placing yourself higher than the accident scene so that you will not be in the path of escaping gases or heated air. Also be alert to the fact that a sewer system can rapidly spread hazardous materials over a large area.

Call for the help that you will need. The support services required at the scene of a hazardous materials accident may include fire services, special rescue personnel, local or state hazardous materials experts, and law enforcement personnel for crowd control. If the accident has taken place at an industrial site or along a railway, the company experts in hazardous materials need to be notified. Much of this can be done by a single call to your dispatcher. (See Table 32-2 and "Sources of Information" below.)

Local backup support will want to know certain facts, including

- Type of hazardous material: gas, liquid chemical, cooled chemical, dry chemical, radioactive liquid, radioactive gases, or solid radioactive materials
- Specific name of the material or its identification number
- How much material is at the scene
- Current state of the material: escaping as a gas, leaking as a liquid, being blown into the air, in flames, or apparently still contained
- When the incident began, or how long you estimate that the scene has been dangerous
- Other hazardous materials near the scene
- Estimated number of possible patients in the danger zone

Sources of Information

Vehicle drivers, plant and railroad personnel, and perhaps even bystanders may be able to tell you the name of the hazardous material. In many cases there will be a colored placard (Figure 32-1) on the vehicle, tank, or railroad car. This placard will have a four-digit identification number. Older placards are usually orange and have an identification number preceded by the letters UN or UA. Your dispatcher may have access to the name of the material through this identification number. There also may be an invoice, shipping manifest (trains), or bill of lading (trucks) that can confirm the identity of the substance.

FIGURE 32-1 Hazardous materials placard.

Warning: *Do not approach the scene to obtain this information. Placard information may be obtained from a safe distance by observation with binoculars.*

The Chemical Transportation Emergency Center (CHEMTREC) has been established in Washington, DC, by the Chemical Manufacturers Association. They can provide your dispatcher or you with information about the hazardous material. They have a 24-hour toll-free telephone number for the continental United States: 800-424-9300. In the DC area the 24-hour number is 202-483-7616. CHEMTREC will accept collect calls in an emergency. When you call, keep the line open so that changes at the scene can be reported to CHEMTREC and the center can confirm that they have contacted the shipper or manufacturer. CHEMTREC will be able to direct you as to your initial course of action.

If there is no identification number and no one knows what is being carried, you may have no other choice than to wait for experts to arrive at the scene.

Warning: Recent studies by the Office of Technology Assessment have shown that some states report 25% to 50% of the identification placards have been found to be incorrect. These same studies indicate that many shipping documents also are inaccurate or incomplete. *Do only what you have been trained to do. Follow the directions of hazardous materials experts.*

TABLE 32-2   Hazardous Materials Hotlines

Organizations	24-Hour Hotline Numbers
CHEMTREC (Chemical Transportation Emergency Center in Washington, DC)	800-424-9300 202-483-7616
REAC/TS (Radiation Emergency Assistance Center/ Training Site in Oak Ridge, TN)	615-482-2441

Initial actions at the scene can be directed according to information sent to you by your dispatcher, hazardous materials expert, or CHEMTREC. Often, this initial action is based on the procedures presented in *Hazardous Materials: The Emergency Response Guidebook* (DOT P 5800.2), published by the U. S. Department of Transportation. When you call your dispatcher or CHEMTREC

1. Give your name and call back number.
2. Explain the nature and location of the problem.
3. Report the identification number, if there is a safe way for you to obtain it.
4. When possible, supply the name of the shipper or manufacturer.
5. Describe the type, size, and shape of container.
6. Report if the container is on rail car, truck, open storage, or housed storage.
7. Give the carrier's name and the name of the consignee.
8. Report local conditions, including the weather.
9. Keep the line of communication open at all times.

Rescue and Care Procedures

During the entire process, you must stay in a safe area. Do not walk in any spilled materials. Do not think that the scene is safe simply because the substances do not have any apparent color or odor. Keep people away from the scene.

As soon as possible, decide who will take charge of the scene. If this has not been decided in planning sessions prior to the incident, you or another professional at the scene should become the incident manager until experts arrive to take over responsibility.

After a safe zone is created, you may do the following if you are trained to do so.

1. Put on 100% full-body protective clothing and a self-contained breathing apparatus (SCBA). *You must know how to check out and properly wear such equipment in order to use it.*
2. Isolate the accident area and keep the danger zone clear of unauthorized and unprotected personnel.
3. Evaluate the scene in terms of possible fire or explosion. *This takes special training.*

Patient Assessment—Hazardous Materials Injuries

Follow normal patient assessment procedures—including patient and bystander interviews—to assess injuries. Do not overlook medical conditions and injuries that may be present in addition to burns and other immediate effects of the hazardous material.

Patient Care—Hazardous Materials Injuries

As soon as it is safe to do so (expert judgment is required to determine this), begin assessment and care of patients.

Emergency Care Steps

1. Move patients to the safe zone as quickly as possible if the scene is still potentially dangerous and if there is no risk to you. Note that this is the kind of situation in which an emergency move of patients may need to be executed before assessment and care can begin. Only if the experts assure you that the scene offers no immediate danger should you begin life support measures within the danger zone.
2. Provide basic life support. For artificial ventilations and CPR, use oxygen from a flow-restricted, oxygen-powered ventilation device or a bag-valve mask and oxygen reservoir so that you do not have to take off your own protective gear.
3. Administer a high concentration of oxygen to any patient having difficulty breathing.
4. Immediately flush with water the skin, clothing, and eyes of anyone who has come into contact with the hazardous material. Retain the run-off.
5. Remove clothing, shoes, and jewelry from all persons who have come into contact with the hazardous material. Continue flushing the patient's skin with water for no less than 20 minutes. Continue to retain run-off.
6. Remove your protective gear as recommended by local guidelines.
7. Transport the patient as soon as possible, providing care for shock, administering oxygen, and taking all steps necessary to maintain normal body temperature.

Warning: Do not neglect to decontaminate or to be sure others with the proper training have decontaminated the patient prior to transport.

Otherwise the ambulance crew may be overcome en route. The contaminated patient and EMT-Bs also can contaminate and even shut down the hospital emergency department.

Remember: Some materials will allow you to act, while others will require experts to respond before you can gain access and provide care. This is why you need to provide your dispatcher with all the information available. Your dispatcher will provide you with the proper information about whether and when to proceed. Remember, you are an EMT-B, not an expert in hazardous materials.

See Appendix C for more information on hazardous materials.

MULTIPLE-CASUALTY INCIDENTS

A **multiple-casualty incident (MCI)**—or in some areas, a multiple-casualty situation (MCS)—is an event that places a great demand on EMS equipment and personnel resources (Figure 32-2). The number of patients required before an MCI can be declared varies in practice. Some jurisdictions will declare an MCI for as few as three patients on the grounds that practice with smaller scale incidents will help prepare for larger ones. Other jurisdictions reserve the MCI designation for five, seven, or more patients. The most common MCI is an automobile crash with three or more patients. You also will likely respond to many incidents with three to 15 potential patients. Incidents with large-scale

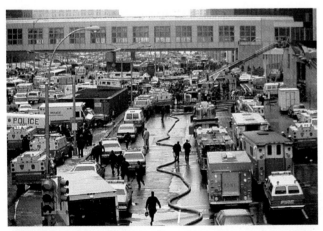

FIGURE 32-2 The scene of a multiple-casualty incident: The World Trade Center bombing, New York City, February 1993.

casualties are rare and apt to be "once in a career" events.

The important ingredient in an MCI is that, for whatever reason, the ability of the EMS system to respond to the situation is challenged or hampered by the situation itself. For any MCI plan to be effective, it must be flexible and expandable enough to be used from small three-patient incidents to large scale incidents of fifteen or more patients. In other words, the plan for "the big one" should be a logical extension of the same plan used to manage smaller incidents.

Multiple-Casualty Incident Operations

Though the principles of managing small- and large-scale MCIs are generally the same, large-scale MCIs unfold over a longer period of time and require greater support from outside agencies. Well-trained and practiced EMT-Bs can usually cope with a small-scale MCI pretty well. However, experience has shown that even the best-trained EMT-Bs have a difficult time managing an incident of greater magnitude.

One way to minimize the operating difficulties of a large-scale MCI is for every EMT-B to be familiar with the local disaster plan. A **disaster plan** is a pre-defined set of instructions that tells a community's various emergency responders what to do in specific emergencies. While no disaster plan can address every problem that could arise, there are several features common to every good disaster plan. The disaster plan should be

- *Written to address the events that are conceivable for a particular location*—Kansas needs to plan for tornadoes, not hurricanes.
- *Well publicized*—Each emergency responder should be familiar with the plan and how it is to be put into operation.
- *Realistic*—The plan must be based on the actual availability of resources.
- *Rehearsed*—Experience has proven that the only way to get a plan to work correctly is to exercise it and, in so doing, work out the unforeseen "bugs."

It is beyond the scope of this text to attempt to teach you how to write a disaster plan or even to impart enough knowledge for you to be in charge of a disaster operation. However, it is important to understand your potential roles in the management of such an incident.

Scene Management

The first EMT-Bs on the scene of an MCI or disaster must be sure to initiate the **incident management system** that is in practice in their jurisdiction. This is a general plan for managing an MCI that assists in the control, direction, and coordination of emergency response resources. It provides a single, orderly means of communication for decision making among all the agencies involved in the incident.

The senior EMT-B will give a radio report on the nature of the emergency, its exact location, and the best estimate of the number of patients. This crucial information will be used by the dispatch center to send additional resources to the scene. The radio report should include a request for any special resources that the EMT-Bs feel may be necessary.

If the disaster plan is to be put into operation, it is critical that other responding units be informed of this fact. The EMT-Bs on the scene must take command of the scene until they are relieved. This will include telling other units what equipment to bring, what they should plan on doing once they arrive, how best to access the scene, and where to park. It is also important to keep uninjured people from becoming injured. This will probably require restricting access to the scene to only those personnel performing triage (explained below), extrication from wreckage, and patient care.

After an incident manager is determined, EMS sectors are established as needed. These include

- Extrication sector
- Treatment sector
- Transportation sector
- Staging sector
- Supply sector
- Triage sector
- Mobile command center

Individuals and agencies on the scene will be assigned particular roles in one or more sectors. Any EMT-B arriving at the scene at this time would be expected to report to a sector officer for assignment of specific duties. Once assigned a specific task, the EMT-B should complete the task and report back to the sector officer.

Usually the crew leader on the first arriving EMS unit will assume medical or **EMS command.** EMS command establishes an EMS command post to oversee the medical aspects of the incident and the safety of all personnel, to designate sector officers, and to work closely with the fire and police commanders. Most systems use brightly colored reflective vests that can be worn over protective clothing to make each incident sector officer easy to identify. Command may be transferred to higher-ranking EMS officers if and as they arrive on the scene. On larger incidents, EMS command may have an aide to assist with communications as well as a safety officer and a public information officer.

Once EMS command has been established, the next task is to quickly assess all the patients and assign each a priority for receiving emergency care or transportation to definitive care. This process is called **triage,** which comes from a French word meaning "to sort." The most knowledgeable EMS provider becomes the **triage officer.** The triage officer calls for additional help if needed, assigns available personnel and equipment to patients, and remains at the scene to assign and coordinate personnel, supplies, and vehicles.

Initial Triage

When faced with more than one patient, your goal must be to afford the greatest number of people the greatest chance of survival. To accomplish this goal, you must provide care to patients according to the seriousness of illness or injury while keeping in mind that spending a lot of time trying to save one life may prevent a number of other patients from receiving the treatment they need.

To properly triage a group of patients, you should quickly classify each patient into one of four groups.

- *Priority 1: Treatable Life-Threatening Illness or Injuries*—Airway and breathing difficulties; uncontrolled or severe bleeding; decreased mental status; patients with severe medical problems; shock (hypoperfusion); severe burns
- *Priority 2: Serious But Not Life-Threatening Illness or Injuries*—Burns without airway problems; major or multiple bone or joint injuries; back injuries with or without spinal cord damage
- *Priority 3: "Walking Wounded"*—Minor musculoskeletal injuries; minor soft tissue injuries
- *Priority 4 (sometimes called Priority 0): Dead or Fatally Injured*—Examples include exposed brain matter, cardiac arrest (no pulse

for over 20 minutes except with cold-water drowning or severe hypothermia), decapitation, severed trunk, and incineration.

Patients in arrest are considered Priority 4 (or 0) when resources are limited. The time that must be devoted to rescue breathing or CPR for one person is not justified when there are many patients needing attention. Once ample resources are available, patients in arrest become Priority 1.

How triage is performed depends on the number of injuries, the immediate hazards to personnel and patients, and the location of backup resources. Local operating procedures will give you more guidance on the exact method of triage for a given situation. Basic principles of triage are presented here.

The first triage cut can be done rapidly by using a bullhorn, PA system, or loud voice to direct all patients capable of walking (Priority 3) to move to a particular area. This has a two-fold purpose. It quickly identifies these individuals who have an airway and circulation, and it physically separates them from patients who will generally need more care.

You must rapidly assess each remaining patient, stopping only to secure an airway or stop profuse bleeding. It is important that you not develop "tunnel vision"—spending time rendering additional care to any one patient and thus failing to identify and correct life-threatening conditions of the remaining patients. If Priority 3 patients are nearby and well enough to help, they may be employed to assist you by maintaining an airway or direct pressure on bleeding wounds of other patients. Priority 3 patients who have been reluctant to leave ill or injured friends or relatives may be permitted to stay near them where they can be of possible help later.

Once all patients have been assessed and treated for airway and breathing problems and severe bleeding, more thorough treatment can be initiated. You will need to render care to the patients who are most seriously injured or ill but who stand the best chance of survival with proper treatment. This requires treating all the Priority 1 patients first, Priority 2 patients next, and Priority 3 patients last. Priority 4 patients do not receive treatment unless no other patients are believed to be at risk of dying or suffering long-term disability if their conditions go unattended.

Usually patients will be immobilized on backboards if necessary and carried by "run-ners" to the appropriate secondary sector (as described below). Extensive treatment does not occur at the incident site since it is in a hazard zone and since it could impede rescue and initial treatment of other patients.

Patient Identification

By now it should be clear that a system will be required to group and identify patients by treatment priority. A widely used system is to color-code patients according to their priority. For example, Priority 1 = red, Priority 2 = yellow, Priority 3 = green, Priority 4 (if a separate category) = black or gray.

Different localities have different systems. It is important that you know and understand the system used in your area. It is equally important that different services in the same region use the same coding system. This is because many MCIs are multiple-agency events. If each agency were to use a different system, there would be no way to correctly coordinate the order in which patients are to receive care.

As you move among patients to conduct initial triage, you should affix a **triage tag** to each patient, indicating the priority group to which that patient has been assigned. Triage tags are color-coded and may have space in which limited medical information can be recorded (Fig-

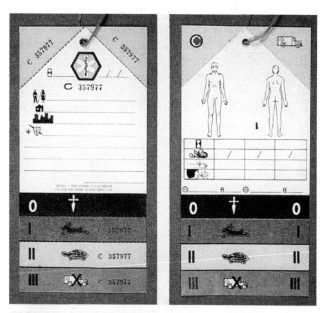

FIGURE 32-3 Typical triage tags used to identify Priority 1, Priority 2, Priority 3, and Priority 0 patients.

ited medical information can be recorded (Figure 32-3).

There are some local variations of the triage tag. Some use adhesive-backed colored shipping labels. Others use colored surveyor's tape or duct tape to classify patients. Surveyor's tape can be quickly tied on as an arm band. Duct tape will stick to just about anything in any kind of weather. For this reason it is particularly useful in an MCI setting. It is also useful to have a laundry marker or wax pencil handy for wet conditions when a standard pen or pencil will not write well.

Whatever system you use, it is vital that the color coding be easily located and identified. Properly done, this allows a later EMT-B to quickly identify which treatment group patients belong to and to institute treatment accordingly.

Secondary Triage and Treatment

As more personnel arrive at the incident scene, they should be directed to assist with the completion of initial triage. If triage has been completed, these EMT-Bs can initiate treatment.

Secondary triage generally begins at this point. In ideal triage systems, patients are gathered into a **triage sector** and, under the direction of the triage officer, are physically separated into treatment groups based on their priority level as designated by a triage tag. Some systems call for vehicles to carry red, yellow, and green tarps, which are used to designate these areas. An area to which patients are removed is referred to as a **treatment sector.** Each treatment sector should have its own **treatment officer,** an EMT responsible for overseeing the triage and treatment within that sector. The treatment officer should again triage the patients in that sector to determine the order in which they will receive treatment.

During secondary triage, it may be necessary to recategorize a patient whose condition has deteriorated or improved or who was incorrectly triaged to a higher or lower priority group than was medically warranted. This will necessitate moving the patient to the proper treatment sector as resources permit. Some systems use a different disaster tag during secondary triage on which more detailed information about the patient can be recorded (Figure 32-4).

The treatment sector EMT-Bs will need supplies and equipment from the ambulances such as bandages, blood pressure cuffs, and oxygen.

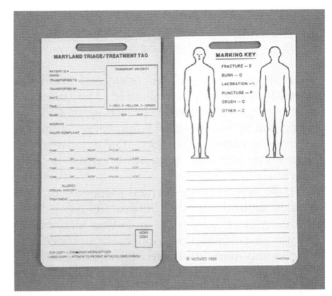

FIGURE 32-4 EMS disaster tag used during secondary triage.

Staging and Transportation

Transportation Logistics

Once patients have been properly assessed and separated, and once treatment for the patients has been initiated according to their priority, consideration must be given to the order in which the patients will be transported to a hospital. Again, this is done according to triage priority.

It is advisable to have a staging sector from which ambulances can be called to transport patients. The **staging sector** will be the responsibility of the **staging officer.** This person must keep track of the ambulance vehicles and personnel. In large-scale incidents, the staging officer may need to arrange to meet human needs, such as rest rooms, meals, and rotation of crews.

No ambulance should proceed to a treatment sector without having been requested by the **transportation officer** and directed by the staging officer. The staging officer is responsible for communicating with each treatment sector to determine the number and priority of the patients in that sector. This information can then be used by the transportation officer to arrange for transport of patients from the scene to the hospital in the most efficient way.

It is vital that no ambulance transport any patient without the approval of the transportation officer. This is because the transporta-

officer is responsible for maintaining a list of patients and the hospitals to which they are transported. This information is relayed from the transportation officer to each receiving hospital. (In a large-scale incident, the transportation officer may actually have an aide who does nothing but speak to hospitals.) In this way the hospitals know what to expect and receive only the patients they are capable of handling. It is critical that the EMT-Bs on the ambulance comply with the instructions of the transportation officer. Failure to do so may result in patients being transported to the wrong facilities.

Once an ambulance has completed a run to a hospital, it will probably be directed to return to the staging area, perhaps bringing needed supplies, to await its next instructions from the staging officer.

Communicating with Hospitals

It is important that receiving hospitals be alerted to the nature of the MCI or disaster as soon as the magnitude of the incident is known. This allows the hospitals to call in additional personnel or to clear beds as necessary to accept the anticipated numbers of patients.

Because radio communication channels will be heavily used, the transportation officer, not individual EMT-Bs, should communicate with the hospitals. This will keep unnecessary radio usage to a minimum. It will also ensure that the proper information is recorded at both ends of the ambulance ride. In large-scale MCIs, it is not necessary to give a patient report for each patient. This is because the transporting and treating EMT-Bs will most likely be different and because there will generally be too many patients to allow EMT-Bs to give a good patient radio report under the circumstances. In these instances, the hospital may be told only that they are receiving a Priority 1 patient with respiratory problems, for example.

Psychological Aspects of MCIs

During MCIs, EMT-Bs often encounter another, frequently overlooked condition: psychologically stressed patients. While they may outwardly exhibit few signs of injury or emotional stress, people involved in MCIs have been subjected to devastating circumstances with which they are normally unprepared to cope. Proper early management of the psychologically stressed patient

can support later treatment and help ensure a faster recovery.

Adequately managing a patient during an MCI may require you to administer "psychological first aid." This may take the form of talking with a terrified parent, child, or witness. You should not attempt to engage in psychoanalysis and should not say things that are untrue in an attempt to calm a patient. However, a caring honest demeanor can reassure a patient, as will listening to the patient and acknowledging his fears and problems. Often this is all the patient will need.

Patients are not the only ones subject to emotional stress during an MCI. So are emergency responders. It is very important that you understand that large-scale or horrific MCIs may affect rescuers as much as, if not more than, non-rescuers.

EMT-Bs who become emotionally incapacitated should be treated as patients and removed to an area where they can rest without viewing the scene. These patients must be monitored by an EMS provider until a clinically competent provider can take over. These EMT-Bs should not be allowed to return to duty without first being evaluated by someone professionally trained to do so.

Critical incident stress debriefing (CISD) teams are a resource that can provide the emotional and psychological support required by this type of incident. Intervention by a CISD team may help to prevent post-traumatic stress disorder. See Chapter 2, The Well-Being of the EMT-Basic, to review information on stressful incidents and CISD.

FYI

Topics included in the FYI—"For Your Information"—section are those that go beyond the chapter objectives. The information in this segment is intended to broaden your understanding of the chapter topic but is not essential to an understanding of your job as an EMT-B.

The Incident Command System

One of the most widely used systems in the country is the federal Incident Command or Management System (ICS). While not specifically a plan designed for MCI management, it provides a clear management framework for all types of incidents. In addition, it is mandated by law for the management of some types of incidents such as those involving hazardous materials.

ICS originated in California, where it was designed as a management plan to handle large-scale fire fighting operations involving multiple agencies and jurisdictions. A flexible tool for managing people and resources, the components of ICS are Command, Operations, Logistics, Planning, and Finance.

The most commonly used components of the plan are Command and Operations. Command is established at all incidents and assumes responsibility for incident management. This individual stays in command unless that function is transferred to another person or the incident is brought to a conclusion. Command handles all functions except those that are delegated to a Sector Officer.

It is recognized by ICS that the manageable span of control is six people. As the MCI escalates and needs become more complex, the number of people and span of control become larger. It is at this point that Command designates Sector Officers to help.

Command

There are two methods of Command—singular and unified. Singular command is used where all resources are specifically under the jurisdiction and control of one agency. In many communities EMS is managed by fire services. Accordingly, singular command is often used at fire and rescue incidents. However, if police agencies have major involvement, if there is a separate EMS provider, or if other agencies are involved, unified command is more appropriate. (See Figure 32-5.)

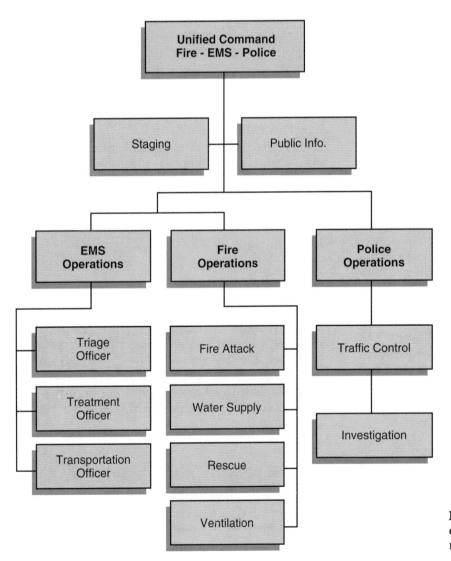

FIGURE 32-5 An organizational chart for a unified command method.

In most communities unified command is the best way to manage resources. It recognizes that incidents tend to grow more complex and that the right agency must take the lead at the right time, with command officers from all agencies cooperating.

Command Functions

There are two modes or phases of an MCI: scene size-up/triage and command/delegation. The most senior person on the first arriving EMS unit establishes EMS Command. Then Command and the crew do an initial scene size-up, start the triage process, and call for back-up. While waiting for help, initial triage is completed and command gets ready for arriving resources.

When reinforcements arrive, there are two options: continue to be in command or transfer command to someone of higher rank. In either case, EMS Command is positioned at a location close enough to allow observation of the scene but secure enough to permit management of incoming resources and communication with others. In many areas where unified command is used, EMS, Police, and Fire Command establish one field command post together and stay there. Some plans call for the field command vehicle or command post to be designated by placing two traffic cones on top of the vehicle being used.

Scene Size-Up

Size up the scene by making a sweep to determine what needs must be met.

1. Arrive at the scene and establish EMS command. Put on the proper identification.
2. Do a quick walk through the scene (or, if it is a hazmat scene, observe from a safe distance) and assess the number of patients, hazards, and degree of entrapment. Identify the number of patients including the "walking wounded," apparent priority of care, need for extrication, number of ambulances needed, other factors affecting the scene and corresponding resources needed to address them, and areas where resources can be staged.
3. Get as calm and composed as possible to radio in an initial scene report and call for additional resources.

Communications

Once scene size-up has been done, an initial scene report usually should be made to the communications center. Keep the report short and to the point. Give only the information necessary for the communications centers and other responders to understand the severity of the situation and react accordingly. Example: *MED-COM, this is Medic 100. We are on the scene of a two-car MVA with severe entrapment of four Priority 1 patients. Dispatch a rescue company and four paramedic ambulances. I will now be called Houston Avenue Command. Police are needed at the scene to assist with traffic and crowd control as soon as possible.*

As help begins to arrive, control of scene communication is important. Once units arrive, as much face-to-face communication as possible should be used, especially between Sector Officers and subordinates. This will help to reduce radio channel crowding. If you feel you are getting too tied up in radio communications, designate a radio aide. Basically, the flow of communications at the scene should correspond to the organizational chart being used. Accordingly, the only unit talking to the communications center and requesting resources is Command. All others talk to their assigned sector officers.

Operations

Getting organized early and aggressively is very important. You must have a plan to deploy resources when they arrive. You must have decided what sector officers will be needed and where resources will be placed. A common mistake is to underestimate the resources that will be needed. Somehow new patients not found during size-up have a way of appearing. Think big. Order big. Put resources in the staging area if they are not needed right away. In urban/suburban incidents, back-up can be fast and overwhelming. Think about a staging area early or you take the chance of being overrun.

Prevention of Freelancing

Freelancing is uncoordinated or undirected activity at the scene. Given the opportunity, most rescuers will arrive on the scene and begin setting their own priorities. Command can prevent this problem. When established early, people and crews are assigned to tasks as they arrive.

EMS Sector Functions

For smaller MCIs, Command may be able to handle all aspects of management without delegating tasks to others. However, as an incident increases in size and complexity, additional staff and sector officers will be needed. (See Figures 32-6 through 32-8.)

General Tactics

The object of incident management is to treat patients and give the best care with the available resources. IMS is simply a tool to be used to help provide organized and appropriate emergency care.

Often it is helpful to have some personal tools to help to get organized. For example,

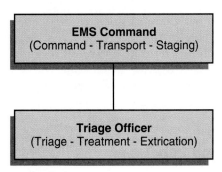

FIGURE 32-6 An organizational chart for a smaller incident.

many organizations have distilled the major points of their plans into a "tactical worksheet" they can use in the field. With enough use, the plan can become committed to memory. (See Figure 32-9.)

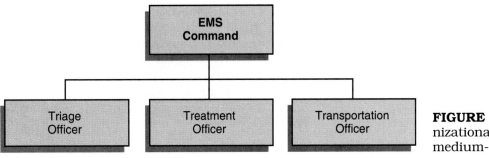

FIGURE 32-7 An organizational chart for a medium-sized incident.

CHAPTER REVIEW

KEY TERMS

You may find it helpful to review the following terms.

disaster plan a predefined set of instructions that tells a community's various emergency responders what to do in specific emergencies.

EMS command the senior EMS person on the scene who establishes an EMS command post and oversees the medical aspects of a multiple-casualty incident.

hazardous material according to the U.S. Department of Transportation, "any substance or material in a form which poses an unreasonable risk to health, safety, and property when transported in commerce."

incident management system a system used for the management of a multiple-casualty incident, involving assumption of responsibility for command and designation and coordination of such elements as triage, treatment, transport, and staging.

multiple-casualty incident (MCI) any medical or trauma incident involving multiple patients.

staging officer the person responsible for overseeing and keeping track of ambulances and ambulance personnel at a multiple-casualty incident. The staging officer will direct ambulances to treatment areas at the request of the transportation officer.

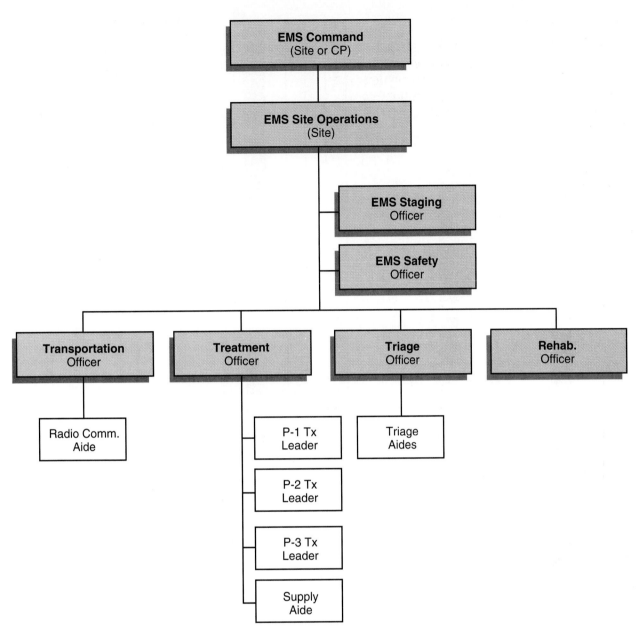

FIGURE 32-8 An organizational chart for a major incident.

staging sector the area where ambulances are parked and other resources are held until needed.

transportation officer the person responsible for communicating with sector officers and hospitals to manage transportation of patients to hospitals from the scene of a multiple-casualty incident.

treatment officer the person responsible for overseeing treatment of patients who have been triaged at a multiple-casualty incident.

treatment sector the area in which patients are treated at a multiple-casualty incident.

triage the process of quickly assessing patients in a multiple-casualty incident and assigning each a priority for receiving treatment according to the severity of their illness or injuries. From a French word meaning "to sort."

triage officer the person responsible for overseeing triage at a multiple-casualty incident.

triage sector the area in which secondary triage takes place at a multiple-casualty incident.

triage tag color-coded tag indicating the priority group to which a patient has been assigned.

COLONIE EMS — Incident Tactical Worksheet

_____ Establish unified command with fire & police
_____ Place 2 cones on command vehicle

_____ Put bib on
_____ Designate triage office

Location _____
Med. Command _____

_____ Advise inbound units where to stage
_____ Advise crews to stay with units until given instructions
_____ Advise units to switch to EMS Admin., 265 or 715

LEVEL 1 (3-10 Patients)

_____ Declare MCI
_____ EMS All Call
_____ Request # of Units Needed
_____ Cover Town/Sr. Medic Act 615
_____ Roll Call Hospitals
_____ Transport Officer?

LEVEL 2 (11-25 Patients)

_____ Declare MCI
_____ EMS All Call
_____ Request # of Units Needed
_____ Cover Town/Sr. Medic Act 615
_____ Roll Call Hospitals
_____ Get Mutual Aid Units
_____ Designate Treatment Officer
_____ Designate Transport Officer
_____ Designate Staging Officer
_____ REMO MD to Scene
_____ Consider Rehab & CISD

(6-13 Amb. Needed)
(2-5 Amb. Needed)

LEVEL 3 (over 25 Patients)

_____ Declare MCI
_____ EMS All Call
_____ Request # of Units Needed
_____ Cover Town/Sr. Medic Act 615
_____ Roll Call Hospitals
_____ Get Mutual Aid Units
_____ Designate Treatment Officer
_____ Designate Transport Officer
_____ Designate Staging Officer
_____ REMO MD to Scene
_____ Request Bus to Scene

(over 13 Amb. Needed)

FIRE

_____ Assess # of Units Needed
_____ EMS All Call Req. 619
_____ Designate Triage
_____ Set up Rehab at Air Bank
_____ Use 619 as ALS Unit

RESCUE

_____ Establish Perimeter
_____ Request Speciality Units
_____ Triage Officer Handles Inner Circle

HAZ-MAT

_____ Req. # of Units Needed
_____ EMS All Call
_____ Est. Command in Cold Zone
_____ Designate Triage
_____ Identify Agent
_____ Research Decontamination
_____ Research Med.

_____ Medical Baseline Assessment of Team
_____ Don Protective Barriers
_____ Assist With Decontamination
_____ Rehabilitate

HOSPITAL ROLL CALL	AMCH	St. PETERS	MEMORIAL	VA	ELLIS	St. CLARE'S	LEONARD	St. MARY'S	SAMARITAN
CAN TAKE									
# PATIENTS SENT									

UNITS RESPONDING

620 621 622
630 631 632
640 641 642
650 651 652
610 611 605
TSU-1 TSU-2
619
Guild. ___
CPHM ___
Albany ___
Mohawk ___
Empire ___

UNITS IN STAGING

620 621 622
630 631 632
640 641 642
650 651 652
610 611 605
TSU-1 TSU-2
619
Guild. ___
CPHM ___
Albany ___
Mohawk ___
Empire ___

OF PATIENTS BY PRIORITY

1 (Red)	2 (Yellow)	3 (Green)	0 (Black)	TOTALS

FIGURE 32-9 An incident tactical worksheet from the Town of Colonie, New York EMS.

702

Become familiar with your local plans for dealing with hazardous materials and multiple casualty incidents. Practice every chance you get. Understand the management systems and triage systems used in your area, and be prepared to do your part. Also, remember: hazardous materials accidents require specialized training beyond your expertise. However, you can learn to recognize them quickly, call for the appropriate assistance, and help to ensure the safety of rescuers, patients, and bystanders.

REVIEW QUESTIONS

1. List the information you need to include in your initial report of a hazardous materials incident.
2. Explain how to identify a hazardous material and to obtain information about that material.
3. Describe the general assessment and emergency care of a patient with a hazardous material injury.
4. Describe the major components and benefits of an incident management system.
5. Define the basic role of the EMT-B at a multiple-casualty incident.
6. Explain why patients are assigned priorities during triage.
7. Identify four priority categories of triage.

Application

- Your call is to a motor vehicle collision with an unknown number of injuries. As your unit approaches the scene, you see that three cars and downed wires are involved. You get a whiff of gasoline as you pass by. The drivers are visible in each vehicle—one appears to be conscious and the other two are bent forward or slumped back. There are passengers visible in two vehicles, one or more of whom may need extrication. How should you proceed?

Module 8 (Elective)

Advanced Airway Management

IN THIS MODULE
Chapter 33   Advanced Airway Management

MODULE OVERVIEW

In Chapter 7 you learned the importance of opening and maintaining a patient's airway. You also learned how to use airway adjuncts such as oral and nasal airways, ventilation devices such as bag-valve masks, flow-restricted, oxygen-powered ventilation devices, and suction devices. All of these devices are useful, but they do not protect the airway directly, as do the methods of advanced airway management.

This module concentrates on two major techniques: orotracheal intubation and insertion of a nasogastric tube in children.

Orotracheal intubation consists of placing an endotracheal tube through the mouth into the patient's trachea and inflating a cuff on the end of it. This seals off the airway and greatly reduces the risk of aspiration into the lungs of stomach contents, blood, or foreign matter. It also makes ventilation much easier since a bag-valve mask can be attached directly to the tube and there is no need to seal the mask on the patient's face. In addition, deep suctioning of the airway to the level of the lungs can be accomplished through the endotracheal tube. Orotracheal intubation is the best method available today to protect a patient's airway.

One of the things that makes children different is how they react to stress. Unlike adults, they frequently swallow large amounts of air. The air distends the stomach, pushing it up against the diaphragm and reducing the amount of space in the chest for the lungs. This prevents the child from breathing adequately. By inserting a tube that goes through the child's nose into the stomach (a nasogastric tube), you will be able to relieve this distention and allow the child to breathe or be ventilated adequately.

Both of these skills—orotracheal intubation and nasogastric insertion—have traditionally been considered advanced life support and, therefore, off limits to EMT-Basics. Because patients often die of airway problems before advanced life support teams can reach the scene, some EMS systems, in an attempt to improve this situation, will have EMT-Bs learn to intubate and insert gastric tubes.

Successful use of these advanced maneuvers, however, will depend on the EMT-B's ability to open and maintain an airway with basic methods first. When confronted with a patient with a difficult airway, as an EMT-Basic you may need to draw on all of the knowledge and skills you have accumulated, both basic and advanced.

Advanced Airway Management

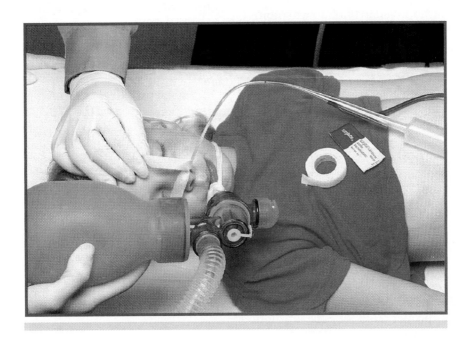

There is no skill more important for the EMT-Basic to master than the ability to assure that a patient has an adequate airway. Mastery of the airway is dependent on two separate skills: first, the ability to assess and recognize airway and breathing problems, and second, the ability to maintain an open airway by using both manual techniques and airway adjuncts. Assuring an adequate airway is the first assessment and treatment priority in both basic and advanced life support. Control of a patient's airway is recognized as so crucial a skill that advanced airway skills are now included as an elective in the EMT-Basic curriculum. The potential benefit of teaching EMT-Bs advanced airway skills cannot be overstated, as EMT-Bs are frequently the first providers on the scene, and rapid and definitive control of the airway is essential to patient survival.

Knowledge and Attitude *At the end of this chapter, you should be able to meet the following objectives.*

1. Identify and describe the airway anatomy in the infant, child, and adult. (pp. 710–713)

2. Differentiate between the airway anatomy in the infant, child, and adult. (pp. 710–713)

3. Explain the pathophysiology of airway compromise. (pp. 710–713)

4. Describe the proper use of airway adjuncts. (p. 713)

5. Review the use of oxygen therapy in airway management. (p. 713)

6. Describe the indications, contraindications, and technique for insertion of nasal gastric tubes. (pp. 725–726, 727)

7. Describe how to perform Sellick's maneuver (cricoid pressure). (pp. 722, 725)

8. Describe the indications for advanced airway management. (pp. 710–713, 718, 726)

9. List the equipment required for orotracheal intubation. (pp. 714–718)

10. Describe the proper use of the curved blade for orotracheal intubation. (p. 715)

11. Describe the proper use of the straight blade for orotracheal intubation. (p. 715)

12. State the reasons for and proper use of the stylet in orotracheal intubation. (p. 717)

13. Describe the methods of choosing the appropriate size endotracheal tube in an adult patient. (pp. 716–717)

14. State the formula for sizing an infant or child endotracheal tube. (p. 724)

15. List complications associated with advanced airway management. (pp. 713–714, 729)

16. Define the various alternative methods for sizing the infant and child endotracheal tube. (p. 724)

17. Describe the skill of orotracheal intubation in the adult patient. (pp. 718–723)

18. Describe the skill of orotracheal intubation in the infant and child patient. (pp. 723–725)

19. Describe the skill of confirming endotracheal tube placement in the adult, infant, and child patient. (pp. 722–723, 725)

20. State the consequence of and the need to recognize unintentional esophageal intubation. (pp. 714, 722–723)

21. Describe the skill of securing the endotracheal tube in the adult, infant, and child patient. (pp. 718, 723)

22. Recognize and respect the feelings of the patient and family during advanced airway procedures. (p. 721)

23. Explain the value of performing advanced airway procedures. (pp. 707, 710, 713)

24. Defend the need for the EMT-Basic to perform advanced airway procedures. (pp. 705–707)

25. Explain the rationale for the use of a stylet. (p. 717)

26. Explain the rationale for having a suction unit immediately available during intubation attempts. (p. 713)

27. Explain the rationale for confirming breath sounds. (p. 722)

28. Explain the rationale for securing the endotracheal tube. (p. 718)

Skills

1. Demonstrate how to perform Sellick's maneuver (cricoid pressure).

2. Demonstrate the skill of orotracheal intubation in the adult patient.

3. Demonstrate the skill of orotracheal intubation in the infant and child patient.

4. Demonstrate the skill of confirming endotracheal tube placement in the adult patient.

5. Demonstrate the skill of confirming endotracheal tube placement in the infant and child patient.

6. Demonstrate the skill of securing the endotracheal tube in the adult patient.

7. Demonstrate the skill of securing the endotracheal tube in the infant and child patient.

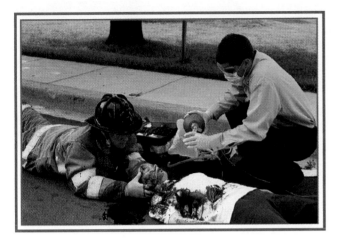

Your rescue squad responds to a motor vehicle crash on a busy street.

On arrival you *size up the scene* and note that the police have traffic safely diverted away from the crash site. There is only one car involved that has sustained extensive damage. The vehicle is upright and stable and there is no apparent fuel leak. Fire department first responders arrive on the scene at the same time as your unit. As the police officer directs your ambulance into the scene, she informs you that there is a single victim who was ejected from the car. No purse or wallet has been found, and the police are in the process of trying to learn her identity by tracing the license plate number.

Approaching the patient to begin *initial assessment,* you and your partner find a female in her twenties, unconscious, face down in the street in a pool of blood. You hear gurgling respirations. While a fire department first responder maintains cervical stabilization, you, your partner, and two first responders log-roll the patient onto her back. You see that she has sustained multiple facial lacerations and there is copious blood in the airway.

You begin suctioning the patient's mouth with a large bore rigid tip suction catheter and note that she has no gag reflex, even with aggressive suctioning. You then insert an oropharyngeal airway, which she tolerates. The patient is not breathing. You assign one of the fire department members to her airway. His responsibility will be to ventilate the patient with a BVM and suction as necessary. Another firefighter will take over manual stabilization of the head and neck. You complete your initial assessment and your partner takes baseline vital signs. Assessment of the circulation has revealed strong radial pulses and no apparent major external

blood loss. The patient remains completely unresponsive to any stimuli.

You quickly discuss the situation with your partner and decide—because of the urgency of getting control of this patient's airway—to delay the rapid trauma exam in order to go to the ambulance to set-up for orotracheal intubation while your partner and a first responder continue ventilation of the patient with the BVM. Meanwhile your partner directs the other first responder and two troopers in maintaining manual stabilization while applying a cervical collar and securing the patient to a backboard.

In the ambulance you select a 7.5 endotracheal tube and a curved laryngoscope blade and assure that both are functioning properly. As you don mask and goggles, the patient is loaded into the ambulance and you see that she is now fully immobilized. Your partner and the first responder continue to ventilate the patient with the BVM. A firefighter volunteers to drive.

You turn on the on-board suction so it will be ready if needed and tuck the rigid catheter between the backboard and the stretcher to the right of the patient's head. Your partner hyperventilates the patient, giving her a series of ventilations at twice the usual rate. This will provide extra oxygen to tide her through the moments when oxygen intake will be interrupted while you insert an endotracheal tube.

You assign one of the first responders to again manually stabilize the patient's head while your partner opens the cervical collar and applies pressure to the cricoid cartilage. This will help suppress potential vomiting and help bring the glottic opening into your view. Using the laryngoscope to help you see what you are doing, you then pass the endotracheal tube through the glottic opening into the trachea. After quickly inflating the endotracheal tube's cuff, you attach the BVM, which is connected to your on-board oxygen, and ventilate. Your partner listens for breath sounds and determines that the tube is properly placed. You secure the tube and initiate transport to the hospital. Your scene time was eleven minutes.

You perform a *focused history and physical exam* en route by conducting a rapid trauma exam and taking vital signs. The need to monitor tube placement and ventilation means that there is no time to conduct a *detailed physical exam.* You frequently auscultate for the presence of breath sounds and reconfirm proper tube placement. Your partner conducts *ongoing assessment* every five minutes en route. The patient begins to respond to pain by the time you arrive at the hospital.

A irway control is the highest priority in managing any critically ill or injured patient, because without an adequate airway the patient will die no matter what other care you provide. Advanced airway management can only be effective and successful if you have already mastered the basic airway techniques discussed in Chapter 7, Airway Management.

ANATOMY AND PHYSIOLOGY

The anatomy and physiology of the respiratory system has already been discussed at length in Chapters 4, the Human Body; 7, Airway Management; and 17, Respiratory Emergencies. There are, however, specific aspects of both airway anatomy and physiology that the EMT-Basic who performs advanced airway skills must understand in greater depth in order to optimize the effectiveness and success of these advanced skills.

Anatomy

Air initially enters the respiratory tract via the nose and the mouth. Air that enters through the nose then passes through the **nasopharynx** and air that enters through the mouth passes through the **oropharynx**. The **hypopharynx** is the area directly above the openings of both the **trachea** (windpipe) and the **esophagus** (the tube to the stomach). The **epiglottis** is a leaf-shaped structure that acts as a covering to the opening of the trachea. The epiglottis protects the airway by covering the entrance to the trachea when food or liquids are being swallowed. Anterior to the epiglottis is a groove-like structure called the **vallecula.**

The epiglottis allows air to pass into the opening of the trachea and through the **larynx,** or voice box. The larynx contains the two **vocal cords.**

Giving support to the larynx and trachea are several rigid pieces of cartilage. The thyroid cartilage is a shield shaped structure that is at the anterior of the larynx. Multiple horseshoe-shaped cartilages give support to the trachea. The **cricoid cartilage** is a cartilage at the lower portion of the larynx. It is unique in that it is the only tracheal cartilage that completely surrounds the windpipe.

Once air has passed through the larynx, it proceeds through the trachea until the trachea

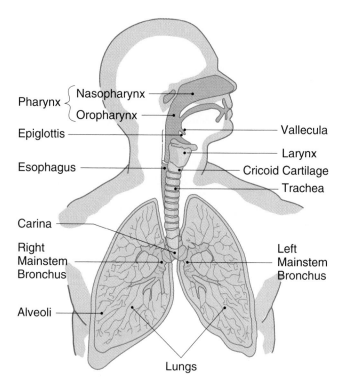

FIGURE 33-1 The airway, anatomical position.

bifurcates, or splits, into the two **mainstem bronchi** at the level of the **carina.** The right mainstem bronchus splits off the carina at less of an angle than the left mainstem bronchus. Because of the angle of the right mainstem bronchus, objects that pass all the way down the trachea (such as aspirated food) tend to lodge in the right rather than the left mainstem bronchus. The mainstem bronchi subsequently divide into smaller air passages until reaching the level of the **alveoli** where the exchange of oxygen and carbon dioxide takes place.

When trying to study and memorize the anatomy of the airway, remember that the majority of the time you are managing a critical airway problem the patient will be supine, or lying flat. For this reason it is important to visualize the anatomy in both the traditional upright "anatomical position" (Figure 33-1) and in the supine position (Figure 33-2).

Physiology

The most important aspect of respiratory physiology for the EMT-B who uses advanced airways is an understanding of what can cause the respiratory system to fail so severely that an advanced airway is necessary.

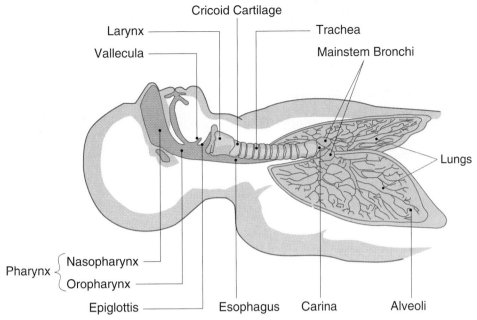

Cricoid Cartilage

Larynx

Trachea

Vallecula

Mainstem Bronchi

Lungs

Pharynx { Nasopharynx
          Oropharynx

Epiglottis   Esophagus   Carina   Alveoli

FIGURE 33-2 The airway, supine position.

When the respiratory system functions properly, adequate breathing is the result of many factors including the following.

- A functioning brainstem where the brain's centers of respiratory control are located
- An open airway
- An intact chest wall
- The ability of gas exchange to take place at the alveoli

Injuries or illnesses that affect any of these components can result in inadequate breathing and respiratory failure. For example, a massive head injury could result in both brainstem injury and an airway obstructed by blood and broken teeth. Similarly, a patient with massive pulmonary edema from congestive heart failure can go into respiratory failure because edema prevents adequate gas exchange at the level of the alveoli.

Assessing the adequacy of a patient's breathing is an essential skill when making decisions about what basic and advanced airway management is indicated. A patient's respiratory status can range anywhere from normal, unlabored breathing to complete cessation of breathing or respiratory arrest. Recognition of adequate breathing or respiratory arrest is rarely a diagnostic challenge for the EMT-B. It is recognizing the more subtle signs and symptoms of inadequate breathing that is an essential skill for the EMT-B.

In general, when assessing the adequacy of breathing you should carefully observe the rate, rhythm, quality, and depth of the patient's respirations. The normal rate of breathing is dependent on the age of the patient (Table 33-1). An adequately breathing patient will normally be breathing in a regular rather than an irregular rhythm. The quality of a patient's breathing should be assessed by listening for breath sounds and observing chest expansion and effort of breathing. The adequately breathing patient will have breath sounds that are equal and present bilaterally. In addition, when observing the patient's chest during normal breathing you will note equal and full expansion of the chest and a lack of any accessory muscle use in the chest or neck during inspiration. Finally, the depth of breathing (tidal volume) will normally be sufficient not only to expand the lungs, but to assure adequate delivery of oxygen and removal of carbon dioxide at the level of the alveoli.

TABLE 33-1   Normal Rates of Breathing

Normal Rates of Breathing
Adult - 12 - 20 breaths per minute
Child - 15 - 30 breaths per minute
Infant - 25 - 50 breaths per minute

When a patient is in respiratory distress because of inadequate breathing the following variations in rate, rhythm, quality, and depth of breathing will be noted.

- Rate—Outside the normal range: either too fast or too slow
- Rhythm—Irregular pattern of breathing
- Quality—
  Breath sounds: diminished, unequal or absent
  Chest expansion: unequal or inadequate
  Effort of breathing: increased effort, use of accessory muscles, and inability to speak in full sentences
- Depth—shallow

In addition, you may also note the following signs and symptoms in the patient with inadequate breathing.

- Cyanosis in the lips, nailbeds, and fingertips
- Cool and clammy skin
- Agonal breathing (gasping breaths just prior to respiratory arrest)

Pediatric Airway Anatomy and Physiology

The pediatric airway is not simply a miniature version of an adult airway. The anatomy and physiology of infants' and children's respiratory systems differ in important respects from those of adults (Figure 33-3). Not suprisingly, these younger patients may also have different signs and symptoms of respiratory failure than adults.

Features that are unique to the anatomy and physiology of the infant and child versus the adult include the following.

- All structures in the mouth and nose are smaller in the child and can be more easily obstructed.
- The tongue is proportionately larger, occupying more of the mouth and pharynx.
- The trachea is softer and more flexible, allowing the airway to be closed off if the neck is too far extended when opening the airway.
- The trachea is narrower, allowing the airway to become more easily obstructed if swelling occurs.
- The narrowest area in the airway is at the level of the cricoid cartilage.

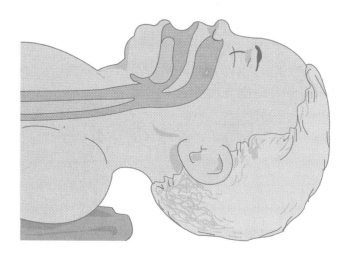

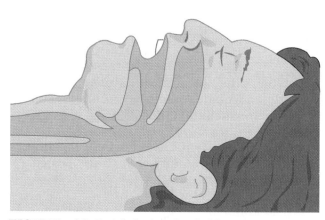

FIGURE 33-3 Adult and child airways compared. In the child, the mouth, nose, pharynx, and trachea are smaller and more easily obstructed.

- Because the chest wall is softer, the diaphragm is relied on heavily for the work of breathing.

Although infants and children may manifest inadequate breathing with the signs and symptoms mentioned above, they also frequently show respiratory distress in other ways, including

- A slower than normal heart rate
- Weak or absent peripheral pulses
- Retractions between and below the ribs, above the clavicles, and sternal notch
- Nasal flaring, in which the nostrils "flare" open with exhalation and clamp almost shut with inhalation

- So-called "seesaw" breathing, in which the chest and abdomen move in opposite directions during breathing

Recognition of respiratory distress and inadequate breathing is especially critical in infants and children, since respiratory failure is the leading cause of cardiac arrest in this age group.

MANAGEMENT OF THE AIRWAY

Although this chapter is about advanced airway management, it cannot be over-emphasized that the primary management of any airway is with basic airway techniques such as opening and suctioning the airway, administration of supplemental oxygen, and using oro- and nasopharyngeal airways. You should review these skills (as taught in Chapter 7) prior to learning the techniques of advanced airway management.

Oropharyngeal Suctioning

The goal of airway management is keeping the airway open and free of obstructions. If the airway is obstructed with secretions, blood, or foreign materials, the airway will have to be suctioned. Suction equipment should always be within easy reach when managing any critically ill patient. If the patient is being managed outside the ambulance, either an electrical or hand-operated suction device should be brought to the patient's side. If the patient is in the ambulance, the on-board suction system should be set up and ready for immediate use. Nothing is more embarrassing for the EMT-B, or harmful for the patient, than fumbling around to get a suction unit working when the airway is filled with vomit or blood.

You will learn that a working rigid-tip suction catheter is an essential piece of equipment. In Chapter 7, Airway Management, you learned the technique for oropharyngeal suctioning—suctioning the mouth and pharynx—with a rigid-tip catheter. This must be done before performing orotracheal intubation.

Orotracheal Intubation

An **endotracheal tube** is a tube designed to be inserted into the trachea (*endo* meaning "into," *tracheal* referring to the trachea). Oxygen, med-ication, or a suction catheter can be directed into the trachea through the endotracheal tube. **Intubation** means the insertion of a tube. **Orotracheal intubation** is the placement of an endotracheal tube orally, that is, by way of the mouth (*oro* means "mouth"), then through the vocal cords and into the trachea.

Orotracheal intubation allows direct ventilation of the lungs through the endotracheal tube, bypassing the entire upper airway. The endotracheal tube is placed through the vocal cords with direct *visualization* of the process (that is, seeing what you are doing). A **laryngoscope** is an illuminating instrument that is inserted into the pharynx and allows you to visualize the pharynx and larynx.

The advantages of orotracheal intubation of the apneic (nonbreathing) patient include

- Complete control of the airway (the tube going directly into the trachea prevents the tongue, blood, or debris that may be present in the upper airway from interfering with the passage of air into the trachea and lungs)
- Minimizes the risk of aspiration (the tube blocks vomitus or foreign matter from being aspirated, or breathed into the lungs)
- Allows for better oxygen delivery (oxygen is fed directly to the lungs via the trachea)
- Allows for deeper suctioning of the airway (a flexible suction catheter can be passed through the endotracheal tube to suction the trachea to the level of the carina)

Complications

Although orotracheal intubation is frequently a life-saving procedure, it has many potential complications. Orotracheal intubation is considered an "invasive" technique because it requires placement of equipment inside the body cavity. Whenever you perform an invasive procedure you must be aware of the potential complications, and be prepared to recognize and treat them should they arise. These concerns about invasive procedures are never more critical than in orotracheal intubation, since improper placement of the endotracheal tube in the apneic patient can rapidly result in the patient's death if it is not immediately detected and corrected.

Specific complications of orotracheal intubation include

- Slowing of the heart rate—Stimulation of the airway with the laryngoscope and the endotracheal tube can lead to a slowing of the heart. The patient's heart rate should be monitored throughout the intubation.

- Soft tissue trauma to the teeth, lips, tongue, gums, and airway structures.
- Hypoxia—Prolonged attempts at intubation may lead to inadequate oxygenation, or oxygen starvation, known as **hypoxia.** To prevent this, you should **hyperventilate** the patient with high concentration oxygen (ventilations provided at about double the normal rate, or 24 ventilations per minute) prior to intubation, and intubation attempts should be limited to 30 seconds from the time ventilations cease until the patient is ventilated through the endotracheal tube.
- Vomiting—Stimulation of the airway may cause the patient to gag and vomit.
- Right main-stem intubation—The endotracheal tube has to remain superior to the carina (before the point where the right and left mainstem bronchi branch off) in order to send air into both lungs. If the tube is advanced too far, the tube is likely to go down the steep right mainstem bronchus. Mainstem intubation results in only one lung being ventilated and the development of hypoxia.
- Esophageal intubation—This is the most serious complication, since the unrecognized placement of the tube in the esophagus rather than the trachea will rapidly result in death.
- Accidental extubation—Even if the endotracheal tube is properly placed initially, the tube can become dislodged while moving the patient, or by the patient himself if he regains consciousness. Be sure to reassess chest wall movement and breath sounds after every major move with the intubated patient, such as down the stairs or from the floor to the stretcher.

Equipment

Orotracheal intubation requires specialized equipment.

BSI Precautions Because of the high risk of splattering of sputum or blood during intubation, it is essential that body substance isolation precautions be taken. This means that a mask and goggles or other protective eye wear be worn in addition to gloves (Figure 33-4). This is mandatory since your face will be in direct line

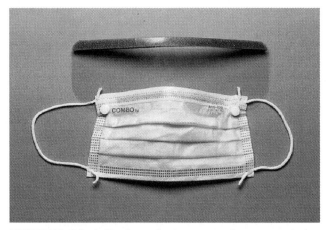

FIGURE 33-4 Body substance isolation precautions must include gloves, mask, and protective eye wear when managing the airway.

with the path of secretions, blood, and vomit coming from the mouth while you attempt to visualize the airway.

Laryngoscope A laryngoscope is made up of two components; the handle that contains the batteries, and the blade that is inserted in the airway and illuminates the airway. In most laryngoscopes the handle and the blades are two separate pieces that need to be assembled with each use. In these devices, the blade is placed parallel to the handle and the notch at the base of the blade is attached to the bar on the handle. The blade is then lifted to a 90 degree angle with the handle and, as the blade locks into place, the light at the tip of the blade illuminates (Figure 33-5). Always check the light at the end of the blade to assure that it illuminates with a bright white color and that the bulb is tightly secured to the blade. It should be noted that some disposable laryngoscopes are preassembled with the handle and blade as a single fixed unit.

No matter what type of laryngoscope you use, it is essential that you conduct a daily check of the device to assure that it is working properly. Spare batteries and bulbs should always be stored with the laryngoscope.

Laryngoscope blades are specifically designed to fit into the anatomy of the airway and provide optimal illumination of the vocal cords to enable you to pass the endotracheal tube between them. Most commercially available blades are designed with the light on the right side of the blade. This requires that the handle of the scope be held in the left hand to provide optimal illumination of the airway.

There are two general types of blades straight and curved. Both types of blades come

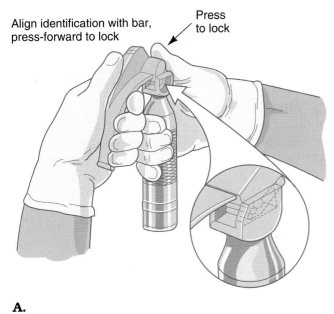

Align identification with bar, press-forward to lock

Press to lock

A.

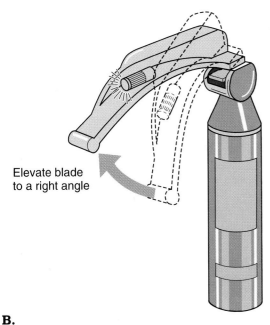

Elevate blade to a right angle

B.

FIGURE 33-5 A. Affix the laryngoscope blade. B. Elevate the laryngoscope blade.

in assorted sizes ranging from the smallest size, 0, to the largest size, 4. The size of the blade used depends on the size of the patient. Most adult patients can be intubated using a size 2 or 3 straight blade or a size 3 curved blade. (Pediatric blade sizes will be discussed later in this chapter.) The decision as to whether to use a straight or curved blade depends on individual preference; however, straight blades are preferred for pediatric orotracheal intubations.

Each blade type is designed to enable you to visualize the cords by taking advantage of different anatomical mechanisms. The straight

blade is designed so that the tip of the blade is placed under the epiglottis to lift the epiglottis upward and bring the **glottic opening** (the opening to the trachea) and the vocal cords into view (Figure 33-6). The curved blade is designed so that the tip of the blade is inserted into the vallecula so that lifting the laryngoscope handle upward brings the glottic opening and the vocal cords into view (Figure 33-7).

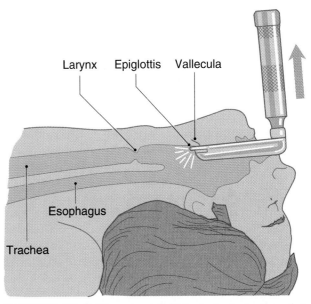

Larynx   Epiglottis   Vallecula

Esophagus

Trachea

FIGURE 33-6 The straight blade brings the glottic opening and vocal cords into view by lifting the epiglottis.

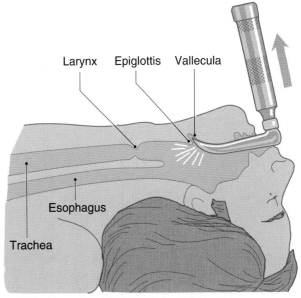

Larynx   Epiglottis   Vallecula

Esophagus

Trachea

FIGURE 33-7 The curved blade brings the glottic opening and vocal cords into view by lifting the vallecula.

Endotracheal Tube The endotracheal tube (Figure 33-8) consists of a single lumen tube through which air and supplemental oxygen are delivered. At the proximal end of the tube (the end that will remain outside the patient, nearer to you) is a standard 15 millimeter adapter for connection to the bag valve.

At the distal end of the tube (the end farther from you, the end that will go into the patient) is a cuff. The cuff is designed to be inflated after the tube is placed to prevent leakage of air and fluid around the tip of the tube. The cuff holds approximately 10 cc's of air and should be inflated only enough to prevent air from leaking around the tube. The cuff of the tube is filled with a 10 cc syringe at the inflation valve. Just below the inflation valve is the pilot balloon, which fills with air when the cuff is inflated. Since the cuff is inside the patient's trachea, you won't be able to see if it is inflated, but the inflation of the pilot balloon will verify that there is air in the cuff. If the pilot balloon does not hold air, then you must assume that the cuff at the end of the tube has also failed.

Endotracheal tubes used on infants and children less than eight years old do not have a cuff (see Orotracheal Intubation of an Infant or Child later in this chapter). Many endotracheal tubes have a small hole on the left side of the tube on the side opposite the bevel, known as a Murphy eye. This feature is designed to lessen the chances of tube obstruction.

Endotracheal tubes come in various diameters, from 2.0 millimeters (used on premature infants) to 10.0 millimeters (used on large adults). The diameter measured is the distance from one internal wall of the tube to the other, called the internal diameter or "i.d." No matter what the internal diameter of the tube, the standard 15 millimeter adapter is affixed to the end of the tube. When determining the proper size of the endotracheal tube for the adult patient, the rule of thumb is: In an emergency use a 7.5 mm tube. For more precise sizing of the endotracheal tube, it is generally accepted that the adult male should receive either an 8.0 or an 8.5 mm tube and the adult female should receive from a 7.0 to an 8.0 mm tube. The sizing of pediatric endotracheal tubes will be discussed later in this chapter.

The adult endotracheal tube has a standard length of 33 centimeters. The side of the tube is marked in centimeters starting from the tip of the tube. The most important number to remember is that, as a general rule, a properly placed endotracheal tube will have the 22 centimeter mark at the teeth. This position assures that the tip of the tube is in the trachea above the carina. (As you will learn, assuring proper placement of the tube is a critical skill, and checking the length marking is only a small part of this procedure.) It may be helpful to envision the depth of tube placement by reviewing the following distances in the average adult.

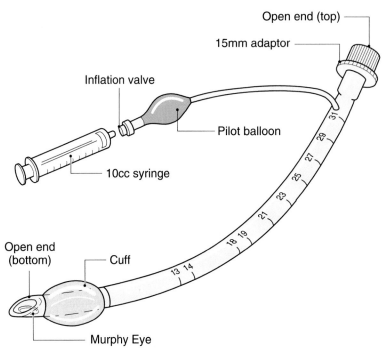

FIGURE 33-8 The endotracheal tube.

- 15 centimeters from the teeth to the vocal cords
- 20 centimeters from the teeth to the suprasternal notch
- 25 centimeters from the teeth to the carina

As you can see, there is very little room for error when placing the endotracheal tube, since only a few centimeters can mean the difference between proper placement and the tube being past the carina into the right main stem bronchus.

Accessories to the Endotracheal Tube There are several accessories to the endotracheal tube with which you need to be familiar. These include the stylet, lubricant, a 10 cc syringe, devices for securing the tube once it is placed, and a suction device.

Because the endotracheal tube is made of relatively flexible plastic, it is generally recommended that a **stylet** (Figure 33-9)—a long, thin, bendable metal probe—be inserted into the tube prior to intubation to help stiffen the tube and provide the tube with a shape that will ease its insertion through the vocal cords. It is recommended that the stylet be lubricated with water-soluble lubricant, such as K-Y jelly, Lubrifax, or Surgilube, prior to insertion into the endotracheal tube to allow for a smooth withdrawal of the stylet once the tube is successfully placed. (A silicone-based lubricant or a petroleum-based lubricant such as Vaseline must not be used.)

Once the lubricated stylet is inserted, the endotracheal tube should be shaped into a "hockey stick" configuration. To avoid trauma to the airway it is essential that the stylet should not be inserted past the tip of the tube. Since the stylet is longer than the endotracheal tube it is easy to inadvertently allow the tip to extend beyond the end of the tube. Such an error, however, could cause a puncture of the trachea. To avoid this complication, the tip of the stylet should not be inserted beyond the proximal end of the Murphy eye and the excess length should be bent over the 15 mm adapter.

When performing orotracheal intubation, it is often a problem that excessive oral secretions obstruct an adequate view of the vocal cords. Paradoxically, airways are sometimes very dry, thus making insertion of the tube difficult because of friction between the end of the tube and the patient's pharynx and glottis. For these reasons, it is important both that a wide bore suction device be operational and within easy

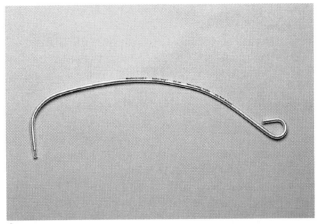

A.

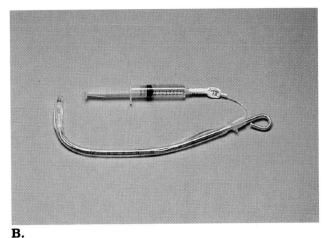

B.

FIGURE 33-9 A. The stylet. B. The stylet in place.

reach during intubation attempts, and that water soluble lubricant be applied to the outside of the distal portion of the tube. The suction device should be turned on and placed by your right hand (since your left hand will be holding the laryngoscope). In general, you can use half a packet of lubricant on the stylet and the other half of the packet on the outside of the tube.

Another piece of essential equipment for use with the endotracheal tube is a 10 cc syringe. As mentioned above, the syringe is used to inflate the cuff through the inflation valve. The syringe should also be used to test that the cuff is intact and holds air prior to inserting the tube. Once the integrity of the cuff has been assured, the air should be withdrawn, but the syringe should remain attached to the tube so that it is easily found when it is time to reinflate the cuff after the patient is intubated. It should be noted that, following final inflation of the cuff, the 10 cc syringe should be detached from the inflation valve to prevent any subsequent leakage of air out of the cuff and back into the syringe.

One of the final steps in orotracheal intubation is securing the tube to the patient so that it does not move or become dislodged. This is especially important in the prehospital setting where the tube can easily be dislodged during patient movement. Prior to securing the endotracheal tube, an oral airway or similar device should be inserted as a bite block in case the patient becomes responsive and gnaws at the tube. There are a number of methods for securing endotracheal tubes. These range from cloth tape to commercially available devices. The manner in which tubes are secured is usually dictated by the medical direction of the EMS system you work in. Whatever system you use to secure the tube, make sure the tube is firmly secured in place and able to withstand the tugs and pulls that are routine during moves of critically ill patients.

Indications

When properly performed, orotracheal intubation is clearly a life-saving technique. It is essential, however, that you know under what conditions a patient needs to be intubated. The following is a listing of indications for when to perform orotracheal intubation.

- Inability to ventilate the apneic patient
- To protect the airway of a patient without a gag reflex or cough
- To protect the airway of a patient unresponsive to any painful stimuli
- Cardiac arrest

Technique of Insertion— the Adult Patient

Orotracheal intubation is the most complicated and difficult procedure the EMT-B is expected to perform. Properly performed, it is truly a life-saving procedure. Incorrectly performed, the EMT-B's actions can easily result in the patient's death. Because many EMT-Bs will only rarely perform orotracheal intubation, it is essential that you not only learn and practice the technique extensively during your training but also practice the technique on a regular basis once you are a certified EMT-B.

The following is a step by step guide to orotracheal intubation of the adult patient (Scan 33-1).

Preparation
1. Assure body substance isolation precautions. This should include gloves, goggles or other protective eye wear, and a mask.
2. Assure that adequate ventilation with a bag-valve mask and high concentration oxygen is being performed.
3. Hyperventilate the patient at a rate of 24 breaths per minute prior to any intubation attempts.
4. Assemble, prepare, and test all equipment including

   - A suction unit with a large bore rigid tip— It should be functional and positioned so that it is within easy reach of the intubater's right hand should it be needed.
   - The cuff on the endotracheal tube—It should be tested and then deflated, with the 10 cc syringe left attached to the inflation valve.
   - The laryngoscope—Assemble and assure that the light is bright and constant.
   - The device that will be used to secure the tube after successful intubation

5. Position yourself at the patient's head so that, during intubation, *left* and *right* are your left and right as well as the patient's left and right.

Visualizing the Glottic Opening and Vocal Cords
6. Position the patient's head to assure good visualization of the vocal cords. Remove the oral airway.

   - If trauma is not suspected, tilt the head, lift the chin, and attempt visualization of the cords. If the cords cannot be seen, raise the patient's shoulders approximately one inch by placing a towel beneath them and attempt visualization again.
   - If trauma is suspected, the patient will have to be intubated with the head and neck in a neutral position with a second rescuer maintaining in-line stabilization of the neck and head.

7. Hold the laryngoscope in your left hand and insert the laryngoscope into the right corner of the patient's mouth.
8. Use a sweeping motion to lift the tongue upward and to the left, out of the way, to enable visualization of the glottis.
9. Insert the blade into the proper anatomical location.

   - Curved blade fits into the vallecula.
   - Straight blade lifts the epiglottis.

Orotracheal Intubation—Adult Patient

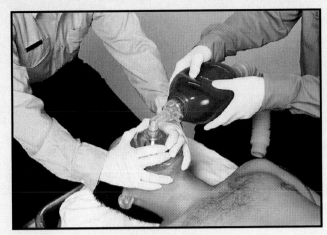

1. Hyperventilate the patient.

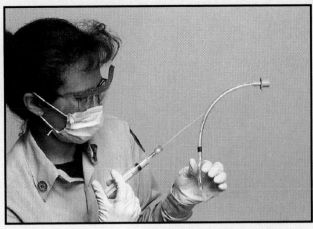

2. Assemble, prepare, and test all equipment.

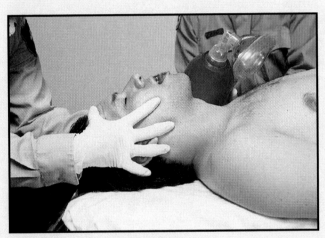

3. Position the patient's head.

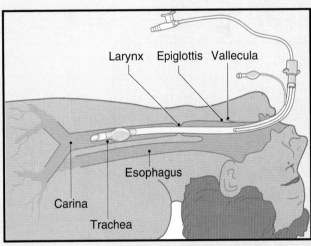

Larynx   Epiglottis   Vallecula

Esophagus

Carina

Trachea

4. Make sure the airway is aligned. (If trauma is suspected, keep patient's head and neck in a neutral position with manual stabilization.)

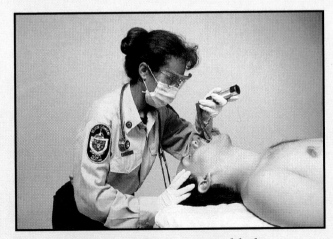

5. Prepare to insert laryngoscope blade.

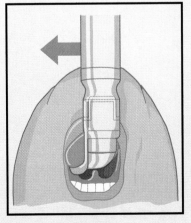

6. Lift the tongue out of the way.

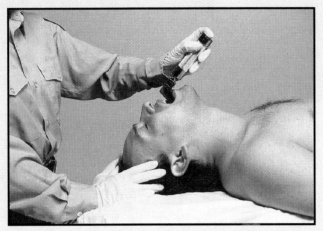

7. Insert the blade (curved blade into vallecula, straight blade under epiglottis) and lift to bring glottic opening into view.

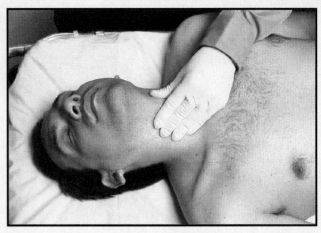

8. A second rescuer may perform Sellick's maneuver (cricoid pressure) during intubation to suppress vomiting and aid visualization.

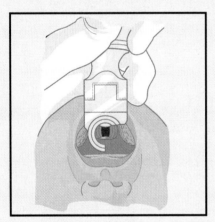

9. Visualize the glottic opening.

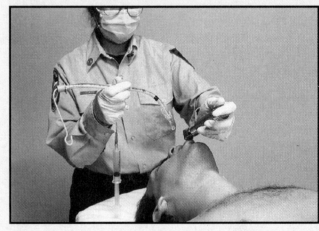

10. Insert endotracheal tube with stylet.

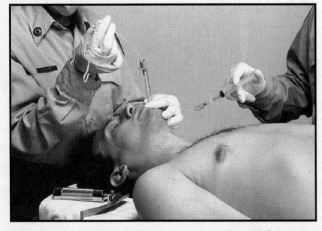

11. Remove laryngoscope and stylet. Inflate the cuff with 5-10 ccs of air.

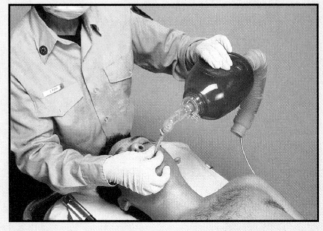

12. Attach bag-valve unit or other ventilation device to tube.

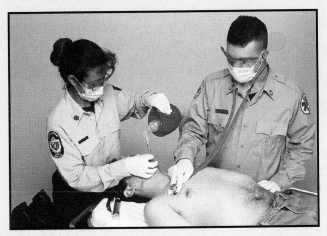

13. Auscultate lung and epigastrium areas to confirm correct placement.

Confirm correct placement of tube.

- Observe rise and fall of chest.
- Auscultate epigastrium for absence of breath sounds.
- Auscultate over both lungs for breath sounds. The sounds should be equal when comparing the left and right sides.
- Observe patient for signs of deterioration, e.g., cyanosis.
- Use measures such as pulse oximetry or end tidal carbon dioxide detectors per local protocols.

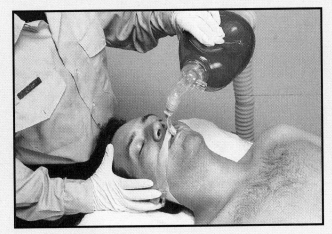

14. If correct placement is confirmed, secure tube in place.

Correct any incorrect placement of tube.

- Breath sounds present on right, diminished or absent on left—right mainstem bronchus probably intubated. Deflate cuff, gently withdraw tube (continue ventilation) until breath sounds are equal right and left.
- Breath sounds in epigastrium—esophagus intubated. Withdraw tube. Hyperventilate 2-5 minutes.

Note: Make only two attempts at intubation. If both attempts fail, insert an oral airway and continue to ventilate with bag-valve mask. Aggressively suction the airway. If tube has been correctly placed and secured, reassess breath sounds and placement after every major move with patient. Offer reassurance and emotional support to the patient and family.

10. Lift the scope up and away from the patient.
11. Avoid using the teeth as a fulcrum.
12. Application of **cricoid pressure** (Sellick's maneuver) during intubation attempts may be beneficial. Sellick's maneuver is performed by a second rescuer who uses his index finger and thumb to exert direct pressure on the patient's cricoid cartilage (Figure 33-10). Since the cricoid cartilage is the only cartilage in the neck that completely encircles the trachea, direct pressure helps to compress the esophagus, which is posterior to the trachea, reducing the risk of vomiting. In addition, the pressure often brings the vocal cords into better view. Cricoid pressure should be maintained until the patient is intubated.
13. Visualize the glottic opening and vocal cords. Once the cords come into view do not lose sight of them!

Inserting the Endotracheal Tube
14. With the right hand, carefully insert the endotracheal tube through the vocal cords. The tube should be inserted just deep enough that the cuff material is past the cords. Verify that the endotracheal tube is at about 22 cm at the gums and teeth.
15. Remove the laryngoscope and extinguish the lamp.
16. Remove the stylet, if used.
17. Inflate the cuff with 5 to 10 cc of air and remove the syringe.
18. Continue to hold onto the endotracheal tube. Never let go of the endotracheal tube until it is secured in place.
19. Have a partner attach the bag valve to the endotracheal tube and deliver artificial ventilations.

Assuring Correct Tube Placement
20. The single most accurate way of assuring proper tube placement is visualizing the endotracheal tube as it passes through the vocal cords. All the following methods are for verification of tube placement.

   • Observe the patient's chest rise and fall with each ventilation.
   • Auscultate for the presence of breath sounds as follows.

     a. Begin over the epigastrium. Breath sounds heard here during ventilations indicate air entering the stomach rather than the lungs.
     b. Listen over the left apex (top of the left lung area). Compare the breath sounds with those at the right apex. Breath sounds should be heard equally on both sides.
     c. Listen over the left base (bottom of the lung area). Compare the breath sounds with those at the right base. Breath sounds should be heard equally on both sides.

The Cricoid Cartilage

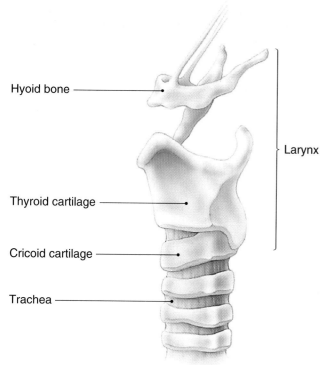

Hyoid bone

Larynx

Thyroid cartilage

Cricoid cartilage

Trachea

A.

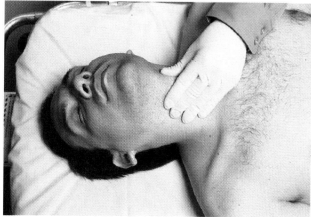

B.

FIGURE 33-10 A. The cricoid cartilage rings the trachea at the lower end of the larynx. B. Sellick's maneuver is placing pressure on the cricoid cartilage to help suppress vomiting and to help bring the vocal cords into view.

- Observe the patient for signs of deterioration after tube placement, for example becoming combative or developing cyanosis. Both are signs of hypoxia and probable incorrect tube placement.
- Use other objective measures such as pulse oximetry or end tidal carbon dioxide detectors if allowed by local protocol.

Detecting and Correcting Incorrect Tube Placements

- If breath sounds are diminished or absent on the left but present on the right, it is likely the tube has advanced beyond the carina and intubated the right main stem bronchus. If this occurs

  —Deflate the cuff and gently withdraw the tube while artificially ventilating and while auscultating over the left apex of the chest.
  —Take care not to completely remove the endotracheal tube.
  —When the breath sounds become equal at both the left and right apex, reinflate the cuff and follow the directions below for securing the tube.

- If breath sounds are only present in the epigastrium, the esophagus has been intubated and air is being sent into the stomach instead of the lungs. Since esophageal intubation is a fatal occurrence, immediately deflate the cuff and withdraw the tube. The patient should then be hyperventilated for at least 2 to 5 minutes prior to your second attempt to intubate.
- The EMT-B should only make two attempts at orotracheal intubation. If both attempts fail, insert an oral airway, continue to ventilate the patient with high concentration oxygen via bag-valve mask, and aggressively suction the airway.

Securing the Tube

21. If breath sounds are heard bilaterally and no sounds are heard over the epigastrium, the endotracheal tube should be secured in place using tape or whatever system is approved by your medical director. An oral airway may be inserted as a bite block to protect the tube. Note the depth of the tube at the teeth both before and after securing it to assure that the tube has not been dislodged during the procedure.

Ongoing Assessment

22. Be sure to assess and reassess the breath sounds following every major move with the patient.

Warning: Although the complications of orotracheal intubation have already been discussed above, it cannot be over-emphasized that inadvertent esophageal intubation will likely result in the patient's death. Because of the magnitude of this complication, if at any time—despite your efforts to properly assess tube placement—you are in doubt of proper tube placement, immediately withdraw the tube, and manage the airway with basic airway adjuncts.

Orotracheal Intubation of an Infant or Child

Although the goal of orotracheal intubation is identical in both adult and pediatric patients, intubation of the infant and child requires special training because of various considerations of anatomy, physiology, and size.

The specific anatomy and physiology of the pediatric airway has been discussed earlier. The importance of these factors as they relate to orotracheal intubation are as follows.

1. In an infant or child, it is often difficult to create a single clear visual plane from the mouth through the pharynx and into the glottis for orotracheal intubation because of such factors as the relatively large size of the tongue.
2. Because of size differences among infants and children as well as the fact that the narrowest portion of the airway is at the level of the cricoid ring, the proper sizing of the endotracheal tube is crucial.
3. Because infants and children tend to develop hypoxia and bradycardia (slowed heartbeat) easily during intubation attempts, pediatric intubations require careful monitoring coupled with swift and accurate technique.

The indications for orotracheal intubation of the infant and child are similar to those for the adult patient.

- When prolonged artificial ventilation is required
- When adequate artificial ventilation cannot be achieved by other means

- To ventilate the clearly apneic patient
- To ventilate the cardiac arrest patient
- To control the airway of an unresponsive patient without a cough or gag reflex

The laryngoscope blades and the endotracheal tubes necessary for the orotracheal intubation of infants and children must be carefully sized to the patient. In general the straight blade, usually a size 1, is preferred in infants and small children because it provides for greater displacement of the tongue and better visualization of the glottis. As in adults, the blade lifts the epiglottis, bringing the vocal cords into view. In older children the curved blade is often preferred because the blade's broad base displaces the tongue better, allowing better visualization of the vocal cords once the blade is placed into the vallecula and lifted.

Assorted sizes of endotracheal tubes should always be stocked in the pediatric airway kit. As previously mentioned, the proper sizing of the tube is essential in children. Ideally a chart should be placed in the airway kit to assist the EMT-B in determining what size tube is generally used for a certain age patient. As an alternative there are commercially available measuring tapes that estimate tube size based on the height of the patient.

A formula—(patient's age + 16) / 4 = tube size—can also be used to estimate the proper size. Finally, using the diameter of the patient's little finger or the diameter of the nasal opening are alternative techniques for estimating correct tube size.

Because infants are often the pediatric patients who require orotracheal intubation, it is helpful to simply memorize that newborns and small infants generally require a 3.0 to a 3.5 tube, and a 4.0 tube can be used for older infants up to the age of one year. No matter what system you use in determining tube size, it is always prudent to have one half-size larger tube and one half-size smaller tube on stand-by, since the size of the glottic structures does vary in infants and children.

Endotracheal tubes come in both cuffed and uncuffed versions. Cuffed tubes are always used in adult patients. In the pediatric population, cuffed tubes are reserved for children 8 years of age and older. For younger children and infants, uncuffed tubes are used since the narrowing at the level of the cartilage serves as a functional cuff, snugging the tube in the airway. Uncuffed tubes (Figure 33-11) should display a vocal cord marker to assure proper placement of

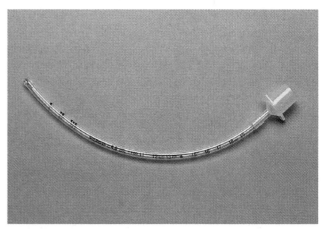

FIGURE 33-11 An uncuffed endotracheal tube is used for patients under 8 years of age.

the tube. This marker is designed so that the vocal cords are at the level of the translucent marker in the tube. If the child is old enough to get a cuffed tube it should be inserted, like the adult tube, just deep enough that the cuff material is distal to the cords.

Proper depth of tube placement can also be approximated by age (Table 33-2). However, direct visualization of the tube being placed at the proper depth is the best measure of tube depth.

The step-by-step procedure for orotracheal intubation of infants and children is very similar to the procedure outlined for adults (above and Scan 33-1).

There are, however, some important differences that you must keep in mind when performing a pediatric intubation.

1. The rate of hyperventilation both before and after intubation must be adjusted to the patient's age.
2. The patient's heart rate must be continuously monitored during intubation attempts,

TABLE 33-2 Length of Endotracheal Tubes in Infants and Children

Measurement of Endotracheal Tube at the Teeth
6 months to 1 year: 12 cm teeth to midtrachea
2 years: 14 cm teeth to midtrachea
4 - 6 years: 16 cm teeth to midtrachea
6-10 years: 18 cm teeth to midtrachea
10 - 12 years: 20 cm teeth to midtrachea

since mechanical stimulation of the airway and hypoxia can both slow the heart rate. If the heart rate is noted to slow during intubation, the blade should immediately be withdrawn and the infant or child reventilated with high concentration oxygen.

3. The optimal manner of positioning the patient's head is to gently tilt the head forward and lift the chin into the "sniffing position" (Figure 33-12).

4. Very little force is needed to intubate the infant or child. Gentle finesse is the rule, not the exception.

5. Sellick's maneuver is also often beneficial, but the landmarks may be difficult to locate in the infant and child. In addition, excessive pressure on the relatively soft cartilage may cause tracheal obstruction.

6. When using a straight blade, realize that the epiglottis in infants and children is not as stiff as in adults and may partially obscure a clear view of the vocal cords.

7. Since distances in the infant and child are small, be certain to hold onto the tube until you are assured that it is well secured. As with adults, reassess tube placement every time you move the patient.

8. In infants and children, the best indicator of tube placement is symmetrical rise and fall of the chest during ventilation.

9. Breath sounds in infants and children can often be misleading since the chest is small and sounds are easily transmitted from one area to another.

10. Observe the patient for increase in heart rate and improving color after intubation. An infant or child who becomes dusky in color and slows his heart rate after intubation is likely not to be properly intubated.

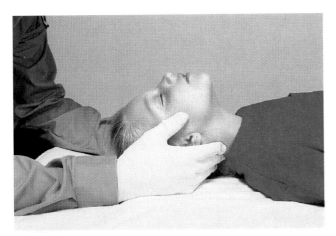

FIGURE 33-12 Place the pediatric patient's head in the "sniffing position" for intubation.

11. Once tube placement is confirmed, the patient should be secured to an appropriate device to prevent any head movement from dislodging the tube.

12. If the tube is properly placed but there is inadequate chest expansion, seek out one of the following causes.

- The tube is too small and there is an air leak around the tube at the glottic opening. This is detected by auscultating over the neck. The tube should be replaced by a larger tube.
- The pop-off valve on the bag-valve device has not been deactivated.
- There is a leak in the bag-valve device.
- The ventilator is delivering an inadequate volume of air/oxygen.
- The tube is blocked with secretions. This can be treated initially with endotracheal suctioning (see later in this chapter). If suctioning fails, the tube should be removed.

13. Infants and children are at risk for the same complications of orotracheal intubation as adult patients. Inadvertent esophageal intubation is perhaps even more rapidly fatal in infants and children than adults. In addition, barotrauma from over inflation of the lungs can result in collapse of the lung, which can further compromise your ability to ventilate the patient.

Nasogastric Intubation of an Infant or Child

An additional procedure the EMT-B may have to master in conjunction with orotracheal intubation of an infant or child is the placement of a **nasogastric tube** (NG tube). A nasogastric tube is inserted through the child's nose into the infant's or child's stomach. The most common use of the NG tube in regard to advanced airway management is that the tube is used to decompress the stomach and proximal bowel of air. In infants and children air frequently fills the stomach and bowel after overly aggressive artificial ventilation or as a result of air swallowing. The NG tube provides a route for escape of the excess air. The NG tube can also be used to drain the stomach of blood or other substances. In the hospital setting, NG tubes can be used to give medication and provide a route for nutrition as well.

The indications for insertion of the NG tube in pediatric patients are as follows.

- Inability to adequately ventilate the patient because of distention of the stomach
- The unresponsive patient with gastric distention

Many experts believe that the NG tube should only be inserted after the trachea has been secured with an endotracheal tube to prevent incorrectly placing the NG tube into the trachea instead of the esophagus. Other possible complications of NG intubation include trauma to the nose, triggering vomiting, and—in very rare cases—passing the tube into the cranium through a basilar skull fracture. *Because of the risk of cranial intubation with the NG tube, the presence of major facial trauma or head trauma is considered a contraindication to the nasogastric tube.* In such cases, the insertion of the tube through the mouth (orogastric technique) is preferred.

The equipment required for nasogastric tube insertion is listed in Table 33-3.

The procedure for insertion of the nasogastric tube as illustrated in Scan 33-2 is

1. Prepare and assemble all equipment.
2. Assure that the patient is well oxygenated prior to the procedure.
3. Measure the tube from the tip of the nose and around the ear to below the xiphoid process. (If the tube will be inserted by the orogastric technique, measure from the lips.) This length will determine the depth the tube will be inserted.

TABLE 33-3 Equipment for Nasogastric Intubation

Equipment for Nasogastric Intubation

Nasogastric tubes of various sizes—
  Newborn/infant: 8.0 French
  Toddler/preschool: 10.0 French
  School age: 12 French
  Adolescent: 14 - 16 French

20 cc syringe
Water soluble lubricant
Emesis basin
Tape
Stethoscope
Suction unit with connecting tubing

4. Lubricate the end of the tube.
5. Pass the tube gently downward along the nasal floor.
6. Confirm that the tube is in the stomach by

- Aspirating stomach contents
- Auscultating a rush of air over the epigastrium while injecting 10-20 cc of air into the tube

7. Aspirate gastric contents by attaching the tube to suction.
8. Secure the tube in place with tape.

Orotracheal Suctioning

In conjunction with your training in advanced airway management, you may also be trained in the techniques of orotracheal suctioning. For this procedure, a flexible soft suction catheter is used to suction the trachea, usually down to the level of the carina in the artificially ventilated patient. This procedure is sometimes referred to as "deep suctioning" to set it apart from the basic airway management procedure, suctioning of the oropharynx, in which suctioning does not advance as far as the trachea.

The indications for orotracheal suctioning are as follows.

- Obvious secretions in the airway—This may be detected by either moist bubbling sounds during ventilation with the bag-valve mask or by visible secretions inside the endotracheal tube after the patient has been intubated.
- Poor compliance with bag-valve-mask ventilation—Resistance to ventilation may be caused by secretions below the level of the larynx in the trachea.

The technique for orotracheal suctioning is shown in Scan 33-3. (**Note:** Although endotracheal suctioning can be performed on an unintubated patient, the procedure is by far most commonly performed through an endotracheal tube.) Specific steps in the procedure include

1. Pre-oxygenate the patient with high concentration oxygen prior to attempting suction.
2. Hyperventilate the patient prior to suctioning.
3. Check that all equipment is operating correctly.
4. Use sterile technique.

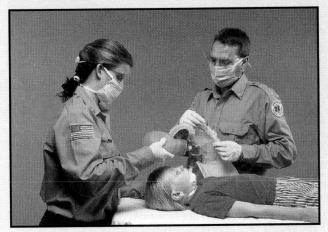

1. Oxygenate patient.

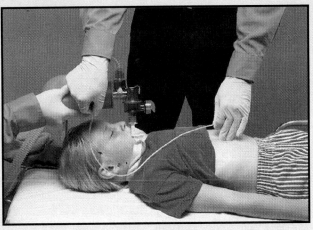

2. Measure tube from tip of nose, over ear, to below xiphoid process.

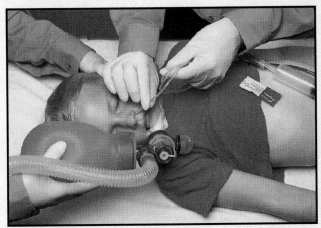

3. Pass lubricated tube gently downward along nasal floor into stomach.

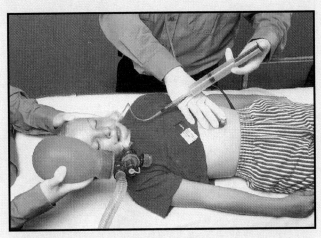

4. To confirm correct placement, auscultate over epigastrium. Listen for bubbling while injecting 10-20 cc air into tube.

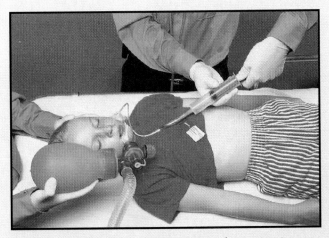

5. Use suction to aspirate stomach contents.

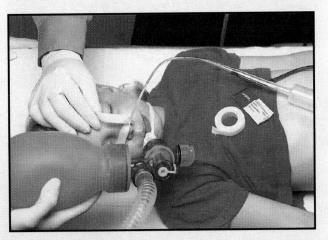

6. Secure tube in place.

727

Orotracheal Suctioning

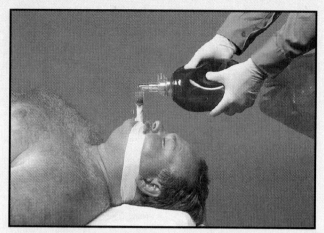

1. Hyperventilate patient.

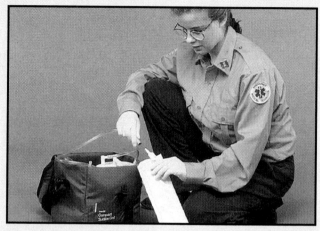

2. Carefully check equipment.

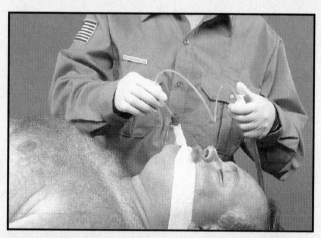

3. Insert catheter without applying suction.

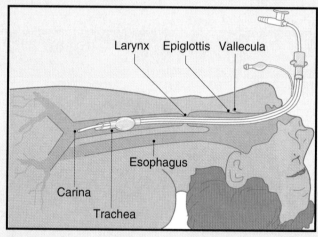

Larynx   Epiglottis   Vallecula

Esophagus

Carina

Trachea

4. Catheter may be advanced as far as carina level.

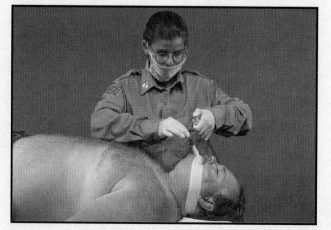

6. Resume ventilation. Suctioning procedure should interrupt ventilation for no more than 15 seconds.

5. Advance catheter to desired level, apply suction, and withdraw catheter with a twisting motion.

5. Observe body substance isolation precautions. Be especially mindful to have eye protection, as splattering during deep suctioning is common.
6. Approximate the desired length of the catheter to be inserted by measuring from the lips to the ear to the nipple line. This will approximate the level of the carina.
7. Advance the catheter to the desired location.
8. Apply suction and withdraw the catheter in a twisting motion.
9. Resume ventilations.
10. Attempts at deep suctioning should not exceed 15 seconds to prevent hypoxia.

Deep suctioning is not without potential complications. Most of the serious complications relate to the fact that the ventilated patient is deprived of oxygen during suctioning. Hyperventilation prior to suctioning, careful technique, and limiting suctioning to 15 seconds can help prevent the following complications of deep suctioning.

- Cardiac arrhythmias
- Hypoxia
- Coughing
- Damage to the lining (mucosa) of the airway
- Spasm of the bronchioles (bronchospasm) if catheter extends past the carina
- Spasm of the vocal cords (laryngospasm) during orotracheal suctioning

FYI

Topics included in the FYI—"For Your Information"—section are those that go beyond the chapter objectives. The information in this segment is intended to broaden your understanding of the chapter topic but is not essential to an understanding of your job as an EMT-B.

Automatic Transport Ventilators

Automatic transport ventilators (ATVs—Figure 33-13) have been used extensively in Europe for a number of years. The devices are rapidly gaining popularity in the United States as recent studies have demonstrated them to be superior in some respects to manual ventilation with the bag-valve mask.

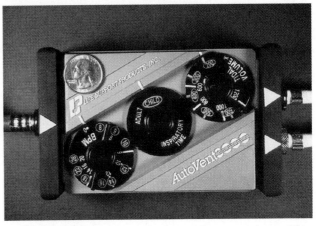

FIGURE 33-13 The automatic transport ventilator (ATV). The coin in the upper left corner is shown for scale.

ATVs are compact devices that have controls that set both the rate of ventilation and the tidal volume. Tidal volumes are determined by the patient's weight. A number of different ATV models are commercially available. The American Heart Association recommends that ATVs should meet certain minimal standards. They should

- Have the ability to deliver 100% oxygen
- Be able to provide at least two rates of ventilation: 10 breaths per minute for adults and 20 breaths per minute for children
- Be lightweight (2 to 5 kg) and rugged
- Be equipped with an audible alarm to alert the user to problems in ventilation
- Have a standard 15 mm/22 mm coupling to connect with a mask or endotracheal tube

Although some units are marketed for pediatric use with controls for lower tidal volumes, the device is not suitable for children less than 5 years of age.

Because ATVs do require some additional training for safe use, the decision to use ATVs in an EMS system and the establishment of ATV protocols should be done by the medical director.

Esophageal and Multilumen Airways

In some EMS systems medical direction may elect to allow the EMT-B to use esophageal and/or multilumen airways such as the PtL® or the Combitube®. Although these devices do not provide the definitive airway control of an endotracheal tube, when properly used they provide superior ventilation of the apneic patient as compared with a simple oral airway adjunct.

The EOA and EGTA

For over twenty years, alternative methods of intubating the patient using the esophageal obturator airway (EOA) and its close cousin the esophageal gastric tube airway (EGTA) have been available. They can be passed "blindly" into the pharynx, eliminating the need to use a laryngoscope to visualize the process as it is happening, and they do not need to be maneuvered between the vocal cords into the trachea, so many of the problems of improper placement are eliminated.

The ease of use and simplicity of both these devices have probably been overemphasized. It is true that they are easier to insert than the endotracheal tube. Nevertheless, they are invasive procedures, and the EMT using either device must be well versed in its complications, indications, and contraindications.

The major feature of the EOA or EGTA is an inflatable cuff that allows the trachea to be open but closes off the esophagus. The device is usually used during CPR or rescue breathing to "seal the meal," or prevent regurgitation (bringing up stomach contents that can be aspirated into the lungs) and prevent gastric distention (blowing air meant for the lungs into the stomach, which in turn tends to cause vomiting or regurgitation).

Both the EOA and the EGTA are usually connected to a bag-valve-mask unit which blows air or oxygen through the mask port. (As noted above, the EOA or EGTA tube doesn't go into the trachea, but since the esophagus is sealed off by the inflatable cuff, the only place for the ventilation to go is into the trachea and the lungs.)

Although the EOA or EGTA is less often misplaced than an endotracheal tube, it does sometimes get pushed into the trachea instead of the esophagus. When this happens—if the error is not quickly recognized through listening for lung sounds—it can be fatal.

There are certain contraindications to the use of the EOA or the EGTA. Neither should be used in

- A patient who is alert, verbally responsive, or who responds to painful stimuli and also still has a gag reflex. Vomiting and aspiration are likely.

- A patient who is under the age of 16 or who is less than 5 feet tall. The devices come in only one size and are too long for the anatomy of a small patient.
- A patient who has ingested a corrosive substance. A corrosive could perforate the tip of the device, or may weaken the esophagus so that the device could perforate the esophagus wall.
- A patient with a known esophageal disease such as cancer or esophageal verices, which weaken the wall of the esophagus and increase the chance for a ruptured esophagus.
- A patient with significant upper airway bleeding. Blood flowing from the nose or mouth will pass directly into the lungs once the inflated cuff has closed off the esophagus.

Although the EOA and EGTA have much in common, the differences are important to learn. Both have an air-cushion-inflatable mask and a 16-inch tube with a 30-35 cc inflatable air cuff on the distal end. The EOA has a closed distal end to the tube and a series of air holes on the proximal end of the tube. As air is ventilated into the tube with the mask sealed against the face, the air exits the holes into the pharynx. Since the tube has a blind end and the cuff is inflated after insertion, no air gets into the esophagus. (Figure 33-14).

The EGTA has an open end to the tube, or a valve at the end through which a tube can be inserted into the esophagus and the stomach. In this way, stomach contents can be suctioned or medications administered to the stomach. Ventilations are not blown through the tube port (indeed, this port is designed so that a BVM coupling will not fit, thus avoiding ventilating the stomach by mistake). Instead, the ventilations enter through a second port which, like the first and only EOA port, is a standard 15 mm ventilation device adapter. These ventilations, of course, do not travel through the tube at all but flow freely under the mask and into the mouth and pharynx on the outside of the tube. In other words, the EGTA provides access to the stomach while still protecting the trachea, while the EOA only protects the trachea.

To attach the mask to the tube of either device, insert the tube into the port 180 degrees from the desired normal anatomical position, then twist the tube 180 degrees until it snaps into place in the mask. To detach the mask from

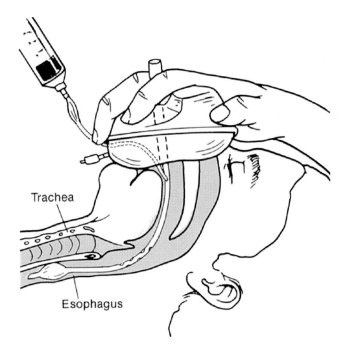

Check the positioning of the EOA by ventilating it by a bag-valve device and then watching for bilateral expansion of the chest and auscultating for bilateral breath sounds. If the chest does not rise on both sides and breath sounds are not heard, withdraw the tube, hyperventilate the patient, and reinsert the EOA. When the tube is correctly positioned, the cuff will lie below the carina. To avert possible esophageal rupture, inflate the cuff in the esophagus with no more than 35 ml of air.

FIGURE 33-14 The esophageal obturator airway (EOA).

the tube, simply squeeze the plastic tips that protrude through the mask and pull out the tube from the opposite direction from which it was inserted. Both devices should be stored in the position of function. They should never be stored flat or rolled into a coil as the shape of the tube will be lost and will decrease your chances of correctly intubating the esophagus.

To insert either device, you will first need to assemble all the correct supplies.

- An EOA or EGTA tube with the proper mask (*the masks are not interchangeable* and will fit only the correct tube)
- A water-soluble lubricant
- A BVM with reservoir
- A stethoscope
- A suction unit and rigid Yankauer tip
- A few 4 × 4 gauze pads
- A 35 cc syringe
- Gloves, mask, and protective eye wear

Then perform the following procedures.

1. Another EMT hyperventilates the patient with the BVM. Meanwhile . . .
2. Lubricate the tube with the water-soluble lubricant.
3. Stop the resuscitation momentarily and lift the jaw and tongue straight upward without hyperextending the neck. This is best accomplished with the neck in the neutral or slightly flexed position.
4. Pass the tube following the pharyngeal curvature until the mask is seated against the face (Figure 33-15).
5. Give one ventilation with the BVM and watch for the chest to rise. This is the way to check that the tube has been correctly placed in the esophagus and has not been incorrectly inserted into the trachea (which would block off the trachea and air pathway into the lungs). Once you are certain that the tube is correctly placed in the esophagus. . .
6. Inflate the cuff using the 35 cc syringe. (You must be certain the tube is in the esophagus. Inflation of the cuff in the trachea could cause serious damage.)
7. Use the stethoscope to listen to both lung fields (sounds of air intake into the lungs should be present) and the epigastrium. Having assured correct placement of the device . . .
8. Ventilate the patient using the BVM or a flow-restricted, oxygen-powered ventilation device.

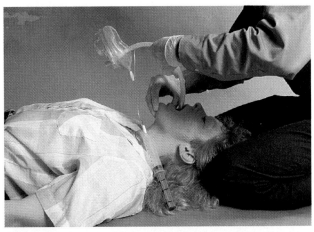

FIGURE 33-15 Advance the EOA or EGTA tube carefully behind tongue and into pharynx and esophagus.

Note: The key point to remember is that the EOA or EGTA mask must be sealed in the same manner as a BVM mask. The American Heart Association Emergency Cardiac Care Guidelines recommend that ventilation with a mask be a two-person, four-handed skill: two hands on the mask attending to the seal, two hands squeezing the bag. Otherwise, a sufficient ventilation is unlikely to be delivered.

When working with the EOA or EGTA, keep the following considerations in mind.

- Remove the bag from the mask prior to each defibrillation to prevent its weight from pulling out the tube.
- Be alert for vomitus in the airway and the need for suction, since regurgitation *can* occur even with the EOA or EGTA in place. If you need to suction, temporarily remove the mask from the tube.
- If a CPR board is used, which has an indentation to hyperextend the neck, be especially careful as hyperextension can increase the chances of misplacing the EOA or EGTA in the trachea. To guard against this possibility it is wise to place a towel in the indentation where the patient's head rests. This places the head in a neutral position. Remove the towel after EOA insertion. The importance of listening to lung sounds to confirm correct placement cannot be over-emphasized.

If the patient becomes conscious, you must remove the tube. Remember that extubation is likely to be followed by vomiting. Follow these guidelines for removing the EOA or EGTA.

- Always have the suction unit with a rigid Yankauer tip standing by.
- Do not deflate the EOA or EGTA cuff until the patient has resumed breathing or an endotracheal tube has been inserted and its cuff is inflated in the trachea. If you are using an EGTA, a gastric tube can be inserted through it to decompress the stomach or evacuate its contents to reduce the chances of regurgitation or vomiting.
- Provided there is no possibility of a spinal injury, or if the patient is secured to a spine board, turn the patient on his side, insert the syringe into the one-way valve, and withdraw air slowly from the EOA or EGTA cuff.

- Carefully remove the tube, staying alert for vomiting.

Warning: Whenever an EOA or EGTA is inserted or extubated, gloves, mask, and protective eye wear should be worn to protect the EMT-B from the potential spraying of body fluids.

The Pharyngeo-tracheal Lumen Airway (PtL®)

One problem with airway devices such as the endotracheal tube, the EOA, and the EGTA is that they must be correctly placed into the intended passageway, the trachea or the esophagus. The Pharyngeo-tracheal Lumen Airway (PtL®) has been constructed to get around this problem. It can easily be inserted into either the trachea or the esophagus with minimum skill, and it will work no matter which passageway it is in.

The PtL® has two lumens (tubes), one inside the other, and for this reason it is sometimes referred to as a double-lumen airway. A long endotracheal-type tube is located within a short, large-diameter tube. The long tube can be inserted into either the trachea or the esophagus, while the shorter tube opens into the pharynx above the epiglottis. Both tubes have low-pressure cuffs at their distal ends. On the long tube, the cuff, when inflated, provides a seal for the trachea or esophagus, depending on which of the two passageways it is resting in. On the short tube, the larger-volume cuff, when fully inflated, seals off the oropharynx.

When the long, inner tube of the PtL® is placed in the esophagus and its cuff is inflated to seal off the esophagus, air delivered through the short outer tube is diverted into the trachea and the lungs. When the long, inner tube is placed in the trachea, air is delivered through that tube, not the short outer tube, to the lungs. Whether it is in the esophagus or the trachea, the longer tube's cuff prevents air from leaking into the esophagus and stomach.

The PtL® also solves the problem of needing extra hands to provide a seal for a face mask. The cuff on the short, outer tube seals the pharynx and prevents delivered air from escaping through the mouth and nose, as well as preventing blood and debris from entering the airway from above. Both tubes of the PtL® have a 15 mm adapter to which a BVM or other ventilation device can be attached.

The PtL® also includes inflation lines so

that the cuffs can be inflated. A metal stylet is provided to facilitate guiding the tubes into position. A plastic bite block prevents the patient's teeth from occluding the airway. A neck strap secures the airway to the patient's head.

As with the EOA or EGTA, the PtL® should *not* be used on

- A conscious patient or one with an active gag reflex
- A patient under the age of 16
- A patient who has swallowed a corrosive substance.
- A patient with a known esophageal disease.

The procedure to insert the PtL® starts with preparing the equipment. Ensure that both cuffs are fully deflated, that the long, clear, inner #3 tube (see Figure 33-16) has a bend in the middle, and that the white cap is securely in place over the deflation port located under the #1 inflation valve. Lubricate the long #3 tube with a water-soluble lubricant.

If the patient has facial trauma, quickly sweep out the mouth with your gloved fingers and remove any broken teeth, dentures, or other debris that could damage the air cuffs or interfere with passing the tube.

When the patient and the airway are ready, insertion should be accomplished quickly between ventilations.

1. Open the airway. In a patient with potential spinal trauma, have a partner stabilize the head in a neutral in-line position while you pass the airway with minimal cervical manipulation. Use a thumb-in-mouth jaw-lift or tongue-lift method to open the airway. If you have ruled out spinal trauma, hyperextend the patient's head with one hand, insert your thumb deep into the patient's mouth, grasp the tongue and lower jaw between your thumb and index finger, and lift straight upward.

2. Hold the PtL® in your free hand so that it curves in the same direction as the natural curvature of the pharynx. Then insert the tip of the airway into the patient's mouth and advance it carefully behind the tongue until the teeth strap contacts the lips and teeth. (Positioning the airway in this manner with the teeth strap against the lips and teeth is proper for an average-sized adult. If the patient is very small, it may be neces-

sary to withdraw the airway so that the teeth strap is as much as one inch from the teeth. When the patient is very large, it may be necessary to insert the airway beyond the normal depth so that the teeth strap is actually inside the patient's mouth, past the teeth.)

3. When the tube is at the proper depth, flip the neck strap over the patient's head and tighten it with the hook-and-tape closures located on both sides of the strap.

4. Inflate the small cuff that seals either the esophagus or the trachea and the large cuff that seals the oropharynx, first making sure that the white cap is in place over the deflation port located under the inflation valve. To inflate both cuffs simultaneously, deliver a sustained ventilation into the inflation valve. Failure to inflate the cuffs properly can be detected by the failure of the exterior pilot balloon to inflate or by hearing or feeling air escaping from the patient's mouth and nose. In this case one of the cuffs, probably the large one, may be torn. Quickly remove the airway, ventilate the patient, then replace it with a new one. When you see by the pilot balloon that the two cuffs are inflated, deliver puffs of air to increase pressure in the cuffs and improve the seal.

5. Is the long, clear #3 tube in the esophagus or the trachea? Determine its location by ventilating the short, green #2 tube. If the chest rises, the long tube is in the esophagus and air is, obviously, being diverted through the trachea into the lungs. In this case, deliver ventilations with breaths or with air or oxygen delivered from a BVM or positive-pressure ventilator through the short, green #2 tube.

6. If the chest does not rise when the short, green #2 tube is ventilated, the long, clear #3 tube is probably in the trachea. In this case, remove the stylet and deliver ventilations through the #3 tube. Verify proper delivery of ventilations by listening to both lung fields (for sounds of air entering both lungs) and the epigastrium (where there should be *no* sounds of air entering the esophagus and stomach). Also verify chest rise with each breath.

7. Continue ventilations through the airway until the patient regains consciousness or protective airway gag reflexes return, or the patient is transferred to the emergency department.

Parts of the PtL® Airway:

A

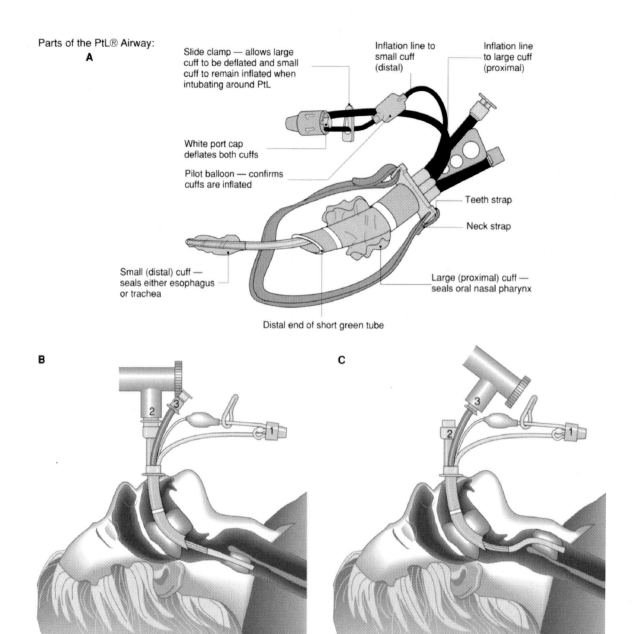

Slide clamp — allows large cuff to be deflated and small cuff to remain inflated when intubating around PtL

Inflation line to small cuff (distal)

Inflation line to large cuff (proximal)

White port cap deflates both cuffs

Pilot balloon — confirms cuffs are inflated

Teeth strap

Neck strap

Small (distal) cuff — seals either esophagus or trachea

Large (proximal) cuff — seals oral nasal pharynx

Distal end of short green tube

B

C

The PtL® airway inserted in the esophagus. Oxygen delivered into the short #2 tube passes into the lungs. An inflated cuff at the end of the long #3 tube seals the esophagus, while another inflated cuff seals the oropharynx and prevents air loss from the mouth and nose.

The PtL® airway inserted in the trachea. Oxygen is delivered into the long #3 tube after the stylet is removed. The inflated cuff at the end of the long tube keeps air from leaking from the trachea into the esophagus. The large cuff that is sealing the oropharynx serves as a secondary seal.

FIGURE 33-16 A. The PtL® airway. B. The PtL® in place in the esophagus. C. The PtL® in place in the trachea.

Continually monitor the appearance of the pilot balloon during ventilation efforts. Loss of pressure in the balloon will signal a loss of pressure in the cuffs. If you suspect that a cuff is leaking, increase cuff pressure by blowing forcefully into the #1 inflation valve, or replace the airway. Repositioning the PtL® to ensure that the teeth strap is snug against the patient's teeth is another way of reducing leakage.

As with the EOA or EGTA, if the patient becomes conscious, you must remove the PtL®. Remember that extubation is likely to be followed by vomiting. Follow these guidelines for removing the PtL®.

- If there is no possibility of trauma, or if the patient is secured to a spine board, turn the patient onto his side and make sure that the stomach has been decompressed and that gastric contents have been evacuated. This can be accomplished by passing a #18 French Levine suction catheter into the non-airway tube.
- Remove the white cap from the deflation port to simultaneously deflate both cuffs.
- Carefully withdraw the airway and discard.
- Stay alert for vomiting.

Warning: Whenever a PtL® is inserted or extubated, gloves, mask, and eye wear should be worn to protect the EMT from the potential spraying of body fluids.

The Esophageal Tracheal Combitube®

The most recent alternative to the EOA, EGTA, and PtL® airways is called the esophageal tracheal combitube or, more commonly, "Combitube®." Like the PtL® airway, the Combitube® is a double lumen airway and functions very much like a PtL®. With the Combitube®, however, one lumen is not inside the other. Rather, the two lumens are separated by a partition wall.

In one lumen of the Combitube®, the distal end is sealed and there are perforations in the area that would be in the pharynx. When the tube is in the esophagus, ventilations are delivered through this tube. The sealed end prevents the ventilations from entering the esophagus and stomach and diverts them through the perforations into the pharynx from which they flow into the trachea and the lungs.

In the other lumen of the Combitube®, the distal end is open. When the tube is in the trachea, ventilations are delivered through this tube.

The Combitube® has a distal cuff that inflates to seal the esophagus or trachea, depending on which passageway it is in. (When the trachea is sealed, the cuff prevents stomach contents from being aspirated, but does not prevent ventilations from entering the trachea via the tube that passes through the cuff.)

There is also a pharyngeal balloon that, as with the PtL® seals the pharynx, preventing air

from escaping the mouth and nose and blood and debris from entering the airway.

As with the EOA or EGTA, the PtL® should not be used on

- A conscious patient or one with an active gag reflex.
- A patient under the age of 16.
- A patient who has swallowed a corrosive substance.
- A patient with a known esophageal disease.

Follow these steps to insert the Combitube®.

1. Insert the device blindly, watching for the two black rings on the Combitube® that are used for measuring the depth of insertion. These rings should be positioned between the teeth and the bony cavities where the teeth have their roots.
2. Use the large syringe to inflate the pharyngeal cuff with 100 cc of air. On inflation, the device will seat itself in the posterior pharynx behind the hard palate.
3. Use the smaller syringe to fill the distal cuff with 10 cc to 15 cc of air.
4. Usually the tube will have been placed in the esophagus. On this assumption, ventilate through the esophageal connector. It is the external tube that is the longer of the two and is marked #1. As with the PtL®, you must listen for the presence of breath sounds in the lungs and the absence of sounds from the epigastrium in order to be sure that the tube is, in fact, placed in the esophagus.
5. If there is an absence of lung sounds and presence of sounds in the epigastrium, the tube has been placed in the trachea. In this case, change the ventilator to the shorter tracheal connector, which is marked #2. Listen again to be sure of proper placement of the tube.

An advantage of the Combitube® over the PtL® is that no stylet must be withdrawn from the open-ended esophageal lumen before suctioning of the stomach can take place, making this process quicker. Another advantage is the automatic seating of the pharyngeal cuff.

The biggest advantage of the Combitube® is that rapid intubation is possible independent of the position of the patient, which is helpful for trauma patients requiring limited cervical spine movement.

As with the EOA, EGTA, or PtL®, if the patient becomes conscious, you must remove the Combitube®. Remember that extubation is likely to be followed by vomiting. Have suction equipment ready. Follow the same guidelines as for removal of the other airway devices.

Warning: Whenever a Combitube® is inserted or extubated, gloves, mask, and protective eye wear should be worn to protect the EMT from the potential spraying of body fluids.

CHAPTER REVIEW

KEY TERMS

You may find it helpful to review the following terms.

alveoli (al-VE-o-li) the microscopic sacs of the lungs where gas exchange with the bloodstream takes place.

bronchi (BRONG-ki) the two large sets of branches that come off the trachea and enter the lungs. There are right and left mainstem bronchi. The singular is *bronchus.*

carina (kah-RI-nah) the fork at the lower end of the trachea where the two mainstem bronchi branch.

cricoid (KRIK-oid) **cartilage** the ring-shaped structure that circles the trachea at the lower edge of the larynx.

cricoid pressure pressure applied to the cricoid cartilage to suppress vomiting and bring the vocal cords into view. Also called *Sellick's maneuver.*

endotracheal (EN-do-TRAY-ke-ul) **tube** a tube designed to be inserted into the trachea. Oxygen, medication, or a suction catheter can be directed into the trachea through an endotracheal tube.

epiglottis (EP-i-GLOT-is) a leaf-shaped structure that prevents food and foreign matter from entering the trachea.

esophagus (eh-SOF-uh-gus) the tube that leads from the pharynx to the stomach.

glottic opening the opening to the trachea.

hyperventilate (HI-per-VEN-ti-late) to provide ventilations at a higher rate to compensate for oxygen not delivered during intubation or suctioning.

hypopharynx (HI-po-FAIR-inks) the area directly above the openings of both the trachea and the esophagus.

hypoxia (hi-POK-se-uh) inadequate oxygenation, or oxygen starvation.

intubation (IN-tu-BAY-shun) insertion of a tube. See also *endotracheal tube; nasogastric tube; orotracheal intubation.*

laryngoscope an illuminating instrument that is inserted into the pharynx to permit visualization of the pharynx and larynx.

larynx (LAIR-inks) the voice box.

mainstem bronchi *See* bronchi.

nasogastric (NAY-zo-GAS-trik) **tube (NG tube)** a tube designed to be passed through the nose, nasopharynx, and esophagus. It is used to relieve distention of the stomach in an infant or child patient.

nasopharynx (NAY-zo-FAIR-inks) the area directly posterior to the nose.

oropharynx (OR-o-FAIR-inks) the area directly posterior to the mouth.

orotracheal (OR-o-TRAY-ke-ul) **intubation** placement of an endotracheal tube through the mouth and into the trachea. See also *endotracheal tube.*

Sellick's maneuver see *cricoid pressure.*

stylet a long, thin, bendable metal probe.

trachea (TRAY-ke-uh) the "windpipe"; the structure that connects the pharynx to the lungs.

vallecula (val-EK-yuh-luh) a groove-like structure anterior to the epiglottis.

vocal cords two thin folds of tissue within the larynx that vibrate as air passes between them, producing sounds.

Airway control is the highest priority in managing any critically ill or injured patient, because without an adequate airway the patient will die no matter what other care you provide. Control of a patient's airway is recognized as so crucial a skill, that advanced airway skills are now included as an elective in the EMT-Basic curriculum. Advanced airway management centers on the skill of orotracheal intubation, the placement of an endotracheal tube through the mouth and into the patient's trachea. This permits complete control of the airway, minimizes the risk of aspiration, allows for better oxygen delivery, and allows for deep suctioning of the trachea.

Endotracheal intubation of infants and children is similar to the procedure for adults with these exceptions: All structures in the mouth and nose are smaller, the tongues are proportionately larger, the trachea is softer, more flexible, and narrower, the airway is especially narrow at the cricoid cartilage, and the chest wall is softer. These differences result in the airways of infants and children being more easily obstructed, in the use of uncuffed endotracheal tubes under the age of 8 because the narrow cricoid acts as a cuff, and in distinctive breathing patterns. Infants and children are more susceptible to damage from incorrect placement of a tube and to interruptions of the supply of oxygen and must be monitored especially carefully during intubation and suctioning procedures.

Nasogastric intubation is performed on infants and children to relieve the pressure of swallowed air in the stomach.

Endotracheal suctioning is performed by inserting a suction catheter—usually through an endotracheal tube—to the level of the carina.

REVIEW QUESTIONS

1. Explain why it is important for EMT-Bs to be able to perform orotracheal intubation.
2. List and explain the errors in intubation that can lead to a patient's death.
3. Explain the procedures for assuring correct placement of an endotracheal tube.
4. Explain reasons and describe the procedure for insertion of a nasogastric tube in an infant or child.
5. Explain how orotracheal suctioning differs from oropharyngeal suctioning. Explain reasons why orotracheal suctioning may be advisable.

Application

- You have successfully intubated a non-breathing patient and transferred him to the ambulance. During your ongoing assessment you ausculate the chest and find that there are breath sounds on the right, but not the left. What does this indicate? What should you do in this situation?

ALS-Assist Skills

Local protocol may require you to assist more highly trained EMS personnel in the administration of advanced life support (ALS) procedures. There are several new skills you can learn to enhance your capability as a "team player" on such calls. Your instructor will discuss the skills that are authorized by your medical director. However, the most common are

- Assisting in the endotracheal intubation of a patient.
- Applying ECG/defibrillator electrodes.
- Using a pulse oximeter.
- Assisting in intravenous (IV) fluid therapy.

Note: The following information is intended as a summary of ALS-assist skills. More detailed information and additional in-service training may be required. Consult with your instructor on local protocols.

ASSISTING IN THE ENDOTRACHEAL INTUBATION OF A PATIENT

Among the highest priorities of patient care is to assure a patent airway and to prevent aspiration. The "gold standard" for airway care is the endotracheal tube. All other airway devices are at best secondary. This is because the endotracheal tube is directly inserted into the trachea, forming an open pathway for air, oxygen, or medications to be blown into the lungs. In addition, adult sizes have an inflatable cuff that seals off the trachea to prevent aspiration. Patients who typically need to have an endotracheal tube inserted are those in pulmonary or cardiopulmonary arrest, trauma patients in need of airway control or supplemental oxygen, and those in respiratory distress or failure due to overdose, fluid in the lungs, asthma, asphyxia, or allergic reaction.

In some areas, EMT-Bs will be trained to perform endotracheal intubation of a patient. The skill is taught as an elective in Chapter 33, Advanced Airway Management. In other areas, only advanced EMTs or paramedics will perform endotracheal intubation, but EMT-Bs may be asked to assist with the procedure. The skills of assisting with endotracheal intubation are presented below.

Preparing the Patient for Intubation

Before the paramedic inserts the endotracheal tube (intubation), you may be asked to give the patient an extra amount of oxygen. This can easily be accomplished by ventilating with a bag-valve-mask once every two seconds. Then the paramedic will place the non-trauma patient in the sniffing position (neck elevated approximately two inches, chin and nose thrust forward, head tilted back—see Chapter 33, Figure 33-12) to align the mouth, throat, and trachea. The paramedic will remove the oral airway and pass the endotracheal tube through the mouth (sometimes the nose) into the throat past the vocal cords and into the trachea. This procedure usually requires a laryngoscope to move the tongue and other obstructions out of the way.

In order to maneuver the tube past the vocal cords correctly, the paramedic will need to see them. You may be asked to gently press on the throat to push the vocal cords into the paramedic's view. You will do this by pressing your thumb and index finger just to either side of the medial throat over the cricoid cartilage (ring-shaped cartilage just below the thyroid cartilage, or Adam's apple—Figure A-1). This procedure is known as cricoid pressure, or Sellick's maneuver.

Once the tube is properly placed, the cuff is inflated with air from a 10 cc syringe. While holding the tube, the paramedic uses a stethoscope to listen for lung sounds on both sides

The Cricoid Cartilage

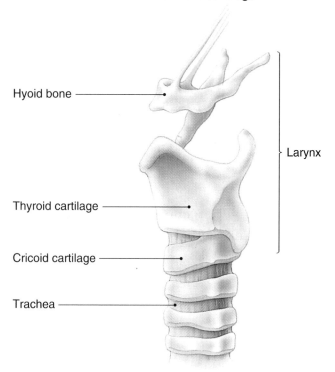

Hyoid bone

Larynx

Thyroid cartilage

Cricoid cartilage

Trachea

FIGURE A-1 The cricoid cartilage is a ring-shaped cartilage just below the Adam's apple.

and over the epigastrium (the area of the upper abdomen just under the xiphoid process). If the tube has been correctly placed, there will be sounds of air entering the lungs but no sounds of air in the epigastrium. Air sounds in the epigastrium indicate that the tube has been incorrectly placed in the esophagus instead of the trachea so that air is entering the stomach instead of the lungs. The tube position must be corrected immediately by removing the tube, reoxygenating the patient, and repeating the process of intubation.

The correctly positioned tube is anchored in place with tape or a commercially made tube restraint. The entire procedure—including the last ventilation, passing the tube, and the next ventilation—should take less than 30 seconds.

Ventilating the Tubed Patient

When asked to ventilate a tubed patient, keep in mind that very little movement can displace the endotracheal tube. Look at the gradations on the side of the tube. In the typical adult male, for example, the 22 cm mark will be at the teeth when the tube is properly placed. If the tube moves, report this to the paramedic immediately.

Note: Be especially careful **not** to disturb the endotracheal tube. If the tube is pushed in, it will most likely enter the right mainstem bronchus, preventing oxygen from entering the patient's left lung. If the tube is pulled out, it can easily slip into the esophagus and send all the ventilations directly to the stomach, denying the patient oxygen. *This is a fatal complication if it goes unnoticed before the tube is anchored in place.*

Hold the tube against the patient's teeth with two fingers of one hand (Figure A2). Use the other hand to work the bag-valve-mask (BVM). A patient with an endotracheal tube offers less resistance to ventilations, so you may not need two hands to work the bag. If you are ventilating a breathing patient, be sure to provide ventilations that are timed *with* the respiratory effort as much as possible so the patient can take full breaths. It is also possible to help the patient increase respiratory rate, if needed, by interposing extra ventilations. There are some cautions to remember.

- Pay close attention to what the ventilations feel like. Report any change in resistance. Increased resistance when ventilating with the bag-valve mask is one of the first signs of air escaping through a hole in the lungs and filling the space around the lungs, an extremely serious problem. A change in

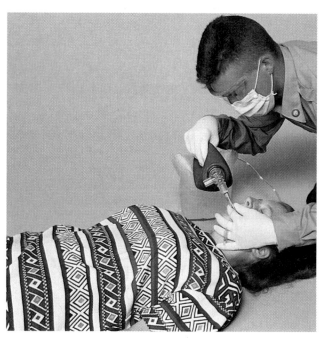

FIGURE A-2 Make sure the endotracheal tube does not move. Hold it with two fingers against the patient's teeth.

resistance can also indicate that the tube has slipped into the esophagus.

- Whenever a patient is to be defibrillated, carefully remove the bag from the tube. If you do not, the weight of the unsupported bag may accidentally displace the tube.
- Watch for any change in the patient's mental status. As the patient becomes more alert, he or she may need to be restrained from pulling out the tube. In addition, an oral airway generally is used as a bite block (a device that prevents the patient from biting the endotracheal tube). If the patient's gag reflex returns along with increased consciousness, you may need to pull the bite block out a bit.

Finally, during a cardiac arrest in the absence of an IV (see Assisting in IV Therapy, below), you may be asked to stop ventilating and remove the BVM. The paramedic may then inject a medication such as epinephrine down the tube. To increase the rate at which medication enters the blood stream through the respiratory system, you then may be asked to hyperventilate the patient for a few minutes (give ventilations at a faster-than-normal rate).

Assisting with a Trauma Intubation

Occasionally you will be asked to assist in the endotracheal intubation of a patient with a suspected cervical-spine injury. Since using the "sniffing position," which involves elevating the neck, risks worsening cervical spine injury, some modifications are necessary. Your role will change as well. You may be required to provide manual in-line stabilization during the whole procedure.

To accomplish this the paramedic will hold manual stabilization while you apply a cervical collar. In some EMS systems, the patient may be intubated without a cervical collar in place but with attention to manual stabilization during and after intubation. Since the paramedic must stay at the patient's head, it will be necessary for you to stabilize the head and neck from the patient's side (Figure A-3). Once you are in position, the paramedic will lean back and use the laryngoscope, which will bring the vocal cords into view. The patient can then be tubed.

After intubation, you will hold the tube against the teeth until placement is confirmed and anchored. At that time you can change your position to a more comfortable one. However,

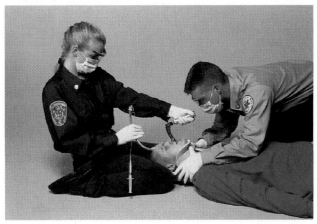

FIGURE A-3 To assist in the intubation of a patient with suspected cervical-spine injury, maintain manual stabilization throughout the procedure.

until the patient is immobilized on a long backboard, it will be necessary to assign another EMS worker to maintain manual stabilization while you ventilate the patient. Never assume that a collar provides adequate immobilization by itself. Manual stabilization must be used in addition to a collar until the head is taped in place on the backboard.

APPLYING ECG/DEFIBRILLATOR ELECTRODES

An electrocardiogram (ECG) provides data on the electrical activity of the heart. In the field, it is used to alert EMS personnel to life-threatening rhythm disturbances. Interpretation of an ECG has traditionally been a paramedic skill. However, to save time on calls you may be asked to assist. Make sure that you review the ECG equipment (Figure A-4). You should know how to turn on the monitor, how to record an ECG strip, how to change the battery, and how to change the roll of ECG paper. (These are the things that most often go wrong when the paramedic is involved with the patient.)

You also may be asked to carry out four steps in the process of applying the electrodes.

1. Turn on the ECG monitor.
2. Plug in the monitoring cables or "leads."
3. Attach the monitoring cables to the electrodes.
4. Apply the electrodes to the patient's body.

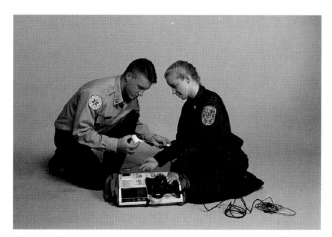

FIGURE A-4 An ECG monitor/defibrillator.

Become familiar with the electrodes used by the paramedics with whom you work. There are two types: monitoring electrodes (with smaller pads) and combination monitoring/defibrillator electrodes (with larger pads). The one most commonly used by paramedics is the monitoring electrode.

If you are asked to apply monitoring electrodes to the patient's body, you will need three—each one giving a different "view" of the heart's electrical activity. First prepare the patient's skin. The best connection is on dry, bare skin, so it may be necessary to dry the area and shave excessive hair. Use a wash cloth to remove oil from the skin and consider using an antiperspirant on patients with very sweaty skin. Become familiar with the monitoring configuration (where to place the electrodes) used by ALS personnel in your system. The most common setup is placing the negative (white) electrode

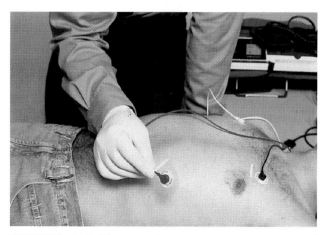

FIGURE A-5 The most common positioning of electrodes for an ECG is shown here. Become familiar with the monitoring configuration used by ALS personnel in your system.

under the center of the right clavicle, the positive (red) electrode on the left lower chest, and the ground (black or green) electrode under the center of the left clavicle or the right lower chest (Figure A-5).

USING A PULSE OXIMETER

A pulse oximeter is a photoelectric device that monitors the amount of oxygen circulating in the blood. It consists of a portable monitor and sensing probe that easily clips onto the patient's finger or earlobe (Figure A-6). The oximeter screen displays a percentage measurement of oxygen saturation.

The oximeter should be used with all patients complaining of respiratory problems. It is useful in assessing the effectiveness of artificial respirations, oxygen therapy, bronchodilator therapy, and bag-valve-mask ventilations.

It is important for you to note that

• Use of a pulse oximeter is helpful because it encourages you to be more aggressive about providing oxygen therapy and ventilations of a patient (in order to get the satu-

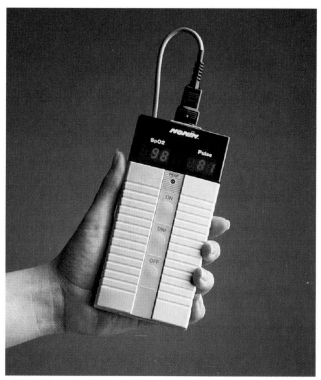

FIGURE A-6 A pulse oximeter is a photoelectric device that monitors the amount of oxygen circulating in the blood.

ration reading up to 95%), especially a conscious patient in respiratory distress. *The reverse situation is not true. That is, oxygen should not be withheld from a patient with signs and symptoms that indicate the need for oxygen, even if the reading is 95% or above.*

- The oximeter is inaccurate with hypothermic patients (those whose body temperatures have been lowered by exposure to cold) and patients in shock.
- The oximeter will produce falsely high readings in patients with carbon monoxide poisoning. This is because carbon monoxide binds with hemoglobin in the blood, producing the red color read by the device. Also note that chronic smokers normally have 10% to 15% more residual carbon monoxide in their blood than nonsmokers, so they may show higher-than-normal readings while still requiring oxygen.
- Excessive movement of the patient can cause inaccurate readings. So can nail polish, if the device is attached to a finger. Carry acetone wipes to quickly remove the nail polish from a patient's fingernail before attaching the oximeter.
- Monitor the oximeter reading every five minutes.
- The accuracy of the unit should be checked by following the manufacturer's recommendations. Remember, the oximeter is just another tool. Do not rely on it solely for indications of the patient's condition. Treat the patient, not the machine.

ASSISTING IN IV THERAPY

Setting Up an IV Fluid Administration Set

IV therapy is an advanced life support procedure. An intravenous (IV) line is inserted into a vein so that blood, fluids, or medications can be administered directly into the patient's circulation. A blood transfusion is almost always given at the hospital. An infusion of other fluids or medications can usually be done in the field.

The bag of fluid that feeds the IV is usually a clear plastic bag that collapses as it empties. The administration set is the clear plastic tubing that connects the fluid bag to the needle, or catheter. There are three important parts to this tubing.

- The *drip chamber* is near the fluid bag. There are two basic types: the mini drip and the macro drip. The mini drip is used when minimal flow of fluid is needed (with children, for example). Sixty small drops from the tiny metal barrel in the drip chamber equal one cubic centimeter (cc) or one milliliter (ml). The macro drip is used when a higher flow of fluid is needed (for a multi-trauma victim in shock, for example). There is no little barrel in the drip chamber of the macro drip, and only 10 to 15 large drops equal one cc or one ml.
- The *flow regulator* is located below the drip chamber. It is a stopcock that can be pushed up or down to start, stop, or control the rate of flow (Figure A-7).
- The *drug or needle port* is below the flow regulator. The paramedic can inject medication into this opening.

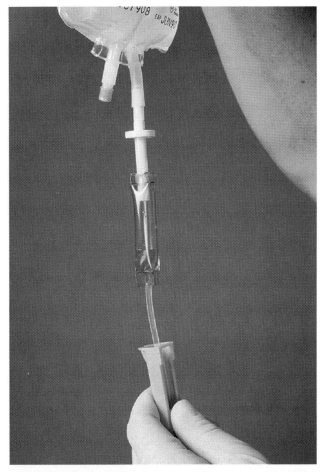

FIGURE A-7 Located below the drip chamber, the flow regulator is a stopcock that can be pushed up or down to start, stop, or control the rate of flow.

An extension set includes an extra length of tubing, which can make it easier to carry or disrobe the patient without accidentally pulling out the IV. Extension sets should not be used with the macro drip set because lengthening tubing reduces the flow rate.

In most cases, a paramedic will insert the IV into the patient's vein. However, you may be enlisted to help set up the IV administration set. You will need to

1. Take out and inspect the fluid bag. The bags come in a protective wrapping to keep them clean. If you are setting up the IV, you must remove the wrapper, then inspect the bag to be sure it contains the fluid that has been ordered. Check the expiration date to make sure the fluid is usable, and look to see that the fluid is clear and free of particles. Squeeze the bag to check for leaks. Occasionally, the fluid comes in a bottle. If so, be sure it is free of cracks. If anything is wrong, report the problem and inspect another bag or bottle (Figure A-8).

2. Select the proper administration set. Uncoil the tubing, and do not let the ends touch the ground.

3. Connect the extension set to the administration set, if an extension set is to be used.

4. Make sure the flow regulator is closed. To do this, roll the stopcock away from the fluid bag.

5. Remove the protective covering from the port of the fluid bag and the protective covering from the spiked end of the tubing (Figure A-9). Insert the spiked end of the

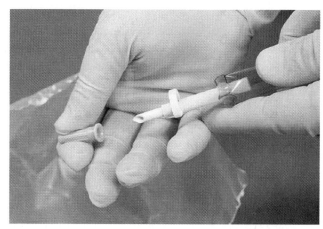

FIGURE A-9 Setting up the IV administration set includes removing the protective coverings from the port of the fluid bag and the spiked end of the tubing.

tubing into the fluid bag with a quick twist. Do this carefully. *Maintain sterility. If these parts touch the ground, they must not be used. Running germs or dirt directly into a patient's bloodstream can be extremely serious, even fatal.*

6. Hold the fluid bag higher than the drip chamber. Squeeze the drip chamber a time or two to start the flow. Fill the chamber to the marker line (approximately one-third full).

7. Open the flow regulator and allow the fluid to flush all the air from the tubing. You may need to loosen the cap at the lower end to get the fluid to flow. Maintain the sterility of the tubing end and replace the cap when you are finished. Most sets can be flushed without removing the cap. Be sure that all air bubbles have been flushed from the tubing to avoid introducing a dangerous air embolism into the patient's vein.

8. Turn off the flow.

Make certain that the setup stays clean until the paramedic removes the needle and connects the IV tubing to the catheter inside the patient's vein. Occasionally, the paramedic will draw blood from the vein to obtain samples before inserting the IV. You may be asked to assist by placing the blood in sample tubes and labeling the tubes with the patient's name and any other information that your hospital requires. Remember that they are potential carriers of pathogens. Be sure to take BSI precautions. Carry the blood tubes to a safe place where they will not be in danger of breaking.

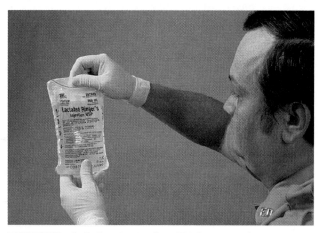

FIGURE A-8 Inspect the IV bag to be sure it contains the solution that was ordered, for clarity, leaks, and to be sure it has not expired.

Do not be surprised if you are asked to hold up the arm for a few minutes during a cardiac arrest. During cardiac arrest, medications can be more effective if the patient's arm is temporarily raised after a drug is injected into the IV.

Maintaining an IV

An IV must continue to flow at the proper rate once it has been inserted into the patient's vein. However, a number of things may interrupt the flow. If you are charged with maintaining an IV, be sure to check for and correct the following problems.

- Flow regulator may be closed.
- Clamp may be closed on the tubing.
- Tubing may kink.
- Tubing may get caught under the patient or on the backboard.
- Constricting band used to raise the vein for insertion of the needle may have been mistakenly left on the patient's arm, perhaps covered by a sleeve.
- Tubing may have pulled out of the catheter.

The position of the IV or of the patient's arm also may need to be adjusted. Some IVs only flow when the patient's arm or IV site is in a certain position. Adjusting or even splinting the arm (Figure A-10) may be helpful as long as the splint is not too tight. Since the IV flow usually depends on gravity, be sure that the bag is held well above the IV site and the patient's heart.

Insufficient flow can cause blood to clot in the catheter. This can be prevented by adjusting the flow to an adequate "keep the vein open" or KVO rate. The KVO rate varies, but it is usually about 30 drops per minute for a micro drip and 10 drops per minute for a macro drip set. If the drip chamber is overfilled, clamp the tubing, invert the drip chamber, and pump some fluid back into the bag.

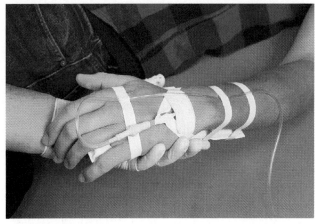

FIGURE A-10 Some IVs only flow when the IV site is in a certain position. Adjust or splint the body part as needed.

An IV with a flow rate that is too fast is called a "runaway IV." It can rapidly overload the patient with fluid and cause serious problems, especially in a infant or child patient.

An *infiltrated* IV is one where the needle has either punctured the vein and exited the other side or has pulled out of the vein. In either case, the fluid is flowing into the surrounding tissues instead of into the vein. An unnoticed infiltrated IV can be very dangerous. Certain high concentration medications (such as 50 ccs of 50% dextrose) can kill the surrounding tissue. In addition to complaining of pain, the patient will show swelling at the site (noticeable in all but some obese patients). The person in charge of maintaining the IV must stop the flow and discontinue the IV according to local protocol. If you are not authorized to do this, report the problem immediately to the paramedic or medical direction.

If you learn how to help advanced life support personnel start an IV, run through an administration set, label blood tubes, and maintain an IV, valuable time can be saved at the scene and during transport.

Infectious Diseases

As an EMT-B you will come into close contact with a wide variety of people, some of whom may be carrying communicable diseases. Because you work in the prehospital setting, you must be concerned with preventing the spread of disease to yourself and to others. Be sure to keep up to date on the methods of protection against disease, including BSI (body substance isolation) precautions such as use of barrier devices, personal protective equipment, and proper procedures for decontaminating and disposing of contaminated equipment and materials. Use these precautions as a matter of course. Follow your agency's exposure control plan at all times.

DISEASES OF CONCERN

The communicable diseases we are concerned with are caused by bloodborne and airborne pathogens, such as viruses, bacteria, and other harmful organisms. Bloodborne pathogens are contracted by exposure to an infected patient's blood, especially exposure through breaks in the noninfected person's skin. Airborne pathogens are spread by tiny droplets sprayed when a patient breathes, coughs, or sneezes. These droplets are inhaled or are absorbed through the noninfected person's eyes, mouth, or nose.

Although there are many communicable diseases, three that are of particular concern are hepatitis B, tuberculosis, and HIV/AIDS.

- Hepatitis is an infection that causes an inflammation of the liver. It comes in at least four forms: hepatitis A, B, C, and Delta. The disease is acquired through contact with blood, stool, or other body fluids. The virus that causes hepatitis is especially hardy. Hepatitis B has been found to live for extended periods (many days) in dried blood spills, so it poses a risk of transmission long after many other viruses would have died. For this reason, it is critical that any body fluid in any form, dried or otherwise, should be assumed to be infectious until proven otherwise. Hepatitis B can be deadly. Hepatitis B virus (HBV) kills approximately 200 health care workers every year in the United States—more than any other infectious disease.

- Tuberculosis (TB) is an infection that sometimes settles in the lungs and can be fatal. It was thought to be largely eradicated, but since the late 1980s it has been making a steady comeback. TB is highly contagious. Unlike many other infectious diseases, TB can be spread easily through the air. Health care workers and others can become infected even without any direct contact with a carrier. Because TB spreads so easily, you need to assume that any person with a cough—especially one who is in an institution such as a nursing home or shelter—may have TB.

- AIDS is the name for a set of conditions that result when the immune system has been attacked by HIV (human immunodeficiency virus) and rendered unable to combat infections adequately. No cure for AIDS has been discovered at the time of publication of this text. However, HIV/AIDS presents far less risk to health care workers than hepatitis and TB because the virus does not survive well outside the human body. This limits the routes of exposure to direct contact with blood by way of open wounds, intravenous drug use, unprotected sexual contact, or blood transfusions. Puncture wounds into which HIV is introduced, such as with an accidental needle stick, are also potential routes of infection. However, less than half of one percent of such incidents result in infection, according

747

to the U. S. Occupational Safety and Health Administration (OSHA), compared to 30% for the hepatitis B virus (HBV). The difference is due to the quantity and strength of HBV compared to HIV.

Hepatitis B, TB, and HIV/AIDS are the communicable diseases of greatest concern because they are life-threatening. However, there are many communicable diseases emergency response and other health care personnel may be exposed to. Table B-1 lists common communicable diseases, their modes of transmission, and their incubation periods (the time between contact and first appearance of symptoms).

PREVENTIVE MEASURES

Human skin is a particularly effective barrier when it is not broken. Pathogens will not cross intact skin. However, they will enter through cuts, and they can cross mucous membranes (tissues such as those that line the mouth and nose or surround the eyes) quite easily. To prevent pathogens from entering the body, the EMT-B should use barrier protection such as disposable gloves, surgical-type masks, eye wear, and gowns as appropriate.

Generally, appropriate BSI (body substance isolation) precautions should be taken at all times. Wearing protective gloves is always

TABLE B-1 Communicable Diseases

Disease	Mode of Transmission	Incubation
AIDS (acquired immune deficiency syndrome)	AIDS or HIV infected blood via intravenous drug use, unprotected sexual contact, blood transfusions, or (rarely) accidental needle sticks. Mothers also may pass the HIV virus to their unborn children.	Several months or years
Chickenpox (varicella)	Airborne droplets. Can also be spread by contact with open sores.	11 to 21 days
German measles (rubella)	Airborne droplets. Mothers may pass the disease to unborn children.	14 to 21 days
Measles (rubeola)	Airborne droplets or secretions from the mouth, nose, and eyes.	10 to 12 days
Meningitis, bacterial	Oral and nasal secretions.	2 to 10 days
Mumps	Droplets of saliva or objects contaminated by saliva.	14 to 24 days
Pneumonia, bacterial and viral	Oral and nasal droplets and secretions.	Several days
Staphylococcal skin infections	Direct contact with infected wounds or sores or with contaminated objects.	Several days
Tuberculosis (TB)	Respiratory secretions, airborne or on contaminated objects.	2 to 6 weeks
Hepatitis	Blood, stool, or other body fluids, or contaminated objects.	Weeks to months, depending on type
Whooping cough (pertussis)	Respiratory secretions or airborne droplets.	6 to 20 days

required when blood or other body fluids are present or likely to be present. Other personal protective equipment such as masks and protective eye wear may be needed when you will be exposed to splashing blood or other body fluids during procedures such as suctioning. Also always use extreme caution around sharp, blood-covered objects such as knives and intravenous needles. Wounds made with these objects may provide a route of infection.

EMT-Bs responding to emergencies should never have to perform direct mouth-to-mouth rescue breathing. Ample equipment is available on an ambulance to provide ventilations for a patient through a pocket mask or other devices designed to prevent cross infection (infection passing from you to the patient or from the patient to you). Many EMT-Bs also carry pocket masks in their cars while off duty.

The oldest recognized method of infection control—hand washing—is still an effective means of reducing or preventing cross-infection. Always wash thoroughly between calls—even when you have worn protective gloves. Wash again before food preparation and consumption.

Finally, EMT-Bs must realize that equipment and supplies that have been contaminated with body fluids must not be left on the scene of an emergency, in the ambulance, or around the station. They may expose other people to infection. Ensure that contaminated equipment and supplies are properly decontaminated or disposed of in accordance with local protocols and operating procedures.

(See Chapter 2 for a more detailed discussion of personal protective equipment and Chapter 30 for procedures for dealing with contaminated equipment and materials.)

INFECTION CONTROL AND THE LAW

Scientists have identified the main culprits in the transmission of many deadly infectious diseases—blood and body fluids. EMT-Bs and other health care workers have been recognized as having a higher than usual exposure and therefore a higher risk of contracting these unwanted infections.

Congress and federal agencies have responded by taking several steps to ensure the safety of people who are in such high-risk positions. In particular, the Occupational Safety and Health Administration (OSHA) of the U. S. De-

partment of Labor and the Centers for Disease Control and Prevention (CDC) of the U. S. Department of Health and Human Services have issued standards and guidelines for the protection of workers whose jobs may expose them to infectious diseases, while the Ryan White CARE Act establishes procedures by which emergency response workers can find out if they have been exposed to life-threatening infectious diseases. These legal protections are described in more detail below.

Occupational Exposure to Bloodborne Pathogens

On March 6, 1992, the OSHA standard on bloodborne pathogens went into effect. It mandates measures employers of emergency responders must take to protect employees who are likely to be exposed to blood and other body fluids. One of the basic principles behind the standard is that infection control is a joint responsibility between employer and employee. The employer must provide training, protective equipment, and vaccinations to employees who are subject to exposure in their jobs. In return, employees must participate in an infection exposure control plan that includes training and proper workplace practices.

Without the active participation of both the employer and the employee, any workplace infection control program is destined to fail. Be sure your system has an active and up-to-date infection exposure control plan and that you and your fellow EMT-Bs follow it carefully at all times. Consult with your state OSHA representative to make sure that specific hazards are identified and corrected.

Contact the U. S. Department of Labor to request the booklet "Occupational Exposure to Bloodborne Pathogens: Precautions for Emergency Responders—OSHA 3130 1992," an overview of the standard. For details regarding how to develop an infection control plan, request Title 29 Code of Federal Regulation 1919.1030 for the complete text of the standard and all requirements regarding occupational exposure to bloodborne pathogens. Critical elements of the standard are summarized below.

- *Infection exposure control plan.* Each emergency response employer must develop a plan that identifies and documents job classifications and tasks in which there is the possibility of exposure to potentially infectious body fluids. The plan must outline a schedule of how and when the bloodborne pathogen standards will be implemented. It must also include identification of the methods used for communicating hazards to employees, post-exposure evaluation, and follow-up.

- *Adequate education and training.* EMT-Bs must be provided with training that includes general explanations of how diseases are transmitted, uses and limitations of practices that reduce or prevent exposure, and procedures to follow if exposure occurs.
- *Hepatitis B vaccination.* Employers must make available free of charge and at a reasonable time and place the hepatitis B vaccination series.
- *Personal protective equipment* must be of a quality that will not permit blood or other infectious materials to pass through or reach an EMT-B's work clothes, street clothes, undergarments, skin, eyes, mouth, or other mucous membranes. This equipment must be provided by the employer to the EMT-B at no cost and includes but is not limited to protective gloves, face shields, masks, protective eye wear, gowns and aprons, plus bag-valve masks, pocket masks, and other ventilation devices.
- *Methods of control.* Engineering controls remove potential infectious disease hazards or separate the EMT-B from exposure. Examples include pocket masks, disposable airway equipment, and puncture-resistant needle containers. Work practice controls improve the manner in which a task is performed to reduce risk of exposure. Examples include the proper and safe use of personal protective equipment; proper handling, labeling, and disposal of contaminated materials; and proper washing and decontamination practices.
- *Housekeeping.* Clean and sanitary conditions of the emergency response vehicles and work sites are the responsibility of both the EMT-B and the employer. Procedures include the proper handling and proper decontamination of work surfaces, equipment, laundry, and other materials.
- *Labeling.* The standard requires labeling of containers used to store, transport, or ship blood and other potentially infectious materials, including the use of the *biohazard symbol* (Figure B-1).

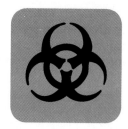

FIGURE B-1 The biohazard symbol (shown here) must be included with warning labels for containers used to ship blood or other potentially infectious materials.

- *Post-exposure evaluation and follow-up.* EMT-Bs must immediately report suspected exposure incidents—including mucous membrane or broken-skin contact with blood or other potentially infectious materials—that result from the performance of an employee's duties. (See Figure B-2 for a model plan based on the Ryan White CARE Act, which is described below.)

Ryan White CARE Act

In 1994, the Centers for Disease Control issued the final notice for the Ryan White Comprehensive AIDS Resources Emergency (CARE) Act Regarding Emergency Response Employees. This federal act, which applies to all 50 states, mandates a procedure by which emergency response personnel can seek to find out if they have been exposed to potentially life-threatening diseases while providing patient care. Emergency response personnel referred to in this act include firefighters, law enforcement officers, paramedics, EMTs, and other individuals such as First Responders who provide emergency aid on behalf of a legally recognized volunteer organization.

CDC has published a list of potentially life-threatening infectious and communicable diseases to which emergency response personnel can be exposed. The list includes airborne diseases such as TB, bloodborne diseases such as hepatitis B and HIV/AIDS, and uncommon or rare diseases such as diphtheria and rabies.

The Ryan White CARE Act requires every state's public health officer to designate an official within every emergency response organization to act as a "designated officer." The designated officer is responsible for gathering facts surrounding possible emergency responder airborne or bloodborne infectious disease exposures. Take time to learn who is the designated officer within your organization.

Two different notification systems for infectious disease exposure are defined in the act.

- *Airborne disease exposure.* You will be notified by your designated officer when you have been exposed to an airborne disease.
- *Bloodborne or other infectious disease exposure.* You may submit a request for a determination as to whether or not you were exposed to bloodborne or other infectious disease.

The difference between the two procedures results from the differences in how an exposure is most likely to be detected. With an airborne disease such as TB, you may not realize that the patient you have cared for and transported was infected. However, a disease like TB will be diagnosed at the hospital. Therefore, the Ryan White Act states that for airborne diseases like TB, the hospital will notify the designated officer who will notify you.

A bloodborne disease such as hepatitis B or HIV/AIDS may or may not be diagnosed at the hospital, but you will know if you have had contact with a patient's blood or body fluids. If so, you can submit a request to your designated officer who will gather the information necessary to request a determination from the hospital on whether you have been exposed and then will notify you of the result.

In either case, once you have been notified of an exposure, your employer will refer you to a doctor or other health care professional for evaluation and follow-up.

Consider how the Ryan White CARE Act would apply in the following example of exposure to an airborne pathogen.

> As an EMT-B, you treat and transport a patient who complains of weakness, fever, and chronic cough. The next day you receive a phone call from your organization's designated officer, who informs you that you have been exposed to a patient with TB. The designated officer helps you arrange an appointment with a doctor who can determine if you have contracted the disease and arrange for early treatment if you have.

According to CDC guidelines, exposure to airborne pathogens may occur when you share "air space" with a tuberculosis patient. So, if a med-ical facility diagnoses that patient as having the airborne infectious disease, it must notify the designated officer within 48 hours. The designated officer must notify the emergency care workers of disease exposure. The employer must schedule a post-exposure evaluation and follow-up (Figure B-2).

Consider another example, this one an incident in which exposure to a bloodborne pathogen occurs.

> As an EMT-B, you are called to treat an unconscious woman. During the scene size-up you put on disposable gloves, mask, gown, and goggles. The patient is lying on the kitchen floor. Pink, frothy sputum trickles from her mouth. Breathing is labored. A hypodermic needle lies beside her. While you are suctioning the patient, fluids from her mouth splash onto your goggles. You report the incident immediately after the call is completed. Your designated officer follows up, and you learn that you have not been exposed to a life-threatening bloodborne disease.

Under CDC guidelines, after contact with the blood or body fluids of a patient you have transported, you may submit a request for a determination to your designated officer. The designated officer must then gather information about the possible exposure. If the information indicates a possible exposure, the officer forwards the information to the medical facility where the patient is being treated. If the patient can be identified, medical records are reviewed to determine if the patient has a life-threatening disease. The medical facility then must notify your designated officer of their findings in writing within 48 hours after receiving the officer's request. The designated officer must notify you, and you will be directed by your employer to a health care professional for a post-exposure evaluation and follow-up as appropriate.

Tuberculosis Compliance Mandate

Thousands of new cases of TB are reported in the U. S. each year. Hundreds of health care workers have been infected. Of particular concern are the rising cases of multi-drug resistant TB (MDR-TB). In 1993 OSHA issued policies and procedures based on the 1990 Centers for Disease Control (CDC) guidelines for treating a suspected or confirmed TB patient, "Guidelines for

INFECTIOUS DISEASE EXPOSURE PROCEDURE

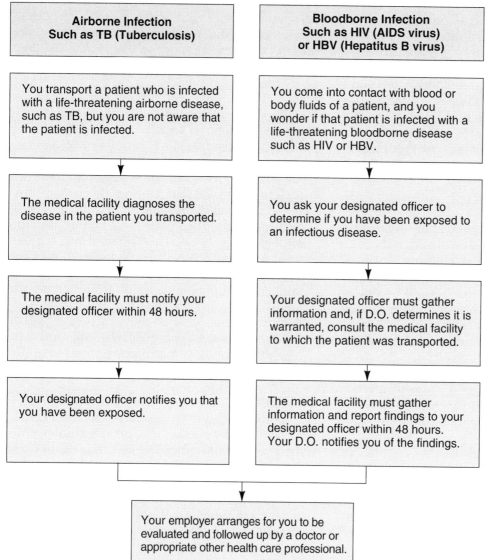

FIGURE B-2 Under the Ryan White CARE Act, there is a procedure for finding out and following up if you have been exposed to a life-threatening infectious disease.

Airborne Infection Such as TB (Tuberculosis)

You transport a patient who is infected with a life-threatening airborne disease, such as TB, but you are not aware that the patient is infected.

↓

The medical facility diagnoses the disease in the patient you transported.

↓

The medical facility must notify your designated officer within 48 hours.

↓

Your designated officer notifies you that you have been exposed.

Bloodborne Infection Such as HIV (AIDS virus) or HBV (Hepatitus B virus)

You come into contact with blood or body fluids of a patient, and you wonder if that patient is infected with a life-threatening bloodborne disease such as HIV or HBV.

↓

You ask your designated officer to determine if you have been exposed to an infectious disease.

↓

Your designated officer must gather information and, if D.O. determines it is warranted, consult the medical facility to which the patient was transported.

↓

The medical facility must gather information and report findings to your designated officer within 48 hours. Your D.O. notifies you of the findings.

↓

Your employer arranges for you to be evaluated and followed up by a doctor or appropriate other health care professional.

Preventing the Transmission of Tuberculosis in Health Care Settings with Special Focus on HIV-Related Issues."

Study the guidelines as summarized below. Learn to recognize situations in which the potential of exposure to TB exists. Those at greatest risk of contracting and transmitting TB are people who have suppressed immune systems, including people with HIV/AIDS. Patients who have TB may have the following signs and symptoms: productive cough (coughing up mucus or other fluid) and/or coughing up blood, weight loss and loss of appetite, lethargy and weakness, night sweats, and fever. *It is safest to assume that any person with a cough may be infected with TB.*

When the potential exists for exposure to exhaled air of a person with suspected or confirmed TB, OSHA requires that you wear a high efficiency particulate air (HEPA) respirator that is approved by the National Institute for Occupational Safety and Health (NIOSH). (See Chapter 2 for photographs.) You are required to wear a HEPA respirator when

- You are caring for patients suspected of having TB. High risk areas include correctional institutions, homeless shelters, long-term care facilities for the elderly, and drug treatment centers.
- Transporting an individual from such a setting in a closed vehicle. If possible, keep the

windows of the ambulance open and set the heating and air conditioning system on the nonrecirculating cycle.

- Performing high-risk procedures such as endotracheal suctioning and intubation.

Remember to take all recommended infection control precautions, including hand washing and using personal protective equipment and barrier devices such as pocket masks or bag-valve masks for rescue breathing. Properly dispose of contaminated equipment and materials, and decontaminate all surfaces, clothing, and equipment.

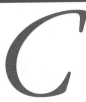

Hazardous Materials

Hazardous materials (hazmats) are everywhere, and EMS responds to incidents involving them frequently. Because many incidents begin as routine EMS calls, it will be up to you to recognize a hazmat early and follow the local Incident Management Plan. In order to accomplish that effectively, you should recognize the levels of training required by law and understand your role at a hazardous materials incident.

TRAINING REQUIRED BY LAW

Two federal agencies—the Occupational Safety and Health Administration (OSHA) and the Environmental Protection Agency (EPA)—have developed regulations to deal with the increasing frequency of hazmat emergencies. These regulations are meant to enhance the knowledge, skills, and safety of emergency response personnel, as well as to bring about a more effective response to hazmat emergencies. The regulations are described in the OSHA publication "29 CFR 1910.120—Hazardous Waste Operations and Emergency Response Standard."

According to the regulations, it is the responsibility of employers to determine, provide, and document the appropriate level of training for each employee. Training is required for "all employees who participate, or who are expected to participate, in emergency response to hazardous substance accidents."

The regulations identify four levels of training.

- First Responder Awareness—Rescuers at this level are likely to witness or discover a hazardous substance release. They are trained only to recognize the problem and initiate a response from the proper organizations. There are no minimum training hours required.
- First Responder Operations—This level of training is for those who initially respond to releases or potential releases of hazardous materials in order to protect people, property, and the environment. They stay at a safe distance, keep the incident from spreading, and protect from any exposures. A minimum of eight hours of training is required.
- Hazardous Materials Technician—This level is for rescuers who actually plug, patch, or stop the release of a hazardous material. A minimum of 24 hours of training is required.
- Hazardous Materials Specialist—This level rescuer is expected to have advanced knowledge and skills and to command and support activities at the incident site. A minimum of 24 hours of additional training is required.

Most of the training levels outlined by OSHA have a fire-service focus. EMS responders should be trained to the awareness level and perhaps the operations level but in different skills. Responding to this difference, the National Fire Protection Association has published Standard #473, which deals with competencies for EMS personnel at hazardous materials incidents.

Regardless of agency affiliation, EMT-Bs play an important role. You are usually among the first on the scene for all types of hazmat calls. Your initial decisions and actions build the crucial groundwork for the remainder of the incident.

RESPONSIBILITIES OF THE EMT-B

Recognize a Hazmat Incident

Whether hazmat incidents are very obvious or very subtle, you must quickly recognize one for what it is. One way is to recognize the locations at which hazmats are likely. They include highway accidents involving common carriers, trucking terminals, chemical plants or places where chemicals are used, delivery trucks, agriculture and garden centers, railway incidents, and laboratories.

Every community has chemical hazards. Identification starts with awareness and knowledge of what exists in the community. Spend some time with local police and fire agencies. Learn about or develop pre-incident plans for common hazardous materials.

When you arrive at a potential incident, as an EMT-B you must restrain your natural impulse to take action. Never assume the scene is safe. After the initial victims, EMT-Bs are the most likely to become injured or killed because they tend to react quickly. So assess the situation first. Take a command position and stay a safe distance from the site before you take action. Once a hazmat is recognized, only those personnel trained to the technician level and equipped with the proper personal protective equipment should enter the immediate site, or the HOT ZONE. All victims leaving the hot zone should be considered contaminated until proven otherwise.

Establish Command and Control Zones

When you arrive at the scene of a hazmat emergency, take a defensive position—a safe place far enough from the site to ensure your safety. Then call for a hazmat team capable of entering the hot zone to rescue the injured and control the incident.

Warning: *Rescue of people from the hot zone should not be attempted by EMT-Bs.*

Implement your agency's Incident Management System and establish command. You will stay in command until you are relieved by someone higher in the chain of command.

The situation must be prevented from becoming worse. Establish a perimeter, evacuate people if necessary, and direct bystanders to a safe area. It cannot be overemphasized that EMT-Bs should not risk personal safety by initiating rescue attempts.

While help is en route, establish control zones. Isolate the hot zone (the area of contamination or the area of danger). Establish a decontamination corridor (area where patients will be decontaminated) in the WARM ZONE, an area immediately adjacent to the hot zone. Equipment and other emergency rescuers should be staged in the next adjacent area—the COLD ZONE. Station yourself in the cold zone.

Identify the Substance

An attempt must be made to identify the hazardous material and assess the severity of the situation. Until that is done, it will be difficult to determine the risk to the public, rescuers, patients, and the environment. You must try to find out what the substance is and what its properties and dangers might be; whether or not there is imminent danger of the contamination spreading; what you can hear, see, and smell; how many victims are involved; and if there is any danger of secondary contamination from the victims. (Secondary contamination occurs when a contaminated person makes contact with someone who previously was "clean.")

An important piece of scene assessment equipment is a simple pair of binoculars (Figure C-1). They will allow a visual inspection of the hot zone from a safe distance, from which you can spot identifying labels, placards, and shipping papers.

Another tool is your ears. Victims leaving the hot zone are usually a good source of information about the substances or materials

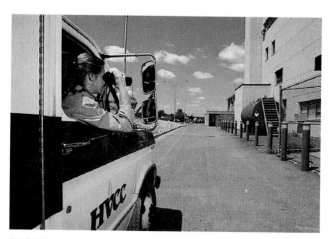

FIGURE C-1 Binoculars will allow a visual inspection of the hot zone from a safe distance.

involved. Take the time to question them and pay careful attention to their answers. The knowledge of workers at a manufacturing site, for example, can make identification very easy. They often understand very well what chemicals are used, the reactions, and processes. However, note that workers may identify a substance by its trade name and not realize that it is a mixture of many chemicals.

All of this makes hazardous materials responses very challenging. When a hazmat team arrives, they have the training needed to identify unknown substances and the necessary computer and textbook resources. EMT-Bs are only expected to make basic identification and understand some of the common substance identifying systems available.

The sources of information already described in Chapter 32, Overviews, include

- The U. S. Department of Transportation's (DOT's) essential publication *Hazardous Materials: The Emergency Response Guidebook*, which provides the names of chemicals and concise but thorough descriptions of the actions that should be taken in case of a hazmat emergency. Be sure to have the latest edition in your vehicle at all times (Figure C-2).
- CHEMTREC is the Chemical Manufacturers Association 24-hour service for identifying hazardous materials and providing instructions for dealing with the specific hazmat emergency. (24-hour toll-free telephone number for the continental United States: 800-424-9300; in Washington, DC 202-483-7616.)
- Placarding, signage, and labeling systems that help to identify the hazard potential of a substance (Figures C-3 and C-4).
- Invoices, bills of lading, and shipping papers identify the exact substance being transported, the exact quantity, its place of origin, and its destination.

One commonly used placarding system is the National Fire Protection Association (NFPA) 704 System. It advises rescuers of the health, reactivity, and fire hazard contained within a fixed facility by way of numerical and color coding (Figure C-5).

Another source of information is dictated by federal regulations: All employees working with hazardous materials have a right to know about the properties and hazards of those materials. Accordingly, all manufacturers are required to

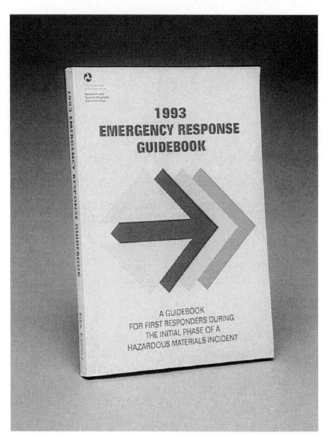

FIGURE C-2 Have the latest edition of DOT's *Hazardous Materials: The Emergency Response Guidebook* in your vehicle at all times.

provide Material Safety Data Sheets (MSDS) on hazardous materials. These sheets must be maintained at the work site by the employer and available to all employees. Unfortunately, there is no standard form or format for the information contained in them. They generally name the

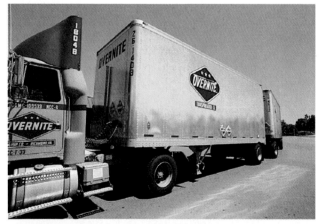

FIGURE C-3 Vehicles carrying hazardous materials are required to display placards that communicate the nature of their cargo.

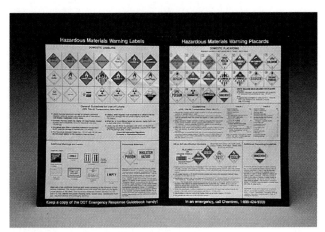

FIGURE C-4 Examples of hazardous materials warning placards.

substance, its physical properties, fire and explosion hazard information, health hazard information, and emergency first aid treatment.

One important source of information that is often overlooked is the regional poison control center. Using their reference and medical resources, they can provide essential guidance

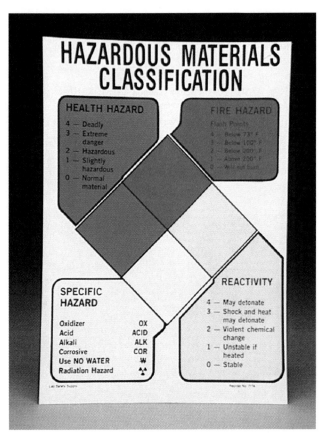

FIGURE C-5 Key to the National Fire Protection Association (NFPA) 704 System of numeric and color codes.

in the decontamination and treatment of patients affected by hazardous materials.

Establish a Medical Treatment Sector

All EMS personnel and equipment must be staged in the cold zone. EMS personnel have two responsibilities at a hazmat incident: *to take care of the injured and to monitor and rehabilitate the hazmat team members.*

Rehabilitation Operations

In order to safely enter the hot zone, the hazmat team members must wear chemical protective clothing and breathing apparatus that slows heat loss and prevents heat stress. Team members must be carefully monitored prior to, during, and after emergency operations. This is done to make sure that their condition does not deteriorate to a point where safety or the integrity of the operation is jeopardized. To address this need, a sector of operations called rehabilitation (rehab) should be established. While the rehab sector officer may not be an EMS provider, all rehab operations include EMT-Bs or Advanced EMTs.

The characteristics of the rehab sector include the following.

- Located in the cold zone
- Protected from weather (shielded from rain or snow, a warm area in a cold environment, a cool area in a warm environment)
- Large enough to accommodate multiple rescue crews
- Easily accessible to EMS units
- Free from exhaust fumes
- Allows for rapid re-entry into the emergency operation

While suiting up in chemical protective equipment, hazmat team members should have their baseline vital signs taken. When the hazmat team members show signs of fatigue or when they have had 45 minutes of work time, they are sent to rehab. As soon as possible after entry, reassess their vital signs. If heart rate exceeds 110 beats per minute, an oral temperature should be taken. If temperature exceeds 100.6°F, the rescuer must stay in rehab until pulse slows and temperature returns to normal. Always follow local protocols and consult medical direction. All pre-entry and exit vitals should be tracked on a flow sheet.

In addition to medical monitoring, rehab should be set up for prehydration and hydration, rest, and in some cases nourishment of hazmat team members. Proper hydration is an important element in preventing heat stress and promoting optimal physical performance. Heat injury is usually caused by imbalances of water and electrolytes during periods of high heat stress and physical exertion. During physical exertion at least one quart of water per hour should be consumed. For short-duration emergency operations, electrolyte sport drinks usually are not necessary. However, if they are used they should be diluted to half strength. Coffee and caffeinated beverages should be avoided because they promote dehydration.

When incidents will be of extended duration, some type of nourishment may be provided in rehab. Foods low in salt and saturated fats are ideal. Bananas, apples, oranges, and other fruits are excellent for the fast nourishment required during emergency operations. In cold environments, soups and stews are more easily eaten and digested than sandwiches.

Care of Injured and Contaminated Patients

EMT-Bs must work with the Incident Manager and hazmat team members to determine the most appropriate course of action. The decision to stay at the scene and decontaminate or to begin evacuation must be made after careful consultation with CHEMTREC, the poison control center, and other reference sources.

EMS is responsible for setting up the medical treatment sector in the cold zone to receive decontaminated patients. In the decontamination (decon) corridor, the hazmat team will decontaminate hazmat team members and any patients rescued. Unless EMS personnel are trained to the hazmat technician level, they must remain in the cold zone.

The field decon process is designed to remove most of the poison and deliver a relatively "clean" patient to EMS personnel for care and transportation (Figure C-6). However, there still may be some chance of secondary contamination from patients to EMS personnel. It is important that EMS personnel work closely with the decon officer and consult with medical direction on both treatment and appropriate protection during transportation.

The following points must be kept in mind about treating and transporting hazmat patients.

- *Field decontaminated patients are not completely "clean."* Chemicals that pose a risk of secondary contamination to rescuers sometimes settle in hard-to-clean areas of the body. These areas are typically the scalp/hair, groin, buttocks, between fingers and toes, and the arm pits.
- *Personal protective equipment is needed to prevent secondary contamination of rescuers.* EMS personnel will need to wear Tyvek coveralls and booties to keep clothing from being contaminated. A double layer of gloves also may need to be worn. Often nitrile or neoprene is best, because these are more resistant to chemicals than standard latex or vinyl gloves. Work with the decon officer to determine if your supplies are appropriate or if they have items that might work better than yours.
- *Vehicles must be protected from contamination.* In the decon process, patients are washed and are usually dripping wet. Since they cannot be completely decontaminated in the field, some of their water run off could contaminate an emergency vehicle. To prevent this, the water run off must be contained by either placing the patient in a disposable decontamination pool or covering the inside of an ambulance vehicle with plastic.
- *Consider any equipment used to be disposable.* When an item such as a spine board, splint, blood-pressure cuff, or stethoscope is used, it may not be able to be decontaminated and may need to be disposed of.

When treating a contaminated patient is unavoidable, identification of the hazardous materials is crucial. Follow the treatment instructions given by DOT's publication *Hazardous Materials: The Emergency Response Guidebook* or by the poison control center.

There are four types of patients likely to be encountered by EMT-Bs.

- Uninjured and not contaminated
- Injured but not contaminated
- Uninjured but contaminated
- Injured and contaminated

Anyone who is not contaminated—whether injured or not—can be treated like any other patient. However, anyone who is contaminated—whether injured or not—poses a risk of secondary contamination and should be decontaminated prior to leaving the scene. Unfortu-

9-Station Decontamination Procedure

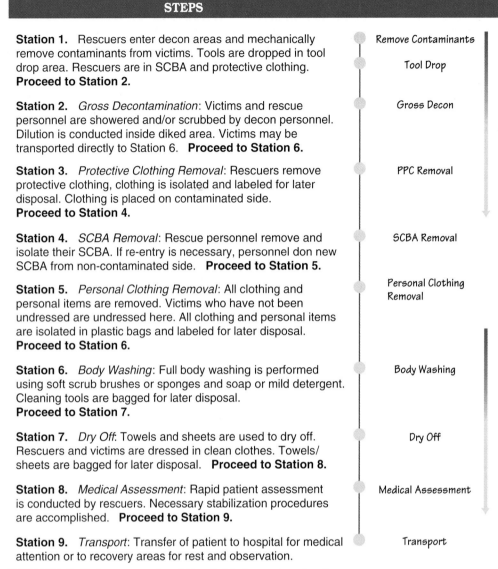

STEPS

Station 1. Rescuers enter decon areas and mechanically remove contaminants from victims. Tools are dropped in tool drop area. Rescuers are in SCBA and protective clothing. **Proceed to Station 2.**

Remove Contaminants

Tool Drop

Station 2. *Gross Decontamination*: Victims and rescue personnel are showered and/or scrubbed by decon personnel. Dilution is conducted inside diked area. Victims may be transported directly to Station 6. **Proceed to Station 6.**

Gross Decon

Station 3. *Protective Clothing Removal*: Rescuers remove protective clothing, clothing is isolated and labeled for later disposal. Clothing is placed on contaminated side. **Proceed to Station 4.**

PPC Removal

Station 4. *SCBA Removal*: Rescue personnel remove and isolate their SCBA. If re-entry is necessary, personnel don new SCBA from non-contaminated side. **Proceed to Station 5.**

SCBA Removal

Station 5. *Personal Clothing Removal*: All clothing and personal items are removed. Victims who have not been undressed are undressed here. All clothing and personal items are isolated in plastic bags and labeled for later disposal. **Proceed to Station 6.**

Personal Clothing Removal

Station 6. *Body Washing*: Full body washing is performed using soft scrub brushes or sponges and soap or mild detergent. Cleaning tools are bagged for later disposal. **Proceed to Station 7.**

Body Washing

Station 7. *Dry Off*: Towels and sheets are used to dry off. Rescuers and victims are dressed in clean clothes. Towels/sheets are bagged for later disposal. **Proceed to Station 8.**

Dry Off

Station 8. *Medical Assessment*: Rapid patient assessment is conducted by rescuers. Necessary stabilization procedures are accomplished. **Proceed to Station 9.**

Medical Assessment

Station 9. *Transport*: Transfer of patient to hospital for medical attention or to recovery areas for rest and observation.

Transport

FIGURE C-6 An example of the field decontamination process.

nately, field decontamination is not always possible because of poor weather, because there is no one at the scene who is trained to perform the decon process, or because the patient is high priority for immediate care, and treatment and transport cannot be delayed for decontamination.

If you are confronted with patients at risk of causing secondary contamination prior to the arrival of the hazmat team, do the following.

1. Take precautions appropriate to the substance as listed in DOT's *Hazardous Materials: The Emergency Response Guidebook*.

This usually means isolation from the substance. Be sure to use personal protective equipment similar to what you would use for splash protection from bloodborne pathogens.

2. Follow the first aid measures listed in DOT's *Hazardous Materials: The Emergency Response Guidebook*.

3. Be sure to manage the patient's critical needs, just as you would any other patient. Do not forget to manage the ABCs.

4. If treatment calls for irrigation with water, remember that water only dilutes most substances. It does not neutralize them. Cut

the patient's clothing off and irrigate with large amounts of water. Try to contain the runoff. If possible, use tepid or warm water to prevent hypothermia. If there are open wounds, try to avoid flushing contaminants directly into them. Pay particular attention to cleaning areas such as dense body hair, ear canals, navel, fingernails, crotch, arm pits, and so on. Also try to use as much disposable equipment as possible. It can be discarded later.

5. After treating the patient, decontaminate yourself. Some of your clothing may also need to be disposed of.

Remember that the severity of any poisoning depends on the substance, route of entry, dosage, and duration of contact. Immediate emergency care measures as listed in DOT's *Hazardous Materials: The Emergency Response Guidebook* may decrease the severity of the poisoning and save lives. Whenever possible, the entire decontamination process should be carried out by qualified personnel from the hazmat team before the EMT-B touches the patient.

When this is not possible—when a contaminated patient who has been brought out of the hot zone requires immediate life-saving care but has not yet been decontaminated—provide the required care, taking as many precautions as possible to protect yourself. Use the proper personal protective clothing and equipment, and decontaminate yourself as soon as you can.

Basic Life Support: Airway, Rescue Breathing, and CPR

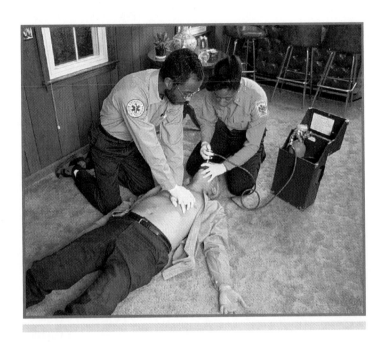

Before beginning your EMT-Basic course, you are required to have completed a course in cardiopulmonary resuscitation (CPR). The elements of CPR are presented here.

◆ ◆

When breathing stops, or when breathing and heartbeat both stop, death will follow unless these basic functions can be quickly restarted. By performing rescue breathing, you can force air into a patient's lungs. By performing CPR, you can both force air into the patient's lungs and also force blood to circulate through his body. These actions can help keep the patient alive until he can receive definitive care or until he recovers breathing and heartbeat on his own.

Rescue breathing and CPR do not always succeed. Often, a patient whose breathing and/or heartbeat have stopped will die despite your best efforts. However, if you have been able to intervene with these basic life-support procedures, you will know that you provided that patient the best possible chance of survival. And sometimes you will experience the thrill of actually saving or helping to save your patient's life.

763

Note: The following are not U.S. Department of Transportation curriculum objectives.

Knowledge

Airway and Breathing

1. Define and compare clinical death and biological death. (p. 765)

2. List the signs of adequate and of inadequate breathing. (p. 768)

3. Describe the steps of the head-tilt, chin-lift and the jaw-thrust maneuvers. (pp. 769–771)

4. Explain the circumstances in which the tongue can cause airway obstruction; in which foreign objects or materials can cause airway obstruction. (pp. 769, 771)

5. List three major signs of partial airway obstruction. (p. 771)

6. State when you must treat a partial airway obstruction as if it were a complete airway obstruction. (p. 772)

7. Describe the signs displayed by a conscious and by an unconscious patient with a complete airway obstruction. (p. 772)

8. Describe step by step the following procedures used to correct airway obstruction:

   • The Heimlich maneuver (pp. 773–774)
   • Chest thrusts (pp. 774–775)
   • Back blows (pp. 775–776)
   • Finger sweeps (pp. 776–777)

9. State the criteria for success in clearing an airway obstruction. (p. 777)

10. State the sequence of procedures for correcting an airway obstruction in an adult, child, and infant who are conscious, who lose consciousness, and who are unconscious when you find them. (pp. 778–783)

Rescue Breathing

11. Explain why mouth-to-mask ventilation is preferred over ventilations with direct contact. (p. 783)

12. List the steps of mouth-to-mask ventilation. (pp. 783–785)

13. Compare mouth-to-mask and mouth-to-nose ventilations. (pp. 785–788)

14. Explain the procedures for mask-to-stoma or mouth-to-stoma ventilations. (pp. 788–789)

15. List the steps of rescue breathing for an infant or a child. (pp. 789–790)

16. Explain how to correct the problems of gastric distention caused by artificial ventilation. (p. 790)

17. Describe the recovery position and explain the circumstances in which a patient should be placed in this position. (p. 791)

CPR

18. Define CPR and explain how CPR works. (pp. 765–792)

19. List the steps that lead to CPR, as defined by the American Heart Association. (p. 793)

20. List, step by step, the procedures for performing CPR on adults. (pp. 793–802)

21. Compare one-rescuer and two-rescuer CPR for adults. (pp. 793–802)

22. Explain how to join CPR in progress. (pp. 802–803)

23. Explain the procedures for changing positions during two-rescuer CPR. (pp. 803, 804)

24. List, step by step, the procedures for performing CPR on infants and children. (pp. 803, 806–807)

25. Compare rates and ratios of compressions and ventilations for one- and two-rescuer CPR for adults, infants, and children. (pp. 797, 800, 802, 805, 807)

26. State how to determine if CPR is effective. (pp. 807–808)

27. State ways to counter deficiency in CPR. (p. 808)

28. List factors that may make CPR ventilations and compressions ineffective. (p. 808)

29. List reasons why CPR may be interrupted. (p. 808)

30. Describe how, while performing CPR, to move a patient down stairs, through narrow hallways and doorways, and while loading on and off the ambulance. (pp. 809, 810)

31. List possible complications of CPR. (pp. 809, 811)

32. Explain circumstances in which, even though a patient has no pulse, CPR should not be started and circumstances in which CPR may be terminated. (pp. 811, 812)

Skills

1. Determine if the patient has adequate or inadequate breathing or is in respiratory arrest.

2. Open a patient's airway using the head-tilt, chin-lift or the jaw-thrust maneuver.

3. Determine if a patient has a partial or complete airway obstruction.

4. Perform the Heimlich maneuver and chest thrusts to relieve airway obstructions in adults and children.

5. Perform back blows and chest thrusts to relieve airway obstructions in infants.

6. Correctly perform rescue breathing with mouth-to-mask, mouth-to-mouth, mouth-to-nose, and mouth-to-stoma ventilations.

7. Correctly perform rescue breathing on infants and children.

8. Identify and prevent gastric distention during rescue breathing.

9. Place a patient in the recovery position.

10. Correctly evaluate a patient to detect cardiac arrest.

11. Perform one-rescuer CPR on adults, infants, and children.

12. Perform two-rescuer CPR, including the proper change of positions.

13. Perform CPR on a patient while he is being moved.

CLINICAL DEATH AND BIOLOGICAL DEATH

When a patient's breathing and heartbeat stop, **clinical death** occurs. This condition may be reversible through CPR and other treatments. However, when the brain cells die, **biological death** occurs. This usually happens within 10 minutes of clinical death, and it is not reversible. In fact, brain cells will begin to die after 4 to 6 minutes without fresh oxygen supplied from air breathed in and carried to the brain by circulating blood (Figure BLS-1). Occasionally, a person who has been without breathing or heartbeat for more than 10 minutes will survive, sometimes without brain damage. However, the patient will have the best chance of survival if CPR begins within 10 minutes—preferably within 4 minutes—after breathing and heartbeat have stopped.

BEFORE BEGINNING CPR: THE ABCS

CPR stands for **cardiopulmonary resuscitation.** Breaking the term down into its parts tells you its meaning: *Cardio* means "heart," *pulmonary* means "lungs," and *resuscitation* means "reviving," or "bringing back to life." So *cardiopulmonary resuscitation* is the actions you take to revive a person—or at least temporarily prevent biological death—by keeping the person's heart and lungs working. You can see why CPR is a key element of what is known as **basic life support,** or basic live-saving procedures.

Before beginning CPR you must assess the ABCs (Airway, Breathing, and Circulation).

- *Is the patient's **airway** (breathing passageway) open?* If the airway is not open, you must open it. You will not be able to ventilate the patient effectively (force air into his lungs) if the airway is not open.
- *Is the patient **breathing**?* If the patient is not breathing, you must provide ventilations.
- *Does the patient have **circulation** of blood (does he have a **pulse**)?* If the heart is pumping blood through the body, the patient will have a pulse. If there is no pulse, you know that the heart has stopped beating, and you must begin CPR, including both ventilations to get air (with oxygen) into the lungs, and chest compressions to force the oxygenated blood to circulate.

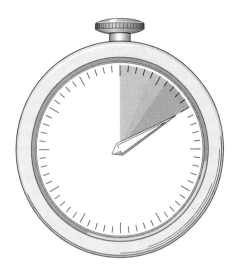

- 0 minutes: cessation of breathing and circulation
- 4-6 minutes: brain damage begins
- 10 minutes: brain cells begin to die

FIGURE BLS-1 Brain cells begin to die within minutes after breathing and heartbeat stop.

Each of the ABCs will be discussed in more detail below.

Respiratory Failure

Sometimes you will encounter a patient who has stopped breathing (also called **respiration)** before you arrived or who stops breathing while you are assessing or treating him. This patient is in **respiratory arrest.** Respiratory arrest can develop during heart attack, stroke, airway obstruction, drowning, electrocution, drug overdose, poisoning, brain injury, severe chest injury, or suffocation.

Sometimes breathing has not stopped but is reduced to the point where not enough oxygen is getting into the lungs to keep the patient alive. Either condition—respiratory arrest or inadequate respiration—can be called **respiratory failure.**

Sometimes the patient's heart also stops beating (or soon will stop beating if breathing continues to be inadequate or stops), and then the patient is also in **cardiac arrest.**

In any of these cases, you will follow the sequence of the ABCs, first assessing and caring for the airway and breathing before you deal with the circulation of blood.

Positioning the Patient

Before you do the assessment and care steps described below, you should make sure that the

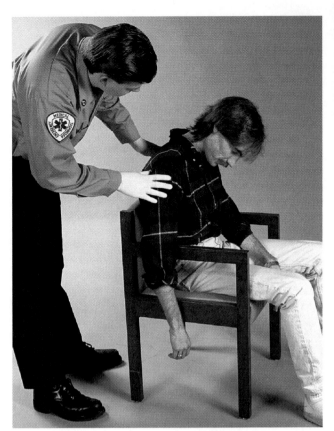

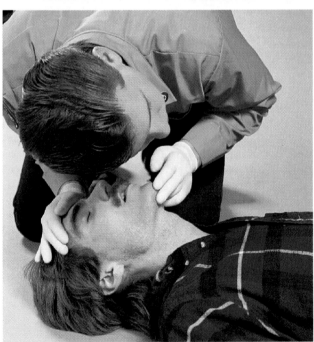

FIGURE BLS-2 Positioning the patient for airway evaluation and care.

patient is lying **supine** (on his back). If you find the patient in some other position, help him to the floor or stretcher (Figure BLS-2). If the patient is already lying on the floor, move him onto his back (Scan BLS-1).

Positioning the Patient for Basic Life Support

Warning: This maneuver is used to initiate airway evaluation, rescue breathing, or CPR when you must act alone. When possible, the four-rescuer log roll (Chapter 28) is preferred.

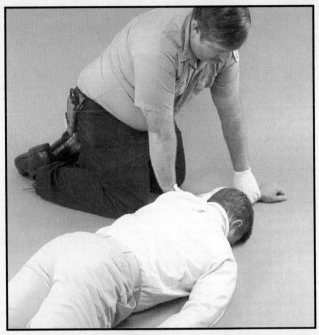

1. Straighten the legs and position the closest arm above the head.

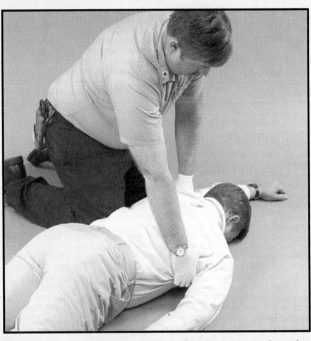

2. Cradle the head and neck. Grasp under the distant armpit.

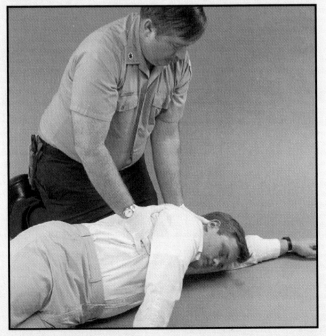

3. Move the patient as a unit onto his side.

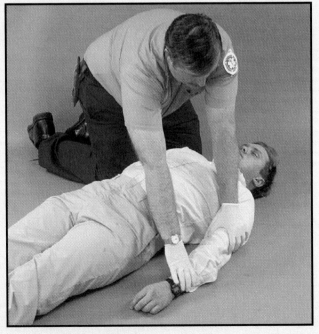

4. Move the patient onto his back and reposition the extended arm.

If you suspect that the patient may have been injured, you or a helper must support the patient's neck and hold the head still and in line with his spine while you are moving, assessing, and caring for him. This is because any serious injury may also have injured the patient's cervical spine (the part of the spine that is in the neck). Allowing the patient's head or neck to move could cause the bones of the injured cervical spine to pinch or sever the spinal cord, causing paralysis or death.

Use the following as indications that spinal injury may have occurred—especially when the patient is unconscious and cannot tell you what happened.

- The mechanism of injury (anything that could cause an injury) was forceful enough that it could have also injured the spine. For example, a patient who is found on the ground near a ladder or stairs may have such injuries. Motor vehicle accidents are another common cause of spinal injuries.
- Any injury at or above the level of the shoulders indicates that neck or spinal injuries may also be present.
- Family or bystanders may tell you that an injury to the head, neck, or spine has occurred or may give you information that leads you to suspect it.
- The patient is unconscious.

In any of these situations, be sure to protect the patient's cervical spine by supporting his head and neck and holding his head still and in line with his spine.

Assessing and Caring for the Patient

Your first task in caring for the patient who seems to be suffering from respiratory failure or cardiac arrest will be to determine whether breathing has, in fact, stopped or is inadequate.

Patient Assessment—Respiratory Failure

Signs

To determine the signs of ADEQUATE BREATHING, you should

☐ LOOK for the rise and fall of the chest associated with breathing. Also watch to see if both sides of the chest are rising and falling evenly (showing that both lungs are filling with air).

☐ LISTEN for air entering and leaving the nose or mouth. The sounds should be typical, free of sounds such as gurgling, gasping, crowing, or wheezing.

☐ FEEL for air moving out of the nose or mouth.

☐ Check for typical skin coloration, which should be pink. There should be no blue or gray colorations. (In a dark-skinned person, look for these colors at the insides of the lower eyelids, the lips, the tongue, or the nail beds. In a light-skinned person you can also look at the ear lobes or any visible skin.)

☐ Note if the person is taking normally deep breaths (neither very shallow breaths nor deep gasps). Note if the breath rate seems normal. (A breath rate of 12 to 20 breaths per minute is normal.)

The following are signs of INADEQUATE BREATHING.

☐ Chest movements are absent, minimal, or uneven.

☐ Movements associated with breathing are limited to the abdomen (abdominal breathing).

☐ No air can be felt or heard at the nose or mouth, or the exchange of air is evaluated as below normal.

☐ Noises such as wheezing, snoring, gurgling, or gasping are heard during breathing.

☐ The rate of breathing is too rapid or too slow. A breath rate slower than 8 per minute or faster than 24 per minute in an unresponsive patient may require rescue breathing; in a responsive patient will require that a trained person put an oxygen mask on the patient. You can count breaths by watching the patient breathe for 30 seconds and multiplying the number of breaths by 2.

☐ Breathing is very shallow, very deep, or appears labored (the patient seems to be working hard to breathe).

☐ The patient's skin shows blue or gray colorations.

☐ Breathing in or breathing out is prolonged (indicating a possible airway obstruction).

☐ The patient is unable to speak, or the patient cannot speak full sentences because of shortness of breath.

Emergency Care Steps

When the patient's signs indicate inadequate or no breathing, you must act quickly, as follows.

1. *Open the airway.* If this does not correct the problem . . .
2. *Clear the airway of foreign body obstructions.* If this does not correct the problem . . .
3. *Perform rescue breathing.*

These procedures are discussed in detail below.

THE AIRWAY

The **airway** (Figure BLS-3) is the passageway by which air enters the body. It is made up of the *nose, mouth, pharynx* (throat), *larynx* (structure that connects the pharynx to the trachea), *trachea* (the windpipe), *bronchi* (the branches that reach from the trachea into the lungs), and *lungs.*

The human body needs oxygen. Oxygen is contained in the air we breathe. Once it reaches the lungs, oxygen is picked up by the blood and circulated to the cells as the heart pumps the blood around the body. When the supply of fresh oxygen is cut off, death quickly follows, as explained under Clinical Death and Biological Death, above.

There will be no point to doing rescue breathing or CPR if the airway is closed or blocked. The air you breathe into the person will not reach his lungs. The blood you force to circulate will not have fresh oxygen to carry to the body's cells. So rescue breathing or CPR will not save a person's life if the airway is not open.

This is why detecting and correcting airway problems comes before all other life-saving steps.

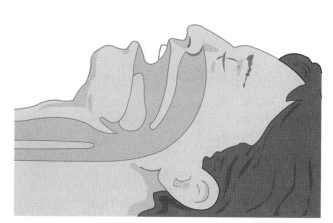

FIGURE BLS-3 Adult and child airways.

Opening the Airway

Most airway problems are caused by the tongue. As the head tips forward, especially when the patient is lying on his back, the tongue may slide into the airway. When the patient is unconscious, the risk of airway problems is worsened because unconsciousness causes the tongue to lose muscle tone and muscles of the lower jaw (to which the tongue is attached) to relax.

Two procedures can help to correct the position of the tongue (Figure BLS-4) and thus open the airway. These procedures are the head-tilt, chin-lift maneuver and the jaw-thrust maneuver.

The Head-Tilt, Chin-Lift Maneuver

The head-tilt, chin-lift maneuver (Figure BLS-5) provides for the maximum opening of the airway. It is useful on all patients who are in need of assistance in maintaining an airway or breathing. It is one of the best methods for correcting obstructions caused by the tongue. However, since it involves changing the position of the head, the head-tilt, chin-lift maneuver

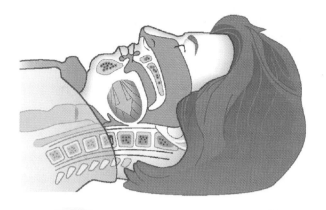

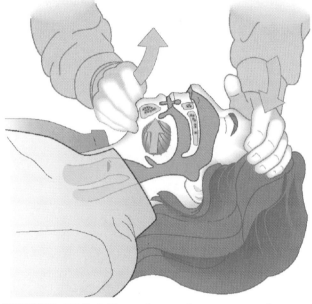

FIGURE BLS-4 Procedures for opening the airway help reposition the tongue.

should be used only on a patient who you can be quite sure has not suffered a spine injury.

Warning: IF ANY INDICATION OF HEAD, NECK, OR SPINE INJURY IS PRESENT, DO NOT USE THE HEAD-TILT, CHIN-LIFT MANEUVER. Instead, use the jaw-thrust maneuver described in the next section. Remember that any unconscious patient and many conscious patients may be suspected of having an injury to the head, neck, or spine.

Follow these steps to perform the head-tilt, chin-lift maneuver.

1.   Once the patient is supine (on his back), place one hand on the forehead and place the fingertips of the other hand under the bony area at the center of the patient's lower jaw.

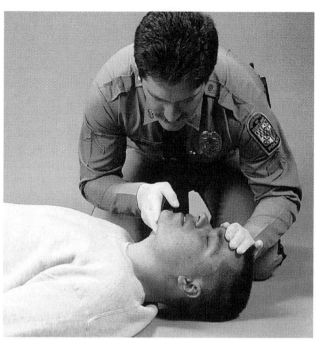

FIGURE BLS-5 The head-tilt, chin-lift maneuver.

2.   Tilt the head by applying gentle pressure to the patient's forehead.
3.   Use your fingertips to lift the chin and to support the lower jaw. Move the jaw forward to a point where the lower teeth are almost touching the upper teeth. Do not compress the soft tissues under the lower jaw, which can press and close off the airway.
4.   Do not allow the patient's mouth to be closed. To provide an adequate opening at the mouth, you may need to use the thumb of the hand supporting the chin to pull back the patient's lower lip. For your own safety (to prevent being bitten), do not insert your thumb into the patient's mouth.

The Jaw-Thrust Maneuver

The jaw-thrust maneuver (Figure BLS-6) is most commonly used to open the airway of an unconscious patient or one with suspected head, neck, or spinal injuries.

Note: THE JAW-THRUST MANEUVER IS THE ONLY WIDELY RECOMMENDED PROCEDURE FOR USE ON UNCONSCIOUS PATIENTS OR PATIENTS WITH POSSIBLE HEAD, NECK, OR SPINAL INJURIES.

Follow these steps to perform the jaw-thrust maneuver.

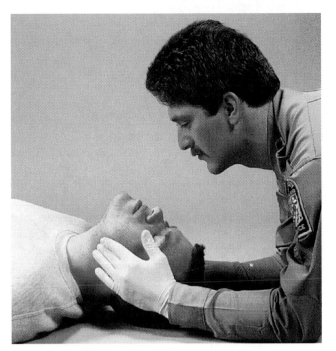

FIGURE BLS-6 The jaw-thrust maneuver.

1. Carefully keep the patient's head, neck, and spine aligned, moving him as a unit, as you place him in the supine position.
2. Kneel at the top of the patient's head, resting your elbows on the same surface on which the patient is lying.
3. Reach forward and gently place one hand on each side of the patient's lower jaw, at the angles of the jaw below the ears.
4. Stabilize the patient's head with your forearms.
5. Using your index fingers, push the angles of the patient's lower jaw forward.
6. You may need to retract the patient's lower lip with your thumb to keep the mouth open.
7. Do not tilt or rotate the patient's head. REMEMBER, THE PURPOSE OF THE JAW-THRUST MANEUVER IS TO OPEN THE AIRWAY WITHOUT MOVING THE HEAD OR NECK.

Clearing Airway Obstructions

Not every airway problem is caused by the tongue (the situation in which you would use the head-tilt, chin-lift maneuver or the jaw-thrust maneuver, described above, to open the airway). The airway can also be blocked by foreign objects or materials. These can include pieces of food, ice, toys, and vomitus. This problem is often seen with children and with patients who have abused alcohol or other drugs. It also hap-

pens when an injured person's airway becomes blocked by blood or broken teeth or dentures or when a person chokes on food.

Airway obstructions are either partial or complete. Partial and complete obstructions have different characteristics that may be noted during assessment, and each type has a different procedure of care. It is important to understand the differences between partial and complete obstruction and the correct care for each.

Patient Assessment— Partial Airway Obstruction

Keep in mind the mechanisms of injury. Look over the scene for clues that tell you to be alert for airway problems. Something as simple as noticing a half-eaten sandwich, or a child's game or toy that has small pieces, may make a difference.

Signs

Suspect partial airway obstruction if you note

☐ Unusual Breathing Sounds—Listen for
Snoring—probably caused by the tongue obstructing the pharynx.
Gurgling—often due to a foreign object or blood or other fluids in the trachea.
Crowing—sharp sounds probably caused by spasms in the larynx.
Wheezing—This may not indicate any major problems or it may indicate a medical problem you cannot do anything about, such as spasms along the airway. However, wheezing should be noted in your report about the patient and is an indication that the patient should be transported to the hospital quickly.

☐ Skin Discoloration—The patient is breathing, but there is a noticeable blue or gray color to the skin, which is caused by a lack of oxygen.

☐ Changes in Breathing—The patient's breathing may keep changing from near normal to very labored and back again.

A conscious patient trying to indicate an airway problem will usually point to his mouth or hold his neck (Figure BLS-7). Many do this even when a partial obstruction does not prevent speech. Ask the patient if he is choking, or ask if he can speak or cough. If he can, then the obstruction is partial.

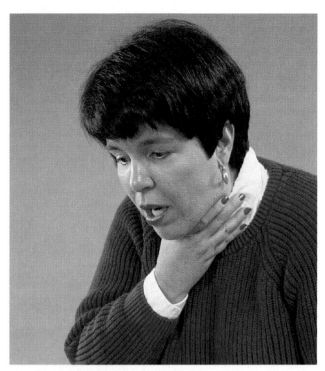

FIGURE BLS-7 The distress signal for choking.

Patient Care—Partial Airway Obstruction

For the conscious patient with an apparent partial airway obstruction, have him cough. A strong and forceful cough indicates he is exchanging enough air. Continue to encourage the patient to cough in the hope that such action will dislodge and expel the foreign object. *Do not* interfere with the patient's efforts to clear the partial obstruction by means of forceful coughing.

Warning: In cases where the patient has an apparent partial airway obstruction but he cannot cough or has a very weak cough, or the patient is blue or gray or shows other signs of poor air exchange, *treat the patient as if there is a complete airway obstruction* (see below).

Patient Assessment—Complete Airway Obstruction

Signs

☐ The Conscious Patient—The conscious patient with a complete airway obstruction will try to speak but will not be able to. He will also not be able to breathe or cough. Usually, he will display the distress signal for choking by clutching the neck between thumb and fingers.

☐ The Unconscious Patient—The unconscious patient with a complete airway obstruction is more difficult to identify. You will find this patient in respiratory arrest. Only when ventilation attempts are unsuccessful does it become apparent that there is an obstruction. (The rescue breather discovers resistance when trying to breathe air into the patient's lungs, and doing a head-tilt, chin-lift or a jaw-thrust maneuver does not correct the problem. The chest will not rise. There is no observable exchange of air.) Clues to an airway obstruction may also be found at the scene. (Bystanders report that the patient collapsed while eating, for example.)

Patient Care—Complete Airway Obstruction

Follow the procedures described under "Techniques for Clearing the Airway" and "Procedures for Clearing the Airway," below.

Techniques for Clearing the Airway

When you have determined that the airway is obstructed, you must take appropriate measures to clear it.

1. *Open the airway.* Since so many obstructions are caused by the tongue, you must first try to open the airway by using a head-tilt, chin-lift or a jaw-thrust maneuver, as described above.

2. *If the patient is unconscious and not breathing, attempt to provide ventilations (rescue breathing).* Once the head-tilt, chin-lift, or jaw-thrust has been performed to open the airway, do not waste time looking for or trying to remove a foreign object. Instead, first attempt to deliver a ventilation (discussed later in this chapter). If unsuccessful, readjust head position and attempt another ventilation. If still unsuccessful, then assume that there is foreign matter in the airway that must be cleared. *If the patient is conscious and indicating that he is choking, do not attempt artificial ventilations, but instead move right to step 3.*

3. *Remove any foreign object.* If the patient is choking, or, for the unconscious patient you have already opened the airway or unsuccessfully tried ventilation, two tech-

niques are recommended for removal of a foreign object.

- Manual thrusts (including the Heimlich maneuver)
- Finger sweeps

On any given patient you may have to use both techniques. These techniques are discussed in detail below.

Note: If the cause of airway obstruction is blood, liquids, or vomitus pooling in the throat, a trained person should perform suctioning.

The Heimlich Maneuver—Abdominal Thrusts
In the **Heimlich maneuver,** developed by Dr. Henry Heimlich, manual thrusts to the abdomen are used to force bursts of air from the lungs that will be sufficient to dislodge an obstructing object (Figure BLS-8).

Warning: Do not use the Heimlich maneuver on patients in late stages of pregnancy (when the uterus is so large that it intrudes into the area of the abdomen where you would apply the thrusts). Also do not use the Heimlich maneuver on infants (from birth to 1 year of age).

For the conscious adult or child (not infant) patient who is standing or sitting

1. While standing behind the patient, reach underneath the patient's arms to his front. Wrap your arms around his waist. Place your feet so that one is a half step in front of the patient's feet and the other a half step behind, so that your feet are apart from each other and set diagonally to the patient.
2. Make a fist and place the thumb side of this fist against the midline of the patient's abdomen, between the waist and rib cage. Avoid touching the patient's chest, especially the area immediately below the breastbone.
3. Grasp your properly positioned fist with your other hand and apply pressure inward and up toward the patient's head in one smooth, quick movement. This will cause your fist to press into the patient's abdomen. Deliver a series of FIVE RAPID INWARD THRUSTS up toward the diaphragm. Each new thrust should be separate and distinct,

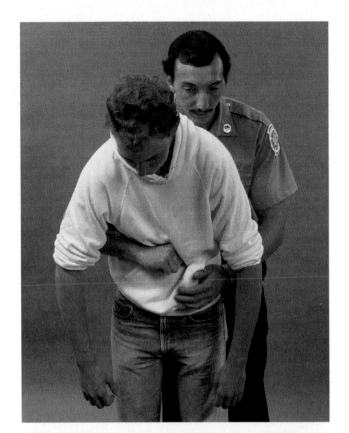

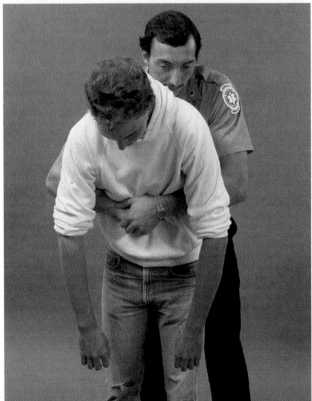

FIGURE BLS-8 The Heimlich maneuver. Place your fist on the patient's midline, between waist and rib cage. Grasp the fist with your other hand and rapidly deliver five inward and upward thrusts.

delivered with the intent of relieving the obstruction.

For the unconscious adult or child (not infant) patient or for a conscious patient who cannot sit up or be seated with your assistance, or if you are too short to reach around the patient and deliver upward thrusts

1. Move the patient into a supine position (Figure BLS-9).
2. Kneel and straddle the patient at the level of the thighs, facing his chest.
3. Place the heel of your hand on the midline of his abdomen, slightly above the navel and well below the breastbone.
4. Now place your free hand over the positioned hand. Your shoulders should be directly over the patient's abdomen. Be sure that you are positioned over the midline of the abdomen so that thrusts will be delivered straight up, not off to one side.
5. Deliver the thrusts by pressing your hands inward and upward toward the patient's diaphragm. Deliver FIVE RAPID THRUSTS. Each new thrust should be separate and distinct, delivered with the intent of relieving the obstruction.

If you complete a series of five thrusts and the obstruction is still present, take one of the following courses of action. If the patient is conscious quickly reassess your hand position and the victim's airway. Repeat the thrusts in series of five until the object is expelled or the patient who could not breathe is now able to breathe. If the patient is unconscious, open the airway, use finger sweeps to attempt to remove the obstruction and attempt to ventilate before repeating thrusts.

If the patient is very large or if you are a small individual, you can deliver more effective thrusts if you straddle one leg of the patient.

Chest Thrusts Chest thrusts are used in place of abdominal thrusts when the patient is in the late stages of pregnancy (Figure BLS-10), or when the patient is too obese for abdominal thrusts to be effective. To follow these steps, you should know two terms: The **sternum** is the breastbone, the flat bone in the center of the chest. The **xiphoid process** is a short, triangular piece of cartilage (tough, elastic gristle) that extends from the bottom of the sternum.

For the conscious adult patient who is standing or sitting

1. Position yourself behind the patient and slide your arms under his armpits, so that you encircle his chest.

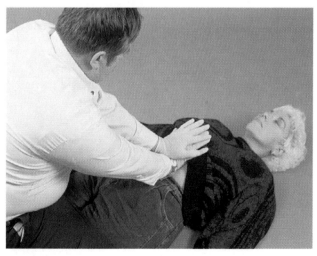

FIGURE BLS-9 The Heimlich maneuver used on supine patient.

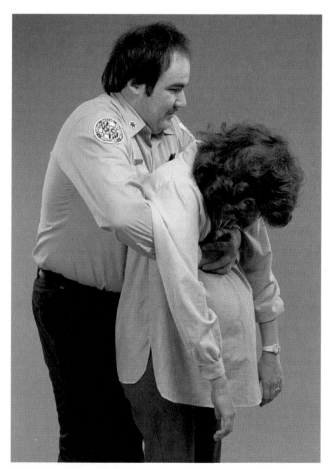

FIGURE BLS-10 The chest thrust applied to a pregnant patient.

2. Form a fist with one hand and place the thumb side of this fist on the patient's sternum. You should make contact with the midline of the sternum, about two to three finger widths above the xiphoid process. This results in the fist being placed over the lower half of the sternum, but not in contact with the edge of the rib cage.

3. Grasp the fist with your other hand and deliver FIVE CHEST THRUSTS directly backward toward the spine until the obstruction is relieved. Do not exert this force in an upward or downward direction or off to one side.

If the obstruction is not relieved, quickly reassess your position and the patient's airway and continue delivering series of five thrusts.

For the unconscious adult patient chest thrusts are best carried out when the patient is supine (Figure BLS-11). In this position, chest thrusts are delivered as you would for CPR (described below). Once the patient is properly positioned, you should

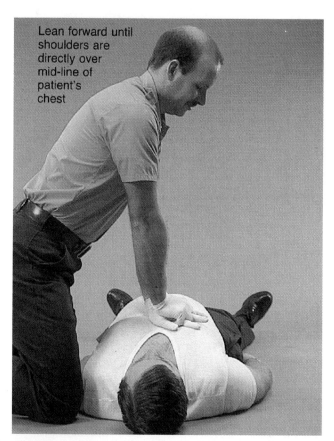

Lean forward until shoulders are directly over mid-line of patient's chest

FIGURE BLS-11 The chest thrust can be used when the patient is lying on his back.

1. Kneel alongside the patient at the level of his chest. Have both of your knees facing the patient's chest.

2. Position the heel of one hand on the midline of the sternum, two to three finger widths above the xiphoid process (your fingers should be perpendicular to the sternum). Lift and spread your fingers to avoid applying too much pressure to the ribs.

3. Place your other hand on top of the first, interlocking your fingers. Lock your elbows and lean forward until your shoulders are directly over the midline of the patient's chest.

4. Deliver FIVE SLOW, DISTINCT THRUSTS in a downward direction, applying enough force to compress the chest cavity. Then open the airway, perform finger sweeps, and attempt to ventilate. Repeat the sequence of thrusts, finger sweeps, and attempts to ventilate until successful.

For an infant, back blows are alternated with chest thrusts (Figure BLS-12).

1. Lay the infant face down along your forearm with the head lower than the trunk. Support the head by placing your hand around the jaw. You may need to add support by resting your forearm on your thigh. Rapidly deliver FIVE BACK BLOWS (in 3 to 5 seconds) using the heel of your hand. Strike forcefully directly between the shoulder blades.

2. Place your free arm on the infant's back. Support the head with your hand and sandwich him between your two arms. Turn the infant over so his back is along your forearm. Place your forearm against your thigh again. The head should be lower than the trunk.

3. Rapidly deliver FIVE CHEST THRUSTS, using the tips of two or three fingers. Apply pressure along the midline of the sternum. The fingers should be placed one finger width below an imaginary line drawn directly between the nipples.

4. If the airway remains obstructed, continue back blows and chest thrusts.

Note: Do not place infants or small children into the head-down position if they have a partial obstruction and can breathe adequately in an upright position. Keep in mind that forceful

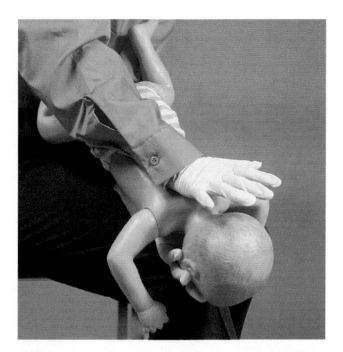

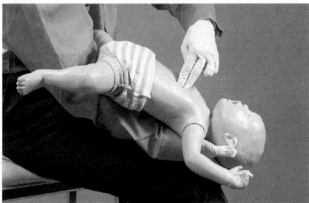

FIGURE BLS-12 To clear an airway obstruction in an infant, alternate back blows with chest thrusts.

coughing is a good sign in cases of partial airway obstruction.

Finger Sweeps A finger sweep is an attempt to manually remove an airway obstruction that has become dislodged or partially dislodged. Using a gloved hand to protect from infectious agents, sweep the mouth from one side to the other. Take care not to force the object farther down the patient's throat. The finger sweep technique should not be used for infants and children unless the object can actually be seen. "Blind" finger sweeps are especially dangerous in these smaller patients; if the obstruction is in sight, use your little finger to remove it.

You can open an unconscious patient's mouth and airway by using the tongue-jaw-lift procedure (Figure BLS-13). This requires you to

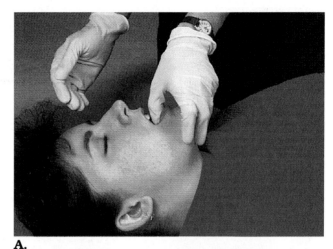

A.

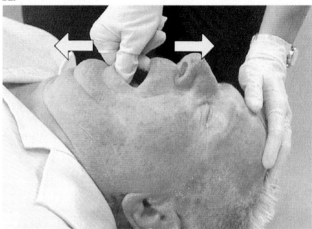

B.

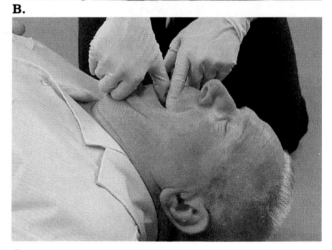

C.

FIGURE BLS-13 Open the patient's mouth using (A) the tongue-jaw lift or (B) the crossed-fingers technique. (C) Use finger sweeps to remove foreign objects from the airway and mouth.

grasp both tongue and lower jaw between your gloved thumb and fingers and lift to move the tongue away from the back of the pharynx. This movement will also move the tongue away from any foreign object that might be lodged in the back of the throat. The procedure may partially solve the problem of obstruction. However, it will be necessary to keep the patient's face up and insert the index finger of your free gloved hand into the patient's mouth and move this finger along the inside of the cheek to the base of the tongue. Using your finger as a hook, attempt to dislodge the object and sweep it into the mouth so it can be removed.

In some cases, it may be necessary to use your index finger to push the foreign object against the opposite side of the patient's throat in order to dislodge and lift the object. During such a procedure, you must take extra care not to push the object farther down the patient's throat.

You can also use the crossed-fingers technique to open the mouth of an unconscious patient (Figure BLS-13). Use one gloved hand to steady the patient's forehead. Place your thumb against the patient's lower teeth and your index finger against his upper teeth. Crossing the thumb and finger will force open the patient's mouth. Once the mouth is open, hold the lower jaw so that it cannot close.

Once you have opened the patient's mouth, release the patient's forehead and use the index finger of this hand to dislodge the foreign object as you would in the tongue-jaw-lift procedure.

Warning: A conscious patient has a gag reflex that can induce vomiting. This vomitus can be aspirated into the lungs. This is why most EMS Systems do not sanction the use of finger sweeps on conscious patients. Some localities believe that there are situations in which aggressive actions must be taken during basic life support. If an obstructing object becomes visible, use a finger sweep to dislodge and remove the object. If you are using a finger sweep method on a conscious patient, or you are trying to grasp a dislodged object, take great care not to induce vomiting or force the object farther down the patient's airway. Stay alert to avoid being bitten by the patient.

Remember: When using the finger sweep technique, if the object comes within reach grasp the object and remove it. Be careful not to push it down the patient's airway. Be aware of a possible gag reflex and be prepared for the patient to vomit.

Procedures for Clearing the Airway

The following pages contain sequences of procedures to use in the event of a complete airway obstruction or a partial airway obstruction with poor air exchange (Table BLS-1). These procedures or combinations of procedures are considered to have been effective if any of the following happens.

- The patient re-establishes good air exchange or spontaneous breathing.
- The foreign object is expelled from the mouth.
- The foreign object is expelled into the mouth where it can be removed by the rescuer.
- The unconscious patient regains consciousness.
- The patient's skin color improves.

The use of the Heimlich maneuver or of chest thrusts requires a little common sense. Even though five thrusts are called for, if the first one works, the remaining thrusts are not needed. You must stay aware of what is happening to the patient when applying the procedure. Remember that each manual thrust should be performed with the intent of relieving the obstruction.

The thrusts are to be delivered rapidly, but some restraint is needed. Too forceful and too rapid a blow may injure the patient. An improperly delivered thrust may cause damage in the chest or abdomen. Trying to do the thrusts as quickly as you can move will probably cause you to lose your balance and deliver an improper and possibly harmful thrust. You must practice these techniques on the manikins provided in your course and keep your skills up to date.

If a person has only a partial airway obstruction and is still able to speak and cough forcefully, do not interfere with his attempts to expel the foreign body. Carefully watch him, however, so that you can immediately provide help if this partial obstruction becomes a complete one.

An unconscious patient, or a conscious patient with total airway obstruction, will present the greatest problems.

Warning: If the patient has no pulse or at any point becomes pulseless, CPR must be initiated.

Remember: Although the Heimlich maneuver is specified in the procedures described below, chest thrusts must be used for very obese patients and for patients in late stages of pregnancy. Alternating back blows and chest thrusts must be used for infants.

TABLE BLS-1 Airway Clearance Sequences

	Adult	Child	Infant
Age	8 yrs and older	1-8 yrs	birth-1 yr
Conscious	Ask, "Are you choking?" Series of 5 Heimlich maneuvers.	Ask, "Are you choking?" Series of 5 Heimlich maneuvers.	Observe signs of choking (small objects or food, wheezing, agitation, blue color, not breathing). Series of: 5 back blows. 5 chest thrusts.
Loses consciousness during procedure	Assist patient to floor. Establish unresponsiveness (ask "Are you OK?") If alone, call for help, then . . . Open airway. Perform finger sweeps. Attempt to ventilate. If unsuccessful, reposition head and attempt to ventilate again. If unsuccessful, perform Heimlich maneuver. (Repeat as needed.)	Assist patient to floor. Establish unresponsiveness (ask "Are you OK?") Open airway. Remove visible objects (NO blind sweeps). Attempt to ventilate. If unsuccessful, reposition head and attempt to ventilate again. If unsuccessful, perform Heimlich maneuver. (Repeat as needed.) After 1 minute, call for help if alone.	Establish unresponsiveness (tap or speak loudly). Open airway. Remove visible objects (NO blind sweeps). Attempt to ventilate. If unsuccessful, reposition head and attempt to ventilate again. If unsuccessful, perform back blows and chest thrusts. (Repeat as needed.) After 1 minute, call for help if alone.
Unconscious when found	Establish unresponsiveness. If alone, call for help, then . . . Open airway. Attempt to ventilate. If unsuccessful, reposition head and attempt to ventilate again. If unsuccessful, Heimlich maneuver. Finger sweeps. (Repeat as needed.)	Establish unresponsiveness. Open airway. Attempt to ventilate. If unsuccessful, reposition head and attempt to ventilate again. If unsuccessful, Heimlich maneuver. Remove visible objects (NO blind sweeps). (Repeat as needed.) After 1 minute, call for help if alone.	Establish unresponsiveness. Open airway. Attempt to ventilate. If unsuccessful, reposition head and attempt to ventilate again. If unsuccessful, back blows and chest thrusts. Remove visible objects (NO blind sweeps). (Repeat as needed.) After 1 minute, call for help if alone.

Procedures for an Adult

The following are procedures for clearing an obstructed airway in an adult (Scan BLS-2).

Conscious Adult If the adult patient is conscious, you should

1. Determine if there is a COMPLETE OBSTRUCTION or a PARTIAL OBSTRUCTION WITH POOR AIR EXCHANGE. Look, listen, and feel for the signs of obstruction. Be certain to ask, "Are you choking?" If the patient can speak, see if he can produce a forceful cough. If the patient has a complete obstruction or poor air exchange . . .
2. Provide FIVE THRUSTS OF THE HEIMLICH MANEUVER in rapid succession. If the manual thrusts have not expelled the obstruction . . .

3. Re-evaluate your hand position and repeat the thrusts until you are successful or the patient loses consciousness.

Adult Loses Consciousness If the patient loses consciousness, you should

1. Protect the patient from possible injury due to falling.
2. Establish unresponsiveness. (Shout, "Are you okay?" If the patient does not react, he is unresponsive.) If you are working alone, call 911, or telephone your local emergency number, or radio the EMS dispatch center immediately. Do this before attempting patient care.
3. Use the tongue-jaw lift to open the mouth. Perform finger sweeps.
4. Open the airway (using the head-tilt, chin-lift maneuver if there is no possible head,

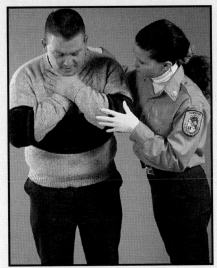

1. Recognize and assess that patient is choking. Ask, "Are you choking?"

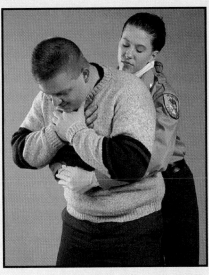

2. Position yourself to perform the Heimlich maneuver.

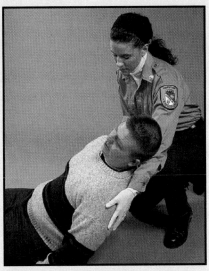

3. If the patient becomes weak or unconscious, assist him to the floor.

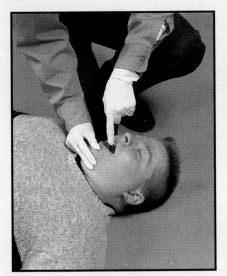

4. Perform finger sweeps.

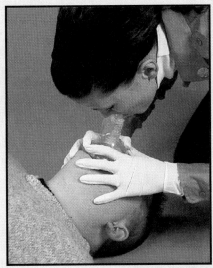

5. Attempt to ventilate. If this fails, reposition head and try again. If you are not successful. . .

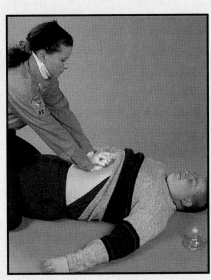

6. Perform the Heimlich maneuver.

neck, or spinal injury—the jaw-thrust maneuver if there is a possibility of injury) and attempt to ventilate. If this fails . . .

5. Reposition the head and attempt to ventilate again. If this fails . . .
6. Deliver FIVE THRUSTS OF THE HEIMLICH MANEUVER.
7. Repeat the tongue-jaw lift and finger sweeps.
8. Open the airway and repeat your attempt to ventilate the patient as described in the section on rescue breathing later in this chapter. If this fails . . .
9. Continue with the following cycle until you are successful.

- 5 thrusts of the Heimlich maneuver
- Finger sweeps
- Attempt to ventilate

Unconscious Adult If the patient is unconscious when you arrive

1. Establish unresponsiveness. If you are working alone, call 911, or telephone your local emergency number, or radio the EMS dispatch center immediately. Do this before attempting patient care.
2. Position the patient on his back.
3. Attempt to open the patient's airway by the head-tilt, chin-lift maneuver (if there is no possible head, neck, or spinal injury) or jaw-thrust maneuver (if there is a possibility of injury). Remember to look, listen, and feel for breathing.
4. Try to give ONE SLOW VENTILATION (1½ to 2 seconds) as described in the section on rescue breathing later in this chapter. If your attempts to ventilate the patient fail, you should . . .
5. Reposition the patient's head to attempt to create an open airway, and try again to ventilate. If this fails . . .
6. Deliver FIVE THRUSTS OF THE HEIMLICH MANEUVER. If this fails . . .
7. Use the tongue-jaw lift and attempt finger sweeps. After removing the object, or if you cannot find and remove the obstruction, you should . . .
8. Open the airway and attempt to ventilate. If attempt to ventilate fails . . .
9. Continue with the cycle of Heimlich maneuver, finger sweeps, and attempts to ventilate until successful.

If you are unable to dislodge the obstruction, you have a critical emergency, requiring transport to a medical facility without delay. You must continue efforts to clear the obstruction, even if you can do no more than partially dislodge the object. The chances of at least partially dislodging the object will improve with time as the muscles of the unconscious patient's jaw and upper airway relax. Once the object is partially dislodged, you should be able to keep the patient alive by artificial ventilations. If the heart stops beating, CPR will be necessary.

Remember: You must persist in your efforts until the airway is clear or until you have dislodged the object enough to allow for you to provide artificial ventilations. If the patient's brain cells do not receive oxygen, they will begin to die within 10 minutes. Keep in mind that procedures used to clear the airway may at first fail, only to be successful later as muscles in the patient's body relax.

Procedures for a Child

The following are procedures for clearing an obstructed airway in a child.

Conscious Child Start by determining if there is an airway obstruction. Ask the child, "Are you choking?" If the child cannot cough or has an ineffective cough, or if the child's breathing problems continue to worsen, perform FIVE THRUSTS OF THE HEIMLICH MANEUVER. Continue with the thrusts until the object is expelled or the child loses consciousness.

Child Loses Consciousness If the child who has an airway obstruction loses consciousness while you are providing care, provide the same care as you would for an adult, but DO NOT ATTEMPT BLIND FINGER SWEEPS. (Look for and remove only *visible* foreign objects.) The Heimlich maneuver is best delivered if you kneel at the child's feet. You may place the child on a table and stand at his feet.

If your attempts to clear the airway fail, continue the cycle of Heimlich maneuver, attempts to remove visible foreign objects, and attempts to ventilate until you are successful.

If you are working alone when the child loses consciousness, stop to telephone or radio for assistance after 1 minute of attempts to clear the airway and ventilate.

Unconscious Child If the child is unconscious when you arrive, carry out the same procedures as you would for an adult patient. The Heimlich maneuver is best delivered if you kneel at the child's feet. You may place the child on a table and stand at his feet.

DO NOT ATTEMPT BLIND FINGER SWEEPS. (Look for and remove only *visible* foreign objects.)

If you fail at your attempts to clear the airway, repeat the cycle of Heimlich maneuver, attempts to remove visible foreign objects, and attempts to ventilate until you are successful.

If you are working alone, stop to telephone or radio for assistance after 1 minute of attempts to clear the airway and ventilate.

Procedures for an Infant

The following are procedures for clearing an obstructed airway in an infant (Scan BLS-3).

Conscious Infant If the patient is a conscious infant who requires your assistance to clear an airway obstruction, you should

1. Determine that there is an airway obstruction. An infant is not yet old enough to display the universal choking sign. Indications that an infant is choking are

   - Evidence such as small objects or food around the infant
   - Wheezing or other unusual airway noises
   - Agitation
   - Blue or gray skin discoloration (cyanosis)
   - Absence of respirations
   - Inability to ventilate

2. Lay the infant face down along your forearm with the head lower than the trunk. Support the head by placing your hand around the jaw. Add support by resting your forearm on your thigh.
3. Deliver FIVE BACK BLOWS in 3 to 5 seconds. Deliver the blows forcefully with the heel of your hand between the infant's shoulder blades. If this fails . . .
4. Support the infant's head and sandwich him between your two hands. Turn the infant over onto his back, keeping the head lower than the trunk.
5. Deliver FIVE CHEST THRUSTS, using the tips of two or three fingers. Apply pressure along the midline of the sternum. The fingers should be placed one finger width

below an imaginary line drawn directly between the nipples.
6. Continue with the sequence of back blows and chest thrusts until the object is expelled or the infant loses consciousness.

Note: The above procedures are recommended only when the infant's problem is a known or strongly suspected obstruction due to a foreign object or substances such as vomitus, or blood. If you have any reason to suspect that the problem is caused by tissue swelling related to an allergy or infection, do not attempt airway clearance but ensure transport to the hospital as quickly as possible.

Infant Loses Consciousness If the infant suffers a loss of consciousness while you are attempting to clear the airway, you should

1. Establish unresponsiveness (the infant does not move or cry when tapped or spoken to loudly. DO NOT SHAKE THE INFANT).
2. Position the patient and use the tongue-jaw lift. Look for and remove any visible foreign objects. DO NOT ATTEMPT BLIND FINGER SWEEPS.
3. Attempt to ventilate. If this fails . . .
4. Reposition the head and attempt to ventilate again. If this fails . . .
5. If working alone, call 911, telephone your local emergency number, or radio the EMS dispatch center after 1 minute of attempts to clear the airway and ventilate.
6. Deliver FIVE BACK BLOWS. If this fails . . .
7. Deliver FIVE CHEST THRUSTS.
8. Employ the tongue-jaw lift and look for and remove any foreign objects. DO NOT ATTEMPT BLIND FINGER SWEEPS.
9. Re-attempt to ventilate. If this fails . . .
10. Continue with the sequence of back blows, chest thrusts, foreign object removal (not "blind"), and attempts to ventilate until you are successful.

Unconscious Infant If the infant is unconscious when you arrive

1. Establish unresponsiveness.
2. Place the infant on its back, supporting the head and neck.
3. Open the airway and establish breathlessness.
4. Attempt to ventilate, using the mouth-to-mouth-and-nose or mouth-to-mask technique (see Rescue Breathing, below). Should this fail . . .

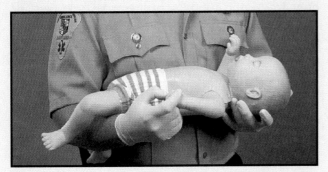

1. Establish unresponsiveness. Position the infant.

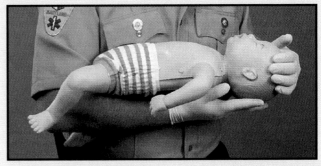

2. Open airway. Establish breathlessness.

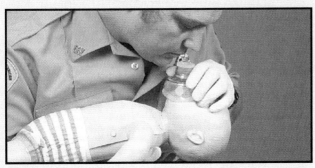

3. Attempt to ventilate. If this fails, reposition head and try again.

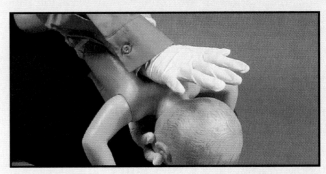

4. Deliver 5 back blows.

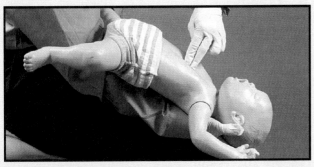

5. Deliver 5 chest thrusts.

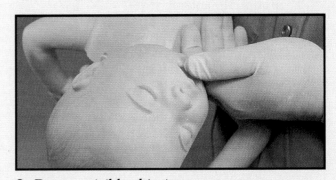

6. Remove visible objects.

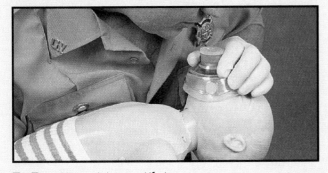

7. Re-attempt to ventilate.

8. Repeat the sequence of

- Back blows
- Chest thrusts
- Removing visible objects
- Re-attempting ventilation

5. If working alone, call 911, telephone your local emergency number, or radio the EMS dispatch center after 1 minute of attempts to clear the airway and ventilate.
6. Reposition the infant's head and attempt to ventilate. If this fails . . .
7. Lay the infant face down along your forearm with the head lower than the trunk. Support the head by placing your hand around the jaw. Support your forearm on your thigh. Deliver FIVE BACK BLOWS in 3 to 5 seconds. If this fails . . .
8. Sandwich the infant between your arms and turn him over onto his back, keeping the head lower than the trunk. Deliver FIVE CHEST THRUSTS. If this fails . . .
9. Insert your gloved thumb into the mouth, over the tongue. Wrap your fingers around the lower jaw and lift the tongue and jaw forward, opening the patient's mouth. Look for any objects causing the obstruction. If you can see the object, remove it using your little finger, but do not attempt "blind" finger sweeps. If you cannot see and remove an object . . .
10. Open the airway and attempt to ventilate using the mouth-to-mouth-and-nose or mouth-to-mask technique.
11. Repeat the following sequence until you are successful.

- Five back blows
- Five chest thrusts
- Looking for and removing visible objects (no "blind" finger sweeps)
- Attempts to ventilate

Should the infant develop respiratory arrest, and you have cleared enough of the obstruction to provide adequate ventilation, provide one breath and check for a pulse to see if CPR must be initiated.

RESCUE BREATHING

Rescue breathing is also called **ventilation** or *artificial ventilation*. The purpose of this technique is to provide oxygen to, and allow carbon dioxide to be removed from, a patient who has stopped breathing or whose breathing is inadequate to sustain life. The procedure may not cause normal breathing to resume, but it will keep the patient alive until more advanced techniques can be applied.

Many people wonder how rescue breathing can provide enough oxygen to the patient, since the air is coming from the rescuer's lungs. Atmospheric air contains 21% oxygen. The air you breathe out contains 16% oxygen—still about three times the amount of oxygen (5%) that would normally be removed from the air by the patient's lungs. In other words, the air you provide contains more than enough oxygen to supply the patient's needs.

To make artificial ventilations more effective, supplemental oxygen should be provided. The use of supplemental oxygen increases the patient's chance of survival. The start of rescue breathing should not be delayed, however, if oxygen is not available. Instead, start ventilations and begin providing oxygen as soon as possible after the start of ventilations. An EMT-B should be able to provide ventilations both with and without supplemental oxygen. (For information on providing supplemental oxygen, see Chapter 7, Airway Management.)

Mouth-to-Mask Ventilation

Mouth-to-mask ventilation is performed using a pocket face mask (Scan BLS-4 and Table BLS-2). The pocket face mask is made of soft, collapsible material and can be carried in your pocket, jacket, or purse. Many rescuers purchase their own pocket face masks for their workplace or automobile first aid kits.

Face masks have important infection control features. Your breaths are delivered through a valve in the mask so that you do not have direct contact with the patient's mouth. Most pocket masks have one-way valves that allow your ventilations to enter but prevent the patient's exhaled air from coming back through the valve and into contact with you.

Some pocket masks have oxygen inlets. When high concentration oxygen is attached to the inlet, an oxygen concentration of approximately 50% is delivered. This is significantly better than the 16% delivered by mouth-to-mask ventilations without oxygen.

Most pocket face masks are made of a clear plastic. This allows observation of the patient's mouth and nose for vomiting or secretions that need to be suctioned and for the color of the lips (a bluish color shows that the patient is not getting enough oxygen). Some pocket face masks may have a strap that goes around the patient's head. This is helpful during one-rescuer CPR since it will hold the mask

Mouth-to-Mask Ventilation

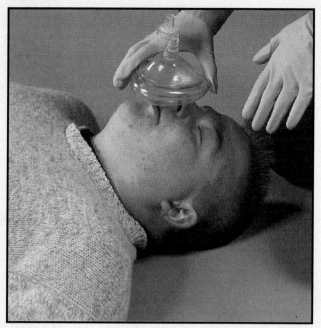

1. Position the patient and prepare to place the mask.

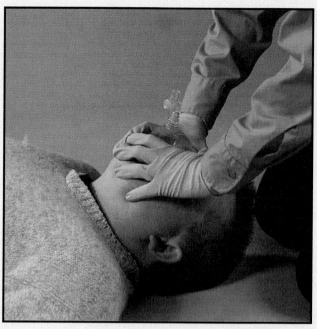

2. Seat the mask firmly on the patient's face.

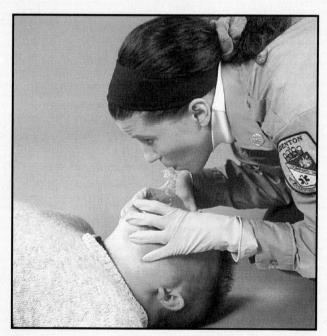

3. Open the patient's airway and watch the chest rise as you ventilate through the one-way valve.

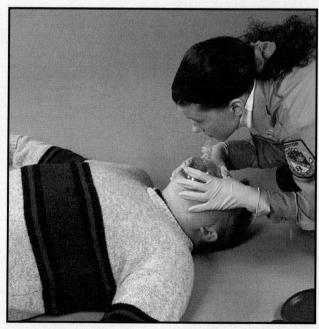

4. Watch the patient's chest fall during exhalation.

TABLE BLS-2   Rescue Breathing and Clearing the Airway

	Adult	Child	Infant
Age	8 yrs and older	1-8 yrs	birth-1 yr
Initial ventilation	1½ to 2 sec.	1 to 1½ sec.	1 to 1½ sec.
Ventilation rate	10-12 breaths/min.	20 breaths/min.	20 breaths/min.
Heimlich maneuver	Series of 5 abdominal thrusts	Series of 5 abdominal thrusts	NOT USED FOR INFANTS
Chest thrusts (if obese or pregnant); back blows and chest thrusts (for infants)	Series of 5 thrusts to chest—arms locked, hands in CPR position	NOT USED FOR CHILDREN	Series of: 5 back blows 5 chest thrusts, using 2-3 fingers
When working alone: Call 911 or emergency dispatcher	After establishing unresponsiveness— before beginning resuscitation	After establishing unresponsiveness and 1 minute of resuscitation	After establishing unresponsiveness and 1 minute of resuscitation

on the patient's face while you are performing chest compressions.

To provide mouth-to-mask ventilation for an adult patient (see also Ventilating Infants and Children later in this chapter), you should

1. Establish if the patient is unresponsive (tap the shoulder and ask, "Are you OK?").
2. If the adult patient is unresponsive and you are working alone, immediately telephone 911 or your designated emergency number, or radio your EMS dispatch center for help, BEFORE BEGINNING ARTIFICIAL VENTILATIONS.
3. Position yourself at the patient's head and open the airway, using the head-tilt, chin-lift maneuver (if no spinal injury is suspected) or the jaw-thrust maneuver (if spinal injury is suspected).
4. Determine if the patient is breathing and if the breathing is adequate (see "Patient Assessment—Respiratory Failure," earlier in this chapter). Take 3 TO 5 SECONDS to determine if the patient is breathing.
5. Position the mask on the patient's face so that the apex (top of the triangle) is over the bridge of the nose and the base is between the lower lip and the prominence of the chin.
6. Hold the mask firmly in place while maintaining the proper head tilt by placing

- Both thumbs on the sides of the mask
- Index, third and fourth fingers of each hand grasping the lower jaw on each side between the angle of the jaw and the ear lobe to lift the jaw forward

7. Take a deep breath and exhale into the mask port or one-way valve at the top of the mask port. The ventilation should be delivered over 1½ to 2 seconds. Watch for the patient's chest to rise.
8. Remove your mouth from the port and allow for passive exhalation.
9. If the attempt to ventilate is unsuccessful, reposition the head and try again.
10. If the patient does not begin spontaneous breathing after these initial breaths, check for a carotid pulse. (See information on the carotid pulse later in this chapter) If the patient has no pulse, begin cardiopulmonary resuscitation (see CPR later in this chapter). If there is a pulse, but no breathing, continue with the following cycle.

- Take a deep breath and exhale air through the valve of the mask.
- Break contact with the mask.
- Air should be passively released from the patient's lungs while you . . .
- Watch the patient's chest fall and listen and feel for the return of air.
- Take another deep breath and begin the cycle again. Provide breaths at the rate of 10-to-12 per minute.

11. When available, supplemental oxygen should be connected to the mask. Then continue rescue breathing as before, but with supplemental oxygen now attached.

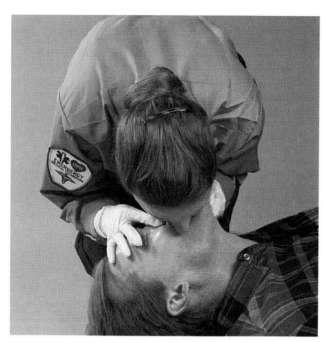

FIGURE BLS-14 Mouth-to mouth ventilation.

Mouth-to-Mouth Ventilation

Mouth-to-mouth ventilation (Figure BLS-14 and Table BLS-2) can be performed by one person with no special equipment.

Warning: When possible, use a barrier device (pocket face mask) for infection control.

Mouth-to-mouth ventilation is used when the patient is in respiratory arrest, that is, when he is no longer breathing. The procedure is also used when a patient's respiratory rate or depth is inadequate to sustain life. When performing mouth-to-mouth ventilations, remember that you will need to open and maintain the airway using the head-tilt, chin-lift method, or, on patients with suspected head, neck or spine injuries, the jaw-thrust maneuver.

When providing mouth-to-mouth ventilations for an adult patient, you should follow the steps below (see also Ventilating Infants and Children later in this chapter). Remember that you will be safer if you employ a pocket face mask with one-way valve.

1. Establish unresponsiveness.
2. If the adult patient is unresponsive and you are working alone, call for help BEFORE BEGINNING VENTILATIONS.
3. Position the patient and open the airway.

4. Determine that breathing is absent or inadequate.
5. Maintain the patient in the optimum head-tilt position and pinch the nose closed with the thumb and forefinger of the hand you are using to hold the patient's forehead.
6. Deliver one slow breath (1½ to 2 seconds) as follows: Open your mouth wide and take a deep breath. Place your mouth around the patient's mouth, making a tight seal with your lips against the patient's face. Exhale into the patient's mouth until you see his chest rise and feel the resistance offered by his expanding lungs. Stop when you see the chest rise so that you do not over-ventilate the patient. Break contact with the patient's mouth (allowing the nostrils to open) to allow him to exhale (breathe out) passively.
7. If the initial breath is unsuccessful, reposition the patient's head and try again.
8. Unless the patient begins spontaneous breathing after these initial breaths, check for a carotid pulse. (See information on the carotid pulse later in this chapter.) If the patient has no pulse, begin cardiopulmonary resuscitation. (See CPR later in this chapter.) If there is a pulse, but no breathing, continue with the following cycle.

- Take a deep breath and pinch the patient's nostrils closed; form a seal with the patient's mouth and exhale air into the patient's airway.
- Break contact with the patient's mouth (allowing the nostrils to open).
- Air should be passively released from his lungs while you . . .
- Turn your head to watch the patient's chest fall and listen and feel for the return of air.
- Take another deep breath and begin the cycle again, providing breaths at the rate of 10-12 per minute.

Note: For artificial respirations provided to the adult patient, after the initial slow breaths, you must deliver breaths to the patient at ONE EVERY 5 OR 6 SECONDS to give a rate of 10 TO 12 BREATHS PER MINUTE. A respiratory cycle—inhalation/exhalation—takes 5 to 6 seconds. Watch the chest rise as you ventilate, then watch the chest fall as the patient exhales, then ventilate again.

Once you are breathing for the patient, you must continue to do so until he starts to breathe on his own (spontaneous breathing) or until you transfer the responsibility to another person who is trained at your level or higher. If you detect cardiac arrest, you must begin cardiopulmonary resuscitation (CPR), continuing to breathe for the patient as part of this procedure.

You will know that you are adequately ventilating the patient if you

- SEE the chest rise and fall
- HEAR and FEEL air leaving the patient's lungs
- FEEL resistance to your ventilations as the patient's lungs expand

You also may note that the patient's color improves or remains normal. In some cases, another rescuer may note that the pupils of the patient's eyes react to light.

The most common problems with mouth-to-mask or mouth-to-mouth ventilation include

- Failure to form a tight seal (with your mouth or pocket face mask)
- Failure to pinch the nose completely closed in mouth-to-mouth procedures
- Failure to establish an open airway because of inadequate head tilt or head positioning
- Failure to have the patient's mouth open wide enough to receive ventilations
- Failure to clear the upper airway of obstructions.

Many students wonder how big the rescue breath should be. The clearest guideline is that it must be big enough to make the patient's chest rise, but not bigger. That is why it is so important to watch the patient's chest rise and feel for resistance to your breaths. The average breath of an adult at rest moves 500 milliliters of air. More air is needed for an effective artificial ventilation. The size should be somewhere between a normal breath and a double-sized breath. You are trying to deliver at least 800 to 1,200 milliliters of air to the adult patient. Often, each breath turns out to be around 500 milliliters if you try to deliver the breaths too quickly. If the volume of air is too great or delivered too quickly, it can also overwhelm the ability of the patient's trachea to accept the breath and cause gastric distention (discussed later in this chapter).

Remember: If there is a possibility of spinal injury, employ the jaw-thrust maneuver to open the airway. If you are using your hands to maintain the jaw thrust, then you must use your cheek to seal the nose if you are doing mouth-to-mouth rescue breathing. This technique is difficult, even when practiced on a regular basis, and is very tiring for the rescuer. If the jaw thrust is used, the mouth-to-nose technique or use of a pocket face mask is preferred.

Mouth-To-Nose-Ventilation

Occasionally, you will not be able to ventilate a nonbreathing patient by the mouth-to-mouth technique. An accident victim may have severe injuries to the mouth and lower jaw. A patient lacking teeth or dentures may make it difficult to get a good seal. For this patient, you may have to use the mouth-to-nose technique (Figure BLS-15). *Remember that a mouth-to-mask procedure is preferred if a pocket mask is available and will accomplish the same objectives as mouth-to-nose ventilation since the mask will cover both the nose and the mouth.*

Most of the mouth-to-nose procedure is very similar to the mouth-to-mouth technique.

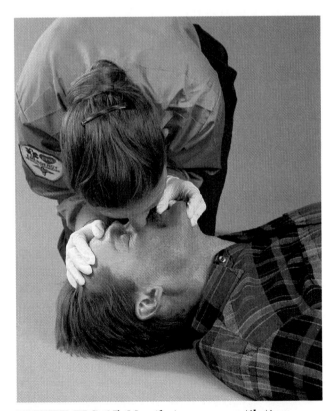

FIGURE BLS-15 Mouth-to-nose ventilation.

The airway must be opened and two slow breaths delivered. As with the mouth-to-mouth procedure, breaths are then delivered ONE EVERY 5 OR 6 SECONDS to give a rate of 10 TO 12 BREATHS PER MINUTE. The following are ways in which the mouth-to-nose procedure differs from the mouth-to-mouth procedure.

- You must keep one hand on the patient's forehead to maintain an open airway and use your other hand to close the patient's mouth.
- The patient's nose is left open.
- To provide breaths, you must seal your mouth around and deliver ventilations through the patient's nose. The patient's mouth must be kept shut during delivery of the ventilation.
- When allowing the patient to exhale passively, you must break contact with his nose and slightly open his mouth. Keep your hand on the patient's forehead to help keep his airway open as he exhales.

Remember: The jaw thrust should be used if there is a possibility of spinal injury. For the mouth-to-nose technique, do not allow the lower lip to retract as you push with your thumbs. Use your cheek to seal the patient's mouth.

Ventilating Neck Breathers

Although such occasions are rare, you may have to ventilate a neck breather, or a patient who has a **stoma** (STO-mah). A stoma is a permanent surgical opening in the neck through which the patient breathes. There may be a metal tube placed within the stoma to help keep it open. Follow these steps for mask-to-stoma ventilation.

1. If the stoma's metal tube has become clogged, quickly clean the neck opening of encrusted mucus and foreign matter using a gauze pad or handkerchief, not a tissue. If EMT-Bs are present and have suctioning equipment, they may suction the tube by passing a sterile suction catheter through the stoma and into the trachea (Figure BLS-16). The catheter should not be inserted more than 3 to 5 inches into the trachea. Suctioning should take place for only a few seconds. Time should not be

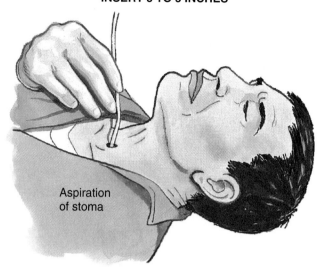

INSERT 3 TO 5 INCHES

Aspiration of stoma

FIGURE BLS-16 Suctioning a neck opening.

wasted in attempting to do a complete suctioning. Once the airway is partially open, start ventilations.

2. Leave the head and neck in a neutral position as it is unnecessary to position the airway prior to ventilations in a neck breather.

3. Use a pediatric-sized pocket mask to establish a seal around the neck opening.

4. Breathe into the mask in the same way as for any mouth-to-mask procedure (Figure BLS-17).

5. Use the same size breaths you normally would during mouth-to-mask or mouth-to-mouth resuscitation, and provide VENTILATIONS AT THE RATE OF ONE EVERY 5 OR 6 SECONDS OR 10 TO 12 BREATHS PER MINUTE.

6. Make certain that you watch for the patient's chest to rise and fall as you provide ventilations. If the patient's chest does not rise, it may mean that the patient is a partial neck breather. This type of patient does take in and expel some air through the mouth and nose. In such cases, you will have to pinch closed the nose and seal the mouth with the palm of one hand, or have an assistant do so, while ventilating through the stoma.

7. If unable to successfully ventilate the patient through the stoma, consider sealing the stoma and attempting artificial ventilation through the mouth and nose. (This will work only if the trachea is still connected to the passageways of the mouth, nose, and

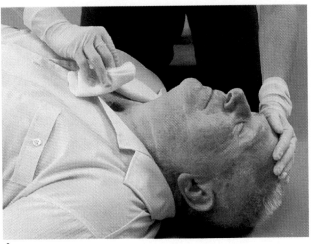

A.

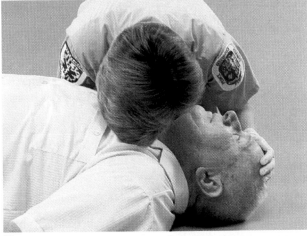

B.

FIGURE BLS-17 For mask-to-stoma ventilations, use a pediatric-sized pocket face mask.

pharynx. In some cases, the trachea has been permanently connected to the neck opening with no remaining connection to the mouth, nose, or pharynx.)

Safety Note:

If no pocket mask or other barrier device is available, mouth-to-stoma ventilation can be performed using the same procedures as mouth-to-mouth ventilation. However, direct mouth-to-stoma ventilation risks exposure to infectious disease. Mask-to-stoma ventilation, which provides barrier protection from the patient's body fluids, should be used whenever possible.

Ventilating Infants and Children

In basic life support, an infant is any patient from birth to 1 year of age, a child is any patient from 1 to 8 years of age, and an adult is any patient older than 8 years of age.

To provide ventilations to the infant or child (Figure BLS-18 and Table BLS-2), you should

1. Establish whether the patient is responsive. (Tap the patient. Ask a child, "Are you OK?" An infant should move or cry when tapped or spoken to loudly.)
2. Lay an infant or child on a hard surface. A small infant may be held in your arms.
3. Open the airway and determine if the patient is breathing. Take 3 TO 5 SECONDS to determine breathlessness.

Warning: A slight head tilt is all that is required to open the airway of an infant or child. Some rescuers provide too great a tilt, which may actually obstruct the airway of a young infant. On the other hand, some rescuers are too cautious with the head tilt. If the patient's chest does not rise when you provide a breath, it may be due to an improper head tilt. Make certain that you do not under-ventilate the patient because of failure to maintain an open airway.

4. Take a breath and cover both the mouth and nose of the infant or small child patient (mouth-to-mouth-and-nose technique). If a pocket face mask is used, it must be the correct size for the patient.
5. Deliver one slow breath (1 to 1½ seconds). Note that only small breaths are required to ventilate infants.
6. If the first breath is not successful, reposition the head and try again.

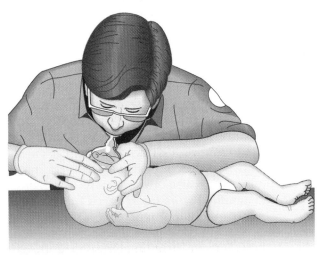

FIGURE BLS-18 Ventilating infants and small children.

Warning: You must stay alert for resistance to your ventilations and for chest movements. If you are too forceful with your ventilations, air will be forced into the patient's stomach. Provide a breath that is just large enough to make the patient's chest rise. If your efforts are met with resistance, there may be an upper airway obstruction (discussed earlier in this chapter). Do not use excessive pressure to force air into the lungs.

7. When allowing the patient to exhale, uncover both mouth and nose. Allow for deflation between breaths.

8. If the infant or child patient is unresponsive and you are working alone, PROVIDE ARTIFICIAL VENTILATIONS FOR 1 MINUTE BEFORE BREAKING to telephone 911 or your local emergency number, or to radio for help.

9. If the patient is not breathing after two initial ventilations, determine pulselessness. If there is no pulse, start cardiopulmonary resuscitation. (See information on determining pulse in infants and children and on CPR for infants and children under CPR later in this chapter). If the patient has a pulse, start rescue breathing and . . .

10. Provide ventilations to infants and children at the rate of ONE BREATH EVERY 3 SECONDS in order to deliver 20 BREATHS PER MINUTE. The volume should be that which makes the patient's chest rise without over-inflating. Watch as the patient exhales, then re-inflate enough to make the chest rise.

Gastric Distention

Rescue breathing can force some air into the patient's stomach, causing the stomach to become distended (bulging). This may indicate that the airway is blocked, that there is improper head position, or that the ventilations being provided are too large or too quick to be accommodated by the lungs or the trachea. This problem is seen more frequently in infants and children but can occur with any patient.

A slight bulge is of little worry, but a major distention can cause two serious problems. First, the air-filled stomach reduces lung volume by forcing up the diaphragm. Second, regurgitation (the passive expulsion of fluids and partially digested foods from the stomach into the throat) or vomiting (the forceful expulsion of the stomach's contents) are strong possibilities. This could lead to additional airway obstruction or the **aspiration** (AS-pir-AY-shun), or breathing in, of vomitus into the patient's lungs. When this happens, lung damage can occur and a lethal form of pneumonia may develop.

The best way to avoid gastric distention, or to avoid making it worse once it develops, is to position the patient's head properly, avoid too forceful and too quickly delivered ventilations, and limit the volume of ventilations delivered. The volume delivered should be limited to the size breath that causes the chest to rise. This is why it is so important to watch the patient's chest rise as each ventilation is delivered and to feel for resistance to your breaths.

When gastric distention is present, be prepared for vomiting (Figure BLS-19). If the patient does vomit, roll the entire patient onto his side. (Turning just the head may allow for aspiration of vomitus as well as aggravating any possible neck injury.) Manually stabilize the head and neck of the patient as you roll him. Be prepared to use suction to clear the patient's mouth and throat of vomitus.

Manually pressing on the abdomen to relieve distention in the prehospital setting is not recommended.

The Recovery Position

Patients who resume adequate breathing and pulse after rescue breathing or CPR are placed in the **recovery position,** lying on the side (Fig-

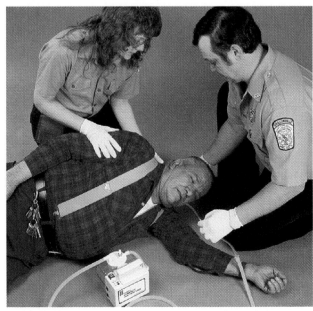

FIGURE BLS-19 Be prepared for vomiting when attempting to relieve gastric distention.

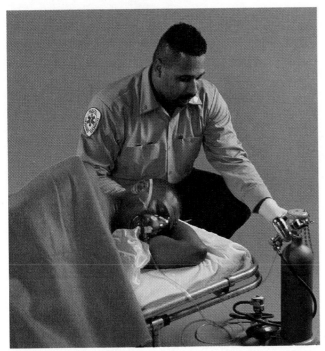

FIGURE BLS-20 Place the breathing but unresponsive patient who has no head, neck, or spine injury in the recovery position to protect the airway.

ure BLS-20). This position is also suitable for patients who are unconscious with adequate pulse and respirations. The recovery position allows for drainage from the mouth and prevents the tongue from falling backward and causing an airway obstruction.

The patient should be rolled onto his side. This should be done moving the patient as a unit, that is, not twisting the head, shoulders, or torso. The patient may be rolled onto either side; however it is preferable to have the patient facing you so that monitoring and suctioning may be more easily performed.

If the patient does not have respirations that are sufficient to support life, the recovery position must not be used. The patient should be placed supine and his ventilations assisted.

Warning: Do not use the recovery position for patients who have possible spinal injuries.

CPR

Assessing Circulation

Cardiac Arrest

The oxygen a patient breathes in is picked up from the lungs by the blood and carried to the body cells as the heart beats and pumps the blood around the body. This **circulation** of blood around the body is necessary to life. *Cardiac arrest* is the term used to mean that the heart has stopped beating and circulating blood. CPR is begun when a patient is in cardiac arrest as an artificial way of circulating blood.

Checking the Carotid Pulse

If a patient has been in respiratory arrest for a few minutes, he may have developed cardiac arrest as well. You can determine if the heart is still beating and circulating blood by feeling for the **carotid pulse** (Figure BLS-21) in the patient's neck.

While stabilizing the patient's head and maintaining the proper head-tilt, use your hand that is closest to the patient's neck to locate his "Adam's apple" (the prominent bulge in the front of the neck). Place the tips of your index and middle fingers directly over the midline of this structure. (Do not use your thumb. It has a pulse that you may feel instead of the patient's pulse.) Slide your fingertips to the side of the patient's neck closest to you. Keep the palm side of your fingertips against the patient's neck. (*Do not* slide your fingertips to the opposite side of the patient's neck which may cause you to put pressure on the trachea and interfere with the patient's airway.) Feel for a groove between the Adam's apple and the muscles located along the side of the neck. Very little pressure needs to be applied to the neck to feel the carotid pulse.

The reason for feeling for the carotid pulse, rather than for a pulse at the wrist or elsewhere, is that a heartbeat that is too faint to be felt at the wrist or other area may still be felt in the

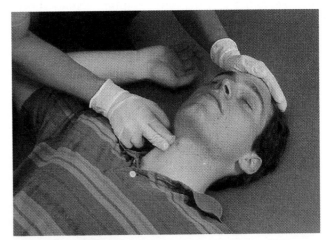

FIGURE BLS-21 Check the carotid pulse to confirm circulation.

neck. IT IS DANGEROUS TO DO CPR ON A PATIENT WHOSE HEART IS STILL BEATING. Therefore, it is the carotid pulse that you must feel in order to determine if cardiac arrest has occurred and CPR should be started. If the patient has a pulse, even a very weak pulse, you may continue rescue breathing, but *you must not perform chest compressions.* In other words, you will begin CPR only if there is *no* carotid pulse.

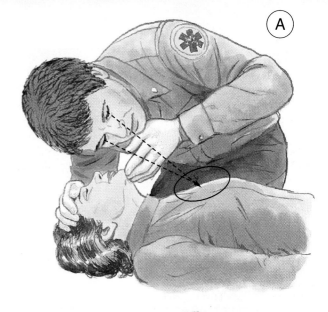

How CPR Works

Cardiopulmonary resuscitation is the basic life support measure applied when a patient's heart and lung actions have stopped. During CPR, you will have to

- Maintain an open airway.
- Breathe for the patient.
- Perform chest compressions to force the patient's blood to circulate.

These steps are related to and follow the sequence of the ABCs in which A = Airway, B = Breathing, and C = Circulation (Figure BLS-22).

CPR is a method of artificial breathing and circulation. When natural heart action and breathing have stopped, we must provide an artificial means to oxygenate the blood and keep it in circulation. This is accomplished by providing *chest compressions* and *ventilations.*

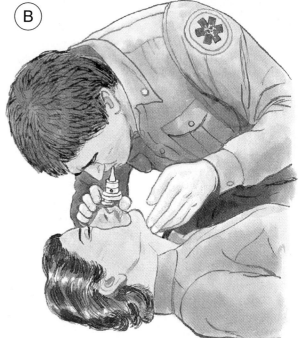

- *To provide chest compressions,* you place the patient supine on a hard surface and compress the chest by applying downward pressure with your hands. This action causes an increase of pressure inside the chest and possible actual compression of the heart itself, one or both of which force the blood out of the heart and into circulation. When pressure is released, the heart refills with blood. The next compression sends this fresh blood into circulation and the cycle continues.
- *To provide ventilations,* you use mouth-to-mask, mouth-to-mouth, mouth-to-nose, or mouth-to-stoma methods as described earlier in this chapter. IT IS HIGHLY RECOMMENDED THAT CPR BE PERFORMED USING A POCKET FACE MASK OR OTHER BARRIER DEVICE AS PROTECTION AGAINST INFECTIOUS DISEASES.

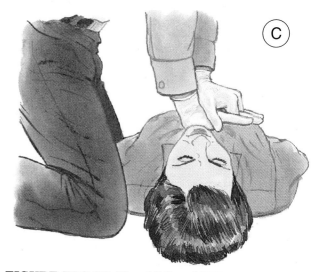

FIGURE BLS-22 The ABCs of CPR.

Remember: Both compressions and ventilations are necessary in CPR. One does little good without the other. Compressions without ventilations would circulate blood without enough oxygen in it to sustain brain or heart function. Ventilations without compressions would force oxygen into the lungs without circulating the blood to pick up the oxygen and deliver it to the body.

Steps Leading to CPR

The American Heart Association has established a series of steps that should be followed before CPR is begun. (The steps described here are for an adult patient. Special steps for infants and children will be described later in this chapter.) These steps are

1. ESTABLISH UNRESPONSIVENESS—Is the patient responsive? Gently shake the patient's shoulder and shout, "ARE YOU OKAY?" If the patient is conscious and able to speak clearly, you know that his ABCs are all right for the present. He would not be conscious or able to speak if he did not have an open airway, breathing, and heartbeat.

Note: If the mechanism of injury suggests possible spinal injury, protect the head and spine while establishing unresponsiveness.

2. CALL FOR HELP—If the patient is unresponsive, you know that he may have an obstructed airway, may be without respirations, and/or may be without circulation (without heartbeat and pulse). If you are working alone, however, DO NOT BEGIN RESUSCITATION BEFORE YOU HAVE CALLED FOR HELP. Call 911 or your local emergency number or radio to your dispatch center, then immediately continue your assessment and care for the ABCs.
3. REPOSITION THE PATIENT, if necessary, placing him supine on a hard surface. Be sure to turn the patient as a unit, protecting the alignment of head and spine.
4. ESTABLISH AN OPEN AIRWAY—This should be done by the head-tilt, chin-lift, or jaw-thrust maneuver (use the jaw thrust if spinal injury is suspected). Usually, at this time, you can easily check to see if the patient is a neck breather.

5. CHECK FOR BREATHING—Use the LOOK, LISTEN, and FEEL method, taking no more than 3 to 5 seconds to determine if the patient is breathing. A patient who is breathing adequately does not immediately need either ventilations or CPR. If the patient is not breathing, you should . . .
6. DELIVER ONE BREATH—Use rescue breathing techniques described earlier in this chapter. The breath should take 1½ to 2 seconds to deliver. Allow time for deflation. If the breath is unsuccessful, REPOSITION THE PATIENT'S HEAD (or jaw if using the jaw-thrust maneuver) to try to correct the airway opening, then DELIVER ANOTHER BREATH. If these initial breaths are unsuccessful and you believe there may be an upper airway obstruction, begin techniques to CLEAR THE AIRWAY (e.g., the Heimlich maneuver or chest thrusts and finger sweeps). If the patient's airway is clear and he is still in respiratory arrest . . .
7. CHECK FOR A CAROTID PULSE—Maintain the head tilt with one hand on the patient's forehead and use your other hand to feel for a carotid pulse in the patient's neck. IF THERE IS A PULSE but the patient is not breathing, continue rescue breathing. IF THERE IS NO PULSE after 5 to 10 seconds of palpation the patient is in cardiac arrest and you should . . .
8. BEGIN CPR.

Remember: DO NOT INITIATE CPR ON ANY PATIENT WHO HAS A CAROTID PULSE.

Note: Bleeding can prevent proper and adequate circulation. If a patient has lost too much blood, then CPR will not be effective. When bleeding is very profuse, as in the case of a severed major artery, CPR might speed up the patient's blood loss. Oxygenated blood would be circulated, but the patient would bleed to death. If CPR accelerates blood loss, the bleeding may have to be quickly controlled. This situation is rare, but it is critical when it occurs.

How to Do CPR

CPR can be done by one or by two rescuers. All of the information below under "Positioning the Patient," "Finding the CPR Compression Site,"

"Providing Chest Compressions," and "Providing Ventilations" applies to both one-rescuer and two-rescuer CPR. Specific information about each type of CPR then follows under "One-Rescuer CPR" and "Two-Rescuer CPR." Scans BLS-5, -6, -7, -8, and -9 can help you follow and review these procedures as they are described below. These procedures are for an adult patient. Procedures for infants and children will be described later in this chapter.

Positioning the Patient

The cardiac arrest patient must be placed supine on a hard surface, such as the floor or ground or a spine board. If the patient is in bed or on an ambulance stretcher, a backboard or similar rigid object should be placed under the patient. *Do not* delay CPR to find a rigid object if one is not at hand. Instead, move the patient to the floor. CPR cannot be delayed because of patient injury. If you are alone, *do not* try to immobilize the spine or splint fractures before initiating CPR. It is critical that CPR be started as soon as possible without regard to injuries or aggravation of injuries that may result—except for taking due care to attempt to keep the head and neck aligned while moving the patient and using the jaw-thrust maneuver to open the airway if spinal injury is suspected. Saving the patient's life is the first consideration.

Finding the CPR Compression Site

First visualize the location of the heart, which lies at about the midline of the body between the **sternum,** or breastbone, and the spinal column. The upper seven pairs of the ribs attach to the sternum. These, along with the **clavicles** (KLAV-i-kulz), or collarbones, support the sternum over the heart.

To be effective and prevent serious injury to the patient, chest compressions must be delivered to the *CPR compression site* on the sternum (Scan BLS-5). Locate the CPR compression site by using the following technique.

1. Kneel alongside the patient. Face the patient with your knees at the level of the patient's shoulders. This will allow you to perform ventilations and chest compressions without having to move your knees. Have your knees shoulder-width apart for balance and stability.
2. Use the index and middle fingers of your hand closest to the patient's feet to locate the lower margin (border) of the rib cage. Do this on the side of the chest closest to your knees.
3. Move your fingers along the rib cage toward the center of the patient's body. Stop when you find the location where the ribs meet the sternum. This area is called the **substernal notch.** Keep your middle finger at this notch and your index finger resting on the lower tip of the sternum.
4. Now move your other hand and place it so the heel of that hand is resting against your index finger and is centered on the sternum. This is the CPR compression site. Your hand is placed over the lower half of the sternum, centered from side to side.
5. The hand that was used to locate the substernal notch is now placed over the hand on the CPR compression site (Figure BLS-23). The fingers of both hands are pointing away from your body. You may interlace or extend your fingers, but you must KEEP YOUR FINGERS OFF THE PATIENT'S CHEST.

This position provides a centered compression and avoids injury to the patient's ribs or

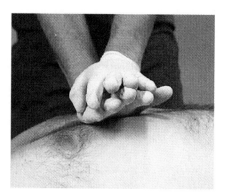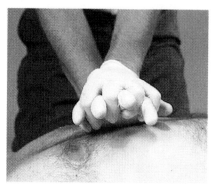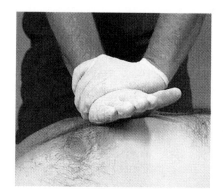

FIGURE BLS-23 Hand placement for compressions.

Locating the CPR Compression Site

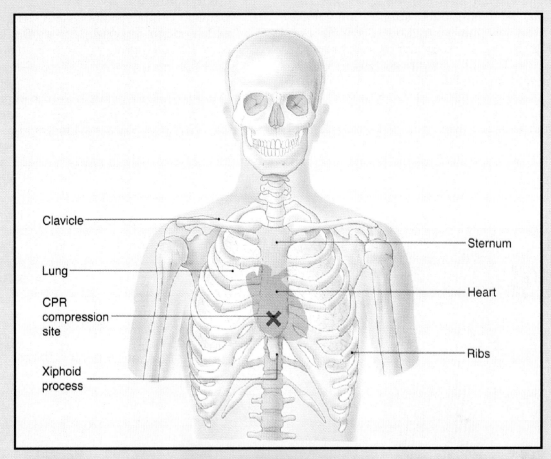

- Clavicle
- Lung
- CPR compression site
- Xiphoid process
- Sternum
- Heart
- Ribs

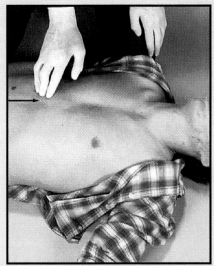

1. Use the index and middle fingers of the hand that is closest to the patient's feet to locate the lower border of the rib cage.

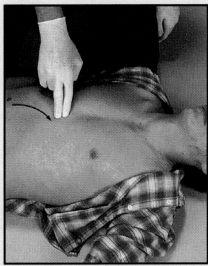

2. Move your fingers along the rib cage to the point where the ribs meet the sternum, the substernal notch. Keep your middle finger at the notch and your index finger resting on the lower tip of the sternum.

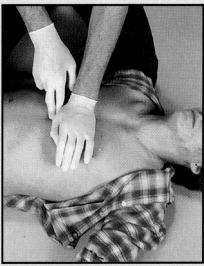

3. Move your hand to the midline. Place its thumb side against the index finger of the lower hand.

795

internal organs. You are now ready to provide compressions.

Providing Chest Compressions

To summarize what has been done so far: The patient has been positioned supine on a hard surface. You are on your knees, which are shoulder-width apart. Your hands are properly positioned on the CPR compression site, which is midline and on the lower half of the sternum. Now . . .

1. Straighten your arms and lock your elbows (Figure BLS-24). You must not bend the elbows when delivering or releasing compressions.

2. Make certain that your shoulders are directly over your hands (directly over the patient's sternum). This will allow you to deliver compressions straight down onto the site. Keep both of your knees on the ground or floor.

3. Deliver compressions STRAIGHT DOWN, with enough force to depress the sternum of a typical adult 1½ to 2 inches (Figure BLS-25).

Note: Monitoring the depth of your compressions is one way to determine if they are adequate—the *only* way, if you are working alone. Another method for determining whether your compressions are adequate is to have someone else feel for a carotid pulse while you perform

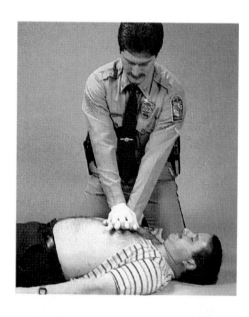

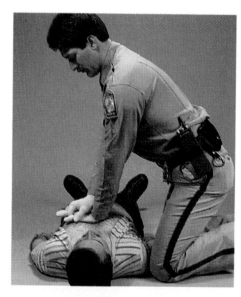

FIGURE BLS-24 The shoulders are placed directly over the compression site.

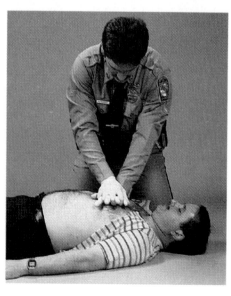

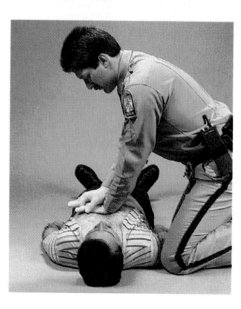

FIGURE BLS-25 Compressions are delivered straight down.

compressions. When CPR compressions are being performed properly, they should produce a carotid pulse. Never try to feel for a carotid pulse during compressions if you are by yourself; rather, perform compressions at 1½ to 2 inches until help arrives.

4. Fully release pressure on the patient's sternum, but *do not* bend your elbows and *do not* lift your hands from the sternum, which can cause you to lose correct positioning of your hands. Your movement should be from your hips, the hips acting as a fulcrum. Compressions should be delivered in a rhythmic, not a "jabbing," fashion. THE AMOUNT OF TIME YOU SPEND COMPRESSING SHOULD BE THE SAME AS THE TIME FOR THE RELEASE. This is known as the **50:50 rule:** 50% compression, 50% release.

Providing Ventilations

Ventilations are given between sets of compressions. You are to use the same techniques that you learned for rescue breathing as described earlier in this chapter. Mouth-to-mask, mouth-to-mouth, mouth-to-nose, mask-to-stoma, or mouth-to-stoma methods can be used as needed. REMEMBER THAT USE OF A POCKET FACE MASK OR OTHER BARRIER DEVICE IS RECOMMENDED AS PROTECTION AGAINST INFECTIOUS DISEASES (Figure BLS-26). Provide each ventilation with enough force so that you observe the patient's chest rise. Breaths provided slowly (at 1½ to 2 seconds for each breath) and with adequate but not too great force, will help prevent gastric distention, which is caused when air is forced into the stomach.

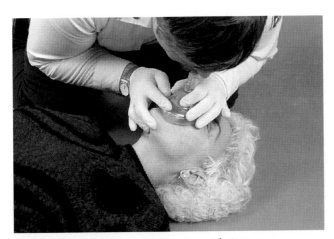

FIGURE BLS-26 Providing ventilations.

One-Rescuer CPR

Refer to Scan BLS-6, which shows the techniques of one-rescuer CPR for the adult patient. Follow this page step by step as you practice on the adult manikins provided for your training.

Compressions and Ventilations: Rates and Ratios

One-rescuer CPR is delivered as follows (see also Table BLS-3).

- COMPRESSIONS—80 to 100 per minute (15 compressions every 10 seconds will put you in the middle of this range)
- VENTILATIONS—2 breaths after every 15 compressions, each breath 1½ to 2 seconds in duration (exhalation takes place naturally; do not delay return to compressions to watch for exhalation)
- RATIO—15 compressions to 2 ventilations (15:2)

During one-rescuer CPR, time is taken away from compressions in order to provide ventilations. Even though you are delivering compressions at the rate of 80 to 100 per minute, usually only 60 compressions are delivered in 1 minute because of the breaks for ventilation. To be certain that you are delivering compressions at the correct rate, you should say "One-and, two-and, three-and, four-and, five-and, . . ." until you reach 15 compressions. Don't take time to say "and" after "fifteen," but immediately deliver two ventilations, relocate the CPR compression site, and begin the next set of 15 compressions.

Once CPR is begun it should not be interrupted unless absolutely necessary. Interruptions in CPR are discussed later in the chapter.

Checking for Pulse and Breathing

CPR should be carried out for approximately ONE MINUTE, or FOUR CYCLES of 15 compressions and 2 ventilations. At this point you should check for a carotid pulse (3 to 5 seconds). At the same time look, listen, and feel for breathing. If there is no pulse, return to CPR. If there is a pulse but no breathing, perform rescue breathing. If there are both pulse and breathing, continue to monitor both carefully, taking care to check every few minutes for a carotid pulse.

CPR should not be delayed for more than a few seconds for a pulse-and-breathing check. If

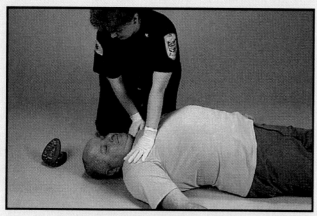

1. Establish unresponsiveness and reposition. (Call for help if you are working alone.)

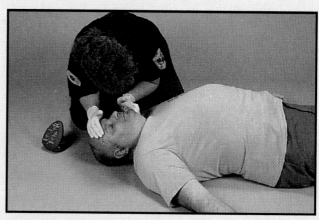

2. Open airway.

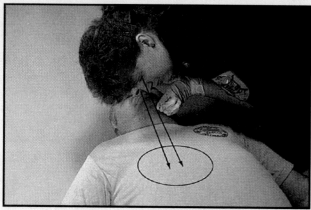

3. Look, listen, and feel for breath (3-5 seconds).

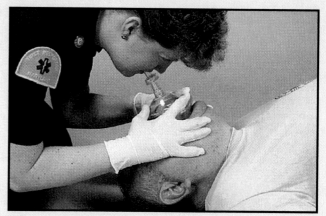

4. Ventilate once (1½ to 2 sec/ventilation). If unsuccessful, reposition patient's head and attempt ventilation again. Clear the airway if necessary.

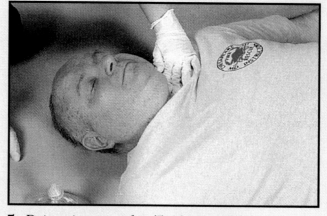

5. Determine no pulse (5-10 seconds).

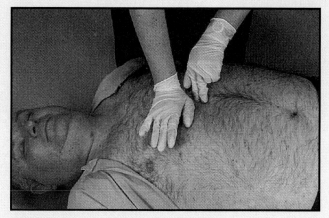

6. Locate compression site.

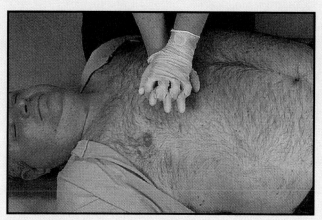

7. Position hands.

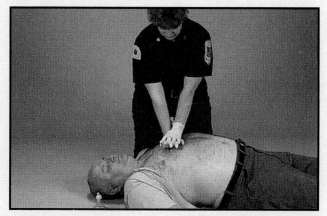

8. Begin compressions (Compressions at depth of 1½ to 2 inches, delivered at a rate of 80-100/minute).

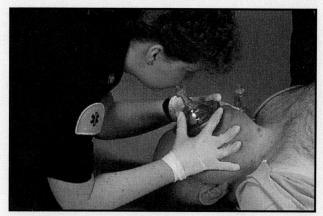

9. Ventilate twice. (Provide 2 ventilations every 15 compressions.)

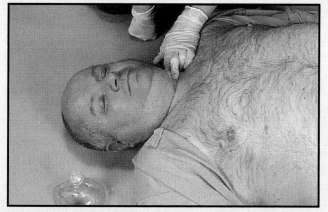

10. Recheck pulse and breathing after 4 cycles, then every few minutes.

Remember: When alone, call for help as soon as unresponsiveness is established.

TABLE BLS-3 CPR for Adults, Children, and Infants

	Adult	Child	Infant
Age	8 yrs and older	1-8 yrs	birth-1 yr
Compression depth	1½ to 2 inches	1 to 1½ inches	½ to 1 inch (newborn ½ to ¾ inch)
Compression rate	80-100/min.	100/min.	at least 100/min. (newborn 120/min.)
Each ventilation	1½ to 2 seconds	1 to 1½ seconds	1 to 1½ seconds
Pulse check location	carotid artery (throat)	carotid artery (throat)	brachial artery (upper arm)
One-rescuer CPR compressions-to-ventilations ratio	15:2	5:1	5:1 (newborn 3:1)
Two-rescuer CPR compressions-to-ventilations ratio	5:1	5:1	Two-rescuer CPR not performed on an infant.
When working alone: Call 911 or emergency dispatcher	After establishing unresponsiveness—before beginning resuscitation	After establishing unresponsiveness and 1 minute of resuscitation	After establishing unresponsiveness and 1 minute of resuscitation

CPR is continued after the first check, break to check for a carotid pulse and the return of spontaneous breathing every few minutes thereafter. After breaking for the pulse-and-breathing check, resume CPR with chest compressions rather than ventilations.

Considerations for the Single Rescuer

Remember, you may be called upon to perform CPR while off duty or even on duty, but by yourself. Begin the sequence for CPR by checking for responsiveness. ONCE YOU FIND THE PATIENT UNRESPONSIVE, ACTIVATE THE EMS SYSTEM BEFORE ANY FURTHER ASSESSMENT OR CPR. Call 911 or your local emergency number. If you have a radio, contact the EMS dispatcher for assistance. Tell the dispatcher

1. The location of the emergency (with cross streets or roads, if possible)
2. The telephone number you are calling from
3. What you believe has happened (e.g., heart attack, fall, vehicle collision)
4. How many persons need help
5. The condition of the patient or patients
6. What aid you are giving or plan to give the patient or patients
7. What additional help is needed (e.g., advanced life support, fire department)
8. Other information dispatcher requests

Relay the information accurately but swiftly and return to the patient.

Remember that it is recommended that CPR be conducted using a pocket face mask or other barrier device as protection against infectious diseases. Any of these devices that have a strap that holds the mask on the patient's face is best for one-rescuer CPR. It will hold the mask in place while you are doing compressions. Devices without a strap will need to be placed on the patient's face after each set of compressions.

Two-Rescuer CPR

Refer to Scan BLS-7, which shows the techniques of two-rescuer CPR for the adult patient. Follow this page step by step as you practice on the adult manikins provided for your training. In the Scan, both rescuers are shown on the same side of the patient to allow you to see what each person is doing. *The procedure goes more smoothly if the rescuers are on opposite sides of the patient.* This is particularly true when position changes are taking place. Once in the ambulance, the procedure will have to be done with one rescuer providing ventilations with supplemental oxygen while positioned at the patient's head.

There are several advantages to two-rescuer CPR. The patient receives more oxygen (since ventilations are given more frequently and by a rescuer whose main responsibility is ventilation rather than chest compressions), circulation and blood pressure improve (since chest compressions, though interrupted more frequently, are

Two-Rescuer CPR

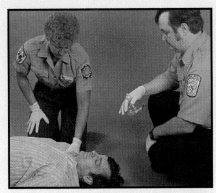

1. Determine unresponsiveness. Position patient.

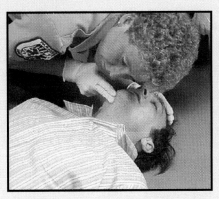

2. Open the airway and look, listen, and feel for breath (3-5 seconds).

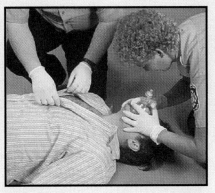

3. Ventilate once (1½ to 2 sec/ventilation). If unsuccessful, reposition head and try again. Clear airway if necessary.

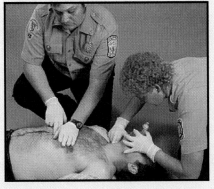

4. Determine pulselessness. Locate CPR compression site.

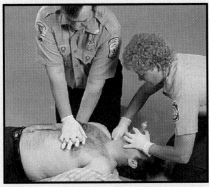

5. Say "no pulse." Begin compressions.

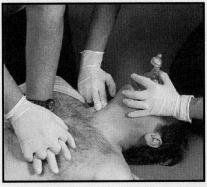

6. Check compression effectiveness. Deliver 5 compressions in 3-4 seconds (80-100/ minute).

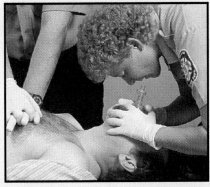

7. Stop for compressions ventilation. Ventilate once (1½ to 2 sec/ ventilation).

8. Continue with 1 ventilation every 5 compressions.

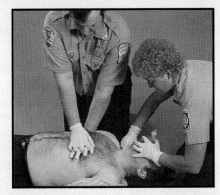

9. After a few minutes, reassess breathing and pulse. No pulse—say "Continue CPR." Pulse—say, "Stop CPR."

Note: Assess for spontaneous breathing and pulse at the end of the first minute, and then every few minutes thereafter.

not interrupted for as long), and the problem of rescuer fatigue is lessened. CPR with two rescuers also makes it easier to use barrier devices such as pocket face masks and bag-valve masks, since there is not the difficulty posed by a single rescuer having to move from ventilations to chest compressions and back again.

Compressions and Ventilations: Rates and Ratios

Two-rescuer CPR is delivered as follows (see also Table BLS-3).

- COMPRESSIONS—80 to 100 per minute (about 5 compressions every 3–4 seconds)
- VENTILATIONS—1 breath after every 5 compressions, each breath 1½ to 2 seconds in duration (exhalation takes place naturally during the next compression)
- RATIO—5 compressions to 1 ventilation (5:1)

The compressor counts out loud saying, "one and two and three and four and five, breathe." The compressor pauses for 1½ to 2 seconds to allow the ventilator to deliver a breath. After the breath has been delivered, the compressor resumes. Between ventilations, the ventilator may check the carotid pulse to determine the effectiveness of compressions.

Note: If the ventilator misses a breath, he should not wait for the next fifth stroke to provide the ventilation. Instead, he should deliver this missed ventilation on the upstroke of the next compression.

Checking for Pulse and Breathing

After the first minute of CPR and every few minutes thereafter, the ventilator should check to see if the patient has a carotid pulse and also to look for spontaneous breathing. Since compressions will cause a pulse, to get a true check of the patient's status (whether spontaneous heartbeats have resumed) compressions must be stopped for pulse checks. A pulse check during CPR should take only 3 to 5 seconds. If a pulse is detected, the ventilator should say, "Stop compressions." Rescue breathing should continue to be provided if needed. If there is no pulse, the ventilator should say, "No pulse. Continue CPR." CPR is then continued, beginning with chest compressions.

How to Join CPR in Progress

If you wish to join another member of the EMS System who has initiated CPR, you should

1. Ask to help.
2. Allow the first rescuer to complete a cycle of 15 compressions and 2 ventilations.
3. Assume the responsibility for compressions and allow the first rescuer to become the ventilator if he wishes, since many rescuers consider ventilation to be less strenuous than compression.

If CPR has been started by someone who is certified to do CPR but is not part of the EMS System and you join this person to start CPR

1. Identify yourself and your training and state that you are ready to perform two-rescuer CPR.
2. While the first rescuer is providing compressions, spend five seconds checking for a carotid pulse produced by each compression. This is to determine if the compressions being delivered are effective. Inform the first rescuer if there is or is not a pulse being produced. (If the first rescuer cannot deliver effective compressions, you will have to take over for him when CPR is resumed.)
3. You should say, "Stop compressions" and check for spontaneous pulse and breathing. This should take only a few seconds.
4. If there is no pulse, you should state, "No pulse. Continue CPR."
5. The switch from one-rescuer to two-rescuer CPR should take place after the first rescuer has completed a cycle of 15 compressions and 2 ventilations.
6. The first rescuer resumes compressions, and the second rescuer provides a ventilation during a brief pause after every fifth compression. If desired, the second rescuer can start compressions and allow the first rescuer to provide the ventilations.

Note: If you are off duty and arrive after CPR has been started, let the first rescuer know that you are trained in CPR. If you find that the first rescuer does not know CPR or is not performing effectively, stop him and take over, providing one-rescuer techniques. Always verify that someone has activated the EMS system.

Should you find yourself providing CPR while off duty, you may be able to have a bystander assist you in the two-rescuer method. However, be certain that the bystander has been trained by the American Heart Association or the American Red Cross in CPR. Too often people wish to help thinking they know the procedure based on what they have seen on television, without the benefit of formal CPR training. If you begin two-rescuer CPR with the aid of a bystander and find that he is unable to perform properly and you cannot quickly correct the problem, stop the two-rescuer procedure and begin one-rescuer CPR. The volunteer may be sent to confirm that EMS is en route or to direct the incoming ambulance crew to the patient.

How to Change Positions

When two rescuers are performing CPR, one of the rescuers may wish to change positions (Scan BLS-8). Often the compressor is the one who becomes fatigued, but the ventilator also may request a change. The most important factor in the change is that it be done in as little time as possible. The compressor controls the change and will signal the pending change at the beginning of a series of compressions as follows: "CHANGE. One and two and three and four and five, BREATHE." The ventilator will provide one full breath, and the two rescuers will quickly change positions.

The rescuer who was previously providing compressions is now the ventilator. This rescuer opens the airway immediately upon reaching the patient's head and checks for a carotid pulse and respirations. These checks should take no more than 3 to 5 seconds. If a change takes place every 2 minutes or less, a check of pulse and breathing does not need to be done on every change.

CPR Techniques for Infants and Children

The techniques of CPR for infants and small children are essentially the same as those used for adults (See Scan BLS-9). You will have to

1. Establish unresponsiveness.
2. Correctly position the patient.
3. Open the airway (head-tilt, chin-lift, or jaw-thrust).
4. Establish respiratory arrest (3 to 5 seconds).

5. Provide artificial ventilations and clear the airway, if necessary.
6. Establish the lack of pulse in 5 to 10 seconds.
7. Provide chest compressions and ventilations.
8. Do frequent assessments of pulse and breathing. This is to be done every few minutes.

Some procedures and rates differ when the patient is an infant or a child. If younger than 1 year of age, the patient is considered to be an infant. Between 1 and 8 years of age, the patient is considered to be a child. Over the age of 8 years, adult procedures apply to the patient. Keep in mind that the size of the patient can also be an important factor. A very small 9-year old may have to be treated as a child.

Positioning the Patient

When CPR must be performed, adults, children, and infants are placed on their backs on a hard surface. For an infant, the hard surface can be the rescuer's hand or forearm.

Opening the Airway

For an infant or a child, use the head-tilt, chin-lift or the jaw-thrust technique, but apply only a slight tilt for an infant. Too great a tilt may close off the infant's airway; however, make certain that the opening is adequate (note chest rise during ventilation). Always be sure to support an infant's head.

Establishing a Pulse

Take these steps to establish a pulse in an infant or a child.

- INFANT—For infants, you should use the **brachial** (BRAY-key-al) **pulse.** This is the pulse that can be felt when compressing the major artery of the upper arm, the brachial artery (Figure BLS-27). Do not use the carotid or radial pulse. To find the brachial pulse

1. Locate the point halfway between the infant's elbow and shoulder.
2. Place your thumb on the outer side of the upper arm at this midway point.

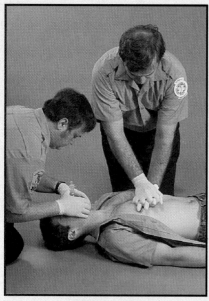

1. When fatigued, the compressor calls for the switch.

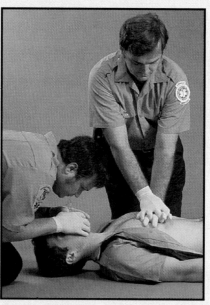

2. Compressor completes fifth compression. Ventilator provides one ventilation.

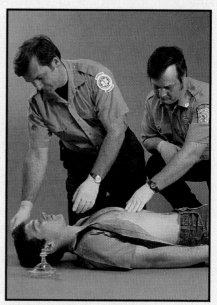

3. Ventilator moves to chest and begins to locate compression site. Compressor moves to head.

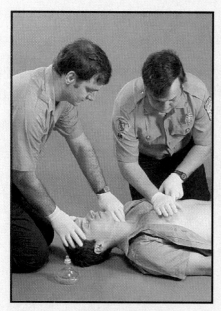

4. New compressor finds site. New ventilator checks carotid pulse.

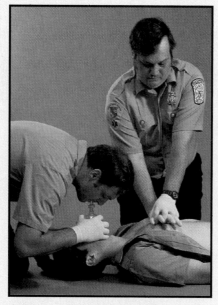

5. New ventilator says, "No pulse." Both rescuers in new position, ready to continue CPR.

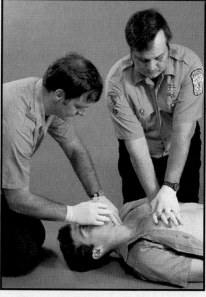

6. New compressor delivers 5 compressions (3-4 seconds) at a rate of 80-100 per minute. New ventilator assesses effectiveness of compressions.

Note: Both rescuers are shown on same side of patient for purpose of clarity. When performing CPR, rescuers should be positioned on opposite sides of patient.

CPR Summary—Adult Patient

ONE RESCUER	FUNCTIONS	TWO RESCUERS
	• Establish unresponsiveness • If there's no response, call 911 • Position patient • Open airway • Look, listen, and feel (for 3-5 seconds)	
	• Deliver 1 breath (1½–2 sec). If unsuccessful, reposition head and try again. Clear airway if necessary.	
	• Check carotid pulse. . . (5-10 seconds) If no pulse. . . • Begin chest compressions	

	DELIVER COMPRESSIONS	
	1½–2 inches 80-100/min (15/9-11 sec)	1½–2 inches 80-100/min (5/3-4 sec)

	DELIVER VENTILATIONS 10-12 breaths/min	
	15:2	5:1 (Pause to allow ventilations)
	• Do 4 cycles • Check pulse	• Ventilator checks effective-ness

CONTINUE PERIODIC ASSESSMENT

Changing Postions

• Compressor—signal to change; provide 5 compressions • Ventilator—1 ventilation	New ventilator checks pulse If no pulse, instructs compressor to begin CPR	Continue CPR sequence

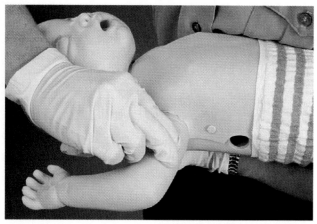

FIGURE BLS-27 For infants, determine circulation by feeling for a brachial pulse.

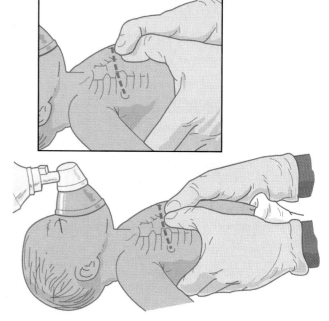

FIGURE BLS-28 Performing chest compressions on a newborn infant.

3. Place the tips of your index and middle fingers at the midway point on the inner surface of the infant's upper arm. You will feel a groove in the muscle at this location.
4. Press your index and middle fingers in toward the bone, taking care not to exert too much pressure. To do so may collapse the artery, stopping circulation to the lower arm and perhaps causing you to miss feeling the pulse.
5. Take 5 to 10 seconds to determine pulselessness. If no pulse is felt after 10 seconds, begin CPR.

    • CHILD—Determine circulation in the same manner as for an adult. Check 5 to 10 seconds at the carotid artery for a pulse. If no pulse is felt in 10 seconds, begin CPR.

If you are acting alone and you find an unresponsive infant or child, check airway, breathing, and circulation. If there is no pulse, start CPR. DO CPR FOR 1 MINUTE BEFORE ACTIVATING THE EMS SYSTEM.

Chest Compressions

Follow these procedures to provide chest compressions to an infant or a child .

    • NEWBORN—Place both thumbs on the middle third of the sternum with your fingers encircling the chest and supporting the infant's back (Figure BLS-28). The thumbs should be positioned on the sternum just below an imaginary line between the nipples. For a very small newborn, you may have to place one thumb over the other

(Figure BLS-28 inset). The infant's sternum should be depressed ½ to ¾ inch. The pulse should be checked periodically and chest compressions discontinued when the infant's spontaneous heartbeat reaches 80 beats per minute or greater.

    • INFANT—Compressions are delivered to an infant (who is older than a newborn or too large for encircling the chest as described above for the newborn) on the midline of the sternum, one finger-width below an imaginary line drawn between the infant's nipples. This position is easily located by placing the index finger of the hand nearest the infant's feet on the imaginary line between the nipples. This places the middle and ring fingers in the proper area for compressions (Figure BLS-29). The infant's sternum should be depressed ½ to 1 inch.

    • CHILD—Compressions are applied using the heel of one hand. The compression site is the lower third of the sternum one finger-width above the substernal notch, located using the same procedure that is applied to the adult patient (Figure BLS-30). The child's sternum should be depressed 1 to 1½ inches.

Ventilations

Follow the procedures below to provide ventilations to an infant or a child. AS WITH ADULTS,

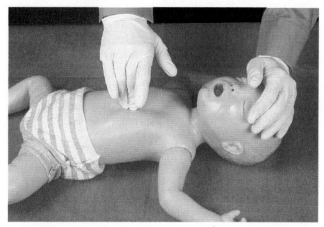

FIGURE BLS-29 Performing chest compressions on an infant.

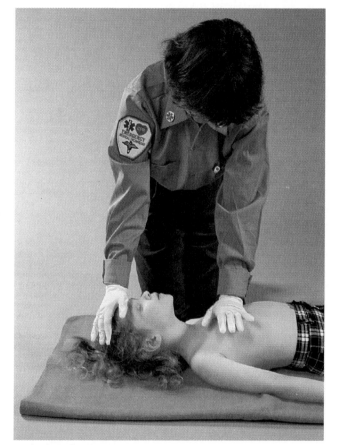

FIGURE BLS-30 Performing chest compressions on a child.

USE A POCKET FACE MASK OR OTHER BAR-RIER DEVICE.

- NEWBORN, INFANT, OR CHILD—Provide a slow, gentle breath (1 to 1½ seconds) using mouth-to-mask, mouth-to-mouth, mouth-to-nose, or (if the patient is small) mouth-to-mouth-and-nose techinique. If a pocket

face mask is to be used, be sure it is the right size for the newborn, infant, or child. Deliver just enough air to cause the patient's chest to rise. It is essential to watch the rise and fall of the patient's chest.

Compressions and Ventilations: Rates and Ratios

For infants and children, deliver compressions and ventilations as follows (see also Table BLS-3).

- NEWBORN—Deliver compressions at the rate of 120 per minute (5 compressions in 2½ seconds). Pause to give a slow (1 to 1½ seconds), gentle breath every 3 compressions for a ratio of 3:1.
- INFANT—Deliver compressions at the rate of at least 100 per minute (5 compressions in no more than 3 seconds). Pause to give a slow (1 to 1½ seconds) gentle breath every 5 compressions for a ratio of 5:1.
- CHILD—Deliver compressions at the rate of 100 per minute (5 compressions every 3 seconds). Pause to give a slow (1 to 1½ seconds) gentle breath every 5 compressions for a ratio of 5:1.

Note: To establish the correct rate for infants and children, count: "One, two, three, four, five, breathe." Provide the ventilation during a pause immediately after "five."

For more about resuscitation of a newborn, see Chapter 24, Obstetrics and Gynecology.

Special Considerations in CPR

How to Know if CPR Is Effective

To determine if CPR is effective

- *If possible have someone else feel for a carotid pulse* during compressions and watch to see the patient's chest rise during ventilations.
- *Listen for exhalation of air,* either naturally or during compressions, as additional veri-fication that air has entered the lungs.

In addition to the above, any of the following indications of effective CPR may be noticed.

- Pupils constrict.
- Skin color improves.
- Heartbeat returns spontaneously.
- Spontaneous, gasping respirations are made.
- Arms and legs move.
- Swallowing is attempted.
- Consciousness returns.

Even at best, the CPR you provide will be only 25% to 33% as effective as normal heart action. To counter this deficiency, you may take several actions.

- Perform CPR as closely as possible to the recommended guidelines.
- Consider using a mechanical-compressor to assist chest compressions if your EMS system provides them and you are trained in their use.
- Avoid stopping CPR or keep interruption of CPR to a minimum.
- Supplemental oxygen should be provided by an EMT-B or other trained person. (Even though supplemental oxygen is significant in basic life support, do not delay or stop CPR in order to set up an oxygen delivery system.)
- Call for assistance from those who can provide defibrillation (electrical shock to the heart) as quickly as possible.
- Call for advanced cardiac life support assistance as quickly as possible.

CPR alone rarely causes the return of spontaneous heartbeat and breathing. The main objective of CPR is to keep a patient who is clinically dead from reaching the irreversible point of biological death. Often defibrillation and advanced life support measures such as medications and advanced airway techniques are required to fully reverse the patient's condition. However, remember, WITHOUT YOUR EFFORTS AT CPR, THERE WOULD BE NO HOPE AT ALL!

If you perform CPR and the patient does not survive, it is most likely because the patient had experienced a severe heart attack with death of heart muscle, had already reached irreversible biological death before CPR could begin, or had injuries too severe to survive. Whether it is your first or your hundredth time, the death of a patient is a traumatic event. Share your feelings with others. Everyone has had similar feelings.

Factors That May Make CPR Ineffective

Ineffective CPR refers to the application of improper resuscitative techniques. The patient's chances for survival greatly improve if CPR is done efficiently. Problems that may decrease the efficiency of CPR include

For ventilations
- The patient's head is not placed in the proper head-tilt, chin-lift or jaw-thrust position for ventilations.
- The patient's mouth is not opened wide enough for air exchange.
- There is not an effective seal made against the patient's face, mouth, or nose.
- The patient's nose is not pinched shut during mouth-to-mouth ventilations.
- The patient's mouth is not closed completely during mouth-to-nose ventilations.
- The ventilations are delivered too rapidly or at too great a volume, and gastric distention develops as air intended for the lungs goes into the stomach.

For chest compressions
- The patient is not lying on a hard surface.
- The rescuer's hands are incorrectly placed.
- There are prolonged interruptions.
- The chest is not sufficiently compressed.
- The compression rate is too rapid or too slow.
- Compressions are jerky, not smooth with 50% of the cycle being compression and 50% being the release of compression.

Interrupting CPR

Once you begin CPR, you may interrupt the process for no more than a few seconds to check for pulse and breathing or to reposition yourself and the patient. The first recommended pulse and breathing check is after the first minute of CPR. You should continue to check for these vital signs every few minutes.

In addition to these built-in interruptions, you may interrupt CPR to

- Move a patient onto a stretcher
- Move a patient down a flight of stairs or through a narrow doorway or hallway, or on and off the ambulance (see "Moving Patients During CPR" following)
- Suction to clear vomitus or airway obstructions
- Allow for defibrillation or advanced cardiac life support measures to be initiated

When CPR is resumed, begin with chest compressions rather than with ventilations.

Moving Patients During CPR

CPR must be continued while the patient is on the stretcher and being transferred to the ambulance, as shown in Scan BLS-10. Ideally, CPR should not be interrupted for more than a few seconds during transfer. When moving the stretcher down stairs or through narrow spaces or in loading it on and off the ambulance, however, interruptions to CPR may take longer than a few seconds. These interruptions can be minimized as follows.

- Stairs—It is difficult to perform CPR on stairs. Perform CPR at the top of the stairs then, on a signal, move the patient down the stairs where CPR is quickly resumed. If there are multiple flights of stairs, stop on each landing to perform CPR before moving to the next level.
- Narrow Hallways and Doors—It is also difficult to maintain a position beside the stretcher while moving through doorways or proceeding down narrow hallways. In these situations, perform CPR until it is time to move through the narrow spot. On signal, discontinue CPR and resume it as quickly as possible when you reach an open area.
- Loading into the Ambulance—Other brief interruptions may be encountered while loading the patient into the ambulance. Delays may be shortened by having a rescuer in the ambulance, ready to start CPR when the stretcher is loaded. The reverse should be done on arrival at the hospital with a rescuer or hospital personnel prepared to begin CPR when the stretcher reaches the ground.

CPR must be continued once the patient is loaded into the ambulance. If you are not an EMT-B or part of the ambulance crew, someone who is will take over CPR aboard the ambulance. The procedures should continue uninterrupted except for suctioning or other essential procedures until the emergency department staff takes over CPR or the physician on duty orders CPR to stop.

Complications of CPR

Injury to the rib cage is the most common complication of CPR. When the hands are placed too high on the sternum, fractures to the upper sternum and the clavicles may occur. If the hands are too low on the sternum, the xiphoid process may be fractured or driven down into the liver, producing severe lacerations (cuts) and profuse internal bleeding. When the hands are placed too far off center, or when they are allowed to slip from their position over the CPR compression site, the ribs or their cartilage attachments may be fractured (Figure BLS-31).

Even when CPR is correctly performed, cartilage attached to the ribs may separate or ribs

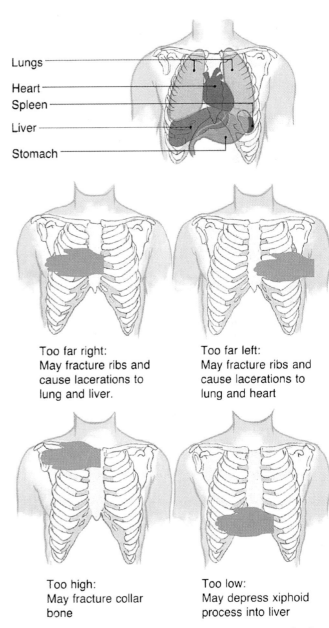

Lungs
Heart
Spleen
Liver
Stomach

Too far right:
May fracture ribs and cause lacerations to lung and liver.

Too far left:
May fracture ribs and cause lacerations to lung and heart

Too high:
May fracture collar bone

Too low:
May depress xiphoid process into liver

FIGURE BLS-31 Improper positioning of the hands during CPR can damage the rib cage and underlying organs.

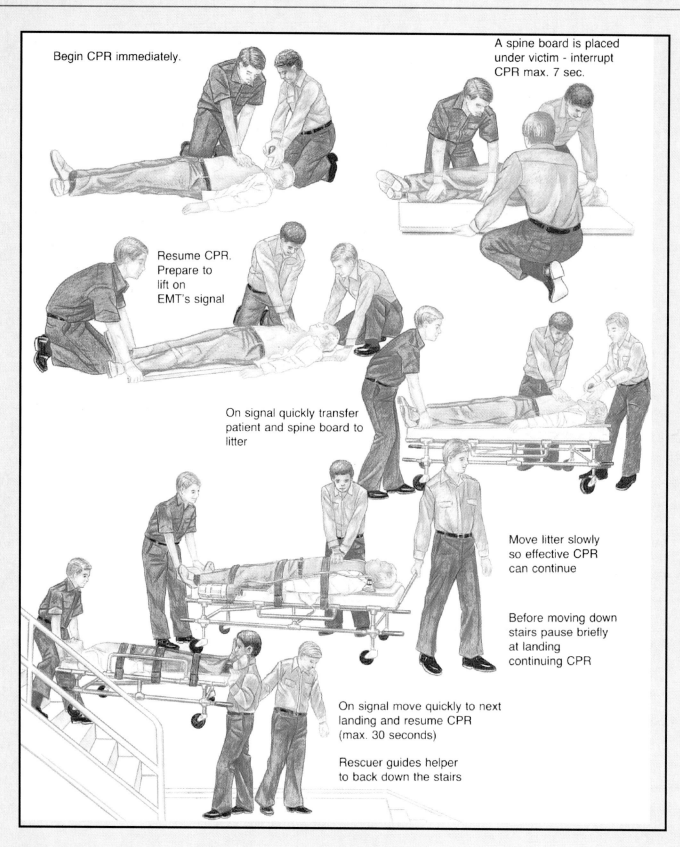

Begin CPR immediately.

A spine board is placed under victim - interrupt CPR max. 7 sec.

Resume CPR. Prepare to lift on EMT's signal

On signal quickly transfer patient and spine board to litter

Move litter slowly so effective CPR can continue

Before moving down stairs pause briefly at landing continuing CPR

On signal move quickly to next landing and resume CPR (max. 30 seconds)

Rescuer guides helper to back down the stairs

may be fractured. In such cases, *do not* stop CPR. Simply reassess your hand position and compression depth and continue CPR. It is far better that the patient suffer a few broken ribs and live than die because you did not continue to perform CPR for fear of inflicting additional injury.

Often when CPR is performed on elderly patients, the first few compressions will separate rib cartilage. When this happens, you may hear a "crunch" as you apply a compression. *Do not stop CPR.* Again, reassess your hand position and the depths of your compressions and continue CPR.

The problem of gastric distention that is associated with artificial ventilations (see earlier in this chapter) also may occur when performing CPR. When performing one-rescuer CPR, the rescuer often rushes to get to the patient's head and ventilate. Ventilations are delivered too fast and too hard. To prevent gastric distention (or ineffective respirations), adequately position the head to open the airway for every ventilation and provide slow (1½ to 2 seconds for adults; 1 to 1½ seconds for infants and children) ventilations that are just adequate to make the chest rise. When gastric distention is present, be alert for vomiting.

Other complications may result from improper CPR efforts, but most are easy to avoid by following American Heart Association guidelines for CPR.

When Not to Begin or to Terminate CPR

As discussed earlier in this chapter, CPR should not be initiated *when you find that the patient— even though unresponsive and perhaps not breathing—does have a pulse.* Usually, of course, you will perform CPR when the patient has no pulse. However, there are special circumstances in which CPR should not be initiated *even though the patient has no pulse.*

- Obvious mortal wounds—These include decapitation, incineration, a severed body, and injuries that are so extensive that CPR cannot be effectively performed (e.g., severe crush injuries to the head, neck, and chest).
- Rigor mortis—This is the stiffening of the body and its limbs that occurs after death, usually within 4 to 10 hours.
- Obvious decomposition.

- A line of lividity—Lividity is a red or purple skin discoloration that occurs when gravity causes the blood to sink to the lowest parts of the body and collect there. Lividity usually indicates that the patient has been dead for more than 15 minutes unless the patient has been exposed to cold temperatures. Using lividity as a sign requires special training.
- Stillbirth—CPR should not be initiated for a stillborn infant who has died hours prior to birth. This infant may be recognized by blisters on the skin, a very soft head, and a strong disagreeable odor.

In all cases, if you are in doubt, seek a physician's advice.

Except in the above instances, when dealing with a patient in cardiac arrest, your duty is to begin CPR immediately. Even though the patient may have a terminal illness or is very old, you cannot decide to withhold CPR. Bystanders may ask you not to begin CPR. Family members may say that the patient would not want your help, but you have no proof of this. Even though many states are now recognizing that resuscitation may violate certain persons' rights to die with dignity, you cannot make such a decision. It would be rare, but it is possible that the people at the scene want the patient to die for less noble reasons.

To refrain from performing resuscitation, you must have written documentation that is accepted by your EMS System. This documentation must be immediately available. You cannot delay starting CPR while someone searches for the document. Once CPR is started, it should be stopped only if the following criteria have been met: At the hospital, the physician's written order sheet can be used to authorize cessation of resuscitation by the professional medical staff. Such an order sheet is often called a "Do Not Resuscitate" or "DNR" order. Your instructor can tell you if DNR orders may be honored by you in your region or state. Become familiar with the form or forms required. In the absence of these regulations, the only person who can tell you not to resuscitate a clinically dead patient is a physician, either on the scene or via radio or telephone. Remember, YOU MUST FOLLOW LOCAL PROTOCOLS.

CPR is most effective if started immediately after cardiac arrest occurs. If a patient has been in arrest for more than ten minutes, resuscitation efforts usually are not effective. However, there are documented cases of adults who were in arrest for more than ten minutes being resuscitated with no major brain damage. Some have survived after being in arrest for well over 30 minutes. Cold air temperatures appear to prolong the time someone can be in arrest before biological death occurs; cold water is even more effective in delaying biological death. Also keep in mind that children and infants may tolerate longer periods of cardiac arrest than adults.

Do not refuse to begin CPR because someone is thought to have been in cardiac arrest for more than 10 minutes. The moment the patient was seen to collapse and the moment of cardiac arrest are not always the same. A patient can be unconscious with minimum effective lung and heart action for quite some time before actual cardiac arrest occurs. Once you have started CPR, you must continue to provide CPR until

- Spontaneous circulation occurs . . . then provide rescue breathing as needed.
- Spontaneous circulation and breathing occur.
- Another trained rescuer can take over for you.
- You turn care of the patient over to a person with a higher level of training.
- You are too exhausted to continue.
- You receive a "no CPR" order from a physician or other authority per local protocols.

If you turn the patient over to another rescuer, this person must be trained to your level or higher. The new rescuer must have certification (American Heart Association or American Red Cross) in basic cardiac life support. If you turn over resuscitation to a person who is certified, but not at your level or higher, it should be because you are exhausted, you need to set up

oxygen delivery or defibrillation equipment, or there are other patients who have life-threatening emergencies. You must supervise the person who has taken over CPR, since you are still responsible for the patient.

Many students have fears of having to stop CPR because of exhaustion. You have to be realistic about patient care and know when you have done all you can for a patient. If you are isolated and have provided CPR for 30 minutes to an hour and are too exhausted to go on, remember that there are physical limitations to the care you can provide. Few patients having received CPR for such a long period of time will survive. You will have done all you could for the patient and should not feel guilty at having to stop CPR.

You lessen the chances of physical exhaustion if you learn to control rescuer hyperventilation. When providing CPR, you establish an irregular pattern of breathing for yourself. This may cause you to begin to breathe very quickly and deeply, unable to regain control. You can help prevent this by keeping in good physical condition and learning not to try to take a breath with each compression. You have to learn to establish a normal breathing rate when delivering chest compressions.

Keeping CPR Skills Current

CPR skills can be quickly lost when not regularly practiced. Be certain to practice CPR on infant, child, and adult manikins. Ideally you should complete a CPR course once every year. One way to stay current in the technique is to become a CPR instructor for the American Heart Association or American Red Cross and teach CPR to the citizens in your community.

CHAPTER REVIEW

KEY TERMS

You may find it helpful to review the following terms.

airway   the passageway for air entering or leaving the body. The structures of the airway are the nose, mouth, pharynx, larynx, trachea, bronchi, and lungs.

aspiration (AS-pir-AY-shun)   the breathing of vomitus or other foreign matter into the lungs.
basic life support   basic live-saving procedures.
biological death   when the brain cells die.
brachial (BRAY-key-al) **pulse**   the pulse measured by feeling the major artery (brachial artery) of the arm. The absence of a brachial

pulse is used as a sign, in infants, that heart-beat has stopped and CPR should begin.

cardiac arrest   when the heart stops beating.

cardiopulmonary resuscitation (KAR-de-o-PUL-mo-ner-e re-SUS-it-TAY-shun), **CPR** a combined effort to provide artificial breathing and circulation of the blood.

carotid pulse   the pulse felt in a person's neck. The absence of a carotid pulse is used as a sign, in adults and children and heartbeat has stopped and CPR should begin.

circulation (SIR-ku-LAY-shun)   the movement of blood as it is pumped throughout the body by the heart.

clavicles (KLAV-i-kulz)   collarbones.

clinical death   when breathing and heartbeat stop.

50:50 rule   the rule that CPR compressions and releases should be equal: 50% compression, 50% release.

Heimlich maneuver   manual thrusts to the abdomen to force bursts of air from the lungs to dislodge an airway obstruction.

recovery position   lying on the side. The recovery position protects the airway by allowing for drainage from the mouth and preventing the tongue from falling backward into the airway.

rescue breathing   providing artificial ventilations to a person who has stopped breathing or whose breathing is inadequate. See also *ventilation*.

respiration (RES-pir-AY-shun)   breathing.

respiratory (RES-pir-uh-tor-e) **arrest** when breathing completely stops.

respiratory failure   the reduction of breathing to the point where not enough oxygen is being taken in to sustain life.

sternum   the breastbone

stoma (STO-mah)   a surgical opening in the neck through which a person breathes.

substernal notch   a general term for the lowest region of the sternum to which the ribs attach.

supine (SOO-pine)   lying on the back.

ventilation Also called *artificial ventillation*. Forcing air or oxygen into the lungs when a patient has stopped breathing or has inadequate breathing. See also *rescue breathing*.

xiphoid (ZIF-oid) **process** a short triangular piece of cartilage (tough, elastic gristle) that extends from the bottom of the sternum.

Reference Section

Skeleton

The skeleton is a living framework made by the joining of bones. It serves to provide support, body movement powered by muscular contractions, protection for the vital organs and other soft structures, blood cell production, and storage for essential minerals. There are 206 bones in the adult body, forming the two divisions of the skeletal system. The axial skeleton is comprised of skull, vertebrae, rib cage, and sternum. The upper and lower extremeties and the shoulder and pelvic girdles form the appendicular skeleton.

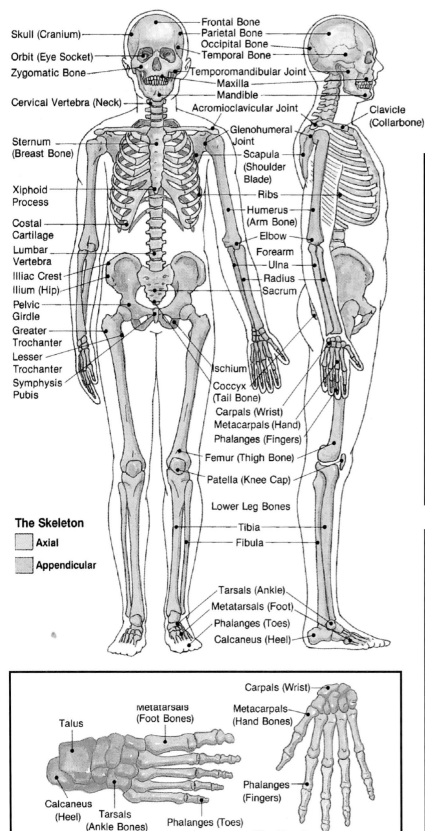

Skull (Cranium)
Orbit (Eye Socket)
Zygomatic Bone
Cervical Vertebra (Neck)
Sternum (Breast Bone)
Xiphoid Process
Costal Cartilage
Lumbar Vertebra
Illiac Crest
Ilium (Hip)
Pelvic Girdle
Greater Trochanter
Lesser Trochanter
Symphysis Pubis

Frontal Bone
Parietal Bone
Occipital Bone
Temporal Bone
Temporomandibular Joint
Maxilla
Mandible
Acromioclavicular Joint
Glenohumeral Joint
Scapula (Shoulder Blade)
Ribs
Humerus (Arm Bone)
Elbow
Forearm
Ulna
Radius
Sacrum
Ischium
Coccyx (Tail Bone)
Carpals (Wrist)
Metacarpals (Hand)
Phalanges (Fingers)
Femur (Thigh Bone)
Patella (Knee Cap)
Lower Leg Bones
Tibia
Fibula

Clavicle (Collarbone)

The Skeleton
☐ Axial
☐ Appendicular

Tarsals (Ankle)
Metatarsals (Foot)
Phalanges (Toes)
Calcaneus (Heel)

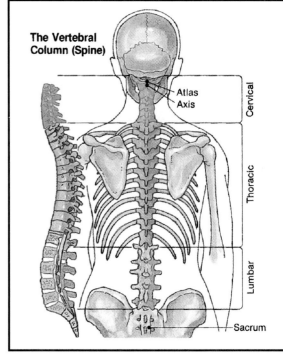

The Vertebral Column (Spine)

Atlas
Axis
Cervical
Thoracic
Lumbar
Sacrum

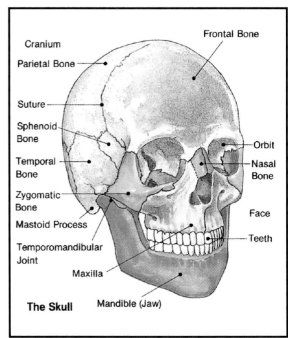

Cranium
Parietal Bone
Suture
Sphenoid Bone
Temporal Bone
Zygomatic Bone
Mastoid Process
Temporomandibular Joint
Maxilla

Frontal Bone
Orbit
Nasal Bone
Face
Teeth
Mandible (Jaw)

The Skull

Talus
Metatarsals (Foot Bones)
Calcaneus (Heel)
Tarsals (Ankle Bones)
Phalanges (Toes)

Carpals (Wrist)
Metacarpals (Hand Bones)
Phalanges (Fingers)

The Hand

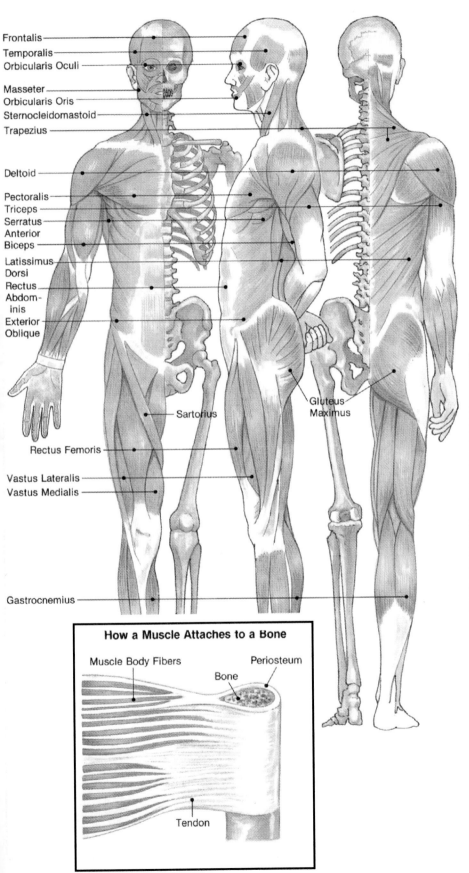

Frontalis
Temporalis
Orbicularis Oculi

Masseter
Orbicularis Oris
Sternocleidomastoid
Trapezius

Deltoid

Pectoralis
Triceps
Serratus
Anterior
Biceps

Latissimus
Dorsi
Rectus
Abdom-
inis
Exterior
Oblique

Sartorius

Gluteus
Maximus

Rectus Femoris

Vastus Lateralis
Vastus Medialis

Gastrocnemius

The tissues of the muscular system comprise 40 to 50% of the body's weight. The skeletal muscles of the body are voluntary muscles, subject to conscious control. They exhibit the properties of excitability; that is, they will react to nerve stimulus. Once stimulated, skeleton muscles are quick to contract and can relax and very quickly be ready for another contraction. There are 501 separate skeletal muscles that provide contractions for movement, coordinated support for posture, and heat production. Muscles connect to bones by way of tendons.

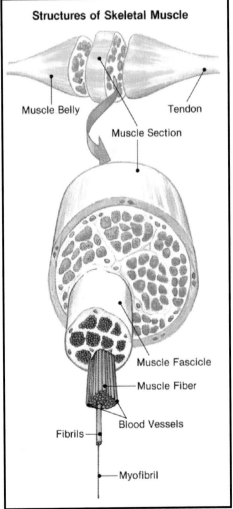

Structures of Skeletal Muscle

Muscle Belly
Tendon
Muscle Section
Muscle Fascicle
Muscle Fiber
Blood Vessels
Fibrils
Myofibril

How a Muscle Attaches to a Bone

Muscle Body Fibers
Periosteum
Bone
Tendon

The Brain

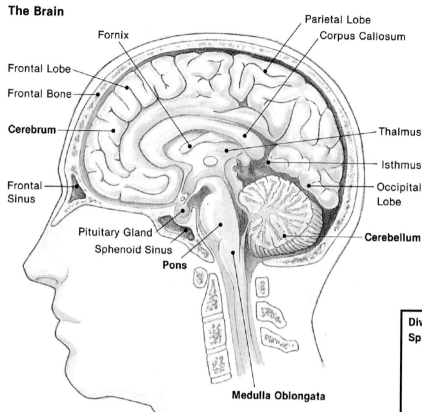

Fornix
Frontal Lobe
Frontal Bone
Cerebrum
Frontal Sinus
Pituitary Gland
Sphenoid Sinus
Pons
Parietal Lobe
Corpus Callosum
Thalmus
Isthmus
Occipital Lobe
Cerebellum
Medulla Oblongata

The nervous system includes the brain, spinal cord, and nerves. Structures within the system may be classified according to divisions: central, peripheral, and autonomic divisions of the nervous system. The central nervous system includes the brain and spinal cord. The sensory (incoming) and motor (outgoing) nerves make up the peripheral nervous system. The autonomic nervous system has structures that parallel the spinal cord and then share the same pathways as the peripheral nerves. This division is involved with motor impulses (outgoing commands) that travel from the central nervous system to the heart muscle, blood vessels, secreting cells of glands, and the smooth muscles of organs. The impulses will stimulate or inhibit certain activities.

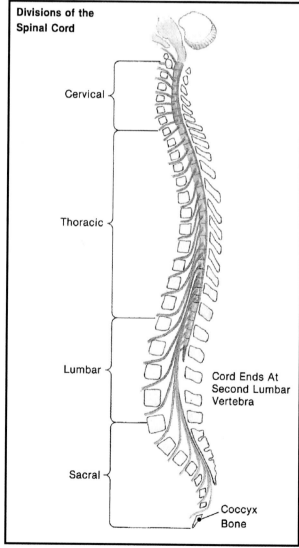

Divisions of the Spinal Cord

Cervical
Thoracic
Lumbar
Sacral
Cord Ends At Second Lumbar Vertebra
Coccyx Bone

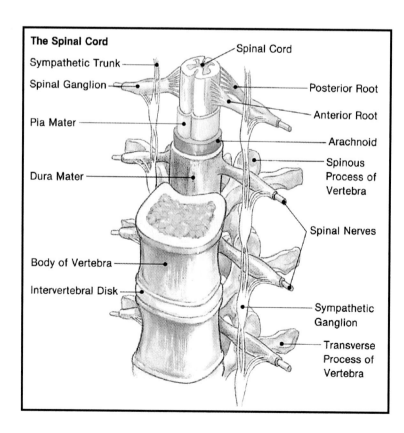

The Spinal Cord

Sympathetic Trunk
Spinal Ganglion
Pia Mater
Dura Mater
Body of Vertebra
Intervertebral Disk
Spinal Cord
Posterior Root
Anterior Root
Arachnoid
Spinous Process of Vertebra
Spinal Nerves
Sympathetic Ganglion
Transverse Process of Vertebra

Nervous System

Nerves

Brain (in Cranial Cavity)

Brachial Plexus

Phrenic

Axillary

Ulnar

Musculo Cutaneous

Radial

Median

Spinal Cord (in Spinal Cavity)

Lateral Femoral Cutaneous

Femoral

Sciatic

Common Peroneal

Superficial Peroneal

Tibial

Deep Peroneal

Saphenous

Sural

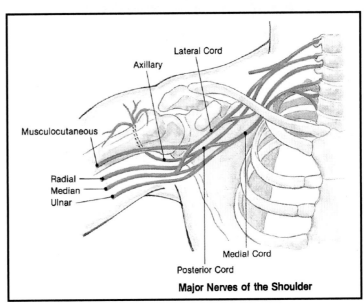

Lateral Cord

Axillary

Musculocutaneous

Radial
Median
Ulnar

Medial Cord

Posterior Cord

Major Nerves of the Shoulder

Autonomic Nervous System

The autonomic nervous system affects the heart, blood vessels, digestive tract, salivary and digestive glands, pancreas, liver, spleen, anal sphincter, kidneys, urinary bladder, urinary sphincter, adrenal glands, thyroid gland, gonads, genitalia, nasal lining, larynx, bronchi, lungs, iris and ciliary muscles of the eyes, tear glands, and hair muscles. Impulses can increase or slow heart rate, stimulate dilation or constriction of blood vessels, cause glands to secrete or decrease secretion, initiate or inhibit contractions in the bladder, stimulate or decrease a wave of muscle contraction along the digestive tract, and many other essential body activities.

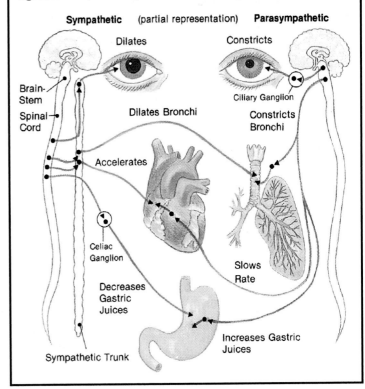

Sympathetic   (partial representation)   Parasympathetic

Dilates

Constricts

Brain-Stem

Spinal Cord

Ciliary Ganglion

Dilates Bronchi

Constricts Bronchi

Accelerates

Celiac Ganglion

Slows Rate

Decreases Gastric Juices

Sympathetic Trunk

Increases Gastric Juices

Heart

The heart is a hollow, muscular organ that pumps 450 million pints of blood in the average lifetime. Its superior chambers, the atria, receive blood. Both atria fill and then contract at the same time. The inferior chambers are the ventricles. They pump blood out of the heart. Both ventricles fill and then contract at the same time. When the atria are relaxing, the ventricles are contracting.

The right side of the heart receives blood from the body and sends it to the lungs (pulmonic circulation). The heart's left side receives oxygenated blood from the lungs and sends it out to the body (systemic circulation).

The heartbeat originates at the sinoatrial node (pacemaker) and spreads across the atria to stimulate contraction. After a slight delay, the impulse is sent from the atrioventricular node, down the bundles of His, and out across the ventricles. This stimulates the ventricles to contract while the atria are relaxing.

The heart muscle (myocardium) receives its blood supply by way of the right and left coronary arteries. These vessels are the first branches of the aorta.

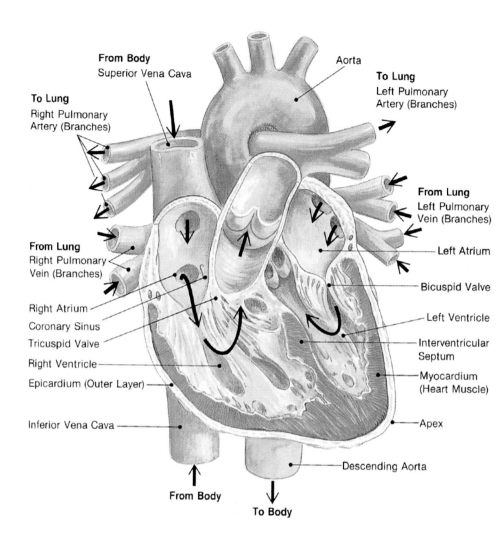

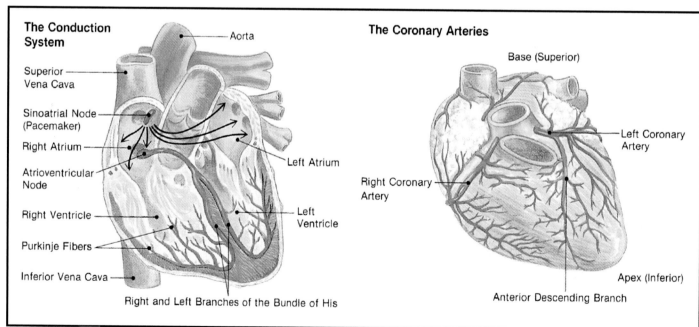

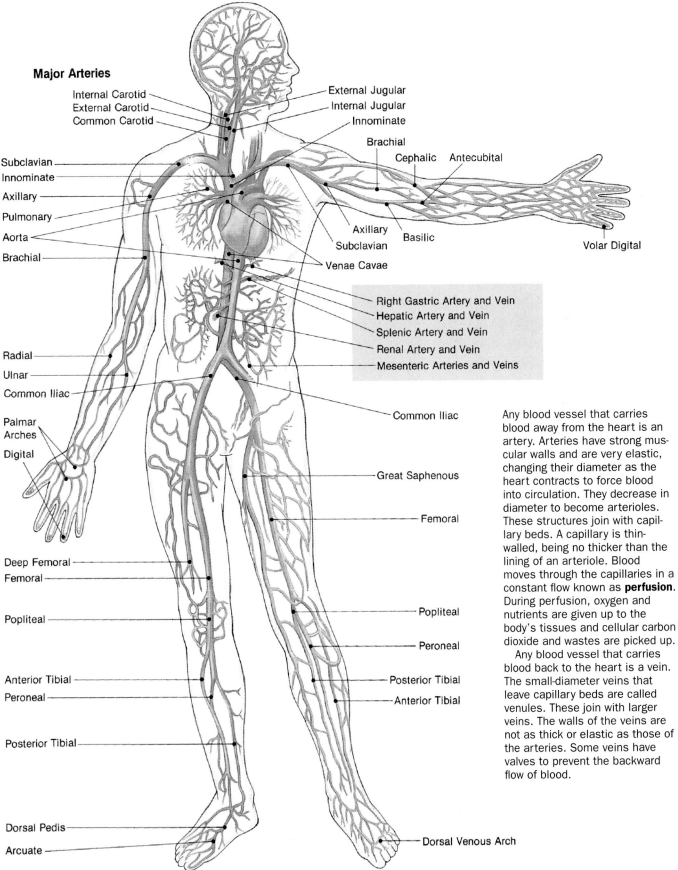

Major Arteries

Internal Carotid
External Carotid
Common Carotid

External Jugular
Internal Jugular
Innominate

Brachial
Cephalic   Antecubital

Subclavian
Innominate
Axillary
Pulmonary
Aorta
Brachial

Axillary
Subclavian   Basilic

Volar Digital

Venae Cavae

Right Gastric Artery and Vein
Hepatic Artery and Vein
Splenic Artery and Vein
Renal Artery and Vein
Mesenteric Arteries and Veins

Radial
Ulnar
Common Iliac

Common Iliac

Palmar
Arches
Digital

Great Saphenous

Femoral

Deep Femoral
Femoral

Popliteal

Popliteal

Peroneal

Anterior Tibial
Peroneal

Posterior Tibial
Anterior Tibial

Posterior Tibial

Dorsal Pedis
Arcuate

Dorsal Venous Arch

Any blood vessel that carries blood away from the heart is an artery. Arteries have strong muscular walls and are very elastic, changing their diameter as the heart contracts to force blood into circulation. They decrease in diameter to become arterioles. These structures join with capillary beds. A capillary is thin-walled, being no thicker than the lining of an arteriole. Blood moves through the capillaries in a constant flow known as **perfusion**. During perfusion, oxygen and nutrients are given up to the body's tissues and cellular carbon dioxide and wastes are picked up.

Any blood vessel that carries blood back to the heart is a vein. The small-diameter veins that leave capillary beds are called venules. These join with larger veins. The walls of the veins are not as thick or elastic as those of the arteries. Some veins have valves to prevent the backward flow of blood.

Respiratory System

The airway consists of structures involved with the conduction and exchange of air. Conduction is the movement of air to and from the exchange levels of the lungs. Air enters through the nose (primary) and mouth (secondary) and travels down the pharynx to enter the larynx. After passing through the larynx, air enters the trachea. At its distal end, the trachea branches into the left and right primary bronchi. These bronchi branch into secondary bronchi, which then branch into the bronchioles. Some of the bronchioles end as closed tubes. Air movement in them helps the lungs expand. The rest of the bronchioles carry the air to the exchange levels of the lungs.

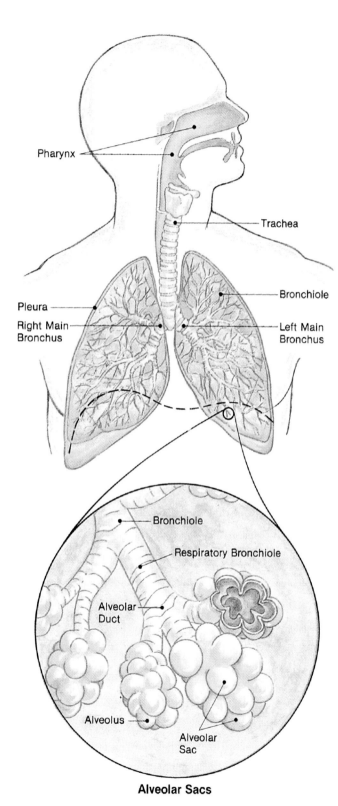

Alveolar Sacs

The respiratory bronchioles turn into alveolar ducts. These form alveolar sacs that are made up of the alveoli. Gas exchange takes place between the alveoli and the capillaries in the lungs.

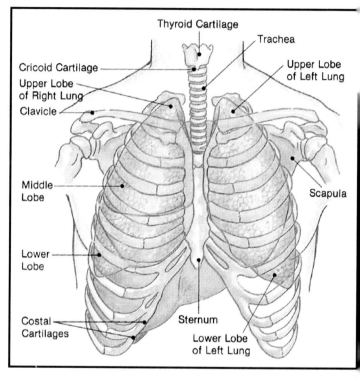

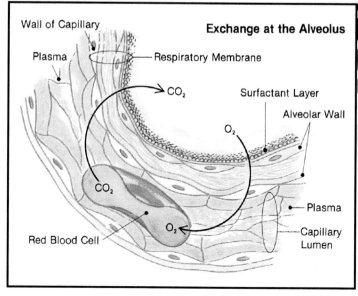

Exchange at the Alveolus

The digestive system includes the digestive tract and various supportive structures and accessory glands. The tract begins at the oral cavity with the teeth and tongue. The salivary glands release saliva into the mouth to moisten food for swallowing. The tract continues down the throat to the esophagus, through the cardiac sphincter, and into the stomach. Acid and digestive enzymes are added to the food to produce chyme. The chyme passes through the pyloric sphincter to enter the small intestine. Digestive enzymes from the pancreas and bile from the liver are added to the chyme. The processes of digestion and absorption are completed in the small intestine. Wastes are carried through the ileocecal valve into the large intestine. The wastes are moved to the rectum, from where they can be expelled through the anus.

Liver, Stomach, and Pancreas

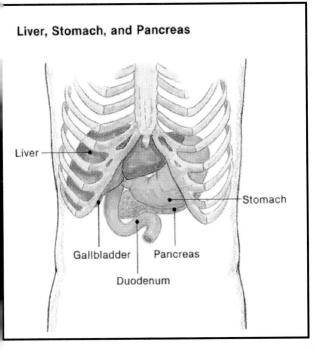

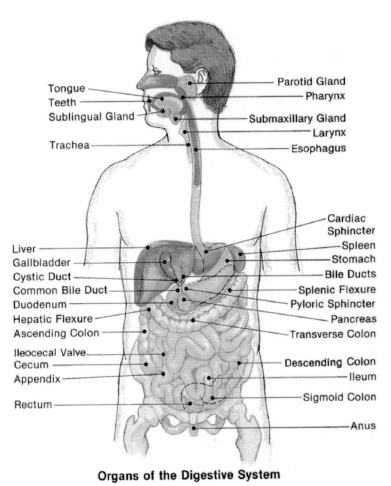

Organs of the Digestive System

Small Intestine

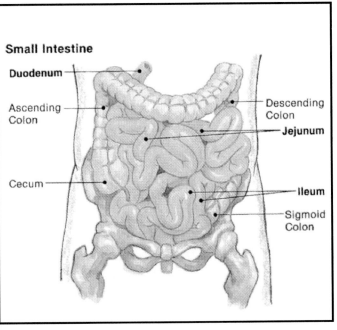

Large Intestine

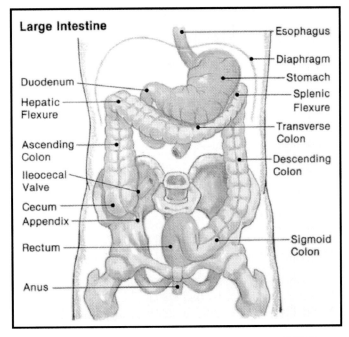

Organs of the Urinary System

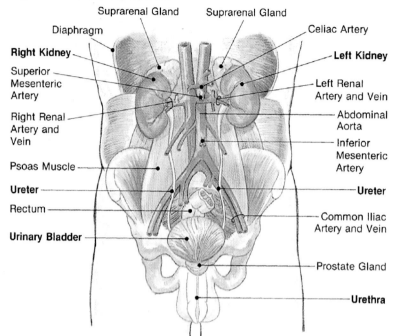

Suprarenal Gland
Suprarenal Gland
Diaphragm
Celiac Artery
Right Kidney
Left Kidney
Superior Mesenteric Artery
Left Renal Artery and Vein
Right Renal Artery and Vein
Abdominal Aorta
Inferior Mesenteric Artery
Psoas Muscle
Ureter
Ureter
Rectum
Common Iliac Artery and Vein
Urinary Bladder
Prostate Gland
Urethra

The urinary system is part of the body's excretory structures (urinary system, lungs, sweat glands, and intestine). The kidneys remove the wastes of chemical activities (metabolism) in the body. These wastes are removed from the blood to produce urine. At the same time, the kidneys remove certain excess compounds, regulate the blood pH (acid–base balance), and the concentration of sodium, potassium, chlorine, glucose, and other important chemicals.

The Nephron

Each kidney is made up of microscopic nephrons. Both wastes and needed chemicals are filtered from the blood. As these materials are passed through the nephron, the needed compounds (including water) are sent back into the blood. Wastes are collected as urine.

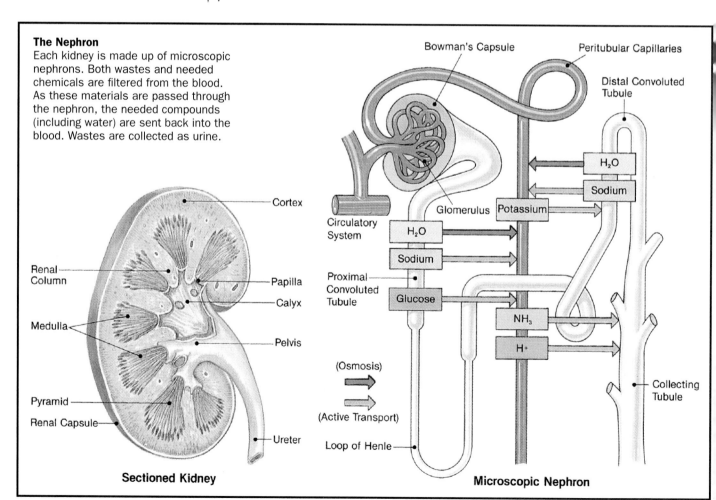

Cortex
Renal Column
Papilla
Calyx
Medulla
Pelvis
Pyramid
Renal Capsule
Ureter

Sectioned Kidney

Bowman's Capsule
Peritubular Capillaries
Distal Convoluted Tubule
H_2O
Sodium
Glomerulus
Potassium
Circulatory System
H_2O
Sodium
Proximal Convoluted Tubule
Glucose
NH_3
H^+
Collecting Tubule
(Osmosis)
(Active Transport)
Loop of Henle

Microscopic Nephron

Female

Fundus
Ovary
Uterus
Cervix
Vagina
Rectum
Fallopian (Uterine) Tube
Urinary Bladder
Symphysis Pubis
Urethra
Labium Minus
Clitoris
Labium Majus

Labium Minus (singular), Labia Minora (plural)
Lablum Majus (singular), Labia Majora (plural)

The reproductive system consists of the organs, glands, and supportive structures that are involved with human sexuality and procreation. In the male, spermatozoa and the hormone testosterone are produced in the testes. The female produces ova (eggs) and the hormones estrogen and progesterone in her ovaries. The union of ovum and sperm produce a single cell called a zygote. Through growth, cell division, and cellular differentiation (the formulation of specialized cells) the new individual develops and matures.

Male

Ductus Deferens
Urinary Bladder
Seminal Vesicle
Rectum
Symphysis Pubis
Prostate Gland
Urethra
Corpus Cavernosum
Corpus Spongiosum
Testis
Ejaculatory Duct
Bulb of Urethra
Epididymis   Duct of Bulbourethral Gland

The Ovary

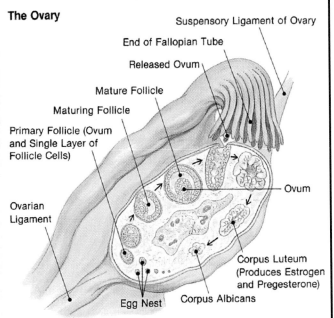

Suspensory Ligament of Ovary
End of Fallopian Tube
Released Ovum
Mature Follicle
Maturing Follicle
Primary Follicle (Ovum and Single Layer of Follicle Cells)
Ovarian Ligament
Ovum
Corpus Luteum (Produces Estrogen and Pregesterone)
Corpus Albicans
Egg Nest

The developing ovum and its supportive cells are called a follicle. Each month, follicle-stimulating hormone (FSH) from the pituitary gland starts the growth of several follicles. Usually, only one will mature and release an ovum (ovula-ion). During its growth, the follicle produces estrogen. After ovulation, the remaining cells of the follicle form a specialized structure that produces both estrogen and progesterone.

The Breast

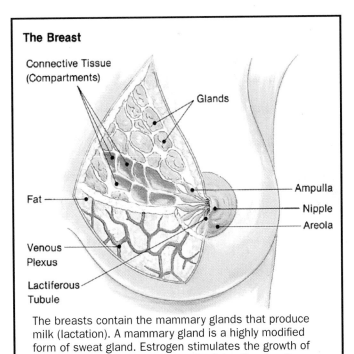

Connective Tissue (Compartments)
Glands
Fat
Ampulla
Nipple
Areola
Venous Plexus
Lactiferous Tubule

The breasts contain the mammary glands that produce milk (lactation). A mammary gland is a highly modified form of sweat gland. Estrogen stimulates the growth of the ducts, while progesterone stimulates the development of the secreting (milk-producing) cells. Lactic hormone from the pituitary stimulates milk production. Another pituitary hormone, oxytocin, stimulates the milk-producing cells to eject their milk into the ducts.

Anatomy and Physiology Illustrations   **825**

Integumentary System
Membranes

The Skin

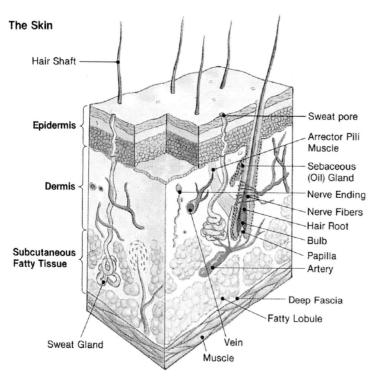

- Hair Shaft
- Epidermis
- Dermis
- Subcutaneous Fatty Tissue
- Sweat Gland
- Sweat pore
- Arrector Pili Muscle
- Sebaceous (Oil) Gland
- Nerve Ending
- Nerve Fibers
- Hair Root
- Bulb
- Papilla
- Artery
- Deep Fascia
- Fatty Lobule
- Vein
- Muscle

The skin is the largest organ of the body. In the adult the skin covers about 3000 square inches (1.75 square meters) and weighs about 6 pounds. It is involved with protection, insulation, thermal regulation, excretion, and the production of vitamin D.

The Peritoneum

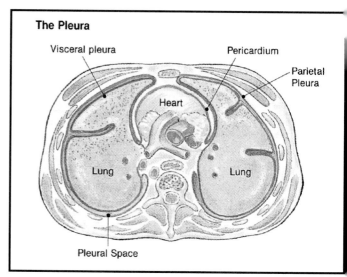

- Peritoneum
- Stomach
- Transverse Colon
- Greater Omentum
- Small Intestine
- Uterus
- Bladder
- Liver
- Lesser Omentum
- Pancreas
- Lesser Omental Sac
- Mesentery
- Rectum

Membranes

Membranes cover or line body structures to provide protection from injury and infection. There are four major classes of membranes. Mucous membranes line those structures that open to the outside world (for example, the mouth, the airway, digestive tract, urinary tract, and vagina). Serous membranes line the closed body cavities and cover the outsides of organs. The cutaneous membrane is the skin. Synovial membranes line joints to reduce friction during movement.

A serous membrane that covers an organ is called a visceral layer. The term parietal layer is used for the part of the serous membrane that lines a cavity. The serous membrane in the thoracic cavity is called pleura (for example, the parietal pleura lines the chest cavity). In the abdominal cavity, it is called peritoneum (for example, the parietal peritoneum). A double layer of peritoneum is called mesentery. The membrane that lines the sac surrounding the heart is pericardium.

Synovial Joint

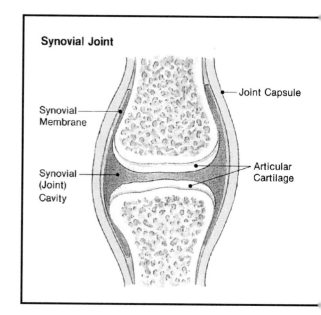

- Synovial Membrane
- Synovial (Joint) Cavity
- Joint Capsule
- Articular Cartilage

The Pleura

- Visceral pleura
- Pericardium
- Parietal Pleura
- Heart
- Lung
- Lung
- Pleural Space

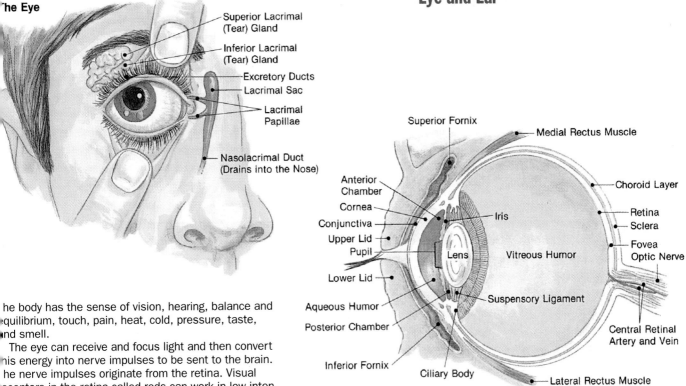

The Eye

- Superior Lacrimal (Tear) Gland
- Inferior Lacrimal (Tear) Gland
- Excretory Ducts
- Lacrimal Sac
- Lacrimal Papillae
- Nasolacrimal Duct (Drains into the Nose)

- Superior Fornix
- Medial Rectus Muscle
- Anterior Chamber
- Choroid Layer
- Cornea
- Iris
- Retina
- Conjunctiva
- Sclera
- Upper Lid
- Pupil
- Fovea
- Lens
- Optic Nerve
- Vitreous Humor
- Lower Lid
- Suspensory Ligament
- Aqueous Humor
- Posterior Chamber
- Central Retinal Artery and Vein
- Inferior Fornix
- Ciliary Body
- Lateral Rectus Muscle

he body has the sense of vision, hearing, balance and equilibrium, touch, pain, heat, cold, pressure, taste, and smell.

The eye can receive and focus light and then convert his energy into nerve impulses to be sent to the brain. he nerve impulses originate from the retina. Visual eceptors in the retina called rods can work in low intenity light. They have no color function. The visual recepors called cones operate in high intensity light and do eceive colors.

The ear's functions include hearing, static equilibrium (balance while standing still), and dynamic equilibrium (balance when moving). The outer and middle ear are responsible for sound gathering and its transmission. The inner ear has the nerve endings for hearing and equilibrium.

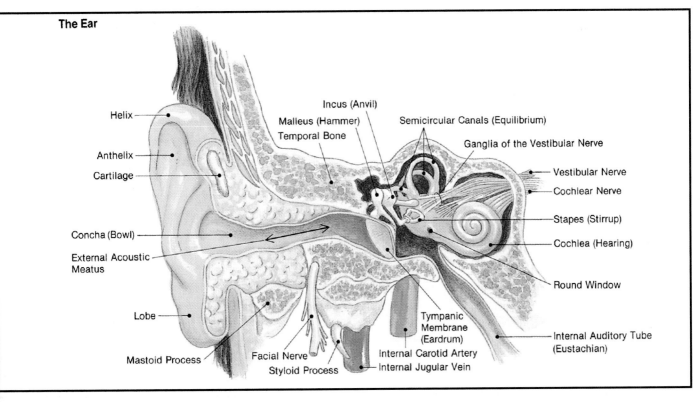

The Ear

- Helix
- Incus (Anvil)
- Malleus (Hammer)
- Semicircular Canals (Equilibrium)
- Temporal Bone
- Ganglia of the Vestibular Nerve
- Anthelix
- Vestibular Nerve
- Cartilage
- Cochlear Nerve
- Stapes (Stirrup)
- Concha (Bowl)
- Cochlea (Hearing)
- External Acoustic Meatus
- Round Window
- Lobe
- Tympanic Membrane (Eardrum)
- Internal Auditory Tube (Eustachian)
- Mastoid Process
- Facial Nerve
- Internal Carotid Artery
- Styloid Process
- Internal Jugular Vein

Atlas of Injuries

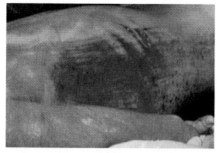

ABRASION (Gravel Roadway)

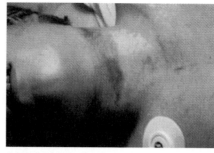

ABRASION (Rope or Cord)

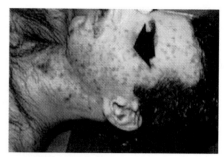

PITTED ABRASION

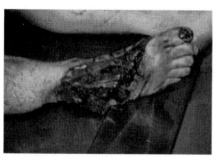

INCISION

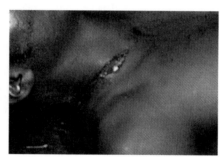

INCISION

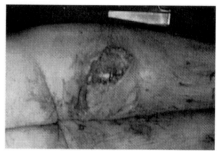

LACERATION (Jagged Margins)

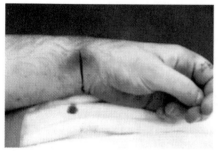

LACERATION (Tendons Still Intact)

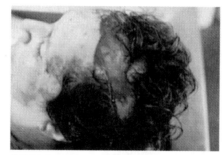

SCALP LACERATION (With Skin Separation)

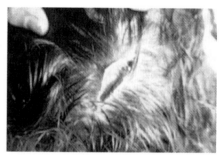

SCALP LACERATION (Minor)

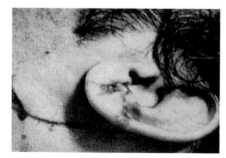

PUNCTURE WOUNDS (Stab Wounds)

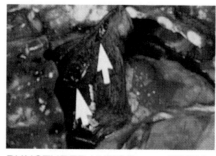

PUNCTURED LUNGS – FROM STAB WOUNDS (Autopsy)

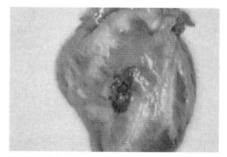

PERFORATED HEART (Bullet Wound)

ALL PHOTOGRAPHS ON THIS PAGE ARE FROM:
Dr. Lee J. Abbott, PO Box 1285, Laxahatchee, FL 33470

Atlas of Injuries

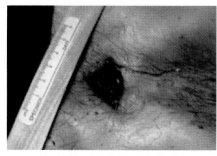

ENTRANCE WOUND (Bullet)

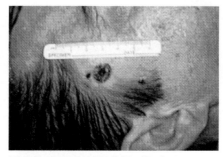

ENTRANCE WOUND (Bullet – Close Range)

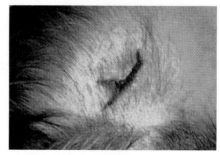

EXIT WOUND (Bullet)

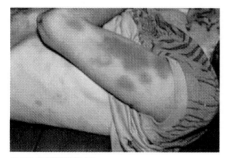

SHOTGUN WOUND

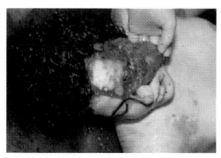

FACIAL AVULSION

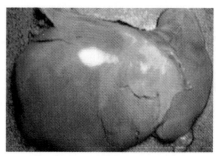

SKIN AVULSION (All Layers)

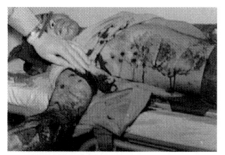

CONTUSIONS

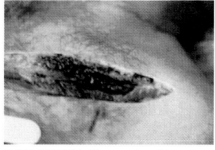

CONTUSION (Opened to Show Blood Accumulation)

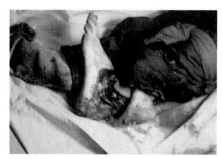

LACERATED LIVER (Abdominal Trauma)

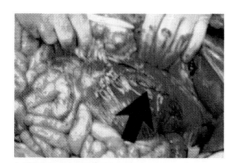

LACERATED SPLEEN

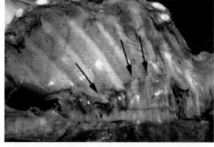

FRACTURED RIBS (Death due to Blood Loss from Lacerated Lungs)

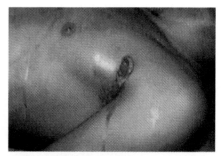

PERFORATED CHEST (Sucking Chest Wound)

ALL PHOTOGRAPHS ON THIS PAGE ARE FROM:
Dr. Lee J. Abbott, PO Box 1285, Laxahatchee, FL 33470

Atlas of Injuries

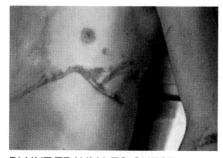

BLUNT TRAUMA TO CHEST

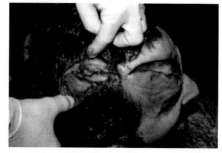

OPEN HEAD WOUND – SKULL FRACTURE

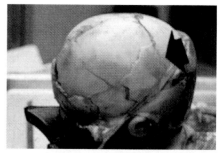

RADIATING SKULL FRACTURE (Blunt Trauma)

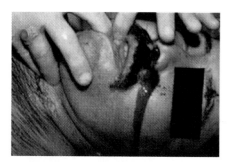

MULTIPLE SKULL FRACTURES (X-ray)

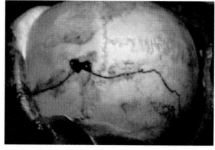

DEPRESSED SKULL FRACTURE (Force from Small Object)

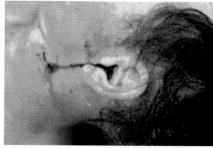

BLEEDING FROM EAR (Possible Skull Fracture)

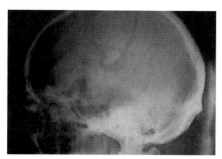

BLEEDING FROM NOSE (Possible Skull Fracture)

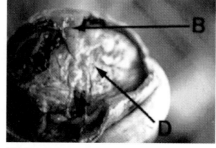

EPIDURAL HEMATOMA (D = Dura, B = Bone Fragment)

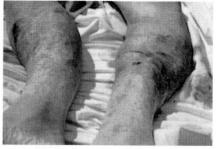

EXTENSIVE BILATERAL INJURY – LOWER EXTREMITIES (Impact with Car)

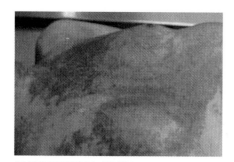

SUPERFICIAL BURN

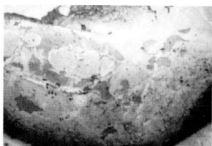

PARTIAL THICKNESS BURN

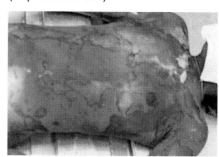

FULL THICKNESS BURN

ALL PHOTOGRAPHS ON THIS PAGE ARE FROM:
Dr. Lee J. Abbott, PO Box 1285, Laxahatchee, FL 33470

Atlas of Injuries

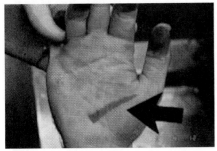

ELECTRICAL BURN
(Contact with Source)
LJA

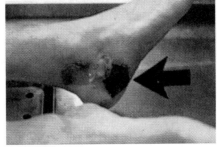

ELECTRICAL BURN (Exit)
LJA

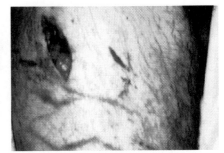

OPEN FRACTURE (Femur)
UT

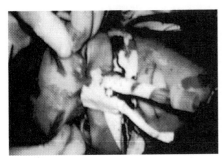

FROSTBITE

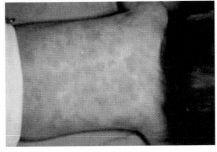

SNAKEBITE
UT

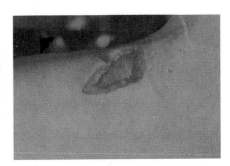

BOWEL EVISCERATION

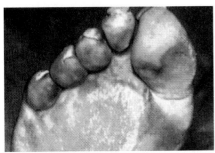

ORBITAL EDEMA

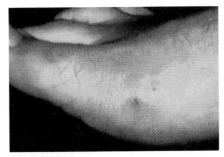

HIVES
AFIP Neg. No. 65-6982-4

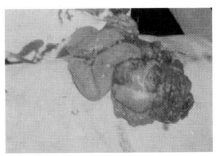

DOG BITE (Leg)
AFIP Neg. No. 62-12291

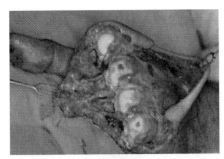

AMPUTATION (Fingers)
AFIP Neg. No. 75-20914

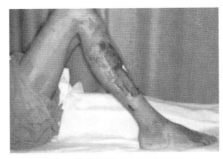

LACERATED LEG
AFIP Neg. No. 68-15269

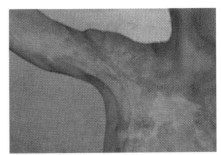

BURN (Hot Water)
AFIP Neg. No. 64-8320

LJA = Dr. Lee J. Abbott   AFJP = Armed Forces Institute of Pathology
UT = University of Tennessee, Memphis, Division of Forensic Pathology

Medical Terminology

As an EMT, you will probably never have to use more than a few medical terms in the course of your prehospital emergency care activities, and most of them will probably deal with parts of the body. Physicians and nurses prefer EMTs to speak in other than medical terms. But if you are an avid reader, much of what you read is likely to be freely sprinkled with medical terms, and if you cannot translate them, you may not understand what you are reading.

Medical terms are comprised of words, word roots, combining forms, prefixes, and suffixes—all little words, if you will, and each with its own definition.

Sometimes medical terms are made up of two whole words. For example, the word SMALL, is joined with the word POX to form the medical term SMALLPOX, the name of a disease. Would that it were all so simple!

Word roots are the foundations of words and are not used by themselves. THERM is a word root that means heat; to use it alone would make no sense. But when a vowel is added to the end of the word root to make it the combining form THERM/O, it can be joined with other words or word roots to form a compound term. THERM/O and METER (an instrument for measuring) combine to form THERMOMETER, an instrument for measuring heat or temperature.

More than one word root or combining form can be joined to form medical terms; ELECTRO-CARDIOGRAM is a good example. ELECTR/O (electric) is joined to CARDI (heart) and the suffix -GRAM (a written record) to form the medical term that means a written record of the heart's electrical activity.

Prefixes are used to modify or qualify the meaning of word roots. They usually tell the reader what kind of, where (or in what direction), or how many.

The term -PNEA relates to breathing, but it says nothing about the quality or kind of breathing. Adding the prefix DYS- qualifies it as difficult breathing.

ABDOMINAL PAIN is a rather broad term; it gives the reader no clue as to exactly where the pain is located either inside or outside the abdomen. Adding the prefix -INTRA to ABDOMINAL pinpoints the location of the pain, for INTRA-ABDOMINAL PAIN means pain within the abdomen. -PLEGIA refers to paralysis of the limbs. The prefix QUADRI informs the reader as to how many limbs are paralyzed. QUADRIPLEGIA means paralysis of all four limbs.

Suffixes are word endings that form nouns, adjectives, or verbs. Medical terms can have more than one suffix, and a suffix can appear in the middle of a compound term affixed to a combining form. A number of suffixes have specialized meanings. -ITIS means inflammation; thus ARTHRITIS means inflammation of a joint. -IAC forms a noun indicating a person afflicted with a certain disease, as for example, HEMOPHILIAC.

Some suffixes are joined to word roots to form terms that indicate a state, quality, condition, procedure, or process. PNEUMONIA and PSORIASIS are examples of medical conditions, while APPENDECTOMY and ARTHROSCOPY are examples of medical procedures. The suffixes in each case are underlined.

Some suffixes combine with word roots to form adjectives, words that modify nouns by indicating quality or quantity or by distinguishing one thing from another. GASTRIC, CARDIAC,

FIBROUS, ARTHRITIC, and DIAPHORETIC are all examples of adjectives formed by adding suffixes (underlined) to word roots.

Some suffixes are added to word roots to express reduction in size, -OLE and -ULE, for example. An ARTERIOLE is smaller than an ARTERY, and a VENULE is smaller than a vein.

When added to word roots, -E and -IZE form verbs. EXCISE and CATHETERIZE are examples.

Finally, some of what are commonly accepted as suffixes are actually the combination of a word root and a suffix. -MEGALY (enlargement) results from the combination of the word root MEGAL (large) and the suffix -Y (which forms the term into a noun). CARDIOMEGALY means enlargement of the heart.

STANDARD TERMS

The following terms are used to denote direction of movement, position, and anatomical posture.

ABDUCTION: movement away from the body's midline.
ADDUCTION: movement toward the body's midline.
AFFERENT: conducting toward a structure.
ANTERIOR: the front surface of the body.
ANTERIOR TO: in front of.
CAUDAD: toward the tail.
CEPHALAD: toward the head.
CIRCUMDUCTION: circular movement of a part.
CRANIAD: toward the cranium.
DEEP: situated remote from the surface.
DISTAL: situated away from the point of origin.
DORSAL: pertaining to the back surface of the body.
DORSIFLEXION: bending backward.
EFFERENT: conducting away from a structure.
ELEVATION: raising a body part.
EXTENSION: stretching, or moving jointed parts into or toward a straight condition.
EXTERNAL: situated outside.
FLEXION: bending, or moving jointed parts closer together.
INFERIOR: situated below.
INTERNAL: situated inside.
LATERAD: toward the side of the body.
LATERAL: situated away from the body's midline.
LATERAL ROTATION: rotating outward away from the body's midline.

LEFT LATERAL RECUMBENT: lying horizontal on the left side.
MEDIAD: toward the midline of the body.
MEDIAL: situated toward the body's midline.
MEDIAL ROTATION: rotating inward toward the body's midline.
PALMAR: concerning the inner surface of the hand.
PERIPHERAL: away from a central structure.
PLANTAR: concerning the sole of the foot.
POSTERIOR: pertaining to the back surface of the body.
POSTERIOR TO: situated behind.
PRONATION: lying face downward or turning the hand so the palm faces downward or backward.
PRONE: lying horizontal, face down and flat.
PROTRACTION: a pushing forward, as the mandible.
PROXIMAL: situated nearest the point of origin.
RECUMBENT: lying horizontal, generally speaking.
RETRACTION: a drawing back, as the tongue.
RIGHT LATERAL RECUMBENT: lying horizontal on the right side.
ROTATION: turning around an axis.
SUPERFICIAL: situated near the surface.
SUPERIOR: situated above.
SUPINATION: lying face upward or turning the hand so the palm faces forward or upward.
SUPINE: lying horizontal, flat on the back and face up.
VENTRAL: the front surface of the body.

PLANES

A plane is an imaginary flat surface that divides the body into sections.

CORONAL OR FRONTAL PLANE: an imaginary plane that passes through the body from side to side and divides it into front and back sections.
MIDSAGITTAL PLANE: an imaginary plane that passes through the body from front to back and divides it into right and left halves.
SAGITTAL PLANE: an imaginary plane parallel to the median plane. It passes through the body from front to back and divides the body into right and left sections.
TRANSVERSE PLANE: an imaginary plane that passes through the body and divides it into upper and lower sections.

WORD PARTS

Prefixes are generally identified by a following dash (AMBI-). Combining forms have a slash and a vowel following the word root (ARTHR/O). Suffixes are generally identified by a preceding dash (-EMIA).

A- **(not, without, lacking, deficient);** *afebrile,* without fever.

AB- **(away from);** *abduct,* to draw away from the midline.

-ABLE, -IBLE (capable of); *reducible,* capable of being reduced (as a fracture).

ABDOMIN/O (abdomen); *abdominal,* pertaining to the abdomen.

AC- **(to);** *acclimate,* to become accustomed to.

ACOU (hear); *acoustic,* pertaining to sound or hearing.

ACR/O (extremity, top, peak); *acrodermatitis,* inflammation of the skin of the extremities.

ACU (needle); *acupuncture,* the Chinese practice of piercing specific peripheral nerves with needles to relieve the discomfort associated with painful disorders.

AD- **(to, toward);** *adduct,* to draw toward the midline.

ADEN/O (gland); *adenitis,* inflammation of a gland.

ADIP/O (fat); *adipose,* fatty; fat (in size).

AER/O (air); *aerobic,* requiring the presence of oxygen to live and grow.

AF- **(to);** *afferent,* conveying toward.

AG- **(to);** *aggregate,* to crowd or cluster together.

-ALGESIA (painful); *hyperalgesia,* overly sensitive to pain.

-ALGIA (painful condition); *neuralgia,* pain that extends along the course of one or more nerves.

AMBI- (both sides); *ambidextrous,* able to perform manual skills with both hands.

AMBL/Y (dim, dull, lazy); *amblyopia,* lazy eye.

AMPHI-, AMPHO- (on both sides, around both); *amphigonadism,* having both testicular and ovarian tissues.

AMYL/O (starch); *amyloid,* starchlike.

AN- (without); *anemia,* a reduced volume of blood cells.

ANA- (upward, again, backward, excess); *anaphylaxis,* an unusual or exaggerated reaction of an organism to a substance to which it becomes sensitized.

ANDR/O (man, male); *android,* resembling a man.

ANGI/O (blood vessel, duct); *angioplasty,* surgery of blood vessels.

ANKYL/O (stiff); *ankylosis,* stiffness.

ANT-, ANTI- (against, opposed to, preventing, relieving); *antidote,* a substance for counteracting a poison.

ANTE- (before, forward); *antecubital,* situated in front of the elbow.

ANTERO- (front); *anterolateral,* situated in front and to one side.

AP- (to); *approximate,* to bring together; to place close to.

APO- (separation, derivation from); *apoplexy,* sudden neurologic impairment due to a cardiovascular disorder.

-ARIUM, -ORIUM (place for something); *solarium,* a place for the sun.

ARTERI/O (artery); *arteriosclerosis,* thickening of the walls of the smaller arteries.

ARTHRIO (joint, articulation); *arthritis,* inflammation of a joint or joints.

ARTICUL/O (joint); *articulated,* united by joints.

AS- (to); *assimilate,* to take into.

AT- (to); *attract,* to draw toward.

AUDI/O (hearing); *audiometer,* an instrument to test the power of hearing.

AUR/O (ear); *auricle,* the flap of the ear.

AUT/O (self); *autistic,* self-centered

BI- (two, twice, double, both); *bilateral,* having two sides; pertaining to two sides.

BI/O (life); *biology,* the study of life.

BLEPHARIO (eyelid); *blepharitis,* inflammation of the eyelid.

BRACHI/O (upper arm); *brachialgia,* pain in the upper arm.

BRADY- (slow); *bradycardia,* an abnormally slow heart rate.

BRONCH/O (larger air passages of the lungs); *bronchitis,* inflammation of the larger air passages of the lungs.

BUCC/O (cheek); *buccal,* pertaining to the cheek.

CAC/O (bad); *cacosmis,* a bad odor.

CALC/O (stone); *calculus,* an abnormal hard inorganic mass such as a gallstone.

CALCANE/O (heel); *calcaneus,* the heel bone.

CALOR/O (heat); *caloric,* pertaining to heat.

CANCR/O (cancer); *cancroid,* resembling cancer.

CAPIT/O (head); *capitate,* head-shaped.

CAPS/O (container); *capsulation,* enclosed in a capsule or container.

CARCIN/O (cancer); *carcinogen,* a substance that causes cancer.

CARDI/O (heart); *cardiogenic,* originating in the heart.

CARP/O (wrist bone); *carpal,* pertaining to the wrist bone.

CAT-, CATA- (down, lower, under, against, along with); *catabasis,* the stage of decline of a disease.

-CELE (tumor, hernia); *hydrocele,* a confined collection of water.

CELI/O (abdomen); *celiomyalgia,* a pain in the muscles of the abdomen.

-CENTESIS (perforation or tapping, as with a needle); *abdominocentesis,* surgical puncture of the abdominal cavity.

CEPHAL/O (head); *electroencephalogram,* a recording of the electrical activity of the brain.

CEREBR/O (cerebrum); *cerebrospinal,* pertaining to the brain and spinal fluid.

CERVIC/O (neck, cervix); *cervical,* pertaining to the neck (or cervix).

CHEIL/O, CHIL/O (lip); *cheilitis,* inflammation of the lips.

CHEIRIO, CHIR/O (hand); *cheiralgia,* pain in the hand.

CHLOR/O (green); *chloroma,* green cancer, a greenish tumor associated with myelogenous leukemia.

CHOL/E (bile, gall); *choledochitis,* inflammation of the common bile duct.

CHONDR/O (cartilage); *chondrodynia,* pain in a cartilage.

CHROM/O, CHROMAT/O (color); *monochromatic,* being of one color.

CHRON/O (time); *chronic,* persisting for a long time.

-CID- (cut, kill, fall); *insecticide,* an agent that kills insects.

CIRCUM- (around); *circumscribed,* confined to a limited space.

-CIS- (cut, kill, fall); *excise,* to cut out.

-CLYSIS (irrigation); *enteroclysis,* irrigation of the small intestine.

CO- (with); *cohesion,* the force that causes various particles to unite.

COL- (with); *collateral,* secondary or accessory; a small side branch such as a blood vessel or nerve.

COL/O (colon, large intestine); *colitis,* inflammation of the colon.

COLP/O (vagina); *colporrhagia,* bleeding from the vagina.

COM- (with); *comminuted,* broken or crushed into small pieces.

CON- (with); *congenital,* existing from the time of birth.

CONTRA- (against, opposite); *contraindicated,* inadvisable.

COR/E, CORE/O (pupil); *corectopia,* abnormal location of the pupil of the eye.

COST/O (rib); *intercostal,* between the ribs.

CRANI/O (skull); *cranial,* pertaining to the skull.

CRY/O (eold); *cryogenic,* that which produces low temperature.

CRYPT/O (hide, cover, conceal); *cryptogenic,* of doubtful origin.

CYAN/O (blue); *cyanosis,* bluish discoloration of the skin and mucous membranes.

CYST/O (urinary bladder, cyst, sac of fluid); *cystitis,* inflammation of the bladder.

-CYTE (cell); *leukocyte,* white cell.

CYT/O (cell); *cytoma,* tumor of the cell.

DACRY/O (tear); *dacryorrhea,* excessive flow of tears.

DACTYL/O (finger, toe); *dactylomegaly,* abnormally large fingers or toes.

DE- (down); *descending,* coming down from.

DENT/O (tooth); *dental,* pertaining to the teeth.

DERM/O, DERMAT/O (skin); *dermatitis,* inflammation of the skin.

DEXTR/O (right); *dextrad,* toward the right side.

DI- (twice, double); *diplegia,* paralysis affecting like parts on both sides of the body.

DIA- (through, across, apart); *diaphragm,* the partition that separates the abdominal and thoracic cavities.

DIPL/O (double, twin, twice); *diplopia,* double vision.

DIPS/O (thirst); *dipsomania,* alcoholism.

DIS- (to free, to undo); *dissect,* to cut apart.

DORS/O (back); *dorsal,* pertaining to the back.

-DYNIA (painful condition); *cephalodynia,* headache.

DYS- (bad, difficult, abnormal, incomplete); *dyspnea,* labored breathing.

-ECTASIA (dilation or enlargement of an organ or part); *gastrectasia,* dilation (stretching) of the stomach.

ECTO- (outer, outside of); *ectopic,* located away from the normal position.

-ECTOMY (the surgical removal of an organ or part); *appendectomy,* surgical removal of the appendix.

ELECTR/O (electric); *electrocardiogram,* the written record of the heart's electrical activity.

-EMIA (condition of the blood); *anemia,* a deficiency of red blood cells.

EN- (in, into, within); *encapsulate*, to enclose within a container.

ENCEPHAL/O (brain); *encephalitis*, inflammation of the brain.

END-, ENDO- (within); *endotracheal*, within the trachea.

ENT-, ENTO- (within, inner); *entopic*, occurring in the proper place.

ENTER/O (small intestine); *enteritis*, inflammation of the intestine.

EP-, EPI- (over, on, upon); *epidermis*, the outermost layer of skin.

ERYTHR/O (red); *erythrocyte*, a red blood cell.

ESTHESIA (feeling); *anesthesia*, without feeling.

EU (good, well, normal, healthy); *euphoria*, an abnormal or exaggerated feeling of well-being.

EX- (out of, away from); *excrement*, waste material discharged from the body.

EXO- (outside, outward); *exophytic*, to grow outward or on the surface.

EXTRA- (on the outside, beyond, in addition to); *extracorporeal*, outside the body.

FACI/O (face, surface); *facial*, pertaining to the face.

FEBR/I (fever); *febrile*, feverish.

-FERENT (bear, carry); *efferent*, carrying away from a center.

FIBR/O (fiber, filament); *fibrillation*, muscular contractions due to the activity of muscle fibers.

-FORM (shape); *deformed*, abnormally shaped.

-FUGAL (moving away); *centrifugal*, moving away from a center.

GALACT/O (milk); *galactopyria*, milk fever.

GANGLI/O (knot); *ganglion*, a knotlike mass.

GASTR/O (stomach); *gastritis*, inflammation of the stomach.

GEN/O (come into being, originate); *genetic*, inherited.

-GENESIS (production or origin); *pathogenesis*, the development of a disease.

-GENIC (giving rise to, originating in); *cardiogenic*, originating in the heart.

GLOSS/O (tongue); *glossal*, pertaining to the tongue.

GLYC/O (sweet); *glycemia*, the presence of sugar in the blood.

GNATH/O (jaw); *gnathitis*, inflammation of the jaw.

-GRAM (drawing, written record); *electrocardiogram*, a recording of the heart's electrical activity.

-GRAPH (an instrument for recording the activity of an organ); *electrocardiograph*, an instrument for measuring the heart's electrical activity.

-GRAPHY (the recording of the activity of an organ); *electrocardiography*, the method of recording the heart's electrical activity.

GYNEC/O (woman); *gynecologist*, a specialist in diseases of the female genital tract.

GNOS/O (knowledge); *prognosis*, a prediction of the outcome of a disease.

HEM/A, HEM/O, HEMAT/O (blood); *hematoma*, a localized collection of blood.

HEMI- (one-half); *hemiplegia*, paralysis of one side of the body.

HEPAT/O (liver); *hepatitis*, inflammation of the liver.

HETER/O (other); *heterogeneous*, from a different source.

HIDR/O, HIDROT/O (sweat); *hidrosis*, excessive sweating.

HIST/O (tissue); *histodialysis*, the breaking down of tissue.

HOM/O, HOME/O (same, similar, unchanging, constant); *homeostasis*, stability in an organism's normal physiological states.

HYDR/O (water, fluid); *hydrocephalus*, an accumulation of cerebrospinal fluid in the skull with resulting enlargement of the head.

HYPN/O (sleep); *hypnotic*, that which induces sleep.

HYAL/O (glass); *hyaline*, glassy, transparent.

HYPER- (beyond normal, excessive); *hypertension*, abnormally high blood pressure.

HYPO- (below normal, deficient, under, beneath); *hypotension*, abnormally low blood pressure.

HYSTER/O (uterus, womb); *hysterectomy*, surgical removal of the uterus.

-IASIS (condition); *psoriasis*, a chronic skin condition characterized by lesions.

IATR/O (healer, physician); *pediatrician*, a physician that specializes in children's disorders.

-ID (in a state, condition of); *gravid*, pregnant.

IDIO (peculiar, separate, distinct); *idiopathic*, occurring without a known cause.

IL- (negative prefix); *illegible*, cannot be read.

ILE/O (ileum); *ileitis*, inflammation of the ileum.

ILI/O (ilium); *iliac*, pertaining to the ilium.

IM- (negative prefix); *immature*, not mature.

IN- (in, into, within); *incise*, to cut into.

INFRA- (beneath, below); *infracostal*, below a rib, or below the ribs.

INTER- (between); *intercostal*, between two ribs.

INTRA- (within); *intraoral*, within the mouth.

INTRO- (within, into); *introspection*, the contemplation of one's own thoughts and feelings; self-analysis.

IR/O, IRID/O (iris); *iridotomy*, incision of the iris.

ISCHI/O (ischium); *ischialgia*, pain in the ischium.

-ISMUS (abnormal condition); *strabismus*, deviation of the eye that a person cannot overcome.

ISO- (same, equal, alike); *isometric*, of equal dimensions.

-ITIS (inflammation); *endocarditis*, inflammation within the heart.

KERAT/O (cornea); *keratitis*, inflammation of the cornea.

KINESI/O (movement); *kinesialgia*, pain upon movement.

LABI/O (lip); *labiodental*, pertaining to the lip and teeth.

LACT/O (milk); *lactation*, the secretion of milk.

LAL/O (talk); *lalopathy*, any speech disorder.

LAPAR/O (flank, abdomen, abdominal wall); *laparotomy*, an incision through the abdominal wall.

LARYNG/O (larynx); *laryngoscope*, an instrument for examining the larynx.

LEPT/O (thin); *leptodactylous*, having slender fingers.

LEUC/O, LEUK/O (white); *leukemia*, a malignant disease characterized by the increased development of white blood cells.

LINGU/O (tongue); *sublingual*, under the tongue.

LIP/O (fat); *lipoma*, fatty tumor.

LITH/O (stone); *lithotriptor*, an instrument for crushing stones in the bladder.

-LOGIST (a person who studies); *pathologist*, a person who studies diseases.

LOG/O (speak), give an account; *logospasms*, spasmodic speech.

-LOGY (study of); *pathology*, the study of disease.

LUMB/O (loin); *lumbago*, pain in the lumbar region.

LYMPH/O (lymph); *lymphoduct*, a vessel of the lymph system.

-LYSIS (destruction); *electrolysis* destruction (of hair, for example) by passage of an electric current.

MACR/O (large, long); *macrocephalous*, having an abnormally large head.

MALAC/O (a softening); *malacia*, the morbid softening of a body part or tissue.

MAMM/O (breast); *mammary*, pertaining to the breast.

-MANIA (mental aberration); *kleptomania*, the compulsion to steal.

MAST/O (breast); *mastectomy*, surgical removal of the breast.

MEDI/O (middle); *mediastinum*, middle partition of the thoracic cavity.

MEGA- (large); *megacolon*, an abnormally large colon.

MEGAL/O (large); *megalomaniac*, a person impressed with his own greatness.

-MEGALY (an enlargement); *cardiomegaly*, enlargement of the heart.

MELAN/O (dark, black); *melanoma*, a tumor comprised of darkly pigmented cells.

MEN/O (month); *menopause*, cessation of menstruation.

MES/O (middle); *mesiad*, toward the center.

META- (change, transformation, exchange); *metabolism*, the sum of the physical and chemical processes by which an organism survives.

METR/O (uterus); *metralgia*, pain in the uterus.

MICR/O (small); *microscope*, an instrument for magnifying small objects.

MON/O (single, only, sole); *monoplegia*, paralysis of a single part.

MORPH/O (form); *morphology*, the study of form and shape.

MULTI- (many, much); *multipara*, a woman who has given two or more live births.

MYC/O, MYCET/O (fungus); *mycosis*, any disease caused by a fungus.

MY/O (muscle); *myasthenia*, muscular weakness.

MYEL/O (marrow, also often refers to spinal cord); *myelocele*, protrusion of the spinal cord through a defect in the spinal column.

MYX/O (mucous, slimelike); *myxoid*, resembling mucous.

NARC/O (stupor, numbness); *narcotic*, an agent that induces sleep.

NAS/O (nose); *oronasal*, pertaining to the nose and mouth.

NE/O (new); *neonate*, a newborn infant.

NECR/O (corpse); *necrotic*, dead (when referring to tissue).

NEPHR/O (kidney); *nephralgia*, pain in the kidneys.

NEUR/O (nerve); *neuritis*, inflammation of nerve pathways.

NOCT/I (night); *noctambulism*, sleep walking.

NORM/O (rule, order, normal); *normotension*, normal blood pressure.

NULL/I (none); *nullipara,* a woman who has never given birth to a child.

NYCT/O (night); *nycturia,* excessive urination at night.

OB- (against, in front of, toward); *obturator,* a device that closes an opening.

OC- (against, in front of, toward); *occlude,* to obstruct.

OCUL/O (eye); *ocular,* pertaining to the eye.

ODONT/O (tooth); *odontalgia,* toothache.

-OID (shape, form, resemblance); *ovoid,* egg-shaped.

OLIG/O (few, deficient, scanty); *oligemia,* lacking in blood volume.

-OMA (tumor, swelling); *adenoma,* tumor of a gland.

O/O- (egg); *ooblast,* a primitive cell from which an ovum develops.

ONYCH/O (nail); *onychoma,* tumor of a nail or nail bed.

OOPHOR/O (ovary); *oophorectomy,* a surgical removal of one or both ovaries.

-OPSY (a viewing); *autopsy,* postmortem examination of a body.

OPTHALM/O (eye); *opthalmic,* pertaining to the eyes.

OPT/O, OPTIC/O (sight, vision); *optometrist,* a specialist in adapting lenses for the correcting of visual defects.

OR/O (mouth); *oral,* pertaining to the mouth.

ORCH/O, ORCHID/O (testicle); *orchitis,* inflammation of the testicles.

ORTH/O (straight, upright); *orthopedic,* pertaining to the correction of skeletal defects.

-OSIS (process, an abnormal condition); *dermatosis,* any skin condition.

OSTE/O (bone); *osteomyelitis,* inflammation of bone or bone marrow.

OT/O (ear); *otalgia,* earache.

OVARI/O (ovary); *ovariocele,* hernia of an ovary.

OV/I, OV/O (egg); *oviduct,* a passage through which an egg passes.

PACHY- (thicken); *pachyderma,* abnormal thickening of the skin.

PALAT/O (palate); *palatitis,* inflammation of the palate.

PAN- (all, entire, every); *panacea,* a remedy for all diseases, a "cure-all."

PARA- (beside, beyond, accessory to, apart from, against); *paranormal,* beyond the natural or normal.

PATH/O (disease); *pathogen,* any disease-producing agent.

-PATHY (disease of a part); *osteopathy,* disease of a bone.

-PENIA (an abnormal reduction); *leukopenia,* deficiency in white blood cells.

PEPS/O, PEPT/O (digestion); *dyspepsia,* poor digestion.

PER- (throughout, completely, extremely); *perfusion,* the passage of fluid through the vessels of an organ.

PERI- (around, surrounding); *pericardium,* the sac that surrounds the heart and the roots of the great vessels.

-PEXY (fixation); *splendopexy,* surgical fixation of the spleen.

PHAG/O (eat); *phagomania,* an insatiable craving for food.

PHARYNG/O (throat); *pharyngospasms,* spasms of the muscles of the pharynx.

PHAS/O (speech); *aphasic,* unable to speak.

PHIL/O (like, have an affinity for); *necrophilia,* an abnormal interest in death.

PHLEB/O (vein); *phlebotomy,* surgical incision of a vein.

-PHOBIA (fear, dread); *claustrophobia,* a fear of closed spaces.

PHON/O (sound); *phonetic,* pertaining to the voice.

PHOR/O (bear, carry); *diaphoresis,* profuse sweating.

PHOT/O (light); *photosensitivity,* abnormal reactivity of the skin to sunlight.

PHREN/O (diaphragm); *phrenic nerve,* a nerve that carries messages to the diaphragm.

PHYSI/O (nature); *physiology,* the science that studies the function of living things.

PIL/O (hair); *pilose,* hairy.

-PLASIA (development, formation); *dysplasia,* poor or abnormal formation.

-PLASTY (surgical repair); *arthroplasty,* surgical repair of a joint.

-PLEGIA (paralysis); *paraplegia,* paralysis of the lower body, including the legs.

PLEUR/O (rib, side, pleura); *pleurisy,* inflammation of the pleura.

-PNEA (breath, breathing); *orthopnea,* difficult breathing except in an upright position.

PNEUM/O, PNEUMAT/O (air, breath); *pneumatic,* pertaining to the air.

PNEUM/O, PNEUMON/O (lung); *pneumonia,* inflammation of the lungs with the escape of fluid.

POD/O (foot); *podiatrist,* a specialist in the care of feet.

-POIESIS (formation); *hematopoiesis,* formation of blood.

POLY- (much, many); *polychromatic*, multicolored.

POST- (after, behind); *postmortem*, after death.

PRE- (before); *premature*, occurring before the proper time.

PRO- (before, in front of); *prolapse*, the falling down, or sinking of a part.

PROCT/O (anus); *proctitis*, inflammation of the rectum.

PSEUD/O (false); *pseudoplegia*, hysterical paralysis.

PSYCH/O (mind, soul); *psychopath*, one who displays aggressive antisocial behavior.

-PTOSIS (abnormal dropping or sagging of a part); *hysteroptosis*, sagging of the uterus.

PULMON/O (lung); *pulmonary*, pertaining to the lungs.

PY/O (pus); *pyorrhea*, copious discharge of pus.

PYEL/O (renal pelvis); *pyelitis*, inflammation of the renal pelvis.

PYR/O (fire, fever); *pyromaniac*, compulsive fire setter.

QUADRI- (four); *quadriplegia*, paralysis of all four limbs.

RACH/I (spine); *rachialgia*, pain in the spine.

RADI/O (ray, radiation); *radiology*, the use of ionizing radiation in diagnosis and treatment.

RE- (back, against, contrary); *recurrence*, the return of symptoms after remission.

RECT/O (rectum); *rectal*, pertaining to the rectum.

REN/O (the kidneys); *renal*, pertaining to the kidneys.

RETRO- (located behind, backward); *retroperineal*, behind the perineum.

RHIN/O (nose); *rhinitis*, inflammation of the mucus membranes of the nose.

-RRHAGE (abnormal discharge); *hemorrhage*, abnormal discharge of blood.

-RRHAGIA (hemorrhage from an organ or body part); *menorrhea*, excessive uterine bleeding.

-RRHEA (flowing or discharge); *diarrhea*, abnormal frequency and liquidity of fecal discharges.

SANGUIN/O (blood); *exsanguinate*, to lose a large volume of blood either internally or externally.

SARC/O (flesh); *sarcoma*, a malignant tumor.

SCHIZ/O (split); *schizophrenia*, any of a group of emotional disorders characterized by bizarre behavior (erroneously called split personality).

SCLER/O (hardening); *scleroderma*, hardening of connective tissues of the body, including the skin.

-SCLEROSIS (hardened condition); *arteriosclerosis*, hardening of the arteries.

SCOLI/O (twisted, crooked); *scoliosis*, sideward deviation of the spine.

-SCOPE (an instrument for observing); *endoscope*, an instrument for the examination of a hollow body, such as the bladder.

-SECT (cut); *transsect*, to cut across.

SEMI- (one-half, partly); *semisupine*, partly, but not completely, supine.

SEPT/O, SEPS/O (infection); *aseptic*, free from infection.

SOMAT/O (body); *psychosomatic*, both psychological and physiological.

SON/O (sound); *sonogram*, a recording produced by the passage of sound waves through the body.

SPERMAT/O (sperm, semen); *spermacide*, an agent that kills sperm.

SPHYGM/O (pulse); *sphygmomanometer*, a device for measuring blood pressure in the arteries.

SPLEN/O (spleen); *splenectomy*, surgical removal of the spleen.

-STASIS (stopping, controlling); *hemostasis*, the control of bleeding.

STEN/O (narrow); *stenosis*, a narrowing of a passage or opening.

STERE/O (solid, three-dimensional); *stereoscopic*, a three-dimensional appearance.

STETH/O (chest); *stethoscope*, an instrument for listening to chest sounds.

STHEN/O (strength); *myasthenia*, muscular-weakness.

-STOMY (surgically creating a new opening); *colostomy*, surgical creation of an opening between the colon and the surface of the body.

SUB- (under, near, almost, moderately); *subclavian*, situated under the clavicle.

SUPER- (above, excess); *superficial*, lying on or near the surface.

SUPRA- (above, over); *suprapubic*, situated above the pubic arch.

SYM-, SYN- (joined together, with); *syndrome*, a set of symptoms that occur together.

TACHY- (fast); *tachycardia*, a very fast heart rate.

-THERAPY (treatment); *hydrotherapy*, treatment with water.

THERM/O (heat); *thermogenesis*, the production of heat.

THORAC/O (chest cavity); *thoracic*, pertaining to the chest.

THROMB/O (clot, lump); *thrombophlebitis*, inflammation of a vein.

-TOME (a surgical instrument for cutting); *microtome*, an instrument for cutting thin slices of tissue.

-TOMY (a surgical operation on an organ or body part); *thoracotomy*, surgical incision of the chest wall.

TOP/O (place); *topographic*, pertaining to special regions (of the body)

TRACHE/O (trachea); *tracheostomy*, an opening in the neck that passes to the trachea.

TRANS- (through, across, beyond); *transfusion*, the introduction of whole blood or blood components directly into the bloodstream.

TRI- (three); *trimester*, a period of three months.

TRICH/O (hair); *trichosis*, any disease of the hair.

-TRIPSY (surgical crushing); *lithotripsy*, surgical crushing of stones.

TROPH/O (nourish); *hypertrophic*, enlargement of an organ or body part due to the increase in the size of cells.

ULTRA- (beyond, excess); *ultrasonic*, beyond the audible range.

UNI- (one); *unilateral*, affecting one side.

UR/O (urine); *urinalysis*, examination of urine.

URETER/O (ureter); *ureteritis*, inflammation of a ureter.

URETHR/O (urethra); *urethritis*, inflammation of the urethra.

VAS/O (vessel, duct); *vasodilator*, an agent that causes dilation of blood vessels.

VEN/O (vein); *venipuncture*, surgical puncture of a vein.

VENTR/O (belly, cavity); *ventral*, relating to the belly or abdomen.

VESIC/O (blister, bladder); *vesicle*, a small fluid-filled blister.

VISCER/O (internal organ); *visceral*, pertaining to the viscera (abdominal organs).

XANTH/O (yellow); *xanthroma*, a yellow nodule in the skin.

XEN/O (stranger); *xenophobia*, abnormal fear of strangers.

XER/O (dry); *xerosis*, abnormal dryness (as of the mouth or eyes).

ZO/O (animal life); *zoogenous*, acquired from an animal.

Glossary

abandonment—to leave an injured or ill patient before the responsibility for care is properly transferred to someone of equal or superior training.

abdominal quadrants—the four zones of the abdominal wall, used for quick reference: the *right upper quadrant, left upper quadrant, right lower quadrant,* and *left lower quadrant.*

abortion—spontaneous (miscarriage) or induced termination of pregnancy.

abrasion (ab-RAY-zhun)—a scratch or scrape.

abruptio placentae (ab-RUPT-si-o plah-SEN-ta)—a condition in which the placenta separates from the uterine wall; a cause of excessive prebirth bleeding.

absorbed poisons—poisons that are taken into the body through unbroken skin.

acetabulum (AS-uh-TAB-yuh-lum)—the socket into which the head of the femur fits to form the hip joint.

acromioclavicular (ah-KRO-me-o-klav-IK-yuh-ler) **joint**—the joint where the acromion and the clavicle meet.

acromion (ah-KRO-me-on)—the highest portion of the shoulder.

activated charcoal—a powder, usually premixed with water, that will absorb some poisons and help prevent them from being absorbed by the body.

active rewarming—application of an external heat source to rewarm the body of a hypothermic patient. See also *central rewarming.*

acute myocardial infarction (MY-o-KARD-e-ul in-FARK-shun) **(AMI)**—occurs when a portion of myocardium (heart muscle) dies when deprived of oxygenated blood; a heart attack.

afterbirth—the placenta, membranes of the amniotic sac, part of the umbilical cord, and some tissues from the lining of the uterus that are delivered after the birth of a baby.

air embolism—gas bubbles in the bloodstream. The more accurate term is *arterial gas embolism (AGE).*

air-inflatable splint—a splint that is classified as a soft splint but becomes rigid when inflated.

airway—the passageway for air entering or leaving the body. The structures of the airway are the nose, mouth, pharynx, larynx, trachea, bronchi, and lungs.

allergen—something to which a person is allergic; something that causes an adverse physical response.

allergic reaction—an exaggerated immune response.

alveoli (al-VE-o-li)—the microscopic air sacs of the lungs where gas exchange with the bloodstream takes place.

amniotic (am-ne-OT-ic) **sac**—the "bag of waters" that surrounds the developing fetus.

amputation—the surgical removal or traumatic severing of a body part. The most common usage in emergency care refers to the traumatic amputation of an extremity or part of an extremity.

anaphylaxis (an-ah-fi-LAK-sis)—a severe or life-threatening allergic reaction in which the blood vessels dilate, causing a drop in blood pressure, and the tissues lining the respiratory system swell, interfering with the airway. Also called *anaphylactic shock.*

anatomical position—the standard reference position for the body in the study of anatomy. The body is standing erect, facing the observer. The arms are down at the sides and the palms of the hands face forward.

anatomy—the study of body structure.

aneurysm (AN-u-rizm)—the dilation, or ballooning, of a weakened section of an arterial wall.

angina pectoris (AN-ji-nah PEK-to-ris)—the sudden pain occurring when a portion of the myocardium is not receiving enough oxygenated blood.

anterior—the front of the body or body part.

aorta (ay-OR-tah)—the largest artery in the body. It transports blood from the left ventricle to begin systemic circulation.

apnea (AP-ne-ah)—the cessation of breathing.

arrhythmia (ah-RITH-me-ah)—a disturbance in heart rate and rhythm.

arteriole (ar-TE-re-ol)—the smallest kind of artery.

arteriosclerosis (ar-TE-re-o-skle-RO-sis)—"hardening of the arteries" caused by calcium deposits.

artery—any blood vessel carrying blood away from the heart.

841

artificial ventilation—forcing air or oxygen into the lungs when a patient has stopped breathing or has inadequate breathing.

ascites (a-SI-tez)—the accumulation of excessive fluids in the abdomen.

asphyxia (as-FIK-si-ah)—suffocation from lack of air.

aspiration (AS-pir-AY-shun)—the breathing in of vomitus or other foreign matter into the lungs.

asystole (ah-SIS-to-le)—a condition in which the heart has ceased generating electrical impulses.

atherosclerosis (ATH-er-o-skle-RO-sis)—a buildup of fatty deposits and other particles on the inner wall of an artery. This buildup is called plaque.

atria (AY-tree-ah)—the two upper chambers of the heart. There is a right atrium (which receives unoxygenated blood returning from the body) and a left atrium (which receives oxygenated blood returning from the lungs).

auscultation (os-skul-TAY-shun)—the process of listening to sounds that occur within the body.

auto-injector—a syringe pre-loaded with medication that has a spring-loaded device that pushes the needle through the skin when the tip of the device is pressed firmly against the body.

automated external defibrillator (AED)—a machine that automatically recognizes shockable chaotic heart rhythms and delivers a shock to the outside of the patient's chest. See also *defibrillation*.

automaticity (AW-to-mat-IS-it-e)—the ability of the heart to generate and conduct electrical impulses on its own.

autonomic nervous system—the division of the peripheral nervous system that controls involuntary motor functions.

AVPU—a memory aid for *alert, verbal response, painful response, unresponsive* as a classification of a patient's level of responsiveness. See also mental status.

avulsion (ah-VUL-shun)—the tearing away or tearing off of a piece or flap of skin or other soft tissue. This term also may be used for an eye pulled from its socket or a tooth dislodged from its socket.

bag-valve mask—a hand-held device with a face mask and self-refilling bag that can be squeezed to provide artificial ventilations to a patient. Can deliver air from the atmosphere or oxygen from a supplemental oxygen supply system.

bandage—any material used to hold a dressing in place.

base station—a two-way radio at a fixed site such as a hospital or dispatch center.

behavior—the manner in which a person acts.

behavioral emergency—when a patient's behavior is not typical for the situation; when the patient's behavior is unacceptable or intolerable to the patient, his family, or the community; or when the patient may harm himself or others.

bilateral—on both sides.

biological death—when the brain cells die.

blood—the fluids and cells that are circulated to carry oxygen and nutrients to and wastes away from the body's tissues.

blood pressure—the pressure caused by blood exerting force against the walls of blood vessels. Usually arterial blood pressure (the pressure in an artery) is measured.

body mechanics—the proper use of the body to facilitate lifting and moving and prevent injury.

body substance isolation—a form of infection control that assumes that all body fluids should be considered potentially infectious.

bones—hard but flexible living structures that provide support for the body and protection to vital organs. Types of bones are *long*, *short*, *flat*, and *irregular*. The typical long bone has a cylindrical *shaft*, and a rounded end, or *head*, which is connected to the shaft by the *neck*.

brachial (BRAY-ke-ul) **artery**—artery of the upper arm; the site of the pulse checked during infant CPR.

brachial pulse—the pulse measured by palpating the major artery (brachial artery) of the arm. This pulse is used to detect heart action and circulation in infants.

bradycardia (BRAY-duh-KAR-de-uh)—a slow pulse; any pulse rate below 60 beats per minute.

breech presentation—when the baby appears buttocks or both legs first during birth.

bronchi (BRONG-ki)—the two large sets of branches that come off the trachea and enter the lungs. There are right and left bronchi.

bronchoconstriction—constriction, or blockage, of the bronchi that lead from the trachea to the lungs.

calcaneus (kal-KAY-ne-us)—the heel bone.

capillary (KAP-i-lar-e)—the thin-walled, microscopic blood vessel where oxygen/carbon dioxide and nutrient/waste exchange with the tissues takes place.

capillary refill—the return of blood to the microscopic blood vessels known as capillaries after blood has been forced out by pressure that is then released. Normal refill time is 2 seconds. Capillary refill time is a measure of distal circulation.

cardiac arrest—when the heart stops circulating blood or stops beating entirely.

cardiac compromise—any heart problem.

cardiac conduction system—a system of specialized muscle tissues that conduct electrical impulses that stimulate the heart to beat.

cardiac muscle—specialized involuntary muscle found only in the heart.

cardiac tamponade (TAM-po-NOD)—condition when a penetrating or blunt injury to the heart causes blood to flow into the surrounding pericardial sac.

cardiopulmonary resuscitation (KAR-de-o-PUL-mo-ner-e re-SUS-i-TA-shun), **CPR**—heart-lung resuscitation. A combined effort is made to restore or maintain respiration and circulation, artificially.

cardiovascular (KAR-de-o-VAS-kyu-ler) **system**—the system made up of the heart (*cardio*) and the blood vessels (*vascular*); the circulatory system.

carina (kah-RI-nah)—the fork at the lower end of the trachea where the two mainstem bronchi branch.

carotid (kah-ROT-id) **arteries**—the large neck arteries, one on each side of the neck, that carry blood from the heart to the head.

carotid pulse—the pulse that can be felt on each side of the patient's neck, over the carotid arteries.

carpals (KAR-pulz)—the wrist bones.

cartilage—tough tissue that covers the joint ends of bones and helps to form certain body parts such as the ear.

central nervous system (CNS)—the brain and spinal cord.

central pulses—the carotid and femoral pulses, which can be felt in the central part of the body.

central rewarming—application of heat to the lateral chest, neck, armpits, and groin of a hypothermic patient. Rewarming of the limbs is avoided to prevent the collection of blood in the extremities and resulting shock.

cephalic (se-FAL-ik) **presentation**—when the baby appears head first during birth. This is the normal presentation.

cerebrospinal (SER-e-bro-SPI-nal) **fluid (CSF)**—the clear, watery fluid that surrounds and protects the brain and spinal cord.

cervical (SER-vi-kal)—in reference to the neck.

cervical spine—the section of the spine in the neck.

cervix (SER-viks)—the neck of the uterus that enters the birth canal.

chief complaint—in emergency medicine, the reason EMS was called, usually in the patient's own words.

chronic obstructive pulmonary disease (COPD)—a general classification for chronic bronchitis, emphysema, black lung, and many undetermined respiratory diseases that cause problems like those of emphysema.

circulatory system—See *cardiovascular system.*

clavicles (KLAV-i-kulz)—the two collarbones.

clinical death—when breathing and heart action stop.

closed wound—an internal injury with no open pathway from the outside.

coccyx (KOK-siks)—the four fused vertebrae that form the terminal bone of the spine; the "tailbone."

colostomy (ko-LOS-to-me)—A colostomy, like an ileostomy, is a surgical opening in the abdominal wall with an external bag in place to receive digestive excretions.

compensated shock—when the patient is developing shock but the body is still able to maintain perfusion. See *shock.*

concussion—mild closed head injury without detectable damage to the brain. Complete recovery is usually expected.

conduction—the transfer of heat from one material to another through direct contact.

confidentiality—the obligation not to reveal information obtained about a patient except to other health care professionals involved in the patient's care, or under subpoena, or in a court of law, or when the patient has signed a release of confidentiality.

congestive heart failure (CHF)—the failure of the heart to pump efficiently, leading to excessive blood or fluids in the lungs, the body, or both.

consent—permission from the patient for care or other action by the EMT-B. See also *expressed consent; implied consent.*

constrict (kon-STRIKT)—get smaller.

contamination—the introduction of disease or infectious materials. See also *decontamination.*

contraindications (KON-truh-in-duh-KAY-shunz)—specific signs or circumstances under which it is not appropriate and may be harmful to administer a drug to a patient.

contusion (kun-TU-zhun)—a bruise; in head injuries, a bruised brain.

convection—carrying away of heat by currents of air or water or other gases or liquids.

COPD—See *chronic obstructive pulmonary disease.*

coronary (KOR-o-nar-e) **arteries**—blood vessels that supply the muscle of the heart (myocardium).

coronary artery disease (CAD)—diseases that affect the arteries of the heart.

cranial floor—the inferior wall of the brain case; the bony floor beneath the brain.

cranium (KRAY-ne-um)—the bony structure making up the forehead, top, back, and upper sides of the skull.

crepitation (krep-uh-TAY-shun)—the grating sound or feeling of broken bones rubbing together.

crepitus (KREP-i-tus)—see *crepitation.*

cricoid (KRIK-oid) **cartilage**—the ring-shaped structure that circles the trachea at the lower edge of the larynx.

cricoid pressure—pressure applied to the cricoid cartilage to suppress vomiting and bring the vocal cords into view. Also called *Sellick's maneuver.*

critical incident stress debriefing (CISD) teams—teams of counselors who provide emotional and psychological support to EMS personnel who are or have been involved in a multiple-casualty incident or disaster.

croup (KROOP)—a group of viral illnesses that cause inflammation of the larynx, trachea, and bronchi.

crowning—when part of the baby is visible through the vaginal opening.

crush injury—an injury that results when an extremity is caught between heavy items or is subjected to great pressure. Blood vessels, nerves, and muscles are damaged. Bones may be fractured.

cyanosis (sigh-ah-NO-sis)—when the skin, lips, tongue, ear lobes, or nailbeds turn blue or gray from lack of oxygen in circulation. The patient is said to be cyanotic (sigh-ah-NOT-ik).

danger zone—the area around the wreckage of a vehicle collision or other accident within which special safety precautions should be taken.

DCAP-BTLS—A memory aid to remember deformities, contusions, abrasions, punctures/penetrations, burns, tenderness, lacerations, and swelling—signs and symptoms of injury found by inspection or palpation during patient assessment.

decompensated shock—occurs when the body can no longer compensate for low blood volume or lack of perfusion. Late signs such as decreasing blood pressure become evident. See *shock.*

decompression sickness—a condition resulting from nitrogen trapped in the body's tissues caused by coming up too quickly from a deep, prolonged dive. A symptom of decompression sickness is "the bends," or deep pain in the muscles and joints.

decontamination—the removal or cleansing of dangerous chemicals and other dangerous or infectious materials.

defibrillation (de-FIB-ri-LAY-shun)—an electrical current applied to the outside of a patient's chest to stop all electrical activity, often enabling the heart to restart in a coordinated fashion.

delirium tremens (de-LEER-e-um TREM-enz) **(DTs)**—a severe reaction that can be part of alcohol withdrawal, characterized by sweating, trembling, anxiety, and hallucinations. Severe alcohol withdrawal with the DTs can lead to death if untreated.

dermis (DER-mis)—the inner (second) layer of skin found beneath the epidermis. It is rich in blood vessels and nerves.

designated agent—an EMT-B or other person authorized by a Medical Director to give medications and provide emergency care. The transfer of such authorization to a designated agent is an extension of the Medical Director's license to practice medicine.

detailed physical exam—an assessment of the head, neck, chest, abdomen, pelvis, extremities, and posterior of the body to detect signs and symptoms of injury. It differs from the rapid trauma assessment only in that it also includes examination of the face, ears, eyes, nose, and mouth during the examination of the head, that it may be done less rapidly than the rapid trauma assessment, and that it may be done en route to the hospital after earlier on-scene assessments and interventions are completed.

diabetes mellitus (di-ah-BEE-tez MEL-i-tus)—also called *sugar diabetes* or just *diabetes*, the condition brought about by decreased insulin production, which prevents the body's cells from taking the simple sugar called glucose from the bloodstream. The person suffering from this condition is a *diabetic*.

diaphragm (DI-ah-fram)—the muscular structure that separates the chest from the abdomen.

diastolic (di-as-TOL-ik) **blood pressure**—the pressure in the arteries when the left ventricle is refilling.

dilate (DI-late)—get larger.

dilution (di-LU-shun)—thinning down or weakening by mixing with something else. Ingested poisons are sometimes diluted by drinking water or milk.

direct carry method—a method of transferring a patient from bed to stretcher in which two or more rescuers curl the patient to their chests, then reverse the process to lower the patient to the stretcher.

direct ground lift—a method of lifting and carrying a patient from ground level to a stretcher in which two or more rescuers kneel, curl the patient to their chests, stand, then reverse the process to lower the patient to the stretcher.

disaster plan—a pre-defined set of instructions that tells a community's various emergency responders what to do in specific emergencies.

dislocation—injury causing the end of a bone to be pulled or pushed from its joint.

distal—away from a point of reference or attachment; used as a comparison with *proximal*.

distal pulse—a pulse taken at the foot or wrist. It is called *distal* because it is at the distal end of the limb.

distention (dis-TEN-shun)—a condition of being stretched, inflated, or larger than normal.

do not resuscitate (DNR) order—a legal document, usually signed by the patient and his physician, which states that the patient has a terminal illness and does not wish to prolong life through resuscitative efforts.

dorsal—referring to the back of the body. A synonym for *posterior*.

dorsalis pedis (dor-SAL-is PEED-is) **artery**—artery supplying the foot, lateral to the large tendon of the big toe.

dorsalis pedis pulse—See *pedal pulse*.

downers—depressants such as barbiturates that depress the central nervous system, often used to bring on a more relaxed state of mind.

draw sheet method—a method of transferring a patient from bed to stretcher by grasping and pulling the loosened bottom sheet of the bed.

dressing—any material (preferably sterile) used to cover a wound that will help control bleeding and help prevent additional contamination.

drowning—death caused by changes in the lungs resulting from immersion in water. See also *near-drowning*.

duty to act—the legal responsibility to provide care.

dyspnea (DISP-ne-ah)—difficult breathing.

embolism (EM-bo-liz-m)—a moving blood clot or foreign body, such as fat or an air bubble inside a blood vessel. (The plural is *emboli*.)

EMS command—the senior EMS person on the scene who establishes an EMS command post and oversees the medical aspects of a multiple-casualty incident.

endocrine (EN-do-krin) **system**—the system that produces the hormones that regulate body functions.

endotracheal (EN-do-TRAY-ke-ul) **tube**—a tube designed to be inserted into the trachea. Oxygen, medication, or a suction catheter can be directed into the trachea through an endotracheal tube.

epidermis (ep-i-DER-mis)—the outer layer of skin.

epidural hematoma (ep-i-DU-ral he-mah-TOH-mah)—formed when blood from ruptured vessels flows between the meninges and the cranial bones.

epiglottis (EP-i-GLOT-is)—a leaf-shaped structure that prevents food and foreign matter from entering the trachea.

epiglottitis (epi-glo-TI-tis)—a potentially life-threatening condition most commonly caused by a bacterial infection that produces swelling of the epiglottis and partial airway obstruction.

epilepsy (EP-uh-lep-see)—a medical condition that sometimes causes seizures.

epinephrine (EP-uh-NEF-rin)—a hormone produced by the body. As a medication it dilates respiratory passages and is used to relieve severe allergic reactions.

esophagus (eh-SOf-uh-gus)—the tubular structure that leads from the pharynx to the stomach.

evaporation—the change from liquid to gas. When the body perspires or gets wet, evaporation of the perspiration or other liquid into the air has a cooling effect on the body.

evisceration (e-VIS-er-AY-shun)—when an organ or part of an organ protrudes through a wound opening.

exhalation (EX-huh-LAY-shun)—a passive process in which the intercostal (rib) muscles and the diaphragm relax, causing the chest cavity to decrease in size and causing air to flow out of the lungs.

expiration—see *exhalation*.

expressed consent—consent given by adults who are of legal age and mentally competent to make a rational decision in regard to their medical well-being. See also *consent*.

extremities (ex-TREM-i-teez)—the portions of the appendicular skeleton that include the clavicles, scapulae, arms, forearms, wrists, and hands (upper extremities); the pelvis, thighs, legs, ankles, and feet (lower extremities).

extremity lift—a method of lifting and carrying a patient in which one rescuer slips hands under the patient's armpits and grasps the wrists, while another rescuer grasps the patient's knees.

femoral (FEM-o-ral) **artery**—the major artery supplying the thigh.

femur (FEE-mer)—the large bone of the thigh.

fetus (FE-tus)—the baby as it develops in the womb.

fibula (FIB-yuh-luh)—the outer and smaller bone of the lower leg.

50:50 rule—the rule that CPR compressions and releases should be equal: 50% compression, 50% release.

first-degree burn—see *superficial burn*.

flail chest—injury in which usually three or more consecutive ribs on the same side of the chest are fractured, each in at least two locations. A flail chest also can occur when the sternum is fractured loose from its attachments with the ribs. This is sometimes referred to as a flailed sternum.

flowmeter—a valve that indicates the flow from an oxygen cylinder in liters per minute.

flow-restricted, oxygen-powered ventilation device (FROPVD)—a device that uses oxygen under pressure to deliver artificial ventilations. Its trigger is placed so that the rescuer can operate it while still using both hands to maintain a seal on the face mask. Has automatic flow restriction to prevent over-delivery of oxygen to the patient.

focused history and physical exam—the step of patient assessment that follows the initial assessment.

Fowler's position—a sitting position.

fracture (FRAK-cher)—any break in a bone.

frostbite—see *local cooling*.

full-thickness burn—a burn in which all the layers of the skin are damaged. There are usually areas that are charred black or areas that are dry and white. Also called a third-degree burn.

gag reflex—vomiting or retching that results when something is placed in the throat.

Glasgow Coma Scale—a detailed measure of level of consciousness.

glottic opening—the opening to the trachea.

glucose (GLU-kos)—a form of sugar, the body's basic source of energy.

Good Samaritan laws—a series of laws, varying in each state, designed to provide limited legal protection for citizens and some health care personnel when they are administering emergency care.

hallucinogens (huh-LOO-sin-uh-jens)—mind-affecting or -altering drugs that act on the central nervous system to produce excitement and distortion of perceptions.

hazardous material incident—the release of a harmful substance into the environment.

head-tilt, chin-lift maneuver—a means of correcting blockage of the airway by the tongue by tilting the head back and lifting the chin. Used when no trauma, or injury, is suspected. See also *jaw-thrust maneuver*.

heart attack—an informal term for acute myocardial infarction (AMI).

Heimlich maneuver—manual thrusts to the abdomen to force bursts of air from the lungs to dislodge an airway obstruction.

hematoma (HE-mah-TO-mah)—a swelling caused by the collection of blood under the skin or in damaged tissues as a result of an injured or broken blood vessel; in a head injury, a collection of blood within the skull or brain.

hemopneumothorax (HE-mo-NU-mo-THOR-aks)—a combination of blood and air in the thoracic cavity.

hemorrhage (HEM-o-rej)—internal or external bleeding.

hemorrhagic (HEM-o-AJ-ik) **shock**—shock resulting from blood loss.

hemothorax (HE-mo-THOR-aks)—blood in the thoracic cavity.

hives—red, itchy bumps on the skin that often result from allergic reactions.

humerus (HYU-mer-us)—the bone of the upper arm, between the shoulder and the elbow.

humidifier—a device connected to the flowmeter to add moisture to the dry oxygen coming from an oxygen cylinder.

hyperglycemia (HI-per-gli-SEE-me-ah)—too much sugar in the blood.

hyperthermia (HI-per-THURM-i-ah)—an increase in body temperature above normal; life-threatening at its extreme.

hyperventilate (HI-per-VENT-i-late)—in suctioning, to provide ventilations at a higher rate to compensate for oxygen not delivered during suctioning.

hypoglycemia (HI-po-gli-SEE-me-ah)—too little sugar in the blood.

hypoperfusion—shock; inadequate perfusion of the cells and tissues of the body caused by insufficient flow of blood through the capillaries. See also *perfusion*.

hypopharynx (HI-po-FAIR-inks)—the area directly

above the openings of both the trachea and the esophagus.

hypothermia (HI-po-THURM-i-ah)—a generalized cooling that reduces the body temperature below normal; life-threatening at its extreme.

hypovolemic (HI-po-vo-LE-mik) **shock**—shock resulting from blood or fluid loss.

hypoxia (hi-POK-se-ah)—an inadequate supply of oxygen in the body's tissues.

ileostomy (il-e-OS-to-me)—See *colostomy*.

iliac (IL-e-ak) **crest**—the upper, curved boundary of the ilium.

ilium (IL-e-um)—the superior and widest portion of the pelvis.

implied consent—a legal concept that assumes an unconscious patient (or one so badly injured or ill that he cannot respond) would consent to receiving emergency care if he or she could do so. In some states, implied consent may apply to children when parents or guardians are not at the scene.

incident management system—a system used for the management of a multiple-casualty incident, involving assumption of responsibility for command and designation and coordination of such elements as triage, treatment, transport, and staging.

indications—specific signs or circumstances under which it is appropriate to administer a drug to a patient.

induced abortion—expulsion of a fetus as a result of deliberate actions taken to stop the pregnancy.

inferior—away from the head; usually compared with another structure that is closer to the head (e.g., the lips are inferior when compared with the nose).

ingested poisons—poisons that are swallowed.

inhalation (IN-huh-LAY-shun)—an active process in which the intercostal (rib) muscles and the diaphragm contract, expanding the size of the chest cavity and causing air to flow into the lungs.

inhaled poisons—poisons that are breathed in.

inhaler—a spray device with a mouthpiece that contains an aerosol form of a medication that a patient can spray into his airway.

initial assessment—the first element in assessment of a patient; steps taken for the purpose of discovering and dealing with any life-threatening problems. The six parts of initial assessment are forming a general impression, assessing mental status, assessing airway, assessing breathing, assessing circulation, and determining the priority of the patient for treatment and transport to the hospital.

injected poisons—poisons that are inserted through the skin, possibly into the bloodstream, for example by needle, snake fangs, or insect stinger.

inspiration (in-spir-AY-shun)—see *inhalation*.

insulin (IN-suh-lin)—a hormone produced by the pancreas or taken as a medication by many diabetics.

interventions—actions taken to correct a patient's problems.

intracerebral hematoma (in-trah-SER-e-bral he-mah-TO-mah)—formed when blood from ruptured vessels pools within the brain.

intubation (IN-tu-BAY-shun)—insertion of a tube. See also *endotracheal tube; nasogastric tube; orotracheal intubation*.

involuntary muscle—muscle that responds automatically to brain signals but cannot be consciously controlled.

ischium (ISH-e-um)—the lower, posterior portions of the pelvis.

jaw-thrust maneuver—a means of correcting blockage of the airway by moving the jaw forward without tilting the head or neck. Used when trauma is suspected to open the airway without causing further injury to the spinal cord in the neck. See also *head-tilt, chin-lift maneuver*.

joints—places where bones articulate, or meet.

jugular (JUG-yuh-ler) **vein distention (JVD)**—bulging of the neck veins.

labor—the stages of delivery that begin with the contractions of the uterus and end with the expulsion of the placenta.

laceration—a cut.

laryngoscope—an illuminating instrument that is inserted into the pharynx to permit visualization of the pharynx and larynx.

larynx (LAR-inks)—the portion of the airway connecting the pharynx and the trachea. It contains the voicebox and vocal cords.

lateral—to the side, away from the midline of the body.

lateral recumbent—lying on the side.

liability—being held legally responsible.

ligaments—tissues that connect bone to bone.

local cooling—cooling or freezing of particular (local) parts of the body.

log roll—a maneuver for changing a patient's position by rolling him as a unit, keeping head, neck, and torso aligned.

lumbar (LUM-bar) **spine**—the section of the spine in the midback.

lungs—the organs where exchange of oxygen and carbon dioxide take place.

malar (MA-lar)—the cheek bone, also called the zygomatic bone.

malleolus (mal-E-o-lus)—protrusion on the side of the ankle. The lateral malleolus is on the outer ankle, the medial malleolus is on the inner ankle.

mandible (MAN-di-bl)—the lower jaw bone.

manual traction—the process of applying tension to straighten and realign a fractured limb before splinting. Also known as *tension*.

manubrium (man-OO-bre-um)—the superior portion of the sternum.

maxillae (mak-SIL-e)—the two fused bones forming the upper jaw.

mechanism of injury—a force or forces that may have caused injury.

meconium staining—amniotic fluid that is greenish or brownish-yellow rather than clear; an indication of possible fetal or maternal distress during labor.

medial—toward the midline of the body.

medical directions—oversight of the patient care aspect of an EMS system by the Medical Director. **Off-line medical direction** consists of standing orders issued by the Medical Director that allow EMTs to give certain medications or perform certain procedures without speaking to the Medical Director or another physician. **On-line medical direction** consists of orders from the on-duty physician given directly to an EMT-B in the field by radio or telephone.

Medical Director—a physician who assumes the ultimate responsibility for the patient care aspects of the EMS system.

meningitis (men-in-JI-tis)—a condition caused by either a bacterial or viral infection of the lining of the brain and spinal cord.

mental status—level of responsiveness. See also *AVPU*.

metacarpals (MET-uh-KAR-pulz)—the hand bones.

metatarsals (MET-un-TAR-sulz)—the foot bones.

mid-axillary (mid-AX-uh-lair-e) **line**—a line drawn vertically from the middle of the armpit to the ankle.

mid-clavicular (mid-clah-VIK-yuh-ler) **line**—the line through the center of each clavicle.

midline—an imaginary line drawn down the center of the body, dividing it into right and left halves.

miscarriage—see *spontaneous abortion*.

mobile radio—a two-way radio that is used or affixed in a vehicle.

multiple birth—when more than one baby is born during a single delivery.

multiple-casualty incident (MCI)—any medical or trauma incident involving multiple patients.

muscles—tissues or fibers that cause movement of body organs and parts.

musculoskeletal (MUS-kyu-lo-SKEL-e-tal) **system**—the system of bones and skeletal muscles that support and protect the body and permit movement.

myocardial infarction (heart attack)—see *acute myocardial infarction*.

myocardium (mi-o-KAR-de-um)—heart muscle.

narcotics—a class of drugs that affect the nervous system and change many normal body activities. Their legal use is for the relief of pain. Illicit use is to produce an intense state of relaxation.

nasal (NAY-zl) **bones**—the nose bones.

nasal cannula (KAN-yuh-luh)—a device that delivers low concentrations of oxygen through two prongs that rest in the patient's nostrils.

nasogastric (NAY-zo-GAS-trik) **tube (NG tube)**—a tube designed to be passed through the nose, nasopharynx, and esophagus. It is used to relieve distention of the stomach in an infant or child patient.

nasopharyngeal (na-zo-fah-RIN-je-al) **airway**—a flexible breathing tube inserted through the patient's nose into the pharynx to help maintain an open airway.

nasopharynx (NAY-zo-FAIR-inks)—the area directly posterior to the nose.

near-drowning—the condition of having begun to drown. The near-drowning patient may be conscious, unconscious with heartbeat and pulse, or with no heartbeat or pulse but still able to be resuscitated.

Only when sufficient time without breathing has passed to render resuscitation useless (sometimes 30 minutes or more if the patient has been in cold water) has *drowning* truly taken place.

negligence—a finding of failure to act properly in a situation in which there was a duty to act, needed care as would be reasonably be expected of the EMT-B was not provided, and harm was caused to the patient as a result.

nervous system—the system of brain, spinal cord, and nerves that govern sensation, movement, and thought.

nitroglycerin (NI-tro-GLIS-uh-rin)—a drug that helps to dilate the coronary vessels that supply the heart muscle with blood.

nonrebreather mask—a face mask and reservoir bag device that delivers high concentrations of oxygen. All of the patient's exhaled air escapes through a valve and is not rebreathed.

occlusion (uh-KLU-zhun)—blockage, as in the blockage of an artery.

occlusive (uh-KLU-siv) **dressing**—any dressing that forms an airtight seal.

ongoing assessment—a procedure for detecting changes in a patient's condition. It involves four steps: repeating the initial assessment, repeating and recording vital signs, repeating the focused history and physical exam, and checking interventions.

open wound—an injury in which the skin is interrupted, exposing the tissue beneath.

OPQRST questions—a memory device for the questions asked to get a description of the present illness: Onset, Provokes, Quality, Radiation, Severity, Time.

oral glucose (GLU-kos)—a form of glucose (a kind of sugar) given by mouth to treat an awake patient with an altered mental status and a history of diabetes.

orbits—the bony structure around the eyes; the eye sockets.

oropharyngeal (or-o-fah-RIN-je-al) **airway**—a curved airway adjunct inserted through the patient's mouth into the pharynx to help maintain an open airway.

oropharynx (OR-o-FAIR-inks)—the area directly posterior to the mouth.

orotracheal (OR-o-TRAY-ke-ul) **intubation**—placement of an endotracheal tube through the mouth and into the trachea. See also *endotracheal tube*.

oxygen—a gas commonly found in the atmosphere. Pure oxygen is used as a drug to treat any patient whose medical or traumatic condition may cause him to be hypoxic, or low in oxygen.

oxygen cylinder—a cylinder filled with oxygen under pressure.

palmar—referring to the palm of the hand.

palpation—to feel any part of the body.

paradoxical (pair-uh-DOKS-i-kal) **motion**—movement of a flailed section in the opposite direction to the rest of the chest during respirations.

partial-thickness burn—a burn in which the epidermis (first layer of skin) is burned through and the dermis (second layer) is damaged. Burns of this type cause reddening, blistering, and a mottled appearance. Also called a second degree burn.

passive rewarming—covering a hypothermic patient and taking other steps to prevent further heat loss and to help the body rewarm itself.

patella (pah-TEL-uh)—the kneecap.

pathogens—the organisms that cause infection.

pedal (PEED-al) **edema**—accumulation of fluid at the feet or ankles.

pedal pulse—a foot pulse. There are two locations used in field emergency care: the *dorsalis pedis* (lateral to the large tendon of the big toe) and the *posterior tibial* (behind the medial ankle).

penetrating trauma—an injury caused by an object that passes through the skin or other body tissue.

perfusion—the supply of oxygen to and removal of wastes from the cells and tissues of the body as a result of the flow of blood through the capillaries.

perineum (per-i-NE-um)—the surface area between the vulva and anus.

peripheral nervous system (PNS)—the nerves that enter and leave the spinal cord and that travel between the brain and organs without passing through the spinal cord.

peripheral pulses—the radial, brachial, posterior tibial, and dorsalis pedis pulses, which can be felt at peripheral (outlying) points of the body.

phalanges (fuh-LAN-jiz)—the toe bones and finger bones.

pharmacology—(FARM-uh-KOL-uh-je) the study of drugs, their sources, characteristics, and effects.

pharynx (FAIR-inks)—the area directly posterior to the mouth and nose. It is made up of the oropharynx and the nasopharynx..

physiology—the study of body function.

placenta (plah-SEN-tah)—the organ of pregnancy where exchange of oxygen, foods, and wastes occurs between mother and fetus.

placenta previa—a condition in which the placenta is formed in an abnormal location (low in the uterus and close to or over the cervical opening) that will not allow for a normal delivery of the fetus; a cause of excessive prebirth bleeding.

plantar—referring to the sole of the foot.

plasma (PLAZ-mah)—the fluid portion of the blood.

platelets—components of the blood; membrane-enclosed fragments of specialized cells.

pneumothorax (NU-mo-THO-raks)—condition resulting when air enters the thoracic cavity from an open wound or from a damaged lung or both.

pocket face mask—a device with a one-way valve for mouth-to-mask resuscitation. It can be used with supplemental oxygen when fitted with an oxygen inlet. It is a barrier device, the one-way valve preventing contact with the patient's breath or fluids.

poison—any substance that can harm the body by altering cell structure or functions.

portable radio—a hand-held two-way radio.

posterior—the back of the body or body part.

posterior tibial (TIB-ee-ul) **artery**—artery supplying the foot, behind the medial ankle.

posterior tibial pulse—See *pedal pulse.*

power grip—gripping with as much hand surface as possible in contact with object being lifted, all fingers bent at the same angle, hands at least 10 inches apart.

power lift—also called the *squat lift position*. It is a lift from a squatting position with weight to be lifted close to the body, feet apart and flat on the ground, body weight on or just behind balls of feet, back locked in. The upper body is raised before the hips.

premature infant—any newborn weighing less than 5.5 pounds or being born before the 37th week of pregnancy.

pressure dressing—a bulky dressing held in position with a tightly wrapped bandage to apply pressure to help control bleeding.

pressure point—a site where a main artery lies near the surface of the body and directly over a bone. Pressure on such a point can stop distal bleeding.

pressure regulator—a device connected to an oxygen cylinder to reduce cylinder pressure to a safe pressure for delivery of oxygen to a patient.

priapism (PRY-ah-pizm)—persistent erection of the penis often associated with spinal injury and some medical problems.

prolapsed umbilical cord—when the umbilical cord presents first during birth and is squeezed between the vaginal wall and the baby's head.

prone—lying face down.

protocols—lists of steps, such as assessment steps and interventions, to be taken in different situations. Protocols are developed by the Medical Director of an EMS system.

proximal—close to a point of reference or attachment; used as a comparison with *distal*.

pubis (PYOO-bis)—the medial, anterior portion of the pelvis.

pulmonary (PUL-mo-nar-e) **arteries**—the blood vessels that carry blood from the right ventricle of the heart to the lungs.

pulmonary edema—fluid in the lungs.

pulmonary veins—the vessels that carry blood from the lungs to the left atrium of the heart.

pulse—the rhythmic beats caused as waves of blood move through and expand the arteries.

pulseless electrical activity (PEA)—a condition in which the heart's electrical rhythm remains relatively normal, yet the mechanical pumping activity fails to follow the electrical activity, causing cardiac arrest.

pulse quality—the rhythm (regular or irregular) and force (strong or weak) of the pulse.

pulse rate—the number of pulse beats per minute.

puncture wound—an open wound that tears through the skin and destroys underlying tissues. A *penetrating puncture wound* can be shallow or deep. A *perforating puncture wound* has both an entrance and an exit wound.

pupil—the adjustable opening that admits light to the eye; the black center of the eye.

quality improvement—a process of continuous self-review with the purpose of identifying and correcting aspects of the system that require improvement.

radial artery—artery of the lower arm. It is felt when taking the pulse at the wrist.

radial pulse—a pulse found in the lateral wrist.

radiation—sending out energy, such as heat, in waves into space.

radius (RAY-de-us)—the lateral bone of the forearm.

rapid trauma assessment—a rapid assessment of the head, neck, chest, abdomen, pelvis, extremities, and posterior of the body to detect signs and symptoms of injury.

reactivity (re-ak-TIV-uh-te)—in the pupils of the eyes, reacting to light by changing size.

recovery positon—lying on the side. The recovery position protects the airway by allowing for drainage from the mouth and preventing the tongue from falling backward into the airway.

red blood cells—components of the blood. They carry oxygen to and carbon dioxide away from the cells.

rescue breathing—providing artificial ventilations to a person who has stopped breathing on his own or whose breathing is inadequate.

respiration (res-pi-RAY-shun)—the act of breathing in and breathing out.

respiratory (RES-pir-uh-tor-e) **arrest**—when a person stops breathing completely.

respiratory failure—the reduction of breathing to the point where not enough oxygen is being taken in to sustain life.

respiratory (RES-puh-ruh-tor-e) **quality**—the normal or abnormal (shallow, labored, or noisy) character of breathing.

respiratory rhythm—the regular or irregular spacing of breaths.

respiratory rate—the number of breaths per minute.

respiratory system—the system of nose, mouth, throat, lungs, and muscles that brings oxygen into the body and expels carbon dioxide.

resuscitation (re-SUS-i-TAY-shun)—any efforts used to artificially restore breathing or breathing and heart function.

Rule of Nines—a method for estimating the extent of a burn. For an adult, each of the following areas represents 9% of the body surface: the head and neck, each upper limb, the chest, the abdomen, the upper back, the lower back and buttocks, the front of each lower limb, and the back of each lower limb. The remaining 1% is assigned to the genital region. For an infant or child the percentages are modified so that 18% is assigned to the head, 14% to each lower limb.

Rule of Palm—a method for estimating the extent of a burn. The palm of the hand, which equals about 1% of the body's surface area, is compared with the patient's burn to estimate its size.

sacrum (SAY-krum)—the five fused vertebrae of the lower back.

SAMPLE history—the current or past history of a patient, so called because the elements of the history begin with the letters of the word *sample*: s̲igns/symptoms, a̲llergies, m̲edications, pertinent past history, l̲ast oral intake, e̲vents leading to the injury or illness.

scapula (SKAP-yuh-luh)—the shoulder blade.

scene size-up—steps taken by an ambulance crew when approaching the scene of an emergency call: taking body substance isolation precautions, checking scene safety, noting the mechanism of injury or nature of the patient's illness, determining the number of patients, and deciding what, if any, additional resources to call for.

scope of practice—a set of regulations and ethical considerations that define the scope, or extent and limits, of the EMT-B's job.

second-degree burn—see *partial thickness burn*.

seizure (SE-zher)—a sudden change in sensation, behavior, or movement. The more severe forms produce violent muscle contractions called convulsions.

Sellick's maneuver—see *cricoid pressure*.

shock—See *hypoperfusion*.

shock position—see *Trendelenburg position*.

side effect—any action of a drug other than the desired action.

sign—an indication of a patient's condition that is objective, or can be observed by another person; an indication that can be seen, heard, smelled, or felt by the EMT-B or others.

sphygmomanometer (SFIG-mo-mah-NOM-e-ter)—the cuff and gauge used in blood pressure determination.

spinous processes—the bony bumps on vertebrae.

spontaneous abortion—when the fetus and placenta deliver before the 28th week of pregnancy; commonly called *miscarriage*.

sprain—a partially torn ligament.

staging officer—the person responsible for overseeing and keeping track of ambulances and ambulance personnel at a multiple-casualty incident. The staging officer will direct ambulances to treatment areas at the request of the transportation officer.

staging sector—the area where ambulances are parked and other resources are held until needed.

standing orders—A policy or protocol that is issued by a Medical Director that authorizes EMT-Bs and others to perform particular skills in certain situations.

status epilepticus (ep-i-LEP-ti-kus)—when a person suffers two or more convulsive seizures without regaining full consciousness. It is a true emergency, requiring immediate transport.

sternum (STER-num)—the breastbone.

stillborn—born dead.

stoma (STO-mah)—the permanent neck opening created in a laryngectomy or tracheostomy.

stroke—blockage or rupture of a blood vessel to the brain.

stylet—a long, thin, bendable metal probe.

subcutaneous layers—the layers of fat and soft tissues found below the dermis.

subdural hematoma (sub-DU-ral he-mah-TOH-mah)—formed when blood from ruptured vessels flows between the brain and the meninges.

substernal notch—a general term for the lowest region on the sternum to which the ribs attach.

sucking chest wound—an open wound to the chest

that draws air from the atmosphere into the chest cavity. This is a form of pneumothorax.

suctioning (SUK-shun-ing)—use of a vacuum device to remove blood, vomitus, and other secretions or foreign materials from the airway.

sudden death—a cardiac arrest that occurs within two hours of the onset of symptoms. The patient may have no prior symptoms or coronary artery disease.

sudden infant death syndrome (SIDS)—an unexplained sudden death of an apparently healthy infant while asleep.

superficial burn—a burn that involves only the epidermis, the outer layer of the skin. It is characterized by reddening of the skin and perhaps some swelling. An example is a sunburn. Also called a first-degree burn.

superior—toward the head; often used in reference with *inferior*.

supine—lying on the back.

supine hypotensive syndrome—dizziness and a drop in blood pressure caused when a pregnant woman is in a supine position and the weight of the uterus, infant, placenta, and amniotic fluid compress the inferior vena cava, reducing venous return to the heart and reducing cardiac output.

symptom—an indication of a patient's condition that cannot be observed by another person but rather is subjective, or felt and reported by the patient.

systolic (sis-TOL-ik) **blood pressure**—the pressure created in the arteries when the left ventricle contracts and forces blood out into circulation.

tachycardia (TAK-uh-KAR-de-uh)—a rapid pulse; any pulse rate above 100 beats per minute.

tarsals (TAR-sulz)—the ankle bones.

temporal bone—bone that forms part of the lateral wall of the skull and the floor of the cranial cavity. There is a right and a left temporal bone.

temporomandibular (TEM-po-ro-man-DIB-u-lar) **joint**—the movable joint formed between mandible and temporal bone, also called the TM joint.

tendons—tissues that connect muscle to bone.

third-degree burn—see *full thickness burn*.

thoracic spine—the section of the spine in the upper back.

thorax (THOR-ax)—the chest.

thrombus (THROM-bus)—a clot formed of blood and plaque attached to the inner wall of an artery.

thyroid (THY-roid) **cartilage**—the Adam's apple.

tibia (TIB-e-uh)—the inner and larger bone of the lower leg.

torso—the trunk of the body; the body without the head and the extremities.

tourniquet (TURN-i-ket)—a device that constricts all blood flow to and from an extremity.

tourniquet shock—a dangerous condition caused when a tourniquet is loosened or released, and toxic substances that have gathered distal to the tourniquet are released in high concentrations to the rest of the body.

toxin—a poisonous substance secreted by bacteria, plants, or animals.

trachea (TRAY-ke-ah)—the windpipe; the tubular structure that carries air to and from the lungs.

tracheostomy (TRAY-ke-OS-to-me)—a surgical incision in the trachea held open by a metal or plastic tube. See also *stoma*.

traction splints—special splints that apply a constant pull along the length of a lower extremity. This helps to stabilize the fractured bone and reduce muscle spasms in the limb. Traction splints are used primarily to treat femoral shaft fractures.

transportation officer—the person responsible for communicating with sector officers and hospitals to prioritize and manage transportation of patients to hospitals from the scene of a multiple-casualty incident.

traumatic (traw-MAT-ik) **asphyxia** (a-SFIKS-e-ah)—a group of signs and symptoms associated with sudden severe compression of the chest and, in some cases, the abdomen. When this occurs, the sternum exerts severe pressure on the heart, forcing blood out of the right atrium up into the jugular veins in the neck.

treatment officer—the person responsible for overseeing treatment of patients who have been triaged at a multiple-casualty incident.

treatment sector—the area in which patients are treated at a multiple-casualty incident.

Trendelenburg (trend-EL-un-berg) **position**—a position in which the patient's feet and legs are higher than the head. Also called *shock position*.

trending—changes in a patient's condition, such as slowing respirations or rising pulse rate, that may show improvement or deterioration, and that can be shown by documenting repeated assessments.

triage—the process of quickly assessing patients in a multiple-casualty incident and assigning each a priority for receiving treatment according to the severity of their illness or injuries. From a French word meaning "to sort."

triage officer—the person responsible for overseeing triage at a multiple-casualty incident.

triage sector—the area in which secondary triage takes place at a multiple-casualty incident.

triage tag—color-coded tag indicating the priority group to which a patient has been assigned.

ulna (UL-nah)—the medial bone of the forearm.

umbilical (um-BIL-i-cal) **cord**—the fetal structure containing the blood vessels that travel to and from the placenta.

universal dressing—a bulky dressing.

uppers—stimulants such as amphetamines that affect the central nervous system to excite the user.

uterus (U-ter-us)—the muscular abdominal organ where the fetus develops; the womb.

vagina (vah-JI-nah)—the birth canal.

vallecula (val-EK-yuh-luh)—a groove-like structure anterior to the epiglottis.

vein—any blood vessel returning blood to the heart.

venae cavae (VE-ne KA-ve)—the *superior vena cava* and the *inferior vena cava*. These two major veins return blood from the body to the right atrium.

venom—a poison (toxin) produced by plants or animals such as certain snakes, spiders, and marine life forms.

ventilation—the breathing in of air or oxygen or providing breaths artificially. See also *artificial ventilation*.

ventral—referring to the front of the body. A synonym for *anterior*.

ventricles (VEN-tri-kulz)—the two lower chambers of the heart. There is a right ventricle (which sends oxygen-poor blood to the lungs) and a left ventricle (which sends oxygen-rich blood to the body).

ventricular fibrillation (ven-TRIK-u-ler fib-ri-LAY-shun) **(VF)**—a condition in which the heart's electrical impulses are disorganized, preventing the heart muscle from contracting normally.

ventricular tachycardia (tak-i-KAR-de-uh) **(V-Tach)**—a condition in which the heartbeat is quite rapid; if rapid enough, ventricular tachycardia will not allow the heart's chambers to fill with enough blood between beats to produce blood flow sufficient to meet the body's needs.

venule (VEN-yul)—the smallest kind of vein.

vertebrae (VERT-uh-bray)—the 33 irregularly shaped bones of the spinal column.

vital signs—outward signs of what is going on inside the body, including respiration; pulse; skin color, temperature, and condition (plus capillary refill in infants and children); pupils; and blood pressure.

vocal cords—two thin folds of tissue within the larynx that vibrate as air passes between them, producing sounds.

volatile chemicals—vaporizing compounds, such as cleaning fluid, that are breathed in by the abuser to produce a "high."

voluntary muscle—muscle that can be consciously controlled.

water chill—chilling caused by conduction of heat from the body when the body or clothing is wet.

white blood cells—components of the blood. They produce substances that help the body fight infection.

wind chill—chilling caused by convection of heat from the body in the presence of currents of cool air.

withdrawal—referring to alcohol or drug withdrawal, in which the patient's body reacts severely when deprived of the abused substance.

xiphoid (ZI-foyd) **process**—the inferior portion of the sternum.

zygomatic (ZI-go-MAT-ik) **bones**—the cheekbones.

Index